DIAGNOSTIC PATHOLOGY
OF
INFECTIOUS DISEASES

Gail L. Woods, M.D.
Associate Professor,
Departments of Pathology and Laboratory Medicine,
Microbiology and Immunology,
  and Internal Medicine,
Medical Director of Laboratories,
Medical College Hospitals,
Philadelphia, Pennsylvania

Yezid Gutierrez, M.D., M.P.H., and T.M., Ph.D.
Associate Professor of Pathology,
Institute of Pathology,
Case Western Reserve University, and
Department of Pathology,
University Hospitals of Cleveland,
Cleveland, Ohio

David H. Walker, M.D.
Professor and Chairman,
Department of Pathology,
The University of Texas Medical Branch at Galveston,
Galveston, Texas

David T. Purtilo, M.D.
Late Professor and Chairman,
Department of Pathology and Microbiology,
University of Nebraska Medical Center,
Omaha, Nebraska

John D. Shanley, M.D.
Professor and Director,
Division of Infectious Diseases,
Department of Internal Medicine,
University of Connecticut Health Center,
Farmington, Connecticut

DIAGNOSTIC PATHOLOGY
OF
INFECTIOUS DISEASES

Lea & Febiger   Philadelphia   London   1993

Lea & Febiger
Box 3024
200 Chester Field Parkway
Malvern, Pennsylvania 19355-9725
U.S.A.
(215) 251-2230

Executive Editor—R. Kenneth Bussy
Developmental Editor—Tanya Lazar
Project Editor—Frances M. Klass
Production Manager—Samuel A. Rondinelli

Library of Congress Cataloging-in-Publication Data

Woods, Gail L.
　　Diagnostic Pathology of infectious diseases / Gail L. Woods.
　　　　p.　　cm.
　　ISBN 0-8121-1604-6
　　1. Communicable diseases—Diagnostic.　2. Diagnosis, Laboratory.
　I. Title.
　　[DNLM: 1. Communicable Diseases—diagnosis.　2. Diagnosis,
Laboratory—methods.　3. Microbiological Techniques.　4. Specimen
Handling.　QY 25 W894d]
RC113.3.W66　1993
616.9'0475—dc20
DNLM/DLC
for Library of Congress　　　　　　　　　　　　　　　　　　92-49695
　　　　　　　　　　　　　　　　　　　　　　　　　　　　　　CIP

Reprints of chapters may be purchased from Lea & Febiger in quantities of 100 or more. Contact Sally Grande in the Sales Department.

NOTE: Although the author(s) and the publisher have taken reasonable steps to ensure the accuracy of the drug information included in this text before publication, drug information may change without notice and readers are advised to consult the manufacturer's packaging inserts before prescribing medications.

Copyright © 1993 by Lea & Febiger. Copyright under the International Copyright Union. All Rights Reserved. This book is protected by copyright. *No part of it may be reproduced in any manner or by any means without written permission from the publisher.*

PRINTED IN THE UNITED STATES OF AMERICA

Print number:　5　4　3　2　1

DEDICATION

*The book is dedicated to my son, Michael Latimer,
who has given special meaning to my life.*

FOREWORD

Despite some notable triumphs in the prevention, eradication, and treatment of infectious diseases, diseases due to well recognized pathogenic microorganisms continue to confront students and practitioners in the field of pathology. The increasing numbers of our population who survive to an older age with a variety of underlying conditions and diseases, the increasing number of immunocompromised patients, including those with the acquired immunodeficiency syndrome, and the increasing number of patients with implanted prosthetic devices have caused us to recognize the clinical importance of many microorganisms previously considered to be purely saprophytic and harmless. Moreover, the advent of every new antimicrobial agent has been met with the emergence of microbial resistance so that previously controllable or treatable diseases now defy rational therapy and challenge our pharmaceutical research colleagues to further investigation and development of new products which, unfortunately, the microbial world will ultimately find ways of defeating. Thus, for example, tuberculosis which was very much controlled and on the wane in the developed world, has now had a resurgence, in part due to susceptible populations with the acquired immunodeficiency syndrome, intravenous drug abusers, the homeless, and those who lack the benefits of good medical care. Confounding this particular picture is the emergence of multidrug resistant *Mycobacterium tuberculosis*. The dynamic nature of the field of infectious diseases, therefore, remains a daily challenge to pathologists who are responsible for implementing procedures for the laboratory diagnosis of infectious diseases and are often called upon for consultation regarding specimen selection and interpretation of laboratory results.

This textbook fills a void between those written for infectious disease practitioners and those written for clinical microbiologists. It provides a reference for pathology residents learning microbiology and for pathologists in practice who may have responsibility for the microbiology laboratory, as well as ancillary responsibility for infection control. After a brief overview of the organization of the text, Dr. Woods and the noted contributors to her textbook have organized their material into two major parts, one of which describes the structure and methods of reproduction of each microorganism, significant aspects of its epidemiology, pathogenesis with emphasis on relevant pathologic features, major clinical manifestations, basic approaches to detection and identification, and when appropriate, a brief description of therapy. This part of the book discusses each microorganism in order of ascending complexity ranging from viruses to parasites.

The other major part of the book reviews in some detail the important aspects of specimen handling and laboratory diagnosis by organ system. Unlike many other areas of the clinical laboratory in which the variety of specimen types is limited and the measurement of analytes can be very specific, the microbiology laboratory is the recipient of an infinite variety of specimens from virtually every body site, source, and orifice. Many of the sites harbor indigenous microorganisms, cultures of which require careful assessment and interpretation. As such, the microbiology laboratory has an obligation to promulgate the appropriate selection of specimens, processing of those specimens for the clinically relevant microorganisms, and the reporting of clincally important information. The last part of this textbook attempts to provide guidelines. It also provides in general outline approaches to the identification of major groups of microorganisms.

This textbook is a valuable reference which is written in an easily readable and comprehensible style for students and practitioners in pathology. It is also a valuable supplement to textbooks in microbiology and infectious diseases.

John A. Washington, M.D.
Vice Chairman,
Division of Pathology and Laboratory Medicine
Chairman, Department of Clinical Pathology
Head, Section of Microbiology
The Cleveland Clinic Foundation
Cleveland, Ohio

PREFACE

I wrote this book to fill a void that I perceived: an ideal reference for pathologists and pathology residents. The information in the text, however, certainly can be utilized by infectious disease clinicians, medical students, and medical technologists.

I organized the book and wrote most of it. Dr. Yezid Gutierrez wrote the parasitology section in Part II and the parasitology portion of each of the chapters in Part III. The Rickettsia chapter in Part II was written by Dr. David Walker, and other contributions were provided by Dr. David Purtilo and Dr. John Shanley. Magnifications shown in the figure legends represent the original magnifications.

In Part I, the role of the clinical pathologist, as it relates to the organization of the text, host-pathogen interactions, and the pathogenesis of infectious diseases are discussed, and an overview of the text is provided.

Part II, Clinical Infection and Laboratory Diagnosis, is divided phylogenetically into four sections: viruses, bacteria, fungi and algae, and parasites. In the introductory chapter of each section classification, structure, replication, and laboratory diagnosis of the type of organism reviewed in that section are presented. The discussion of laboratory diagnosis includes an overview of methods used for detection of the organisms and, if appropriate, antimicrobial susceptibility testing. The remaining chapters in each section are divided into three parts: clinical infection, which includes epidemiology, pathogenesis (and pathology where applicable), and clinical manifestations; laboratory diagnosis; and treatment and prevention.

In Part III, specimen handling (collection, transport, and processing) is reviewed by organ system. The Appendix includes procedures for tests that are used frequently in the clinical microbiology laboratory and with which, therefore, the clinical pathologist should be familiar.

Philadelphia, PA   GAIL L. WOODS

ACKNOWLEDGMENTS

I thank Dr. Gerri Hall and Ann Morrissey for their help with the artwork, and the following persons for their secretarial assistance: Arlene Reichart, Dottie Bathe, and Val Rementer at The Medical College Hospitals; Sara Chesnic at Case Western Reserve University; and Michelle Fisher and Lisa Karnish at the University of Nebraska Medical Center, where the book was begun. I am grateful for the encouragement and support of Dr. David Purtilo, who died unexpectedly while the book was in the final stages of proof; he will be missed by many. I also appreciate the expert advice and technical assistance of Tanya Lazar and Samuel Rondinelli.

CONTENTS

PART I. OVERVIEW

Chapter 1. General Introduction 3
Chapter 2. Host-Pathogen Relationships and Pathogenesis of Infectious Disease 5

PART II. CLINICAL INFECTION AND LABORATORY DIAGNOSIS

Section I. Viruses

Chapter 3. Introduction to Viruses 33
Chapter 4. Poxviruses 43
Chapter 5. Herpesviruses 46
Chapter 6. Adenoviruses 65
Chapter 7. Papovaviruses 70
Chapter 8. Parvoviruses 75
Chapter 9. Hepatitis B Virus and the Delta Agent 77
Chapter 10. Paramyxoviruses 85
Chapter 11. Orthomyxoviruses 97
Chapter 12. Coronaviruses 102
Chapter 13. Picornaviruses 105
Chapter 14. Reoviruses 116
Chapter 15. Caliciviruses 122
Chapter 16. Rhabdoviruses 123
Chapter 17. Togaviruses 129
Chapter 18. Flaviviruses 134
Chapter 19. Bunyaviruses 138
Chapter 20. Arenaviruses 141
Chapter 21. Filoviruses 144
Chapter 22. Retroviruses 146
Chapter 23. Unclassified and Unconventional Viruses 163

Section II. Bacteria

Chapter 24. Introduction to Bacteria 173
Chapter 25. Chlamydias 184
Chapter 26. Rickettsias 194
Chapter 27. Mycoplasmas 214
Chapter 28. Aerobic and Facultative Gram-Positive Cocci 218
Chapter 29. Aerobic and Facultative Gram-Positive Bacilli 239
Chapter 30. Anaerobic Gram-Positive Bacteria 253
Chapter 31. Neisseria and Branhamella 268
Chapter 32. Aerobic, Nonfermentative Gram-Negative Bacilli and Coccobacilli 281
Chapter 33. Fastidious Aerobic Gram-Negative Bacilli and Coccobacilli 293

xiii

Chapter 34.	Enterobacteriaceae	307
Chapter 35.	Vibrionaceae	329
Chapter 36.	Haemophilus and Other Facultative Gram-Negative Bacilli	336
Chapter 37.	Campylobacter and Helicobacter	350
Chapter 38.	Anaerobic Gram-Negative Bacteria	357
Chapter 39.	Spirochetes	361
Chapter 40.	Mycobacteria	378
Chapter 41.	Other Gram-Negative Bacteria	399

Section III. Fungi and Algae-like Organisms

Chapter 42.	Introduction to Fungi and Algae-like Organisms	407
Chapter 43.	Yeasts	415
Chapter 44.	Moulds	426
Chapter 45.	Dimorphic Fungi	447
Chapter 46.	Miscellaneous Fungi	460
Chapter 47.	Algae-like Organisms	463

Section IV. Animal Parasites

Chapter 48.	Introduction to Animal Parasites	469
Chapter 49.	Intestinal, Oral, and Vaginal Protozoa	472
Chapter 50.	Intestinal Helminths	482
Chapter 51.	Blood and Tissue Protozoa	497
Chapter 52.	Blood and Tissue Helminths	512
Chapter 53.	Arthropods	530

PART III. SPECIMEN HANDLING AND LABORATORY DIAGNOSIS, BY ORGAN SYSTEM

Chapter 54.	Introduction to Specimen Handling and Laboratory Diagnosis	539
Chapter 55.	Central Nervous System	544
Chapter 56.	Head and Neck: Eye, Sinuses, Ear, and Oral Cavity	551
Chapter 57.	Respiratory Tract	561
Chapter 58.	Cardiovascular and Hematopoietic Systems	573
Chapter 59.	Gastrointestinal Tract	585
Chapter 60.	Liver, Biliary Tract, and Pancreas	595
Chapter 61.	Genitourinary Tract	600
Chapter 62.	Skin, Adenexa, and Subcutaneous Tissues	610
Chapter 63.	Body Cavities	619
Chapter 64.	Musculoskeletal System	623

Appendix ... 631

Index ... 639

Part I

Overview

Chapter 1

GENERAL INTRODUCTION

The role of the clinical pathologist in the diagnosis of infectious diseases and the organization of the text in relation to this role are discussed in this chapter.

ROLE OF THE CLINICAL PATHOLOGIST

Clinical pathologists today function as fulcrums for a variety of medical disciplines, and it is through their offices and the laboratories they direct that the agents of infectious diseases are identified. Moreover, their efforts help determine appropriate therapy for many bacteria and some fungal and viral diseases.

To serve effectively as a consultant for the clinician caring for a patient suspected of having an infectious disease, the clinical pathologist must understand the epidemiology, pathogenesis, and clinical manifestations of the diseases caused by the various groups of organisms: viruses, bacteria, fungi, algae, and parasites. It is only with this knowledge that the clinical pathologist confidently can discuss cases with clinicians, help develop a list of potential pathogens, and ensure that appropriate steps are taken to reach a diagnosis. Working from the differential diagnosis in each case, the clinical pathologist must determine which specimens should be obtained to identify the most likely pathogens and must know how and when to collect the sample, how it should be transported to the laboratory, and if necessary, proper storage conditions. The clinical pathologist also must know how to process the specimen to identify the organism responsible for the illness.

When direct examination of the clinical specimen is critical to patient management—samples obtained by an invasive procedure (tissue, bronchoalveolar lavage fluid, protected specimen brush, aspirates), sterile body fluids, peripheral blood smears—the clinical pathologist reviews preparations of the sample stained with the Gram stain or another appropriate stain and issues a formal report. When culture is indicated, the clinical pathologist must know what cell lines (for viruses and, occasionally, for chlamydia) and agar media (for bacteria, fungi, algae, and, rarely, parasites) should be inoculated. The clinical pathologist must know when rapid diagnostic tests such as those for monoclonal antibodies, enzyme immunoassays, and nucleic acid probes would be useful and when serologic tests are indicated. Moreover, the clinical pathologist must know the limitations of all these diagnostic techniques, in order to provide an accurate interpretation of the results.

When tissue must be obtained for diagnosis, the clinical and the anatomic pathologist should function as a team to ensure appropriate handling of the sample. The clinical pathologist should indicate what portion of the specimen is used and how much is required to optimize the chances of making the correct diagnosis. Together, the clinical and the anatomic pathologist review the histologic findings in tissue sections and stained smears and the culture results, consider the data, and jointly provide the clinician with an interpretation that incorporates all information.

In addition to determining what tests to perform for optimal diagnosis, the clinical pathologist is responsible for providing the results of those tests within a period of time that will allow appropriate patient management. For this reason, test selection often is based on a turnaround time that affords the best quality of patient care.

The clinical pathologist must have a general understanding of the chemotherapeutic agents that are effective against infectious agents. This is especially true for infections caused by aerobic, facultative, and, to a lesser extent, anaerobic bacteria, because methods for susceptibility testing of these organisms currently are standardized, and recommended guidelines must be followed to ensure appropriate patient care (see Chapter 24). The clinical pathologist must be aware of the potential advantages and disadvantages of each method of susceptibility testing and must know the special requirements for evaluating certain organisms, in order to select the system most appropriate for the laboratory and for the patient population it serves. In consultation with the medical staff and the pharmacists, the clinical pathologist must choose panels of antimicrobial agents to test against different types of bacteria (gram-positive, gram-negative, fastidious, anaerobic). Then based on the knowledge of the expected susceptibility of the various species of bacteria to the antimicrobial agents tested, the clinical pathologist can recognize potential errors in susceptibility test results before they leave the laboratory. Moreover, when an unusually resistant isolate is identified, the pathologist can alert the clinician quickly, thus allowing more rapid intervention in patient management and optimal care.

TEXT ORGANIZATION

This text is divided into three parts. The first provides an overview of the topics discussed in the bulk of the book. The second part addresses the clinical infections caused by each group of organisms and how those infections are diagnosed in the microbiology laboratory. The third part is a guide for handling (collection, transport, and processing) specimens from each organ system for detection of all pathogens that might be present. This organizational design reflects a logical approach to the study of the clinical pathology of infectious diseases. Because any organ can be attacked by many infectious agents, an understanding of the structure and function of the individual organisms provides the foundation for a discussion of the laboratory diagnosis of infections involving the various organ systems.

The book begins with an overview of host-pathogen relationships because the interactions that occur between a host and an infectious agent form the core of the study of infectious diseases. The outcome of an encounter between host and micro-organism depends on the immune response of the host and the virulence of the microbe. The host and infectious agent may have a symbiotic relationship; the organism may cause an inapparent infection; or the interaction between the two may progress to disease. In the latter situation, the clinical pathologist plays an essential role in diagnosis, which ultimately is based on an understanding of the pathogenesis of the particular disease.

The discussion of infectious agents in the second portion of the text is divided into sections, arranged phylogenetically in order of ascending complexity: viruses, the simplest agents, are presented first, followed by bacteria, fungi, and algae, and then parasites. In addition to the differences in complexity between each group of organisms, the laboratory diagnoses of infections caused by each group, in general, are different and frequently are performed in separate sections of the laboratory.

Each chapter in Part II includes a review of the epidemiology, pathogenesis, and clinical manifestations of the diseases caused by the respective organisms, followed by a discussion of the laboratory diagnosis and a brief overview of treatment and, if appropriate, prevention. This organizational structure reflects the role of the clinical pathologist as a consultant for the practicing clinician. To effectively communicate and advise, the pathologist must be able to develop a differential diagnosis. An accurate laboratory diagnosis requires collecting an appropriate specimen and performing a reliable test. What specimens are recommended for diagnosis depends on the clinical manifestations, and, in some cases, the pathogenesis, of the particular disease. Tests to detect an infectious agent are selected according to the biologic characteristics of the suspected pathogens, the pathogenic mechanisms of the disease process, and, frequently, turnaround time.

After the fundamental background information on the clinical infection and laboratory diagnosis of each group of organisms is provided, data on specimens required for diagnosis, which are presented in the laboratory diagnosis section of each chapter in Part II, are expanded in the last part of the book, which addresses specimen handling (collection, transport, and processing) and laboratory diagnosis by organ system. In this way, essential information used constantly by clinical pathologists is presented in a readily accessible format.

As medical director of the microbiology laboratory, the clinical pathologist must ensure that specimens are processed in a way that allows detection of all pathogens that might be present. Each chapter in the last part of the book is organized according to the specimens associated with the respective organ system, and for each specimen, specific guidelines are presented for detection of viruses, bacteria, fungi, algae, and parasites.

Chapter 2

HOST-PATHOGEN RELATIONSHIPS AND PATHOGENESIS OF INFECTIOUS DISEASE

The interaction between host and infectious agent has several possible outcomes that depend on the ability of the organism to produce infection (replication of micro-organisms in or on body tissues), the host's response to the infection, and the virulence of the invading microbe. For example, organisms that comprise the host's normal flora do not produce infection unless the host's defenses are compromised. For some organisms the outcome of the host-pathogen relationship is subclinical (inapparent) infection: the encounter is limited to an immune response detectable only by serologic testing. In other cases, the interaction may progress to disease, which is the clinical expression of infection and indicates that the replicating organisms are disrupting the host to a degree that signs and symptoms are manifested. Disease varies from mild to severe and may be fatal. In this chapter the host defense mechanisms and the microbial factors involved in disease production are reviewed. The pathogenesis and epidemiology of infectious diseases are described briefly and are discussed in more detail for individual organisms in Part II of the book.

HOST DEFENSE MECHANISMS

Host defense mechanisms may be categorized as nonspecific or specific. Nonspecific responses protect against a wide range of infectious agents, whereas specific responses are directed against one particular micro-organism.

NONSPECIFIC DEFENSES

Nonspecific defense mechanisms include physical barriers to invasion, secretions at potential portals of entry, complement, and phagocytic cells (granulocytes and monocytes). Monocytes also are an essential component of the specific cell-mediated immune response and, therefore, are discussed in the section on specific defenses.

Physical Barriers and Secretions

The integrity of the body surfaces is the first line of defense against invading micro-organisms. The normal flora of the skin and mucous membranes, the normal anatomy, and substances in secretions at potential portals of entry for micro-organisms—the eyes and the respiratory, gastrointestinal, and genitourinary tract—are other barriers to infection.

Normal Flora

Bacteria that comprise the normal flora (Table 2–1) protect the host from invasion by pathogenic micro-organisms in several ways (1,2). They inhibit the growth of invading bacteria by competing for the same nutrients and for the same receptors on host cells and by producing bacteriocins, substances that are toxic to other bacteria. Members of the normal flora stimulate the host's immune system to maintain a constant, low level of expression of class II major histocompatibility complex (MHC) molecules on macrophages and other antigen-presenting cells. This allows the immune system to respond more efficiently to invading micro-organisms, because T lymphocytes recognize antigens only after they are processed by an antigen-presenting cell and presented on the surface of that cell in physical association with a class II MHC molecule (described under Cell-Mediated Immunity). Moreover, some members of the normal bacterial flora share antigens with certain pathogenic bacteria and thus stimulate the production of cross-protective immune factors such as natural antibodies. These organism-specific antibodies are detected in healthy persons who have no history of infection with that particular pathogen. They help protect against disease caused by some bacteria, especially Neisseria meningitidis and Haemophilus influenzae type b (see Chapters 31 and 36).

Skin

In general, micro-organisms do not penetrate intact skin but enter the body through breaks in it produced by minor or major trauma, a surgical procedure, a primary skin condition such as eczema or dermatitis, or placement of an intravascular catheter or an arthropod vector. In addition to the physical barrier, other properties of the skin protect against infection. Frequent desquamation eliminates organisms, and fatty acids on the skin surface, derived from partial hydrolysis of triglycerides by the normal flora, create a mildly acidic environment (pH 5 to 6) that has an antibacterial effect.

Eyes

In the eyes, tears provide protection by diluting and washing away micro-organisms. Moreover, tears contain lysozyme, an enzyme that lyses bacteria, especially gram-positive ones, by disrupting the cell wall.

Respiratory Tract

The upper airways—nasal turbinates, epiglottis, and larynx—are the initial physical barrier to inhalation of micro-organisms. Turbulent air flow in these sites forces large particles to adhere to mucosal surfaces, and the

Table 2–1. The Normal Flora of Healthy Humans

Site	Organisms	Relative Frequency of Isolation	Site	Organisms	Relative Frequency of Isolation
Skin	Staphylococcus aureus	++			
	Staphylococcus epidermidis	++++			
	Viridans streptococci	+	Large intestine†	Staphylococcus aureus	+
	Corynebacterium spp	++++		Staphylococcus epidermidis	+
	Propionibacterium acnes	++++		Group B streptococci	+
	Malassezia furfur	++++		Viridans streptococci	++
	Candida spp	+		Enterococcus spp	++
Mouth and oropharynx	Staphylococcus aureus	+		Lactobacillus spp	+++
	Staphylococcus epidermidis	+++		Clostridium spp	++++
	Streptococcus pneumoniae	++		Actinomyces spp	+
	Viridans streptococci	++++		Peptostreptococcus spp	++++
	Enterococcus spp	+		Pseudomonas spp	+
	Lactobacillus spp	++		Other nonfermenters	+
	Actinomyces spp	+		Enterobacteriaceae	++++
	Peptostreptococcus spp	+		Bacteroidaceae	++++
	Neisseria spp	++		Treponema spp	+
	Haemophilus influenzae	+		Mycobacterium spp	+
	Haemophilus spp	+		Candida spp	+
	Bacteroides spp	++	Vagina	Mycoplasma spp	±
	Porphyromonas spp	++		Ureaplasma urealyticum	±
	Prevotella spp	++		Staphylococcus epidermidis	+
	Fusobacterium spp*	++++		Group B streptococcus	+
	Veillonella spp	++++		Viridans streptococci	+
	Treponema spp*	+++		Enterococcus spp	+
	Candida spp	++		Lactobacillus spp	++++
Nose	Staphylococcus aureus	++		Clostridium spp	++
	Staphylococcus epidermidis	++++		Actinomyces spp	+
	Streptococcus pneumoniae	+		Bifidobacterium spp	+
	Viridans streptococci	++		Propionibacterium acnes	+
	Neisseria spp	+		Peptostreptococcus spp	+
	Haemophilus spp	+		Neisseria spp	±
Outer ear	Staphylococcus epidermidis	++++		Acinetobacter spp	+
	Pseudomonas spp	+		Enterobacteriaceae	+
	Enterobacteriaceae	+		Gardnerella vaginalis	+
Conjunctivae	Staphylococcus aureus	+		Bacteroidaceae	+
	Staphylococcus epidermidis	++++		Candida spp	++
	Haemophilus spp	+	External genitalia and anterior urethra	Skin flora (see above)	
Esophagus and stomach	Surviving bacteria from upper respiratory tract and food	+		Mycoplasma spp	±
Small intestine	Enterococcus spp	++		Ureaplasma urealyticum	±
	Lactobacillus spp	+++		Enterococcus spp	+
	Clostridium spp	++		Peptostreptococcus spp	+
	Enterobacteriaceae	++		Enterobacteriaceae	±
	Bacteroidaceae	+++		Bacteroidaceae	+
	Mycobacterium spp	++		Mycobacterium spp‡	++

* Less prevalent in edentulous persons.
† At least 95% are obligate anaerobes. Protozoa may be present in inhabitants of underdeveloped countries.
‡ Especially common in smegma of uncircumcised males.
Key: ++++, almost always present; +++, usually present; ++, frequently present; +, occasionally present; ±, infrequently present.
(Adapted from Tramont EC: General or nonspecific host defense mechanisms. In Principles and Practice of Infectious Diseases. 3rd ed. Edited by GL Mandell, RG Douglas Jr, and JE Bennett. New York, Churchill Livingstone, 1990.)

humid atmosphere causes organisms to increase in size, promoting their phagocytosis.

The dichotomously branching conducting airways located between the upper airways and the terminal bronchioles and alveoli provide an additional anatomic barrier. Their mucosal surfaces are protected by mucociliary clearance and coughing, both of which propel organisms orad. Bronchial secretions also contain lysozyme, lactoferrin, which has antibacterial activity, and secretory immunoglobulin (Ig) A, which may prevent attachment of certain bacteria and viruses to the ciliated epithelial cells (discussed later).

Host defenses of the alveolar spaces are activated when the upper and conducting airways fail to eliminate inspired pathogens. Surfactant (secreted by type II pneumocytes) and transferrin have some antibacterial activity. IgG, complement, and phagocytic cells are discussed in later sections.

Defects in any one of these factors predispose to infection and disease. For example, bypassing the upper airways with an endotracheal tube affords pathogens direct access to the lungs, placing patients who require assisted ventilation at increased risk of pneumonia. Malnutrition may disrupt the integrity of the mucosal epithelial cells, enhancing bacterial adherence, which is often the first step in microbial invasion (discussed later). The ciliated epithelium may be damaged by cigarette smoke, other noxious fumes, and several viruses (influenza and parainfluenza viruses, respiratory syncytial virus, rhinovirus, coronavirus); such insults promote bacterial colonization. Congenital structural defects of cilia predispose to recurrent or chronic otitis media, sinusitis, and bronchiectasis. Loss of consciousness and anesthesia suppress the cough reflex; consequently, oral secretions (which contain about 10^5 aerobic and 10^6 anaerobic bacteria per 0.01 ml of fluid) accumulate in the airways, increasing the risk of aspiration pneumonia. Pulmonary congestion, edema, and emphysema interfere with bacterial clearance by mechanisms that are currently unknown.

Gastrointestinal Tract

Nonspecific defenses of the gastrointestinal tract are the acid pH of the stomach, pancreatic enzymes, bile, intestinal secretions, peristalsis, normal shedding of epithelial cells, and normal bowel flora. These defenses, however, may be overwhelmed if a large inoculum of the invading pathogen is ingested. Moreover, alteration of any of these defense mechanisms increases the likelihood of disease. For example, infections with salmonellae, Yersinia enterocolitica, and Mycobacterium tuberculosis are more common in persons with achlorhydria and in those who have undergone gastrectomy. Disruption of the normal flora by broad-spectrum antimicrobial therapy allows infection with Clostridium difficile, and possibly disease (3).

Genitourinary Tract

Several factors in the genitourinary tract protect against infection. The acid pH of urine may be bactericidal, and voiding washes most bacteria from the lower urinary tract unless they can attach firmly to the epithelium, an attribute of Neisseria gonorrhoeae and uropathogenic strains of Escherichia coli (4). In males, the length of the urethra provides some protection against infection. The hypertonic environment of the renal medulla inhibits the growth of most bacteria, and Tamm-Horsfall glycoprotein produced by the kidneys and excreted in the urine binds certain bacteria, possibly preventing colonization and subsequent disease (5). The acid environment of the vagina inhibits most pathogenic bacteria, and cervical mucus and prostatic fluid contain the antibacterial substance lysozyme.

Complement

The complement system is a complex series of proteins (Table 2–2) that form two inter-related enzyme cascades: the more recently evolved classical pathway and the alternative pathway. Complement activation and its role in host defense are discussed in this section.

Activation

The sequence of events in the two complement pathways (Figs. 2–1, 2–2) interact at the level of C3, forming a final common pathway composed of the terminal complement components C5 through C9, also called the membrane attack complex (reviewed in detail in reference 6). Activation of the classical pathway, which occurs predominantly on target surfaces, requires a specific antigen-antibody interaction. In contrast, activation of the alternative pathway occurs in the fluid phase and on surfaces and does not require antibodies. Without antibodies to direct complement activation, however, the process is less efficient because C3b is deposited randomly over the surface of the particle.

Role in Host Defense

Complement functions in host defense in several ways (7). First, the cleavage fragments of the classical pathway—C3a, C4a, C5a, referred to as anaphylatoxins—are stimuli for local inflammation. The biologic functions of these molecules are listed in Table 2–3. Second, complement is important in clearing immune complexes, thus preventing excessive tissue injury associated with their deposition (8). A third effect of complement, predominantly C3, in host defense is modulation (enhancement or inhibition, depending on the concentration of the particular C3 fragment) of T and B lymphocytes (9,10). Fourth, cell-bound fragments of C3 (primarily C3b and C3bi) act as bifunctional opsonic ligands that link target particles to effector cells that possess receptors for these fragments (11). For bacteria, opsonization with C3b or C3bi, especially in conjunction with IgG, promotes phagocytosis of the organisms and activates microbicidal mechanisms, and the terminal complement components C7 and C8 may facilitate neutrophil-dependent intraphagosomal bacterial killing (12). Finally, assembly and insertion of the membrane attack complex disrupts cell membranes and kills cells (13). For bacteria, these events occur only with gram-negative organisms. For viruses, deposition of the early components of the classical pathway may result in viral neutralization, with or without lysis, and activation of the alternative pathway in conjunction with IgG can result in lysis of different virus-infected human cells (14).

The degree to which the complement system is activated depends on various microbial factors (6,7,15,16). Certain surfaces are better activators of complement than others, so activation is to some extent controlled by the composition of the cell wall or capsule of the invading bacteria. Organisms that contain sialic acid (Neisseria meningitidis group B, Escherichia coli K-1, and serotype III of group B streptococci) are poor activators of the alternative complement pathway, whereas those with polysaccharide capsules (especially Streptococcus pneumoniae) are efficient activators. Some organisms (Trypanosoma cruzi) readily activate the complement cascade but also contain surface proteins that degrade essential

Table 2–2. Components of the Complement System

Pathway/Function	Complement Component
Classical pathway	C1q, C1r, C1s, C2, C4, C3
Alternative pathway	D, C3, B
Membrane attack complex	C5, C6, C7, C8, C9
Positive control proteins	Properdin
Negative control proteins	C1 inhibitor, C4bp, factor H, factor I, anaphylatoxin inhibitor, S protein

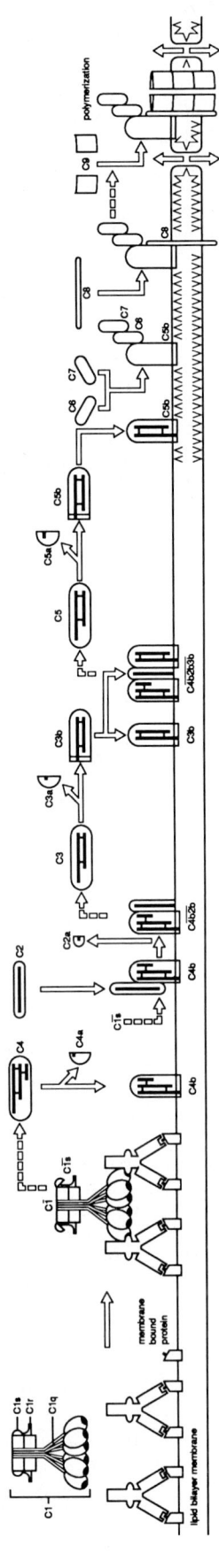

Fig. 2–1. Sequence of events in the classical complement pathway. (Drawn from Roitt IM, Brostoff J, and Male DK (eds.): Immunology. St. Louis, CV Mosby, 1985.)

Activation   Inactivation

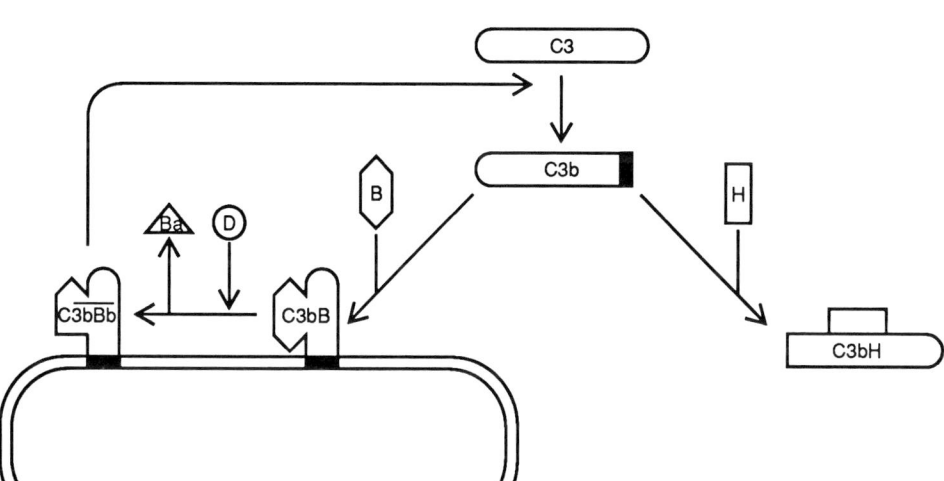

Fig. 2–2. Sequence of events in the alternative complement pathway.

complement components, thus inhibiting completion of the pathway.

The thickness and structure of the cell wall determine the susceptibility of the microbe to the membrane attack complex. The thick cell wall of gram-positive bacteria and fungi protects the cell membrane from complement-mediated lysis. Gram-negative organisms, on the other hand, lack thick cell walls and are susceptible to the bactericidal and lytic effects of complement, though the structure of the cell wall may provide some protection. Long O-antigen side chains (see Chapter 24) cause complement activation to occur at a distance from the outer membrane, inhibiting insertion of the membrane attack complex. Some gram-negative bacteria (Haemophilus influenzae, Neisseria meningitidis, and Neisseria gonorrhoeae) with short O-antigen side chains require specific antibodies for effective sensitization and complement activation. These organisms therefore, are effectively resistant to the bactericidal effect of serum under conditions in which specific antibodies are absent.

Deficiencies, inherited or acquired, of the complement proteins most commonly are manifested by recurrent infections with encapsulated bacteria, although certain disorders—hereditary angioedema and paroxysmal nocturnal hemoglobinuria—are not associated with infectious complications. Inherited deficiencies of complement proteins are uncommon in the general population (prevalence about 0.03%) but are about 10 times more common among persons with rheumatic disease, particularly systemic lupus erythematosus (7,11,17). Features of conditions associated with increased risk of infection are summarized in Table 2–4.

Granulocytes

Granulocytes normally comprise 60 to 70% of the total blood leukocytes and also are found in extravascular sites. These cells are classified by the reaction of their granules when stained with various dyes as neutrophils, eosinophils, or basophils.

Neutrophils

Polymorphonuclear neutrophils (PMN) are essential in host defense against infections with bacteria and some viruses and fungi, but they also mediate tissue damage in certain noninfectious diseases. In this section, the development, structure, and activation of neutrophils and their role in host defense are discussed.

Development, Structure, and Activation. Neutrophils originate from stem cells in the bone marrow. Normally, about 5% of the total body population of neutrophils circulate in the blood, and of the circulating PMN, about half comprise the marginating pool, which adheres to the endothelium of the small vessels. Neutrophils have a half-life of about 6 to 8 hours in the circulation. Then they enter the tissues and function for a few days before they die or are shed from a mucosal surface.

PMN contain three types of granules (Table 2–5) (18,19). Primary granules are released into the phagosome after phagocytosis, and secondary granules discharge much of their contents to the exterior of the cell. Neutrophil surface glycoproteins, which in part mediate adherence to other cells and surfaces, include the C3bi receptor (C3R), lymphocyte function–associated antigen

Table 2–3. Biologic Functions of the Anaphylatoxins

Anaphylatoxin	Function
C4a	Promotes vasodilation
C3a	Stimulates histamine release from mast cells, promotes vasodilation, increases vascular permeability
C5a	Same as C3a, plus is the major factor stimulating neutrophil chemotaxis, adhesiveness, degranulation, and oxidative burst; causes margination of neutrophils and smooth muscle contraction

Table 2–4. Features of Complement Deficiency States

Deficient Component	Functional Defect	Clinical Manifestations
C1, C4, C2	↓ complement activation, ↓ immune complex metabolism, ↓ immune response	Rheumatic disease; systemic infection with Streptococcus pneumoniae, Neisseria meningitidis, Haemophilus influenzae
Properdin, factor B	↓ complement activation	Infection with Neisseria meningitidis
C3	↓ immune response, ↓ chemotaxis, ↓ opsonization, ↓ serum bactericidal activity, ↓ immune complex metabolism	Severe, recurrent infections (sinuses, respiratory tract, blood, meninges) with Streptococcus pneumoniae, Neisseria meningitidis, Haemophilus influenzae
C5, C6, C7, C8	↓ serum bactericidal activity	Recurrent infections with Neisseria meningitidis, especially group Y*

* The mortality rate for meningococcal disease is lower for persons deficient in late complement components than for healthy persons, suggesting that the severity of the disease may be associated with complement activation and an intact membrane attack complex.

1 (LFA-1), and p150,95 (20). C3R also is found on monocytes, natural killer cells, and some lymphocytes, and LFA-1 and p150,95 also are present on monocytes and lymphocytes. C3R binds C3b fixed to the surface of micro-organisms during complement activation and acts synergistically with receptors for the Fc portion of IgG (described later) to enhance adherence and phagocytosis of opsonized organisms. Neutrophils also have receptors for the Fc fragment of IgG, the C5a fragment generated during complement activation, the chemotactic agent leukotriene B_4, and formylmethionylpeptides (chemotactic substances generated by bacteria).

Exposure to stimuli such as bacterial lipopolysaccharide and cytokines (granulocyte/monocyte colony–stimulating factor, tumor necrosis factor [TNF], interferon [IFN]γ, and interleukin [IL] 1, described later) causes neutrophils to become primed: they show increased oxidative metabolism and increased secretory capacity and, therefore, are more effective in protecting against invading bacteria. The mechanism for the enhanced response of primed PMN, however, is unknown. Priming is inhibited by certain bacterial toxins, such as those produced by Bacillus anthracis (21).

Role in Host Defense. The primary function of neutrophils is ingestion and destruction of invading pathogens, a process that involves several steps (Fig. 2–3). One of the first steps in the neutrophil's response to inflammatory stimuli is adherence to endothelial surfaces, an event mediated by the cell surface glycoproteins. Neutrophils then migrate to sites of infection or inflammation in response to chemotactic substances generated by invading bacteria, by phagocytic cells at the involved site, or by activation of the classical complement pathway and release of C5a. Neutrophils sense these substances in nanomolar concentrations and migrate toward them with directed movement.

In general, for phagocytosis by neutrophils to occur, bacteria must be coated by opsonins, of which IgG and complement are the most important. The Fab portion of IgG binds to a bacterium, and the Fc portion interacts with the Fc receptor on the PMN. Complement activation by either pathway generates C3b, which can undergo hydrolysis to C3bi and bind to C3R on PMN. Actin, myosin, and actin-binding proteins provide the force needed for phagocytosis; however, the mechanisms of phagocytosis are not completely understood.

Two events are responsible for killing ingested organisms. Degranulation, an oxygen-independent process, involves the release of primary and secondary granules. Contents of primary granules (such as lysozyme, cathepsin G, and defensins) have antibacterial and antifungal activity, and defensins are active against some enveloped viruses (19). Primary granules also contain substances that enhance the penetration of PMN into tissues and promote abscess formation. Secondary granules contain substances that are important for chemotaxis and substances that have antimicrobial activity. For example, lactoferrin chelates iron and so limits the amount available to microorganisms for growth. The respiratory burst is an oxygen-dependent event during which substances with potent antimicrobial activity (hydrogen peroxide and hypochlorous acid) are generated.

The antimicrobial oxidative and nonoxidative processes described above are important in the pathogenesis of several noninfectious diseases such as gout, rheumatoid arthritis, immune vasculitis, glomerulonephritis, neutrophil dermatoses, inflammatory bowel disease, myocardial infarction, adult respiratory distress syndrome, emphysema, asthma, and thermal injury–associated hemolysis (20,22). Potential mechanisms of tissue injury include the proteolytic enzymes of the primary granules—elastase, collagenase, and gelatinase—and toxic oxygen metabolites.

Qualitative and quantitative disorders of neutrophils

Table 2–5. Contents and Function of Neutrophil Granules

Granule Type	Contents	Function
Primary (azurophilic)	Myeloperoxidase, acid hydrolases, lysozyme, cationic proteins (bactericidal/permeability-increasing factor), cathepsin G, neutral proteases (collagenase, gelatinase, elastase), defensins	Localized microbicidal activity
Secondary (specific)	Lactoferrin, lysozyme, vitamin B_{12}-binding protein, cytochrome b, collagenase, receptor molecules	Regulatory function in inflammatory response, chemotaxis
Tertiary	Gelatinase, cytochrome b, MAC-1 glycoprotein receptor	Not known

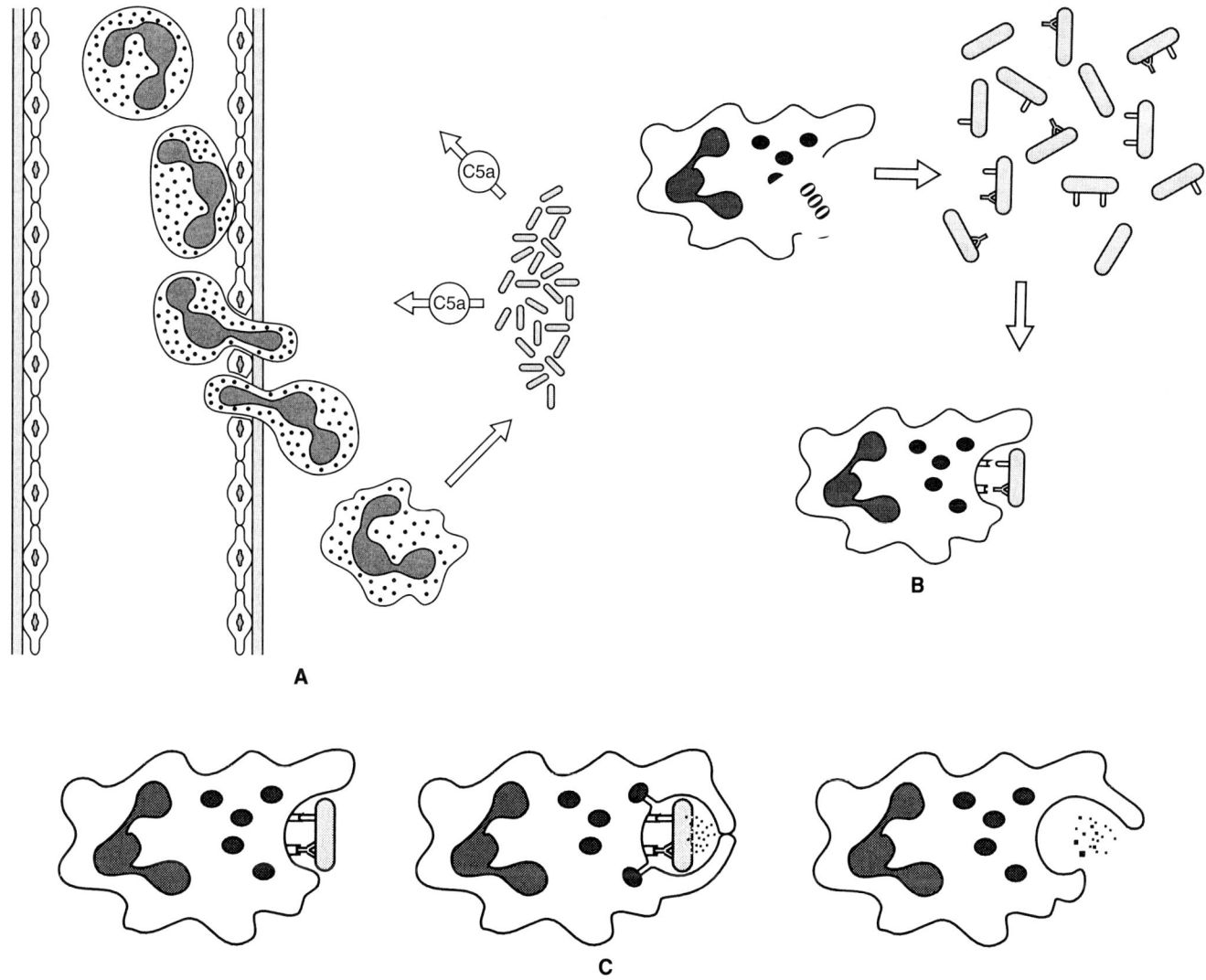

Fig. 2–3. Bacteria activate the complement system, generating C5a, which causes margination of neutrophils and stimulates neutrophil chemotaxis. B, Bacteria coated with IgG and C3b bind to receptors on neutrophils. C, Bacteria bound to neutrophils are phagocytosed and destroyed by the contents of the granules.

are associated with increased risk of infection by organisms that are typically eliminated by these phagocytic cells, pyogenic bacteria and fungi. Features of these disorders are summarized in Table 2–6 (20,22–27).

Eosinophils

Eosinophils are found primarily in tissues, especially those that have an epithelial interface with the environment: the respiratory, gastrointestinal, and lower genitourinary tract. In this section, the development and structure of eosinophils and their role in host defense are reviewed.

Development and Structure. Eosinophils develop and differentiate in the bone marrow (28). Their exact life span is not known, but they live longer than neutrophils and may survive weeks in tissues. Eosinophils have at least three types of granules: specific granules (Table 2–7) responsible for the tinctorial properties of eosinophils visualized by light microscopy, primary granules, and smaller granules that contain arylsulfatase and other enzymes (28,29). Eosinophils have surface receptors for IgG, IgE, and IgA. Binding of immunoglobulins to receptors for IgA—and, to a lesser extent, IgG and IgE—induces degranulation (28). Eosinophils also have receptors for complement components, for cytokines (described under Cell-Mediated Immunity), and for two lipid mediators, platelet-activating factor and leukotriene B_4, both of which are chemoattractants for eosinophils and stimulate eosinophil degranulation and the formation of superoxide anion and other oxidant derivatives. Eosinophil cell surface adhesion proteins involved in cell-cell interactions are integrins, which enable eosinophils to emigrate from blood to tissues, and the neutrophil adhesion proteins C3R, LFA-1, and p150,95.

Role in Host Defense. The predominant role of eo-

Table 2-6. Neutrophil Disorders

Disorder	Laboratory Abnormalities	Clinical Manifestations
Qualitative disorders		
C3bi receptor deficiency	↓ chemotaxis, abnormal antibody-dependent cell-mediated cytotoxicity, ↓ respiratory burst and degranulation	Delayed separation of umbilical cord, delayed wound healing, recurrent bacterial skin infections, mucositis, otitis, gingivitis, periodontitis; severe pneumonia
Chronic granulomatous diseases	Abnormal oxidative metabolism and absent or decreased generation of oxygen metabolites (O_2, H_2O_2, HOCl)	Recurrent severe infections with catalase-positive bacteria and fungi
Specific granule deficiency	Absent or ↓ specific granules; ↓ bactericidal activity; bilobed PMN nuclei	Recurrent, severe bacterial infections of skin and soft tissues
Myeloperoxidase deficiency	↓ killing of Candida in vitro	None
Chediak-Higashi syndrome	↓ chemotaxis, degranulation, and intracellular killing; large intracytoplasmic granules in all circulating leukocytes	Recurrent bacterial (especially Staphylococcus aureus) and fungal infections of skin, mucous membranes, and respiratory tract; oculocutaneous albinism; death in first decade
Actin dysfunction	↓ chemotaxis	Recurrent pyogenic infections
Quantitative disorders		
Neutropenia, acquired* or hereditary†	<1500 PMN/µl (risk increases significantly below 500/µl³)	Bacterial and fungal infections

* Acquired neutropenia most commonly is drug induced but may be associated with bacterial sepsis, hypersplenism, or, occasionally, malnutrition.
† Includes severe and benign familial neutropenia, cyclic neutropenia, and neutropenia associated with other disorders such as orotic aciduria, dyskeratosis congenita, hypoglobulinemia, and pancreatic insufficiency.
Key: ↓, decreased; PMN, polymorphonuclear neutrophil.

sinophils in host defense is protection against large organisms that are not easily phagocytosed, particularly multicellular helminths in the larval stage (Fig. 2-4). Initial binding of eosinophils to parasites may be mediated by specific IgG or IgE or by C3b deposited on the helminth's surface. Bound eosinophils then release potent helminthotoxins—major basic protein, eosinophil cationic protein, and eosinophil peroxidase (28).

In addition to their antihelminthic properties, cationic proteins may damage host cells. For example, they can damage trachael epithelial cells, and major basic protein can augment the contraction of the trachea induced by acetylcholine and can damage the nasal epithelium (30,31). The two lipid mediators produced by eosinophils (described earlier) are involved in allergic diseases. They cause contraction of bronchial smooth muscle, promote mucus secretion, alter vascular permeability, and stimulate eosinophil and neutrophil infiltration (28). Moreover, major basic protein can stimulate release of histamine from basophils and mast cells, and eosinophil peroxidase stimulates histamine release from mast cells.

Basophils

Basophils, which are found predominantly in tissues, have randomly distributed granules that contain heparin, histamine, slow-reacting substance of anaphylaxis (SRS-A), and eosinophil chemotactic factor of anaphylaxis (ECF-A). The small percentage of basophils that circulate in the blood have IgE bound to their surface, and recognition of antigen by this immunoglobulin triggers release of the contents of the granules into the external environment. Basophils do not have a major role in protecting against infection but may be involved in immunity to ticks (32).

SPECIFIC DEFENSES

Specific host defenses include the humoral immune response and the specific cell-mediated immune response.

Humoral Immunity

The humoral immune response is mediated by antibodies, or immunoglobulins, produced by activated B lymphocytes that differentiate into plasma cells. These molecules have binding specificity for a wide range of antigens, including micro-organisms. Antibodies may be involved in the elimination of invading pathogens; they may be useful in diagnosis; and they may have a role in the pathogenesis of certain aspects of some infectious diseases such as tissue injury resulting from immune complex deposition. In this section, immunoglobulin structure, B-cell activation, and the role of the humoral immune response in host defense are discussed.

Table 2-7. Contents and Function of Eosinophil-specific Granules

Contents	Function
Crystalloid core	
Major basic protein	Toxic to helminths, tumor cells, host cells
Eosinophil cationic protein	Bactericidal, toxic to helminths
Eosinophil peroxidase	In presence of hydrogen peroxide and halide ions, toxic to helminths, protozoa, bacteria, tumor cells, and host cells
Eosinophil-derived neurotoxin	Ribonuclease

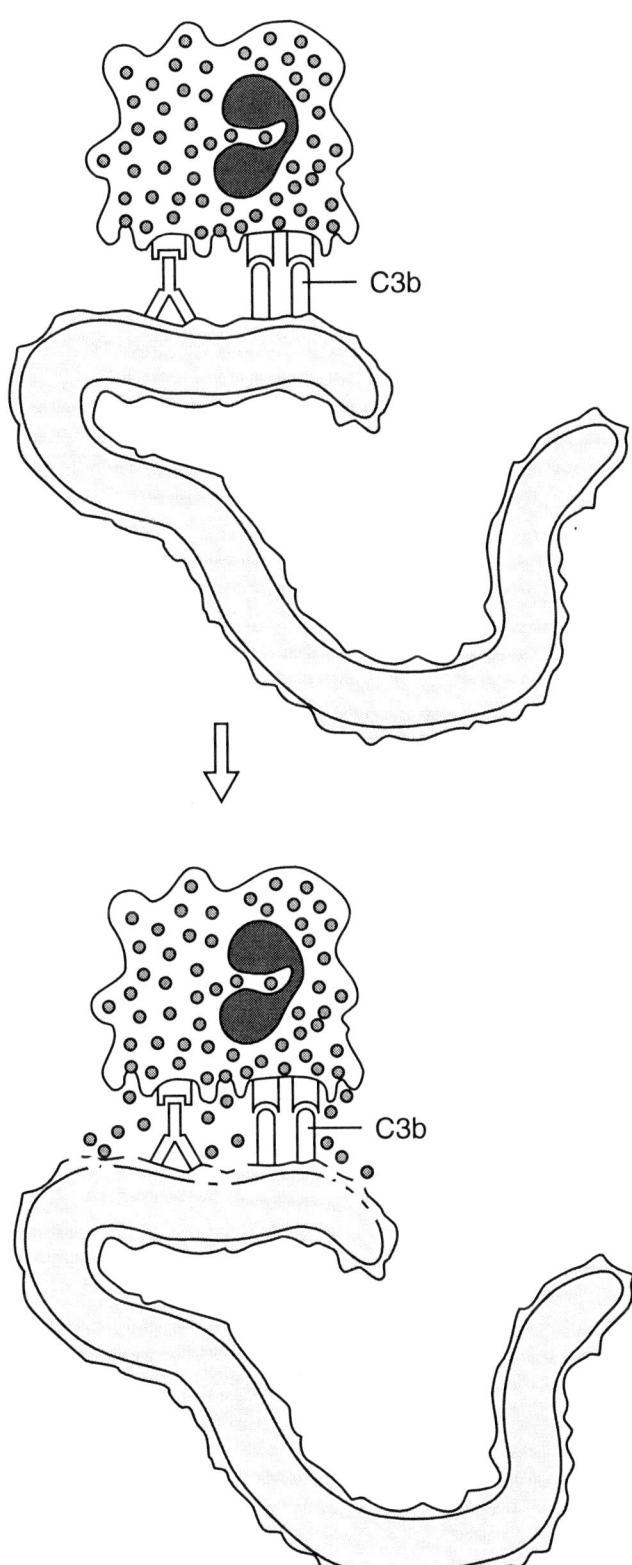

Fig. 2–4. Eosinophil binds to IgG and C3b deposited on the surface of a larval worm and releases helminthotoxins (predominantly major basic protein) that injure the invading helminth.

Immunoglobulin Structure

Five distinct classes of immunoglobulin molecules with different chemical, metabolic, and biologic properties are recognized (Table 2–8). IgG accounts for about 70 to 75% of the total immunoglobulin population and is equally prevalent in intra- and extravascular spaces. IgM, which comprises approximately 10% of the immunoglobulin pool, is confined to the intravascular space and often is the predominant early antibody directed against invading micro-organisms. IgA accounts for 15 to 20% of the serum immunoglobulins and is the predominant immunoglobulin in secretions. IgD comprises less than 1% of the total serum immunoglobulins but is found in large quantities on the membranes of circulating B lymphocytes; and IgE, which accounts for less than 0.01% of the serum immunoglobulins, is present on surface membranes of basophils and mast cells.

Each immunoglobulin molecule, regardless of its class, has the same basic unit structure: two heavy or H chains linked to two shorter light or L chains (Fig. 2–5). Each light chain has one constant (C_L) and one variable (V_L) region; heavy chains contain one variable (V_H) and three or four constant (C_H) regions, depending on the immunoglobulin class. Different portions of the immunoglobulin molecule are associated with specific functions (Table 2–9). These have been evaluated most extensively for IgG, and to a lesser extent for the other classes (6,33–41).

B-Cell Activation

During B-cell differentiation a series of translocations, which differ in every cell, occur in the genes that code for the variable regions of the heavy and light chains (42,43). After the translocation process is completed, IgM molecules are formed and transported to the cell surface. When all possible combinations of heavy-chain and light-chain genes are used, about 1 million clones of B cells, each with different antibody specificity, are created. B cells emerge from the bone marrow soon after they are formed, enter the circulation, and travel to the spleen, lymph nodes, and other organs. Those that are not stimulated by an antigen or nonspecific mitogen die within a few days, but B lym-

Table 2–8. Properties of Human Immunoglobulins

Immunoglobulin Class	Biologic Functions
IgG (1–4)	Opsonic activity, viral neutralization, complement activation (classical pathway predominantly), parasite neutralization, lysis (with the aid of complement), inhibit microbial adherence, antibody-dependent cell-mediated cytotoxicity
IgM	Complement activation (classical pathway predominantly), lysis, viral neutralization, opsonic activity (with the aid of complement)
IgA	Inhibit microbial adherence, viral neutralization, complement activation (alternative pathway)
IgD	Complement activation (alternative pathway)
IgE	Reaginic activity, complement activation (alternative pathway)

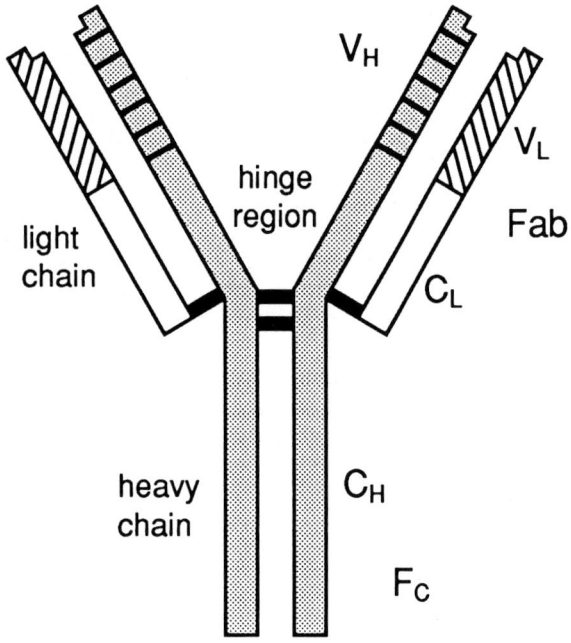

Fig. 2-5. The basic structure of immunoglobulins. Key: V_H, variable region of the immunoglobulin heavy chain; V_L, variable region of the immunoglobulin light chain; Fab, antigen binding site; C_L, constant region of the immunoglobulin light chain; C_H, constant region of the immunoglobulin heavy chain; Fc, crystallizable fragment of the immunoglobulin molecule.

Table 2-9. Function of Immunoglobulin Fragments and Domains

Fragment (Domain)	Function
Fab fragment—IgG, IgM (V_H and V_L)	Bind antigen
Fc fragment	
IgG (C_H2), IgM	Bind C1q, activating classical complement pathway
IgG (C_H1)	Bind C4b fragment of complement
IgG (C_H3)	Bind Fc receptors on monocytes; associated with antibody-dependent cell-mediated cytotoxicity and phagocytosis
IgG (C_H2, C_H3)	Bind neutrophils, inducing phagocytosis; bind CD3-positive T cells associated with antibody-dependent cell-mediated cytotoxicity; bind placental syncytiotrophoblasts, associated with placental transmission
IgG	Bind receptors on lymphocytes, inhibiting activation and proliferation
IgE	Bind mast cells and basophils, releasing vasoactive amines; bind macrophages and eosinophils, associated with cytotoxicity against parasites; bind platelets, associated with cytotoxic activity against Schistosoma mansoni; bind T lymphocytes, involved in regulating IgE production

phocytes that encounter antigens complementary to their surface immunoglobulin receptors are stimulated to enter the cell cycle, enlarge, and begin DNA synthesis in preparation for division.

Bound antigen molecules are internalized, partially digested, and recycled to the B cell surface, where they are expressed in association with class II molecules of the MHC (discussed later). This antigen-MHC complex on the surface of B cells engages receptors of an appropriate CD4-positive helper T cell (discussed later with Cell-Mediated Immunity), which produces factors that promote proliferation and differentiation of the antigen-presenting B cell. The activated B cell enters one of two pathways. It may enlarge, divide, and differentiate into a mature plasma cell that produces thousands of antibody molecules per second before it dies a few days later. Alternatively, the progeny of activated B cells become long-lived memory cells, which over time develop the ability to produce antibodies with greater affinity for the specific antigen.

Role in Host Defense

Immunoglobulins are essential for protection against infection, especially by extracellular organisms. Antibodies of the IgG1, IgG3, and IgM classes bind via their Fab fragments to extracellular pathogens and act as opsonins, preparing the organism for recognition and ingestion by phagocytic cells. This may occur directly by binding of the Fc fragment to Fc receptors on monocytes and neutrophils, indirectly by activating complement (which also is an opsonin), or both mechanisms may be involved. Microbial antigens recognized as targets for these antibodies are capsular polysaccharides, proteins (such as the M protein of group A streptococci), and peptidoglycans. Opsonic antibodies are most important in defense against bacteria and protozoa. Virus- and fungus-specific opsonic antibodies are produced, but their role in protection against infection with these agents is unclear (44,45).

In addition to acting as opsonins, immunoglobulins of the IgM and IgG classes that can initiate complement activation via the terminal component membrane attack mechanism (see Complement, above) may cause lysis of susceptible organisms (46). These antibodies are especially important in protecting against infection with species of Neisseria and Haemophilus influenzae type b. Immunoglobulins of the IgG class may provide protection by neutralizing bacterial toxins. Secretory IgA and, to a lesser extent, IgG may bind to bacterial cell wall components involved in adherence to host cells, blocking their attachment to cellular receptors and, consequently, preventing infection (47). Similarly, immunoglobulins may neutralize a protozoon by blocking its attachment to a new host cell; this occurs with merozoites of Plasmodium organisms. Moreover, neutralizing antibodies (IgG, IgM, and IgA) directed against viruses may inhibit infection by preventing attachment to cellular receptors or interfering with entry or uncoating (44,48).

In infections with helminths, IgG and IgE are involved in antibody-dependent cytotoxicity. In the presence of antibodies, macrophages, neutrophils, and eosinophils adhere to worms via receptors for Fc and the C3 component of complement. Neutrophils injure the worm by releasing hydrogen peroxide and other oxygen metabolites, and eosinophils release major basic protein (described in the Granulocyte section).

Disorders, inherited or acquired, that predominantly affect antibody production are associated primarily with increased risk of infection with pyogenic (extracellular) bacteria, although in some conditions persistent infections with parasites or viruses also are a problem. Features of these disorders, and of conditions that include deficiencies of the humoral immune response and other defects, are summarized in Table 2–10 (49–66).

Cell-Mediated Immunity

The term "cell-mediated immunity" originally was used to describe localized reactions to micro-organisms (typically intracellular pathogens) mediated by lymphocytes and mononuclear phagocytes rather than by antibodies. Now, it generally refers to those aspects of the immune response in which antibodies have a subordinate role. The cell-mediated and humoral arms of the immune response cannot be considered completely separate entities, however, because immune cells are involved in initiating antibody responses and antibodies are essential links in certain cell-mediated reactions. In this section, the cellular components of the cell-mediated immune re-

Table 2–10. Features of Immune Disorders that Affect Antibody Production

Disorder	Laboratory Abnormalities	Clinical Manifestations
X-linked (Bruton's) agammaglobulinemia	Panhypogammaglobulinemia, ↑ T cells; absence of germinal centers and plasma cells in lymphoid tissue	Recurrent pyogenic infections beginning in childhood; persistent parasitic infections, persistent viral infections (enterovirus-induced meningoencephalitis)
Common variable agammaglobulinemia	Panhypogammaglobulinemia	As for X-linked agammaglobulinemia, but less severe
Immunodeficiency with increased IgM	Low IgG and IgA, ↑ IgM	Recurrent pyogenic infections (otitis, sinusitis, pneumonia, tonsillitis); autoimmune disorders are common
Selective IgA deficiency	Secretory IgA <10 mg/dl	Frequent bacterial infections, autoimmune disease in 25%
Selective deficiency of other immunoglobulins		
IgM	Absent IgM	Meningococcemia, severe or recurrent infections with other bacteria
IgG_2, IgG_3	↓ IgG_2, ↓ IgG_3, may have ↓ IgA (inability to mount antibody response to polysaccharides)	Recurrent sinopulmonary infections
Transient hypogammaglobulinemia of infancy	Markedly ↓ IgG, depressed response of B cells to T-cell stimulation in vitro	Usually minimal; severe, recurrent infections are rare
Antibody deficiency with near normal immunoglobulins	Deficient antibody responses	Unexplained recurrent infections
X-linked lymphoproliferative disease	Impaired ability to produce antibodies to EBV nuclear antigen, low ADCC against EBV-infected cells, ↓ NK function, deficient long-lived T-cell immunity to EBV, ↑ suppressor T cells, ↓ Ig synthesis in response to polyclonal B-cell mitogen stimulation	Fatal EBV-induced infections, hypogammaglobulinemia, B-cell lymphoma
Wiskott-Aldrich syndrome	Impaired humoral immune response to polysaccharide antigens; ↓ lymphocyte response to mitogens; cutaneous anergy; ↓ CD3, CD4, and CD8 cells; thrombocytopenia	Eczema, thrombocytopenia; recurrent infections with encapsulated bacteria (early); (later) opportunistic infections (Pneumocystis carinii, herpesviruses)
Ataxia-telangiectasia	Absent IgA; ↓ IgE, ↓ IgG_2 or total IgG; depressed proliferative responses to T- and B-cell mitogens; ↓ CD3 and CD4 cells	Progressive cerebellar ataxia, oculocutaneous telangiectasias, recurrent sinopulmonary infections
Immunodeficiency with thymoma	Panhypogammaglobulinemia, ↓ pre-B and B cells, ↑ suppressor T cells	Recurrent bacterial infections, thymoma (spindle cell), autoimmune disease; resolution of humoral defect with removal of thymoma
Hyperimmunoglobulin E (Job's syndrome)	Markedly ↑ IgE; blood and tissue eosinophilia	Recurrent, severe Staphylococcus aureus-induced abscesses
Acquired disorders*	↓ IgG or ↓ in normally functioning IgG	Recurrent infections with bacteria (Streptococcus pneumoniae, Haemophilus influenzae, Neisseria spp)

* Include lymphomas, thymomas, chronic lymphocytic leukemia, multiple myeloma, Waldenström's macroglobulinemia, heavy-chain disease, severe burns, protein-losing enteropathies, nephrotic syndrome, absent spleen, a spleen that does not function properly, acquired immune deficiency syndrome.
Key: Ig, immunoglobulin; EBV, Epstein-Barr virus; ADCC, antibody-dependent cell-mediated cytotoxicity; NK, natural killer cell; ↓, decreased; ↑, increased.

sponse—mononuclear phagocytes, other accessory cells, T lymphocytes, and natural killer (NK) cells—are reviewed individually (although important interactions occur among them) and the role of cell-mediated immunity in host defense is discussed.

Mononuclear Phagocytes

Mononuclear phagocytes constitute the monocyte/macrophage system, so called because the cells have a common origin, similar structure, and common functions. These cells have a pivotal role in the immune response, presenting antigens to lymphocytes during the development of specific immunity and acting as supportive cells to lymphocytes. Macrophages also protect against infection by ingesting and killing invading pathogens, and they release many factors involved in host defense and inflammation. In this section, the development, structure, and activation of cells of the monocyte/macrophage system and their role in host defense are reviewed (67).

Development, Structure, and Activation. The monocyte/macrophage cell originates and matures in the bone marrow and then enters the circulation. The half-life of circulating monocytes is approximately 3 days. From the blood, monocytes migrate into different tissues, where they transform in response to tissue-specific stimuli into tissue macrophages with morphologic and occasionally functional properties typical of the tissue in which they are located. Macrophages are believed to live months, but their exact life span is unknown.

The monocyte/macrophage cell has many intracytoplasmic lysosomes that contain peroxidase, which is important in the intracellular killing of micro-organisms, and acid hydrolases. These cells have surface receptors for the Fc portion of IgG and for the C3b fragment of complement, both of which bind opsonized micro-organisms.

Macrophages are activated during infection via macrophage-activating cytokines (proteins that serve as molecular signals for communication between cells of the immune system and as systemic mediators of the host's response to infection, see Table 2–8), such as IFN-γ and granulocyte/monocyte colony–stimulating factor, released from T lymphocytes specifically sensitized to antigens of the infecting pathogen. This interaction constitutes the basis of cell-mediated immunity (67). Moreover, macrophages exposed to endotoxin release the cytokine TNF-α (also called cachectin), which can activate macrophages in vitro, and possibly in vivo (68). Activated macrophages have an enhanced capacity for adherence and spreading on surfaces, show increased pseudopod formation, have increased numbers of pinocytotic vesicles and certain IgG Fc receptors, and have enhanced microbicidal activity (69).

Role in Host Defense. A key function of macrophages is ingestion and killing of intracellular parasites such as Listeria monocytogenes, Nocardia asteroides, Pseudomonas pseudomallei, Pseudomonas mallei, Francisella tularensis, species of Brucella, Legionella, Salmonella, and Yersinia, some fungi, species of Leishmania, Toxoplasma gondii, and Trypanosoma cruzi and of such extracellular pathogens as Streptococcus pneumoniae, species of Aspergillus, and some protozoa. To perform this protective function, the monocyte moves by diapedesis through the blood vessel endothelium and migrates to the site of microbial invasion in tissues. Activated macrophages migrate more vigorously in response to chemotactic factors (the complement fragment C5a and chemoattractants derived from neutrophils and lymphocytes) and, therefore, probably enter sites of inflammation more efficiently than normal macrophages. Phagocytosis of invading pathogens is influenced primarily by the presence or absence of opsonins and the surface properties of the micro-organism rather than by the state of activation of the macrophage. Activated macrophages, however, have increased microbicidal activity, reflecting enhanced activity in the respiratory burst associated with phagocytosis (similar to that described earlier for neutrophils) and enhanced ability to synthesize and release hydrolytic enzymes.

Macrophages also are important in the cellular immune response. They process antigens and present them in a biochemically modified form to lymphocytes, serve as accessory cells in lymphocyte replication, and produce essential cytokines (Table 2–11) (70,71).

Other Accessory Cells

Other accessory (or antigen-presenting) cells include dendritic and Langerhans cells. Dendritic cells are derived from bone marrow precursors and are found predominantly in T lymphocyte–rich areas of lymphoid tissue, and in very small numbers in the blood. They express class II MHC molecules but do not have surface receptors for the Fc portion of IgG or for the C3 component of complement. Langerhans cells are abundant in skin and are found in the thymus and lymph nodes. They express class II MHC molecules, receptors for the Fc portion of IgG and for C3, and CD1 and S100 antigens, which are not found on other antigen-presenting cells (72).

T Lymphocytes

T lymphocytes mediate specific immune functions and modulate the functions of other immune cells. They possess specific cell surface receptors, structurally similar to immunoglobulin, for antigen recognition. Antigen-induced activation of T cells stimulates their replication or their action as immune mediators in one of three ways. Helper functions—stimulating B-cell responses, inducing other T cells to suppress immune responses, and, uncommonly, acting as cytotoxic cells—are mediated by the subset of T cells that express the CD4 surface antigen and recognize class II MHC molecules. Suppression, which inhibits the immune responses of other cells, is mediated predominantly by the subset of T cells that express the CD8 surface antigen and recognize MHC class I molecules. CD8-positive T cells also are cytotoxic, directly killing target cells (Fig. 2–6). In this section, an overview of the MHC is presented; the development, structure, and activation of T cells are described; and the role of T cells in host defense is reviewed.

Major Histocompatibility Complex. Initially "major histocompatibility antigens" described the anti-

Table 2–11. Biologic Properties of Common Cytokines

Cytokine	Source	Biologic Effect
IFN-α	MM, nonimmune lymphocytes	Antiviral activity; induces MHC class I antigen expression; ↑ NK activity; fever
IFN-β	Fibroblasts, epithelial cells	As for IFN-α
IFN-γ	Sensitized T lymphocytes, NK cells	As for IFN-α, plus induces class II antigen expression; activates macrophages and endothelial cells; ↑ IgG production; ↑ or ↓ activity of other cytokines
IL-1	MM	Activates T cells; cofactor in promoting proliferation of hematopoietic stem cells; mediator of acute-phase response; ↑ leukocyte adherence and procoagulant properties of endothelial cells; induces release of ACTH, cortisol, and insulin; induces release of PMN from bone marrow; induces catabolic state and fever; ↑ production of other cytokines
IL-2	T lymphocytes	Proliferation of activated T cells; ↑ production and differentiation of cytotoxic T cells; ↑ NK cytotoxicity; induces synthesis of other T-cell cytokines; cofactor for B-cell proliferation and Ig secretion
IL-3	T lymphocytes	Promotes growth of pluripotent bone marrow stem cells; growth factor for mast cells
IL-4	T lymphocytes	↑ B-cell proliferation; ↑ cytotoxic T-cell production and differentiation; induces IgE synthesis
IL-5	T lymphocytes	↑ eosinophil production and function; induces IgA and IgM synthesis
IL-6	MM, fibroblasts, T lymphocytes	Induces Ig production, fever, synthesis of acute-phase reactants and ACTH release
TNF-α (cachectin)	MM, NK cells, T lymphocytes	Mediates septic shock; antiviral and antitumor activity; ↑ leukocyte adherence and procoagulant properties of endothelial cells; ↑ microbicidal activity of PMN; ↑ B-cell proliferation and Ig synthesis; ↑ MHC class I antigen expression; ↑ production of other cytokines; induces catabolic state, fever, and synthesis of acute-phase reactants
TNF-β (lymphotoxin)	T lymphocytes	Same as TNF-α but has less effect on PMN microbicidal activity and cytokine production
GM-CSF	T lymphocytes, MM, endothelial cells, fibroblasts	Promotes differentiation and maturation of PMN, MM, and eosinophil precursors in the bone marrow; activates mature PMN and MM

Key: IFN, interferon; MM, monocyte/macrophage cells; MHC, major histocompatibility complex; NK, natural killer cell; Ig, immunoglobulin; IL, interleukin; TNF, tumor necrosis factor; PMN, polymorphonuclear neutrophil; GM, granulocyte/monocyte; CSF, colony-stimulating factor; ↑, increased; ↓, decreased.

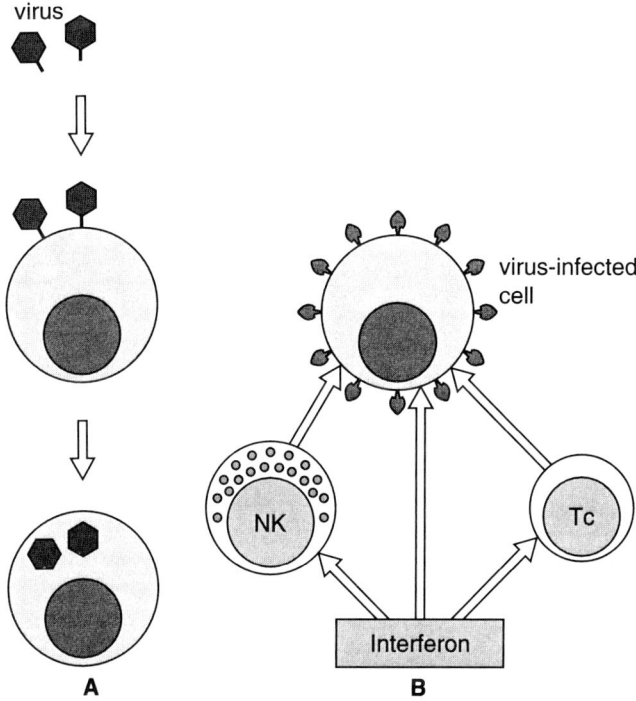

Fig. 2–6. A. Virions bind to specific host cell receptors and enter the host cell. B. Virus-infected cells are eliminated by the action of the cellular immune system: cytokines (such as interferon) have a direct effect and stimulate cytotoxic T lymphocytes (Tc) and natural killer (NK) cells.

gens involved in graft rejection in mice. Subsequently, the products of one particular region of the mouse genome, the MHC, were found to be of predominant importance in the rejection process. Analogous major histocompatibility systems have been identified in all mammalian species studied. In humans the MHC is the human leukocyte antigen (HLA) gene cluster.

Three different types of MHC proteins, determined by their structure and function, are recognized (6). Class I molecules are found in varying amounts on almost all nucleated cells. Class II proteins, which are found on B lymphocytes, cells of the monocyte/macrophage system, and activated T lymphocytes, facilitate cooperation and interaction between immune cells. Class III proteins—the MHC-coded complement components—are not involved in cell-mediated immunity.

Development, Structure, and Activation. T cells originate from bone marrow precursors (prothymocytes) that migrate to the thymus, where they mature. The stages of thymocyte differentiation and the mechanisms responsible for each stage, however, are not clearly established.

Several markers are found on the T-cell surface. The T-cell antigen receptor is expressed in association with the CD3 complex, which probably acts as the signal transduction mechanism, facilitating activation when an antigen is bound (73). Mature T lymphocytes also express on their surface accessory molecules that enhance T-cell recognition of other cells. The CD4 and CD8 molecules probably act as stabilizing ligands for T-cell binding to MHC class

II (for CD4) or class I (for CD8) molecules (Figs. 2–7, 2–8) (74,75). The CD2 molecule may play a role in T-cell activation, thymocyte differentiation and selection, and NK cell activation (76).

The process of T-cell activation involves binding of an antigen-MHC complex to the T-cell receptor. The signal for activation is mediated by the CD3 complex, and perhaps is modulated by CD4 and CD8 molecules. A series of biochemical events ensue, culminating in cytokine production and replication of the T cell, stimulated predominantly by binding of IL-2 to its receptor or in lysis of the target cell (77–81).

Role in Host Defense. T-cell immune functions, which correlate in part with surface expression of CD4 and CD8 molecules, are divided into three categories, helper, cytotoxic, and suppressor, although occurrence, characterization, and specificity of suppressor T cells is a subject of considerable controversy (82–86). T-cell help, performed by helper T cells, includes at least two functions, enhancement of immunoglobulin synthesis by B cells (a function of helper/inducer T cells) and stimulation of CD8-positive cells or macrophages to differentiate into more competent antigen-presenting or effector cells. How cytotoxic T cells function in vivo is not known; but cytotoxic T cells differentiated in vitro have cytoplasmic granules containing perforin, a protein that polymerizes to form pores resembling those produced by the terminal complement components in membranes of target cells and micro-organisms (87). Differentiated cytotoxic T cells also have granules that contain serine esterases, and they may secrete TNF-α and TNF-β, but the precise role of these substances in cytotoxic function is unclear (88).

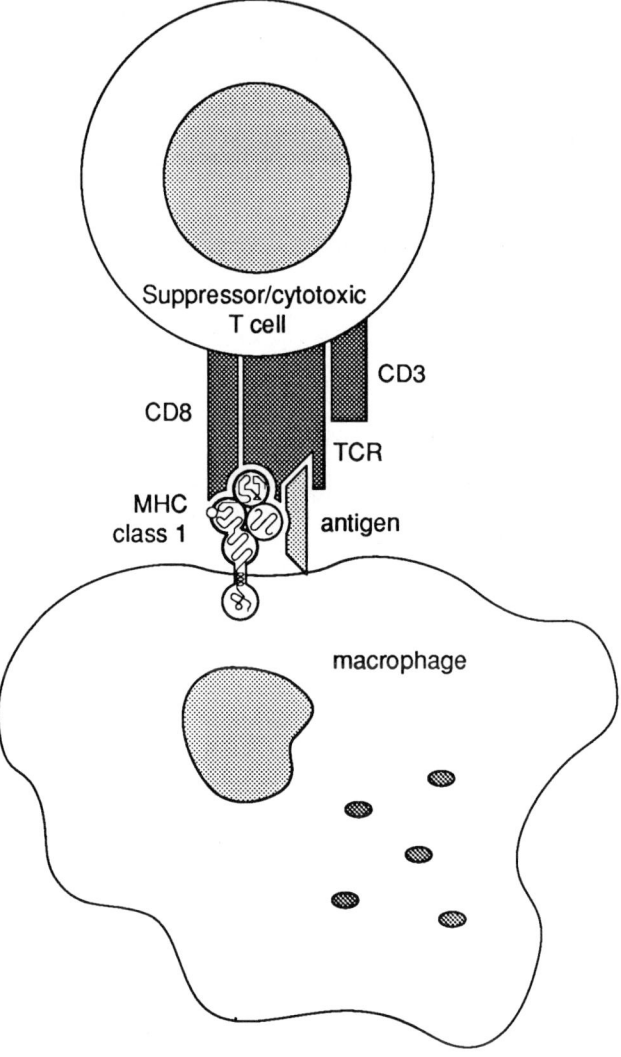

Fig. 2–8. Binding of a suppressor T cell to a macrophage via the CD8 receptor of the suppressor cell and the MHC class I molecule of the macrophage.

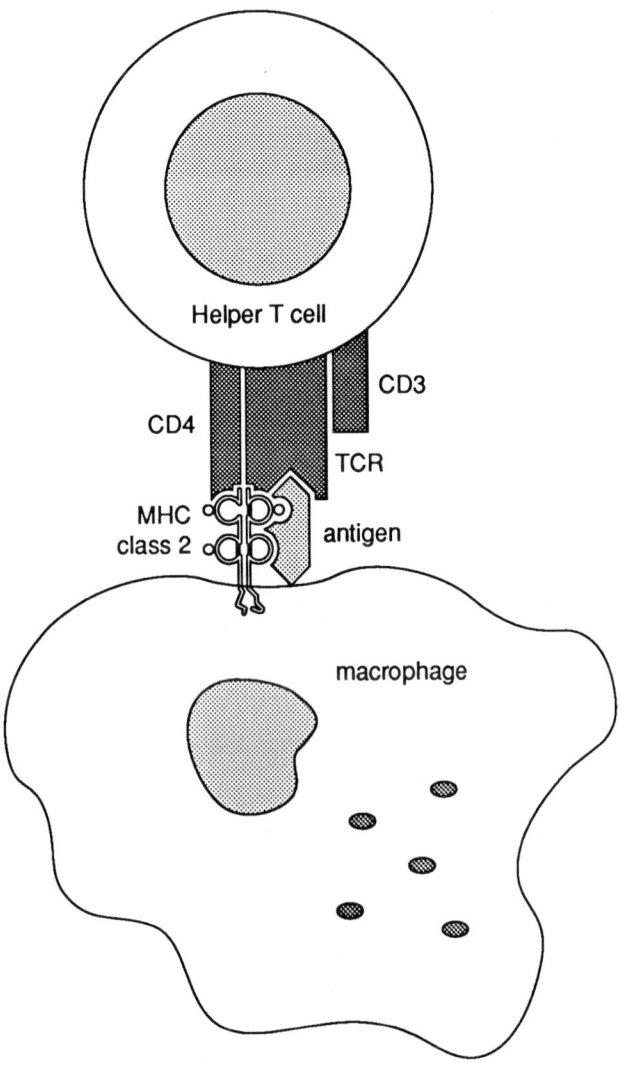

Fig. 2–7. Binding of a helper T cell to a macrophage via the CD4 molecule of the helper cell and the MHC class II molecule of the macrophage.

Natural Killer Cells

NK cells are large, granular lymphocytes that account for 10 to 15% of circulating lymphocytes in healthy adults. They express an NK cell–specific antigen and some surface antigens common to T cells, monocytes, and granulocytes (89). Originally, NK cells were defined by their ability to lyse target cells in a manner not restricted by HLA antigens or requiring antigen presensitization. However, recent observations suggest that cells with missing or abnormal surface HLA antigens, such as virus-infected cells, are preferentially lysed by NK cells, whereas cells with abundant normal HLA antigens are not affected (90,91). The leukocyte cell adhesion molecule family is involved in NK cell binding to targets, but the mechanism is not fully understood (92).

NK cells have a role in protecting against infection with viruses (see Fig. 2–6) such as cytomegalovirus and herpes simplex virus, and perhaps other micro-organisms, such as Toxoplasma gondii (93–95). The cytolytic mechanisms of NK cells, augmented by IFN-α, IFN-β, or IFN-γ and IL-2, resemble those of cytotoxic T cells (86). NK cells are one of the mediators of antibody-dependent cell-mediated cytotoxicity (granulocytes and monocytes also may be involved), a more efficient process than antibody-independent NK cell lysis (90). Moreover, NK cells produce cytokines that augment cytolytic T-cell responses, inhibit growth and differentiation of T and B cells, and inhibit growth and maturation of hematopoietic cells (86,96).

Role in Host Defense

Cell-mediated immunity is an important part of host defense against a variety of intracellular micro-organisms (Table 2–12). The immune response to many viral infections is cell mediated, especially for those transmitted by cell-to-cell contact. Specific defense mechanisms may include mobilization and activation of macrophages to ingest and clear extracellular viruses, lysis (mediated by cytotoxic T or NK cells) of virus-infected cells, and production and release of IFN-α and -β by macrophages, fibroblasts, and nonimmune lymphocytes and of IFN-γ by specifically sensitized lymphocytes to inhibit viral replication in infected cells (97,98).

Infection with nonviral intracellular pathogens is controlled predominantly by monocyte/macrophage cells, T lymphocytes, and cytokine-mediated interactions between them (86). The cytokines IFN-γ, IL-2, granulocyte/monocyte colony–stimulating factor, and TNF-α enhance macrophage activation, an event important in controlling infection with Listeria monocytogenes, salmonellae, mycobacteria, some fungi, species of Leishmania, and Trypanosoma cruzi. Lysis of infected cells or extracellular organisms by cytotoxic T cells or by NK cells may be important in defense against Listeria monocytogenes, Nocardia asteroides, mycobacteria, Cryptococcus neoformans, species of Leishmania, Trypanosoma cruzi, and Toxoplasma gondii. Moreover, IFN-γ may have microbistatic or microbicidal activity against species of Chlamydia and Rickettsia.

Cell-mediated immunity also has a role in defense against certain extracellular helminths and bacteria. For example, activated macrophages are active against schistosomes, and in vitro cytokines enhance killing of these organisms by eosinophils (99,100). In murine models of infection with Bacteroides fragilis and with Pseudomonas aeruginosa, T cells have an important role in the immune response to the infecting organism (101,102). Moreover, in other murine models, cytokines (IL-1 and -2) enhance resistance to infection with pyogenic bacteria (103,104).

In addition to protecting against invading micro-organisms, cell-mediated immunity may contribute to tissue damage via direct cytotoxicity or cytokine production. Events of the cell-mediated immune response are responsible for tissue damage that occurs during infection with some herpesviruses, hepatitis B virus, enteroviruses, arenaviruses, probably human immunodeficiency virus (HIV) and rabies virus, Mycobacterium tuberculosis, Treponema pallidum (tertiary syphilis), and certain fungi, and they probably are critical to the development of cerebral malaria (105–110).

Disorders—physiologic, congenital, or acquired—of cell-mediated immunity are associated with increased risk of infection with intracellular pathogens (Table 2–12). The features of these conditions are summarized in Table 2–13 (23–25,111–122).

MICROBIAL FACTORS IN DISEASE

Microbial factors are critical in determining whether an encounter with a specific organism results in disease. The pathogenicity of an infectious agent describes its ability to produce pathologic changes or cause disease. Some organisms, such as influenza A virus, are very pathogenic, and infection of a susceptible host almost always progresses to disease. The human carrier state for influenza A virus is rare. Other organisms, such as Staphylococcus epidermidis and viridans streptococci, have low pathogenicity. They are associated with a high colonization rate and almost never cause disease unless the normal host defenses are altered. The virulence of an organism describes the degree of its pathogenicity and is indicated by

Table 2–12. Pathogens Controlled Predominantly by Cell-Mediated Immunity

Type of Organism	Specific Pathogens
Virus	Herpes simplex virus, varicella-zoster virus, cytomegalovirus, Epstein-Barr virus, measles and influenza viruses
Bacterium	Species of Chlamydia, Rickettsia, Brucella, Legionella, Salmonella, Yersinia, and Mycobacterium; Listeria monocytogenes, Pseudomonas pseudomallei and -mallei; Treponema pallidum.
Fungus	
Intracellular	Candida spp, Cryptococcus neoformans, Blastomyces dermatitidis, Histoplasma capsulatum, Coccidioides immitis, Paracoccidioides brasiliensis
Extracellular	Aspergillus, Zygomycetes
Parasite	
Intracellular	Toxoplasma gondii, Leishmania spp, Trypanosoma cruzi
Extracellular	
Protozoon	Entamoeba histolytica, Plasmodium spp
Helminths	Strongyloides spp, Trichinella spiralis, Schistosoma spp

Table 2-13. Features of Cell-Mediated Immune Disorders

Disorder	Defect	Clinical Manifestations
Physiologic disorders		
Of infants	↓ production of IFN-γ and IL-4, less efficient migration of monocytes, ↓ NK and antibody-dependent cell-mediated cytotoxicity	Infection with intracellular pathogens (see Table 2-12)
Of Elders	↓ production and response to IL-2, ↓ production of cytotoxic T cells	As for infants' disorder
Congenital disorders		
Thymic hypoplasia (DiGeorge's syndrome)	↓ T cells, ↓ IgA, ↑ IgE	Hypocalcemic seizures; infections with opportunistic pathogens (viruses, fungi, Pneumocystis carinii); congenital anomalies
Cellular immunodeficiency with immunoglobulins (Nezelof's syndrome)	Lymphopenia, normal to ↑ immunoglobulins, ↓ lymphocyte responses to mitogens, neutropenia, eosinophilia	Recurrent infections of lung, skin, urinary tract; mucocutaneous candidiasis; gram-negative sepsis; chronic diarrhea; severe progressive varicella; failure to thrive
Nezelof's syndrome with purine nucleoside phosphorylase deficiency	As for Nezelof's syndrome, plus ↓ serum and urine uric acids	Generalized vaccinia, varicella, lymphoma, graft-versus-host disease
Severe combined immunodeficiency disorders	Marked lymphopenia, ↓ Ig, lack of T- and B-cell function	Recurrent otitis, pneumonia, sepsis, diarrhea, and cutaneous infections; wasting; death from infection with opportunistic pathogens
Defective expression of MHC antigens	Moderate lymphopenia, ↓ T-cell function; variable hypogammaglobulinemia with ↓ IgM and ↓ IgA	Persistent diarrhea, oral candidiasis, bacterial pneumonia, P. carinii-induced pneumonia, infections with enteroviruses and herpesviruses
Severe combined immunodeficiency with leukopenia (reticular dysgenesis)	Absent or marked ↓ of lymphocytes and granulocytes in peripheral blood and bone marrow	Overwhelming infection
Cartilage-hair hypoplasia	↓ T cells, defective lymphocyte proliferation, ↑ NK function	Severe varicella, progressive vaccinia, vaccine-associated poliomyelitis, abnormal physical features
Acquired disorders		
Hodgkin's disease, some lymphomas	Lymphopenia, ↓ NK activity, ↓ delayed-type hypersensitivity, ↓ in vitro lymphocyte functions	Infection with intracellular pathogens (see Table 2-12)
Chemotoxic agents, irradiation	↓ lymphocytes, ↓ cytokines, ↓ monocyte killing	As for Hodgkin's disease
Malnutrition*	↓ T lymphocyte function	As for Hodgkin's disease

* Includes chronic protein-calorie malnutrition and prolonged deficiencies of copper, zinc, thiamine, or folate.
Key: IFN, interferon; IL, interleukin; NK, natural killer cell; Ig, immunoglobulin; MHC, major histocompatibility complex; ↓, decreased; ↑, increased.

the ability of the organism to invade host tissues, by case fatality rates, or both. Virulence, however, often depends on the immune status of the host. For example, an infectious agent such as cytomegalovirus (CMV), which usually has low virulence in a healthy individual, often causes serious disease in an immunocompromised person such as a premature infant or the recipient of an organ transplant.

Microbial factors associated with pathogenicity—infective dose, penetration of anatomic barriers, surface characteristics, endotoxin, elaboration of toxins and enzymes, disruption, evasion or inactivation of host defenses, and the acquisition of resistance to antimicrobial agents—are discussed in this section.

Infective Dose

The infective dose, the number of organisms required to produce disease, varies for different organisms and depends on the route and the condition of transmission and on the age and the immune status of the host. For organisms that cause gastroenteritis the infective dose varies considerably. The "critical mass" of inoculum, however, can be reduced significantly by neutralizing the normal gastric acid barrier or by gastric resection (123–125). The infective dose also can be reduced by transporting the organisms in milk, which protects them against the acidic environment of the stomach. The role of age in the development of infectious diarrhea is evident for disease caused by rotavirus, enteropathogenic Escherichia coli, and species of Shigella and Salmonella, which occur predominantly, and usually are most severe, in infants and young children. Age-related changes in gastrointestinal mucus, cell surface factors, microbial flora, environmental exposure, and specific immunity may be involved.

Penetration of Anatomic Barriers

Many micro-organisms enter the body through breaks in the skin or mucous membranes or via the bite of an arthropod, but most cannot penetrate intact body surfaces. Exceptions are the cercariae of species of Schistosoma and larvae of Strongyloides stercoralis, Ancylostoma duodenale, and Necator americanus, which enter a host by crossing intact skin or mucous membranes. Moreover, some bacteria (species of Salmonella and Shigella, enteroinvasive strains of Escherichia coli, and Yersinia enterocolitica) have the ability to penetrate intact cells, a trait associated with large plasmids in enteroinvasive Escherichia coli and species of Shigella (126–128).

Surface Characteristics

Microbial surface characteristics enhance pathogenicity by allowing an organism to adhere to the host body surfaces or by providing protection from host defenses. Adherence, or binding, is the first stage of invasion for viruses, many bacteria, some fungi, and some parasites. For viruses, specific receptors on the virion surface bind to specific receptors on host cells, which are known for only a few viruses (see Chapter 3). Adhesins or adhesive surface structures, which are important pathogenic elements of bacteria, fungi, and parasites, are listed in Table 2–14 and discussed in more detail in the individual chapters (4,129–138).

Various bacterial structures provide protection against phagocytic host cells. For example, the M protein of group A Streptococcus, its major virulence antigen, exerts an antiphagocytic effect by preventing an interaction between the streptococcal cell wall and complement components, a protective effect overcome by the presence of adequate concentrations of type-specific antibodies (139). The sialic acid residues in the capsules of Neisseria meningitidis group B, Escherichia coli K-1, and serogroup III of group B Streptococcus render these organisms poor activators of the alternative complement pathway. The slime layer of Staphylococcus epidermidis is responsible for adherence and for resistance to phagocytosis, and the envelope antigen of Yersinia pestis is associated with relative resistance to phagocytosis (140,141). Moreover, capsules are important antiphagocytic components of many bacteria: Streptococcus pneumoniae, Neisseria meningitidis, Pseudomonas aeruginosa, Escherichia coli K-1, Klebsiella pneumoniae, Haemophilus influenzae type b, Pasteurella multocida, and Bacteroides fragilis.

Endotoxin

Endotoxin is a component of the core region of the outer membrane of all gram-negative bacteria. The portion of the core region called lipid A exhibits the hemodynamic, pyrogenic, and inflammatory properties associated with "endotoxicity." Slight alterations in the architecture of lipid A cause significant changes in biologic activity, suggesting that expression of endotoxicity depends on several factors, including three-dimensional configuration, rather than on a single constituent of the lipid A molecule.

The biologic effects of endotoxin are the end result of several events. Endotoxin triggers cells of the monocyte/macrophage system to release IL-1, IFN-γ, and TNF-α, the latter of which probably is the most potent mediator of the pathophysiologic events of gram-negative sepsis (the biologic effects of these cytokines are listed in Table 2–11) (142,143). Endotoxin also activates Hageman factor, which in turn activates the intrinsic clotting, fibrinolytic, kinin, and complement pathways. Simultaneous activation of the coagulation and fibrinolytic systems results in acute disseminated intravascular coagulation, and activation of the kinin and complement (via generation of anaphylatoxins) pathways causes vasodilatation and increases vascular permeability. Moreover, endotoxin can injure vascular endothelium, thus triggering or enhancing clotting and bleeding, an event probably mediated by TNF-α (144).

Histopathologic findings in fatal cases of gram-negative sepsis include fibrin thrombi (especially in small vessels of the lung and the intestines, in the glomeruli, and occasionally in the hepatic vessels) accompanied by tissue necrosis and hemorrhage. Bilateral hemorrhages in the adrenal cortex are a potential complication of septicemia caused by Neisseria meningitidis (see Chapter 31) or other gram-negative bacteria and may occur in other shock states.

Elaboration of Toxins and Enzymes

Toxins (also called exotoxins) are proteins that are released by gram-positive and gram-negative bacteria during exponential growth and affect host cells at a distance. Bacteria that cause disease or are pathogenic by virtue of toxin production are listed in Table 2–15 and are discussed in more detail in Part II of the text (145–153).

Some bacteria produce enzymes such as protease, hyaluronidase, neuraminidase, elastase, and collagenase that may contribute to their invasiveness, their ability to spread through tissues. For example, Staphylococcus aureus and group A Streptococcus produce hyaluronidase, an enzyme that degrades hyaluronic acid in the ground substance of connective tissue. Pseudomonas aeruginosa produces elastase and alkaline protease, which are necrotizing in the skin, lung, and cornea, and several species of

Table 2–14. Adhesins That Act as Pathogenic Mechanisms of Infectious Agents

Adhesin	Micro-organism
Bacteria	
Protein P-1	Mycoplasma pneumoniae
Lipoteichoic acid	Staphylococcus aureus
Slime	Staphylococcus epidermidis
Lipoteichoic acid	Group A Streptococcus
Glucans	Streptococcus mutans
Pili	Neisseria gonorrhoeae, Neisseria meningitidis, Pseudomonas aeruginosa
Type 1 fimbriae, colonization factor antigens	Escherichia coli
Fimbriae, cholera lectin	Vibrio cholerae
Fungus	
Mannan	Candida albicans
Parasites	
Cell surface lectin	Entamoeba histolytica
Gripping disk	Giardia lamblia
Apical complex	Plasmodium spp

Table 2–15. Pathogenic Bacterial Toxins

Toxins	Organism
Enterotoxins (A–E), exfoliatin (A, B)	Staphylococcus aureus
Pyrogenic exotoxins (A–C)	Group A Streptococcus
Edema factor, lethal factor, protective antigen	Bacillus anthracis
Diphtheria toxin	Corynebacterium diphtheriae
Botulism toxin (A, B, E, F)	Clostridium botulinum
Tetanus toxin	Clostridium tetani
Enterotoxin, α-toxin, β-toxin	Clostridium perfringens
Toxin A, toxin B	Clostridium difficile
Exotoxin A	Pseudomonas aeruginosa
Pertussis toxin	Bordetella pertussis
Labile- & stable toxin, verotoxin	Escherichia coli
Cholera toxin	Vibrio cholerae

Clostridium produce proteases and collagenases, which probably play a role in gas gangrene (146,154).

Disruption, Evasion, and Inactivation of Host Defenses

Several microbial virulence factors interfere with normal host defenses. Neisseria gonorrhoeae, Neisseria meningitidis, Streptococcus pneumoniae, and Haemophilus influenzae produce IgA-specific proteases that cleave and inactivate secretory IgA on mucosal surfaces; however, the exact role of these enzymes in the pathogenesis of disease is unclear (155,156). Isolates of Neisseria gonorrhoeae from persons with disseminated disease are resistant to the bactericidal effect of serum, whereas isolates from persons with infection limited to the genital tract usually are serum sensitive (157). CMV evades virus-specific antibodies by becoming coated with the host protein β_2-microglobulin, whereas influenza A virus escapes neutralizing antibodies by frequently undergoing antigenic variation (158,159).

Micro-organisms have several mechanisms for evading or inactivating phagocytic cells. The antiphagocytic nature of bacterial capsules was discussed earlier. Some organisms, such as Listeria monocytogenes, Legionella pneumophila, Toxoplasma gondii, and species of Leishmania are ingested by phagocytic cells but evade killing by not eliciting or by actively suppressing the oxidative response associated with phagocytosis (160,161). Many infectious agents produce enzymes such as catalase, glutathione peroxidase, and superoxide dismutase that inactivate the reactive oxygen metabolites generated in the oxygen burst (discussed in the Granulocyte section) (161,162). Some organisms survive within cells by inhibiting fusion of the phagosome with lysosomes, and others (Mycobacterium leprae, some species of Salmonella, and species of Leishmania) appear to have innate resistance to lysosomal enzymes and, therefore, survive phagosome-lysosome fusion and degranulation (163,164). Species of Schistosoma alter their surface proteins to resemble host proteins, thus avoiding recognition by immune effector cells (165).

Some viruses depress neutrophil numbers and function and so increase the risk of secondary bacterial infections (166). For example, influenza virus induces neutropenia, and in vitro neutrophils infected with influenza virus have depressed oxidative, secretory, and chemotactic activity. In animals with primary CMV-induced infection, neutrophil mobilization and function are depressed. Infection with herpes simplex virus (HSV) depresses neutrophil chemotaxis in humans and animals, and hepatitis B virus may decrease neutrophil chemotactic and bactericidal activity.

In addition to altering neutrophil function, viruses also may suppress cell-mediated immunity (117). Immunosuppression may be a direct result of viral replication in lymphocytes, causing cell lysis or functional impairment, as occurs during infection with CMV, Epstein-Barr virus (EBV), measles virus, and HIV. Immunosuppression may result from the activity of soluble factors of viral origin, such as glycoprotein (gp) 120 of HIV, or of cytokines such as IFN-γ released from infected cells (97,98). The cellular immune response may be suppressed when viruses such as influenza virus, CMV, and HSV infect and injure cells involved in phagocytosis, antigen presentation, and the nonspecific effector aspects of cell-mediated immunity. Moreover, suppressed immunity may be caused by a virus-induced imbalance in immune regulation that results in overactivity of suppressor T cells, as in infection with HSV, CMV, and EBV.

Resistance to Antimicrobial Agents

Antimicrobial resistance may be an inherent (natural) property of an organism, or it may be acquired (167). Inherent resistance typically is a characteristic of a species, such as the resistance of most gram-negative bacilli to vancomycin and penicillinase-resistant penicillins, the resistance of enterococci to cephalosporins, and the resistance of anaerobes to aminoglycosides. Acquired resistance results from mutations in existing DNA, which may involve structural or regulatory genes of chromosomes, plasmids, or transposons, or from the acquisition of new DNA.

New DNA is acquired via transformation, transduction, or conjugation. Transformation—intercellular transfer of a small portion of the total DNA of one bacterium to a related bacterium and incorporation of that fragment into the genetic constitution of the recipient—has been important in the development of penicillin resistance in Neisseria meningitidis and Streptococcus pneumoniae and may occur in Haemophilus influenzae and Neisseria gonorrhoeae. Transduction, in which DNA from one bacterium is transferred to another bacterium by a bacteriophage, is best described for the antibiotic resistance plasmids of Staphylococcus aureus.

Transfer of plasmids (extracellular fragments of DNA that cannot be inserted into the chromosome) by conjugation, a form of sexual reproduction in which a donor bacterium contributes some or all of its DNA to a recipient bacterium, probably is the most common mechanism for transferring antimicrobial resistance in nature. Plasmids, however, have limitations in host range. They do not transfer from gram-positive to gram-negative organisms and may not transfer to other organisms of the same family. Transposons (nucleotide sequences that can be transferred from one position to another within a chromosome or plasmid or from one to another chromosome or plasmid), in contrast, are less restrictive in host range, thus providing an additional mechanism for expanding the range of antibiotic resistance genes.

PATHOGENESIS OF INFECTIOUS DISEASES

Pathogenesis, the development of disease, includes all events and reactions involved in the process. The pathogenesis of an infectious disease, therefore, encompasses the events that occur during the interaction between a susceptible host and an infectious agent.

The first steps in the development of disease are entrance of the potential pathogen into the host tissues and initiation of infection. To accomplish this the organism must overcome the physical barriers of the host and the nonspecific antimicrobial substances in secretions at portals of entry. The invading organisms may be transported from an external source (mechanisms of transmission are described later in the Epidemiology section), inciting exogenous infection, or they may be members of the host's normal flora, in which case the infection is endogenous and results from a disruption of the normal relationship between host and infectious agent. For example, an ulcerating adenocarcinoma of the colon affords entry into the circulation for organisms such as Escherichia coli, enterococci, and Streptococcus bovis, all part of the normal colonic flora (see Table 2-1); placement of an intravascular catheter provides a portal of entry for the normal skin flora, especially Staphylococcus epidermidis.

Once infection (defined earlier) occurs, the ultimate balance between microbial factors (endotoxin, production of toxins and enzymes that promote invasiveness, and mechanisms of disruption, evasion or inactivation of the host immune response) and the host defense against those factors (complement, granulocytes, immunoglobulins, and cell-mediated immunity) determines whether the infection remains subclinical or progresses to disease. If disease develops, the balance between the host immune defenses plus antimicrobial therapy and the ability of the invading organism to evade the host defenses and to resist the action of antimicrobial agents determines the outcome of the host-pathogen encounter.

In general, the events of the initial interaction between host and pathogen in healthy persons depend on the virulence of the invading organism. For many organisms, subsequent encounters favor the host because the immune system is primed for defense. The nature of the primary encounter with specific organisms may be altered to benefit the host by immunization. If a defect in any one of the host immune defenses exists, however, the balance of the encounter often favors the infectious agent, regardless of its virulence.

EPIDEMIOLOGY OF INFECTIOUS DISEASES

Epidemiology is the study of the distribution, occurrence, cause (including source and mechanism of transmission), and control of health and disease in a population. The occurrence of an infectious disease may be described by its prevalence, the number of cases of the disease that are active at a specific point in time or that occur during a specified period of time, or by the incidence, which is a rate reflecting the number of new cases of the disease identified in a specified period of time within a specific population.

To identify factors that influence the development of an infectious disease and to devise mechanisms to control its occurrence, an understanding of its transmission is essential. Infectious agents are transmitted from the source to the host by four exogenous routes: contact, common vehicle, airborne, and vector-borne (168). Different types of contact are described. Direct (also called person-to-person) contact means that the source and the host physically touch. During indirect contact organisms are transferred passively, usually on an inanimate object, from the source to the host. Droplet contact occurs when the source produces an aerosol of particles larger than 5 μm in diameter while coughing, sneezing, or talking close to the host. In common vehicle spread, the infectious agent is transmitted via one inanimate vehicle (usually food or water, but blood products and intravenous fluids have been implicated) to multiple hosts. Airborne transmission involves transport of droplet nuclei less than 5 μm in diameter (representing the residua of larger droplets that have evaporated) on dust or skin squames. Vector-borne transmission may occur by passive transport (organisms are transmitted externally or mechanically), by harborage (the organism is ingested by the vector but undergoes no changes); or by biologic transmission (the organism changes physiologically within the vector).

Finally, the environment must be considered when evaluating possible causes of an infectious disease. This is especially important when investigating outbreaks of nosocomial (hospital-acquired) infections. For example, equipment used to monitor hemodynamic status, potable water, respiratory equipment, intravenous fluids, and ventilation systems are recognized sources of infection (169-173). Because hospitalized patients frequently are immunocompromised and at increased risk of infection with a wide variety of pathogens, timely identification of the source of the responsible organism is critical to implementation of measures to control its spread.

REFERENCES

1. Mackowiak PA: The normal microbial flora. N Engl J Med, *307*:83, 1982.
2. Tramont EC: General or nonspecific host defense mechanisms. *In* Principles and Practice of Infectious Diseases. 3rd ed. Edited by GL Mandell, RG Douglas Jr, and JE Bennett. New York, Churchill Livingstone, 1990.
3. Lyverly, DM, Krivan HC, and Wilkins TC: Clostridium difficile: It's disease and toxins. Clin Microbiol Rev, *1*:1, 1988.
4. Johnson JR: Virulence factors in Escherichia coli urinary tract infection. Clin Microbiol Rev, *4*:80, 1991.
5. Israde V, Darabi A, and McCracken GH: The role of bacterial virulence factors and Tamm-Horsfall protein in the pathogenesis of E. coli urinary tract infections in infants. Am J Dis Child, *147*:1230, 1987.
6. Roitt IM, Brostoff J, and Hale DK (eds): Immunology. St. Louis, CV Mosby, 1985.
7. Figueroa JE and Densen P: Infectious diseases associated with complement deficiencies. Clin Microbiol Rev, *4*:359, 1991.

8. Schifferli JA, Ng YC, and Peters DK: The role of complement and its receptor in the elimination of immune complexes. N Engl J Med, 315:488, 1986.
9. Laham MN, Caldwell JR, and Panush RS: Modulation of lymphocyte proliferative responses to mitogens and antigens by complement components Cl, C4, and C2. J Clin Lab Immunol, 9:39, 1982.
10. Weiler J, et al: Complement fragments suppress lymphocyte immune responses. Immunol Today, 3:236, 1982.
11. Densen P: Complement. In Principles and Practice of Infectious Diseases. 3rd ed. Edited by GL Mandell, RG Douglas Jr, and JE Bennett. New York, Churchill Livingstone, 1990.
12. Tedesco F, et al: Bactericidal activities of human polymorphonuclear leukocyte proteins against Escherichia coli O111:B4 coated with C5 or C8. Infect Immun, 54:250, 1986.
13. Taylor PW: Bactericidal and bacteriolytic activity of serum against gram-negative bacteria. Microbiol Rev, 47:46, 1983.
14. Cooper NR and Nemerow GR: Complement-dependent mechanisms of virus neutralization. In Immunobiology of the Complement System. Edited by GD Ross. Orlando, Academic Press, 1986.
15. Fearon DT and Austen KF: Current concepts in immunology: The alternative pathway of complement—a system for host resistance to microbial infection. N Engl J Med, 303:259, 1980.
16. Frank MM, Joiner K, and Hammer C: The function of antibody and complement in the lysis of bacteria. Rev Infect Dis, 9:537, 1987.
17. Densen P: Infectious consequences of complement deficiency states. Clin Immunol Newslett, 11:1, 1991.
18. Sawyer DW, Donowitz GR, and Mandell GL: Polymorphonuclear neutrophils: An effective antimicrobial force. Rev Infect Dis, 11(S7):S1532, 1989.
19. Lehrer RI, et al: Neutrophils and host defense. Ann Intern Med, 109:127, 1988.
20. Malech HL and Gallin JI: Neutrophils in human disease. N Engl J Med, 317:687, 1987.
21. Wright GG and Mandell GL: Anthrax toxin blocks priming of neutrophils by lipopolysaccharide and by muramyl dipeptide. J Exp Med, 164:1700, 1986.
22. Weiss S: Tissue destruction by neutrophils. N Engl J Med, 320:365, 1989.
23. Parry MF, et al: Myeloperoxidase deficiency: Prevalence and clinical significance. Ann Intern Med, 95:293, 1981.
24. Densen P and Mandell GL: Granulocytic phagocytes. In Principles and Practice of Infectious Diseases. 3rd ed. Edited by GL Mandell, RG Douglas Jr, and JE Bennett. New York, Churchill Livingstone, 1990.
25. Bryan HG and Nixon RK: Dyskeratosis congenita and familial pancytopenia. JAMA, 192:203, 1965.
26. Schwachman H, Diamond LK, Oski FA, and Khav KT: The syndrome of pancreatic insufficiency and bone marrow dysfunction. J Pediatr, 65:645, 1964.
27. Morley AA, Carew JP, and Baikie AG: Familial cyclical neutropenia. Br J Haematol, 13:719, 1967.
28. Weller PF: The immunobiology of eosinophils. N Engl J Med, 324:1110, 1991.
29. Gleich GJ and Adolphson CR: The eosinophilic leukocyte: structure and function. Adv Immunol, 39:177, 1986.
30. Brofman JD, et al: Epithelial augmentation of trachealis contraction caused by major basic protein of eosinophils. J Appl Physiol, 66:1867, 1989.
31. Ayars GH, et al: Injurious effect of the eosinophil peroxide–hydrogen peroxide–halide system and major basic protein on human nasal epithelium in vitro. Am Rev Respir Dis, 140:125, 1989.
32. Brown SJ, et al: Ablation of immunity to Amblyomma americanum by antibasophil serum. Cooperation between basophils and eosinophils in expression of immunity to ectoparasites (tubo) in guinea pigs. J Immunol, 129:790, 1982.
33. Shen L, Guyre PM, and Fanger MW: Polymorphonuclear leukocyte function triggered through the high-affinity Fc receptor for monomeric IgG. J Immunol, 139:534, 1987.
34. Willis HE, et al: Monoclonal antibody to human IgG Fc receptors: Cross-linking of receptors induces lysosomal enzyme release and superoxide generation by neutrophils. J Immunol, 140:234, 1988.
35. Ryan JL and Henkart PA: Fc receptor mediated inhibition of murine B-lymphocyte activation. J Exp Med, 144:768, 1976.
36. Clarkson SB and Ory PA: Developmentally regulated IgG Fc receptors on cultured human monocytes. J Exp Med, 167:408, 1988.
37. Lanier LL and Phillips JH: Evidence for three types of human cytotoxic lymphocytes. Immunol Today, 7:132, 1986.
38. Metzger H, et al: The receptor with high affinity for immunoglobulin E. Annu Rev Immunol, 4:419, 1986.
39. Spiegelberg HL, et al: Characterization of the IgE Fc receptors on monocytes and macrophages. Fed Proc, 42:124, 1983.
40. Ishizaka K: Twenty years with IgE: From the identification of IgE to regulatory factors for the IgE response. J Immunol, 135:i, 1985.
41. Joseph M, et al: A new function for platelets: IgE-dependent killing of schistosomes. Nature, 303:810, 1983.
42. Nossal GJU: The basic components of the immune system. N Engl J Med, 316:1320, 1987.
43. Cooper MD: B lymphocytes. Normal development and function. N Engl J Med, 317:1452, 1987.
44. Sissons JGP and Oldstone MBA: Killing of virus-infected cells: The role of antiviral antibody and complement in limiting virus infection. J Infect Dis, 142:442, 1980.
45. Davies SF, et al: Opsonic requirements for the uptake of Cryptococcus neoformans by human polymorphonuclear leukocytes and monocytes. J Infect Dis, 145:870, 1982.
46. Frank MM, Joiner K, and Hammer C: The function of antibody and complement in the lysis of bacteria. Rev Infect Dis, 9:S537, 1989.
47. Williams RC and Gibbons RJ: Inhibition of bacterial adherence by secretory immunoglobulin A: Mechanism of antigen disposal. Science, 177:697, 1972.
48. Dimmock NJ: Mechanisms of neutralization of animal viruses. J Gen Virol, 65:1015, 1984.
49. Buckley RH: Immunodeficiency diseases. JAMA, 258:2841, 1987.
50. Rosen FS, Cooper MD, and Wedgewood RJP: The primary immunodeficiencies (First of two parts). N Engl J Med, 311:235, 1984.
51. Rosen FS, Cooper MD, and Wedgewood RJP: The primary immunodeficiencies [second of two parts]. N Engl J Med, 311:300, 1984.
52. Umetsu DT, et al: Recurrent sinopulmonary infection and impaired antibody response to bacterial capsular polysaccharide in children with selective IgG-subclass deficiency. N Engl J Med, 313:1247, 1985.
53. Bjorkander J, Blake B, Oxelius V-A, and Hanson LA: Impaired lung function in patients with IgA deficiency and low levels of IgG2 or IgG3. N Engl J Med, 313:720, 1985.
54. Purtilo DT: Epstein-Barr virus–induced diseases in the

x-linked lymphoproliferative syndrome and related disorders. Biomed Pharmacother, *39*:52, 1985.
55. Miller DG: Patterns of immunologic deficiency in lymphomas and leukemias. Ann Intern Med, *57*:703, 1972.
56. Weitzman SA, et al: Impaired humoral immunity in treated Hodgkin's disease. N Engl J Med, *297*:245, 1977.
57. Paglieroni T and MacKenzie MR: Studies on the pathogenesis of an immune defect in multiple myeloma. J Clin Invest, *59*:1120, 1977.
58. Heinzel FP and Root RK: antibodies. *In* Principles and Practice of Infectious Diseases. 3rd ed. Edited by GL Mandell, RG Douglas Jr, and JE Bennett. New York, Churchill Livingstone, 1990.
59. Martone WJ, Zuehl RW, and Minson GE: Postsplenectomy sepsis with DF-2: Report of a case with isolation of the organism from the patient's dog. Ann Intern Med, *93*:457, 1980.
60. Chilcote RR, et al: Septicemia and meningitis in children splenectomized for Hodgkin's disease. N Engl J Med, *295*:802, 1976.
61. Bisno AL, and Gopol V: Fulminant pneumococcal infection in "normal" asplenic hosts. Arch Intern Med, *137*:1526, 1977.
62. Pearson HA, Spencer RP, and Cornelius EA: Functional asplenia in sickle-cell anemia. N Engl J Med, *281*:923, 1969.
63. Rosner F, et al: Babesiosis in splenectomized adults: Review of 22 reported cases. Am J Med, *76*:696, 1984.
64. Bernstein LJ, et al: Defective humoral immunity in pediatric acquired immune deficiency syndrome. J Pediatr, *107*:352, 1985.
65. Lane HC, et al: Abnormalities of B-cell activation and immunoregulation in patients with the acquired immunodeficiency syndrome. N Engl J Med, *309*:453, 1983.
66. Buckley RH: Humoral immunodeficiency. Clin Immunol Immunopathol, *40*:25, 1986.
67. Johnston RB: Monocytes and macrophages. N Engl J Med, *318*:747, 1988.
68. de Titto EH, Catteral JR, and Remington JS: Activity of recombinant tumor necrosis factor on Toxoplasma gondii and Trypanosoma cruzi. J Immunol, *137*:1342, 1986.
69. Adams DO and Hamilton TA: The cell biology of macrophage activation. Annu Rev Immunol, *2*:283, 1984.
70. Nathan CF: Secretory products of macrophages. J Clin Invest, *79*:319, 1987.
71. Allen PM: Antigen processing at the molecular level. Immunol Today, *8*:270, 1987.
72. Braathen LR, Bjercke S, and Thorsby E: The antigen-presenting function of human Langerhans cells. Immunobiology, *168*:301, 1984.
73. Davis MM and Bjorkman PJ: T-cell–antigen receptor genes and T-cell recognition. Nature, *334*:395, 1988.
74. Maddon MJ, et al: The isolation and nucleotide sequence of a cDNA encoding the T-cell surface protein T4: A new member of the immunoglobulin gene family. Cell, *42*:93, 1985.
75. Littman DR, et al: The isolation and sequence of the gene encoding T8: A molecule defining functional classes of T lymphocytes. Cell, *40*:237, 1985.
76. Wallner BP, et al: Primary structure of lymphocyte function-associated antigen 3 (LFA-3). The ligand of the T-lymphocyte CD2 glycoprotein. J Exp Med, *166*:923, 1987.
77. Imboden JB, Weiss A, and Stobo JD: The antigen receptor on a human T-cell line initiates activation by increasing cytoplasmic free calcium. J Immunol, *134*:663, 1985.
78. Manger B, et al: The role of protein kinase C in transmembrane signaling by the T-cell–antigen receptor complex. J Immunol, *139*:2755, 1987.
79. MacDonald HR: T-cell activation. Annu Rev Cell Biol, *2*:231, 1986.
80. Dinarello CA and Mier JW: Lymphokines. N Engl J Med, *317*:940, 1987.
81. Isakov N and Altman A: Interleukin 2, an immunoregulatory hormone. Clin Immunol Newslett, *7*:1, 1986.
82. Damle NK: Suppressor T lymphocytes in man. Year Immunol, *2*:60, 1986.
83. Damle NK, Childs AL, and Doyle LV: Immunoregulatory T lymphocytes in man. Soluble antigen-specific suppressor-inducer T lymphocytes are derived from the CD4 CD45R p80 subpopulation. J Immunol, *139*:1501, 1987.
84. Espevik T, et al: Inhibition of cytokine production by cyclosporin A and transforming growth factor-beta. J Exp Med, *166*:571, 1987.
85. Lee G, et al: β-Transforming growth factors are potential regulators of B lymphopoiesis. J Exp Med, *166*:1290, 1987.
86. Wilson CB: The cellular immune system and its role in host defense. *In* Principles and Practice of Infectious Diseases. 3rd ed. Edited by GL Mandell, RG Douglas Jr, and JE Bennett. New York, Churchill Livingstone, 1990.
87. Young JDE, et al: Purification and characterization of a cytolytic pore-forming protein from granules of cloned lymphocytes with natural killer activity. Cell, *44*:849, 1986.
88. Young JDE and Liu C-C: How do cytotoxic T lymphocytes avoid self-lysis? Immunol Today, *9*:14, 1988.
89. Lanier LL, et al: The relationship of CD16(LEU-11) and LEU-19(NKH-1) antigen expression on human peripheral blood NK cells and cytotoxic T lymphocytes. J Immunol, *136*:4480, 1986.
90. Herberman RB and Ortaldo JR: Natural killer cells: Their role in defenses against disease. Science, *214*:24, 1981.
91. Bellan AH, et al: Natural killer susceptibility of human cells may be regulated by genes in the HLA region on chromosome 6. Proc Natl Acad Sci USA, *83*:5688, 1986.
92. Springer TA and Anderson DC: The importance of the Mac-1, LFA-1, glycoprotein family in monocyte and granulocyte adherence, chemotaxis, and migration into inflammatory sites: Insights from an experiment of nature. Ciba Found Symp, *118*:102, 1986.
93. Bukowski JF, et al: Adoptive transfer studies demonstrating the antiviral effect of natural killer cells in vivo. J Exp Med, *161*:40, 1985.
94. Kohl S: Herpes simplex virus immunology: Problems, progress and promises. J Infect Dis, *152*:435, 1985.
95. Hauser WE and Tsai V: Acute Toxoplasma infection of mice induces spleen NK cells that are cytotoxic for T. gondii in vitro. J Immunol, *136*:313, 1986.
96. Callewaert DM: Purification and characterization of NK cells. *In* Mechanisms of Cytotoxicity by NK Cells. Edited by R Herberman. New York, Academic Press, 1985.
97. Tyrrell DAJ: Interferons and their clinical value. Rev Infect Dis, *9*:243, 1987.
98. Stiehm ER, et al: Interferon: Immunobiology and clinical significance. Ann Intern Med, *96*:80, 1982.
99. Ellner JJ: Immunology of human schistosomiasis. Clin Immunol Newslett, *4*:108, 1983.
100. Silberstein DS and David JR: Tumor necrosis factor enhances eosinophil toxicity to Schistosoma mansoni larvae. Proc Natl Acad Sci USA, *83*:1055, 1986.
101. Onderdonk AB, et al: Evidence for T cell–dependent immunity to Bacteroides fragilis in an intraabdominal abscess model. J Clin Invest, *69*:9, 1982.
102. Powderly WG, et al: T cells recognizing polysaccharide-

specific B cells function as contrasuppressor cells in the generation of T-cell immunity to Pseudomonas aeruginosa. J Immunol, 140:2746, 1988.
103. Ozaki Y, et al: Enhanced resistance of mice to bacterial infection induced by recombinant human interleukin-alpha. Infect Immun, 55:1436, 1987.
104. Iizawa Y, et al: Effect of recombinant human interleukin-2 on the course of experimental chronic respiratory tract infection caused by Klebsiella pneumoniae in mice. Infect Immun, 56:45, 1988.
105. Bowden RA, et al: Increased cytotoxicity against cytomegalovirus-infected target cells by bronchoalveolar lavage cells from bone marrow transplant recipients with cytomegalovirus pneumonia. J Infect Dis, 158:773, 1988.
106. Naumov NV, et al: Relationship between expression of hepatitis B virus antigens in isolated hepatocytes and autologous lymphocyte cytotoxicity in patients with chronic hepatitis B infection. Hepatology, 4:63, 1984.
107. Leslie K, et al: Clinical and experimental aspects of viral myocarditis. Clin Microbiol Rev, 2:191, 1989.
108. Oldstone MBA, Tishon A, and Buchmeier MJ: Virus-induced alterations in homeostasis and differentiated functions of infected cells in vivo. Science, 218:1125, 1982.
109. Hemachudha T, et al: Immunologic study of human encephalitic and paralytic rabies. Am J Med, 84:563, 1988.
110. Grau GE, et al: Tumor necrosis factor (cachectin) as an essential mediator in murine cerebral malaria. Science, 237:1210, 1987.
111. Wilson CB, et al: Decreased production of interferon-gamma by human neonatal cells. J Clin Invest, 77:860, 1986.
112. Lewis DB and Wilson DB: Molecular basis for decreased interleukin-4(IL4) and interferon-gamma (IFN-gamma) production by neonatal T cells. Pediatr Res, 23:356A, 1988.
113. Kohl S, et al: Interferon induction of natural killer cytotoxicity in human neonates. J Pediatr, 98:379, 1979.
114. Gillis S, et al: Decreased production of and response to T-cell growth factor by lymphocytes from aged humans. J Clin Invest, 67:937, 1981.
115. Gardner ID: The effect of aging on susceptibility to infection. Rev Infect Dis, 2:801, 1980.
116. Weinberg K and Parkman R: Severe combined immunodeficiency due to a specific defect in the production of interleukin-2. N Engl J Med, 322:1718, 1990.
117. Rouse BT and Horohov DW: Immunosuppression in viral infections. Rev Infect Dis, 8:850, 1986.
118. Twomey JJ, et al: Hodgkin's disease: An immunodepleting and immunosuppressive disorder. J Clin Invest, 56:467, 1975.
119. Fauci AS, Dale DC, and Balow JE: Glucocorticosteroid therapy: Mechanisms of action and clinical considerations (NIH conference). Ann Intern Med, 84:304, 1976.
120. Schaffner A and Schaffner T: Glucocorticoid-induced impairment of macrophage antimicrobial activity: Mechanisms and dependence on the stage of activation. Rev Infect Dis, 9:S620, 1987.
121. Britton S and Palacios R: Cyclosporin A: Usefulness, risks and mechanism of action. Immunol Rev, 65:5, 1982.
122. Sugarman B: Zinc and infection. Rev Infect Dis, 5:137, 1983.
123. Hornick RB, et al: The Broad Street pump revisited: Response of volunteers to ingested cholera vibrios. Bull NY Acad Med, 47:1181, 1971.
124. Gitelson S: Gastrectomy, achlorhydria and cholera. Isr J Med Sci, 7:663, 1971.
125. Giannella RA, Broitman SA, and Zamcheck N: Influence of gastric acidity on bacterial and parasitic enteric infections: A perspective. Ann Intern Med, 78:271, 1973.
126. Zink DL, et al: Plasmid-mediated tissue invasiveness in Yersinia enterocolitica. Nature, 283:224, 1980.
127. Hale TL, et al: Characterization of virulence plasmids and plasmid-associated outer membrane proteins in Shigella flexneri, Shigella sonnei, and Escherichia coli. Infect Immun, 40:340, 1983.
128. Harris JR, et al: High–molecular weight plasmid correlates with Escherichia coli enteroinvasiveness. Infect Immun, 37:1295, 1982.
129. Ofek I, et al: Cell membrane–binding properties of group A streptococcal lipoteichoic acid. J Exp Med, 141:990, 1975.
130. Gaastra W and de Graaf FK: Host-specific fimbrial adhesins of noninvasive enterotoxigenic Escherichia coli strains. Microbiol Rev, 46:129, 1982.
131. Krause DC and Baseman JB: Inhibition of Mycoplasma pneumoniae hemadsorption and adherence to respirtory epithelium by antibodies to a membrane protein. Infect Immun, 39:1180, 1983.
132. Stephens DS and McGee ZA: Attachment of Neisseria meningitidis to human mucosal surfaces: Influence of pili and type of receptor cell. J Infect Dis, 143:525, 1981.
133. Nelson ET, Clements JD, and Finkelstein RA: Vibrio cholerae adherence and colonization in experimental cholera: Electron microscopic studies. Infect Immun, 14:527, 1976.
134. Carruthers MM and Kabat WJ: Mediation of staphylococcal adherence to mucosal cells by lipoteichoic acid. Infect Immun, 40:444, 1983.
135. Christensen GD, Simpson WA, Bisno AL, and Beachy EH: Adherence of slime-producing strains of Staphylococcus epidermidis to smooth surfaces. Infect Immun, 37:318, 1982.
136. Maisch PA and Calderone RA: Role of surface mannan in the adherence of Candida albicans to fibrin-platelet clots formed in vitro. Infect Immun, 32:92, 1981.
137. Baddour LM, Christensen GD, Simpson WA, and Beachey EH: Microbial adherence. In Principles and Practice of Infectious Diseases. 3rd ed. Edited by GL Mandell, RG Douglas Jr, and JE Bennett. New York, Churchill Livingstone, 1990.
138. Johnson AP, Taylor-Robinson D, and McGee ZA: Species specificity of attachment and damage to oviduct mucosa by Neisseria gonorrhoeae. Infect Immun, 18:833, 1977.
139. Bisno AL: Alternate complement pathway activation of group A streptococci: Role of M protein. Infect Immun, 26:1172, 1979.
140. Pfaller MA and Herwaldt LA: Laboratory, clinical, and epidemiological aspects of coagulase-negative staphylococci. Clin Microbiol Rev, 1:281, 1988.
141. Gutman LT: Yersinia. In Zinsser Microbiology. 19th ed. Edited by WK Joklik, HP Willett, DB Amos, and CM Wilfert. Norwalk, Appleton & Lange, 1988.
142. Beutler B, Milsark IW, and Cerami A: Passive immunization with cachectin/tumor necrosis factor (TNF) protects mice from the lethal effects of endotoxin. Nature, 229:869, 1985.
143. Tracey KJ, Lowry SF, and Cerami A: Cachectin: A hormone that triggers acute shock and chronic cachexia. J Infect Dis, 157:413, 1988.
144. Remick DG, et al: Acute in vivo effects of human recombinant tumor necrosis factor. Lab Invest, 56:583, 1987.
145. Uchida T: Diphtheria toxin. In Pharmacology of Bacterial Toxins. Edited by F Dorner and J Drews. Oxford, Pergamon Press, 1986.

146. Hatheway CL: Toxigenic clostridia. Clin Microbiol Rev, *3*: 66, 1990.
147. Levine MM: Escherichia coli that cause diarrhea: Enterotoxigenic, enteropathogenic, enteroinvasive, enterohemorrhagic, and enteroadherent. J Infect Dis, *155*:377, 1987.
148. Friedman RL: Pertussis: The disease and new diagnostic methods. Clin Microbiol. Rev, *1*:365, 1988.
149. Leppla SH: Bacillus anthracis calmodulin–dependent adenylate cyclase: Chemical and enzymatic properties and interactions with eucaryotic cells. Adv Cyclic Nucleotide Prot Phos Res, *17*:189, 1984.
150. Parsonnet J: Mediators in the pathogenesis of toxic shock syndrome: Overview. Rev Infect Dis, *11*:S263, 1989.
151. Betley MJ, Miller VL, and Mekalanos JJ: Genetics of bacterial enterotoxins. Annu Rev Microbiol, *40*:577, 1986.
152. Middlebrook JL and Dorland RB: Bacterial toxins: Cellular mechanisms of action. Microbiol Rev, *48*:199, 1984.
153. Pollack M and Taylor NS: Exotoxin production by clinical isolates of Pseudomonas aeruginosa. Infect Immun, *15*:776, 1977.
154. Morihara K: Production of elastase and proteinase by Pseudomonas aeruginosa. J Bacteriol, *88*:745, 1964.
155. Mulks MH and Knapp JS: Immunoglobulin A1 protease types of Neisseria gonorrhoeae and their relationship to auxotype and serovar. Infect Immun, *55*:931, 1977.
156. Plaut AG, et al: Neisseria gonorrhoeae and Neisseria meningitidis: Extracellular enzyme cleaves human immunoglobulin A. Science, *190*:1103, 1975.
157. Heckels JE: Molecular studies on the pathogenesis of gonorrhea. J Med Microbiol, *18*:293, 1984.
158. Griffiths PD and Grundy JE: Molecular biology and immunology of cytomegalovirus. Biochem J, *241*:313, 1987.
159. Webster RG, Laver WG, and Air GM: Antigenic variation among type A influenza viruses. *In* Genetics of Influenza Viruses. Edited by P. Palese and D. W. Kingsbury. New York, Springer-Verlag, 1983.
160. Wilson CW, Tsai V, and Remington JS: Failure to trigger the oxidative metabolic burst by normal macrophages. J Exp Med, *151*:328, 1980.
161. Murray HW: How protozoa evade intracellular killing. Ann Intern Med, *98*:1016, 1983.
162. Murray HW, Nathan CF, and Cohn ZA: Macrophage oxygen-dependent antimicrobial activity IV. Role of endogenous scavengers of oxygen intermediates. J Exp Med, *152*:1601, 1980.
163. Goren MB: Phagocyte lysosomes: Interactions with infectious agents, phagosomes, and experimental perturbations in function. Annu Rev Microbiol, *31*:507, 1977.
164. Lewis DH and Peters W: The resistance of intracellular Leishmania parasites to digestion by lysosomal enzymes. Ann Trop Med Parasitol, *71*:295, 1977.
165. Sher A, Hall BF, and Vadas MA: Acquisition of murine major histocompatibility complex gene products by schistosomula of Schistosoma mansoni. J Exp Med, *148*:46, 1978.
166. Abramson JS and Mills EL: Depression of neutrophil function induced by viruses and its role in secondary microbial infections. Rev Infect Dis, *10*:326, 1988.
167. Murray BE: New aspects of antimicrobial resistance and the resulting therapeutic dilemmas. J Infect Dis, *163*:1185, 1991.
168. Brachman PS: Transmission and principles of control. *In* Principles and Practice of Infectious Diseases. 3rd ed. Edited by GL Mandell, RG Douglas Jr, and JE Bennett. New York, Churchill Livingstone, 1990.
169. Weinstein RA, et al: Pressure monitoring devices: Overlooked source of nosocomial infection. JAMA, *236*:936, 1976.
170. Kirby BD, et al: Legionnaires' disease: Report of sixty-five nosocomially acquired cases and review of the literature. Medicine, *59*:188, 1980.
171. Reinarz JA, et al: The potential role of inhalation therapy equipment in nosocomial pulmonary infection. J Clin Invest, *44*:831, 1965.
172. Maki DG, et al: Nationwide epidemic of septicemia caused by contaminated intravenous products. I. Epidemiologic and clinical features. Am J Med, *60*:471, 1976.
173. Lentino JR, et al: Nosocomial aspergillosis: A retrospective review of airborne disease secondary to road construction and contaminated air conditioners. Am J Epidemiol, *116*:430, 1982.

Part II

Clinical Infection and Laboratory Diagnosis

Section I

VIRUSES

Chapter 3

INTRODUCTION TO VIRUSES

Viruses, the smallest infectious agents (Fig. 3–1), are obligate intracellular parasites with several unique characteristics: their genome is either DNA or RNA, but not both; they are incapable of independent protein synthesis; they replicate by synthesizing and assembling subunits into infectious particles within a host cell; and they are resistant to antimicrobial agents that interrupt specific steps in the metabolic pathways of other micro-organisms (1). In this chapter, viral classification, structure and replication, laboratory diagnosis, and antiviral agents and susceptibility testing are discussed.

CLASSIFICATION

Viruses are classified according to five major criteria:

The nature of the nucleic acid (DNA or RNA)
The nucleic acid structure
The nucleocapsid's symmetry (icosahedral or helical)
The presence or absence of an envelope
The number of capsomers or helix diameter.

Family delineation is based on the mature virus' (virion's) morphology (determined by electron microscopy), the nature of the genome, and the strategy of its replication. Criteria used to identify genera differ among families, but the most common is antigenic cross-reactivity. Usually genera are subdivided into species on the basis of serologic differences, but this is controversial because no consensus has been reached on quantification of differences in nucleic acid sequences.

The general properties of DNA and RNA virus families (Fig. 3–2) are listed in Tables 3–1 and 3–2 (2). Certain viruses such as hepatitis C and E virus, the δ agent, astroviruses, the Norwalk agent, and Norwalk-like viruses remain unclassified, and the pathogens of the transmissible neurodegenerative diseases (spongiform encephalopathies) are still unknown.

STRUCTURE

The general structure of a virus is diagrammed schematically in Figure 3–3 (3). The mature virus particle, the virion, has at least two components: the DNA or RNA genome and an outer symmetric protein coat called the capsid, which protects the genome from cellular nucleases, facilitates virus attachment to susceptible host cells, gives the virion structural symmetry, and confers antigenicity. The viral capsid is composed of many protein subunits called capsomers (visible with the electron microscope), which in turn are composed of one or more virus-encoded polypeptide chains, the protomers. Because the number and the electron microscopic appearance of capsomers are specific for each virus, they are useful for identification. Together, the genome and capsid make up the nucleocapsid. Surrounding the nucleocapsid of the virus is the envelope, which can be disrupted by detergents, and solvents such as ether, resulting in viral inactivation.

Genome. Except for some retrovirus genomes, viral genomes are haploid: they contain only one copy of each gene. The genome of all DNA viruses, excluding the single-stranded parvoviruses, consists of a circular or linear, double-stranded molecule. The molecular weight of viral DNA ranges from 1.5 million (parvoviruses) to 150 million (poxviruses), which corresponds to about 4000 nucleotides or base pairs (4 kilobases) for the parvoviruses and more than 200 kilobase pairs for poxviruses. A group of about one thousand base pairs codes for one protein; therefore, different DNA virus genomes code for 4 to 200 proteins.

The linear, single- or double-stranded genome of RNA viruses is a single or a segmented molecule. Single-stranded RNA viruses are further classified according to the polarity (or sense) of the genome: genomes of RNA viruses that act as messenger RNA (mRNA) have positive polarity (positive sense), whereas those with a nucleotide sequence complementary to mRNA have negative polarity (negative sense). The single-stranded RNA viral genomes have a molecular weight of 2.5 million to 7.5 million and code for fewer than 10 proteins.

Capsid. Nucleocapsid symmetry is icosahedral or helical. The rigid icosahedral capsid, formed by capsomers arranged in 20 equilateral triangular planes with twelve vertices, varies in size, depending on the number of capsomers. Except for the complex poxviruses, all animal viruses that have a DNA genome are icosahedral; viruses with an RNA genome may be icosahedral or helical. The flexible capsid of helical viruses is composed of identical protomers arranged in a helix with the nucleic acid coiled between the turns of the helix. The diameter and length of the helix are determined, respectively, by the size and shape of the protomer and the length of the enclosed RNA molecule.

Envelope. All helical, and some icosahedral, virions are surrounded by a lipid envelope derived from the host cell's plasma membrane or cytoplasmic organelle membranes and acquired as the nucleocapsid is released from the infected cell, in a process termed "budding." The envelope is composed of many copies of a few virus-encoded polypeptide chains that are inserted into the existing cellular membrane during intracellular viral replication, replacing cell-specified proteins. The individual polypep-

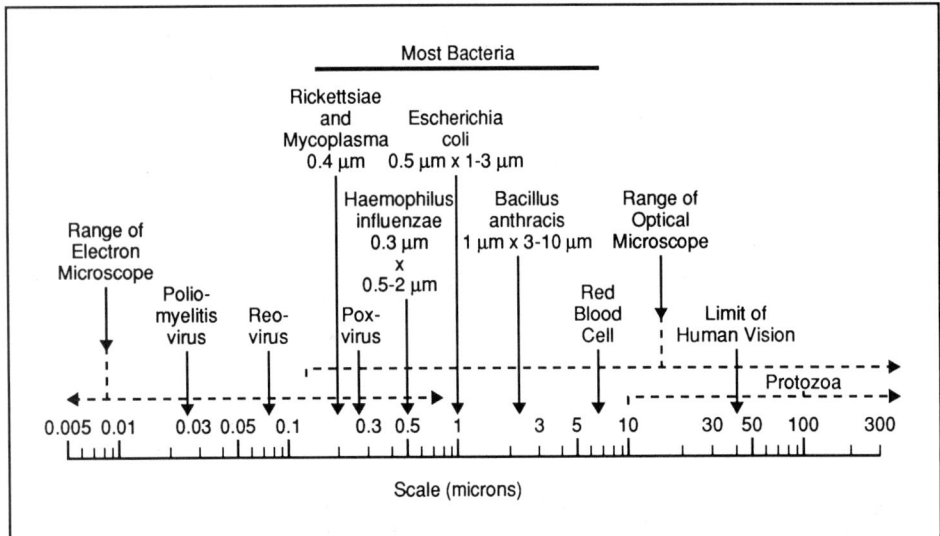

Fig. 3–1. Relative sizes of viruses and bacteria. (From Joklik WK, Willett HP, Amos DB, and Wilfert CM (eds.): Zinsser Microbiology. 19th ed. Norwalk, Appleton and Lange, 1988.)

Table 3–1. Features of the DNA Virus Families

Family	Virion			Genome*	
	Nucleocapsid	Size (nm)	Envelope	Structure	Mol. Wt. (×10⁶)
Poxviridae	Complex, brick-shaped	300 × 240 × 100	±	Linear	85–140
Herpesviridae	Icosahedral	Capsid, 100–110; envelope, 120–200	+	Linear	100–150
Adenoviridae	Icosahedral	70–90	−	Linear	20–25
Papovaviridae	Icosahedral	45–55	−	Circular	3–5
Hepadnaviridae	Spherical	42	+	Circular	~2
Parvoviridae	Icosahedral	18–26	−	Linear	1.5–2.0

* All genomes are double-stranded except the parvovirus genome, which is single stranded and has negative sense. The hepadnavirus genome has a small single-stranded region.
Key: +, present; −, absent; ±, membranes of viral origin, not a true envelope.
(Modified from White DO and Fenner F (eds): Medical Virology. 3rd ed. Orlando, Academic Press, 1986.)

Table 3–2. Features of the RNA Virus Families

Family	Genome*			Virion†			Diameter (nm)
	Mol. wt. (×10⁶)	Molecules	Sense	Shape	Size (nm)	Symmetry	
Picornaviridae	2.3	1	+	Icosahedral	25–30	Icosahedral	25–30
Caliciviridae	2.6	1	+	Icosahedral	35–40	Icosahedral	35–40
Togaviridae	4	1	+	Spherical	60–70	Icosahedral	28–35
Flaviviridae	4	1	+	Spherical	40–50	Icosahedral	25–30
Orthomyxoviridae	5	8	−	Spherical	80–120	Helical	9–15
Paramyxoviridae	5–7	1	−	Spherical	150–300	Helical	12–17
Coronaviridae	6	1	+	Spherical	60–220	Helical	11–13
Arenaviridae	3–5	2	−	Spherical	50–300	Helical	?
Bunyaviridae	4–7	3	−	Spherical	90–100	Helical	2–2.5
Retroviridae	4–6	1	+	Spherical	80–110	Helical	?
Rhabdoviridae	4	1	−	Bullet	180 × 75	Helical	5
Filoviridae	4	1	−	Filament	800 × 80	Helical	?
Reoviridae	11–15	10–12		Icosahedral	60–80	Icosahedral	45–60

* All molecules are linear; all genomes are haploid except that of the retrovirus, which is diploid, and are single stranded except for reoviruses, which have a double-stranded genome.
† All virions except Picornaviridae, Caliciviridae, and Reoviridae are enveloped.
Key: +, positive; −, negative; ?, unknown.
(Modified from White DO and Fenner F (eds): Medical Virology. 3rd ed. Orlando, Academic Press, 1986.)

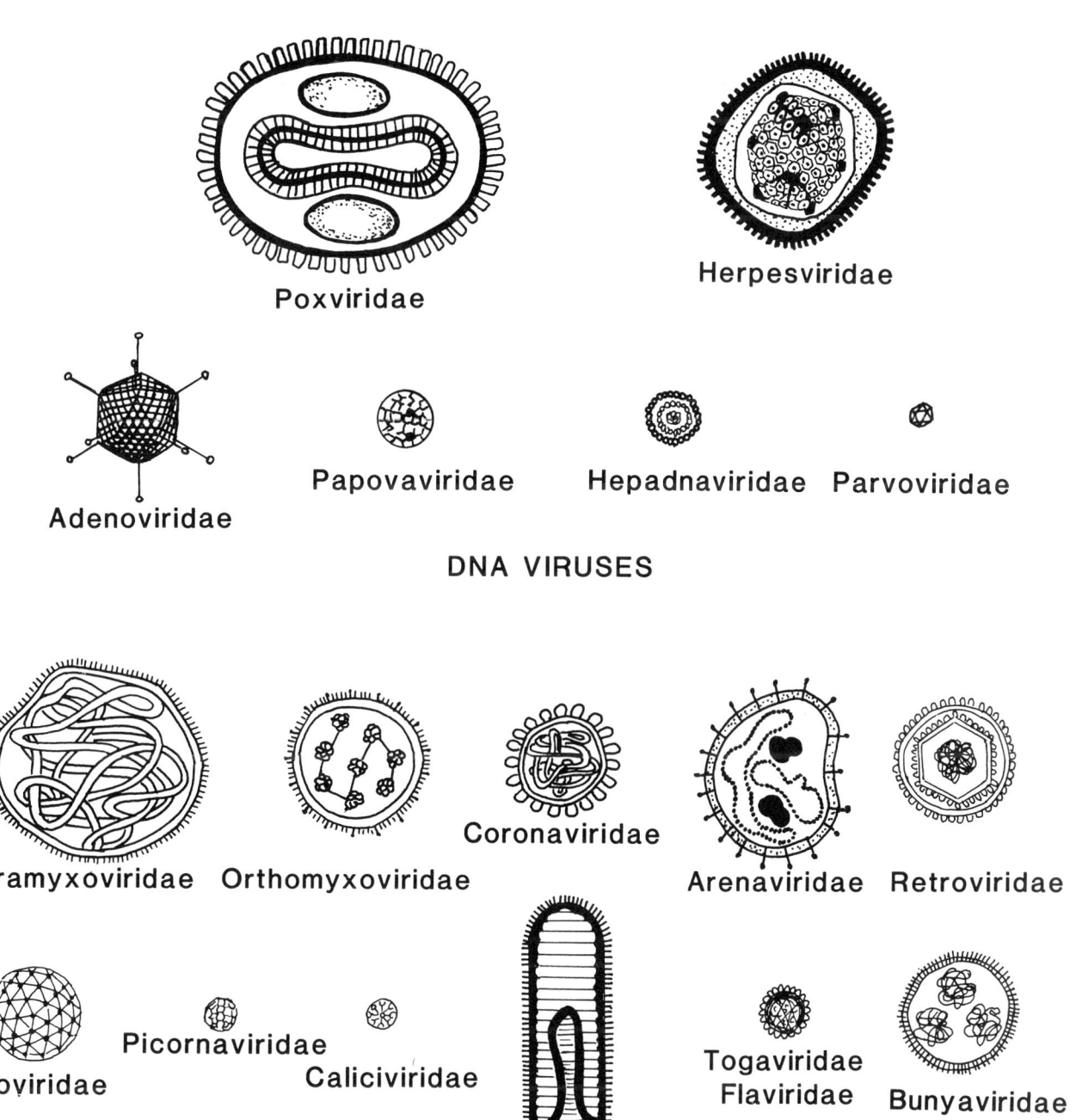

Fig. 3–2. Diagram of the relative sizes and shapes of the DNA and RNA virus families. (From White DO, and Fenner F (eds.): Medical Virology. 3rd ed. Orlando, Academic Press, 1986.)

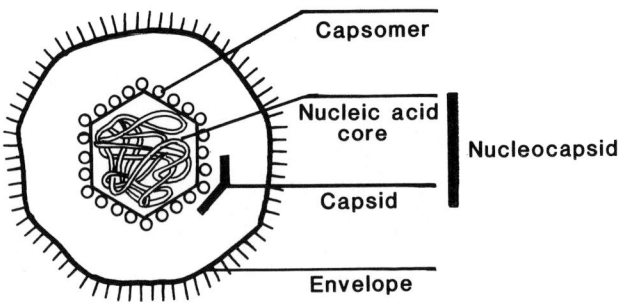

Fig. 3-3. Diagram of a virion. (From Rapp F: Nature and classification of viruses. In Virology. Edited by DA Stringfellow. Kalamazoo, MI, The UpJohn Company, 1983.)

tides, called peplomers, are anchored at one end in the lipid bilayer. The other end usually protrudes as a spike from the membrane and provides a site for virus attachment to host cells. Located on the inside of the envelope of many viruses is a matrix protein that provides structural rigidity, may direct the insertion of viral glycoproteins into host cell membranes or facilitate viral budding, and for several viruses appears to make specific contact with both the internal regions of the spike glycoproteins and nucleocapsid proteins. Viruses that have no matrix protein, such as the arenaviruses, bunyaviruses, and coronaviruses, are pleomorphic and fragile. Those that lack an envelope are called naked viruses.

REPLICATION

Productive Infections

Viral replication occurs only within host cells, relying upon cellular metabolism for support. In a productive viral infection the stages of the replication cycle are adsorption, penetration, uncoating, transcription, nucleic acid synthesis, virus particle assembly, and egress (Fig. 3-4) (2). The first three stages are similar for DNA and RNA viruses; the remaining stages differ and are discussed separately for each virus family.

Adsorption. Adsorption, the initial interaction between virus and host cell, involves attachment of specific sites on the virus to specific host cell surface receptors, which for most viruses range in number from 100,000 to 500,000 per cell. For enveloped viruses receptors are glycoprotein peplomers and for naked viruses, specific capsid proteins. Putative receptors on host cells are known for some viruses (Table 3-3), but for most they have not been determined.

Table 3-3. Putative Host Cell Receptors for Human Viruses

Virus	Host Cell Receptor
Cytomegalovirus	β_2-microglobulin
Epstein-Barr virus	C3d receptor
Human immunodeficiency virus	CD4 molecule
Influenza virus	Sialic acid
Rabies virus	Acetylcholine receptor
Vaccinia virus	Epidermal growth factor receptor

Penetration. Penetration, or entry of the virus particle into the host cell cytoplasm, is accomplished by one of at least three mechanisms: endocytosis, fusion, and translocation. Most naked viruses enter by endocytosis, a process normally used by the cell for uptake of receptor-bound molecules such as hormones. Enveloped viruses are internalized by endocytosis or by direct fusion with the plasma membrane, depending on the optimal pH for fusion. Virions that enter by endocytosis attach to specific cell receptors and move down into pits, which fold inward, producing coated vesicles that enter the cell cytoplasm and fuse with a lysosome to form a lysosomal vesicle (also called a secondary lysosome or phagosome). In the acid environment of the lysosome, the envelope of the endocytosed virus and the lysosomal membrane fuse, releasing the viral nucleocapsid into the cytoplasm. Enveloped viruses that fuse at the neutral pH of the cell surface may do so by virtue of a viral attachment protein. For example, some members of the Paramyxoviridae possess a surface F (fusion) glycoprotein, by which the viral envelope fuses directly with the plasma membrane of host cells, thus allowing direct release of the nucleocapsid into the cytoplasm. Certain naked icosahedral viruses apparently can translocate directly through the plasma membrane; however, whether this is a usual entry mechanism or an atypical event is unknown.

Uncoating. After entering the cell, virions are uncoated, an event that marks the beginning of the eclipse phase of replication, when infectious virus cannot be detected. Uncoating occurs in one of several ways: Enveloped viruses that fuse with the cell membrane are uncoated upon internalization. Capsids of naked viruses are dispersed in the cytoplasm by cellular proteases. Picornavirus capsids are weakened when the cellular receptor is inserted into the viral attachment site, releasing a key structural protein (VP_4). Herpesvirus nucleocapsids "dock" with the nuclear membrane and release the genome directly into the nucleus. Poxviruses are only partially uncoated and must synthesize immediate early proteins, including an uncoating enzyme that allows release of the DNA core into the cytoplasm.

Transcription, DNA Synthesis, Particle Assembly, and Egress. The DNA viruses that replicate in the nucleus employ cellular DNA-dependent RNA polymerase for transcription, whereas DNA viruses that replicate in the cytoplasm (the poxviruses) carry a DNA-dependent RNA polymerase for this purpose. Transcription of the DNA virus genome occurs sequentially: the "early" genes, which are read first, usually encode enzymes required for viral nucleic acid replication; the "late" genes, are read later in the cycle and encode structural proteins required for assembly of new virions. The transcribed mRNA is processed, transported from the nucleus to the cytoplasm, and translated into proteins by cellular ribosomes and transfer RNA (tRNA). Newly synthesized viral polypeptides then migrate to the cellular membranes or to the nucleus, depending on where they are needed. The DNA is replicated, and concurrently capsid proteins are synthesized in the cytoplasm, migrate into the nucleus, and aggregate into capsomers to form capsids, into which viral DNA is inserted. Virion assembly, which for all DNA vi-

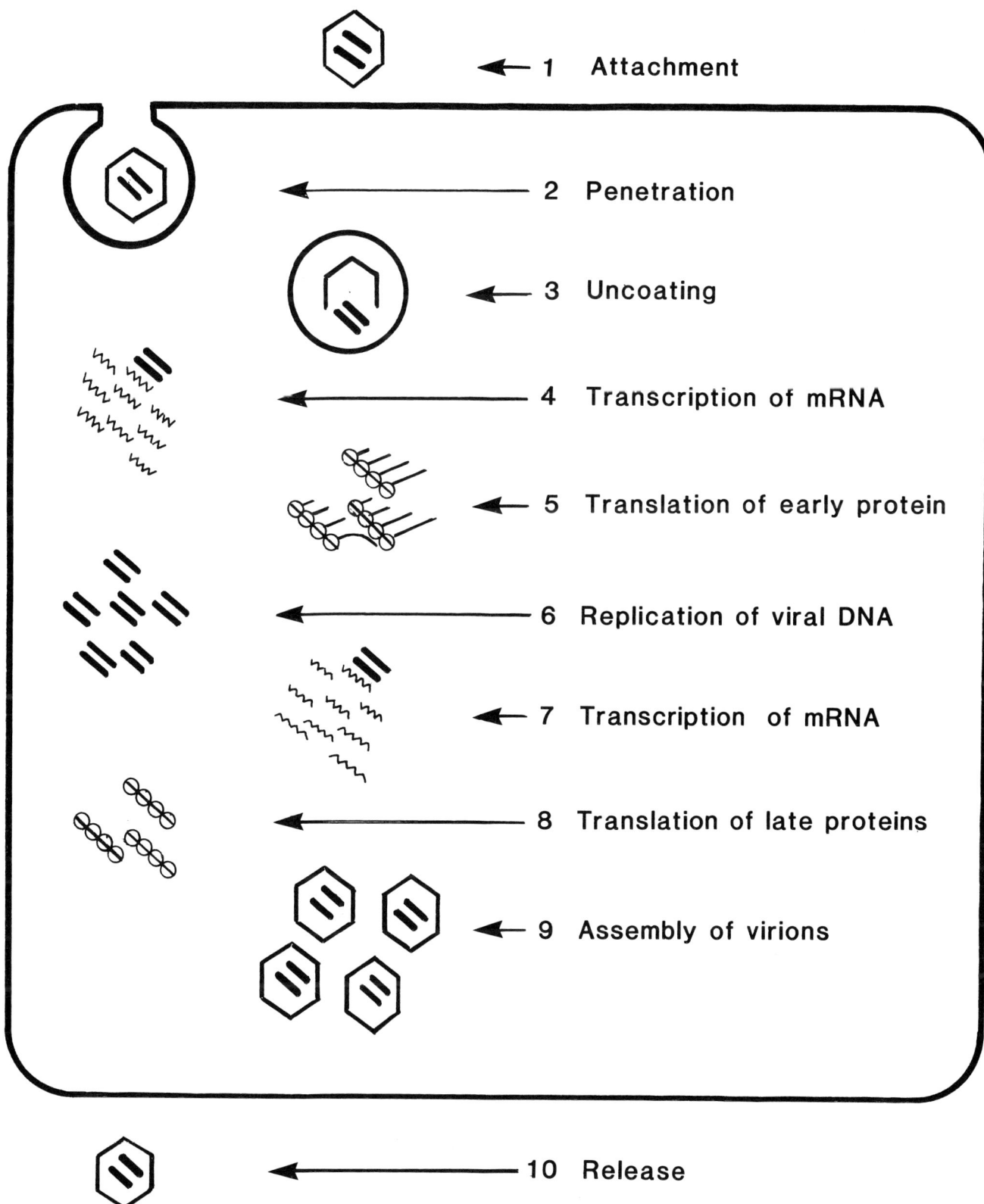

Fig. 3–4. Schematic diagram of the events that occur during viral replication in a productive infection. (From White DO, and Fenner F (eds.): Medical Virology. 3rd ed. Orlando, Academic Press, 1986.)

ruses except the poxviruses occurs in the host nucleus, is very inefficient: for example, only 5 to 10% of herpesvirus DNA molecules are encapsidated. Excess protein capsid production causes localized accumulation of viral components in infected cells, a phenomenon recognized microscopically as eosinophilic or Feulgen-positive masses called inclusion bodies.

Egress of the enveloped viruses occurs by a form of exocytosis called budding. First, newly synthesized viral proteins are glycosylated by cellular enzymes, forming rod-shaped spikes that are inserted into host cellular membranes by displacing cellular proteins. Multivalent attachment of many spikes, each to an underlying molecule on the icosahedron surface, molds the membrane around the nucleocapsid and forces it to bulge outward until it completely surrounds the nucleocapsid, causing the new virion to bud from the cell surface. Different viruses bud from domains in the plasma membrane, from the smooth endoplasmic reticulum, or from the nuclear membrane. Naked DNA viruses, on the other hand, are synthesized until the host cell is incapable of producing new virions. Virions are released from the nucleus following disintegration of the nuclear membrane, and from the cell after it dies.

Transcription, RNA Synthesis, Particle Assembly, and Egress. For RNA viruses, except orthomyxoviruses and retroviruses, the entire replication cycle occurs in the cytoplasm, without involving the nucleus. With single-stranded, positive-sense viruses, the parental genomic RNA acts as mRNA and is translated into RNA-dependent RNA polymerase and into capsid proteins. The RNA-dependent RNA polymerase initiates synthesis and displacement of new positive strands of RNA, which act as additional copies of mRNA or are encapsidated to produce new virions. The single-stranded, negative-sense RNA viruses bring a single-stranded RNA-dependent RNA polymerase into the cell. New polymerase molecules bound to RNA are synthesized using the viral message and incorporated into newly produced virions. Retroviruses have genetic information that codes for an RNA-dependent DNA polymerase, reverse transcriptase, that catalyzes the synthesis of double-stranded DNA complementary to viral RNA. This virus-specified DNA enters the nucleus, integrates into the host chromosome, and acts as a template for transcription of viral RNA, which subsequently is translated into viral proteins.

The nucleocapsid of all RNA viruses except orthomyxoviruses is assembled in the cytoplasm. Naked RNA viruses are released from the cell after it dies, whereas most enveloped helical RNA viruses bud through a segment of the plasma membrane that contains viral envelope proteins on its inner surface. The nucleocapsid binds specifically to a matrix protein attached to the cytoplasm side of the membrane beneath patches of viral glycoproteins, and budding proceeds by outfolding and pinching off of the membrane segment, which surrounds the nucleoprotein. Orthomyxoviruses, paramyxoviruses, rhabdoviruses, arenaviruses, alphaviruses, and rubiviruses bud through the plasma membrane, whereas coronaviruses and the flaviviruses bud through intracytoplasmic membranes.

Nonproductive Infections

Not all virus–host cell interactions result in a productive infection. Occasional infections are abortive, and new infectious virions are not synthesized. Abortive infections may have negligible consequences to the host cell; they may cause cell injury and death; or the virus may become latent or induce transformation. In latent infections, the virus enters a cell and persists without replicating or harming the cell; however, the viral genome is conserved and may be reactivated later to replicate, a process that does not necessarily destroy the cell that harbors the latent virus. Transformation, a virus-cell interaction involving the entire viral genome or only a segment, produces a heritable change in the cell that is transferred to cell progeny.

LABORATORY DIAGNOSIS

The first steps in laboratory diagnosis of a viral infection are collecting an appropriate specimen and transporting it to the laboratory. The sample then is processed for virus detection according to the technique used. The reference method for detecting viruses in clinical specimens is cell culture, but direct detection methods are useful for certain viruses (discussed later). Moreover, infections with viruses that are not easily cultured in the clinical virology laboratory, including Epstein-Barr virus, human herpesvirus 6, the hepatitis viruses, measles virus, rubella virus, parvovirus B19, retroviruses, and most of the viruses transmitted by arthropods, generally are diagnosed serologically.

Specimen Collection and Transport. Specimens useful in diagnosing viral infections are outlined in Table 3–4 and are discussed in more detail in the following chapters. Collection, transport, and processing of individual types of specimens is reviewed in Part III of the text, and the general principles are discussed briefly here.

In most cases, specimens should be collected early in the acute phase of the infection; however, the duration of viral shedding depends on the infecting virus and the host immune response. Various systems and media (Table 3–5) may be used to transport specimens to the laboratory (reviewed in reference 4). Liquid media systems, typically composed of buffers to control osmolality or onto which viruses can adsorb, are valuable for transporting viruses in active form for isolation, particularly if the specimen is collected on a swab. Of the transport media available, Hanks balanced salt solution containing 0.5% gelatin and antibiotics (penicillin, 100,000 U/ml; gentamicin, 50 µg/ml; and amphotericin, 40 µg/ml are recommended) probably is used most. Cell culture medium is acceptable only for short-term transport when the virus is in the medium for a limited time; skimmed milk is used principally as a holding medium for prolonged storage at −70° C. When specimens must be transported far, virus recovery appears to be increased and the time to detection decreased by using a commercially available system consisting of a centrifuge tube containing a monolayer of human fibroblasts and maintenance medium (5).

Specimens should be delivered to the laboratory as rap-

Table 3–4. Specimens Recommended for Diagnosis of Common Viral Syndromes

Clinical Syndrome	Likely Agents	Specimens
Upper respiratory tract infection	Rhinovirus, RSV, PIV	Nasopharyngeal swab/wash
	Adenovirus, enterovirus	Throat swab/wash, stool
	HSV	Throat swab/wash
	EBV	Serum
Pneumonia	Influenza viruses, RSV	Nasopharyngeal swab/wash, BAL, lung tissue
	CMV	BAL, lung tissue, buffy coat (anticoagulated blood)
	Measles	Serum, nasopharyngeal swab/wash, lung tissue
	Adenovirus	Throat swab/wash, BAL, lung tissue, stool, buffy coat (anticoagulated blood)
Rash		
Maculopapular	Rubella virus, measles virus, parvovirus B19	Serum
	Enteroviruses	Throat swab/wash and stool/rectal swab
Vesicular	HSV, VZV	Swab of lesion, aspirate of vesicular fluid, smear of cells
	Enteroviruses	Swab of lesion, aspirate of vesicular fluid, throat swab/wash and stool/rectal swab
Meningitis	Enteroviruses	CSF, blood (anticoagulated), throat swab/wash and stool/rectal swab
	Mumps	CSF, urine, serum
	HSV type 2	CSF
	Arthropod-borne viruses	CSF (for serologic testing), serum
	HIV	CSF, serum, peripheral blood mononuclear cells
Encephalitis	Arthropod-borne viruses	CSF (for serologic testing), serum, brain tissue
	HSV	Brain biopsy
	Enteroviruses	CSF, blood (anticoagulated), throat swab/wash and stool/rectal swab, brain tissue
	HIV	Brain tissue, CSF, serum, peripheral blood mononuclear cells
Hepatitis	Hepatitis A, B, C viruses, δ agent	Serum
	Hepatitis E virus	Stool
	HSV, CMV, adenovirus	Liver tissue, buffy coat (anticoagulated blood)
	EBV	Serum
Diarrhea	Rotavirus, adenovirus, Norwalk agent, Norwalk-like agents, astrovirus, calicivirus	Stool
Conjunctivitis/keratitis	HSV, VZV	Conjunctival scrapings
	Adenovirus enteroviruses	Conjunctival scrapings, throat swab/wash, stool/rectal swab
Genital infection	HSV	Endocervical swab, urethral swab, swab of lesion or vesicular fluid
Congenital/perinatal infection	CMV	Urine, throat swab, serum (test for specific IgM)
	HSV	Throat swab, rectal swab, swab of vesicular lesions, CSF, serum (test for specific IgM)
	Rubella	Serum (test for specific IgM)
	Enterovirus	Throat swab, stool/rectal swab

Key: RSV, respiratory syncytial virus; PIV, parainfluenza virus; HSV, herpes simplex virus; EBV, Epstein-Barr virus; CMV, cytomegalovirus; VZV, varicella-zoster virus; HIV, human immunodeficiency virus; BAL, bronchoalveolar lavage fluid; CSF, cerebrospinal fluid; Ig, immunoglobulin.

idly as possible. For short-term transit (less than 5 days), specimens should be maintained at 4° C (not frozen) and transported on wet ice; if longer transit is anticipated, freezing at −70° C is recommended.

Cell Culture. Three types of cultured cells may be used to recover viruses from clinical specimens: (1) Primary cell cultures, established from tissue taken freshly from animals, are capable of very limited growth in vitro. (2) Diploid cell cultures, consisting of a single cell type, can undergo 20 to 50 divisions in vitro before dying and always retain their original diploid chromosome number. (3) Continuous cell cultures, which consist of a single cell type, are capable of indefinite propagation in vitro. After multiple passages, however, diploid and continuous cell lines often become less permissive to viral infection, viral replication, or both. Cell lines commonly used in the clinical virology laboratory (Table 3–6) may be obtained from the American Type Culture Collection (ATCC) and passaged in the laboratory, or tissue culture tubes seeded with these cells may be purchased from various manufacturers.

The culture medium most commonly used for growth of cells and maintenance of the monolayer is Eagle's Minimum Essential Medium (commercially available) supplemented with fetal bovine or calf serum (10% for growth and 2 to 3% for maintenance). Because a physiologic pH must be maintained, buffering compounds should be added to the medium. If cultures are incubated in ambient air, a buffering compound not dependent on carbon dioxide–bicarbonate, such as HEPES buffer (N-2-hydroxyethylpiperazine-N'-2-ethanesulfonic acid), may be used. Inoculation and incubation of cell cultures is discussed in Chapter 54.

Many of the viruses commonly encountered in the clini-

Table 3-5. Composition of Viral Transport Media

Medium	Components
Swab-tube combination*	
Culturette	Swab-tube combination containing modified Stuart medium, antibiotics
Virocult	Collection swab, plastic transtube, small sponge saturated with phosphate buffer, D-glucose, lactalbumin hydrolysate, antibiotics
Cell culture medium	MEM with amino acids, fetal bovine serum, buffers, antibiotics
BSS, charcoal, protein additives	
Buffered BSA	Hanks BSS, 1% BSA, sodium bicarbonate, phenol red, antibiotics
Buffered gelatin	Hanks BSS, 0.5% gelatin
HH	Hanks BSS, BSA, HEPES and bicarbonate buffers, antibiotics
CVTM	Phosphate-buffered saline, potassium chloride, charcoal, ionagar (or agar)
Modified Leibovitz-Emory	Similar to CVTM except agarose is substituted for agar
Modified Stuart (Amies transport medium)	Phosphate-buffered saline, agar, sodium thioglycolate, charcoal, magnesium chloride, calcium chloride
Skimmed milk	50% phosphate-buffered saline, 50% skimmed milk
Skimmed milk	Phosphate-buffered saline, 10% skimmed milk, sodium bicarbonate, phenol red, antibiotics
Stuart medium	Agar, thioglycolic acid, sodium glycerophosphate, calcium chloride, methylene blue
YLE20CS	Yeast extract, lactalbumin, Earls BSS, 20% calf serum
Broth-based media	
Nutrient broth	Beef extract, peptone
Tryptic soy broth	Tryptone, soytone, dextrose, sodium chloride, dipotassium phosphate
Tryptose phosphate broth	Tryptose phosphate broth, 0.5% BSA or 0.5% gelatin, antibiotics
Veal infusion broth	Veal infusion, proteose peptone, sodium chloride
Bentonite-containing media	
Bentonite transport	HB597 tissue culture powder, Tris buffer, EDTA, bentonite, antibiotics; rabbit serum-coated bentonite may be added
Buffered sucrose-based solutions	
Carr-Scarborough viral/chlamydial transport	Phosphate-buffered sucrose, L-15 medium, glutamic acid, bovine albumin, antibiotics
Leibovitz-SPG	Leibovitz #15, sucrose, phosphate buffer, BSA, antibiotics
Richards Viral Transport	Phosphate buffer, organic buffer, sucrose, amino acids, bovine serum, phenol red, antibiotics
2SP	0.2 M sucrose, phosphate buffer, fetal bovine serum, antibiotics
SPG	Sucrose, phosphate buffer, glutamate
Transporters	
Transporter	MEM, buffers, fetal bovine serum, antibiotics, human diploid fibroblasts

* Components listed according to manufacturers's data sheet.
Key: MEM, minimum essential medium; BSS, balanced salt solution; BSA, bovine serum albumin.
(Modified from Johnson FB: Transport of viral specimens. J Clin Microbiol, 3:120, 1990.)

Table 3-6. Cell Lines Commonly Used to Detect Viruses in Clinical Specimens

Cell Line/Type	Source	Viruses Detected	Days to Detection*: Average (range)
MRC-5[†]/diploid	Human lung fibroblast	CMV	12 (5-28)
		HSV	2 (1-7)
		VZV	7 (5-14)
		Enterovirus	5 (3-14)
		Rhinovirus	7 (4-14)
		±Adenovirus	7 (2-21)
A-549/Continuous	Human squamous cell carcinoma	HSV	2 (1-7)
		VZV	7 (5-14)
		Adenovirus	5 (2-14)
Rhesus monkey kidney[‡]/primary	Monkey kidney	Enterovirus	5 (3-14)
		Influenza A, B	5 (2-14)
		Parainfluenza	9 (5-14)
HEp-2/continuous	Human squamous cell carcinoma	RSV	7 (3-14)
		Adenovirus	5 (2-14)

* Numbers in parentheses correspond to the range of days to detection.
† Human foreskin fibroblasts or WI-38 cells may be substituted.
‡ Cynomolgus monkey kidney cells may be substituted.
Key: CMV, cytomegalovirus; HSV, herpes simplex virus; VZV, varicella-zoster virus; RSV, respiratory syncytial virus; ±, may or may not be detected, other cell lines are preferred.

cal virology laboratory (see Table 3-6) are named presumptively by the light-microscopic appearance of the cytopathic effect induced in the cell monolayer, its rate of progression, and the cell lines in which it occurred (described for individual viruses in the following chapters) (6,7). The assumption is then confirmed by staining the infected cells with different virus-specific monoclonal antibodies. Some isolates of influenza A and B viruses and most parainfluenza and mumps virus isolates do not induce a distinctive cytopathic effect. They do, however, possess hemagglutinins with an affinity for red blood cells, so they can be detected by hemadsorption (see Appendix, Procedure 1). Adsorption of the erythrocytes indicates that one of the hemadsorbing viruses is present, and the specific virus is identified by staining the infected cells with monoclonal antibodies.

A major drawback to conventional cell culture is the prolonged time often required for the cytopathic effect to develop (see Table 3-6). Because effective antiviral therapy is available for several viruses (Table 3-7), more rapid detection methods are essential. Centrifugation culture, introduced in 1984, significantly shortens the time required to detect cytomegalovirus (see Appendix, Procedure 2) and may be used to detect other viruses (8-15). Sterile circular glass coverslips, placed in individual wells of a 24-well plate or in shell vials, are seeded with cells permissive to the suspected virus and inoculated with the clinical specimen. Vials or plates are centrifuged, and after incubation overnight (or longer, depending on the virus) in 5% carbon dioxide at 37° C, the cell monolayer on the coverslip is fixed, stained with monoclonal antibodies against the suspected virus, washed, and stained with a fluorescein isothiocyanate-labeled conjugate. Coverslips

Table 3–7. Antiviral Agents with Proven Efficacy

Drug	Viruses Inhibited	Mechanism of Action
Acyclovir	HSV, VZV	Inhibits viral DNA polymerase
Vidarabine	HSV, VZV	Inhibits viral DNA polymerase
Ganciclovir	CMV	Inhibits viral DNA polymerase
Foscarnet*	HSV, VZV, CMV	Inhibits viral DNA polymerase
Amantadine	Influenza A	Interferes with the interaction of the M1 protein and the viral hemagglutinin, blocking viral assembly
Ribavirin	RSV, lassa fever virus†	Alters cellular nucleotide pools and viral mRNA formation (exact mechanism unknown)
Zidovudine	HIV	Inhibits viral reverse transcriptase

* Does not require phosphorylation for antiviral activity (acyclovir, vidarabine, and ganciclovir do); useful for acyclovir-resistant HSV and VZV and for ganciclovir-resistant CMV.
† In vitro, ribavirin also has activity against the following viruses: Influenza A and B, measles, parainfluenza, mumps, reoviruses, some coxsackie virus strains, Venezuelan equine encephalitis, Japanese encephalitis, yellow fever, herpes simplex types 1 and 2, hepatitis A, and human immunodeficiency virus.
Key: HSV, herpes simplex virus; VZV, varicella-zoster virus; CMV, cytomegalovirus; RSV, respiratory syncytial virus; HIV, human immunodeficiency virus.

are mounted on microscope slides and viewed with an epifluorescent microscope; fluorescent inclusions indicate that the virus is present.

Direct Detection Methods. Several methods allow direct detection of virus in clinical samples. Herpes simplex virus, varicella-zoster virus, and cytomegalovirus induce characteristic cytologic changes in infected cells that may be visualized in Papanicolaou-stained smears of endocervical or esophageal scrapings, scrapings of cutaneous or mucocutaneous vesicles, and preparations of bronchoalveolar lavage fluid or urine (see Chapter 5). Commercially available specific monoclonal antibodies may be used to stain specimens such as endocervical smears, skin scrapings, nasopharyngeal washings or smears, and preparations of bronchoalveolar lavage fluid or buffy coats. This method of diagnosis is recommended for detection of varicella-zoster and respiratory syncytial virus (see Chapters 5 and 10) but should supplement, not replace, conventional cell culture for detection of other viruses. Enzyme-linked immunosorbent assays (ELISA) commonly are used to detect rotavirus and respiratory syncytial virus, and latex agglutination tests for direct detection of rotavirus in stool samples are commercially available but appear less sensitive than enzyme immunoassay (see Chapter 14). Electron microscopy is most valuable for diagnosis when the titer of virus in the specimen is high—at least 10^6 to 10^7 virus particles per milliliter. It is the only method for detection of many of the viruses associated with gastroenteritis such as Norwalk agent, Norwalk-like agents, coronaviruses, caliciviruses, and astroviruses, and it can provide rapid identification of herpesviruses in vesicle fluid, biopsy tissue, or urine.

Techniques such as nucleic acid hybridization and gene amplification via polymerase chain reaction (PCR) currently are used as research tools for virus detection (16,17). A nucleic acid hybridization assay to detect certain serotypes of human papillomavirus is commercially available, however, and in the next few years these technologies likely will be utilized more extensively in the clinical virology laboratory.

ANTIVIRAL AGENTS AND ANTIVIRAL SUSCEPTIBILITY TESTING

During the past several years specific antiviral drugs have been developed that are minimally toxic to normal human cells. Agents of proven efficacy work by interacting with viral enzymes and proteins that affect viral assembly (see Table 3–7) (18–21). With the increasing number of agents effective against several viruses and the emergence of virus strains resistant to first-line therapy, antiviral susceptibility testing is becoming more important (22–24). These tests, however, are not standardized and currently are offered only in specialized reference laboratories. Therefore, susceptibility testing is reviewed briefly here; a more detailed description can be found elsewhere (25–27).

The plaque reduction assay, based on inhibition of viral plaque formation, is the standard technique for determining the susceptibility of cytopathogenic viruses to antiviral agents. Briefly, a known amount of virus is inoculated onto several culture plates seeded with a monolayer of cells permissive to that virus, is adsorbed, and an overlay medium is added that contains a range of concentrations of the antiviral agent plus agar, methylcellulose, or serum immunoglobulin. Plates are incubated 72 hours, stained with crystal violet, and plaques are counted. A dose-response curve is generated, and the drug concentration that inhibits 50% of the viral cytopathic effect (the 50% inhibitory dose, ID_{50}) is calculated. This method is reliable but is tedious, time consuming, and costly.

The dye uptake assay is based on preferential uptake by viable cells of a vital dye. This semiautomated quantitative colorimetric test performed in 96-well microtiter plates, developed to determine the susceptibility of multiple clinical isolates of herpes simplex virus to acyclovir, has been modified for use with other drugs and viruses (27). Other methods of antiviral susceptibility testing are the ELISA, which measures a decrease in production of viral proteins; a DNA hybridization assay, which measures a decrease in viral DNA synthesis; and a modification of the centrifugation-culture technique developed for virus detection (described earlier) (28–30).

REFERENCES

1. Joklik WF, Willet HP, Amos DB, and Wilfert, CM (eds.): Zinsser Microbiology. 19th ed. Norwalk, Appleton & Lange, 1988.
2. White DO, and Fenner F (eds.): Medical Virology. 3rd ed. Orlando, Academic Press, 1986.
3. Rapp F: Nature and classification of viruses. *In* Virology. Edited by DA Stringfellow. Kalamazoo, MI, The Upjohn Company, 1983.
4. Johnson FB: Transport of viral specimens. J Clin Microbiol, 3:120, 1990.
5. Smith TF: Specimen requirements: selection, collection, transport, and processing. *In* Clinical Virology Manual. Ed-

ited by S Spector and GJ Lancz. New York, Elsevier Science Publishing, 1986.
6. Landry ML, and Hsiung GD: Primary isolation of viruses. *In* Clinical Virology Manual. Edited by S Spector and GJ Lancz. New York, Elsevier Science Publishing, 1986.
7. Lennette EH, and Schmidt NJ: Diagnostic procedures for viral, rickettsial and chlamydial infections. 5th ed. Washington, DC, American Public Health Association, 1979.
8. Gleaves CA, Smith TF, Shuster EA, and Pearson GR: Rapid detection of cytomegalovirus in MRC-5 cells inoculated with urine specimens by using low-speed centrifugation and monoclonal antibody to an early antigen. J Clin Microbiol, *19*:917, 1984.
9. Gleaves CA, Smith TF, Shuster EA, and Pearson GR: Comparison of standard tube and shell vial culture techniques for the detection of cytomegalovirus in clinical specimens. J Clin Microbiol, *21*:217, 1985.
10. Paya CV, Wold AD, and Smith TF: Detection of cytomegalovirus infections in specimens other than urine by shell vial assay and conventional tube cell cultures. J Clin Microbiol, *25*:755, 1987.
11. Woods GL, Young A, Johnson A, and Thiele GM: Detection of cytomegalovirus by 24-well plate centrifugation assay using a monoclonal antibody to an early nuclear antigen and by conventional cell culture. J Virol Methods, *18*:207, 1987.
12. Woods GL, and Mills RD: Conventional tube cell culture compared with centrifugal inoculation of MRC-5 cells staining with monoclonal antibodies for detection of herpes simplex virus in clinical specimens. J Clin Microbiol, *26*:570, 1988.
13. Woods GL, Yamamoto M, and Young A: Detection of adenovirus by rapid 24-well plate centrifugation and conventional cell culture with dexamethasone. J Virol Methods *20*:109, 1988.
14. Woods GL, and Johnson AM: Rapid 24-well plate centrifugation assay for detection of influenza virus in clinical specimens. J Virol Methods, *24*:35, 1989.
15. Mills RD, Cain KJ, and Woods GL: Detection of influenza virus by centrifugal inoculation of MDCK cells and staining with monoclonal antibodies. J Clin Microbiol, *27*:2505, 1989.
16. Eisenstein BI: The polymerase chain reaction. A new method of using molecular genetics for medical diagnosis. N Engl J Med, *322*:178, 1990.
17. Persing DH: Polymerase chain reaction: Trenches to benches. J Clin Microbiol, *29*:1281, 1991.
18. Reines ED, and Gross PA: Antiviral agents. Med Clin North Am, *72*:691, 1988.
19. Hermans PE, and Cockerill FR III: Antiviral agents. Mayo Clin Proc, *62*:1108, 1987.
20. Crumpacker CS II: Molecular targets of antiviral therapy. N Engl J Med, *321*:163, 1989.
21. Hayden FG, and Douglas RG Jr: Antiviral agents. *In* Principles and Practice of Infectious Diseases. 3rd ed. Edited by GL Mandell, RG Douglas, Jr, and JE Bennett. New York, Churchill Livingstone, 1990.
22. Ellis MN, et al.: Clinical isolates of herpes simplex virus type 2 that induce a thymidine kinase with altered substrate specificity. Antimicrob Agents Chemother, *31*:1117, 1987.
23. Hirsch MS, and Schooley RT: Resistance to antiviral drugs: The end of innocence. N Engl J Med, *320*:313, 1989.
24. Jacobson MA, et al.: Acyclovir-resistant varicella-zoster virus infection after chronic oral acyclovir treatment in patients with acquired immunodeficiency syndrome. Ann Intern Med, *112*:187, 1990.
25. Newton AA: Tissue culture methods for assessing antivirals and their harmful effects. *In* Antiviral Agents: The Development and Assessment of Antiviral Chemotherapy. Vol. 1. Edited by HJ Field. Boca Raton, FL, CRC Press, 1988.
26. Hill EL, Ellis MN, and Nguyen-Dinh P: Antiviral and antiparasitic susceptibility testing. *In* Manual of Clinical Microbiology. 5th ed. Edited by A Balows, et al. Washington, DC, American Society for Microbiology, 1991.
27. McLauren C, Ellis MN, and Hunter GA: A colorimetric assay for the measurement of the sensitivity of herpes simplex viruses to antiviral agents. Antiviral Res, *3*:223, 1983.
28. Rabalais GP, Levin MJ, and Berkowitz FE: Rapid herpes simplex virus susceptibility testing using an enzyme-linked immunosorbent assay performed in situ on fixed virus-infected monolayers. Antimicrob Agents Chemother, *31*:946, 1987.
29. Swierkosz EM, et al.: Improved DNA hybridization methodology for detection of acyclovir-resistant herpes simplex virus. Antimicrob Agents Chemother, *31*:1465, 1987.
30. Telenti A, and Smith TF: Use of shell vial assay for antiviral susceptibility testing of cytomegalovirus. *In* Abstracts of the Annual Meeting of the American Society for Microbiology. Washington, DC, American Society for Microbiology, 1988.

Chapter 4

POXVIRUSES

Poxvirus infections of vertebrates, which in humans and animals primarily cause cutaneous lesions, are infrequently diagnosed by tests performed in the clinical laboratory. Usually, they are diagnosed on the basis of clinical presentation alone or histologic findings in a biopsy specimen from a lesion.

CLASSIFICATION

Poxviruses belong to the large Poxviridae family of complex DNA viruses, which has two subfamilies: Entemopoxviridae, viruses that infect invertebrates, and Chordopoxviridae, viruses that infect vertebrates. Members of the latter are classified in general as follows:

Subfamily: Chordopoxviridae
Genus: Orthopoxvirus
Members: Variola, vaccinia, monkeypox, cowpox
Genus: Parapoxvirus
Members: Orf, paravaccinia
Unclassified: Molluscum contagiosum, tanapox, yabapox

The medically important Chordopoxviridae—variola, vaccinia, and molluscum contagiosum virus—are discussed in this chapter. The epidemiology and clinical features of those that primarily infect animals and rarely cause human disease are summarized in Table 4–1.

STRUCTURE AND REPLICATION

Poxviruses, 200 to 400 nm in diameter, are the largest of all animal viruses. The oval or brick-shaped virions, surrounded by a lipoprotein bilayer, contain a linear double-stranded DNA genome of some 130,000 to 300,000 base pairs.

The replication cycle of the poxviruses is initiated by viral attachment to the host cell receptor, which for vaccinia virus probably is epidermal growth factor (1,2). The virus then enters the host cell by fusion with the plasma membrane, is released into the cell cytoplasm and uncoated, and within minutes transcription is initiated and functional messenger RNA is produced. Unique to the poxviruses, DNA replication occurs within discrete cytoplasmic foci, termed factory areas, whence mature virus particles are transported to the cell periphery and enveloped by additional membranes, possibly derived from the Golgi apparatus (3). The virion, enclosed by one layer of Golgi membrane, then fuses with the plasma membrane and is liberated from the cell.

VARIOLA (SMALLPOX) VIRUS

Smallpox, first recognized more than 2000 years ago, was successfully eradicated from the world in 1977 (4,5). The first attempt at prevention was variolation: vesicle fluid or scab material from a person with a nonfatal infection was inoculated into the skin of a person susceptible to infection. A mild infection was produced that had a case-fatality rate of 1 to 2%, rather than the 20 to 30% associated with naturally acquired infection. In 1798, Edward Jenner showed that smallpox could be prevented by inoculation with material from cowpox lesions; in 1967, the World Health Organization Smallpox Eradication Unit was established; and the last naturally occurring case of smallpox was reported from Somalia in October, 1977.

Epidemiology and Pathogenesis

Humans were the only natural host for variola virus. Person-to-person transmission of the virus occurred primarily by the respiratory route during the first week of the rash; direct contact with sloughed scabs was a less important mode of spread. The virus initially lodged

Table 4–1. Clinical and Epidemiologic Features of Zoonotic Infections Caused by Poxviruses

Virus	Animal Host	Epidemiologic Characteristics	Clinical Features
Monkeypox	Monkey	West & Central Africa; transmitted by direct animal contact, rarely person to person	Generalized pustular rash, 15% mortality
Cowpox	Rodents; may be spread to other animals	Europe, Russia; transmitted by direct animal contact	Localized vesicle(s) on hands, arms
Paravaccinia*	Cattle	Worldwide; transmitted by direct animal contact	Localized vesicle(s) on hands
Orf	Sheep	Worldwide; transmitted by direct animal contact	Localized vesicle on hand, forearm, occasionally face
Yabapox	Monkey	Africa; occupational hazard of monkey handlers	Localized vesicle
Tanapox	Wild animals	Africa; transmitted by arthropod bite	Localized vesicles, fever, headache, prostration

* Also called milkers' nodules.

somewhere in the upper or lower respiratory tract, producing neither symptoms nor a local lesion. Macrophages soon became infected and reached the regional lymph nodes about 3 days after infection. Virions replicated for a brief period, then entered the blood and travelled to the spleen, bone marrow, and distant lymph nodes. During a second episode of viremia, macrophages infected with the virus localized in small vessels of the dermis and migrated to the epidermis. Virions in the macrophages then infected cells of the basal layer, producing necrosis, edema, and separation from the dermis. Later, neutrophils accumulated in the developing vesicle, and cytoplasmic inclusions called Guarnieri's bodies appeared in infected epithelial cells at the base of vesicles or pustules.

Viral antigens produced by infected macrophages and lymphocytes stimulated cytotoxic T lymphocytes to destroy infected cells, often before mature virions were released, and stimulated production of interferon and neutralizing antibodies. The extent of the cellular immune response determined the clinical presentation: a vigorous response inhibited viral replication, limiting the skin rash, whereas a defective immune response permitted unrestricted viral replication, resulting in megakaryocyte destruction and subsequent coagulation defects, clinically manifested as hemorrhagic smallpox.

VACCINIA VIRUS

Epidemiology and Pathogenesis

Vaccinia virus (from Latin *vacca*, cow) is the name given to the agent Jenner used for intradermal "vaccination" against smallpox. Three or 4 days after vaccine was administered to a susceptible individual, a papule appeared at the site of inoculation, became pustular by day 8 to 10, crusted, and resolved at about 3 weeks. In persons with partial immunity the stages progressed more rapidly. Complications of vaccination included progressive vaccinia in persons with a cellular immune deficiency, eczema vaccinatum in eczematous children, and postvaccinial encephalitis, a demyelinating disease of unpredictable incidence (estimated to be about 1 in 300,000 vaccinations in the United States in 1968).

Since global eradication of smallpox, vaccination has been discontinued except for members of the armed forces, who may develop one of the above complications. For example, disseminated vaccinia occurred in a military recruit infected with human immunodeficiency virus (6). In the future, vaccinia virus may be used as a vector for genes specifying antigens of other infectious agents (7).

MOLLUSCUM CONTAGIOSUM

Epidemiology and Pathogenesis

Molluscum contagiosum infects only humans, most often children and young adults. It is transmitted by direct personal contact or by indirect contact with fomites such as towels or washcloths, although the source of the infection often is unknown.

Clinical Manifestations

After an incubation period of 14 to 50 days, multiple painless, discrete, domed, white, pink, or yellow nodules, 2 to 5 mm in diameter, appear, typically on the trunk, face, or extremities of children and the genitalia of adults, although any body site except the palms and soles may be involved. The disease is self-limited, but lesions may persist several months.

LABORATORY DIAGNOSIS

Specimens necessary for diagnosis of infections caused by poxviruses are vesicle fluid or tissue of involved skin. Molluscum contagiosum and orf, however, frequently are diagnosed by their clinical presentation and history alone or by histologic examination of a skin biopsy specimen. The microscopic appearance of molluscum contagiosum is diagnostic: the central umbilication of the hyperplastic epidermis is composed of squamous cells, each containing a large, hyaline, acidophilic intracytoplasmic granular mass—the molluscum body—composed of virions (Fig. 4–1). Lesions of orf show ballooning degeneration and

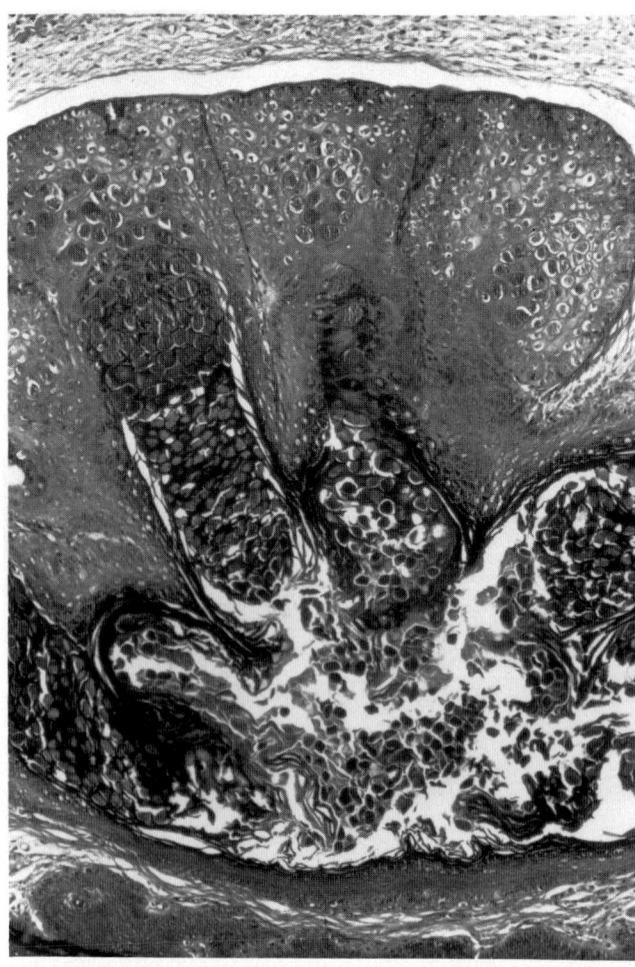

Fig. 4–1. Photomicrograph of a lesion of molluscum contagiosum (hematoxylin and eosin, ×40).

pale eosinophilic inclusions in the epidermal cells, accompanied by a perivascular infiltrate of monocytes and lymphocytes, and occasionally endothelial proliferation.

Infections with orthopoxviruses are diagnosed by identifying characteristic virions in negatively stained preparations of vesicle fluid or skin by electron microscopy. The species of orthopoxvirus is determined by what type of pocks is produced on the chorioallantoic membrane of a developing chick embryo (described elsewhere) (8). Virions of orthopoxviruses, molluscum contagiosum, and tanapox are not distinguished by electron microscopy; however, in contrast to the orthopoxviruses, the unclassified viruses do not grow on chorioallantoic membranes of chick embryos. Parapoxviruses have a distinct electron microscopic appearance and do not grow on chorioallantoic membranes. Orthopoxviruses grow in conventional cell culture (primary rhesus and African green monkey, Vero, and LLC-MK2 cells), parapoxviruses and tanapoxvirus grow poorly, and molluscum contagiosum virus cannot be cultivated.

TREATMENT AND PREVENTION

The chemotherapeutic agent methisazone (*N*-methylisatin β-thiosemicarbazone) has some activity against the orthopoxviruses and appeared to be of some value in treating progressive vaccinia (9). Vaccinia immune globulin should be given to persons with eczema vaccinatum and progressive vaccinia (10). The smallpox vaccine has been discontinued, except for persons in the military.

REFERENCES

1. Moss B: Poxviridae and their replication. *In* Fields Virology. 2nd ed. Edited by BN Fields and DM Knipe. New York, Raven Press, 1990.
2. Marsh YV, and Eppstein DA: Vaccinia virus and the EGF receptor: A portal of entry for infectivity? J Cell Biochem, *34*:239, 1987.
3. Hiller G, and Weber K: Golgi-derived membranes that contain an acylated viral polypeptide are used for vaccinia virus envelopment. J Virol, *55*:651, 1985.
4. Fenner F, et al.: Smallpox and its eradication. Geneva, World Health Organization, 1988.
5. World Health Organization: The Global Eradication of Smallpox. [Final report of the global commission for the certification of smallpox eradication; (History of International Health Publication, No. 4). Geneva, World Health Organization, 1980.
6. Redfield RR, et al.: Disseminated vaccinia in a military recruit with human immunodeficiency virus (HIV) disease. N Engl J Med, *316*:673, 1987.
7. Hruby, DE: Vaccinia virus vectors: New strategies for producing recombinant vaccines. Clin Microbiol Rev, 3:153, 1990.
8. Fenner F, and Nakano JH: Poxviridae: The poxviruses. *In* Laboratory Diagnosis of Infectious Diseases. Principles and Practice. Vol 2. Edited by EH Lennette, P Halonen, and FA Murphy. New York, Springer-Verlag, 1988.
9. Brainerd HD, Hanna L, and Jawetz E: Methisazone in progressive vaccinia. N Engl J Med, *276*:620, 1967.
10. Kempe CH: Studies on smallpox and complications of smallpox vaccination. Pediatrics, *26*:176, 1960.

Chapter 5

HERPESVIRUSES

Infections caused by the herpesviruses are among the most common infections of humans. Clinical manifestations range from asymptomatic infection to rapidly progressive disseminated disease. Moreover, because all herpesviruses become latent in the host, recurrent disease is common. In this chapter, the classification, general structure, and replication of the herpesviruses are reviewed briefly, and specific features of individual viruses are discussed.

CLASSIFICATION

Herpesviruses are classified in the family Herpesviridae, which is divided on the basis of biologic properties into three subfamilies: (1) Alphaherpesvirinae have a variable host range and a short reproductive cycle, spread rapidly in culture, efficiently destroy infected cells, and establish latent infections primarily, but not exclusively, in sensory ganglia. (2) Betaherpesvirinae have a restricted host range and a long reproductive cycle, produce a slowly progressing infection in culture, and can become latent in secretory glands, cells of the monocyte/macrophage system, kidneys, and other tissues. (3) Gammaherpesvirinae, specific for either T or B lymphocytes, replicate in vivo only in the natural host and in vitro in lymphoblastoid cells, and become latent in lymphoid tissue. Human herpesvirus 6 has not been classified, and human herpesvirus 7 has been proposed; however, whether the latter organism represents a new herpesvirus or a serotype of human herpesvirus 6 has not been determined (1). Herpesviruses of medical importance are classified in general as follows:

Family: Herpesviridae
Subfamily: Alphaherpesvirinae
Genus: Simplexvirus
Members: Herpes simplex type 1 (human herpesvirus 1), herpes simplex type 2 (human herpesvirus 2), cercopithecine herpesvirus 1 (B virus)
Genus: Varicellavirus
Members: Varicella-zoster virus (human herpesvirus 3)
Subfamily: Betaherpesvirinae
Genus: Cytomegalovirus
Members: Human cytomegalovirus (human herpesvirus 5)
Subfamily: Gammaherpesvirinae
Genus: Lymphocryptovirus
Members: Epstein-Barr virus (human herpesvirus 4)
Unclassified: Human herpesvirus 6

STRUCTURE

Herpesviruses are large particles, 150 to 250 nm in diameter (Fig. 5–1), composed of four structural elements: (1) a linear double-stranded DNA core with a molecular weight of 96 to 145 million and 120 to 230 kilobase pairs, (2) an icosahedral capsid 100 to 110 nm in diameter, containing 162 hexameric capsomers, (3) an amorphous, occasionally asymmetric assemblage of virus-encoded proteins of variable thickness, called the tegument, and (4) an envelope with viral glycoprotein spikes projecting from its surface.

REPLICATION

All herpesviruses replicate in the nucleus. During the first stage of replication viral envelope glycoproteins bind to specific host cell receptors. The envelope fuses with the plasma membrane, releasing the nucleocapsid into the cytoplasm, where it is uncoated. The viral DNA genome enters the nucleus and is transcribed by cellular DNA-dependent RNA polymerase II. The "immediate early" transcripts produce messenger RNAs (mRNA) that are translated into immediate early (α) proteins, which regulate their own synthesis and stimulate synthesis of proteins from the early genes. Thereafter, the whole genome is available for transcription, yielding "early" mRNAs that are translated into β proteins essential for genome replication: thymidine kinases, DNA polymerases, ribonucleotide reductases, and exonucleases. Replication of viral DNA is begun, and "late" mRNAs are transcribed and translated into structural γ proteins. Newly synthesized DNA is spooled into preformed immature nucleocapsids, which leave the nucleus by budding through the inner lamella of the nuclear membrane. Virions then accumulate between the inner and outer lamellae and are transported to the cell surface via the endoplasmic reticulum. Following primary infection, all herpesviruses become latent in specific host cells and may be reactivated at various times during the person's life.

HERPES SIMPLEX VIRUS

Herpes simplex viruses (HSV) were the first human herpesviruses to be discovered. The infectious nature of herpetic lesions was demonstrated between 1910 and 1920; the virus was isolated in tissue culture in the 1920s; and in the 1960s, two serotypes, now known as herpes simplex virus type 1 (HSV-1) and type 2 (HSV-2) were recognized (2,3).

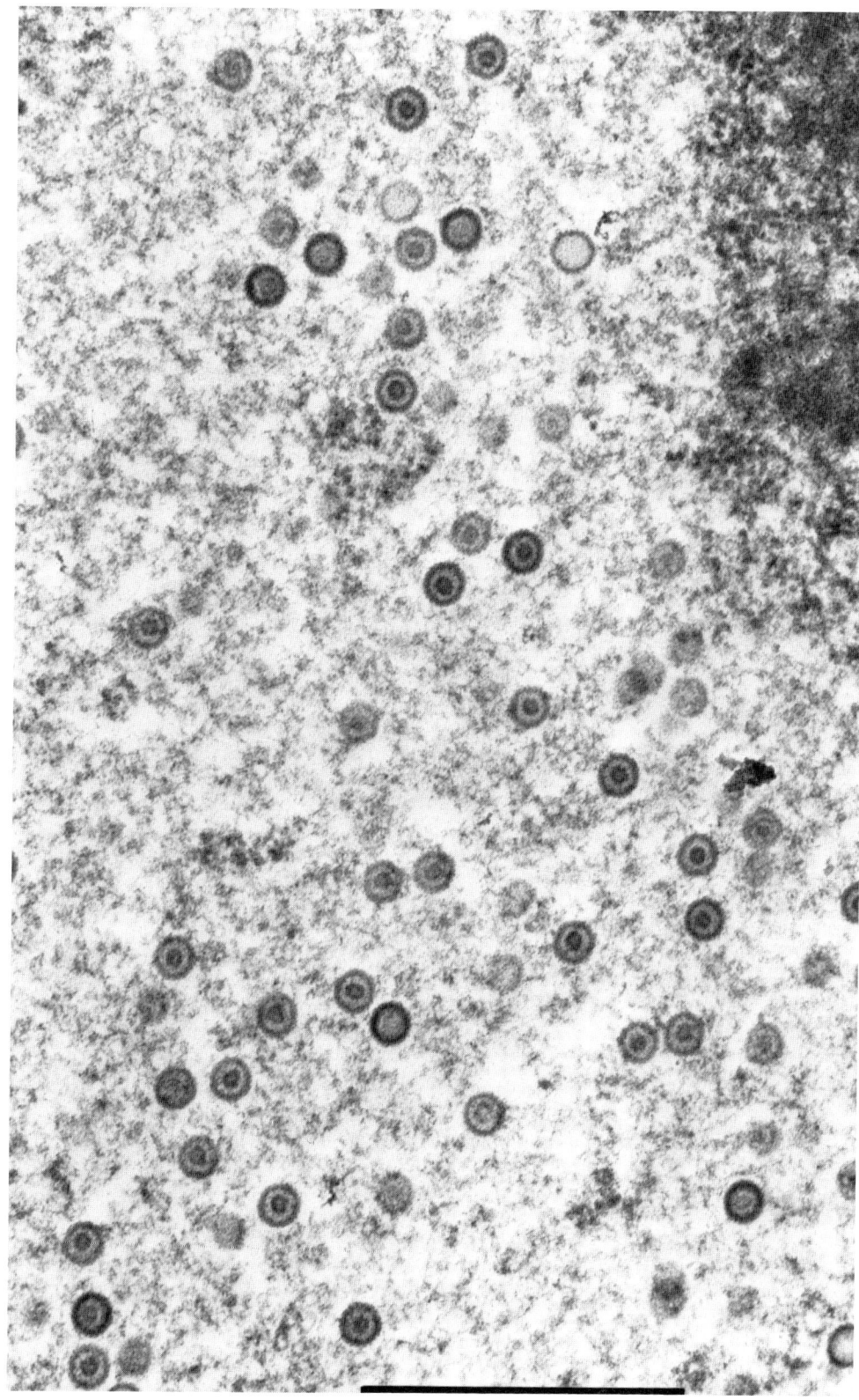

Fig. 5–1. Electron micrograph of virions of herpes simplex virus in vesicle fluid (×80,932).

Structure

The linear, double-stranded DNA genome of HSV consists of 150 kilobase pairs in two covalently linked components, termed L (long) and S (short). Eight viral glycoproteins are known: gB, gC, gD, gE, gG, gH, gI, and gJ. Glycoproteins B, D, and H are essential for viral attachment and penetration into the host cell. Glycoprotein C binds to the C3b component of complement, and if it is deleted viral pathogenicity appears to be enhanced. Glycoprotein E, and perhaps gI, binds to the Fc fragment of immunoglobulin G. Glycoprotein G is different for HSV-1 and HSV-2, allowing differentiation of the two virus types.

Epidemiology

HSV occurs worldwide. Humans are the only natural hosts, but animals are easily infected in the laboratory. Transmission occurs via direct contact with infected secretions of asymptomatic individuals shedding the virus or persons with active disease. HSV-1 is transmitted principally by contact with oral secretions and HSV-2, principally by contact with genital secretions. Antibody studies indicate that HSV-1 is acquired during childhood, whereas infection with HSV-2 occurs after puberty. Other modes of infection include autoinoculation to other body sites and transmission from mother to infant during passage through an infected birth canal or via retrograde spread of the virus from a maternal genital infection.

Pathogenesis

HSV enters the body through breaks in the skin or mucous membranes and replicates locally in the parabasal and intermediate epithelial cells, causing lysis of infected cells and eliciting a local inflammatory response, both of which are responsible for the characteristic vesicular lesion. Microscopically, uninucleate and multinucleate cells with Cowdry type A intranuclear inclusions (Fig. 5–2) are seen. From the site of inoculation, the virus travels through the lymphatics to regional lymph nodes, and if the infection is not controlled at this point by cellular immune mechanisms such as local interferon production, cytokine production by macrophages and T lymphocytes, and natural killer cell and antibody-dependent lymphocyte cytotoxicity (see Chapter 2), unrestricted viral replication may result in viremia and spread to multiple sites. From the primary site of infection virions travel along sensory nerve pathways to the trigeminal, sacral, and vagal sensory nerve ganglia, where the virus becomes latent. Viral DNA, and possibly some mRNA transcripts, localize within neurons, although the precise intracellular form of latent HSV DNA is unclear. During times of stress, the virus or viral genome is reactivated and travels via sensory nerves to cutaneous or mucocutaneous sites, where it spreads from cell to cell causing recurrent disease manifested as vesicle formation or is shed into secretions without producing a visible lesion.

Clinical Manifestations

HSV causes a spectrum of clinical manifestations. In neonates, 60 to 70% of infections are due to HSV-2, which

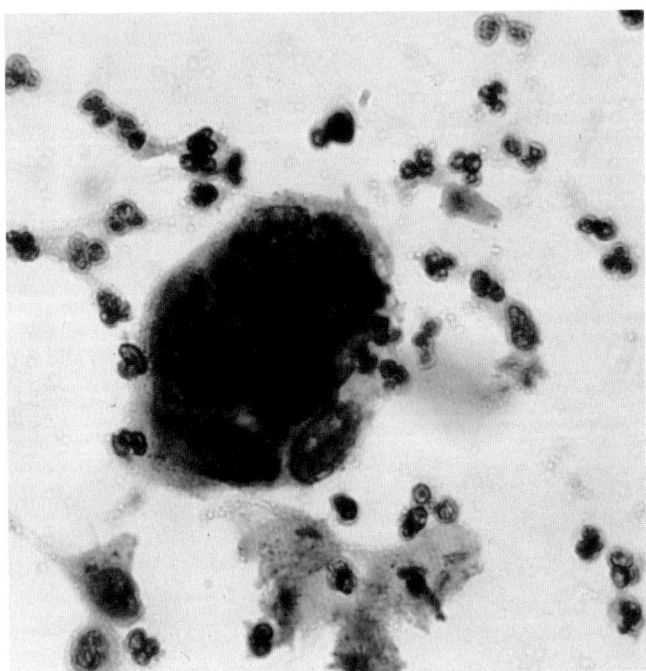

Fig. 5–2. Multinucleate giant cell of herpes simplex virus in a smear of endocervical cells stained with Papanicolaou stain (×201.6).

is acquired during delivery or via retrograde spread from the mother, who usually is asymptomatic (4). Infants, however, may acquire HSV-1 from the mother or other immediate family members who have symptomatic or asymptomatic orofacial infection or via nosocomial transmission. Neonatal disease, categorized according to its extent as disseminated, central nervous system, or skin, eye, and mouth, becomes apparent sometime before age 4 weeks, depending on the time of infection. Disseminated disease, usually manifest at birth or soon thereafter by seizures, irritability, jaundice, hepatosplenomegaly, bleeding disorders, chorioretinitis, pneumonitis, and skin vesicles, if untreated is associated with a mortality rate of 70 to 85%. Localized central nervous system disease, characterized by tremors, lethargy, irritability, paralysis, seizures, and coma, has a mortality rate of about 50% if untreated. Of the babies who survive disseminated and central nervous system infection, fewer than 10% develop normally (5). Infection apparently limited to the skin, eyes, and mouth usually is not fatal, but 20 to 30% of babies later develop severe neurologic impairment. During the past decade, the frequency of disseminated disease has decreased from about 50% to about 23%; the frequency of disease limited to the skin, eye, and mouth increased from 18% to about 43%; and the frequency of localized central nervous system disease remained relatively constant at 32 to 34% (6).

Primary infection with HSV-1 frequently is asymptomatic but may cause gingivostomatitis and pharyngitis, most often in children younger than 5 years but occasionally in older persons. After an incubation period of 2 to 12 days, fever and sore throat develop, followed shortly by the appearance on the pharyngeal and oral mucosa of vesicles that rapidly ulcerate. In young adults, primary HSV infection may cause posterior pharyngitis or tonsillitis. Lesions generally resolve in 10 to 14 days with no sequelae.

Recurrent orofacial lesions caused by HSV, termed herpes labialis, are more often caused by HSV-1. Vesicles develop, typically at the vermilion border of the outer lip (Plate IA), with variable frequency. Potential precipitating factors include sunlight, fever, local trauma, trigeminal nerve manipulation, menstruation, and emotional stress. A prodrome of pain, burning, tingling, or itching frequently precedes the appearance of vesicles, which soon ulcerate and then heal within 7 to 10 days.

Ocular infection caused by HSV-1 is the most common cause of corneal blindness in the United States. Usually the infection is unilateral, presenting as follicular conjunctivitis or blepharitis with regional adenopathy, occasionally involving the cornea. When the stroma is not affected, lesions heal without scarring in 1 to 3 weeks; when it is involved, scarring may result. Ocular disease recurs, most commonly as dendritic keratitis but sometimes as unilateral keratoconjunctivitis or blepharitis, within 2 years in 25 to 50% of patients.

Primary genital infection, due to HSV-2 in 70 to 95% of cases, is most common in adolescents and young adults (7). After an incubation period of 2 to 7 days, painful vesicles, associated with fever, malaise, anorexia, and tender bilateral inguinal adenopathy, appear on the glans penis or penile shaft of men and on the vulva, perineum, buttocks, cervix, or vagina of women. Lesions rapidly ulcerate, becoming covered with a grayish white exudate, and heal in 10 to 14 days. Potential accompanying manifestations include sacral radiculomyelitis with urinary retention, neuralgias, or loss of anal tone; in fewer than 10% of cases aseptic meningitis has been documented. Recurrent genital disease is milder and shorter lived than the primary infection and is more common in males and persons infected with HSV-2.

Primary perianal and anal infection due to HSV-2, most common in homosexual males, is characterized by confluent vesicles and ulcers in the perianal and anal areas that usually heal in 1 to 3 weeks but may persist and progress in persons with the acquired immunodeficiency syndrome (AIDS) (8). Symptoms include itching, tenesmus, discharge, fever, malaise, and possibly difficulty urinating and sacral paresthesias.

Primary cutaneous infections with HSV result from a break in the integrity of the skin. Young children with eczema are at risk of eczema herpeticum, an uncommon but severe illness characterized by high fever, irritability, and crops of vesicles. Fever usually subsides in 7 to 10 days, and the cutaneous lesions heal by the end of the third week unless complicated by bacterial superinfection. Primary infection of the finger, herpetic whitlow, is characterized by vesicle formation deep under the skin of one digit, accompanied by intense local pain and itching, axillary adenopathy, and neuralgias. Among medical and dental personnel, whitlow most commonly is due to HSV-1, whereas HSV-2 is the more frequent cause in the general population. Infection of superficial abrasions with HSV, in wrestlers termed herpes gladiatorum, can occur sporadically or in epidemics (9).

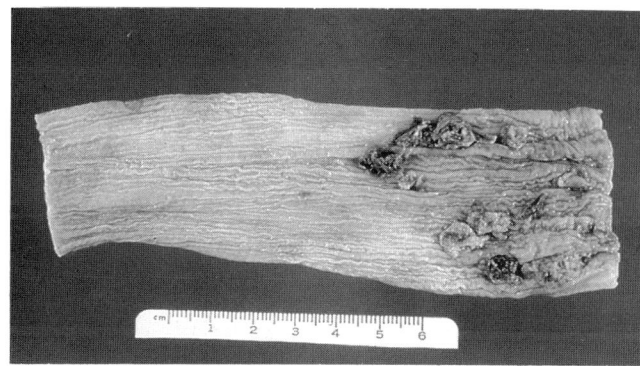

Fig. 5–3. Esophagitis caused by herpes simplex virus.

Infection of the brain with HSV is the most common cause of fatal sporadic encephalitis in the United States, where the estimated incidence is one case per million population annually. Encephalitis caused by HSV, almost always type 1 except in neonates, occurs year-round, affecting persons of all ages. The virus is believed to reach the brain by neural routes during primary or recurrent infection, localizing principally in the temporal lobe, where necrotizing hemorrhagic encephalitis ensues (10). The clinical illness begins abruptly or after an influenza-like prodrome (see Chapter 11) with fever, headache, stiff neck, behavior disorders, speech difficulties, focal seizures, and occasionally olfactory hallucinations. Cerebrospinal fluid examination often shows moderate pleocytosis with mononuclear cells and neutrophils, slightly elevated protein levels, and normal glucose concentration, but findings may be completely normal. The mortality rate for untreated cases is 60 to 80%, and more than 90% of survivors have significant neurologic sequelae (11,12).

Other manifestations of infection with HSV include esophagitis (Fig. 5–3), tracheobronchitis, pneumonia, and in persons with defective cell-mediated immunity, disseminated disease that tends to involve the liver (Fig. 5–4) and adrenals (13–18).

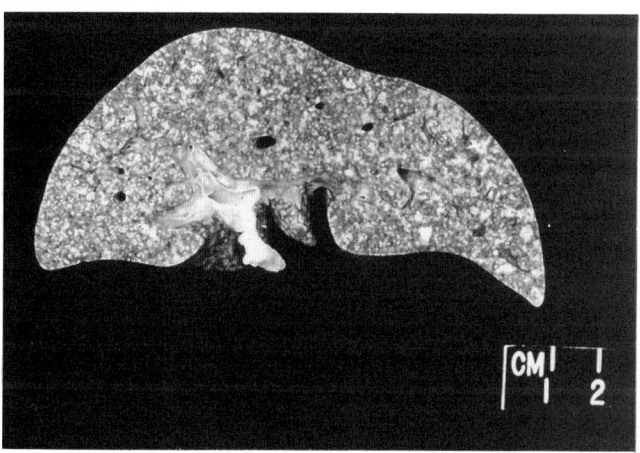

Fig. 5–4. Hepatic lesions caused by herpes simplex virus in a patient with disseminated disease.

VARICELLA-ZOSTER VIRUS

Varicella-zoster virus (VZV) produces two distinct clinical syndromes: primary infection, called varicella (chickenpox), mainly in children; and reactivated latent infection, herpes zoster (shingles), predominantly in elders or immunocompromised persons. The infectious nature of chickenpox was demonstrated in 1875 by transmitting the disease to volunteers inoculated with fluid from another person's vesicles; in 1943, the possibility that herpes zoster resulted from reactivation of a latent infection with VZV was suggested; and the virus was isolated in cell culture in 1958 (19).

Structure

The intact enveloped, 180- to 200-nm diameter VZV particle consists of a capsid, 90 to 95 nm in diameter and a DNA genome of molecular weight 80 to 87 million that contains 125 kilobase pairs encoding about 75 proteins. Five families of VZV glycoproteins are known: gpI, gpII, gpIII, gpIV, and gpV. Monoclonal antibodies specific for gpI, gpII, and gpIII, which represent the primary targets of humoral and cell-mediated immunity, neutralize viral infectivity.

Epidemiology

Humans are the only known reservoir for VZV. Chickenpox occurs worldwide, yearly causing later winter and early spring epidemics, predominantly in children younger than 3 years. Transmission, assumed to occur via respiratory droplet aerosols produced by infected persons, is possible for about 48 hours before vesicles erupt and until all vesicles have crusted.

Zoster occurs sporadically at all ages but is most common after age 50 years and in immunocompromised persons (20–22). The illness results from reactivation of a latent infection with VZV and apparently depends on an interaction between the virus and the host. About 4% of persons who have had zoster experience a second episode.

Pathogenesis

Following transmission, VZV replicates in the nasopharynx or upper respiratory tract, enters the blood, and seeds the monocyte/macrophage system. A second episode of viremia occurs, during which virions infect capillary endothelial cells, spread to epithelial cells of the epidermis or mucosal surface, and replicate, causing ballooning degeneration and cell lysis, which is manifested clinically as vesicles. The latter typically appear in crops, reflecting cyclic episodes of viremia. As neutrophils, degenerated cells, and fibrin accumulate, vesicles become pustules, which eventually rupture, releasing infectious fluid, or are resorbed. In persons with deficient cell-mediated immunity, failure to limit virus replication may result in pneumonia or disseminated disease.

After the primary infection, VZV becomes latent, presumably in the dorsal root ganglions, by a mechanism that currently is unknown. Histologic examination of the dorsal root ganglia after recent infection with VZV shows lymphocytic infiltrate in the nerve route, ganglion cell degeneration, and intranuclear inclusions in ganglion cells. Virions are visualized by electron microscopy, but the virus cannot be cultivated in cell culture.

Clinical Manifestations

After an incubation period of 10 to 23 days (mean 14 days), the vesicular, pruritic eruption of chickenpox appears in crops, usually beginning on the scalp and trunk and spreading to involve the extremities; this is associated with low-grade fever and malaise. Lesions vary in number from a few to many hundreds, may continue to appear for up to 1 week, and generally heal 1 to 2 weeks after the onset of the illness. The mortality rate is less than 2 per 100,000 cases for normal children but it increases by more than 15-fold for adults, whose illness is more severe: higher fever, more diffuse rash, and greater risk of primary viral pneumonia. Chickenpox also is more severe in immunocompromised children, especially those with leukemia: lesions are more numerous and often hemorrhagic, healing takes longer, and visceral involvement occurs in 30 to 50% of cases and is fatal in up to 15% (21). Potential complications of chickenpox in healthy children include acute cerebellar ataxia, a benign condition that complicates an estimated 1 in 4000 cases in children under 15 years of age; encephalitis, a potentially fatal complication occurring in 0.1 to 0.2% of cases; pneumonitis, a life-threatening illness that primarily affects adults; Reye's syndrome; Guillain-Barré syndrome; and bleeding disorders such as Henoch-Schönlein purpura and purpura fulminans (23–26).

Congenital varicella, an uncommon infection transmitted to the fetus from a mother who develops primary varicella during the first trimester of pregnancy, is characterized by skin scarring, hypoplastic extremities, ocular abnormalities, and evidence of central nervous system impairment (27). Perinatal varicella is associated with a high mortality rate when maternal disease occurs within 4 days before or after delivery, owing to the immature immune system of the neonate and the absence of protective transplacental maternal antibodies (28,29).

Herpes zoster is a painful, vesicular eruption with a dermatomal distribution, most commonly thoracic and lumbar. Involvement of the ophthalmic division of cranial nerve V is a sight-threatening complication occurring most frequently among elders. In a normal host the illness lasts 10 to 15 days, but complete healing may take up to 1 month. Cutaneous lesions often are accompanied by acute neuritis, and as many as 50% of persons older than 50 years experience postherpetic neuralgia, debilitating pain that persists over a month. Extracutaneous manifestations include meningoencephalitis, encephalitis, granulomatous angiitis of the internal carotid artery, motor paralysis secondary to involvement of the dorsal root ganglia, transverse myelitis, and myositis. Immunocompromised persons develop more severe herpes zoster than normal ones (30). The total duration of the illness is longer and the risk of cutaneous dissemination and visceral involvement is increased, especially in those with lymphoproliferative malignancies. Even in immunocompromised persons, however, disseminated herpes zoster rarely is fatal.

CYTOMEGALOVIRUS

In the late 1800s, infection with the agent now known as cytomegalovirus (CMV) was termed "cytomegalic inclusion disease" to describe the cellular changes (large "protozoon-like" cells) in tissues of persons with fatal disease, although the specific cause of the illness was unknown (31,32). In the early 1920s, investigators noticed these large cells in the parotid glands of infants who died from a variety of diseases. The viral agent responsible for these cellular changes was demonstrated in guinea pigs in 1926, after which it became known as "salivary gland virus" (33,34). In 1932, Farber and Wolbach described large inclusion–bearing cells in tissues of 12% of more than 180 infants who died from various unrelated diseases (35). This suggested that infection with salivary gland virus was relatively common and probably caused minimal or no symptoms.

Human salivary gland virus was isolated in cell culture in 1956, and in 1960 the term cytomegalovirus was adopted to replace salivary gland virus (36–39). CMV was recognized as one cause of infectious mononucleosis in normal, healthy adults in 1965, and over the next 5 years its transmission by blood and leukocyte transfusions was demonstrated (40–42). By using virus culture and serologic testing, infection with CMV was shown to be very common and subclinical in most cases but potentially severe in neonates and immunosuppressed individuals.

Structure

The pleomorphic enveloped CMV virions, 150 to 300 nm in diameter, are composed of a double-stranded DNA genome with a molecular weight of 150 million (240 kilobase pairs) and a 100-nm diameter naked capsid surrounded by a tegument of variable thickness. Five genes coding for matrix-tegument viral proteins have been identified: two—pp 65 and pp 64—are associated with protein kinase activity and may play a role in regulating transcription, viral DNA synthesis, or viral assembly. Two proteins have a similar molecular mass of about 150,000; one (pp 150) is the major capsid protein, and the other may be a targeting signal for virion morphogenesis. The function of the 28-kd protein is unknown. Antibodies specific for matrix-tegument proteins do not neutralize viral infectivity, but the gene products may be important in the cell-mediated immune response. The principal intranuclear capsid, the B capsid, is involved in capsid assembly and DNA packaging. One CMV gene, termed the gB homolog (gp55) for its homology to the gB gene of HSV, codes for a major envelope glycoprotein that might participate in membrane fusion. The gH homolog, a CMV gene with slight homology to the HSV gH gene, may code for an important immunologic determinant on the CMV envelope, because monoclonal antibodies specific for the glycoprotein gene product neutralize viral infectivity (43). A potential CMV glycoprotein called the α-chain homolog may bind to β_2-microglobulin, the postulated host cell receptor, facilitating attachment and subsequent endocytosis during infection.

Epidemiology

Infection with CMV is species specific and occurs worldwide throughout the year. The prevalence of antibodies to CMV in adults depends on the socioeconomic conditions of the population, ranging from 40% in Europe, Australia, and some parts of North America to 100% in developing areas of Africa and Southeast Asia (44). Infection with CMV is acquired with increased frequency during the perinatal period and during the reproductive years. Transmission occurs by direct or indirect person-to-person contact with infected secretions such as saliva, urine, cervical and vaginal excretions, seminal fluids, breast milk, tears, and feces; by transfusion of blood and blood products and transplantation of organs and tissues procured from persons seropositive for CMV; and in utero.

Pathogenesis

CMV possesses low virulence but is clearly cytopathic and capable of tissue destruction. Viral replication in vitro is slow, yielding more cell-associated than extracellular virions and many more defective than infectious ones, and this is likely the case with replication in vivo, which would allow host immune mechanisms to contain the destructive effects of the virus (45). In addition to the direct cytopathic effects of CMV, the host immune response and the vasculitis that frequently develops contribute to the organ dysfunction that characterizes CMV disease (46).

CMV has evolved intrinsic and extrinsic mechanisms that ensure its survival and latency in the host. Once it leaves an infected cell CMV can bind to host β_2-microglobulin, present in most body fluids, which coats the virus to protect it from neutralizing antibodies (47). Cell-associated CMV induces production of a protein, localized in the perinuclear area and on the surface of the infected cell, that acts as an Fc receptor, binding the Fc portion of immunoglobulin, which could protect the infected cell from the host immune system. Moreover, CMV itself is immunosuppressive: lymphocyte proliferative responses are impaired during acute infection, and this may promote persistence of the viral infection (45,47).

The virologic and immunologic events that occur during primary infection with CMV in normal adults are described best for the infectious mononucleosis syndrome. After entering the host, the virions enter the blood and disseminate throughout the body. Viruria and viremia persist for a few weeks to a few months (48,49). In blood CMV is found predominantly in neutrophils but also in mononuclear cells (50,51). Specific immunoglobulin (Ig) M peaks early in the infection and usually disappears 12 to 16 weeks after the onset of subclinical infection, but it may be detected for longer periods following symptomatic infection and, by highly sensitive techniques, during recurrent infections. IgG peaks during the first 2 months after infection and persists for life. Cell-mediated immunity is depressed during symptomatic primary infections. The number of activated CD8 (cytotoxic/suppressor) cells is increased and CD4 (helper/inducer) cells are slightly decreased. However, during subclinical infections, the cell-mediated immune system appears to be activated, although the information available is limited (52).

At least three outcomes of primary infection with CMV are possible: (1) A low-grade chronic infection during which virus excretion occasionally reaches detectable levels may be established. (2) Immune persons may be reinfected with a different strain of CMV. (3) CMV may become latent in various organs, perhaps in macrophages or dendritic cells, though the exact site is unknown, to be repeatedly reactivated in response to different stimuli throughout life (53,54).

In immunosuppressed persons, such as solid organ and bone marrow transplant recipients and those with AIDS, primary and recurrent infections caused by CMV are more frequent, virus titers usually are higher, virus is excreted longer, and specific IgM may persist as long as a year; however, severely immunocompromised persons may be unable to mount an antibody response (55–64). Cell-mediated immunity generally is more depressed in the immunocompromised host, and the degree to which it is depressed at least in part determines the outcome of the infection (65).

The likelihood of intrauterine transmission of CMV and the outcome of the fetal infection probably are influenced by currently undefined maternal factors. CMV may be transmitted in utero during both a primary or reactivated maternal infection; however, severe cytomegalic inclusion disease rarely is associated with recurrent maternal infection, possibly because maternal antibodies are protective (66,72). The source of the virus in reactivated infection is unknown, but it may be leukocytes, endometrial or endocervical cells, or maternal or paternal germinal cells. CMV may be transmitted to the fetus throughout gestation, but fetal infection acquired during the first half generally is more severe (67).

The major determinant of the severity of congenital and early postnatally acquired infections with CMV is the immune response of the fetus or infant. Given the immaturity of the infant's immune system, the virologic and immunologic features of symptomatic congenital infections most closely resemble those of immunocompromised adults. Large quantities of virus are excreted continuously in the urine for 5 years or longer and in the saliva for 2 to 4 years (68,69). Even children with subclinical infection shed more virus than do ill, immunocompromised adults. IgM, present in cord blood at delivery, persists weeks to months. IgG production by the infant begins as maternal IgG declines, and it continues for life. In response to the high titers of viral antigens, serum immunoglobulin production, especially IgM, is accelerated, and antibodies may combine with viral antigens to form immune complexes, which may be deposited in renal glomeruli, causing glomerulonephritis (70). The only cell-mediated immune defect of symptomatic and asymptomatic infants is persistent inability of lymphocytes to elicit a blastogenic response and induce interferon production in vitro when challenged with CMV antigens (52,69,71).

Natal infections with CMV and those transmitted via breast milk most often result from reactivated latent maternal infection. Transplacental maternal antibodies in the infant's serum protect against infection in about half these cases, and infants who become infected generally are asymptomatic, suggesting that maternal antibodies protect against disease (72,73). Transfusion-acquired infection in young infants is more severe in seronegative than in seropositive infants, further supporting the protective role of maternal antibodies (74).

Clinical Manifestations

The prevalence of intrauterine or congenital infection with CMV is 0.5 to 2.0% of all live births (75). Some 90 to 95% of infected infants are asymptomatic at birth, but more than 10% of them develop sensorineural hearing loss later in childhood (76,77). Infants with classic fulminant congenital cytomegalic inclusion disease have multiple-system and -organ involvement manifested by jaundice, hepatosplenomegaly, petechial rash, microcephaly, motor disability, chorioretinitis, cerebral calcifications, and inner ear abnormalities. Many infants with severe disease die shortly after birth, and almost all who survive suffer neurologic sequelae. Perinatally and postnatally acquired infections with CMV usually are inapparent, but infants are at increased risk of sensorineural hearing loss during childhood, and rarely diffuse visceral or central nervous system involvement occurs. Serious disease, however, can result from exchange transfusion, primarily in CMV-seronegative infants given blood from a seropositive donor (74).

Infections caused by CMV in immunocompetent adults usually are asymptomatic but may produce a wide range of clinical manifestations. In adults, CMV is the most common cause of heterophile-negative infectious mononucleosis (not caused by Epstein-Barr virus [EBV], discussed later). Clinically, infectious mononucleosis caused by CMV is difficult to distinguish from that caused by EBV; however, in general, the former affects older persons (mean age 28 years for CMV; peak age 15 to 19 years for EBV) and is associated with longer duration of fever (mean 18 days versus 1 to 2 weeks for EBV) (78). Uncom-

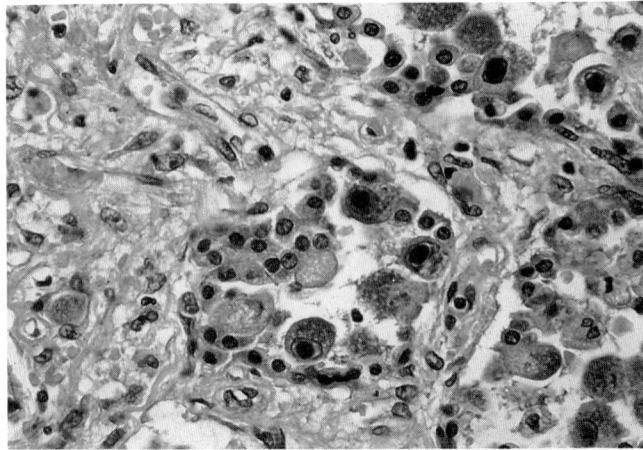

Fig. 5–5. Section of lung from a patient with AIDS shows pneumonitis caused by cytomegalovirus (hematoxylin and eosin, ×100).

mon manifestations of infection with CMV in immunocompetent adults include rash, granulomatous hepatitis, Guillain-Barré syndrome, interstitial pneumonitis, meningoencephalitis, myocarditis, hemolytic anemia, and thrombocytopenia (79–87).

In immunosuppressed persons, infections caused by CMV may be asymptomatic, but often they produce protean clinical manifestations. The most common presentation is a febrile infectious mononucleosis syndrome clinically identical to this disease in immunocompetent adults, but more extensive organ involvement may develop, such as interstitial pneumonitis (Fig. 5–5), hepatitis, gastrointestinal ulcerations, sight-threatening retinitis, encephalopathy, and endocrine disturbances, which rarely occur in otherwise healthy persons (57, 59,66,88–95).

EPSTEIN-BARR VIRUS

EBV is the pathogen of heterophile-positive infectious mononucleosis and is associated with African Burkitt's lymphoma and nasopharyngeal carcinoma. Infectious mononucleosis was recognized as a clinical entity in 1921 by Sprunt and Evans, who described six previously healthy young adults with fever, lymphadenopathy, and prostration associated with lymphocytosis and "pathologic"-looking lymphocytes (96). In 1932, Paul and Bunnell discovered high titers of spontaneously occurring sheep erythrocyte agglutinins, termed heterophile antibodies, in sera of persons with infectious mononucleosis, and a few years later Davidsohn improved the specificity of heterophile antibody detection for infectious mononucleosis by differential absorption of serum with guinea pig kidney and with beef red blood cells (97,98).

Epstein and his colleagues described virus particles resembling herpesviruses in tissue cultures of biopsy specimens of Burkitt's lymphoma in 1964 (99). By using an indirect immunofluorescent antibody test developed by Werner and Gertrude Henle to identify persons infected with this virus, now called Epstein-Barr virus, high titers of the antibodies were demonstrated in sera of persons with African Burkitt's lymphoma, and antibodies were found in 90% of adults in the United States (100). Data from further epidemiologic studies established EBV as the cause of heterophile-positive infectious mononucleosis (101,102).

Structure

EBV has the characteristic morphology of the herpesvirus group (described earlier). Individual virions, 180 to 200 nm in diameter, appear as hexagonal 100-nm diameter nucleocapsids surrounded by a complex envelope. The linear double-stranded DNA genome of approximately 170 kilobase pairs encodes for about 100 genes.

Replication

Receptors for EBV, identified as the d region of the third component of complement (C3d, also known as CR2) are present on B lymphocytes and nasopharyngeal epithelial cells (103,104). Virions attach to the receptor, enter the cell, and initiate the synthesis of EBV nuclear antigens within the cell nucleus. The synthesis of viral early antigens is followed by DNA replication and then production of late membrane antigens. In oral epithelial cells virions assemble and are released from the cell by budding, but in B lymphocytes infection with EBV produces a transforming replication cycle, during which viral DNA remains in a circular nonintegrated form (an episome) or becomes incorporated into host-cell DNA, but mature virus particles are not produced. As a result, the host B lymphocyte gains the property of immortality. In addition, EBV-transformed lymphocytes produce or secrete immunoglobulin, principally IgM (105). EBV usually remains in the latent form in circulating lymphocytes, but occasionally the virus is activated to enter a lytic cycle. The mechanisms that maintain EBV in the latent state and permit activation of a lytic cycle are unknown.

Epidemiology

EBV, distributed worldwide with no sex predilection, is transmitted by close contact with oral secretions of a person who is shedding the virus, by transfusion of blood from a seropositive donor, and possibly by sexual contact (106–108). Infection occurs at an earlier age in developing countries than in developed countries, but by adulthood 90 to 95% of all persons have antibodies to EBV (109,110). In the United States and Great Britain about half of all children younger than 5 years are EBV seropositive, and a second peak of seroconversion occurs between age 15 and 20 years (110,111). The prevalence of seropositivity is higher among lower socioeconomic groups than among affluent age-matched controls. Clinically apparent infection with EBV is most common when the primary exposure occurs during adolescence or early adulthood (112).

Pathogenesis

The most likely port of entry for EBV is the oropharynx, as EBV DNA can be detected in oropharyngeal epithelial cells. The virus also infects susceptible B lymphocytes in the pharyngeal lymphoid tissue, and during the 30- to 50-day incubation period replicates and disseminates throughout the monocyte/macrophage system.

Infection with EBV induces production of specific antibodies, unrelated heterophile antibodies, and antibodies that bind platelets, lymphocytes, neutrophils, nuclear antigens, and ampicillin (113–118). The specific role of these antibodies in the pathogenesis of infectious mononucleosis or its complications is unknown. During the first few weeks of infectious mononucleosis nonspecific cell-mediated immune functions are depressed, evidenced by a relative and absolute increase in the numbers of cytotoxic/suppressor T lymphocytes, which account for the atypical lymphocytosis typically associated with the illness (119). After the peak of atypical lymphocytosis, T lymphocytes capable of suppressing immunoglobulin synthesis appear in the peripheral blood, blastogenic responses and migration inhibitory factor are produced in response to EBV antigens, and interferon production and natural killer cell activity are increased.

With recovery from infectious mononucleosis caused

by EBV, the atypical lymphocytosis resolves and the functional abnormalities of T lymphocytes subside, but EBV is not eliminated from the host. The virus can be cultured from oropharyngeal secretions for 12 to 18 months after recovery from infectious mononucleosis, and intermittently from the oropharynx and blood of healthy and immunosuppressed persons infected with EBV. Moreover, immunosuppressive illnesses or drugs may reactivate EBV and its associated abnormalities of T-lymphocyte functions.

Clinical Manifestations

Infection with EBV causes a broad spectrum of manifestations, influenced by the age of the host. Typical infectious mononucleosis is an acute illness characterized by sore throat, fever, lymphadenopathy, and malaise lasting 2 to 3 weeks. A macular, petechial, "scarlatinaform," urticarial, or erythema multiforme–like rash develops in about 5% of all cases and in 90 to 100% of persons treated with ampicillin. Complications of infectious mononucleosis are listed in Table 5–1. In children primary EBV infection frequently is asymptomatic, and children who become symptomatic are more likely to develop rashes, neutropenia, and pneumonitis. Rarely, EBV produces a chronic or persistent infection with ongoing organ system dysfunction manifested by fever, pulmonary parenchymal involvement, pancytopenia, or ophthalmic or neurologic abnormalities (120–122).

The association between infection with EBV and African Burkitt's lymphoma and nasopharyngeal carcinoma is supported by the following data: Persons with these malignancies have higher titers of antibodies to EBV than do matched controls, and the EBV genome has been demonstrated in neoplastic tissue (109,123,124). EBV also can induce lymphoproliferative syndromes in recipients of organ transplants and in persons with immune deficiencies such as the X-linked lymphoproliferative syndrome, ataxia telangiectasia, Wiskott-Aldrich syndrome, Chediak-Higashi syndrome, and AIDS (125–134). In the setting of immune deficiency, EBV has been associated with B-cell lymphomas, and rarely, fatal T-cell lymphomas (135,136).

HUMAN HERPESVIRUS 6

Human herpesvirus 6 (HHV-6), first isolated in 1986 from peripheral blood mononuclear cells of patients with AIDS and those with various lymphoproliferative disorders, initially was believed to infect only freshly isolated B lymphocytes and, therefore, tentatively was named human B-lymphotropic virus (HBLV) (137). Further investigation, however, demonstrated that the major cell type supporting viral growth expresses T-cell markers; consequently, the virus was renamed human herpesvirus 6 (138,139).

Structure

The mature enveloped HHV-6 virion, 160 to 210 nm in diameter, consists of a 95- to 106-nm diameter nucleocapsid and a linear double-stranded DNA genome estimated to contain 160 to 170 kilobase pairs. Unique among the herpesviruses, HHV-6 nucleocapsids apparently are enveloped by budding into cytoplasmic vesicles. Mature enveloped virions accumulate in cytoplasmic vacuoles and at the extracellular surface of infected lymphocytes. To date, major antigenic proteins with molecular weights of 200, 120, 80, 72, 30 and 19 kd have been identified (140). Because much remains to be learned about the biologic properties of HHV-6 it is not yet classified.

Epidemiology

The mechanism of transmission of HHV-6 currently is unknown. Data from serologic studies in Sweden, the United States, Germany, and Great Britain indicate that infection occurs at an early age: 60% of children under age 1 year are seropositive (140–143). Most primary infections apparently are asymptomatic, and symptoms occur during reactivated latent infection or delayed primary infection. In adults the prevalence of antibody varies from 60 to 80%, depending on hygienic conditions and age, because the titer usually drops after age 40 years (144). The antibody titer is significantly higher in immunosuppressed persons than in normal healthy controls; this may reflect immunosuppression-induced virus reactivation (145).

Clinical Manifestations

Acute infection with HHV-6 may be asymptomatic or may manifest as exanthema subitum (also called roseola infantum) in children and infectious mononucleosis in teenagers and young adults. Exanthema subitum begins abruptly with fever for 3 to 4 days, followed by a rubelliform eruption of the chest, abdomen, face, and extremities that lasts a few hours to 2 days and occasionally is accompanied by lymphadenopathy and splenomegaly. Infectious mononucleosis caused by HHV-6 is indistinguishable from that caused by EBV, except for the absence of heterophile antibodies.

A subacute disease associated with HHV-6 in Japan is histiocytic necrotizing lymphadenitis (146). The illness

Table 5–1. Complications of Acute Infectious Mononucleosis Caused by EBV

Complications	Prevalence (%)
Autoimmune hemolytic anemia	0.5–3
Thrombocytopenia	
Mild (<140,000/μl)	50
Profound (with bleeding)	Rare
Splenic rupture	Rare
Neurologic	<1
Encephalitis	
Aseptic meningitis	
Guillain-Barré syndrome	
Myelitis	
Bell's palsy	
Hepatitis	
Elevated transaminases	80–90
Pericarditis, myocarditis	Rare
Pneumonitis	Rare
Death	Rare

preferentially affects young adults and is manifested by cervical, axillary, or systemic lymphadenopathy, fatigue, and fever, all of which eventually resolve spontaneously. HHV-6 has been associated with chronic fatigue syndrome, a protracted illness characterized by extreme persistent fatigue, fever, myalgias, and depression, and with nonmalignant and malignant lymphoproliferative diseases; however, a causal relationship between active infection with HHV-6 and lymphoproliferative diseases has not been proven (140,147–149).

CERCOPITHECINE HERPES VIRUS 1 (B VIRUS)

The first human infection with herpes B virus was recognized in 1932. Since then fewer than 25 human cases have been reported worldwide.

Structure, Epidemiology, and Pathogenesis

The morphogenesis of B virus is similar to that of other herpesviruses. Its genome has an estimated molecular weight of 107 ± 8 million and is composed of 162 ± 12 kilobase pairs.

B virus is indigenous to Old World monkeys, most commonly rhesus, cynomolgus, and other Asiatic species of Macaca. The virus, present in the saliva, conjunctiva, vesicle fluids, and possibly stool, of infected animals, is transmitted by direct contact (most commonly a bite) or indirect contact with virus-bearing fomites, and person-to-person transmission has been documented (150,151). The frequency of transmission of the virus among animals is unknown, but seroprevalence studies in rhesus monkeys demonstrate that infection with B virus is common.

Clinical Manifestations

Disease in animals is uncommon; vesicular lesions of the tongue and buccal mucosa occur, but systemic infection is unusual. Human infection with B virus is characterized by ascending myelitis, encephalomyelitis, or both. Approximately 3 to 5 days after a bite from an infected monkey localized vesicles appear at the site of virus inoculation. Lymphangitis and regional lymphadenopathy, accompanied by fever, myalgia, vomiting, meningeal irritation, nystagmus, and diplopia ensue. Three to seven days after the rash appears, neurologic findings develop: altered sensation with hyperesthesia, paresthesias, or both precede weakness, areflexia, and flaccid paralysis. Disease progression results in decreased consciousness, altered mentation, seizures, and death, which can occur as early as 10 to 14 days after onset of symptoms.

A few cases of human infection with B virus following presumed exposure to infected secretions by the respiratory route have been documented (152,153). Disease was manifested by fever, coryza, cough, laryngitis, pharyngitis, respiratory distress, neurologic symptoms, and death. Recurrent lesions similar to those of herpes zoster (described earlier) also may occur. The overall mortality of infection with B virus in humans is 75%, and those who survive infections of the nervous system have mild to severe neurologic impairment.

Laboratory Diagnosis

Specimens useful for diagnosis of infections caused by herpesviruses are listed in Table 5–2. Specimen collection, transport, and processing are discussed in Part III. Identification of the herpesviruses is described here.

Herpes Simplex Virus. Techniques available for detecting HSV in clinical specimens are summarized in Table 5–3. Characteristic uninucleate or multinucleate cells with intranuclear inclusions (see Fig. 5–2) may be observed in Tzanck preparations or smears of endocervical cells, cells from cutaneous or mucocutaneous lesions, or alveolar cells collected by bronchoalveolar lavage stained with the Papanicolaou stain. This method of diagnosis, however, has drawbacks. First, the sensitivity for detection of HSV depends on the type and the location of the lesion (154,155). In general, the sensitivity is only 50 to 70% for a vesicle and much lower if the lesion has crusted. In one study of women with genital HSV infections the sensitivity for all types of external lesions was 41%, compared to 23% for cervical lesions (155). Second, cellular changes caused by HSV and VZV look identical and cannot be distinguished. To confirm the diagnosis, these same specimens may be stained with monoclonal antibodies directed against an antigen common to both HSV-1 and HSV-2 or against type-specific antigens (gG-1 and gG-2); however, the sensitivity of staining specimens directly with monoclonal antibodies is only 70 to 80%.

A 15-minute monoclonal antibody–based filtration enzyme immunoassay for detection of HSV directly in clinical specimens recently became available. Data regarding

Table 5–2. Infections Produced by Herpesviruses and Specimens Required for Diagnosis

Infection	Virus	Specimen
Congenital, perinatal	HSV	Vesicle fluid or scrapings, throat swab, rectal swab, CSF
	CMV	Throat swab, urine
Cutaneous, mucocutaneous	HSV, VZV, B virus	Vesicle fluid or scrapings
	CMV	Tissue biopsy
	EBV	Serum
Genital	HSV	Vesicle fluid or scrapings; urethral, rectal, or endocervical swab
	CMV	Endocervical swab, semen
GI ulcers	HSV, CMV	Mucosal brushings, biopsy tissue
Pneumonitis	CMV, HSV, VZV	BAL, lung biopsy tissue, blood
Hepatitis	EBV	Serum, liver biopsy tissue
	CMV, HSV	Blood, liver biopsy tissue
Infectious mononucleosis syndrome	EBV, HHV-6	Serum
	CMV	Serum, blood, urine, saliva
Encephalitis	HSV, CMV B virus	Brain biopsy tissue
Retinitis	CMV	Blood
Exanthem subitum	HHV-6	Serum

Key: CMV, cytomegalovirus; HSV, herpes simplex virus; VZV, varicella-zoster virus; EBV, Epstein-Barr virus; HHV-6, human herpesvirus 6; BAL, bronchoalveolar lavage fluid; GI, gastrointestinal; CSF, cerebrospinal fluid.

Table 5-3. Methods for Diagnosis of Herpesvirus Infections

Test	Virus	Comments
Tzanck smear	HSV, VZV	Rapid; does not differentiate HSV and VZV; sensitivity 50–70% for vesicle (lower if crusted)
Papanicolaou smear	HSV, VZV, CMV	As for Tzanck smear: useful for diagnosing CMV pneumonia (see text)
Staining cell preparations with monoclonal antibodies	HSV, VZV, CMV	Rapid; preferred method for diagnosing VZV cutaneous lesions; useful for detecting CMV in alveolar cells and in WBC
Enzyme immunoassay	HSV	Rapid; may be valuable in high risk persons with vesicles
Cell culture	HSV, CMV, VZV, B virus	Reference method; requires 1–4 days for HSV, up to 14 days for VZV, and up to 4–6 weeks for CMV
Serology	HSV, VZV, CMV, EBV, HHV-6	Used to determine immune status to HSV, VZV, CMV; useful in diagnosing EBV infection
Polymerase chain reaction, nucleic acid hybridization	HSV, VZV, CMV, EBV	Currently research tools

Key: HSV, herpes simplex virus; VZV, varicella-zoster virus; CMV, cytomegalovirus; EBV, Epstein-Barr virus; WBC, peripheral white blood cells.

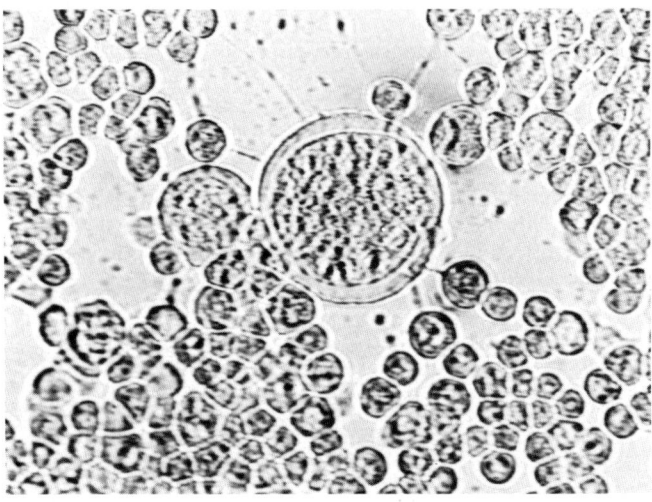

Fig. 5-6. Cytopathic effect produced by herpes simplex virus in A-549 cells (×40).

its reliability are limited, but in one study of persons attending a sexually transmitted disease clinic the sensitivity was 100% for vesicular lesions and about 75% for nonvesicular ones (156). Another technique that may become valuable in the future is the polymerase chain reaction (PCR), especially for detecting HSV DNA in cervical or vaginal samples from pregnant women who have asymptomatic genital infection at delivery (157).

The reference method (and the most sensitive technique) for detection of HSV is conventional cell culture, using A-549 cells, MRC-5 or WI-38 cells, human foreskin fibroblasts, HEp-2 cells, and primary rabbit kidney cells (the latter are specific for HSV). Incubation of cells in minimum essential medium containing 10^{-5} M dexamethasone for at least 24 hours before specimen inoculation decreases the time to appearance of cytopathic effect (CPE) (158). One to three days after inoculation, CPE typically begins focally and progresses to involve the entire monolayer, often within 24 hours. Infected cells are enlarged, rounded, and often multinucleate (Fig. 5-6). Cells may clump together, forming clusters termed syncytia, a phenomenon more commonly associated with HSV-2 than HSV-1. Moreover, HSV-2 may produce CPE in primary monkey kidney cells, whereas HSV-1 generally does not. An isolate may presumptively be called HSV based on the time to development of CPE, its microscopic appearance, and the cell lines in which it occurred. However, occasionally the CPE is not distinct (for example, the CPE of HSV and adenovirus [see Chapter 6] may appear similar), and identification must be confirmed by staining the infected cells with monoclonal antibodies specific for HSV and for other suspect viruses (such as adenovirus). In addition, an isolate of HSV may be typed by staining with type-specific monoclonal antibodies.

Centrifugation culture (discussed in more detail later for CMV), staining with specific monoclonal antibodies, may be used to detect HSV. As a replacement for culture, however, it is controversial, because in some studies the sensitivity for detection of HSV is as low as 80% (159,160).

The presence of HSV does not always indicate active disease, because asymptomatic persons may shed the virus in respiratory or genital secretions. Therefore, HSV in a specimen such as saliva, throat swabs or washings, and bronchoalveolar lavage fluid must be interpreted with caution: the person may have an active infection with HSV, or the virus may have been reactivated during an unrelated illness. Detection of HSV in a genital specimen, however, indicates that the individual may transmit the virus via sexual contact or, in the case of a pregnant woman, to the fetus or to the infant during delivery.

Varicella-Zoster Virus. The most sensitive method for detecting VZV in a vesicular skin lesion is staining a smear of cells scraped from the base of the lesion with fluorescein-conjugated monoclonal antibodies. Alternatively, VZV may be recovered by conventional cell culture using A-549 cells or human lung or foreskin fibroblasts that is maintained at least 14 days before the result is considered negative. CPE, characterized by focal patches of enlarged, rounded refractile cells (Fig. 5-7), appears, on average, in 7 days and does not progress as the CPE associated with HSV does. An isolate is confirmed by staining infected cells with monoclonal antibodies.

Detection of antibodies to HSV or VZV is used to determine immune status and to document primary infection

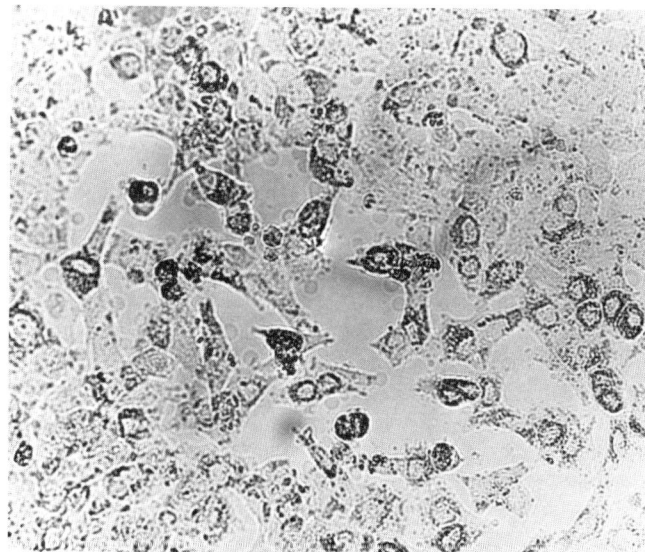

Fig. 5-7. Cytopathic effect produced by varicella-zoster virus in A-549 cells (×40).

by seroconversion, meaning a change from the absence of specific antibodies to a measurable titer. Documenting a fourfold rise or fall in titer of antibodies to HSV or VZV is not sufficient evidence to diagnose recent or reactivated infection. Moreover, measuring HSV or VZV IgG titers in the cerebrospinal fluid should not be used to diagnose infection of the central nervous system by either of these viruses.

Cytomegalovirus. The reference method for detection of CMV is conventional cell culture using human diploid lung or foreskin fibroblasts. Typical evidence of CPE—discrete foci of rounded cells (Fig. 5-8)—develops, on average, 12 days after inoculation and progresses slowly, but it may not appear for 4 to 6 weeks. The time to development of CPE may be shortened by incubating the cell monolayer in minimum essential medium containing 10^{-5} M dexamethasone for at least 24 hours before inoculation (161). Although the appearance of CPE is distinct in most cases, staining infected cells with monoclonal antibodies confirms the identification.

Because in immunocompromised persons CMV may cause severe disease that often can be controlled effectively by early administration of the antiviral agent ganciclovir, a diagnosis must be made more rapidly than is possible with conventional cell culture. Centrifugation culture (see Appendix, Procedure 2), using either shell vials or individual wells of a 24-well plate containing coverslips seeded with MRC-5 cells and staining with monoclonal antibodies to the early nuclear antigen (Fig. 5-9), provides rapid detection (16 to 18 hours) of CMV in clinical specimens but should be used in conjunction with conventional cell culture because it does not detect all CMV-positive specimens (162-165).

Pneumonitis and congenital infection caused by CMV may be diagnosed cytologically by observing characteristic enlarged cells with intranuclear or intracytoplasmic inclusions, or both, (Fig. 5-10) in cytospin preparations of bronchoalveolar lavage fluid and urine, respectively, stained with the Papanicolaou stain. The major disadvantage of this method for diagnosis of CMV-induced pneumonitis is its low sensitivity, ranging from 20 to 60% (166). The sensitivity of detecting CMV-infected cells in bronchoalveolar lavage fluid may be increased to about 80% by using a cytocentrifuge to prepare preparations smears and staining with specific monoclonal antibodies, and CMV viremia can be detected by using a cytocentrifuge to prepare smears of peripheral blood leukocytes and staining with a mixture of monoclonal antibodies directed against immediate early and early nuclear antigens (167,168). CMV also may be detected in clinical specimens by in situ hybridization and gene amplification using PCR; however, currently these are predominantly research tools and they offer no advantage over the techniques that are routinely available in most clinical virology laboratories (169-171).

Detection of CMV in a specimen does not distinguish

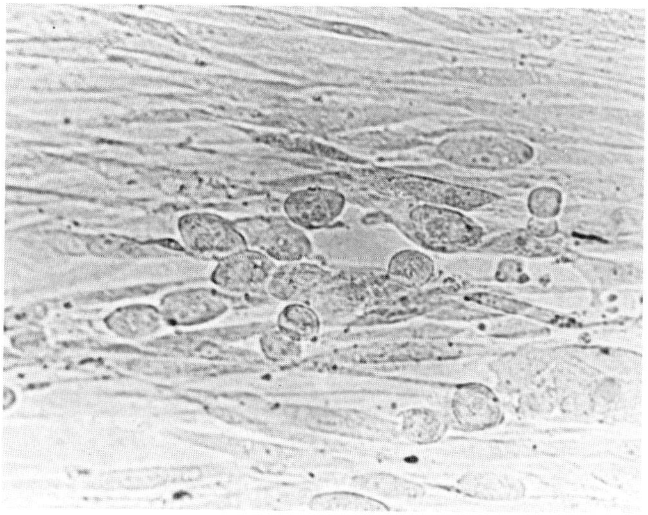

Fig. 5-8. Cytopathic effect produced by cytomegalovirus in MRC-5 cells (×40).

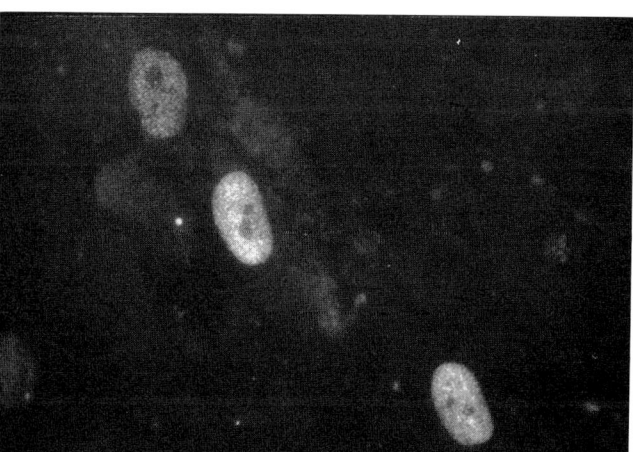

Fig. 5-9. Centrifugation culture shows the typical intranuclear inclusions associated with the early nuclear antigen of cytomegalovirus (×256).

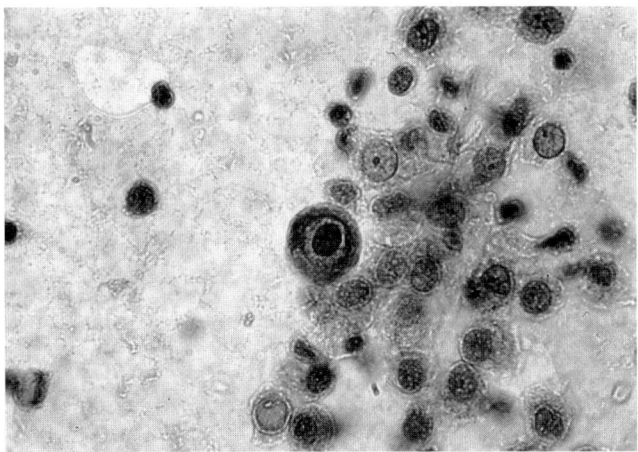

Fig. 5–10. Enlarged alveolar cell shows cytologic changes of cytomegalovirus in a cytospin preparation of bronchoalveolar lavage fluid (Papanicolaou stain, ×201.6).

asymptomatic shedding of the virus during reactivation from active disease. As mentioned earlier, CMV may be excreted in urine and saliva for several months after primary infection in adults or for years following congenital or perinatal infection. Moreover, during reactivation of a latent infection in normal individuals and, perhaps more frequently in those who are immunocompromised, CMV may be shed in urine or respiratory tract secretions such as saliva or bronchoalveolar lavage fluid without causing disease (166). In contrast, CMV infrequently is detected in the blood of asymptomatic persons, so viremia is a better predictor of active disease.

Serologic tests for IgG to CMV are used principally to determine immune status. Specific IgM, most commonly detected following primary infection, has potential diagnostic value; however, problems are associated with its use as a marker of recent infection. For example, in some persons specific IgM is detected for prolonged periods following primary infection, in immunocompromised persons IgM production may be delayed, and IgM occasionally is produced during reactivation.

Epstein-Barr Virus. Infectious mononucleosis syndrome due to EBV often is suspected on the basis of clinical presentation plus circulating lymphocytosis, which peaks during the second or third week of illness in about 70% of cases. Monocytes and lymphocytes comprise 60 to 70% of the total white blood cell count, which generally ranges from 12,000 to 50,000 leukocytes per microliter. The hematologic hallmark of infectious mononucleosis, the atypical lymphocyte, usually accounts for about 30% of the total differential, ranging from fewer than 5% to more than 90% of the circulating lymphocytes. Atypical lymphocytes, however, are not diagnostic of infection with EBV, because they may be present with drug reactions and during infections with other organisms: CMV, hepatitis viruses, rubella virus, mumps virus, human immunodeficiency virus, measles virus, and Toxoplasma gondii. Other hematologic findings include a relative and absolute neutropenia and thrombocytopenia.

Heterophile antibodies, present in about 90% of primary infections with EBV at the onset of symptoms or later in the illness, are distinguished from naturally occurring Forssman antibodies and those of serum sickness by testing for sheep or horse red blood cell agglutination after absorbing the serum with guinea pig kidney and beef red blood cells (Table 5–4). A heterophile antibody titer of 40 or greater after absorption with guinea pig kidney is strong evidence for EBV-induced infectious mononucleosis. Detection of horse red blood cell agglutinins is more sensitive than sheep red blood cell agglutinins; however, the former persist as long as a year in 75% of persons with infectious mononucleosis, whereas the latter are detected at one year in only 30% of cases. Differential absorption forms the basis of the commercially available Monospot tests, whose results generally correlate well with those of the classic heterophile tube test, although false-positive results have been reported uncommonly in persons with lymphoma and hepatitis.

To diagnose heterophile-negative infectious mononucleosis caused by EBV, titers of antibodies directed against EBV-specific antigens should be determined (Table 5–5). Antibody responses to three different antigens are measured: IgG and IgM specific for the viral capsid antigen (VCA), IgG specific for the early antigen (EA), and IgG specific for Epstein-Barr nuclear antigen (EBNA). No specific antibodies are detected in an individual who is susceptible to infection. During the early acute-phase of primary infection, serum contains IgG and IgM against VCA, and in most patients IgG against EA, which peaks 3 to 4 weeks after onset of symptoms. Titers of anti-VCA IgM and anti-EA IgG then gradually decline, becoming indetectable in 4 to 8 weeks and 3 to 6 months, respectively, although as many as 40% of normal persons have a low anti-EA titer, depending on the detection method used. Anti-EBNA antibodies appear 1 to 6 months after primary infection. Anti-VCA IgG and anti-EBNA antibodies persist lifelong; however, immunosuppressive therapy may depress the anti-EBNA titer. As with other herpesviruses, EBV may be reactivated at various times during an individual's life and is detected serologically by a fourfold or greater rise in the anti-EA titer.

Burkitt's lymphoma, nasopharyngeal carcinoma, and

Table 5–4. Interpretation of the Heterophile Antibody Test

	Heterophile Antibody Titer		
		After Absorption with:	
Condition	Unabsorbed	Guinea Pig Kidney	Beef Erythrocytes
Healthy (Forssman antibody)	+	–	+
Infectious mononucleosis (caused by EBV)	+ + + +	+ + +	–
Serum sickness	+ + +	–	–

Key: –, not detected; +, low level; + + +, high level; + + + +, very high level; EBV, Epstein-Barr virus.

Table 5–5. Interpretation of EBV-Specific Antibodies

Condition/Disease	Antibodies			
	VCA			
	IgM	IgG	EA	EBNA
Susceptible (not infected)	−	−	−	−
Acute, primary infection	+	+	+/−	−
Recent infection	+/−	+	−/+	+*
Past infection	−	+	−	+†
Reactivation	−	+	+	+

* Titer generally is >1:2 but <1:10.
† Titer generally is >1:10.
Key: VCA, viral capsid antigen; EA, early antigen; EBNA, Epstein-Barr nuclear antigen; +, positive; −, negative.

progressive lymphoproliferative disease associated with EBV are diagnosed by demonstrating EBNA in frozen tissue sections or acetone-fixed cell imprints of involved tissue by anticomplement immunofluorescent staining or by detecting EBV DNA in involved tissue by Southern blot hybridization or gene amplification using the PCR. Moreover, individuals with Burkitt's lymphoma and nasopharyngeal carcinoma frequently have a high serum titer of IgG to the viral capsid antigen and the early antigen, and those with nasopharyngeal carcinoma also have high IgA titers against the same antigens.

EBV may be recovered from oropharyngeal washings or peripheral blood lymphocytes of 80 to 90% of persons with infectious mononucleosis by cocultivation with cord blood leukocytes. However, because EBV frequently is present in oropharyngeal secretions of normal healthy persons and of those with unrelated illnesses, culturing the virus has limited clinical value and is not routinely available in most clinical virology laboratories.

Human Herpesvirus 6. Primary infection with HHV-6 most often is diagnosed by demonstrating seroconversion. In immunocompromised persons, virus detection in peripheral blood or bone marrow lymphocytes by cocultivation with cord blood cells, hybridization in situ, or gene amplification may be necessary. However, as with all herpesviruses, isolation of HHV-6 alone, in the absence of associated clinical symptoms, does not indicate disease because reactivation and shedding of the virus can occur in healthy persons who have a latent infection.

Cercopithecine Herpes Virus (B Virus). Infections caused by B virus are diagnosed by recovering the virus in cell culture.

Treatment

Herpes Simplex Virus. Idoxuridine, trifluorothymidine, and vidarabine are used topically to treat keratitis caused by HSV. The antiviral agent acyclovir is indicated for treatment of disseminated and central nervous system infections caused by HSV, and in an immunocompromised host acyclovir is used to treat recurrent mucocutaneous lesions (172–174). Acyclovir is not recommended for most episodes of recurrent lesions in immunocompetent persons but may be indicated for suppression or prophylaxis in persons who suffer frequent and severe recurrences and when recurrences are associated with severe complications such as erythema multiforme, meningitis, or eczema herpeticum. Strains of HSV resistant to acyclovir, once extremely uncommon, are being reported with increased frequency (175,176). Preliminary data suggest that infections caused by acyclovir-resistant strains of HSV may respond to foscarnet therapy (177).

Varicella-Zoster Virus. Treatment of chickenpox or zoster in an immunocompetent host is supportive, including acetaminophen for fever, and does not require antiviral agents. Recently, however, acyclovir was shown to reduce the duration and severity of chickenpox in normally healthy children when treatment was begun during the first 24 hours of the rash (178). Whether acyclovir therapy can reduce the rare, serious complications of chickenpox is unknown. Currently, routine administration of acyclovir to normal children with chickenpox is not recommended, but this may change in response to the new data. Acyclovir is indicated for infections caused by VZV in immunocompromised hosts and for visceral complications in immunocompetent persons. Isolates of VZV that are resistant to acyclovir have emerged in persons with AIDS who received longterm oral acyclovir therapy (179).

Cytomegalovirus. Two antiviral agents are active against CMV: ganciclovir and foscarnet. Ganciclovir is effective therapy for most serious infections caused by CMV in immunosuppressed persons, except interstitial pneumonitis in recipients of allogeneic bone marrow transplants (180–184), though for them treatment with ganciclovir plus immune globulin appears promising (185). Moreover, in a recent study of persons with AIDS and retinitis caused by CMV, the survival rate was significantly better for those treated with foscarnet than for those treated with ganciclovir (186). The role of ganciclovir in the treatment of congenital infections caused by CMV has not been determined. Infections due to CMV in immunocompetent hosts are treated supportively; antiviral therapy is not indicated.

Epstein-Barr Virus. Treatment of EBV-induced infectious mononucleosis is supportive. Corticosteroids are used when the illness is complicated by impending airway obstruction, severe thrombocytopenia, or hemolytic anemia, and perhaps for central nervous system involvement, myocarditis, and pericarditis. What antiviral regimen is effective against life-threatening infections caused by EBV in immunosuppressed individuals has not been determined definitively. Acyclovir inhibits replication of EBV in vitro but has not been uniformly effective in vivo. Lymphoproliferative lesions in recipients of organ transplants may respond favorably to withdrawal of immunosuppressive drugs or to large doses of immune globulin plus interferon-α.

Human Herpesvirus 6. Treatment of infections with HHV-6 is symptomatic.

Cercopithecine Herpes Virus (B Virus). Human infections with B virus are treated with acyclovir.

Prevention

Herpes Simplex Virus. Infections caused by HSV can be prevented by avoiding direct contact with lesions. Medical and dental personnel should avoid direct contact with potentially infectious lesions by wearing gloves. Condom use is recommended to prevent genital spread when one partner has active lesions or a history of recurrent genital infections. Patients with eczema herpeticum should be spatially isolated. Preventing neonatal disease in the offspring of mothers with genital infection is problematic. If an active cervical infection is recognized at parturition before rupture of membranes, cesarean section is indicated, but if membranes have ruptured it probably is no safer than rapid vaginal delivery. Most infants who develop congenital disease are born to mothers without active lesions who often have no history of genital infection. Effective prophylaxis via cesarean section in these cases awaits the development of a rapid and sensitive test to detect HSV at the onset of labor (potentially PCR, see reference 157). In the immunocompromised host, acyclovir is used to prevent recurrent herpetic lesions. Vaccines against HSV have shown promise in animal models, but their efficacy in humans has not been determined (187).

Varicella-Zoster Virus. Persons who require hospitalization for VZV infection should be spatially isolated. Administration of varicella-zoster immune globulin (VZIG) within 96 hours of exposure to VZV is useful for preventing or ameliorating symptomatic chickenpox in persons at high risk of infection. Guidelines for the use of VZIG are outlined in Table 5–6 (188). A vaccine developed for preventing chickenpox in immunocompromised and immunocompetent hosts is licensed in Japan and currently under evaluation in the United States (189–191).

Cytomegalovirus. Infection with CMV acquired via transfusion can be prevented by giving persons who are seronegative for CMV blood, platelets, or both collected from CMV-seronegative donors. The risk of serious infection due to CMV in recipients of organ transplants can be significantly reduced by prophylactic administration of immune globulin plus acyclovir (192,193). A live attenuated vaccine against CMV (the Towne vaccine), evaluated in recipients of renal transplants, appears to have minimal effect in preventing primary infection with the virus (194).

REFERENCES

1. Frenkel N, et al: Isolation of a new herpesvirus from human $CD4^+$ T cells. Proc Natl Acad Sci USA, 87:748, 1990.
2. Hirsch MS: Herpes simplex virus. *In* Principles and Practice of Infectious Diseases. 3rd ed. Edited by GL Mandell, RG Douglas Jr, and JE Bennett. New York, Churchill Livingstone, 1990.
3. Roizman B, and Sears AE: Herpes simplex viruses and their replication. *In* Fields' Virology. 2nd ed. Edited by BN Fields and DM Knipe. New York, Raven Press, 1990.
4. Prober CG, et al: Use of routine viral cultures at delivery to identify neonates exposed to herpes simplex virus. N Engl J Med, *318*:887, 1988.
5. Whitley RJ, et al: The natural history of herpes simplex virus infection of mother and newborn. Pediatrics, *66*:489, 1980.
6. Whitley RJ, et al: Changing presentation of herpes simplex virus infection in neonates. J Infect Dis, *158*:109, 1988.
7. Corey L, et al: Genital herpes simplex virus infections: Clinical manifestations, course, and complications. Ann Intern Med, 98: 958, 1983.
8. Siegal FP, et al: Severe acquired immunodeficiency in male homosexuals manifested by chronic perianal ulcerative herpes simplex lesions. N Engl J Med, *305*:1439, 1981.
9. Centers for Disease Control: Herpes gladiatorum at a high school wrestling camp—Minnesota. MMWR, *39*:69, 1990.
10. Nahmias AJ, et al: Herpes simplex virus encephalitis: Laboratory evaluations and their diagnostic significance. J Infect Dis, *145*:829, 1982.
11. Whitley RJ, et al: Adenine arabinoside therapy of biopsy-proven herpes simplex encephalitis. NIAID collaborative antiviral study. N Engl J Med, *297*:289, 1977.
12. Whitley RH, et al: Herpes simplex encephalitis. Vidarabine therapy and diagnostic problems. N Engl J Med, *304*:313, 1981.
13. Agha FP, Lee HH, and Nostrant TT: Herpetic esophagitis: A diagnostic challenge in immunocompromised patients. Am J Gastroenterol *81*:246, 1986.
14. Legge RH, et al: Acyclovir-responsive herpetic tracheobronchitis. Am J Med, *85*:561, 1988.
15. Ramsey PG, Fife KH, Hackman RC, and Corey L: Herpes simplex virus pneumonia: Clinical, virologic, and pathologic features in 20 patients. Ann Intern Med, *97*:813, 1982.
16. Holdsworth SR, Atkins RC, Scott DF, and Hayes K: Systemic herpes simplex infection with fulminant hepatitis post-transplantation. Aust NZ J Med, *6*:588, 1976.
17. Mozes MF, et al: Jaundice after renal allotransplantation. Ann Surg, *188*:783, 1978.
18. Sutton AL, Smithwick EM, Seligman SJ, and Kim D-S: Fatal disseminated herpesvirus hominis type 2 infection in an

Table 5–6. Guidelines for the Use of Varicella-Zoster Immune Globulin

Exposure criteria
One of the following exposures to persons with chickenpox or zoster:
  Continuous household contact
  Playmate contact (generally more than 1 hour of indoor play)
  Hospital contact (in same two- to four-bed room or adjacent beds of large ward, or prolonged face-to-face contact with infectious staff member)
  Newborn contact (newborn of mother who had onset of chickenpox less than 6 days before or less than 2 days after delivery) and
  Time elapsed after exposure is such that varicella-zoster immune globulin can be administered within 96 hours
Persons for whom use is indicated
  Susceptible to varicella
  Significant exposure
  One of these underlying illnesses or conditions:
    Leukemia or lymphoma
    Cellular immune deficiency
    Newborn of mother who had onset of chickenpox less than 6 days before or less than 2 days after delivery
    Premature infant (greater than 28 weeks' gestation) whose mother lacks previous history of chickenpox
    Premature infant (less than 28 weeks' gestation or birth weight less than 1000 g) regardless of maternal history
    Pregnant women
    Normal adults on an individual basis

From Straus SE, et al: Varicella-zoster virus infections. Biology, natural history, treatment, and prevention. Ann Intern Med, *108*:221, 1988.

adult with associated thymic dysplasia. Am J Med, 56:545, 1974.
19. Whitley RJ: Varicella-zoster virus. In Principles and Practice of Infectious Diseases. 3rd ed. Edited by GL Mandell, RG Douglas Jr, and JE Bennett. New York, Churchill Livingstone, 1990.
20. Ragozzino MW, et al: Population-based study of herpes zoster and its sequelae. Medicine (Baltimore), 51:310, 1982.
21. Feldman S, Hughes WT, and Daniel CB: Varicella in children with cancer: Seventy-seven cases. Pediatrics, 56:388, 1975.
22. Arvin AM, et al: Cellular and humoral immunity in the pathogenesis of recurrent herpes viral infection in patients with lymphoma. J Clin Invest, 68:869, 1980.
23. Preblud SR: Varicella: Complications and costs. Pediatrics, 78:728, 1986.
24. Johnson R, and Milbourne PE: Central nervous system manifestations of chickenpox. Can Med Assoc J, 102:831, 1970.
25. Underwood EA: The neurological complications of varicella. A clinical and epidemiological study. Br J Child Dis, 32:83, 1935.
26. Linnemann CC Jr, et al: Reye's syndrome: Epidemiologic and viral studies, 1963–1974. Am J Epidemiol, 101:517, 1975.
27. Paryani SG, and Arvin AM: Intrauterine infection with varicella-zoster virus after maternal varicella. N Engl J Med, 314:1542, 1986.
28. Brunell PA: Fetal and neonatal varicella-zoster infections. Semin Perinatol, 7:47, 1983.
29. Preblud SR, Bregman DJ, and Vernon LL: Deaths from varicella in infants. Pediatr Infect Dis, 4:503, 1985.
30. Whitley RJ: Varicella-zoster infections. In Antiviral Agents and Viral Infections of Man. Edited by G Galasso, T Merigan, and R Buchanan. New York, Raven Press, 1984.
31. Jesionek A, and Kiolemenoglou B: Uber einen Befund von protozoenartigen Gebilden in den Organen eines heriditarluetischen Fotus. Munch Med Wochenschr, 51:1905, 1904.
32. Ribbert D: Uber protozoenartige Zellen in der Niere eines syphilitischen Neugeborenen und in der Parotis von Kindern. Zentralbl Allg Pathol, 15:945, 1904.
33. Goodpasture EW, and Talbot FB: Concerning the nature of "protozoon-like" cells in certain lesions of infancy. Am J Dis Child, 21:415, 1921.
34. Cole R, and Kuttner AG: A filtrable virus present in the submaxillary glands of guinea pigs. J Exp Med, 44:855, 1926.
35. Farber S, and Wolbach SB: Intranuclear and cytoplasmic inclusions ("protozoan-like bodies") in the salivary glands and other organs of infants. Am J Pathol Child 8:123, 1932.
36. Rowe WP, et al: Cytopathogenic agents resembling human salivary gland virus recovered from tissue cultures of human adenoids. Proc Soc Exp Biol (NY), 92:418, 1956.
37. Smith MG: Propagation in tissue cultures of a cytopathogenic virus from human salivary gland virus disease. Proc Soc Exp Biol (NY), 92:424, 1956.
38. Weller TH, Macauley JE, Craig JM, and Wirth P: Isolation of intranuclear inclusion producing agents from infants with illnesses resembling cytomegalic inclusion disease. Proc Soc Exp Biol (NY), 94:424, 1957.
39. Weller TH, Hanshaw JB, and Scott DE: Serologic differentiation of viruses responsible for cytomegalic inclusion disease. Virology, 12:130, 1960.
40. Klemola E, and Kaariainen L: Cytomegalovirus as a possible cause of a disease resembling infectious mononucleosis. Br Med J, 5470:1099, 1965.
41. Kaariainen L, Klemola E, and Paloheimo J: Rise of cytomegalovirus antibodies in an infectious mononucleosis–like syndrome after transfusion. Br Med J, 5498:1270, 1966.
42. Winston DJ, et al: Cytomegalovirus infections associated with leukocyte transfusions. Ann Intern Med, 93:671, 1980.
43. Rasmussen LE, Nelson RM, Kelsall DC, and Merigan TC: Murine monoclonal antibody to a single protein neutralizes the infectivity of human cytomegalovirus. Proc Natl Acad Sci USA, 81:876, 1984.
44. Krech U: Complement-fixing antibodies against cytomegalovirus in different parts of the world. Bull WHO, 49:103, 1973.
45. Alford CA, and Britt WJ: Cytomegalovirus. In Fields Virology. 2nd ed. Edited by BN Fields and DM Knipe. New York, Raven Press, 1990.
46. Ho M: Pathology of cytomegalovirus infection. In Cytomegalovirus, Biology and Infection: Current Topics in Infectious Disease. Edited by WB Greenough III and TC Merigan. New York, Plenum Press, 1982.
47. Griffiths PD, and Grundy JE: Molecular biology and immunology of cytomegalovirus. Biochem J, 241:313, 1987.
48. Klemola E: Cytomegalovirus infection in previously healthy adults. Ann Intern Med, 79:267, 1973.
49. Klemola E, et al: Cytomegalovirus mononucleosis in previously healthy individuals. Ann Intern Med, 71:11, 1969.
50. Rinaldo CR Jr, Black PH, and Hirsch MS: Virus-leukocyte interactions in cytomegalovirus mononucleosis. J Infect Dis, 136:667, 1977.
51. Rinaldo CR Jr, et al: Mechanisms of immunosuppression in cytomegalovirus mononucleosis. J Infect Dis, 141:488, 1980.
52. Reynolds DW, Dean PH, Pass RF, and Alford CA Jr: Specific cell-mediated immunity in children with congenital and neonatal cytomegalovirus infection and their mothers. J Infect Dis, 140:493, 1979.
53. Rinaldo CR, Black PH, and Hirsch MS: Interactions of cytomegalovirus with leukocytes from patients with mononucleosis due to cytomegalovirus. J Infect Dis, 136:667, 1977.
54. Rice GPA, Schrier RD, and Oldstone MBA: Cytomegalovirus infects human lymphocytes and monocytes: Virus expression is restricted to immediate early antigen products. Proc Natl Acad Sci, 81:6134, 1984.
55. Peterson PK, and Andersen RC: Infection in renal transplant recipients. Am J Med, 81(suppl 1A):2, 1986.
56. Rakela J, et al: Incidence of cytomegalovirus infection and its relationship to donor-recipient serologic status in liver transplantation. Transplant Proc, 19:2399, 1987.
57. Zaia JA: The biology of human cytomegalovirus infection after bone marrow transplantation. Int J Cell Cloning, 4(suppl 1):135, 1986.
58. Dummer JS, Hardy A, Poorsattar A, and Ho M: Early infections in kidney, heart, and liver transplant recipients on cyclosporine. Transplantation, 36:259, 1983.
59. Kusne S, et al: Infections after liver transplantation—an analysis of 101 consecutive cases. Medicine, 67:132, 1988.
60. Blaser MK, and Cohn DL: Opportunistic infections in patients with AIDS: Clues to the epidemiology of AIDS and the relative virulence of pathogens. Rev Infect Dis, 8:21, 1986.
61. Lerner CW, and Tapper ML: Opportunistic infections complicating acquired immune deficiency syndrome. Medicine, 63:155, 1984.
62. O'Neill HJ, et al: Cytomegalovirus-specific antibody responses in renal transplant patients with primary and recurrent CMV infections. J Med Virol, 24:461, 1988.
63. Neiman PE, et al: A prospective analysis of interstitial pneu-

monia and opportunistic viral infection among recipients of allogenic bone marrow grafts. J Infect Dis, *136*:754, 1977.
64. Rasmussen L, et al: Virus-specific IgG and IgM antibodies in normal and immunocompromised subjects infected with cytomegalovirus. J Infect Dis, *145*:191, 1982.
65. Quinnan GV Jr, et al: HLA-restricted T-lymphocyte cytotoxic responses correlate with recovery from cytomegalovirus infection in bone marrow–transplant recipients. N Engl J Med, *307*:7, 1982.
66. Ho M: Cytomegalovirus: Biology and Infection. New York, Plenum Press, 1982.
67. Stagno S, et al: Primary cytomegalovirus infection in pregnancy. Incidence, transmission to fetus, and clinical outcome. JAMA, *256*:1904, 1986.
68. Stagno S, et al: Comparative, serial virologic and serologic studies of symptomatic and subclinical congenital and natally acquired cytomegalovirus infection. J Infect Dis, *132*:568, 1987.
69. Pass RF, Stagno S, Britt WJ, and Alford CA: Specific cell-mediated immunity and the natural history of congenital infection with cytomegalovirus. J Infect Dis, *148*:953, 1983.
70. Stagno S, et al: Immune complexes in congenital and natal cytomegalovirus infections of man. J Clin Invest, *60*:838, 1977.
71. Starr SE, et al: Impaired cellular immunity to cytomegalovirus in congenitally infected children and their mothers. J Infect Dis, *140*:500, 1979.
72. Reynolds DW, et al: Maternal cytomegalovirus excretion and perinatal infection. N Engl J Med, *289*:1, 1973.
73. Simmons RL, et al: Clinical characteristics of the lethal cytomegalovirus infection following renal transplantation. Surgery, *82*:537, 1977.
74. Yeager AS, et al: Prevention of transfusion-acquired cytomegalovirus infections in newborn infants. J Pediatr, *98*:281, 1981.
75. Stagno S, et al: Congenital and perinatal cytomegalovirus infections. Semin Perinatol, 7:31, 1983.
76. Stagno S, et al: Auditory and visual defects resulting from symptomatic and subclinical congenital cytomegalovirus and toxoplasma infections. Pediatrics, *59*:669, 1977.
77. Hanshaw JB, et al: School failure and deafness after "silent" congenital cytomegalovirus infection. N Engl J Med, *295*:468, 1976.
78. Cohen JI, and Corey R: Cytomegalovirus infection in the normal host. Medicine, *64*:100, 1985.
79. Klemola E: Hypersensitivity reactions to ampicillin in cytomegalovirus mononucleosis. Scand J Infect Dis, *2*:29, 1970.
80. Carter AR: Cytomegalovirus disease presenting as hepatitis. Br Med J, *3*:786, 1968.
81. Bonkowsky HL, Lee RV, and Klatskin G: Acute granulomatous hepatitis: Occurrence in cytomegalovirus mononucleosis. JAMA, *233*:1284, 1984.
82. Leonard JC, and Tobin JOH: Polyneuritis associated with cytomegalovirus infections. Quart J Med, *40*:435, 1971.
83. Klemola E, Stenstrom R, and von Essen R: Pneumonia as a clinical manifestation of cytomegalovirus infection in previously healthy adults. Scand J Infect Dis, *4*:7, 1972.
84. Klemola E, et al: Further studies on cytomegalovirus mononucleosis in previously healthy individuals. Acta Med Scand, *182*:311, 1967.
85. Tiula E, and Leinikki P: Fatal cytomegalovirus infection in a previously healthy boy with myocarditis and consumption coagulopathy as presenting signs. Scand J Infect Dis, *4*:57, 1972.
86. Waris E, et al: Fatal cytomegalovirus disease in a previously healthy adult. Scand J Infect Dis, *4*:61, 1972.
87. Chanarin I, and Walford DM: Thrombocytopenic purpura in cytomegalovirus mononucleosis. Lancet, *i*:238, 1973.
88. Demetris AJ, et al: Pathology of hepatic transplantation. Am J Pathol, *116*:151, 1985.
89. Petersen PK, et al: Cytomegalovirus disease in renal allograft recipients. A prospective study of the clinical features, risk factors and impact on renal transplantation. Medicine (Baltimore), *59*:283, 1980.
90. Egbert PR, et al: Cytomegalovirus retinitis in immunosuppressed hosts. II. Ocular manifestations. Ann Intern Med, *93*:664, 1980.
91. Holland GN, et al: Ocular disorders associated with a new severe acquired cellular immune deficiency syndrome. Am J Ophthalmol, *93*:393, 1982.
92. Munoz DG, Perl DP, and Pendlebury WW: Comparison of cytomegalovirus infection of brain and lung in a patient with subacute encephalopathy of acquired immunodeficiency syndrome. Arch Pathol Lab Med, *111*:234, 1987.
93. Ward KP, Galloway WH, and Auchterlonie IA: Congenital cytomegalovirus infection and diabetes. Lancet, *i*:497, 1979.
94. Glasgow BJ, et al: Adrenal pathology in the acquired immune deficiency syndrome. Am J Clin Pathol, *84*:594, 1985.
95. Parham DM: Post-transplantation pancreatitis associated with cytomegalovirus (report of a case). Hum Pathol, *12*:663, 1981.
96. Sprunt TP, and Evans FA: Mononuclear leukocytosis in reaction to acute infections ("infectious mononucleosis"). Johns Hopkins Hosp Bull, *31*:410, 1921.
97. Paul JR, and Bunnell WW: The presence of heterophile antibodies in infectious mononucleosis. Am J Med Sci, *183*:90, 1932.
98. Davidsohn I: Serologic diagnosis of infectious mononucleosis. JAMA, *108*:289, 1937.
99. Epstein MA, Achong BA, and Barr YM: Virus particles in cultured lymphoblasts from Burkitt's lymphoma. Lancet, *i*:702, 1964.
100. Henle G, and Henle W: Immunofluorescence in cells derived from Burkitt lymphoma. J Bacteriol, *91*:1248, 1966.
101. Niederman JC, et al: Infectious mononucleosis: Clinical manifestations in relation to EB virus antibodies. JAMA, *203*:205, 1968.
102. Evans AS, Niederman JC, and McCollum RW: Seroepidemiologic studies of infectious mononucleosis with EB virus. N Engl J Med, *279*:1121, 1968.
103. Young LS, et al: Epstein-Barr virus receptor on human pharyngeal epithelia. Lancet, *i*:240, 1986.
104. Sixbey JW, et al: Human epithelial cell expression of an Epstein Barr virus receptor. J Gen Virol, *68*:805, 1987.
105. Kirchner H, et al: Polyclonal immunoglobulin secretion by human B lymphocytes exposed to Epstein-Barr virus in vitro. J Immunol, *122*:1310, 1979.
106. Hoagland RJ: The transmission of infectious mononucleosis. Am J Med Sci, *229*:262, 1955.
107. Gerber P, et al: Association of EB virus infection with the postperfusion syndrome. Lancet, *i*:593, 1969.
108. Portnoy J, et al: Recovery of Epstein-Barr virus from genital ulcers. N Engl J Med, *311*:966, 1984.
109. Henle G, et al: Antibodies to Epstein-Barr virus in Burkitt's lymphoma and control groups. J Natl Cancer Inst, *43*:1147, 1969.
110. Pereira MS, Blake JM, and Macrae AD: EB virus antibody at different ages. Br Med J, *4*:526, 1969.
111. Porter DD, Wimberly I, and Benyesh-Melnick M: Prevalence of antibodies to EB virus and other herpesviruses. JAMA, *208*:1675, 1969.
112. Heath CW Jr, Brodsky AL, and Potolsky AI: Infectious

mononucleosis in a general population. Am J Epidemiol, 95:46, 1972.
113. Kaplan ME, and Tan EM: Antinuclear antibodies in infectious mononucleosis. Lancet, i:561, 1968.
114. McKenzie H, Parratt D, and White RG: IgM and IgG antibody levels to ampicillin in patients with infectious mononucleosis. Clin Exp Immunol, 26:214, 1976.
115. Charlesworth JA, et al: Complement, lymphocytotoxins, and immune complexes in infectious mononucleosis: Serial studies in uncomplicated cases. Clin Exp Immunol, 34:241, 1978.
116. Ellman L, et al: Platelet autoantibody in a case of infectious mononucleosis presenting as thrombocytopenic purpura. Am J Med, 55:723, 1973.
117. Kernoff LM: Demonstration of increased platelet bound IgG in infectious mononucleosis complicated by severe thrombocytopenia. Scand J Infect Dis, 12:67, 1980.
118. Schooley RT, et al: Antineutrophil antibodies in infectious mononucleosis. Am J Med, 76:85, 1984.
119. Haider S, et al: Tuberculin anergy and infectious mononucleosis. Lancet, ii:74, 1973.
120. Schooley RT, et al: Chronic Epstein-Barr virus infection associated with fever and interstitial pneumonitis. Ann Intern Med, 104:636, 1986.
121. Miller G, et al: Selective lack of antibody to a component of EB nuclear antigen in patients with chronic active Epstein-Barr virus infection. J Infect Dis, 156:26, 1987.
122. Okano M, et al: Epstein-Barr virus and human diseases: Advances in diagnosis. Clin Microbiol Rev, 1:300, 1988.
123. Henle W, et al: Antibodies to Epstein-Barr virus in nasopharyngeal carcinoma, other head and neck neoplasms, and control groups. J Natl Cancer Inst, 44:225, 1970.
124. Zur Hausen H, et al: EBV DNA in biopsies of Burkitt's tumors and anaplastic carcinomas of the nasopharynx. Nature, 228:1056, 1970.
125. Grierson H, and Purtilo DT: Epstein-Barr virus infections in males with the X-linked lymphoproliferative syndrome. Ann Intern Med, 106:538, 1987.
126. Harrington DS, Weisenburger DD, and Purtilo DT: Malignant lymphoma in the X-linked lymphoproliferative syndrome. Cancer, 59:1419, 1987.
127. Saemundsen AK, et al: Epstein-Barr virus carrying lymphoma in a patient with ataxia telangiectasia. Br Med J, 282:425, 1981.
128. Okano M, et al: Wiskott-Aldrich syndrome and Epstein-Barr virus–induced lymphoproliferation. Lancet, ii:933, 1984.
129. Merino F, et al: Elevated antibody titers to Epstein-Barr virus and low natural killer cell activity in patients with Chediak-Higashi syndrome. Clin Immunol Immunopathol, 27:326, 1983.
130. Sumaya CV, et al: Enhanced serological and virological findings of Epstein-Barr virus in patients with AIDS and AIDS-related complex. J Infect Dis, 154:864, 1986.
131. Joshi VV, et al: Polyclonal polymorphic B-cell lymphoproliferative disorder with prominent pulmonary involvement in children with acquired immune deficiency syndrome. Cancer, 59:1455, 1987.
132. Hanto DW, Frizzera G, Gajl-Peczalska KJ, and Simmons RL: Epstein-Barr virus, immunodeficiency, and B cell lymphoproliferation. Transplantation, 39:461, 1985.
133. Hanto DW, et al: Epstein-Barr virus (EBV)–induced polyclonal and monoclonal B-cell lymphoproliferative diseases occurring after renal transplantation. Ann Surg, 198:356, 1983.
134. Shearer WT, et al: Epstein-Barr virus–associated B-cell proliferations of diverse clonal origins after bone marrow transplantation in a 12-year-old patient with severe combined immunodeficiency. N Engl J Med, 312:1151, 1985.
135. Hochberg FG, et al: Central nervous system lymphoma related to Epstein-Barr virus. N Engl J Med, 309:745, 1983.
136. Jones JF, et al: T-cell lymphomas containing Epstein-Barr viral DNA in patients with chronic Epstein-Barr virus infections. N Engl J Med, 318:733, 1988.
137. Salahuddin SZ, et al: Isolation of a new virus, HBLV, in patients with lymphoproliferative disorders. Science, 234:596, 1986.
138. Josephs SF, et al: Genomic analysis of the human B-lymphotropic virus (HBLV). Science, 234:601, 1986.
139. Lusso P, et al: Diverse tropism of human B-lymphotropic virus (human herpesvirus-6). Lancet, ii:743, 1987.
140. Krueger GRF, and Sander C: What's new in human herpesvirus-6? Clinical immunopathology of the HHV-6 infection. Pathol Res Pract, 185:915, 1989.
141. Briggs M, Fox J, and Tedder RS: Age prevalence of antibody to human herpesvirus-6. Lancet, i:1058, 1988.
142. Linde A, et al: IgG antibodies to human herpesvirus-6 in children and adults both in primary Epstein-Barr virus and cytomegalovirus infections. J Virol Methods, 21:117, 1988.
143. Morris DJ, Littler E, Jordan D, and Arrand JR: Antibody responses to human herpesvirus 6 and other herpesviruses. Lancet, ii:1425, 1988.
144. Brown NA, et al: Fall in human herpesvirus-6 seropositivity with age. Lancet, ii:396, 1988.
145. Lawrence GL, et al: Human herpesvirus-6 is closely related to human cytomegalovirus. J Virol, 64:287, 1990.
146. Eizura Y, et al: Human herpesvirus 6 in lymph nodes. Lancet, i:40, 1989.
147. Becker WB, et al: New T-lymphotropic human herpesviruses. Lancet, i:41, 1989.
148. Krueger GRF, and Ablashi DV: Human B-lymphotropic virus in Germany. Lancet, ii:694, 1987.
149. Krueger GRF, Ablashi DV, Salahuddin SZ, and Josephs SF: Diagnosis and differential diagnosis of progressive lymphoproliferation and malignant lymphoma in persistent active herpesvirus infection. J Virol Methods, 21:255, 1988.
150. Centers for Disease Control: B virus infection in humans—Pensacola, Florida. MMWR, 36:289, 1987.
151. Holmes GP, et al: B virus (Herpesvirus simiae) infection in humans: Epidemiologic investigation of a cluster. Ann Intern Med, 112:833, 1990.
152. Hull RN: The simian herpesviruses. In The Herpesviruses. Edited by AS Kaplan. New York, Academic Press, 1973.
153. Nagler FP, and Klotz M: A fatal B virus infection in a person subject to recurrent herpes labialis. Can Med Assoc J, 79:743, 1958.
154. Moseby RC, et al: Comparison of viral isolation, direct immunofluorescence and indirect immunoperoxidase techniques for detection of genital herpes simplex virus infection. J Infect Dis, 143:913, 1981.
155. Vontver LA, et al: Clinical course and diagnosis of genital herpes virus infection and evaluation of topical surfactant therapy. Am J Obstet Gynecol, 135:548, 1979.
156. Dorian KJ, Beatty E, and Atterbury KE: Detection of herpes simplex virus by the Kodak SureCell herpes test. J Clin Microbiol, 28:2117, 1990.
157. Hardy DA, et al: Use of polymerase chain reaction for successful identification of asymptomatic genital infection with herpes simplex virus in pregnant women at delivery. J Infect Dis, 162:1031, 1990.
158. Woods GL, and Mills RD: Effect of dexamethasone on detection of herpes simplex virus in clinical specimens by conventional cell culture and rapid 24-well plate centrifugation. J Clin Microbiol, 26:1233, 1988.
159. Gleaves CA, Wilson DJ, Wold AD, and Smith TF: Detection and serotyping of herpes simplex virus in MRC-5 cells by

use of centrifugation and monoclonal antibodies 16 h post-inoculation. J Clin Microbiol, 21:29, 1985.
160. Woods GL, and Mills RD: Conventional tube cell culture compared with centrifugal inoculation of MRC-5 cells and staining with monoclonal antibodies for detection of herpes simplex virus in clinical specimens. J Clin Microbiol, 26:570, 1988.
161. Thiele GM, and Woods GL: The effect of dexamethasone on detection of cytomegalovirus in tissue culture and by immunofluorescence. J Virol Methods, 22:319, 1988.
162. Gleaves CA, Smith TF, Shuster EA, and Pearson GR: Rapid detection of cytomegalovirus in MRC-5 cells inoculated with urine specimens by using low-speed centrifugation and monoclonal antibody to an early antigen. J Clin Microbiol, 19:917, 1984.
163. Gleaves CA, Smith TF, Shuster EA, and Pearson GR: Comparison of standard tube and shell vial cell culture techniques for the detection of cytomegalovirus in clinical specimens. J Clin Microbiol, 21:217, 1985.
164. Woods GL, Young A, Johnson A, and Thiele GM: Detection of cytomegalovirus by 24-well plate centrifugation assay using a monoclonal antibody to an early nuclear antigen and by conventional cell culture. J Virol Methods, 18:207, 1987.
165. Woods GL, and Thiele GM: Rapid detection of cytomegalovirus by 24-well plate centrifugation using a monoclonal antibody to an early nuclear antigen. Am J Clin Pathol, 91:695, 1989.
166. Woods GL, Thompson AB, Rennard SI, and Linder J: Detection of cytomegalovirus in bronchoalveolar lavage specimens by spin amplification and staining with a monoclonal antibody to the early nuclear antigen for diagnosis of cytomegalovirus pneumonia. Chest, 98:568, 1990.
167. Gleaves CA, and Meyers JD: Rapid detection of cytomegalovirus virus in bronchoalveolar lavage specimens from marrow transplant patients: Evaluation of a direct fluorescent-conjugated monoclonal antibody reagent. J Virol Methods, 26:345, 1989.
168. van der Bij W, et al: Rapid immunodiagnosis of active cytomegalovirus infection by monoclonal antibody staining of blood leucocytes. J Med Virol, 25:179, 1988.
169. Wolber RA, and Lloyd RV: Cytomegalovirus detection by in situ DNA hybridization and viral antigen immunostaining using a two-color technique. Hum Pathol, 19:736, 1988.
170. Dankner WM, et al: Localization of human cytomegalovirus in peripheral blood leukocytes by in situ hybridization. J Infect Dis, 161:31, 1990.
171. Jiwa NW, et al: Rapid detection of human cytomegalovirus DNA in peripheral blood leukocytes of viremic transplant recipients by the polymerase chain reaction. Transplantation, 48:72, 1989.
172. Straus SE, et al: Herpes simplex virus infection—biology, treatment, and prevention. Ann Intern Med, 103:404, 1985.
173. Meyers JD, et al: Multicenter collaborative trial of intravenous acyclovir for treatment of mucocutaneous herpes simplex virus infection in the immunocompromised host. Am J Med, 73(1A):229, 1982.
174. Shepp DH, et al: Oral acyclovir therapy for mucocutaneous herpes simplex virus infections in immunocompromised marrow transplant recipients. Ann Intern Med, 102:783, 1985.
175. Erlich KS, et al: Acyclovir resistant herpes simplex virus infections in patients with the acquired immunodeficiency syndrome. N Engl J Med, 320:293, 1989.
176. Hirsch MS, and Schooley RT: Resistance to antiviral drugs: The end of innocence. N Engl J Med, 320:313, 1989.
177. Safrin S, Assaykeen T, Follansbee S, and Mills J: Foscarnet therapy for acyclovir-resistant mucocutaneous herpes simplex virus infection in 26 AIDS patients: Preliminary data. J Infect Dis, 161:1078, 1990.
178. Dunkle LM, et al: A controlled trial of acyclovir for chickenpox in normal children. N Engl J Med, 325:1539, 1991.
179. Jacobson MA, et al: Acyclovir-resistant varicella-zoster virus infection after chronic oral acyclovir therapy in patients with the acquired immunodeficiency syndrome. Ann Intern Med, 112:187, 1990.
180. Buhles WC Jr, et al: Ganciclovir treatment of life or sight-threatening cytomegalovirus infection: Experience in 314 immunocompromised patients. Rev Infect Dis, 10(S3):S495, 1988.
181. Erice A, et al: Ganciclovir treatment of cytomegalovirus disease in transplant recipients and other immunocompromised hosts. JAMA, 257:3082, 1987.
182. Collaborative DHPG Treatment Study Group: Treatment of serious cytomegalovirus infections with 9-(1,3,dihydroxy-2-propoxymethyl) guanine in patients with AIDS and other immunodeficiencies. N Engl J Med, 314:801, 1986.
183. Winston DJ, et al: Ganciclovir therapy for cytomegalovirus infections in recipients of bone marrow transplants and other immunosuppressed patients. Rev Infect Dis, 10(S3):S547, 1988.
184. Shepp DH, et al: Activity of 9-[2-hydroxy-1-(hydroxymethyl) ethoxymethyl] guanine in the treatment of cytomegalovirus pneumonia. Ann Intern Med, 103:368, 1985.
185. Reed EC, et al: Treatment of cytomegalovirus pneumonia with ganciclovir and intravenous cytomegalovirus immunoglobulin in patients with bone marrow transplants. Ann Intern Med, 109:738, 1988.
186. Studies of Ocular Complications of AIDS Research Group, et al: Mortality in patients with the acquired immunodeficiency syndrome treated with either foscarnet or ganciclovir for cytomegalovirus retinitis. N Engl J Med, 326:213, 1992.
187. Rooney JF, et al: Immunization with a vaccinia virus recombinant expressing herpes simplex virus type I glycoprotein D: Long-term protection and effect of revaccination. J Virol, 62:1530, 1988.
188. Straus SE, Ostrove JM, and Inchauspe G: Varicella-zoster virus infections: Biology, natural history, treatment and prevention. Ann Intern Med, 108:221, 1988.
189. Weibel RE, et al: Live attenuated varicella virus vaccine: Efficacy trial in healthy children. N Engl J Med, 310:1409, 1984.
190. Asano Y, et al: Long-term protective immunity of recipients of the OKA strain of live varicella vaccine. Pediatrics, 75:667, 1985.
191. Lawrence R, et al: The risk of zoster after vaccination in children with leukemia. N Engl J Med, 318:543, 1988.
192. Einsele H, et al: Significant reduction of cytomegalovirus (CMV) disease by prophylaxis with CMV hyperimmune globulin plus oral acyclovir. Bone Marrow Transplant, 3:607, 1988.
193. Balfour HH Jr, et al: A randomized, placebo-controlled trial of oral acyclovir for the prevention of cytomegalovirus disease in recipients of renal allografts. N Engl J Med, 320:1381, 1989.
194. Balfour HH Jr, Welo PK, and Sach GW: Cytomegalovirus vaccine trial in 400 renal transplant candidates. Transplant Proc, 17:81, 1985.

Chapter 6

ADENOVIRUSES

Adenoviruses were first identified as latent viruses in spontaneously degenerating adenoid tissue surgically removed from asymptomatic children in 1953; the same year they were established as the cause of an outbreak of acute respiratory disease among military recruits (1,2). Subsequently, adenoviruses have been recognized as an important cause of ocular, gastrointestinal, genitourinary tract and, occasionally, disseminated disease.

CLASSIFICATION

Adenoviruses are classified in the family Adenoviridae, which includes two genera: Mastadenovirus, adenoviruses that are isolated from mammals and share a common complement-fixing antigen; and Aviadenovirus, adenoviruses that infect fowl and lack the common complement-fixing antigen. Human adenoviruses are divided into six subgenera and 42 serotypes based on DNA homology and antigenicity, respectively (Table 6–1). Recently, putative serotypes 43 through 47 have been identified (3).

STRUCTURE

Adenovirus virions are nonenveloped perfect icosahedrons, 70 to 90 nm in diameter (Fig. 6–1) (4). The nucleocapsid consists of a linear, double-stranded DNA genome of molecular weight 23 million, surrounded by a protein capsid containing 252 capsomeres of three morphologic types: hexons, with six nearest neighbors, account for 240 capsomeres; pentons, with five nearest neighbors, occupy the 12 vertices; and rodlike fibers project from the penton base. The hexon has antigenic sites common to all human adenoviruses and sites with type specificity against which neutralizing antibodies are directed; the fiber has type specificity and some group specificity; and the penton base antigen is common to the adenovirus family.

Table 6–1. Classification of Human Adenoviruses

Subgenus	Serotypes	Percent of Guanine and Cytosine in DNA
A	12,18,31	48–49
B	3,7,11,14,16,21,34,35	50–52
C	1,2,5,6	57–59
D	8,9,10,13,15,19,20,22–30,32, 33,36–39,42	57–61
E	4	57–59
Fastidious (F)	40,41	

REPLICATION

Adenovirus replication is initiated by attachment of the viral fiber protein to the host cell receptor. Virions enter the cell by endocytosis or by direct translocation across the plasma membrane, and in the cytoplasm the pentons are removed and the DNA core migrates to the nucleus, where transcription and translation into early proteins ensue. The DNA is replicated, late transcription units are expressed, and translation of structural proteins follows. Capsomeres are produced in the cytoplasm and transported to the nucleus, where virions are assembled and released following cell lysis.

Adenoviruses induce different types of infection depending on the species and cell type infected. For example, in human epithelial cells, adenoviruses initiate a replicative cycle that results in cell lysis and the release of 10,000 to 1 million virions, of which 1 to 5% are infectious. In human lymphoid cells (such as the adenoids) adenoviruses establish latent infection by an unknown mechanism, producing small numbers of virions. In some animals oncogenic transformation is induced: viral DNA integrates into and replicates with host cellular DNA without producing infectious virions.

EPIDEMIOLOGY

Infections with adenoviruses, recognized worldwide, usually occur in the first few years of life, and by the end of the first decade most persons have been infected with one or more serotypes. Adenoviruses are transmitted principally via the fecal-oral route, which is facilitated by prolonged fecal shedding of the virus. Respiratory spread, via aerosol droplets or contact, is responsible for outbreaks of acute respiratory tract disease, especially among military recruits. Transmission also may occur by close contact with infected secretions such as urine or semen; and ocular infections are acquired by swimming in contaminated pools or ponds and by transfer of infected secretions via hands, fomites, and contaminated ophthalmic solutions (5–9).

PATHOGENESIS AND PATHOLOGIC CHANGES

During the lytic replicative cycle of many adenovirus serotypes, cellular DNA and protein synthesis are severely inhibited and normal processing of host messenger RNA is interrupted, events incompatible with cell survival. Degeneration of infected cells produces morphologic changes useful for diagnosis when they are observed in sections of biopsy or autopsy tissue. An infected respiratory epithelial cell has an enlarged nucleus that contains an amphophilic or basophilic intranuclear inclusion sur-

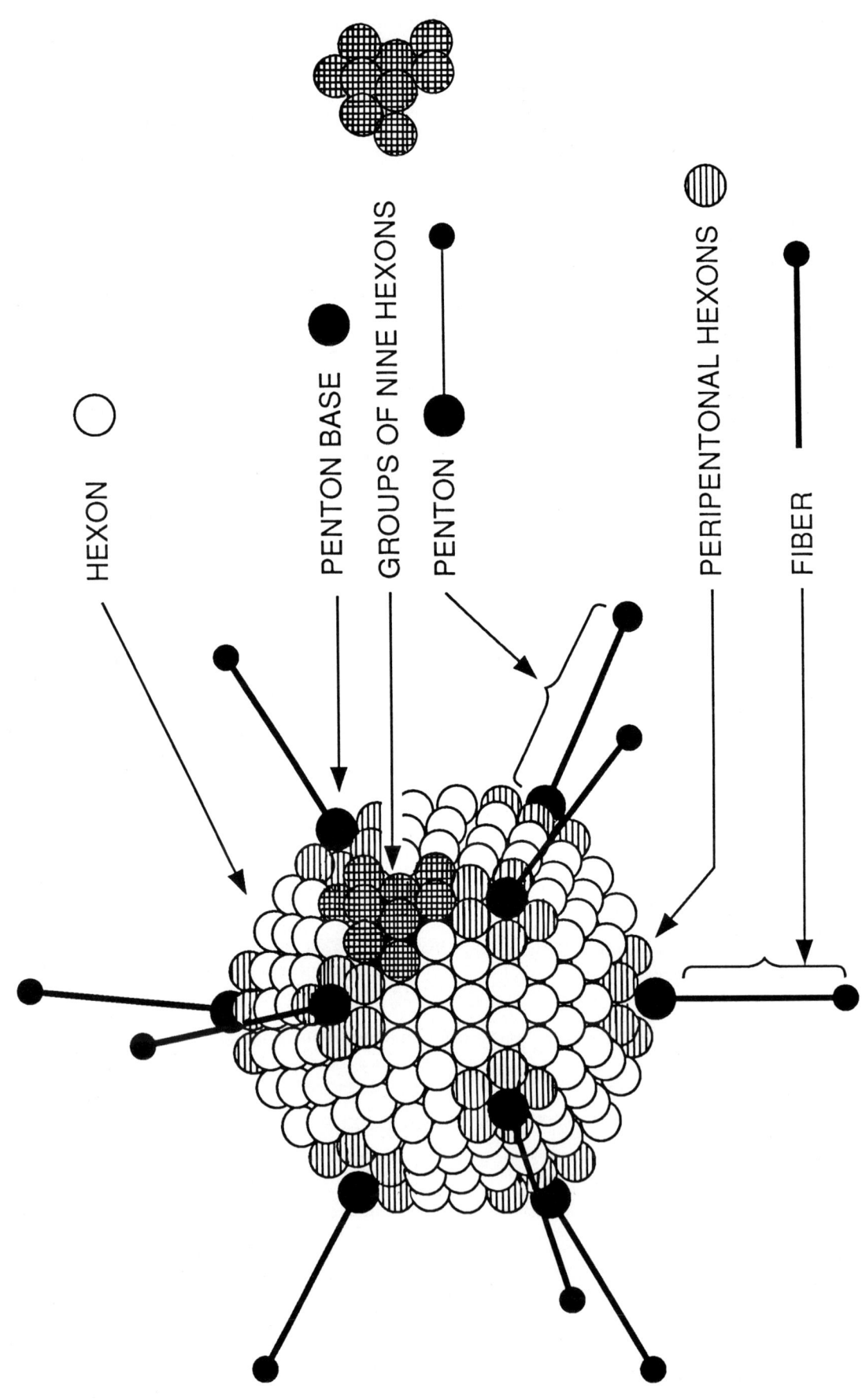

Fig. 6–1. Diagram illustrates the components of an adenovirus virion. (From Philipson L, Pettersson U, and Lindberg U: Molecular biology of adenoviruses. *In* Virology Monographs 14. New York, Springer-Verlag, 1975.)

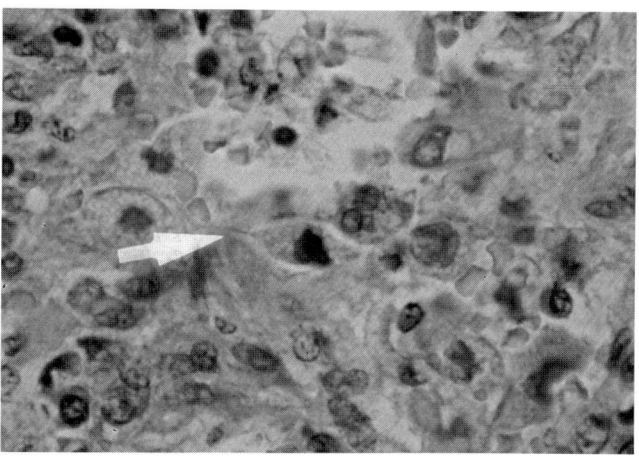

Fig. 6–2. Intranuclear inclusion of adenovirus (smudge cell) in lung tissue of a patient with pneumonia (hematoxylin and eosin, ×400).

rounded by a thin rim of cytoplasm, termed a smudge cell (Fig. 6–2), or an intranuclear inclusion with an intact nuclear membrane, resembling a cell infected with cytomegalovirus (see Chapter 5).

The penton structural protein of adenovirus is directly toxic to cells other than those infected with replicating adenovirus in vitro (10,11). The importance of the penton in human disease is unknown, but it has been detected in the blood of persons with fatal pneumonia caused by adenovirus (12). Serious infections with adenovirus cause considerable injury to the involved organs; for example, pneumonia is characterized by necrotizing bronchitis, bronchiolitis, interstitial infiltrates, and hyaline membranes.

CLINICAL MANIFESTATIONS

The clinical manifestations of infections caused by adenoviruses depend on the infecting serotype and the age of the person (Table 6–2). In nonepidemic situations, at least half of infections are subclinical. In children infection of the upper respiratory tract with adenovirus may produce pharyngitis or tracheitis with cough, fever, sore throat, and rhinorrhea lasting 3 to 5 days, and less frequently, croup (see Chapter 10). Infants infected with serotype 7 may develop fulminant bronchiolitis and pneumonia, and in young adults adenoviruses may cause "atypical" pneumonia. Epidemics of acute respiratory disease produced by adenovirus, characterized by fever, pharyngitis, cervical adenitis, cough, and malaise, occur predominantly among military recruits. Ocular infections caused by adenovirus include pharyngoconjunctival fever—unilateral conjunctivitis, pharyngitis, fever, rhinitis, and cervical adenitis, commonly in children at summer camps—and, in adults, epidemic keratoconjunctivitis, which begins insidiously as bilateral conjunctivitis, gradually resolves, and is followed by keratitis.

Adenoviruses, especially serotypes 11 and 21, have been associated with hemorrhagic cystitis in healthy children and adults and in recipients of renal allografts and bone marrow transplants (13–17). The "enteric" or "fastidious" adenoviruses are the second most common agents (after rotavirus) of gastroenteritis in young children, causing diarrhea lasting 9 to 12 days and occasionally accompanied by vomiting and low-grade fever. Central nervous system infections due to adenoviruses are uncommon but have developed in persons with epidemic respiratory disease and in those with hypogammaglobulinemia (18). In immunocompromised persons infections caused by adenoviruses may become disseminated (19,20).

LABORATORY DIAGNOSIS

Specimens necessary to diagnose infections caused by adenoviruses are listed in Table 6–2. Specimen collection, transport, and processing are discussed in Part III of the text. Identification of the adenoviruses is reviewed below.

The reference method for detection of adenovirus is conventional cell culture, preferably using human embryonic kidney cells (which are difficult to obtain), A-549 cells, or HEp-2 cells. Adenoviruses also grow in human fibroblasts, but in fibroblasts the cytopathic effect (CPE)

Table 6–2. Diseases Caused by Adenoviruses and Specimens Required for Diagnosis

Disease	Frequently Associated Serotypes	Most Frequent Hosts	Specimens
Upper respiratory infection	1,2,3,5,6,7	Infants, young children	Throat swab or wash
Pharyngoconjunctival fever	1,2,3,4,6,7,14	Children (summer epidemics)	Throat swab or wash, conjunctival scrapings
Acute respiratory disease	3,4,7	Young adults (military recruits)	Throat swab or wash, sputum, BAL, lung biopsy tissue, feces
Pneumonia	1,2,3,7,21	Young children	Throat swab or wash, BAL, lung tissue
Keratoconjunctivitis	8,11,19,37	Persons of any age, most often adults	Conjunctival scrapings
Hemorrhagic cystitis	11,21	Young children, immunocompromised persons	Urine
Diarrhea	2,3,5,40,41	Young children	Feces, rectal swab
Cervicitis, urethritis	37	Adults	Endocervical swab, urethral swab, urine
Meningoencephalitis	2,6,7,12,32	Children, immunocompromised host	CSF, brain tissue
Disseminated disease	5,34,35,39	Immunocompromised host	Blood, sputum, BAL, urine, tissue (liver, lung, brain)

Key: BAL, bronchoalveolar lavage fluid; CSF, cerebrospinal fluid.

usually becomes apparent several days later than in A-549 or HEp-2 cells. The Graham 293 cell line, derived from transformation of human embryonic kidney cells by adenovirus 5 DNA, is required to recover the fastidious enteric adenoviruses (serotypes 40 and 41) (21,22). The typical CPE usually is recognized 4 to 7 days after inoculation of A-549 cells as foci of swollen, rounded, refractile cells, often forming clusters that resemble bunches of grapes (Fig. 6–3). An isolate may be called adenovirus presumptively, based on the appearance of the CPE; identification is confirmed by staining infected cells with specific monoclonal antibodies.

More rapid techniques for adenovirus detection are centrifugation and short-term culture, direct staining of the clinical specimen with monoclonal antibodies, and enzyme-linked immunosorbent assay (ELISA). The sensitivity of centrifugation-culture using A-549 cells and staining with monoclonal antibodies directed against the adenovirus hexon after incubation for 40 hours is about 90%; however, this approach may not be cost effective for laboratories with a low prevalence of adenovirus isolates (23). Monoclonal antibodies marketed for direct staining of cell smears prepared from nasal wash or nasal swab specimens and an enzyme-linked immunosorbent assay (ELISA) for detecting adenovirus in stool specimens are commercially available, but data on their sensitivity and specificity are limited. Moreover, the polymerase chain reaction recently has been shown to be a fast, sensitive, and reliable method for detecting adenoviruses in stool samples (24).

The presence of an adenovirus in a respiratory secretion or stool specimen is not evidence that the virus is responsible for disease, because adenoviruses may colonize the respiratory tract without causing symptoms, and they may be shed in feces for up to 18 months after primary infection. Detecting an adenovirus in a throat specimen from a person with pharyngitis usually indicates a viral infection if other common pathogens such as group A streptococci (see Chapter 28) are excluded; however, detecting an adenovirus in a stool specimen but not in a throat specimen from a person with respiratory symptoms is insufficient evidence that the adenovirus is responsible for the clinical illness.

Serologic tests to detect specific immunoglobulin G are available, but interpretation of the results may be difficult. Seroconversion or a fourfold rise in titer between acute- and convalescent-phase serum usually is evidence of active infection; however, recrudescent shedding of adenovirus may be accompanied by a fourfold or greater rise in antibody titer, and young children often do not produce antibody after infection with adenovirus. Therefore, serologic testing is not the best method for diagnosing adenovirus-induced disease.

TREATMENT AND PREVENTION

Treatment of infections caused by adenoviruses is supportive because no effective antiviral therapy is available. In the United States, live, oral, enteric-coated vaccines are used only for military recruits to prevent outbreaks of acute respiratory disease with adenovirus serotypes 4 and 7.

REFERENCES

1. Rowe WP, et al: Isolation of a cytopathogenic agent from human adenoids undergoing spontaneous degeneration in tissue culture. Proc Soc Exp Biol Med, 84:570, 1953.
2. Hilleman MR, and Werner JH: Recovery of new agents from patients with acute respiratory illness. Proc Soc Exp Biol Med, 85:183, 1954.
3. Hierholzer JC, et al: Adenoviruses from patients with AIDS: A plethora of serotypes and a description of five new serotypes of subgenus D (types 43–47). J Infect Dis, 158:804, 1988.
4. Philipson L, Pettersson U, and Lindberg U: Molecular Biology of Adenoviruses. In Virology Monographs 11. New York, Springer-Verlag, 1975.
5. Vastine DW, et al: Simultaneous nosocomial and community outbreak of epidemic keratoconjunctivitis with types 8 and 19 adenovirus. Trans Am Acad Ophthalmol Otolaryngol, 81: 826, 1976.
6. Hendley JO: Epidemic keratoconjunctivitis and hand washing. N Engl J Med, 289:1368, 1973.
7. D'Angelo LJ, Hierholzer JC, Holman RC, and Smith JD: Epidemic keratoconjunctivitis caused by adenovirus type 8: Epidemiologic and laboratory aspects of a large outbreak. Am J Epidemiol, 113:44, 1981.
8. Sprague JB, et al: Epidemic keratoconjunctivitis: A severe industrial outbreak due to adenovirus type 8. N Engl J Med, 289:1341, 1973.
9. Warren D, et al: A large outbreak of epidemic keratoconjunctivitis: Problems in controlling nosocomial spread. J Infect Dis, 160:938, 1989.
10. Pettersson U, and Hoglund S: Structural proteins of adenoviruses. Virology, 39:90, 1969.
11. Valentine RC, and Periera HG: Antigens and structure of the adenovirus. J Molec Biol, 13:13, 1965.
12. Ladisch S, et al: Extrapulmonary manifestations of adenovirus type 7 pneumonia simulating Reye syndrome and the possible role of an adenovirus toxin. J Pediatr, 95:348, 1979.

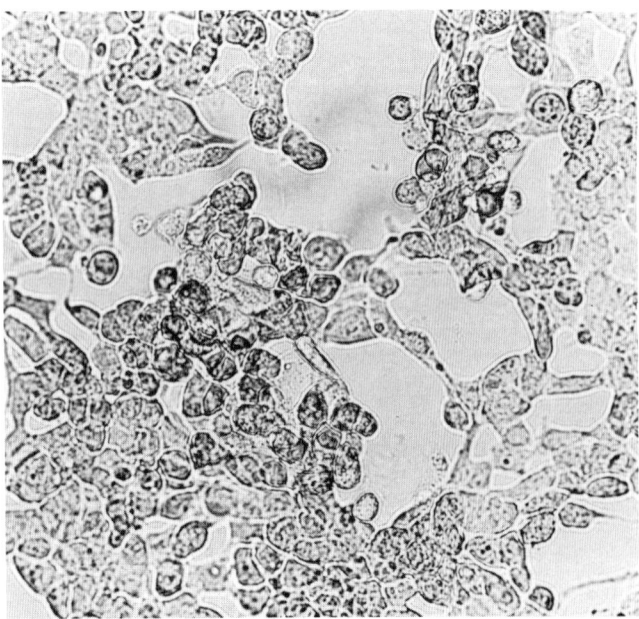

Fig. 6–3. Cytopathic effect produced by adenovirus in A-549 cells (×40).

13. Numazaki Y, et al: Acute hemorrhagic cystitis in children: Isolation of adenovirus type 11. N Engl J Med, *278*:700, 1968.
14. Mufson MA, and Belshe RB: A review of adenoviruses in the etiology of acute hemorrhagic cystitis. J Urol, *115*:191, 1976.
15. Harnett GB, et al: Acute haemorrhagic cystitis caused by adenovirus type 11 in a recipient of a transplanted kidney. Med J Aust, *1*:565, 1982.
16. Fiala M, et al: Role of adenovirus type 11 in hemorrhagic cystitis secondary to immunosuppression. J Urol, *112*:595, 1974.
17. Ambinder RF, et al: Hemorrhagic cystitis associated with adenovirus infection in bone marrow transplantation. Arch Intern Med, *146*:1400, 1986.
18. Simila S, Jouppila R, Salmi A, and Pohjonen R: Encephalomeningitis in children associated with an adenovirus type 7 epidemic. Acta Paediatr Scand, *59*:310, 1970.
19. Keller EW, Rubin RH, Black PH, and Hirsch MS: Isolation of adenovirus type 34 from a renal transplant recipient with interstitial pneumonia. Transplantation, *23*:188, 1977.
20. Landry ML, et al: Disseminated adenovirus infection in an immunocompromised host: Pitfalls in diagnosis. Am J Med, *83*:555, 1987.
21. Takiff HE, Straus SE, and Garon CF: Propagation and in vitro studies of previously non-cultivable enteric adenoviruses in 293 cells. Lancet, *ii*:832, 1981.
22. Shinozaki T, et al: Use of graham 293 cells in suspension for isolating enteric adenoviruses from stools of patients with acute gastroenteritis. J Infect Dis, *156*:246, 1987.
23. Woods GL, Yamamoto M, and Young A: Detection of adenovirus by rapid 24-well plate centrifugation and conventional cell culture with dexamethasone. J Virol Method, *20*:109, 1988.
24. Allard A, Girones R, Juto P, and Wadell G: Polymerase chain reaction for detection of adenoviruses in stool samples. J Clin Microbiol, *28*:2659, 1990.

Chapter 7

PAPOVAVIRUSES

The Papovaviruses are classified in the family Papovaviridae, which has two genera: Papillomavirus and Polyomavirus. These small, nonenveloped viruses have an icosahedral capsid and a double-stranded circular DNA genome, and they replicate in the host cell nucleus.

PAPILLOMAVIRUS

The highly species-specific papillomaviruses have a tropism for squamous epithelial cells. Human papillomaviruses (HPV) produce benign epithelial tumors of the skin and mucous membranes and have been associated with malignancies of the genital tract. Over 60 different types are identified by DNA homology, and to a large extent each is associated with a distinct histopathologic process (Table 7–1) (1).

Structure

The 52- to 55-nm diameter papillomavirus virion is composed of a 72-capsomere capsid and a DNA genome of about 8000 base pairs and molecular weight of 5.2 million. The genome is divided functionally into three regions: the "early" region of five to seven open reading frames (E1 through E7) that codes for proteins essential for transformation and replication, open reading frames L1 and L2, the "late" region that codes for the major and minor capsid proteins, and a noncoding region essential for regulatory functions of the genome. A species-specific antigenic determinant is located on the virion surface and a genus-specific determinant on the major viral polypeptide.

Replication

The mechanism of papillomavirus attachment and entry into host cells is unknown, but the replication cycle probably begins with the virus' entry into cells of the stratum germinativum. As basal cells differentiate and move toward the epithelial surface, replication progresses. Virions are assembled in the nucleus of keratinized cells and released when dead keratinocytes are shed.

Epidemiology

Papillomaviruses occur worldwide with little gender preference. As many as 50% of school-aged children have common skin warts, and such warts are more prevalent among meat- and fish handlers than in the general population. Juvenile, or flat, warts develop less frequently but predominantly in younger children. Persons with epidermodysplasia verruciformis, a rare, probably autosomal recessive, condition, develop disseminated cutaneous flat warts early in life that frequently undergo malignant transformation. Recurrent respiratory papillomatosis, an uncommon disease (estimated prevalence, 1500 new cases per year in the United States) affects preschool children and adults. Genital warts, an infection of sexually active persons, have been associated epidemiologically with genital tract malignancies; however, the virus has not been proven to be the cause (2–5).

The exact mode of transmission of cutaneous warts is unknown, but close personal contact, perhaps associated with local minor trauma, probably is important. Anogenital warts are transmitted venereally. Recurrent respiratory papillomatosis in young children probably is acquired during passage through the birth canal of a woman who has genital HPV infection, but the mode of transmission to adults has not been determined. The incubation period of naturally acquired infection with HPV is unknown, but it ranges from 6 weeks to 2 years (mean, 3 to 4 months) after inoculation of extracts of warts in the laboratory (6).

Pathogenesis

Viral replication induces excessive proliferation of all epidermal layers except the basal layer, resulting in acanthosis, parakeratosis, hyperkeratosis, and elongation of the rete ridges (Fig. 7–1). Some infected cells transform into koilocytes, large polygonal squamous cells with a shrunken nucleus within a cytoplasmic vacuole (Fig. 7–2), and some contain cytoplasmic keratohyalin inclusion bodies (Fig. 7–3). However, squamous epithelium that appears normal on histologic examination may contain papillomavirus DNA, which may explain disease recurrence after treatment.

Warts usually disappear within a few years. An effective host immune response probably is important in their resolution, because warts are more numerous in persons with primary and secondary immunodeficiencies such as Wiskott-Aldrich syndrome, common variable immunodeficiency, acquired immune deficiency syndrome (AIDS), lymphoproliferative disorders, and in those treated with immunosuppressive drugs (7–10). The specific immune mechanism, however, is unknown.

Infection of cervical cells by specific types of HPV is not sufficient by itself to induce malignant change; however, data from studies of HPV genomes in high-grade carcinoma in situ and invasive cancers support the strong association between certain serotypes of HPV and cervical cancer. Human papillomavirus types 16 and 18 are found in invasive cancers and can immortalize human keratinocytes in vitro (11,12). In lesions caused by HPV the viral genome is always transcriptionally active, and the transcription pattern changes as the lesions increase in sever-

Table 7–1. Human Papillomavirus Types Most Often Associated With Disease

Lesion	HPV Type
Cutaneous warts	
Plantar	1
Common and flat	1,2,3,4,7,10
Epidermodysplasia verruciformis	5*,8*,9,17,20,36
Anogenital lesions	
Condyloma acuminatum	6,11
Buschke-Lowenstein tumor	6,11
Bowen's disease	16*,31
Bowenoid papulosis	16*,34,39,42
Low-grade dysplasia	6,11,31
High-grade dysplasia	16*,18*
Cervical carcinoma	16*,18*
Penile carcinoma	6,16*,18*
Vaginal carcinoma	6,16*,18*
Papillomas	
Conjunctival	6,11
Oral	6,11
Laryngeal	6,11,30*,53

* Types believed to have high malignant potential.

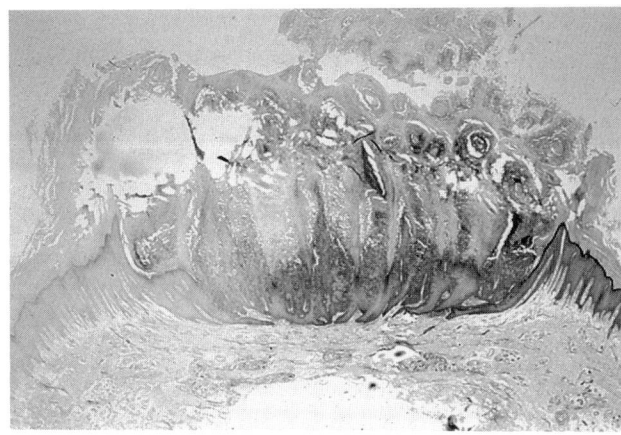

Fig. 7–1. Histologic appearance of a skin wart (hematoxylin and eosin, ×3.2).

ity: all open reading frames are expressed in mild lesions, but open reading frames $E4$ and $E5$ are absent in many invasive cancers (13,14). In tissues from malignancies containing HPV the viral genome may be episomal or integrated with host cell DNA (15,16). For integration to occur, the viral genome becomes linear by a nonrandom break in the $E1/E2$ region, interrupting the integrity of the $E1$ and $E2$ genes (17,18). The $E2$ gene codes for transcriptional regulatory factors that can affect viral transcription positively and negatively (19,20). In HPV types 16 and 18 $E2$ appears to repress expression from the promoter that regulates expression of $E6$ and $E7$ genes (21,22). Consequently, viral genome integration causes deregulation of the viral transforming genes $E6$ and $E7$, which could induce malignant change.

Clinical Manifestations

The common wart (verruca vulgaris) is a painless, firm, raised, rough-surfaced lesion that can measure up to 5 mm in diameter. Such warts may occur at any site on the skin, but most often are found on areas subject to abrasion. A flat wart (verruca plana) is smaller, flatter and smoother, than common warts and has a predilection for the face and knees of young children. Plantar and palmar warts (verruca plantaris) are painful, deep endophytic lesions of weight-bearing areas, especially the heels and soles of the foot. Genital warts (condyloma acuminatum) are moist, soft, pedunculated lesions of variable size found in the genital tract, or flat, often inconspicuous lesions located inside the urethra or vagina or on the cervix.

Warts associated with epidermodysplasia verruciformis appear on the torso and upper extremities, usually before age 10 years. Lesions initially resemble flat warts but often become hypertrophic and coalescent over the extensor surfaces; and in about a third of persons, beginning in young adulthood, lesions, especially those in sun-exposed areas, undergo malignant transformation into invasive squamous cell carcinoma. Respiratory papillomatosis

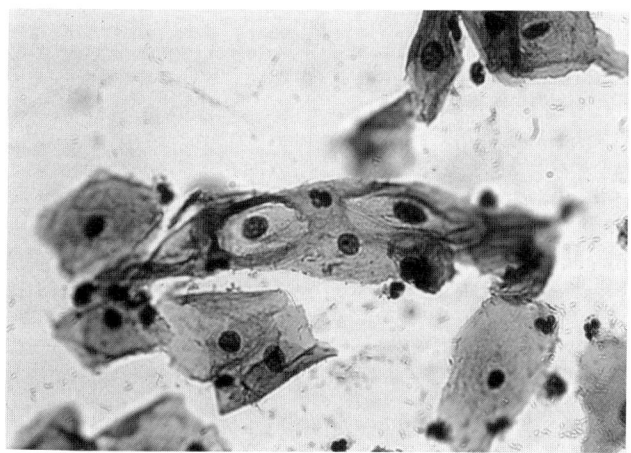

Fig. 7–2. Koilocytotic change caused by human papillomavirus infection in a smear of endocervical cells stained with Papanicolaou stain (×201.6).

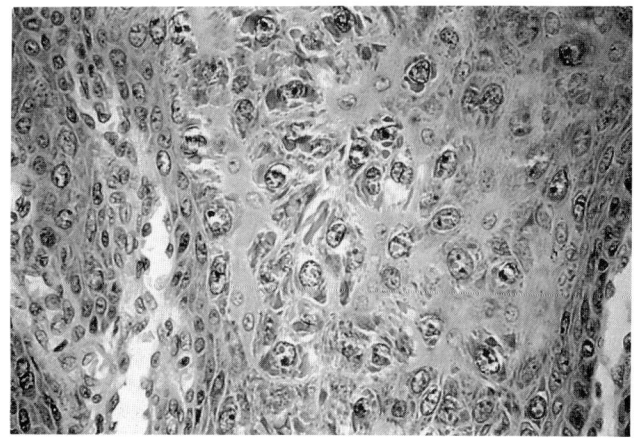

Fig. 7–3. Histologic section biopsy of a skin wart shows intracytoplasmic keratohyalin inclusion bodies (hematoxylin and eosin, ×100).

causes hoarseness in adults and an altered cry, occasionally accompanied by respiratory distress and stridor, in infants. Spread of the papillomas to the trachea and lungs may cause obstruction, infection, and respiratory failure.

POLYOMAVIRUS

The human polyomaviruses include JC virus, the agent responsible for almost all cases of the demyelinating disease progressive multifocal leukoencephalopathy (PML); SV40 (simian vacuolating agent-40)-PML viruses, isolated from the brain of two persons with PML; and BK virus, first isolated in 1971 from the urine of a recipient of a renal allograft (23).

Structure and Replication

The naked, icosahedral polyomavirus virions have a circular, supercoiled double-stranded DNA genome (molecular weight 3 million) divided into early, late, and noncoding regions. The early region codes for nonstructural T (transformation) proteins; the late region codes for three viral capsid proteins (VP1, VP2, VP3); and the noncoding region, the site of origin of DNA replication, contains the transcription control sequences. The replicative cycle includes virion attachment to the host cell, penetration by pinocytosis, uncoating, and viral replication in the host cell nucleus.

The 39- to 42-nm diameter JC virions multiply in human fetal glial cells, possess a hemagglutinin that mediates agglutination of human, guinea pig, and chicken erythrocytes, and are strongly oncogenic in brain and moderately oncogenic in other tissues. SV40-PML virions, 34 to 36 nm in diameter, are very closely related to SV40, lack a hemagglutinin, multiply moderately well in human fetal glial cells and poorly in human and monkey kidney cells, and are moderately oncogenic in brain and strongly oncogenic in other tissues. The 44-nm diameter BK virions have a hemagglutinin, multiply in human fetal glial cells and human and monkey kidney cells, and are weakly oncogenic in brain and other tissues.

Epidemiology

Asymptomatic infections caused by polyomaviruses are common worldwide. Antibody studies conducted in the United States indicate that the prevalence of infection with JC virus increases with age: 10% of persons are seropositive by age 4 years, 65% by 10 to 14 years, and 75% by 50 to 59 years (24). Antibodies to BK virus appear in early childhood and are present in 60 to 70% of adults (25). Respiratory transmission of these viruses is postulated but not proven. JC virus has been cultured from the urine of persons with PML and recipients of renal allografts (26). The JC virus genome has been detected in spleen, lymph node, lung, bone marrow, and brain of persons with PML, and in the urine of about 50% of elderly persons who have no evidence of PML (27–29). BK virus has been isolated from urine of recipients of renal and bone marrow transplants, from the urine and a reticulum cell sarcoma of a child with Wiskott-Aldrich syndrome, and from brain tumors and other human neoplasms (26,30–33).

Pathogenesis and Histologic Appearance

PML predominantly affects adults who have a chronic systemic disease such as sarcoidosis, tuberculosis, Whipple's disease, or systemic lupus erythematosus; a lymphoproliferative or myeloproliferative neoplasm such as Hodgkin's disease or chronic lymphocytic leukemia; or AIDS. The disease may result from reactivation of latent virus in the brain when the host immune system becomes impaired, or it may occur as a primary infection in an immunocompromised person who did not acquire immunity to the virus during childhood. Within an affected brain multiple discrete foci of myelin destruction develop and become confluent, producing large plaques that spare the axons. The oligodendrogliocytes in involved areas have enlarged nuclei with basophilic, eosinophilic, or amphophilic intranuclear viral inclusions (Fig. 7–4); astrocytes are enlarged and have pleomorphic, hyperchromatic nuclei; and inflammatory cells are rare. Papovavirus-like particles are visualized by electron microscopy in affected oligodendrogliocyte nuclei (Fig. 7–5), and rarely in oligodendrogliocyte cytoplasm or astrocyte nuclei.

Clinical Manifestation

PML begins insidiously with multifocal neurologic deficits such as hemiplegia, monoplegia, and cortical blindness, and with changes in higher cortical function, including personality changes, memory loss, apathy, emotional lability, and cognitive difficulties. Dementia is common early and progresses throughout the illness. Terminally, the individual is often comatose and quadriplegic. Death from intercurrent infection or complications of the underlying disease usually occurs within 3 to 6 months of the onset of neurologic signs; though the two persons with disease caused by SV40-PML virus survived for over 1 year (34). Infection with BK virus has been associated

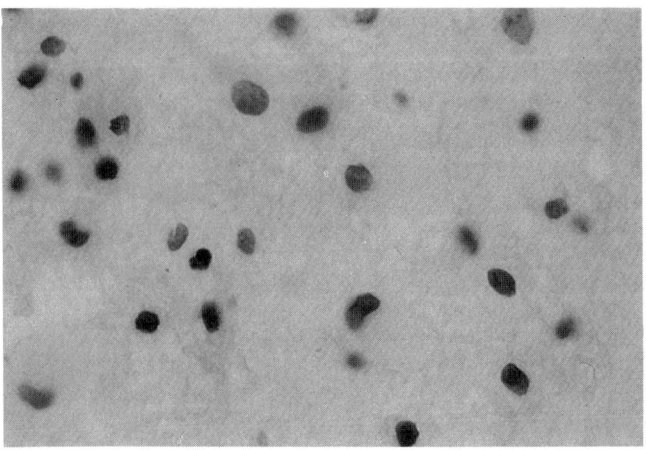

Fig. 7–4. Intranuclear inclusions in oligodendrogliocytes in the brain of a patient with AIDS and progressive multifocal leukoencephalopathy (hematoxylin and eosin, ×400).

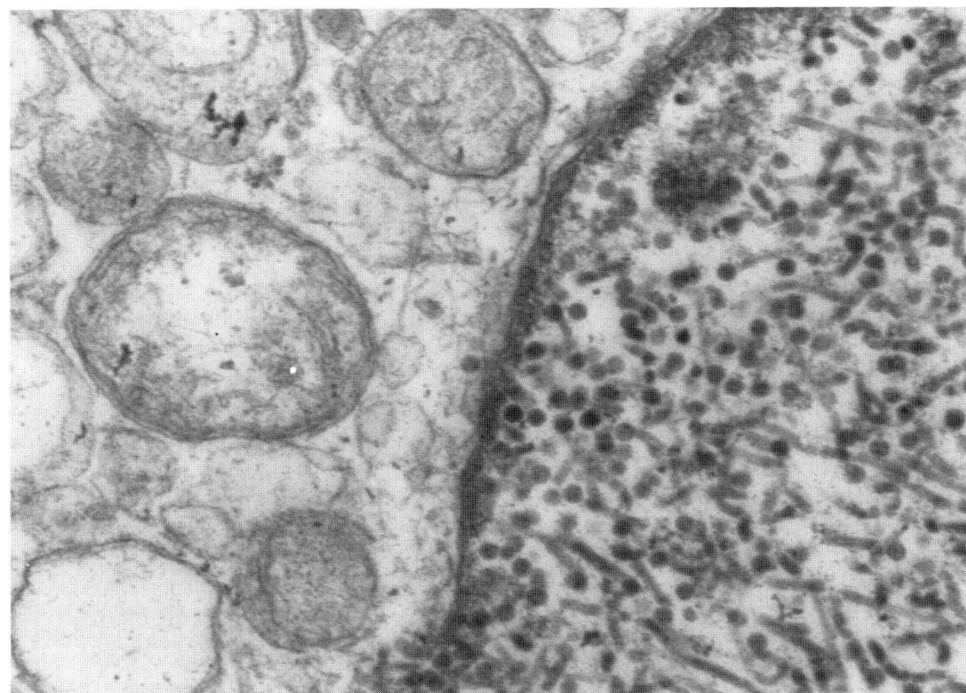

Fig. 7–5. Electron photomicrograph of papovavirus-like particles in the brain of a person with progressive multifocal leukoencephalopathy (×105,000).

with ureteral stenosis and hemorrhagic cystitis in immunosuppressed persons (26,30,31).

LABORATORY DIAGNOSIS

Human Papillomavirus. Infection with HPV is usually diagnosed by the clinical appearance of a lesion, cytologic examination of cells scraped from a lesion, histologic examination of biopsy tissue, or a combination of these. Papillomaviruses can be detected in tissues or exfoliated cells by nucleic acid hybridization or by gene amplification using the polymerase chain reaction (35–37). A nucleic acid hybridization assay for detecting HPV types 6, 11, 16, 18, 31, 33, 35 in tissues or endocervical or urethral swab specimens is commercially available, but its usefulness in managing persons suspected to have infection with HPV has not been established. Human papillomaviruses cannot be cultivated, and reliable serologic tests are not commercially available.

Polyomaviruses. Brain tissue white matter is required to diagnose PML. The histologic changes described earlier are characteristic, and virions can be visualized by electron microscopy. JC virus antigens can be detected by immunofluorescence and immunoperoxidase staining, and JC virus DNA can be detected by nucleic acid hybridization; assays to perform these tests, however, are not commercially available. JC virus can be cultivated in primary human fetal glial cells; but because these cells are not readily available, culture is performed only in a few research laboratories.

Urine is the preferred specimen for diagnosing infections caused by BK virus. The presence of enlarged cells with dense basophilic intranuclear inclusions in cytologic preparations of urine sediment is suggestive of BK virus (Fig. 7–6). BK virus can be recovered from urine in conventional cell culture using human diploid fibroblasts or Vero monkey kidney cells, and recently centrifugation-culture using shell vials seeded with human embryonic kidney cells and staining with monoclonal antibodies to the T antigen of simian virus 40 has been shown to provide rapid detection of BK virus in urine specimens (38).

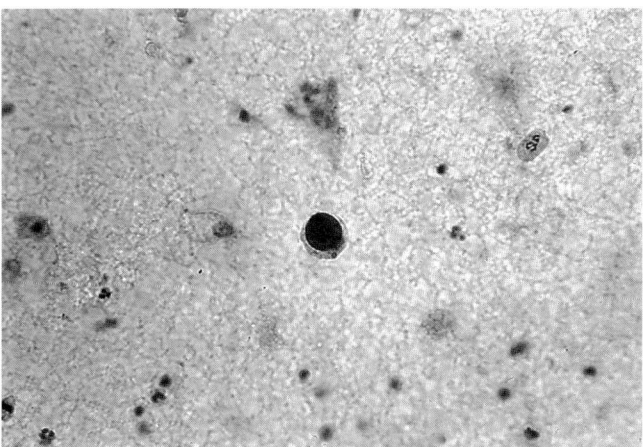

Fig. 7–6. Intranuclear inclusion in a cytocentrifuge preparation of urine sediment stained with the Papanicolaou stain is suggestive of infection with BK virus (×128).

TREATMENT AND PREVENTION

Warts spontaneously disappear after many months to years, but they can be removed surgically by cryotherapy or electrocautery, by applying podophyllin or salicylic acid with formalin or glutaraldehyde, or by injecting interferon. The best way to prevent warts is to avoid direct contact with infected tissue.

No specific treatment is available for PML. One patient with AIDS and biopsy-proven PML appeared to respond to therapy with zidovudine (39).

REFERENCES

1. Pfister H: Papovaviridae: The papillomaviruses. In Laboratory Diagnosis of Infectious Diseases Principles and Practice. Vol II. Edited by EH Lennette, P Halonen, and FA Murphy. New York, Springer-Verlag, 1988.
2. Franchesci S, et al: Genital warts and cervical neoplasm: An epidemiological study. Br J Cancer, 48:621, 1983.
3. Graham S, et al: Genital cancer in wives of penile cancer patients. Cancer, 44:1870, 1979.
4. Fraumeni JF, et al: Cancer mortality among nuns: Role of the marital status in etiology of neoplastic disease in women. J Natl Cancer Inst, 42:455, 1969.
5. zur Hausen H: Genital papillomavirus infections. Prog Med Virol, 32:15, 1985.
6. Goldschmidt H, and Klingman AM: Experimental inoculation of humans with ectodermotropic viruses. J Invest Dermatol, 31:175, 1958.
7. Kirchner H: Immunobiology of human papillomavirus infection. Prog Med Virol, 33:1, 1986.
8. Matis WL, et al: Dermatologic findings associated with human immunodeficiency virus infection. J Am Acad Dermatol, 17:746, 1987.
9. Boyle J, et al: Cancer, warts, and sunshine in renal transplant patients. A case-control study. Lancet, i:702, 1986.
10. Sillman F, et al: The relationship between human papillomavirus and lower genital intraepithelial neoplasm in immunosuppressed women. Am J Obstet Gynecol, 150:300, 1984.
11. Durst M, et al: Molecular and cytogenetic analysis of immortalized human primary keratinocytes obtained after transfection with human papilloma virus type 16 DNA. Oncogene, 1:251, 1987.
12. Kaur P, and McDougall JK: Characterization of primary human keratinocytes transformed by human papillomavirus type 18. J Virol, 62:1917, 1988.
13. Shirasawa H, et al: Integration and transcription of human papillomavirus type 16 and 18 sequences in cell lines derived from cervical carcinomas. J Gen Virol, 68:583, 1987.
14. Stoler MH, and Broker TR: In situ hybridization detection of human papillomavirus DNAs and messenger RNAs in genital condylomas and a cervical carcinoma. Hum Pathol, 17:1250, 1986.
15. Fuchs PG, Girardi F, and Pfister H: Human papillomavirus DNA in normal, metaplastic, preneoplastic and neoplastic epithelia of the cervix uteri. Int J Cancer, 41:41, 1988.
16. Fuchs PG, Girardi F, and Pfister H: Human papillomavirus 16 DNA in cervical cancers and in lymph nodes of cervical cancer patients; a diagnostic marker for early metastases? Int J Cancer, 43:41, 1989.
17. Baker CC, et al: Structural and transcriptional analysis of human papillomavirus type 16 sequences in cervical carcinoma cell lines. J Virol, 61:962, 1987
18. Schwarz E, et al: Structure and transcription of human papillomavirus sequences in cervical carcinoma cells. Nature, 314:111, 1985.
19. Spalholz BA, Zang Y-C, and Howley PM: Transactivation of a bovine papillomavirus transcriptional regulatory element by the E2 gene product. Cell, 42:183, 1985.
20. Lambert PF, Spalholz BA, and Howley PM: A transcriptional repressor encoded by BPV-1 shares a common carboxy terminal domain with the E2 transactivator. Cell, 50:68, 1987.
21. Thierry F, and Yaniv M: The BPV1-E2 trans-acting protein can be either an activator or a repressor of the HPV 18 regulatory region. EMBO J, 6:3391, 1987.
22. Cripe TP, et al: Transcription regulation of the human papillomavirus-16 E6-E7 promoter by a keratinocyte-dependent enhancer, and by viral E2 trans-activator and repressor gene products: implications for cervical carcinogenesis. EMBO J, 6:3745, 1987.
23. Gardner SD, et al: New human papovavirus (BK) isolated from urine after renal transplantation. Lancet, i:1253, 1971.
24. Padgett BL, and Walker DL: Prevalence of antibodies in human sera against JC virus, an isolate from a case of progressive multifocal leukoencephalopathy. J Infect Dis, 127:467, 1973.
25. Brown P, Tsai T, and Gajdusek C: Seroepidemiology of human papovaviruses. Am J Epidemiol, 102:331, 1975.
26. Hogan TF, et al: Human polyomavirus infections with JC virus and BK virus in renal transplant patients. Ann Intern Med, 92:373, 1980.
27. Grinnell BW, Padgett BL, and Walker DL: Distribution of nonintegrated DNA from JC papovavirus in organs of patients with progressive multifocal leukoencephalopathy. J Infect Dis, 147:669, 1983.
28. Houff SA, et al: Involvement of JC virus–infected mononuclear cells from the bone marrow and spleen in the pathogenesis of progressive multifocal leukoencephalopathy. N Engl J Med, 318:301, 1988.
29. Kitamura T, et al: High incidence of urinary JC virus excretion in nonimmunosuppressed older patients. J Infect Dis, 161:1128, 1990.
30. Arthur RR, Shah KV, Charache P, and Saral R: BK and JC virus infections in recipients of bone marrow transplants. J Infect Dis, 158:563, 1988.
31. Gardner SD, MacKenzie EFD, Smith C, and Porter AA: Prospective study of the human polyomaviruses BK and JC and cytomegalovirus in renal transplant recipients. J Clin Pathol, 37:578, 1984.
32. Takemoto KK, et al: Isolation of papovavirus from brain tumor and urine of a patient with Wiskott-Aldrich syndrome. J Natl Cancer Inst, 53:1205, 1974.
33. Corallini A, et al: Association of BK virus with human brain tumors and tumors of pancreatic islets. Int J Cancer, 39:60, 1987.
34. Weiner LP, et al: Isolation of virus related to SV40 from patients with progressive multifocal leukoencephalopathy. N Engl J Med, 286:385, 1972.
35. Beckmann AM, et al: Detection and localization of human papillomavirus DNA in human genital condylomas by in situ hybridization with biotinylated probes. J Med Virol, 16:265, 1985.
36. Gupta J, et al: Specific identification of human papillomavirus type in cervical smears and paraffin sections by in situ hybridization with radioactive probes: A preliminary communication. Int J Gynecol Pathol, 4:211, 1985.
37. Shibata DK, Arnheim N, and Martin WJ: Detection of human papillomavirus in paraffin-embedded tissue using the polymerase chain reaction. J Exp Med, 167:225, 1988.
38. Marshall WF, et al: Rapid detection of polyomavirus BK by a shell vial cell culture assay. J Clin Microbiol, 28:1613, 1990.
39. Conway B, Halliday WC, and Brunham RC: Human immunodeficiency virus–associated progressive multifocal leukoencephalopathy: Apparent response to 3′-azido-3′-deoxythymidine. Rev Infect Dis, 12:479, 1990.

Chapter 8

PARVOVIRUSES

Parvoviruses, the smallest of all viruses, infect many animals and insects, but only the medically important members are discussed here. In this chapter, an overview of the classification, structure, and replication of the parvoviruses is presented, and parvovirus B19 and the adeno-associated viruses are discussed.

CLASSIFICATION

Parvoviruses belong to the family Parvoviridae, which has three genera: Parvovirus, Dependovirus, and Densovirus. Members of the first two genera infect a wide range of warm-blooded animals, and densoviruses infect insects. Parvovirus B19 is a member of the genus Parvovirus, and adeno-associated viruses belong to the genus Dependovirus.

STRUCTURE AND REPLICATION

The 18- to 26-nm diameter nonenveloped parvovirus virions consist of an icosahedral 32-capsomere capsid surrounding a single-stranded linear DNA genome. The latter has a molecular weight of 1.5 to 2 million and codes for three structural and one nonstructural protein. Most virions contain negative-sense DNA, but in occasional virions the DNA has positive sense. Virions require at least one cellular function generated during the late S or early G2 phase of the mitotic cycle for replication and therefore multiply preferentially in actively dividing cells such as erythroid precursors. Transcription, replication, and assembly occur in the host cell nucleus, and virions are released following degeneration of the nuclear and cytoplasmic membranes.

PARVOVIRUS B19

Parvovirus B19 was discovered in 1974 by Cossart and his colleagues, who were evaluating tests to detect hepatitis B virus surface antigen (1). Electron microscopic examination of serum samples that were positive for hepatitis B surface antigen by counterimmunoelectrophoresis but negative by the more sensitive reverse passive hemagglutination technique revealed 23-nm diameter virus particles morphologically similar to parvoviruses. In 1981, infection with parvovirus B19 was associated with aplastic crisis in persons with sickle cell anemia, and in 1984 it was shown to be responsible for erythema infectiosum (2,3).

Epidemiology

Respiratory droplet spread probably is the natural route of transmission of parvovirus B19, and parenteral transmission by transfusion of blood-clotting factor concentrates has been documented (4). Outbreaks among school-aged children are common, especially in late winter and spring, and secondary attack rates in schools and families are high. Serologic surveys indicate that up to 65% of adults have antibodies to parvovirus B19.

Pathogenesis

Susceptible volunteers infected by intranasal inoculation with parvovirus B19 in the laboratory develop transient viremia and begin shedding virus in respiratory secretions 6 to 8 days after challenge; both signs persist 4 to 7 days (5). Virions initiate a lytic infection in erythrocyte precursors, causing reticulocytopenia and a steadily declining hemoglobin concentration of about 0.2g/dl per day for 7 to 10 days. Moderate lymphopenia, thrombocytopenia, and neutropenia also develop but are not clinically important. During the viremia, patients experience fever, malaise, myalgias, and chills, lasting 1 to 4 days. Specific immunoglobulin (Ig) M and G, detected soon after the onset of viremia, are associated with the return of circulating reticulocytes. Some 17 or 18 days after virus challenge a maculopapular rash develops that is accompanied by arthralgias and joint swelling. The mechanism is probably an interaction between the virus and the host immune response, such as immune complex formation. The rash fades in 2 to 3 days, and the joint symptoms subside a few days later.

Clinical Manifestations

The most common presentation of natural infection with parvovirus B19 is erythema infectiosum, a mild, self-limited illness of children 4 to 15 years of age, manifested after a 1- to 2-week incubation period by a facial rash with a "slapped-cheek" appearance accompanied by or followed in 1 to 4 days by a morbilliform, annular, or confluent rash on the extremities. The rash generally resolves in about a week, but late in the illness it may come and go. Up to 25% of children have mild fever, headache, sore throat, and abdominal pain. A prominent feature of natural infection in adults, especially women, is arthropathy without rash. Any joint may be affected, but the wrist, hand, knee, and ankle are involved most often (6,7). Symptoms usually resolve in several weeks but may persist months to years.

Infection with parvovirus B19 may cause aplastic crisis in persons who have chronic hemolytic anemias such as sickle cell disease, hereditary spherocytosis, pyruvate kinase deficiency, and β thalassemia intermedia by infecting and destroying erythroid precursors in the bone marrow (8). Parvovirus B19 acquired during pregnancy may be transmitted to the fetus, producing a persistent fetal infection with anemia and subsequent congestive heart failure, generalized edema (hydrops fetalis), and death. This, however, is rare; maternal infection with parvovirus B19 usually does not cause fetal demise (9,10). In immunocompromised persons, infection with parvovirus B19 may become chronic, causing continuous lysis of red blood cell precursors and, eventually, severe, persistent anemia (11–14). During the infection the level of viremia fluctuates, and intermittent fever and rheumatic symptoms remit and recur.

ADENO-ASSOCIATED VIRUSES

Five serotypes of human adeno-associated viruses have been described: serotypes 1 through 4 were recovered from throat or feces, and serotype 5 from a genital papilloma. These defective viruses require coinfection of cells with adenovirus to replicate, although herpes viruses and vaccinia virus also can provide a helper function. Adeno-associated viruses contain a single-stranded DNA genome of molecular weight 1.4 million that is integrated into the host cell's genome, where it persists indefinitely. These viruses have not yet been associated with any disease, but data from seroepidemiologic surveys indicate that most people are infected by 10 years of age (15).

Laboratory Diagnosis

Infection with parvovirus B19 is diagnosed by detecting the virus or specific antibodies in serum. Currently, diagnostic tests are not commercially available, in part because the virus has not been cultivated in conventional systems. The most useful diagnostic test, performed only in special reference laboratories, is the detection, by radioimmunoassay or enzyme-linked immunosorbent assay, of specific IgM, which is present early in the illness, declines 1 to 2 months after the onset, and generally disappears 2 to 3 months later. During viremia, the virus can be detected in serum by radioimmunoassay, enzyme-linked immunosorbent assay or polymerase chain reaction (16–18). The latter may be required to diagnose B19 infection in immunocompromised persons because antibody assays are not diagnostic in this population.

Infection with parvovirus B19 causes specific changes in the bone marrow of persons with aplastic crisis and in the tissues of congenitally infected fetuses (19,20). In bone marrow the number of erythroid precursors is significantly decreased, and those that are present show megaloblastoid changes with intranuclear alterations (called lantern cells). Nuclei are eosinophilic, enlarged, ballooned, and have marginal inclusions. Identical-looking erythroblasts are found in many tissues of congenitally infected fetuses, predominantly in the small capillaries but also in the stroma of the liver, spleen, and bone marrow. Localization of parvovirus B19 in the lantern cells can be demonstrated by immunohistochemistry and in situ hybridization (20).

Infection with adeno-associated viruses is diagnosed serologically. This test is not available commercially and must be performed in a reference laboratory.

Treatment and Prevention

No antiviral agent effective against the parvoviruses is available. Transient aplastic crisis caused by parvovirus B19 in persons with chronic hemolytic anemia may require transfusion. Intravenous immunoglobulin therapy may control or cure persistent infection in immunocompromised persons (13,19). Immunoglobulin might be effective prophylaxis for an exposed pregnant woman and treatment of the infected fetus; however, this requires further study.

REFERENCES

1. Cossart YE, Cant B, Field AM, and Widdows D: Parvovirus-like particles in human sera. Lancet, *i*:72, 1975.
2. Pattison JR, et al: Parvovirus infections and hypoplastic crises in sickle cell anaemia. Lancet, *i*:664, 1981.
3. Anderson MJ, et al: An outbreak of erythema infectiosum associated with human parvovirus infection. J Hyg Camb, *92*:85, 1984.
4. Mortimer PP, Luban NLC, and Kelleher JF: Transmission of serum parvovirus-like virus by clotting factor concentrates. Lancet, *ii*:482, 1983.
5. Anderson MJ, et al: Experimental parvoviral infection in humans. J Infect Dis, *152*:257, 1985.
6. White DG, et al: Human parvovirus arthropathy. Lancet, *i*:419, 1985.
7. Reid DM, et al: Human parvovirus–associated arthritis: A clinical and laboratory description. Lancet, *i*:422, 1985.
8. Serjeant GR, and Goldstein AR: B19 virus infection and aplastic crisis. *In* Parvoviruses and Human Disease. Edited by JR Pattison. Boca Raton, FL, CRC Press, 1988.
9. Centers for Disease Control: Risks associated with human parvovirus B19 infection. MMWR, *38*:81, 1989.
10. Kinney JS, et al: Risk of adverse outcomes of pregnancy after human parvovirus B19 infection. J Infect Dis, *157*:663, 1988.
11. Kurtzman GJ, et al: Chronic bone marrow failure due to persistent B19 parvovirus infection. N Engl J Med, *317*:287, 1987.
12. Van Horn DK, Mortimer PP, Young N, and Hanson GR: Human parvovirus–associated red cell aplasia in the absence of underlying hemolytic anemia. Am J Pediatr Hematol Oncol, *8*:235, 1986.
13. Kurtzman G, et al: Pure red-cell aplasia of ten years' duration due to persistent parvovirus B19 infection and its cure with immunoglobulin therapy. N Engl J Med, *321*:519, 1989.
14. Weiland HT, et al: Prolonged parvovirus B19 infection with severe anaemia in a bone marrow transplant recipient [letter]. Br J Haematol, *71*:300, 1989.
15. Parks WP, et al: Seroepidemiological and ecological studies of the adenovirus associated satellite viruses. Infect Immun, *2*:716, 1970.
16. Salimans MMM, et al: Rapid detection of human parvovirus B19 DNA by dot hybridization and the polymerase chain reaction. J Virol Methods, *23*:19, 1989.
17. Anderson MJ, Jones SE, and Minson AC: Diagnosis of human parvovirus infection by dot-blot hybridization using cloned viral DNA. J Med Virol, *15*:163, 1985.
18. Anderson LJ: Human parvoviruses. J Infect Dis, *161*:603, 1990.
19. Frickhofen N, et al: Persistent B19 parvovirus infection in patients infected with human immunodeficiency virus type 1 (HIV-1): A treatable cause of anemia. Ann Intern Med, *113*:926, 1990.
20. Schwartz TF, et al: Parvovirus B19 infection of the fetus. Histology and in situ hybridization. Am J Clin Pathol, *96*:121, 1991.

Chapter 9

HEPATITIS B VIRUS AND THE DELTA AGENT

Human hepatitis B virus (HBV) is a member of the Hepadnaviridae, adopted as a new family in 1984. Delta hepatitis virus, an RNA virus not yet classified, also is discussed in this chapter because it requires HBV for replication and possesses an envelope composed of hepatitis B surface antigen (HBsAg).

HEPATITIS B VIRUS

The first component of HBV was detected in 1965, when Blumberg discovered an antigen in the serum of an Australian aborigine that reacted with antibodies in sera of American hemophiliacs who had received multiple blood transfusions (1). That antigen, subsequently named the Australia antigen, has since been identified as HBsAg.

Structure

Two types of HBV particles exist (Fig. 9–1): (1) incomplete viral envelope particles, small heterogeneous spheres (22-nm particles) and filaments 22 nm wide and up to several hundred nanometers long consisting of protein, carbohydrate, and lipid without nucleic acid, and (2) the complete hepatitis B virion, termed the Dane particle, which is a 42-nm diameter enveloped sphere with an electron-dense, 28-nm spherical nucleocapsid composed of a partially double-stranded circular DNA genome with a molecular weight of about 2 million (2,3). The single-stranded portion of the DNA varies in size, comprising some 15 to 60% of the total length of the genome. It is repaired by viral DNA polymerase to make a completely double-stranded molecule of 300 base pairs. Four open reading frames in the complete strand of the genome have been identified: S specifies the major surface antigen–reactive polypeptide and C the major polypeptide and the virion core, P likely encodes viral DNA polymerase, and X encodes a protein that can transactivate some heterologous viral and cellular transcriptional control sequences but its role in HBV replication is unknown.

HBsAg, found in the envelope of the Dane particle and on the surface of the spherical and filamentous 22-nm particles, has at least five antigenic specificities: a group-specific determinant (a) shared by all HBsAg preparations and two pairs of subtype determinants (d, y and w, r) that usually behave as alleles. Antigenic heterogeneity of the (w) determinant and determinants named q, x, and g have been described (4, 5). Eight HBsAg subtypes: ayw, ayw2, ayw3, ayw4, ayr, adw2, adw4, and adr have been identified, and individual isolates of HBV subtypes awr, adwr, adyw, adyr, and adywr have been reported from the Far East (5).

The HBV core or nucleocapsid bearing the hepatitis B core antigen (HBcAg) circulates only as an internal component of HBV virions. Hepatitis B e antigen (HBeAg) is a soluble antigen contained in a cleavage product of the viral core, and its presence in the serum correlates with high concentrations of infectious HBV, indicating that HBV virions and HBeAg are produced together.

Replication

Replication of HBV is initiated by attachment of a portion of the HBsAg complex to unique receptors on the surface of hepatocytes (and perhaps pancreatic cells) (6). After penetrating into the cell, the nucleocapsid and genome are delivered to the nucleus, where replication ensues. The entire HBV genome may be integrated into host cellular DNA. The significance of this to viral replication is unknown, but integrated HBV DNA is present is some hepatocellular carcinomas (7).

Epidemiology

Worldwide, up to 200 million people, or about 5% of the population, have chronic HBV infection. The prevalence of infection with HBV and the mode of transmission vary in different parts of the world. In the United States, Western Europe, and Australia, where infection with HBV occurs primarily in adults, 0.2 to 0.5% of the population is chronically infected. Of the estimated 300,000 persons infected with HBV in the United States each year, 25% become ill with jaundice, more than 10,000 require hospitalization, 6 to 10% develop persistent infection, and an average of 250 die from fulminant disease. The incidence of reported acute hepatitis B in the United States peaked in 1985 (about 12 cases per 100,000 population), despite the availability of hepatitis B vaccine since 1982, and decreased by 18% in 1988 though it was still higher than it had been in 1978 (8).

According to data from serologic surveys, infection caused by HBV is uncommon among the general adult population of the United States but is highly prevalent in certain risk groups (Table 9–1), especially homosexually active men, heterosexual partners of persons with acute hepatitis B or of HBV carriers (described later), and intravenous drug users (9). Prior to 1986 homosexual males were the single largest group infected with HBV in the United States, but in recent years, the proportion of cases reported in this group decreased from about 20 to 10% (10). In contrast, the proportion of reported cases due to heterosexual transmission has increased to 22%. Intravenous drug users account for 28% of reported cases of hepatitis B, and in about one third of cases no source of infection is identified. For all persons aged 12 to 74 years

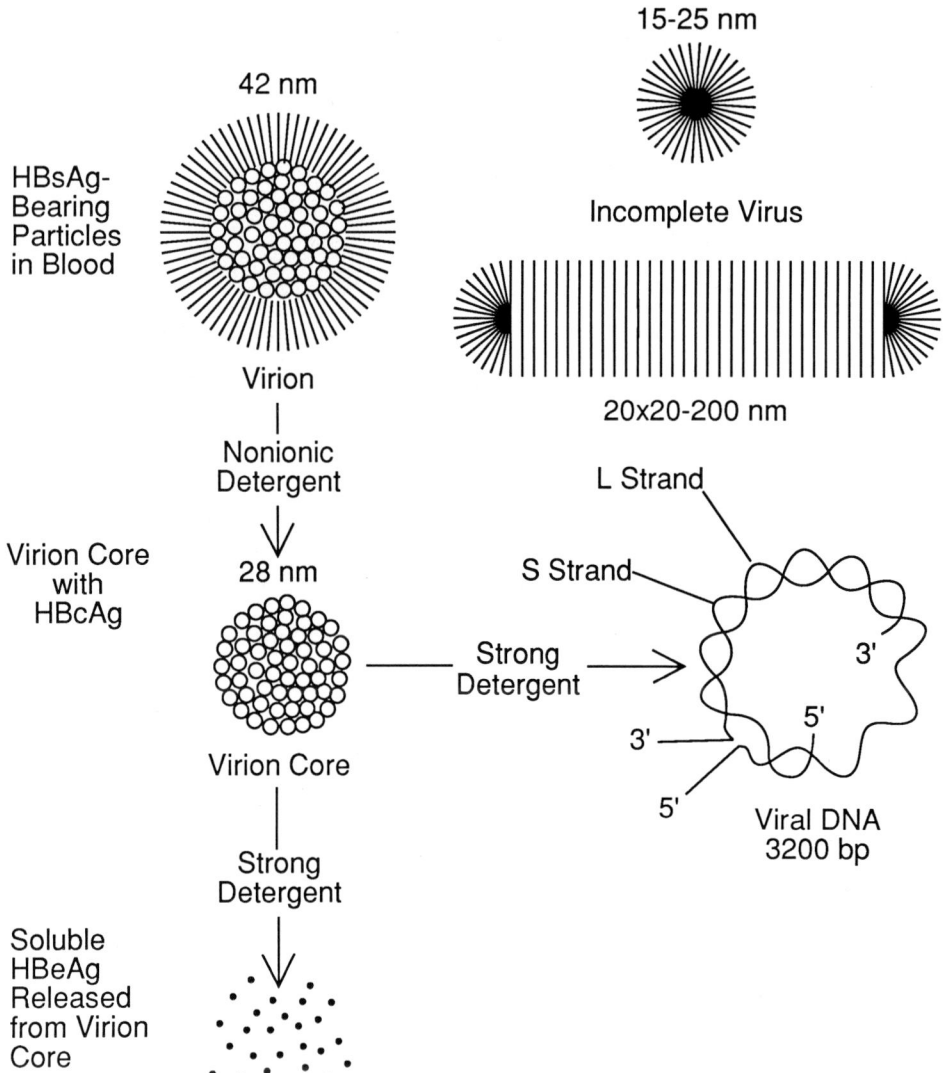

Fig. 9–1. Size and structure of different types of hepatitis B virus particles. (From Hollinger FB, Melnick JL, and Robinson WS: Viral Hepatitis: Biological and Clinical Features, Specific Diagnosis, and Prophylaxis. New York, Raven, 1985.)

rates of HBV seropositivity, among males and females, are significantly higher for blacks than for whites (Fig. 9–2) (11).

In China, Southeast Asia, much of Africa, most Pacific Islands, parts of the Middle East, and the Amazon Basin, infection with HBV is highly endemic: 8 to 15% of the population are chronically infected. In the Far East, the predominant mode of spread of HBV is perinatal transmission, principally from mothers who are HBV carriers or mothers who develop acute hepatitis B during the third trimester of pregnancy or the early postpartum period. Although the precise mechanism of perinatal transmission is unknown, evidence suggests that infection occurs at or just after delivery and that transplacental infection is uncommon. The likelihood of transmission is not reduced by cesarean section or by refraining from breast-feeding, but the rate of vertical transmission of HBV from mothers with antibodies to HBeAg is significantly lower than from "HBeAg-positive" mothers (12). In areas of Africa where HBV is endemic perinatal transmission may be less efficient, because infection is acquired most frequently in early childhood, possibly from close contact with infected siblings and playmates.

Humans are the only important source of HBV. The major reservoir of infection is the HBV carrier, a person who is HBsAg positive at least twice when tested at minimal intervals of 6 months or HBsAg-positive without detectable immunoglobulin (Ig)M against HBcAg when a single serum specimen is tested; but those with acute hepatitis B are a potential source of infection. The virus is transmitted via percutaneous or permucosal contact with serum, saliva, or semen containing infectious HBV (13,14). HBsAg has been found in urine, bile, sweat, tears, breast milk, vaginal secretions, and cerebrospinal and synovial fluid, but infection rarely, if ever, is transmitted by contact with these fluids. Rather, it is acquired by contact with infective blood or body fluids at birth, through sexual contact, by contaminated needles, and in situations of continuous close personal contact, as occur in households or among children in institutions for developmentally dis-

Table 9-1. Prevalence of Hepatitis B Virus (HBV) Serologic Markers in Various Population Groups

Population Group	Prevalence of Serologic Markers of HBV Infection	
	HBsAg (%)	Any Marker (%)
Immigrants/refugees from areas of high HBV endemicity	13	70–85
Alaskan natives/Pacific Islanders	5–15	40–70
Clients in institutions for developmentally disabled persons	10–20	35–80
Users of illicit parenteral drugs	7	60–80
Sexually active homosexual men	6	35–80
Household contacts of HBV carriers	3–6	30–60
Patients of hemodialysis units	3–10	20–80
Health care workers who have frequent blood contact	1–2	15–30
Prisoners (male)	1–8	10–80
Staff of institutions for the developmentally disabled	1	10–25
Heterosexuals with multiple partners	0.5	5–20
Health care workers who have infrequent blood contact or none	0.3	3–10
General population		
Blacks	0.9	14
Whites	0.2	3

(From Centers for Disease Control: Protection against viral hepatitis. MMWR, 39(S-2):1, 1990.)

abled persons, presumably by inapparent contact of infective secretions with skin lesions or mucosal surfaces (15). Transmission via transfusion of blood or blood products is uncommon where donors are routinely screened. HBV is infrequently transmitted by infected health care workers to patients, and never via the fecal-oral route (16,17).

Pathogenesis

The mechanism of hepatocyte injury during infection with HBV is unknown, but the host immune system is probably involved. Given that viral replication not cytopathic and continues for long periods without producing liver damage or symptoms, the virus alone is probably not responsible for the liver cell injury. Of the two arms of the immune system, the humoral response specific for HBV antigens probably does not induce hepatic injury, because persons with agammaglobulinemia may develop severe acute or chronic hepatitis (18). However, data suggest that the cellular immune response, especially that directed against HBcAg, may be responsible for the hepatic injury (19,20). Extrahepatic manifestations of infection with HBV, such as the serum sickness-like syndrome (fever, rash, urticaria, and arthralgias or arthritis), periarteritis nodosa, and membranous glomerulonephritis, are due to immune complex formation.

Host and viral factors appear to influence the development of persistent infection with HBV. The likelihood of infection becoming chronic varies inversely with the age at which it is acquired: as many as 90% of infants infected at birth, 25 to 50% of children infected before age 5 years, and 6 to 10% of adults become carriers. An association has been reported between persistent infection and certain HLA types, but it is not confirmed (21,22). The increased prevalence of HBV carriers among persons undergoing renal dialysis and those with Down's syndrome, lepromatous leprosy, and chronic lymphocytic leukemia suggests that immunosuppression may be a risk factor (23,24). Persistent infection more frequently follows initial anicteric than initial icteric disease; and in chimpanzees infected with HBV in the laboratory, a smaller inoculum results in chronic infection more often than a larger one (25).

Clinical Manifestations

Approximately one third of adults infected with HBV are asymptomatic, about a third have a mild flulike illness without jaundice that probably is not diagnosed as hepatitis, and the remainder have the symptoms and signs described below. In young children, infection with HBV al-

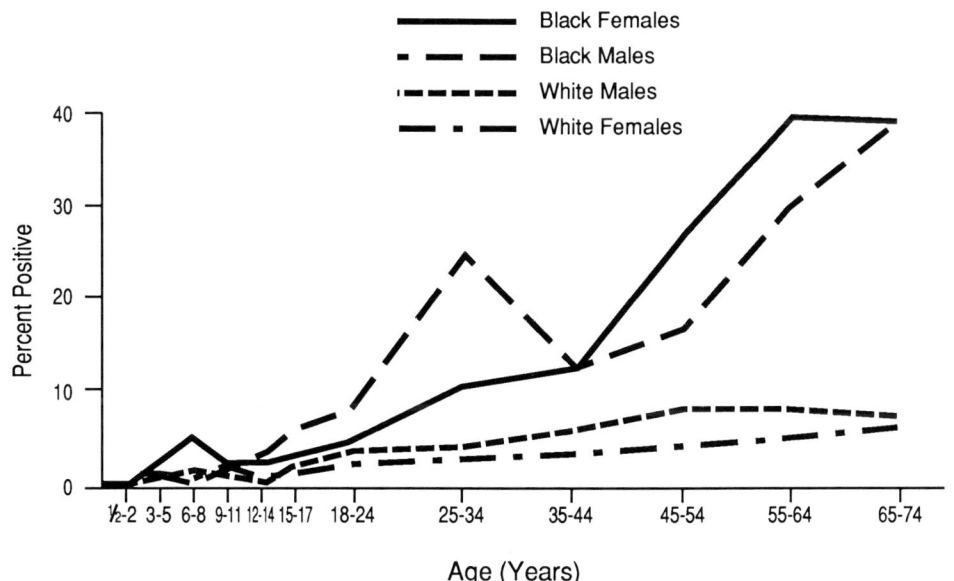

Fig. 9-2. Age-specific prevalence of hepatitis B virus markers by race, sex, and age in the United States, 1976–1980. (From Centers for Disease Control: Racial differences in rates of hepatitis B virus infection—United States, 1976–1980. MMWR, 38:818, 1989.)

most always is asymptomatic and, therefore, unlikely to be diagnosed.

Symptomatic infection with HBV typically begins insidiously after an incubation period of 4 to 28 weeks (60 to 110 days is usual). Headache, malaise, anorexia, nausea, vomiting, abdominal discomfort or right side upper quadrant pain, fever, and chills are followed in 2 to 7 days by jaundice, dark urine, and light or clay-colored stools. Among persons with icteric disease, 10 to 20% have a serum sickness–like illness with an erythematous maculopapular rash, urticaria, arthralgias, and occasionally arthritis and fever several days to weeks before liver disease becomes clinically apparent. Children usually recover in 2 weeks, and adults in 4 to 6 weeks.

Laboratory abnormalities include a significant elevation in serum transaminase activity that peaks in the first week of symptoms and gradually returns to normal as the illness subsides, and a bilirubin value that increases for 10 to 14 days and then gradually drops over 2 to 4 weeks. Mild anemia, relative lymphocytosis, mild proteinuria, and mildly elevated alkaline phosphatase activity also may occur. Urobilinogen and bilirubin are found in the urine before jaundice and the concentrations decrease as jaundice progresses.

The appearance in the serum of the markers of HBV infection during asymptomatic and acute self-limited symptomatic disease is shown in Figure 9-3 (26). HBsAg, indicative of active infection, is detected in the serum between 1 and 12 weeks after exposure to HBV and persists 1 to 6 weeks. Clinical evidence of hepatitis follows the appearance of HBsAg by 1 to 7 weeks (mean 4 weeks), and as symptoms and jaundice resolve the HBsAg titer drops until several weeks later it is indetectable. HBeAg usually appears simultaneously or within a few days after the appearance of HBsAg, peaks and falls in parallel with HBsAg, and disappears just before HBsAg disappears. Concurrent with or soon after the disappearance of HBeAg, antibodies specific for the e antigen (anti-HBe) are detected and persist 1 to 2 years.

Antibodies specific for the core antigen (anti-HBc) appear 3 to 5 weeks after HBsAg is detected and before hepatitis is clinically apparent. The anti-HBc titer rises during the period when HBsAg is detectable, levels off, and eventually falls after HBsAg disappears, dropping three- to fourfold in the first year and more slowly over the next 5 years. Most of the anti-HBc is IgG, but IgM specific for the core is detected in most persons with acute hepatitis B. The anti-HBc IgM titer falls rapidly in about 40% of cases of acute self-limited hepatitis B, declines more slowly in the remaining 60%, and is still positive in 2 years in about 20% (27).

In most persons with self-limited hepatitis B, antibodies specific for HBsAg (anti-HBs) appear some time after HBsAg disappears from the blood and persist for years, protecting against reinfection. In the 10 to 20% of persons who develop arthritis and rash associated with immune complex formation, anti-HBs and HBsAg circulate simultaneously. In approximately 50% of cases anti-HBs does not appear for several months (the "window") after the disappearance of HBsAg, and in about 10% of persons with transient antigenemia it is never detected.

Some asymptomatic persons with serologic evidence of acute self-limited primary hepatitis B never have detectable levels of HBsAg in their blood. Antibodies to the surface antigen typically appear 4 to 12 weeks after exposure to HBV, and IgM and IgG directed against the core are detected in low titer and may disappear sooner than in persons with "surface antigenemia."

Variants of hepatitis B include fulminant infection and persistent disease. Fulminant hepatitis, a severe, frequently fatal illness accompanied by hepatic failure with encephalopathy, develops in a small proportion of cases. In 3 to 5% of persons with acute icteric hepatitis the abnormal laboratory findings and mild symptoms persist beyond 3 to 4 months. About 5 to 10% of acutely infected persons, especially those who are positive for HBeAg for 10 weeks or more, develop chronic persistent or chronic active hepatitis. Persistent infection is most often asymptomatic, whereas chronic active hepatitis may be associated with jaundice, development of cirrhosis, and increased risk (12 to 300 times) of hepatocellular carcinoma.

Serologic markers of persistent HBV infection are shown in Figure 9–4 (28). Persons who exhibit this pattern, termed chronic carriers, by definition test positive for HBsAg, though there is evidence that a small fraction of persons with persistent infection do not have detectable surface antigen (29). Complete virions (Dane particles), DNA polymerase activity, HBcAg, or virion DNA can be detected in the blood of many persistently infected persons, and almost all have high serum titers of IgG and IgM directed against the core antigen (30–32). Using sensitive assays, 25 to 50% of carriers have detectable HBeAg in blood, and antibodies against the e antigen are present in the remainder; but with less sensitive assays about 50% of carriers are seronegative for both of these markers. In

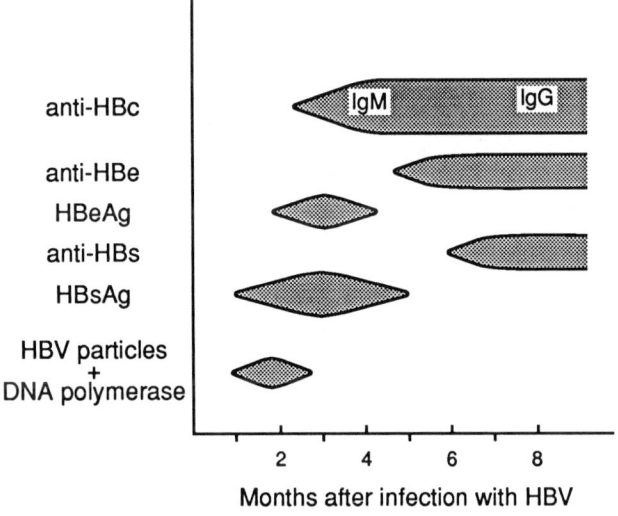

Fig. 9–3. Appearance of serologic markers of hepatitis B virus–induced infection during acute disease. Key: HBsAg, hepatitis B surface antigen; anti-HBs, antibody against hepatitis B surface antigen; anti-HBc, antibody against hepatitis B core antigen; HBe, hepatitis B e antigen; anti-HBe, antibody against hepatitis B e antigen.

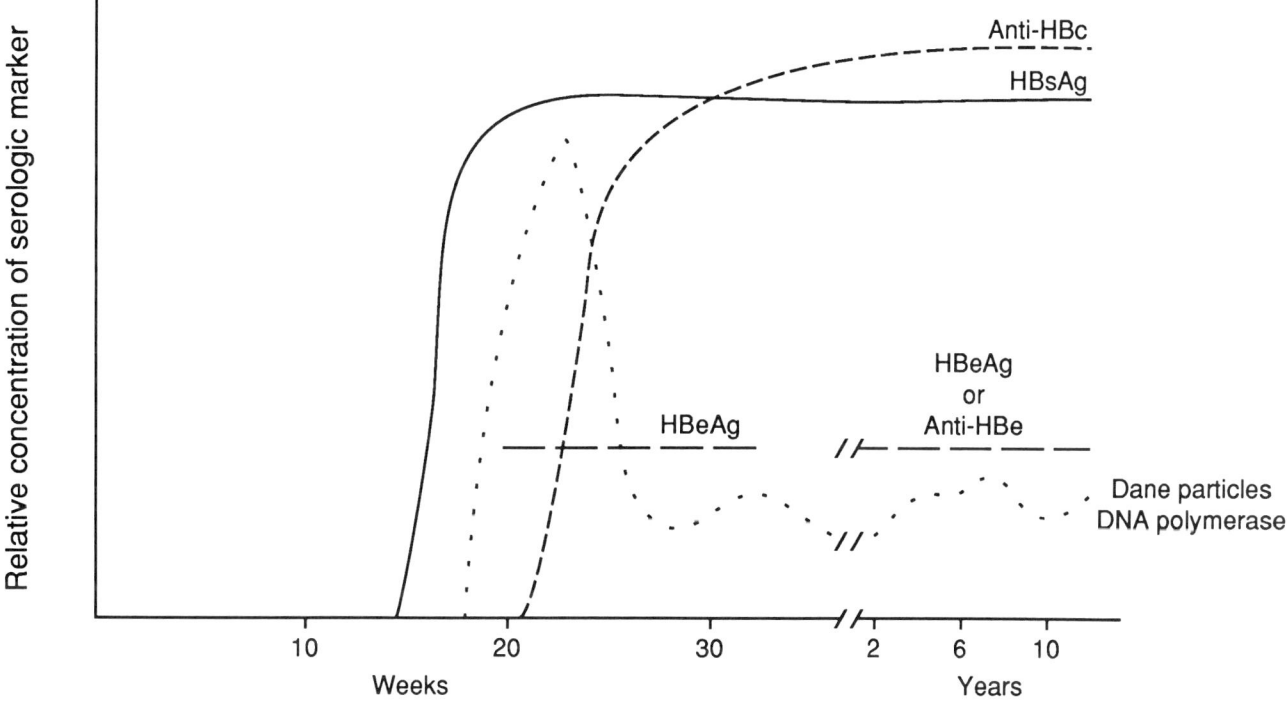

Fig. 9–4. Diagram of serologic markers of hepatitis B virus–induced infection that becomes persistent. Key: HBsAg, hepatitis B surface antigen; anti-HBs, antibody against hepatitis B surface antigen; anti-HBc, antibody against hepatitis B core antigen; HBe, hepatitis B e antigen; anti-HBe, antibody against hepatitis B e antigen.

general, persons with the highest titers of infectious virus and detectable virion DNA polymerase activity, HBeAg, or both have the highest HBsAg titers. Moreover, the highest titers of infectious virus are found in those with HBeAg, virion DNA polymerase activity, or both.

Anti-HBs is not detected in the serum of chronic carriers; however, HBsAg–anti-HBs complexes may form in these persons, suggesting that, at least in some carriers, anti-HBs is produced despite persistent infection (33). The long-term natural history of persistent infection with HBV is unknown, but such infections have subsided spontaneously over months to years, with slowly falling HBsAg and HBeAg titers and virion DNA polymerase activity (34–37).

HEPATITIS δ VIRUS

The hepatitis δ virus antigen (HDAg) was discovered in Italy in 1977 by immunofluorescent staining of hepatocytes of some carriers of HBsAg (38). Hepatitis δ virus is a defective virus that requires intercurrent infection with HBV for replication and expression. Delta virus (HDV) virions are composed of a core of HDAg, a 68,000-dalton protein, and a small, single-stranded, circular RNA genome surrounded by an envelope containing HBsAg. Serologic surveys show a high prevalence of antibodies specific for HDAg (anti-HD) in residents of southern Italy and other Mediterranean regions, especially North Africa (39–41). In the United States the prevalence of anti-HD is low in the general population but high among intravenous drug users and hemophiliacs, and in one study seroprevalence was high among residents of a facility for developmentally disabled persons (42–45).

Simultaneous infection with HBV and δ viruses may result in severe or fulminant hepatitis more frequently than infection with HBV alone; however, in areas where the prevalence of the δ agent is low, the agent generally is not an important factor in the progression to fulminant hepatitis (46,47). In geographic regions where the prevalence of HDV infection is high HDV plays a significant role in the development of chronic liver disease and in the rate of progression to cirrhosis (48–50).

Laboratory Diagnosis

Infections with HBV alone and with HBV and the δ agent are diagnosed by measuring viral antigens or antibodies specific for those antigens in the serum. The stage of infection with HBV is determined by the pattern of HBV serologic markers (Table 9–2). Sensitive test kits (commercially available) for detection of HBsAg, HBeAg, antibodies to the surface, core, and e antigens; and IgM to the core antigen are specific for infection with HBV. Recently, a probe for detection of HBV DNA in serum became commercially available, but studies of its diagnostic usefulness are few (51). A sensitive, commercially available test for detection of antibodies against δ virus antigen is diagnostically useful for identifying persons infected with HDV.

Table 9–2. Serologic Markers of Hepatitis B Virus Detected During Infection

Condition	Marker
Incubation period	HBsAg, ± HBeAg
Acute infection*	HBsAg, HBeAg, anti-HBc (IgG and IgM)
Recent infection	Anti-HBs (↑), anti-HBc IgG (↑), anti-HBe, ± anti-HBc IgM
Remote infection	± anti-HBs, ± anti-HBc IgG
Carrier	HBsAg, anti-HBc IgG (↑), anti-HBe, ± anti-HBc IgM
Chronic infection	HBsAg, HBeAg, anti-HBc IgG (↑), ± anti-HBc IgM
Recent immunization†	anti-HBs

* Some asymptomatic persons with serologic evidence of acute, self-limited hepatitis B (anti-HBc IgG and IgM) have no detectable HBsAg or HBeAg.
† Anti-HBs may become undetectable over time.
Key: HBsAg, hepatitis B surface antigen; HBeAg, hepatitis B e antigen; anti-HBc, antibody to hepatitis B core antigen; anti-HBs, antibody to hepatitis B surface antigen; anti-HBe, antibody to hepatitis B e antigen; ± may or may not be present; ↑, elevated titer.

Tests for detection of HBV DNA polymerase–containing virions and δ virus antigen and RNA in liver and serum currently are available only in research laboratories.

Treatment and Prevention

No specific antiviral agent effective against HBV or δ agent is available. Treatment of acute infection is supportive, including transplantation for fulminant disease. The progression of chronic active hepatitis has been controlled by corticosteroids and azathioprine, and results of uncontrolled trials indicate that interferon α and adenine arabinoside may be beneficial (52–54).

HBV infection can be prevented by interrupting the route of transmission between infected and susceptible persons and by prophylaxis. Mandatory screening of blood donors for HBsAg reduced the frequency of post-transfusion hepatitis B by over 80%, to 0.5% or less (55). Nosocomial transmission can be minimized by enforcing universal precautions (using gloves and gown when handling body fluids); adequately sterilizing blood-contaminated instruments; when possible using disposable instruments, syringes, and needles; and disinfecting contaminated surfaces with formalin or hypochlorite.

Two types of products are available for prophylaxis against hepatitis B. Hepatitis B immune globulin (HBIG), prepared from plasma preselected to contain a high titer of antibodies to the surface antigen, provides temporary, passive protection and is indicated only in certain postexposure situations (described later). Hepatitis B vaccines, first licensed in the United States in 1981, provide active immunization against infection with HBV and are recommended for pre- and postexposure prophylaxis. Two types of hepatitis B vaccine currently are licensed in the United States: A plasma-derived vaccine consisting of a suspension of inactivated 22-nm HBsAg, no longer produced in the United States, is administered to persons receiving hemodialysis, other immunocompromised hosts, and persons with a known allergy to yeast. Recombinant hepatitis B vaccines contain more than 95% surface antigen protein, which is produced by Saccharomyces cerevisiae into which a plasmid containing the gene for the surface antigen is inserted. The recommended series of three intramuscular doses of hepatitis B vaccine (at intervals of 1 and 6 months) induces an adequate antibody response (>10 milli-international units [mIU] measured 1 to 6 months after completion of the vaccination series) in more than 90% of healthy adults and more than 95% of infants, children, and adolescents. Larger doses or more doses (at intervals of 1, 2, and 12 months) are necessary to induce protective antibodies in many persons receiving hemodialysis, and perhaps in those receiving immunosuppressive therapy or those infected with human immunodeficiency virus.

The efficacy of the vaccines licensed in the United States in preventing infection or clinical hepatitis among susceptible persons is 80 to 95%, and protection is complete for those who develop an adequate antibody response following vaccination (8). However, the duration of protection and the need for booster doses is not yet determined. Vaccine-induced antibody levels decline steadily with time, and as many as 50% of adults who develop an adequate antibody response after vaccination have no detectable antibodies after 7 years, though protection against viremic infection and clinical disease appears to persist (8). Booster doses currently are not routinely recommended within 7 years after vaccination, nor is routine serologic testing to assess antibody levels necessary during this period (8). Booster doses are recommended when the antibody level of persons receiving hemodialysis falls below 10 mIU/ml.

Pre-exposure vaccination is recommended for persons at substantial risk of infection with HBV and for those judged likely to be susceptible:

Health care and public safety workers
Clients and staff of institutions for developmentally disabled persons
Persons receiving hemodialysis
Sexually active homosexual males
Intravenous drug users
Persons with disorders that require therapy with clotting factor concentrates
Household and sexual contacts of HBV carriers (if susceptible)
Adoptees from countries where the prevalence of endemic HBV is high (Alaskan natives, Pacific Islanders, immigrants and refugees from Africa and eastern Asia)
Populations in which the prevalence of endemic HBV infection is high
Inmates of long-term correctional facilities
Sexually active heterosexual persons
International travelers who plan to reside longer than 6 months in areas with a high prevalence of endemic HBV and who will have close contact with the population.

Postexposure prophylaxis should be considered after perinatal exposure of an infant born to a mother who tests positive for HBsAg, accidental percutaneous or permu-

Table 9–3. Recommendations for Hepatitis B (HB) Prophylaxis Following Percutaneous or Permucosal Exposure

Exposed Person	Status of Source		
	HBsAg-positive	HBsAg-negative	Unknown
Unvaccinated	HBIG × 1 and initiate HB vaccine	Initiate HB vaccine	Initiate HB vaccine
Previously vaccinated Known responder	Test exposed for anti-HBs 1. If adequate, no treatment 2. If inadequate, HB vaccine booster dose	No treatment	No treatment
Known nonresponder	HBIG × 2 or HBIG × 1 plus 1 dose HB vaccine	No treatment	If known high-risk source, may treat as if source were HBsAg-positive
Response unknown	Test exposed for anti-HBs 1. If inadequate, HBIG × 1 plus HB vaccine booster dose 2. If adequate, no treatment	No treatment	Test exposed for anti-HBs 1. If inadequate, HB vaccine booster dose 2. If adequate, no treatment

Key: HBIG, hepatitis B immune globulin; anti-HBs, antibody against the hepatitis B surface antigen; HBsAg, hepatitis B surface antigen.
(From Centers for Disease Control: Protection against viral hepatitis. MMWR, 39(S-2):1, 1990.)

cosal exposure to HBsAg-positive blood, sexual exposure to a person who tests positive for HBsAg, and household exposure of an infant younger than 1 year to a primary caregiver who has acute hepatitis B. After perinatal exposure to a mother who is positive for HBsAg and HBeAg, administration of HBIG at birth and of the first dose of the vaccine series within 12 hours after birth is 85 to 95% effective in preventing the HBV carrier state (8). Recommended measures after accidental percutaneous or mucosal exposure are outlined in Table 9–3. For greatest effectiveness, HBIG should be given as soon as possible after exposure, because when it is given beyond 7 days after exposure its value is unclear. The first dose of hepatitis B vaccine should be given at a separate site, simultaneously with HBIG or within 7 days of exposure. If a person who has received a single dose of vaccine is exposed, a single dose of HBIG is indicated and the vaccine series should be completed; if a person who has received two doses of vaccine is then exposed, no treatment is necessary if the anti-HBs titer is adequate (>10 mIU) (56). To sexual partners of a person who is HBsAg positive, a single dose of HBIG should be given within 14 days of exposure, and the first dose of vaccine should be administered simultaneously at a different site. Infants exposed to a primary caregiver with acute hepatitis B should be given HBIG and hepatitis B vaccine.

Because HDV is dependent on HBV for replication, HBV prophylaxis of susceptible persons prevents HDV infection. Exposure to both HBV and the δ agent should be treated exactly as exposure to HBV alone.

REFERENCES

1. Blumberg BS, Alter HJ, and Visnich S: A "new" antigen in leukemia sera. JAMA, *191*:541, 1965.
2. Hollinger FB: Serologic evaluation of viral hepatitis. Hosp Pract, *22*:101, 1987.
3. Bayer ME, Blumberg GS, and Werner B: Particles associated with Australia antigen in the sera of patients with leukemia, Down's syndrome and hepatitis. Nature (Lond), *218*:1057, 1968.
4. Courouce-Pauty AM, and Soulier JP: Further data on HBs antigen subtypes—geographical distribution. Vox Sang, *27*:533, 1974.
5. Courouce AM, et al: HBsAg antigen subtypes. Proceedings of the International Workshop on HBs antigen subtypes. Bibl Haematol, *42*:1, 1976.
6. Karasawa T, et al: Light microscopic localization of hepatitis B virus antigens in the human pancreas: Possibility of multiplication of hepatitis B virus in the human pancreas. Gastroenterology, *81*:998, 1981.
7. Miller RH, et al: Hepatitis B viral DNA in infected liver and hepatocellular carcinoma. J Infect Dis, *151*:1081, 1985.
8. Centers for Disease Control: Protection against viral hepatitis: Recommendations of the Immunization Practices Advisory Committee. MMWR, *39*(S-2):1, 1990.
9. Kane MA, Alter MJ, Hadler SC, and Margolis HS: Hepatitis B infection in the United States: Recent trends and future strategies for control. Am J Med, *87*(S-3A):11S, 1989.
10. Centers for Disease Control: Changing patterns of groups at high risk for hepatitis B in the United States. MMWR, *37*:429, 1988.
11. Centers for Disease Control: Racial differences in rates of hepatitis B virus infection—United States, 1976–1980. MMWR, *38*:818, 1989.
12. Beasley RP, Trepo C, Stevens CE, and Szmuness W: The e antigen and vertical transmission of hepatitis B surface antigen. Am J Epidemiol, *105*:94, 1977.
13. Alter JH, Purcell RH, and Gerin JL: Transmission of hepatitis B to chimpanzees by hepatitis B surface antigen–positive saliva and semen. Infect Immun, *16*:928, 1977.
14. Bancroft WH, et al: Transmission of hepatitis B virus to gibbons by exposure to human saliva containing hepatitis B surface antigen. J Infect Dis, *135*:79, 1977.
15. Alter MJ, et al: Importance of heterosexual activity in the transmission of hepatitis B and non-A, non-B hepatitis. JAMA, *262*:1201, 1989.
16. Garibaldi RA, Rasmussen CM, Holmes AW, and Gregg MB: Hospital-acquired serum hepatitis: Report of an outbreak. JAMA, *219*:1577, 1972.
17. Syndmen DR, et al: Nosocomial viral hepatitis B: A cluster among staff with subsequent transmission to patients. Ann Intern Med, *85*:573, 1976.
18. Good RA, and Page AR: Fatal complications of viral hepatitis in two patients with agammaglobulinemia. Am J Med, *29*:804, 1960.
19. Naumov NV, et al: Relationship between expression of hepatitis B virus antigens in isolated hepatocytes and autologous

lymphocyte cytotoxicity in patients with chronic hepatitis B virus infection. Hepatology, 4:63, 1984.
20. Eddleston ALWF, Mondelle M, Mieli-Vergani G, and Williams R: Lymphocyte cytotoxicity to autologous hepatocytes in chronic hepatitis B virus infection. Hepatology, 2:122S, 1982.
21. Hillis WD, Hillis A, Bias WB, and Walker WG: Association of hepatitis B surface antigenemia with HLA locus B specificities. N Engl J Med, 296:1310, 1976.
22. Patterson MJ, Hourani MR, and Mayor GH: HLA antigens and hepatitis B virus. N Engl J Med, 297:1124, 1977.
23. London WT, et al: Host response to hepatitis B infection in patients in a chronic hemodialysis unit. Kidney Int, 12:51, 1977.
24. Blumberg BS, et al: Sex distribution of Australia antigen. Arch Intern Med, 130:231, 1972.
25. Barker LF, and Murray R: Relationship of virus dose to incubation time of clinical hepatitis and time of appearance of hepatitis-associated antigen. Am J Med Sci, 263:27, 1972.
26. Swenson PD: Hepatitis viruses. In Manual of Clinical Microbiology. 5th ed. Edited by A Balows, et al. Washington, DC, American Society for Microbiology, 1991.
27. Gocke DJ: Extrahepatic manifestations of viral hepatitis. Am J Med Sci, 270:49, 1975.
28. Robinson WS: Hepatitis B virus and hepatitis delta virus. In Principles and Practice of Infectious Diseases. 3rd ed. Edited by GL Mandell, RG Douglas Jr, and JE Bennett. New York, Churchill Livingstone, 1990.
29. Hoofnagle JH, et al: Serologic responses in hepatitis B. In Viral Hepatitis: A Contemporary Assessment of Etiology, Epidemiology, Pathogenesis and Prevention. Edited by GN Vyas, SN Cohen, and T Schmid. Philadelphia, Franklin Institute, 1978.
30. Nielsen JO, Nielsen MH, and Elling P: Differential distribution of Australia antigen–associated particles in patients with liver disease and normal carriers. N Engl J Med, 288:484, 1973.
31. Robinson WS: DNA and DNA polymerase in the core of Dane particles. Am J Med Sci, 270:151, 1975.
32. Bonino F, et al: Hepatitis B virus DNA in the sera of HBsAg carriers: A marker of active HBV replication in the liver. Hepatology, 1:386, 1981.
33. Lambert PH, et al: Quantitation of immunoglobulin-associated HBs antigen in patients with acute and chronic hepatitis, in healthy carriers, and in polyarteritis nodosa. J Clin Lab Immunol, 3:1, 1980.
34. Realdi G, et al: Seroconversion from hepatitis B e antigen to anti-HBe in chronic hepatitis B virus infection. Gastroenterology, 79:195, 1980.
35. Aikawa T, et al: Seroconversion from hepatitis B e antigen to anti-HBe in acute hepatitis B virus infection. N Engl J Med, 298:439, 1978.
36. Perrillo RP, et al: Spontaneous clearance and reactivation of HBV infection among male homosexuals with chronic type B hepatitis. Ann Intern Med, 100:43, 1984.
37. Norkrans G, Nordenfeldt E, Hermodsson S, and Iwarson S: Long-term follow-up of chronic hepatitis patients with HBsAg, HBeAg and Dane particle–associated DNA polymerase. Scand J Infect Dis, 12:159, 1980.
38. Rizzetto M, Canese MG, and Arico S: Immunofluorescence detection of a new antigen system (delta/anti-delta) associated to the hepatitis B virus in the liver and the serum of HBsAg carriers. Gut, 18:997, 1977.
39. Rizzetto M, Purcell RH, and Gerin JL: Epidemiology of HBV-associated delta agent: Geographical distribution of anti-delta and prevalence of polytransfused HBsAg carriers. Lancet, i:1215, 1980.
40. Hadziyannis S, Hatzakis A, and Karamanos B: Clinical features of chronic delta infection. In Viral Hepatitis. Edited by GN Vyas. Philadelphia, Franklin Institute, 1984.
41. Ponzetta A, Forzani E, and Shafi MS: Delta agent infection in Saudi Arabia: A general population study. In Viral Hepatitis. Edited by GN Vyas. Philadelphia, Franklin Institute, 1984.
42. Shiels MT, et al: Frequency and significance of delta antibody in acute and chronic hepatitis B. A United States experience. Gastroenterology, 89:1230, 1985.
43. Jacobson IM, et al: Epidemiology and clinical impact of hepatitis D virus (delta) infection. Hepatology, 5:188, 1985.
44. Rosina F, Saracco G, and Rizzetto M: Risk of post-transfusion infection with the hepatitis delta virus. A multicenter study. N Engl J Med, 312:1488, 1985.
45. Hershow RC, et al: Hepatitis D virus infection in Illinois state facilities for the developmentally disabled: Epidemiology and clinical manifestations. Ann Intern Med, 110:779, 1989.
46. Smedile A, Farci P, and Verme G: Influence of delta infection on severity of hepatitis B. Lancet, ii:945, 1982.
47. Tabor E, et al: Does delta agent contribute to fulminant hepatitis? Lancet, i:765, 1983.
48. Caredda F, et al: Hepatitis B virus–associated coinfection and superinfection with delta agent: Indistinguishable disease with different outcome. J Infect Dis, 151:925, 1985.
49. Govindarajan S, De Cock KM, and Redeker AG: Natural course of delta superinfection in chronic hepatitis B virus–infected patients: Histopathologic study with multiple liver biopsies. Hepatology, 6:640, 1986.
50. Fattovich G, et al: Influence of hepatitis delta virus infection on progression to cirrhosis in chronic hepatitis type B. J Infect Dis, 155:931, 1987.
51. Valentine-Thon E, Steinmann J, and Arnold W: Evaluation of the commercially available HepProbe kit for detection of hepatitis B virus DNA in serum. J Clin Microbiol, 28:39, 1990.
52. Soloway RD, et al: Clinical, biochemical and histological remission of severe chronic active liver disease: A controlled study of treatments and early prognosis. Gastroenterology, 63:820, 1972.
53. Murray-Lyon IM, Stern RB, and Wiliams R: Controlled trials of prednisone and azathioprine in active chronic hepatitis. Lancet, i:735, 1973.
54. Scullard GH, et al: Antiviral treatment of chronic hepatitis B virus infection. I. Changes in viral markers with interferon combined with adenine arabinoside. J Infect Dis, 143:772, 1981.
55. Aach RD, and Kahn RA: Post-transfusion hepatitis: Current perspectives. Ann Intern Med, 92:539, 1980.
56. Centers for Disease Control: Postexposure prophylaxis of hepatitis B. MMWR, 33:285, 1984.

Chapter 10

PARAMYXOVIRUSES

Members of the family Paramyxoviridae are significant pathogens in infants and children and may cause disease in adults, especially those who are immunocompromised. In this chapter, classification, structure, and replication of the paramyxoviruses in general are reviewed, and features of the individual viruses are discussed.

CLASSIFICATION

Paramyxoviruses of medical importance are classified in general as follows:

Family: Paramyxoviridae
Genus: Paramyxovirus
Species: Parainfluenza viruses (1 to 4), mumps virus
Genus: Morbillivirus
Species: Measles virus
Genus: Pneumovirus
Species: Respiratory syncytial virus

Classification into three genera is based on antigenic cross-reactivities among members of each genus and differences in the hemagglutinin and neuraminidase surface glycoproteins of members of the respective genera. Members of the genus Paramyxovirus have hemagglutinin and neuraminidase, members of the genus Morbillivirus have hemagglutinin only, and members of the genus Pneumovirus lack both glycoproteins.

STRUCTURE

Paramyxovirus virions (Fig. 10–1) consist of a helical nucleocapsid, 1 μm in length and 18 nm in diameter, that has a nonsegmented, single-stranded, negative-sense RNA genome and is surrounded by a lipoprotein envelope derived from the cytoplasmic membrane of the host cell, from which glycoprotein complexes, or "spikes," project (1). Most virions are 150 to 250 nm in diameter, but larger particles and filaments may be seen.

The major nucleocapsid proteins involved in RNA transcription and replication are the gigantic L protein and the smaller P (polymerase-associated) proteins. Surface viral glycoproteins called H (hemagglutinin) proteins agglutinate avian and mammalian erythrocytes and mediate attachment to host cells by binding to cellular receptors containing sialic acid. Glycoproteins with both hemagglutinating and neuraminidase activity are termed HN, and the homologous attachment protein, which lacks both activities, is designated G (glycoprotein). The surface glycoprotein termed F facilitates fusion of the viral lipoprotein envelope with the lipoprotein surface membrane of the host cell and the subsequent delivery of the nucleocapsid into the host cell cytoplasm. A nonglycoslyated M protein lining the inner surface of the virion envelope may be involved in nucleocapsid-envelope recognition during virion assembly, envelope formation, or both.

REPLICATION

Paramyxoviruses replicate in the cytoplasm of infected cells. Viral glycoproteins replace endogenous cellular proteins in the plasma membrane, and M-protein molecules aggregate on the inner surface of the nascent envelope. Nucleocapsids are assembled in the cytoplasm and transported to the cell surface, and they become enveloped by budding from the plasma membrane at sites where viral glycoproteins are inserted. Activation of F molecules on the cell surface mediates fusion with contiguous cells, allowing cell-to-cell spread of viral genomes without encountering antiviral antibodies.

PARAINFLUENZA VIRUSES

The human parainfluenza viruses, first isolated in the late 1950s, are important respiratory tract pathogens of infants and children. They are responsible for most cases of croup and are the second most common cause (after respiratory syncytial virus) of severe lower respiratory tract disease in infants (2). Four types of parainfluenza viruses (numbered 1 through 4) are known, which are differentiated on the basis of complement fixation and hemagglutinating antigens.

Structure

Pleomorphic, enveloped virions, 150 to 200 nm in diameter, possess HN and F surface glycoprotein spikes. The HN glycoprotein mediates viral attachment to host cell receptors containing sialic acid and functions late in the infection, enzymatically cleaving sialic acid (neuraminic acid) residues on the virus to prevent self-aggregation of virions during egress from infected cells.

Epidemiology

Parainfluenza viruses are distributed worldwide. They are transmitted by direct person-to-person contact or by large-droplet aerosol spread. Each type can cause acute respiratory tract disease, though type 4 is difficult to recover in cell culture and therefore is encountered less frequently in the clinical laboratory. The epidemiologic and clinical manifestations of infection with parainfluenza virus types 1, 2, and 3 differ: type 1, the predominant cause of croup in children, is responsible for epidemics in the fall of odd-numbered years; type 2 also causes croup

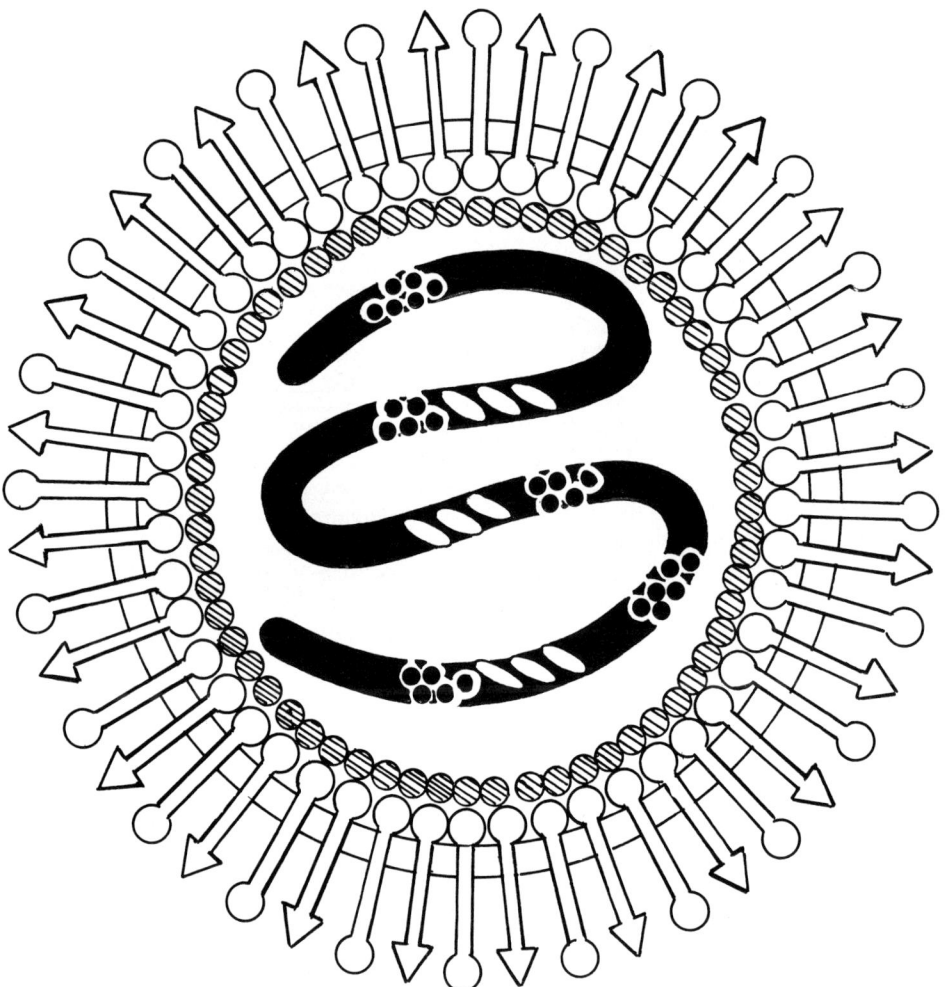

Fig. 10–1. Diagram of a typical paramyxovirus particle. The internal nucleocapsid (black serpentine) contains genomic RNA complexed with the nucleocapsid structural unit and the auxiliary nucleocapsid proteins: L (solid white ovals) and P (dark circles with white circumference). Surrounding the nucleocapsid is the lipid envelope (outer white circle), lined by the M protein (shaded circles), and penetrated by the viral attachment glycoprotein, HN (rounded tips), and the fusion protein, F (pointed tips). (From Kingsbury DW: Paramyxoviridae and their replication. In Fields Virology. 2nd ed. Edited by BN Fields, and DM Knipe. New York, Raven, 1990.)

in a seasonal pattern synchronous with type 1; type 3, the second most common cause of pneumonia and bronchiolitis in infants under age 6 months, was endemic for many years but during the past decade has been associated with yearly spring epidemics (3–6). Reinfection with the parainfluenza viruses occurs, but the resulting illness usually is less severe than the primary infection.

Primary infection with parainfluenza virus generally occurs early in life. Antibody studies indicate that by ages 2 and 4 years respectively, approximately 60 and 80% of children have been infected with parainfluenza virus type 3 (7,8). Infection with types 1 and 2 occurs later, but by age 5 years 75% of children have been infected with type 1, and the majority with type 2. Parainfluenza virus type 3 often causes illness during the first months of life, whereas infection with type 1 or 2 is rare before 4 months of age, apparently owing to protective maternal antibodies. Lower respiratory tract infection with types 1 and 2 occurs less frequently after school age and is uncommon during adolescence and adult life.

Pathogenesis

Parainfluenza viruses first infect the mucous membranes of the nose and throat; obstruction of the paranasal sinuses and eustachian tubes is possible, as is limited bronchial involvement. In more extensive infections, types 1 and 2 involve the larynx and upper trachea and may extend to the lower trachea and bronchi, causing accumulation of inspissated mucus with subsequent atelectasis and pneumonia. Severe infection with parainfluenza virus type 3 causes compromise of the small air passages with bronchitis, bronchiolitis, or bronchopneumonia.

The mechanisms responsible for localization of parainfluenza viruses and the severity of the resultant infection presently are unknown; however, properties of the virus and the host immune response may be important. Because the F glycoprotein of the viral envelope must be cleaved by a cellular protease to become biologically active, interplay between the susceptibility of the viral F glycoprotein to cleavage and the ability of host cells to effect cleavage may influence localization of the virus in the respiratory tract and the intensity of the resulting infection (9,10).

A possible role for the host immune response in the pathogenesis of the infection is supported by the following observations: The specific cell-mediated immune response is more intense in infants with bronchiolitis than in those with localized upper respiratory tract infection (11). Lower respiratory tract involvement is uncommon during reinfection with parainfluenza virus, which suggests that primary infection confers relative resistance to subsequent severe illness. Moreover, individuals with croup produce local specific immunoglobulin (Ig) E earlier and in higher titers than those with infection limited to the upper respiratory tract, and they are more likely to have detectable histamine in nasopharyngeal secretions (12). Although the rapid and increased production of specific IgE may mediate histamine release in the trachea and subglottic region, which subsequently produces the symptoms of croup, it may simply reflect an increased antibody response to more extensive production of viral antigens.

Clinical Manifestations

Infection with parainfluenza virus may be asymptomatic or cause a range of symptoms. Infected children and adults usually present with a "cold-like" illness: rhinorrhea, pharyngeal erythema without cervical adenopathy, cough, and low-grade fever lasting 2 to 3 days. The most common severe manifestation of primary infection is the croup syndrome: barking cough and hoarseness with or without respiratory stridor.

Reinfection with parainfluenza viruses occurs frequently, from a few months to several years after the primary infection. Generally, symptomatic reinfection is manifest as a cold-like illness; severe disease is rare.

MUMPS VIRUS

The clinical manifestations of mumps—parotitis, occasionally accompanied by orchitis—were described by Hippocrates in the fifth century B.C. That a virus is the cause was demonstrated in 1934, by reproducing the disease in monkeys inoculated in the laboratory with filtered saliva from persons with mumps (13). Mumps virus was cultivated in chick embryos in 1945, and in 1966 an effective live-virus vaccine was developed (14,15).

Structure

Mumps virions are pleomorphic, though typically spherical, enveloped particles, 100 to 600 nm in diameter, with HN and F glycoproteins projecting from the outer membrane. The functions of these glycoproteins are identical to those described earlier for the virus family. Mumps virion proteins L (large), NP (nucleocapsid), and P (polymerase) are associated with the nucleocapsid, and the protein M (matrix) is associated with the membrane.

Epidemiology

Mumps is endemic worldwide; infection rates peak in winter and spring. Mumps virus is transmitted by droplet spread, direct contact with contaminated secretions, or indirectly by contact with contaminated fomites; it enters through the nose or mouth. Peak contagion is just before and at the onset of parotitis. In developing countries where infants are not fully immunized, clinically evident infections predominate in children 5 to 9 years of age. The infection probably is less communicable than measles and varicella, though this is difficult to prove because 25 to 30% of mumps cases are subclinical.

A live mumps vaccine, introduced in the United States in 1967, was recommended for routine use in 1977, and between 1967 and 1985 the reported number of cases of mumps steadily declined—from almost 200,000 to fewer than 3,000 per year (16). The number of reported cases rose over the next 2 years, to about 8,000 in 1986 and about 13,000 in 1987, and then declined to fewer than 5,000 in 1988. Before 1986 most mumps patients were children aged 5 to 14 years, but in 1986 and 1987 the age of peak incidence shifted upward from the 5- to 9-year-olds, and adolescents aged 15 years or older accounted for more than a third of the total. This increase in susceptible adolescents and young adults was shown in recent outbreaks of mumps in high schools, on college campuses, and in occupational settings (17–19). The shift of risk to older groups and the recent relative resurgence of reported mumps are attributed to the relatively underimmunized cohort of children born between 1967 and 1977 rather than to waning immunity in vaccinated persons (19).

Pathogenesis

Mumps virus replicates first in the mucosa of the nose or upper respiratory tract, then spreads to regional lymph nodes, and subsequently enters the blood, reaching tissues such as the salivary glands, meninges, testes, pancreas, ovaries, thyroid, heart, and kidneys, where secondary replication occurs. The virus is excreted in the saliva for a few days and in the urine for about 2 weeks after the onset of clinical disease.

In the salivary glands mumps virus replicates in the ductal epithelium, eliciting a local lymphohistiocytic response, interstitial edema, and an accumulation of neutrophils and necrotic debris in duct lumens. In the kidneys the virus replicates in the epithelial cells of the distal tubules, calyces, and ureters, despite the presence of circulating neutralizing antibodies; but renal abnormalities are minimal or absent. In the testicular seminiferous tubules and in the pancreas the virus replicates in the ductal epithelium, eliciting interstitial edema and a local lymphocytic infiltrate. In the testes, foci of interstitial hemorrhage occasionally occur.

Mumps virus frequently invades the central nervous system, presumably across the choroid plexus, an event evidenced by the presence of cerebrospinal fluid pleocytosis in about half of infected persons (20). Occasionally, virions penetrate the brain tissue, and in the rare fatal cases of meningoencephalitis, histologic examination of brain tissue shows a perivascular mononuclear cell inflammatory infiltrate, scattered foci of neuronophagia, microglial cell proliferation, and perivascular demyelination typical of parainfectious encephalitis, which probably is an autoimmune response.

In other organs, for example the heart, viral invasion is characterized histologically by an interstitial lymphocytic infiltrate of the myocardium and mild pericarditis. In the joints, migratory polyarticular arthritis occasionally develops, but the pathogenesis remains obscure; the virus has not been recovered from joint fluid or synovial tissue, and no evidence of immune complex formation has been demonstrated. Mumps virus acquired in the first trimester of pregnancy can infect the fetus, but subsequent congenital anomalies have not been documented (21,22).

The first humoral immune response to infection with mumps virus is IgM production, which gradually declines over 2 to 6 months. Immunoglobulin G peaks about 3 weeks after infection and persists for life. Two types of complement-fixing IgG antibodies are detected: those directed against the soluble (S) or nucleoprotein antigen generally are present at the onset of illness, peak at about 10 days, and are no longer detectable after 8 to 9 months; and antibodies to the viral (V) or surface antigen appear about day 10 and persist for life. Assays for specific IgG class antibodies correlate with complement fixation titers but may cross-react with antigens of parainfluenza virus. Once established, natural immunity to mumps is long lived; reinfection is rare, if, indeed, it occurs.

Clinical Manifestations

After an incubation period of 2 to 4 weeks (average, 16 to 18 days) persons infected with mumps virus experience a prodrome of low-grade fever, headache, anorexia, and malaise. Within a day, earache and enlargement and tenderness of the ipsilateral parotid gland ensue. Pain, fever, and tenderness generally resolve within a week. Other salivary glands are affected concurrently in 10% of cases, but rarely are they involved alone.

Extra–salivary gland manifestations of mumps are listed in Table 10–1. Males experience central nervous system involvement three times as often as females. Clinical meningitis occurs in 1 to 10% of those with mumps parotitis, but only 40 to 50% of persons with proven mumps meningitis have parotitis (23). Meningeal symptoms—headache, vomiting, fever, and nuchal rigidity—generally appear about 4 days after salivary gland involvement, but can develop before, up to 2 weeks after, or in the absence of parotitis; they resolve completely with no sequelae in 10 days or less.

Epididymo-orchitis, the most common extra–salivary gland manifestation in adult males with mumps, affects 20 to 30% of postpubertal males and rarely occurs before puberty. Most cases develop during the first 2 weeks of parotitis, but infection may precede or occur in the absence of parotitis. The illness begins abruptly with fever, chills, headache, vomiting, and testicular pain and enlargement (bilateral in one of six cases), and resolves in about 1 week. Although some degree of testicular atrophy occurs in about 50% of those with orchitis, infertility is uncommon.

MEASLES (RUBEOLA) VIRUS

Measles, a highly contagious disease that usually affects children, was first described by the tenth-century Persian physician Abu Beer, and its contagiousness and transmission from person to person were confirmed by Peter Panum, a Danish physician, in 1846 (24). Measles was first transmitted to monkeys in 1898; in 1911 the pathogen was demonstrated to be a virus by reproducing the disease in monkeys inoculated in the laboratory with a filtrate of respiratory secretions from infected persons; and in 1954, measles virus was isolated in cell culture (25–27). Although the prevalence of measles has decreased dramatically in countries where immunization is widespread, in developing countries it remains a major cause of childhood morbidity and mortality, responsible for an estimated 2 million deaths each year.

Structure

The spherical, pleomorphic, 100- to 250-nm diameter virions of measles virus have an RNA genome with an estimated molecular weight of 4.5 million. Projecting from the virion lipid bilayer envelope are H and F glycoprotein spikes. Six virion structural proteins have been identified: nucleoprotein (N), the predominant internal protein, protects the viral genome; polymerase (phospho) protein (P), an internal protein associated with N, probably is part of the transcription complex; large protein (L), also associated with N, is part of the transcription complex; matrix (M), located inside the virion envelope, functions in virion assembly; hemagglutinin, a transmembrane envelope glycoprotein, is necessary for viral attachment to a host cell; and fusion factor, an envelope glycoprotein, is active in fusion to host cells and virus entry.

Epidemiology

Humans are the only natural host for measles virus, which is transmitted via aerosolized infected droplets produced in the catarrhal stage when an infected person talks, coughs, or sneezes. Measles occurs worldwide, and in developing countries such as Africa more than half the children are infected by age 2 years, and nearly all by age 5 years. In developed countries where immunization is not widespread, most measles cases occur in children 5 to 9 years of age, and 95% of patients are younger than 15 years. In temperate climates where measles vaccine is not used, epidemics lasting 3 to 4 months generally occur every 2 to 3 years in winter and spring.

Since a measles vaccine was licensed in the United States in 1963, the reported incidence of measles has been reduced by 99% (28). Prior to 1963, more than 400,000

Table 10–1. Extra–salivary Gland Manifestations of Mumps*

Manifestation	Prevalence (%)
Cerebrospinal fluid pleocytosis[†]	50
Clinical meningitis	1–10
Encephalitis	0.1
Transient high-frequency deafness	4
Postpubertal epididymo-orchitis	20–30
Postpubertal oophoritis	5
Electrocardiographic changes[‡]	15

* Permanent unilateral deafness, migratory polyarthritis, and pancreatitis are uncommon; thyroiditis, mastitis, prostatitis, hepatitis, and thrombocytopenia are rare.
† 10–2000 WBC/μl with lymphocyte predominance.
‡ Depressed ST segment, flattened or inverted T wave or prolonged PR interval.

measles cases were reported annually in the United States, whereas between 22,000 and 75,000 cases per year were reported during the late 1960s and early 1970s (29). Because the greatest decline occurred in children younger than 10 years, the proportion of total cases in the different age groups has changed. Children 10 years of age and older accounted for 58% of reported measles cases between 1984 and 1988, but for only 10% of cases between 1960 and 1964 (28).

In 1989, almost 18,000 cases of measles were reported in the United States, an increase of 423% over the number reported in 1988 (Fig. 10–2) (30). Cases were reported in 47 states and the District of Columbia, compared with 36 states in 1988. Illinois, Texas, California, and Ohio each reported more than 2,500 cases, accounting for almost 70% of the total. The estimated incidence rates were higher for all age groups in 1989 than in 1988. The largest increases occurred among those aged 25 to 29 years, those younger than 1 year, and those aged 1 to 4 years; and the incidence was highest among children under age 1 year. Outbreaks involving predominantly preschool-aged children, predominantly school-aged children, and predominantly post–school-aged persons accounted for 45%, 32%, and 3% of cases, respectively. Forty per cent of persons who developed measles were vaccinated at or after age 12 months, and of the remaining ones, routine vaccination was indicated but not carried out for almost 60% (or 34% of the total). This increase in unvaccinated persons with measles primarily reflected the increasing number of cases reported among unvaccinated inner-city preschool-aged children. Complications of measles—diarrhea, otitis media, pneumonia, and encephalitis—occurred in almost 20% of cases, and 41 measles-associated deaths were reported, the largest number in a single year since 1971. Most deaths were attributed to pneumonia, and most of those who died were unvaccinated preschool-aged children and adults.

In the first 20 weeks of 1990, over 7,500 cases of measles were reported from 48 states and the District of Columbia, a 40% increase over the number reported for the same period in 1989 (30). Of the persons for whom vaccination status was reported, 70% were unvaccinated, and of those, routine vaccination was indicated for almost 50% (35% of the total). Thirty-five measles-associated deaths were reported, most in unvaccinated preschool-aged children.

Pathogenesis

Virions replicate locally in the respiratory mucosa for 2 to 4 days, spread to regional lymph nodes, where further replication occurs, and then enter the blood and are transported within leukocytes to sites throughout the monocyte/macrophage system. Virions again replicate, causing death of infected cells and release of more virions. During the ensuing secondary viremia, virions circulate in monocytes and lymphocytes, which may account for the temporary depression of cell-mediated immunity associated with the disease. The virus is widely disseminated, involving mucosal surfaces of the respiratory and gastrointestinal tract and the endothelial cells of small vessels in the lamina propria and the dermis. Extensive involvement of the tracheobronchial mucosa accounts for the cough of the prodrome, and mucosal damage may predispose to superinfection with bacteria such as Staphylococcus aureus. Infection of the endothelial cells of the superficial capillaries and small veins causes swelling and proliferation of the cells, vascular congestion, edema, and a perivascular lymphohistiocytic inflammatory infiltrate with multinucleate giant cells. The infiltrate appears after the cellular immune system is activated, which coincides with the onset of the rash. Eventually a minute vesicle forms under the epidermis or mucosal surface, followed by desquamation of the skin or mucosal sloughing.

With the onset of the rash, specific antibodies are detected in the serum, and T lymphocytes are activated to destroy virus-infected cells in lymphoid tissue and endothelial cells. Infectious virus subsequently disappears from the blood and respiratory secretions. Cell-mediated immunity is essential for clearance of the virus and may be responsible for the rash (31). Therefore, in persons with deficiencies of cell-mediated immunity virus replication

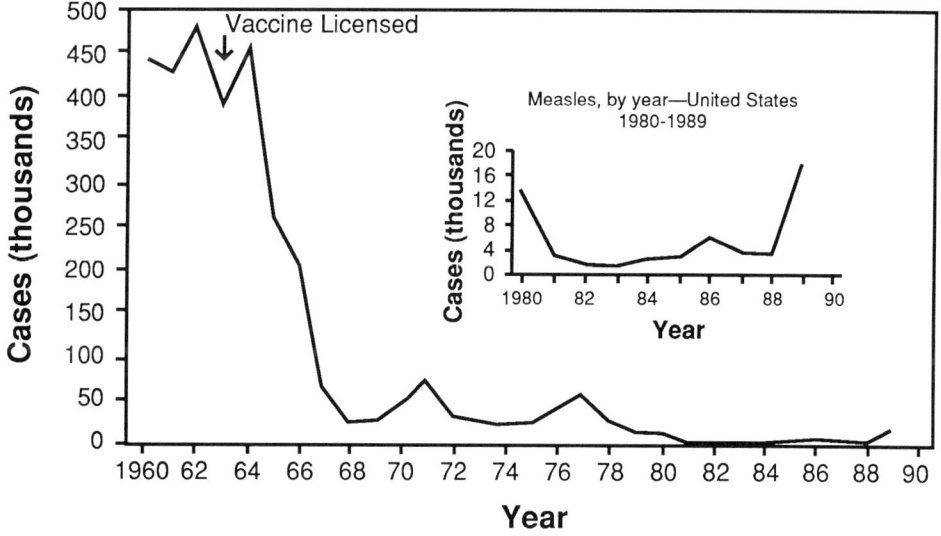

Fig. 10–2. Reported measles cases, by year—United States, 1960–1989 (data for 1989 are provisional). (From Centers for Disease Control: Measles—United States, 1989 and first 20 weeks 1990. MMWR, 39:353, 1990.)

continues unabated, and giant cell pneumonia, characterized histologically by giant cells in the tracheobronchial mucosa and alveoli (Fig. 10–3), ensues without the typical prodrome or rash.

Clinical Manifestations

During the 10- to 14-day incubation period, persons infected with measles virus experience a prodrome of malaise, fever, anorexia, conjunctivitis, cough, and coryza. Pathognomonic Koplik spots (gray specks on an erythematous base involving the buccal mucosa, most commonly opposite the second molars) appear just before the rash, which begins on the face and spreads downward to involve the entire body, including the palms and soles. The rash, initially maculopapular, becomes confluent and may desquamate before clearing about 5 days after it appears.

Persons immunized with the killed measles vaccine and later exposed to wild measles virus may develop atypical measles, an illness believed to represent a hypersensitivity reaction in a partially immune host. The rash (urticarial, maculopapular, hemorrhagic, and/or vesicular) begins peripherally and is accompanied by high fever, peripheral edema, interstitial pulmonary infiltrates, and hepatitis.

The most common complications of measles are pneumonia and central nervous system manifestations. Pneumonia, resulting from direct viral invasion of the lungs (giant cell pneumonia) or bacterial superinfection secondary to local virus-induced tissue damage and depressed cellular immunity, is the immediate cause of death in about 60% of infants who succumb to measles (32,33). Central nervous system manifestations include acute postinfectious encephalitis, which develops in about 0.1% of cases 5 to 7 days after the appearance of the rash, and subacute sclerosing panencephalitis (SSPE), a late complication in about 1 in 300,000 measles cases. An autoimmune mechanism is postulated to cause postinfectious encephalitis, because infectious virus is not detected in the brain and the neuropathologic findings—perivascular lymphocytic inflammation and demyelination—are consistent with an autoimmune response; however, this has not been proven.

SSPE, first recognized in 1933, was incorrectly attributed to chronic infection with influenza virus (34). The true cause was determined in 1969, when measles virus was identified in the brain of a person who had SSPE (35,36). In SSPE the virus persists in the central nervous system in a nonproductive state. Owing to defects in H and F gene expression of the virus, budding cannot occur and extracellular virus is not produced (37,38). Rather, the virus spreads by direct cell-to-cell transmission. Moreover, infected cells are not destroyed by the host immune system because they do not express foreign (viral) antigens. Infected neurons, astrocytes, and oligodendroglial cells contain intranuclear and intracytoplasmic inclusions composed of measles nucleocapsids; and as the disease progresses, gliosis, microglial proliferation, and demyelination due to oligodendroglial cell destruction appear.

SSPE occurs worldwide (incidence, 0.12 to 0.14 per million population), affecting males three times as frequently as females. The clinical manifestations, which reflect steady destruction of gray and white matter, begin an average of 7 years (range, 2 to 32 years) after primary measles. Stage 1 disease is characterized by a subtle psychological and intellectual decline. During the second stage, disturbed motor function (cerebellar ataxia, dystonia, apraxias, and myoclonic jerks) predominates and intellectual deterioration continues. In stage 3 affected persons are in a stuporous, rigid state, and in stage 4, comatose. In most persons, the disease evolves over 1 to 3 years, ending in death, generally from an intercurrent infection of the urinary or respiratory tract.

RESPIRATORY SYNCYTIAL VIRUS

Respiratory syncytial virus (RSV) is the most important cause of viral lower respiratory tract disease in infants and young children (39,40). The virus, first isolated in 1956 from a laboratory chimpanzee with a "cold-like" illness and named the "chimpanzee coryza agent," in 1957 was recovered in cell culture from children with pneumonia and croup (41,42).

Structure

The pleomorphic 150- to 300-nm diameter RSV virions lack the paramyxovirus HN surface glycoprotein and have in its place the G glycoprotein. The RNA genome (molecular weight 5 million) codes for several proteins. The surface glycoproteins G and F are responsible for attachment to host cell receptors and for fusion of the viral envelope with the host cell envelope and syncytium formation, respectively. Dimorphism linked to the G glycoprotein determines the antigenic subgroup, A or B; in different years the two circulate in varying proportions in a community (43,44). The nucleocapsid proteins are nucleoprotein (N), which serves a structural function, and phosphoprotein (P) and large (L) protein, which probably are involved in transcription and replication of viral RNA. Located on the inner lining of the viral envelope are a matrix (M) protein and a putative matrix protein (M2), the exact location in the viral envelope and function of which are not known. Three proteins of unknown function are NS1, NS2, and SH.

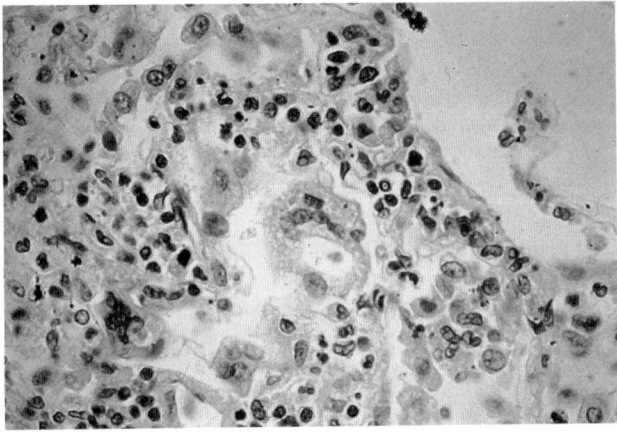

Fig. 10–3. Section of lung from a patient with giant cell (measles) pneumonia (hematoxylin and eosin, ×157.5).

Epidemiology

Infection with RSV occurs worldwide, causing yearly epidemics that frequently alternate between winter and spring in temperate regions and predominate during the rainy season in the tropics. Serious disease, most common in male infants, peaks at 2 months of age (range, 6 weeks to 6 months) (45). Data from serologic studies indicate that infection with RSV occurs frequently during the first few years of life and that nearly all children have been infected by age 5 years (45–47). Reinfection is common but generally results in less severe illness (48,49). Although often subclinical, infection with RSV in adults may be symptomatic; outbreaks among institutionalized young adults and the elderly and serious disease in immunocompromised adults have been reported (50–56).

Pathogenesis

RSV is transmitted by close contact with infected respiratory tract secretions (predominantly large droplets) or with contaminated fomites. During outbreaks of nosocomial infections among newborns and children, hospital staff play a significant role in viral transmission (57–60). After entry into the host via eye or nose, RSV replicates in the upper respiratory tract and may spread in aspirated secretions to involve the entire lower respiratory tract. Early in the infection, lower respiratory tract involvement is characterized by bronchiolitis with a peribronchiolar lymphocytic infiltrate and minimal edema of the bronchiolar walls and surrounding interstitium. As the disease progresses, the bronchial mucosa becomes necrotic and sloughs, causing airway obstruction and subsequent hyperinflation and atelectasis of the distal pulmonary parenchyma. With pneumonia, a mononuclear cell infiltrate develops in the interstitium. The pathogenesis of these changes is not fully understood, but local intrapulmonary immune mechanisms, mediated by the cellular immune system or IgE, may be involved (61–63). Alternatively, severe disease in young infants may result from the combination of an exposure to large doses of virus and an airway system that is unable to adequately compensate for virus-induced physiologic changes.

Naturally acquired specific IgG, IgM, and IgA provide incomplete protection against reinfection. The role of serum antibodies to RSV is unknown, because, in general, the titer does not predict risk of infection, severity of illness, or chances of recovery (45,64). Resolution of the infection, however, appears to depend on an intact cellular immune system, because disease is more severe and viral shedding more prolonged in immunocompromised persons (65–67).

Clinical Manifestations

Primary infection with RSV is manifested as upper or lower respiratory tract disease; subclinical infection is uncommon. Lower respiratory tract involvement (bronchiolitis or pneumonia) develops in about 30 to 70% of infected infants, and in closed populations of infants the proportion may be greater (45,68–71). The illness, which lasts 1 to 3 weeks, generally begins with nasal congestion, pharyngitis, fever, and cough and is followed in several days by dyspnea, increased respiratory rate, and retractions of the intercostal muscles. Typically, the chest roentgenogram shows areas of interstitial infiltration and hyperinflation. A common complication in young children is otitis media.

Reinfection with RSV in older children produces nasal congestion, cough, fever, and earache, lasting 1 to 32 days (mean, 9 days). In young, healthy adults, symptomatic infection with RSV causes a "cold" syndrome; but in adults with chronic bronchitis, the infection may exacerbate bronchitis, and RSV has been associated with bronchitis, pneumonia, and influenza-like illnesses (see Chapter 11) in hospitalized adults and with bronchopneumonia in elders (52,54,72–75).

Complications of infection with RSV are most likely to develop in young infants, children with cardiopulmonary and congenital disorders, and immunocompromised persons of all ages (55,56,65,67,76–78). Acute complications in infants include apnea, respiratory failure, and, occasionally, secondary bacterial infection and sudden infant death syndrome. Longterm complications are not well delineated, but residual small airway disease is possible.

Laboratory Diagnosis

Specimens useful for diagnosis of infection with the paramyxoviruses are listed in Table 10–2. Specimen collection, transport, and processing are discussed in Part III (79). Identification of the viruses is reviewed here.

Parainfluenza Viruses. The most sensitive method for detecting parainfluenza viruses is conventional cell culture using primary rhesus or cynomolgus monkey kidney cells. Cultures are maintained in minimum essential medium without serum (because influenza viruses [Chapter 11], which also replicate in these cells, are very sensitive to inhibitors that might be present in serum) and incubated 14 to 21 days at 33° to 35° C. The continuous rhesus kidney cell line LLC-MK2 with added trypsin (2 μg/ml) also may be used for culture (80). Parainfluenza virus types 1 and 3 rarely produce sufficient cytopathic

Table 10–2. Infections Caused by Paramyxoviruses and Specimens for Diagnosis

Infection	Virus	Specimen
Upper respiratory tract infection	RSV, PIV	Nasal aspirate or wash, nasopharyngeal swab
Pneumonia	RSV	Nasal aspirate or wash, nasopharyngeal swab, BAL, lung biopsy tissue
	Measles virus	Serum, lung tissue
Measles	Measles virus	Serum, nasal wash, nasopharyngeal swab
Parotitis	Mumps virus	Serum, urine, saliva
Meningitis	Mumps virus	Serum, urine, CSF
Orchitis	Mumps virus	Serum, urine
SSPE	Measles	CSF, brain tissue

Key: RSV, respiratory syncytial virus; PIV, parainfluenza virus; BAL, bronchoalveolar lavage fluid; CSF, cerebrospinal fluid; SSPE, subacute sclerosing panencephalitis.

effect (CPE) to permit recognition, although type 3 may cause stretching of the cells at the edge of the cell monolayer. Type 2, on the other hand, induces the formation of dark, granular, irregular syncytia, which retract, giving a "Swiss cheese" appearance to the monolayer. Because CPE is uncommon, most parainfluenza virus isolates are detected by hemadsorption with guinea pig erythrocytes (see Appendix, Procedure 1) on day 9 or 10 after inoculation. A hemadsorption reaction (Fig. 10–4) indicates the presence of a hemadsorbing virus: influenza, parainfluenza, or mumps virus. Infected cell monolayers are scraped from the tube, placed on microscope slides, fixed in acetone, and stained with monoclonal antibodies specific for influenza and for parainfluenza viruses. For the latter, panparainfluenza (directed against antigens common to types 1, 2, and 3) and type-specific reagents are commercially available. Cells infected with parainfluenza virus exhibit cytoplasmic staining. Monoclonal antibodies to parainfluenza virus may also be used to stain smears prepared directly from nasal aspirate, nasal wash, or nasopharyngeal swab specimens; however, data on the sensitivity of this method of detecting parainfluenza viruses are limited.

Serologic tests measuring IgG to parainfluenza viruses are used principally for epidemiologic surveys. Acute and convalescent sera must be tested concurrently; a fourfold rise in titer indicates acute infection. Neither a single high titer nor a fourfold fall in titer is sufficient evidence of recent infection. Moreover, because antigens of mumps and parainfluenza viruses are similar, a heterotypic antibody response to parainfluenza virus may develop after infection with mumps virus.

Mumps Virus. Infection with mumps virus is diagnosed serologically or by isolating the virus. For recovery of the virus in conventional cell culture, primary monkey kidney cell lines are optimal. The best specimen to collect is urine, because the virus is excreted in urine as long as 2 weeks after symptoms begin, but in saliva only during the first few days of the illness. Mumps virus does not induce CPE in the cell monolayer, but can be detected by hemadsorption. Because antibodies specific for mumps virus are not commercially available, an isolate of a hemadsorbing virus is called mumps virus presumptively when smears of infected cells stained with monoclonal antibodies to influenza and parainfluenza viruses are negative. For serologic testing, acute- and convalescent-phase serum samples must be evaluated concurrently; a fourfold or greater rise in IgG titer indicates acute disease.

Measles Virus. Measles virus can be isolated from nasal wash or nasopharyngeal swab specimens in cell culture, a lengthy process that generally is not performed in the clinical virology laboratory, or detected in smears of nasopharyngeal cells stained with monoclonal antibodies (81). Most often, however, the clinical diagnosis of measles is confirmed serologically. Detection of specific IgM in acute-phase serum or a fourfold or greater rise in IgG titer between the acute and the convalescent phase indicates acute disease.

If clinical manifestations are consistent with SSPE, the presence of measles complement–fixing antibodies in the cerebrospinal fluid is diagnostic of the disease. Oligoclonal bands are detected in cerebrospinal fluid in most cases, but their absence does not exclude the diagnosis. Measles virus antigens can be detected in brain biopsy tissue by immunofluorescence, but brain biopsy is not required for diagnosis.

Respiratory Syncytial Virus. Several methods are available for detection of RSV in clinical specimens. In conventional cell culture RSV grows best in HEp-2 cells, although human diploid fibroblasts such as MRC-5 and WI-38 cells, A-549 cells, and rhesus monkey kidney cells will support its growth. Culture tubes are incubated 14 to 21 days at 33° to 36° C. Typical CPE in HEp-2 cells is characterized by syncytium formation: adjacent cells fuse into irregular, refractile masses or large sheets of cells with indistinct borders and multiple nuclei (Fig. 10–5). Infected fibroblast monolayers have a lacy appearance, but the cells are not destroyed and syncytia do not form. In primary monkey kidney cells infected with RSV, clusters of enlarged cells develop. Identification is confirmed by staining infected cells with specific monoclonal antibodies. Disadvantages of cell culture are two: After inoculation, CPE generally is not apparent until day 5 to 7 or even later, and because an effective antiviral agent is available, more rapid detection is essential. Moreover, RSV is relatively unstable and may become nonviable during specimen transport.

Direct and indirect immunofluorescence techniques

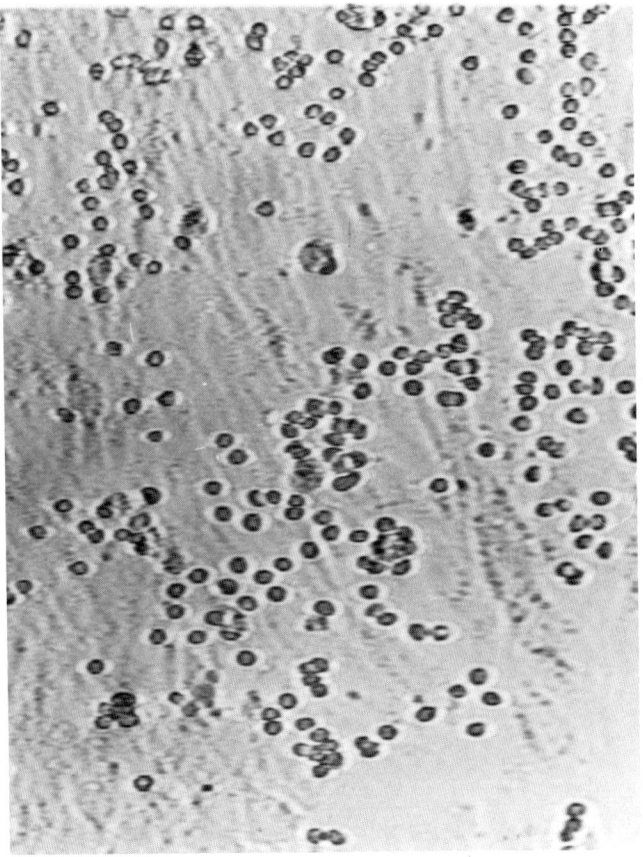

Fig. 10–4. Positive hemadsorption test result in primary monkey kidney cells infected with parainfluenza virus type 3 (×40).

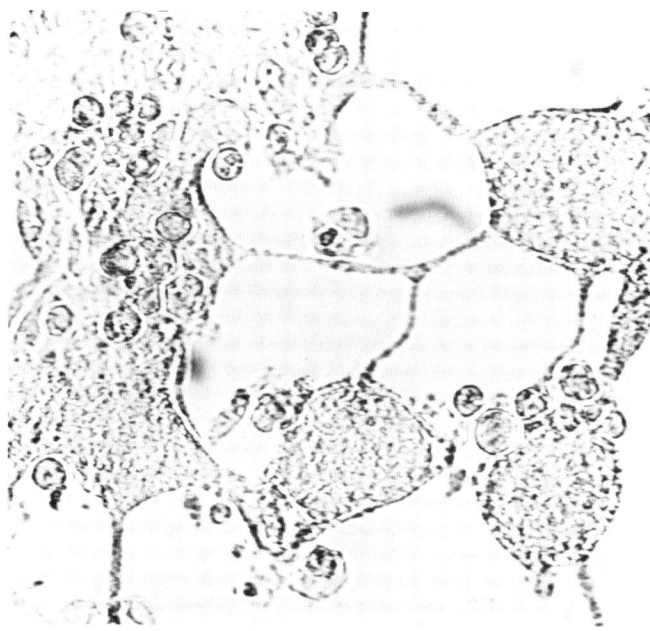

Fig. 10–5. Cytopathic effect produced by respiratory syncytial virus in HEp-2 cells (×40).

Enzyme-linked immunosorbent assays (ELISA) effectively detect RSV antigens in nasopharyngeal secretions within 2 to 3 hours after the specimen is received. If an ELISA is to be used to detect RSV the specimen should be transported in a medium containing no more than 0.5% serum, because larger amounts interfere with some tests. The sensitivities and specificities of commercially available kits have ranged from 79 to 95% and from 72 to 99%, respectively (82,84,86). The ELISA involves less specimen handling than immunofluorescence but does not allow the adequacy of the sample to be assessed. Moreover, with some ELISA kits the results are valid only for nasal and nasopharyngeal specimens because sputum, tracheal aspirate, and bronchoalveolar lavage specimens may yield false-positive results. Recent modifications of the ELISA technology—antibody-coated microparticles, biotinylated antibodies, a focuser to concentrate the reaction, and enzyme-labeled antibiotin antibodies—have allowed reliable detection of RSV antigens in about 30 minutes (83,87).

Serologic tests for detection of IgG to RSV antigens are available, but this approach is not recommended for diagnosis of acute infection, because very young children may not exhibit an elevated antibody titer, and acute- and convalescent-phase sera must be collected. Results are interpreted in the same manner as for parainfluenza viruses.

using commercially available reagents are useful for detecting RSV antigens, which in smears of exfoliated nasopharyngeal epithelial cells appear as distinct intracytoplasmic inclusions (Fig. 10–6). Aspirate and wash samples that contain mucus must be washed before smears are prepared and stained, because the nonspecific fluorescence of mucus interferes with interpretation. The sensitivity of immunofluorescence techniques has ranged from 44 to 92%; results generally are available 3 to 4 hours after the specimen is received (or less with direct fluorescence); and the adequacy of the specimen, determined by the quantity of respiratory epithelial cells present, can be assessed (82–85). The main disadvantage is that nonspecific fluorescence may make interpretation difficult.

Treatment

No specific antiviral agent is available for treating parainfluenza, mumps, or measles virus infection. The mainstay of management for each of these infections, and for most infections caused by RSV, is good supportive care. Recently, vitamin A has been shown to reduce the morbidity and mortality of measles and, so, is recommended for all children with severe measles (88). Ribavirin, a virostatic agent administered as a small-particle aerosol into a tent, oxygen hood, mask, or ventilator 12 to 18 hours a day for 2 to 5 days, is approved treatment for hospitalized infants with severe RSV-induced lower respiratory tract disease.

Prevention

Mumps Virus. The live attenuated mumps vaccine is recommended for all susceptible persons at least 12 months of age, unless a contraindication (pregnancy, severe febrile illness, egg allergy, immunosuppression) exists. Mumps vaccine, usually given in combination with measles and rubella vaccines at 15 months of age, has an estimated clinical efficacy of 95%, inducing a protective, long-lasting antibody response in more than 97% of persons who are susceptible to mumps (89–92).

Measles Virus. In 1963, inactivated and live attenuated (Edmonston B strain) measles vaccines were licensed for use in the United States. The inactivated vaccine was no longer distributed after 1967, and the Edmonston B vaccine was discontinued in 1975. Live, further attenuated measles vaccines, both associated with fewer reactions than the Edmonston B vaccine but equally effective, were introduced in 1965 (Schwartz strain) and in 1968 (Moraten strain). The Moraten vaccine, used cur-

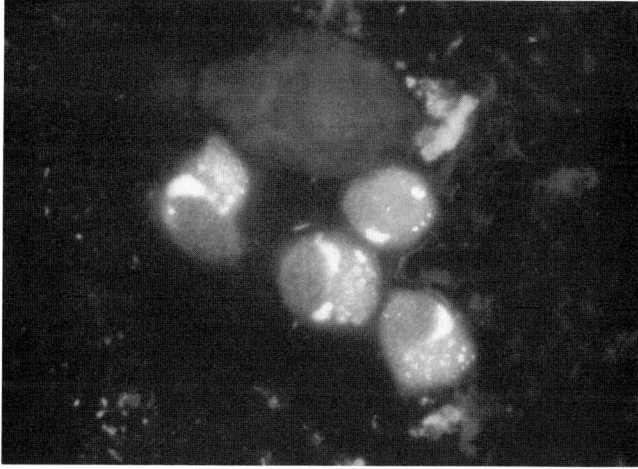

Fig. 10–6. Direct fluorescent antibody–stained nasopharyngeal epithelial cells reflect the presence of respiratory syncytial virus (×400).

rently in the United States, produces an inapparent or mild, noncommunicable infection, induces antibodies in more than 95% of susceptible children vaccinated at age 15 months or older, and provides long-lasting protection for most.

When the measles vaccine was licensed in 1963 a single dose was recommended. Then, the suggested age for vaccination was 9 months, but it was changed to 12 months in 1965, and to 15 months in 1976, because later vaccination was more efficacious. In 1989, the Immunization Practices Advisory Committee recommended a two-dose measles vaccination schedule (Tables 10-3 and 10-4) (28). Live measles vaccine is contraindicated for pregnant women and those who are considering becoming pregnant in the next 3 months, for children with moderate or severe febrile illnesses, for persons who received immune globulin, whole blood, or other antibody-containing blood products within the previous 6 weeks, and for immunocompromised persons.

Respiratory Syncytial Virus. For hospitalized patients measures to prevent nosocomial RSV infection should be implemented. Infected infants should be separated from other infants on a ward, and during an RSV outbreak hospital staff who have a respiratory illness should not care for infants at high risk of complications. Careful hand-washing technique practiced by all personnel is imperative, and using eye-nose goggles and complying with glove and gown isolation precautions decreases the nosocomial infection rate (59,93,94). Research to develop a vaccine to prevent infection with RSV in infancy currently is under way.

Table 10-3. 1989 Recommendations for Measles Vaccination in the United States

Routine childhood schedule	
In most areas	Two doses[*,†]: first at 15 mo, second at 4-6 yrs (on entry to kindergarten or first grade)[‡]
In high-risk areas[§]	Two doses[*,†]: first at 12 mo, second at 4-6 yrs (on entry to kindergarten or first grade)[‡]
Colleges and other educational institutions post-high school	Documentation of two doses of measles vaccine after the first birthday[†] or other evidence of measles immunity[ǁ]
Medical personnel beginning employment	Documentation of two doses of measles vaccine after the first birthday[†] or other evidence of measles immunity[ǁ]

[*] Preferably, both doses should be given as combined measles, mumps, rubella vaccine (MMR).
[†] At least 1 month apart. If no documentation of any vaccination, vaccine should be given on entry to school or employment and no sooner than 1 month later.
[‡] Healthcare personnel in some areas may elect to administer the second dose at a later age or to multiple age groups.
[§] A county with more than five cases among preschool-aged children during each of the last 5 years, a county with a recent outbreak among unvaccinated preschool-aged children, or a county with a large inner-city population. These recommendations may be applied to an entire county or to identified risk areas within a county.
[ǁ] Prior physician-diagnosed measles disease, laboratory evidence of measles immunity, or birth before 1957.
(From Centers for Disease Control: Measles prevention: Recommendations of the Immunization Practices Advisory Committee. MMWR, 38(S-9):1, 1989.)

Table 10-4. Recommendations for Measles Outbreak Control[*]

Population	Measures
Preschool-aged children	Reduce age for vaccination as low as 6 months in outbreak area if cases are occurring in children <1 year of age.[†]
Populations of day-care centers, K-12th grade, colleges, other institutions	Revaccinate all students and their siblings and school personnel born in or after 1957 who do not have documentation of immunity to measles[‡]
Medical caregivers	Revaccinate all medical workers born in or after 1957 who have direct patient contact and no proof of immunity to measles.[‡] Vaccination may also be considered for workers born before 1957. Susceptible persons who have been exposed should be barred from direct patient contact from 5th to 21st day after exposure (regardless of whether they received measles vaccine or immunoglobulin). Workers who become ill should have no patient contact for 7 days after they develop rash.

[*] Revaccination of entire populations is not necessary. Revaccination should be limited to populations at risk, such as students attending institutions where cases occur.
[†] Children initially vaccinated before the first birthday should be revaccinated at 15 months of age. A second dose should be administered at the time of school entry or according to local policy.
[‡] Documentation of physician-diagnosed measles disease, serologic evidence of immunity to measles, or documentation of receipt of two doses of measles vaccine on or after the first birthday.
(Modified from Centers for Disease Control: Measles prevention: Recommendations of the Immunization Practices Advisory Committee. MMWR, 38(S-9):1, 1989.)

REFERENCES

1. Kingsbury DW: Paramyxoviridae and their replication. In Fields' Virology. 2nd ed. Edited by BN Fields and DM Knipe. New York, Raven Press, 1990.
2. Monto AS: The Tecumseh study of respiratory illness. V. Patterns of infection with the parainfluenza viruses. Am J Epidemiol, 97:338, 1973.
3. Brandt CD, Kim HW, Chanock RM, and Parrott RH: Parainfluenza virus epidemiology. Pediatr Res, 8:422, 1974.
4. Downham MAPS, McQuillin J, and Gardner PS: Diagnosis and clinical significance of parainfluenza virus infections in children. Arch Dis Child 49:8, 1974.
5. Denny FW, et al: Croup: An 11-year study in a pediatric practice. Pediatrics, 71:871, 1983.
6. Glezen WP, Frank AL, Taber LH, and Kasel JA: Parainfluenza virus type 3: Seasonality and risk of infection and reinfection in young children. J Infect Dis 150:851, 1984.
7. Parrott RH, et al: Myxoviruses. III. Parainfluenza. Am J Public Health, 52:907, 1962.

8. Parrott RH, et al: Clinical features of infection with hemadsorption viruses. N Engl J Med, 260:731, 1959.
9. Nagai Y, Klenk H-D, and Rott R: Proteolytic cleavage of the viral glycoproteins and its significance for the virulence of Newcastle disease virus. Virology, 72:494, 1976.
10. Rott R: Molecular basis of infectivity and pathogenicity of myxovirus. Arch Virol, 59:285, 1979.
11. Welliver RC, Wong DT, Sun M, and McCarthy N: Parainfluenza virus bronchiolitis: Epidemiology and pathology. Am J Dis Child, 140:3440, 1986.
12. Welliver RC, et al: Role of parainfluenza virus–specific IgE in pathogenesis of croup and wheezing subsequent to infection. J Pediatr, 101:889, 1982.
13. Johnson CD, and Goodpasture EW: An investigation of the etiology of mumps. J Exp Med, 59:1, 1934.
14. Habel K: Cultivation of mumps virus in the developing chick embryo and its application to the studies of immunity to mumps in man. Pub Health Rep, 60:201, 1945.
15. Buynak EB, and Hilleman MR: Live attenuated mumps virus vaccine. I. Vaccine development. Proc Soc Exp Biol Med, 123:768, 1966.
16. Centers for Disease Control: Mumps prevention. MMWR, 38:388, 1989.
17. Wharton M, et al: A large outbreak of mumps in the postvaccine era. J Infect Dis, 158:1253, 1988.
18. Cochi SL, Preblud SR, and Orenstein WA: Perspectives on the relative resurgence of mumps in the United States. Am J Dis Child, 142:499, 1988.
19. Kaplan KM, Marder DC, Cochi SL, and Preblud SR: Mumps in the workplace: Future evidence of the changing epidemiology of a childhood vaccine preventable disease. JAMA, 260:1434, 1988.
20. Bang HO, and Bang J: Involvement of the central nervous system in mumps. Acta Med Scand, 113:487, 1943.
21. Siegal M, Fuerst H, and Peress NG: Comparative fetal mortality in maternal virus diseases. N Engl J Med 274:768, 1966.
22. Ylinen O, and Jarvinen PA: Parotitis during pregnancy. Acta Obstet Gynecol, 32:121, 1953.
23. Johnstone JA, Ross CAC, and Dunn M: Meningitis and encephalitis associated with mumps infection. Arch Dis Child, 47:647, 1972.
24. Panum PL: Observations made during the epidemic of measles on the Faroe Islands in the year 1846. Med Classics, 3:839, 1939.
25. Josias A: Recherches experimentales sur la transmissibilite de la rugeole aux animaux. Med Mod 9:158, 1898.
26. Goldberger J, and Anderson JF: An experimental demonstration of the presence of the virus of measles in the mixed buccal and nasal secretions. JAMA, 57:476, 1911.
27. Enders JF, and Peebles TC: Propagation in tissue cultures of cytopathic agents from patients with measles. Proc Soc Exp Biol Med 86:277, 1954.
28. Centers for Disease Control: Measles prevention: Recommendations of the Immunization Practices Advisory Committee. MMWR, 38(S9):1, 1989.
29. Measles Surveillance Report No. 11, 1977–1981. Atlanta, Centers for Disease Control, 1982.
30. Centers for Disease Control: Measles—U.S., 1989 and first 20 weeks 1990. MMWR, 39:353, 1990.
31. Lachmann PJ: Immunopathology of measles. Proc R Soc Med, 67:12, 1974.
32. Barkin RM: Measles mortality: A retrospective look at the vaccine era. Am J Epidemiol, 102:341, 1975.
33. Barkin RM: Measles mortality. Analysis of the primary cause of death. Am J Dis Child, 129:307, 1975.
34. Dawson JR: Cellular inclusions in cerebral lesions of lethargic encephalitis. Am J Pathol, 9:7, 1933.
35. Horta-Barbosa L, Sever J, and Zeman W: Subacute sclerosing panencephalitis: Isolation of measles virus from a brain biopsy. Nature, 221:974, 1969.
36. Payne FE, Baublis JV, and Itabashi HH: Isolation of measles virus from cell cultures of brain from a patient with subacute sclerosing panencephalitis. N Engl J Med, 281:585, 1969.
37. Cattaneo R, et al: Multiple viral mutations rather than host factors cause defective measles virus gene expression in a subacute sclerosing panencephalitis cell line. J Virol 62:1388, 1988.
38. Cattaneo R, et al: Accumulated measles virus mutations in a case of subacute sclerosing panencephalitis: Interrupted matrix protein–reading frame and transcription alteration. Virology, 154:97, 1986.
39. Chanock RM, and Parrott, RH: Acute respiratory disease in infancy and childhood: Present understanding and prospects for prevention. Pediatrics, 36:21, 1965.
40. Glezen WP, and Denny FW: Epidemiology of acute lower respiratory disease in children. N Engl J Med, 288:498, 1973.
41. Morris JA, Blount RE, and Savage RE: Recovery of cytopathogenic agent from chimpanzees with coryza. Proc Soc Exp Biol Med, 92:544, 1956.
42. Chanock R, Roizman B, and Myers R: Recovery from infants with respiratory illness of a virus related to chimpanzee coryza agent (CCA): I. Isolation, properties and characterization. Am J Hyg 66:281, 1957.
43. Johnson PR, et al: The G glycoprotein of human respiratory syncytial viruses of subgroups A and B: Extensive sequence divergence between antigenically related proteins. Proc Natl Acad Sci USA 84:5625, 1987.
44. Mufson MA, et al: Respiratory syncytial virus epidemics: Variable dominance of subgroups A and B strains among children, 1981–1986. J Infect Dis 157:143, 1988.
45. Parrott RH, et al: Epidemiology of respiratory syncytial virus infection in Washington, DC. II. Infection and disease with respect to age, immunologic status, race and sex. Am J Epidemiol 98:289, 1973.
46. Parrott RH et al: Respiratory syncytial virus. II. Serologic studies over a 34-month period of children with bronchiolitis, pneumonia, and minor respiratory diseases. JAMA, 176:653, 1961.
47. Suto T, et al: Respiratory syncytial virus infection and its serologic epidemiology. Am J Epidemiol, 82:211, 1965.
48. Glezen WP, et al: Risk of primary infection and reinfection with respiratory syncytial virus. Am J Dis Child, 140:543, 1986.
49. Henderson FW, et al: Respiratory syncytial virus infections, reinfections, and immunity. A prospective, longitudinal study in young children. N Engl J Med, 300:530, 1979.
50. Vikersfors T, Grandien M, and Olcen P: Respiratory syncytial virus infections in adults. Am Rev Respir Dis, 136:561, 1987.
51. Hall WJ, Hall CB, and Speers DM: Respiratory syncytial virus infection in adults. Clinical, virologic, and serial pulmonary function studies. Ann Intern Med, 88:203, 1978.
52. Finger R, et al: Epidemic infections caused by respiratory syncytial virus in institutionalized young adults. J Infect Dis, 155:1335, 1987.
53. Hart RJC: An outbreak of respiratory syncytial virus infection in an old people's home. J Infect, 8:259, 1984.
54. Sorvillo FJ, et al: An outbreak of respiratory syncytial virus pneumonia in a nursing home for the elderly. J Infect 9:252, 1984.
55. Englund JA, et al: Respiratory syncytial virus infection in

55. immunocompromised adults. Ann Intern Med, *109*:203, 1988.
56. Hertz MI, et al: Respiratory syncytial virus–induced acute lung injury in adult patients in bone marrow transplants: A clinical approach and review of the literature. Medicine, *68*:269, 1989.
57. Hall CB, et al: Nosocomial respiratory syncytial virus infections. N Engl J Med, *293*:1343, 1975.
58. Hall CB, Kopelman A, and Douglas RG Jr: Neonatal respiratory syncytial viral infections. N Engl J Med, *300*:393, 1979.
59. Agah R, et al: Respiratory syncytial virus (RSV) infection rate in personnel caring for children with RSV infection. Am J Dis Child, *141*:695, 1987.
60. Hall CB: The nosocomial spread of respiratory syncytial virus infections. Annu Rev Med, *34*:311, 1983.
61. Kim, HW, et al: Cell-mediated immunity to respiratory syncytial virus induced by inactivated vaccine or by infection. Pediatr Res, *10*:75, 1976.
62. Welliver RC, Kaul TN, and Ogra PL: The appearance of cell-bound IgE in respiratory-tract epithelium after respiratory syncytial virus infection. N Engl J Med, *303*:1198, 1980.
63. Welliver RC, et al: The development of respiratory syncytial virus–specific IgE and the release of histamine in nasopharyngeal secretions after infection. N Engl J Med, *305*:841, 1981.
64. Toms GL, and Scott R: Respiratory syncytial virus and the infant immune response. Arch Dis Child, *62*:544, 1987.
65. Hall CB, et al: Respiratory syncytial virus infection in children with compromised immune function. N Engl J Med, *315*:77, 1986.
66. Fishaut M, Tubergen D, and McIntosh K: Cellular response to respiratory viruses with particular reference to children with disorders of cell-mediated immunity. J Pediatr, *96*:179, 1980.
67. Ogra PL, and Patel J: Respiratory syncytial virus infection and the immunocompromised host. Pediatr Infect Dis J, *7*:246, 1988.
68. Kapikian AZ, et al: An outbreak of febrile illness and pneumonia associated with respiratory syncytial virus infection. Am J Hyg, *74*:234, 1961.
69. Denny FW, and Clyde WA: Acute lower respiratory tract infections in nonhospitalized children. J Pediatr, *108*:635, 1986.
70. Lee, GC-Y, et al: An outbreak of respiratory syncytial virus infection in an infant nursery. J Formosan Med Assoc, *72*:39, 1973.
71. Sterner G, et al: Respiratory syncytial virus. An outbreak of acute respiratory illness in a home for infants. Acta Paediatr Scand, *55*:273, 1966.
72. Carilli AD, Gohd RS, and Gordon W: A virologic study of chronic bronchitis. N Engl J Med, *270*:123, 1964.
73. Sommerville RG: Respiratory syncytial virus in acute exacerbations of chronic bronchitis. Lancet, *ii*:1247, 1963.
74. Mathur U, Bentley DW, and Hall CB: Concurrent outbreaks of respiratory syncytial virus and influenza A/Texas/77 infection in the institutionalized elderly and chronically ill. Ann Intern Med, *93*:49, 1980.
75. Garvie DG, and Gray J: Outbreak of respiratory syncytial virus infection in the elderly. Br Med J, *281*:1253, 1980.
76. Gardner PS, et al: Deaths associated with respiratory tract infection in childhood. Br Med J, *4*:316, 1967.
77. Brugman S, and Hutter JJ: Respiratory syncytial virus (RSV) pneumonitis in acute leukemia. Am J Hematol Oncol, *2*:271, 1980.
78. Craft QW, et al: Virus infections in children with acute lymphoblastic leukemia. Arch Dis Child, *54*:755, 1979.
79. Johnson FB: Transport of viral specimens. Clin Microbiol Rev, *3*:120, 1990.
80. Frank AL, Couch RB, Griffis CA, and Baxter BD: Comparison of different tissue cultures for isolation and quantitation of influenza and parainfluenza viruses. J Clin Microbiol, *10*:32, 1979.
81. Minnich LL, Goodenough F, and Ray G: Use of immunofluorescence to identify measles virus infections. J Clin Microbiol, *29*:1148, 1991.
82. Masters HB, et al: Comparison of nasopharyngeal washings and swab specimens for diagnosis of respiratory syncytial virus by EIA, FAT, and cell culture. Diagn Microbiol Infect Dis, *8*:101, 1987.
83. Waner JL, et al: Comparison of Directigen RSV with viral isolation and direct immunofluorescence for the identification of respiratory syncytial virus. J Clin Microbiol, *28*:480, 1990.
84. Halstead DC, Todd S, and Fritch G: Evaluation of five methods for respiratory syncytial virus detection. J Clin Microbiol, *28*:1021, 1990.
85. Welliver RC: Detection, pathogenesis, and therapy of respiratory syncytial virus infections. Clin Microbiol Rev, *1*:27, 1988.
86. Ahluwalia GS, and Hammond GW: Comparison of cell culture and three enzyme-linked immunosorbent assays for the rapid diagnosis of respiratory syncytial virus from nasopharyngeal aspirate and tracheal secretion specimens. Diagn Microbiol Infect Dis, *9*:187, 1988.
87. Swierkosz EM, et al: Evaluation of the Abbott TESTPACK RSV enzyme immunoassay for detection of respiratory syncytial virus in nasopharyngeal swab specimens. J Clin Microbiol, *27*:1151, 1989.
88. Hussey GD, and Klein M: A randomized, controlled trial of vitamin A in children with severe measles. N Engl J Med, *323*:160, 1990.
89. Sugg WC, Finger JA, Levine RH, and Pagano JS: Field evaluation of live virus mumps vaccine. J Pediatr, *72*:461, 1968.
90. Hilleman MR, et al: Live, attenuated mumps-virus vaccine: 4. Protective efficacy as measured in a field evaluation. N Engl J Med, *276*:252, 1967.
91. Weibel RE, Buynak EB, McLean AA, and Hilleman MR: Follow-up surveillance for antibody in human subjects following live attenuated measles, mumps, and rubella virus vaccines. Proc Soc Exp Biol Med, *162*:328, 1979.
92. Weibel RE, et al: Persistence of antibody in human subjects for 7 to 10 years following administration of combined live attenuated measles, mumps, and rubella virus vaccines. Proc Soc Exp Biol Med, *165*:260, 1980.
93. Gala CL, et al: The use of eye-nose goggles to control nosocomial respiratory syncytial virus infection. JAMA, *256*:2706, 1986.
94. Leclair JM, et al: Prevention of nosocomial respiratory syncytial virus infections through compliance with glove and gown isolation precautions. N Engl J Med, *317*:329, 1987.

Plate I

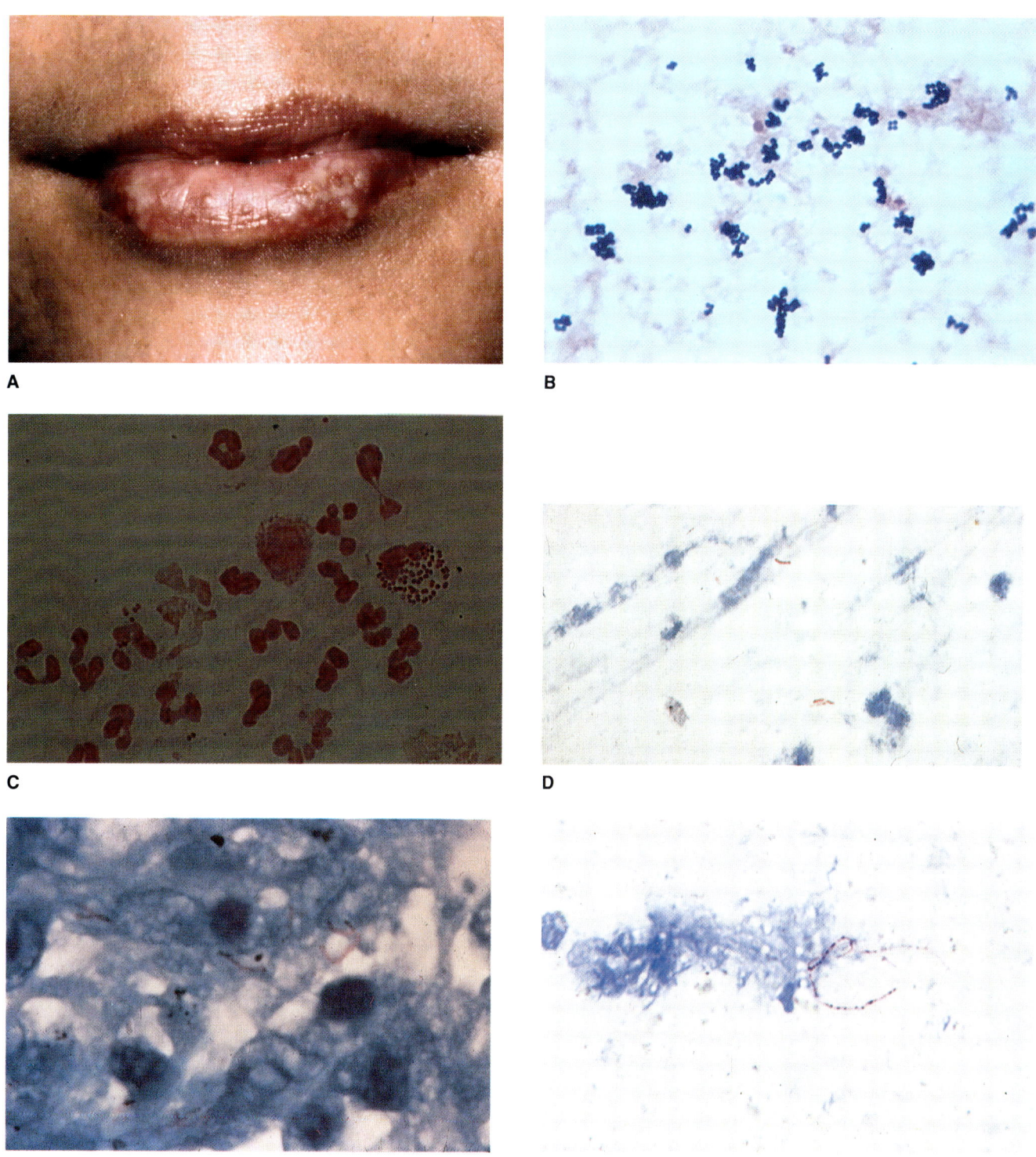

Plate I. *A*, The lesions of herpes labialis. *B*, Gram-positive cocci in clusters (Staphylococcus aureus) in a smear of a blood culture broth (Gram stain, ×400). *C*, Smear of urethral exudate shows intracellular gram-negative diplococci (Neisseria gonorrhoeae, Gram stain, ×400). *D*, Acid-fast bacilli (Mycobacterium tuberculosis) in a smear of sputum (Ziehl-Neelsen stain, ×400). (Courtesy of Gerri Hall, PhD, Cleveland Clinic Foundation.) *E*, Smear of stool shows large, barred, acid-fast bacilli (Mycobacterium kansasii; Ziehl-Neelsen stain, ×512). (Courtesy of Gerri Hall, MD, Cleveland Clinic Foundation.) *F*, Smear of exudate from a subcutaneous abscess contains cells of Nocardia asteroides (partial acid-fast stain, ×400).

Plate II

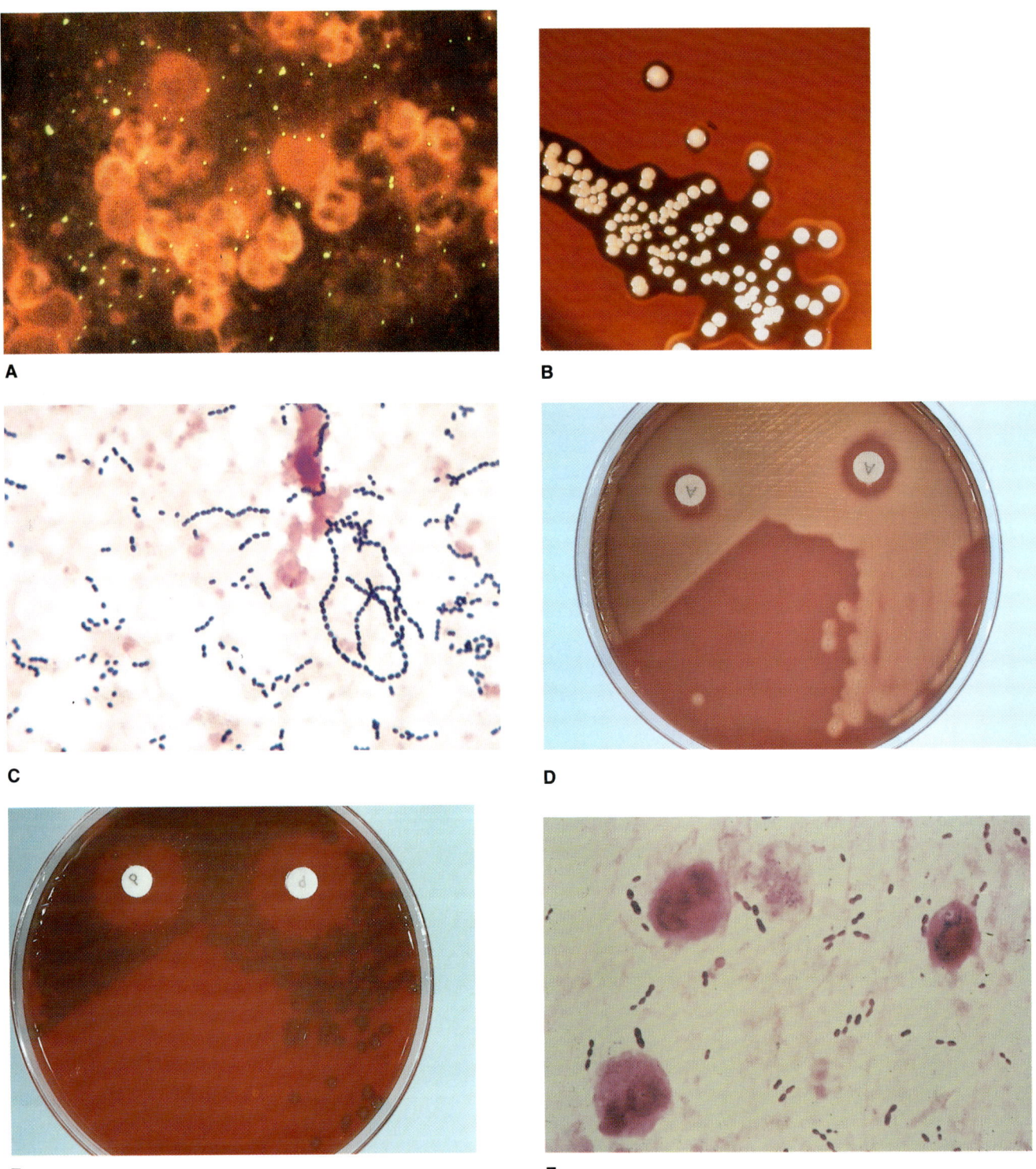

Plate II. *A*, Smear of exudate from the endocervix demonstrates elementary bodies of Chlamydia trachomatis (direct fluorescent antibody, ×320). *B*, Colonies of Staphylococcus aureus on sheep blood agar. *C*, Gram-positive cocci in pairs and chains (Streptococcus pneumoniae) in a smear of a blood culture broth (Gram stain, ×400). *D*, Colonies of group A Streptococcus, susceptible to bacitracin, on sheep blood agar. *E*, Colonies of Streptococcus pneumoniae, susceptible to optochin, on sheep blood agar. *F*, Smear of sputum contains gram-positive, lancet-shaped diplococci (Streptococcus pneumoniae; Gram stain, ×400).

Plate III

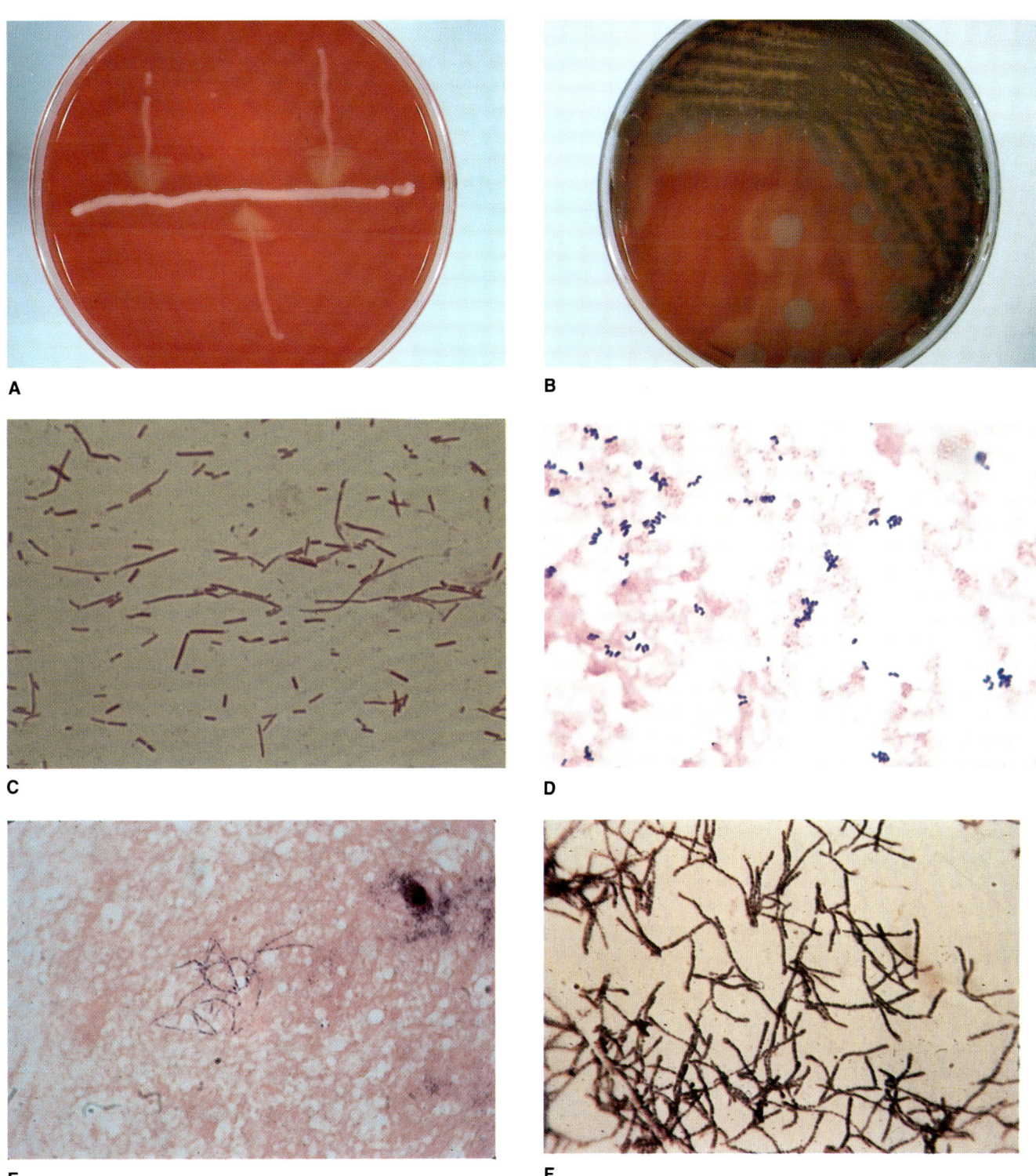

Plate III. *A*, Positive CAMP test result (group B Streptococcus). *B*, Colonies of Bacillus species on sheep blood agar. *C*, Cells of lactobacilli (Gram stain, ×400). *D*, Diphtheroids in a smear of a blood culture broth (Gram stain, ×400). *E*, Branching, beaded, thin gram-positive bacilli of Nocardia asteroides in a smear of exudate from a brain abscess (Gram stain, ×400). *F*, Cells of Actinomyces israelii in a smear of growth from colonies on sheep blood agar (Gram stain, ×400).

Plate IV

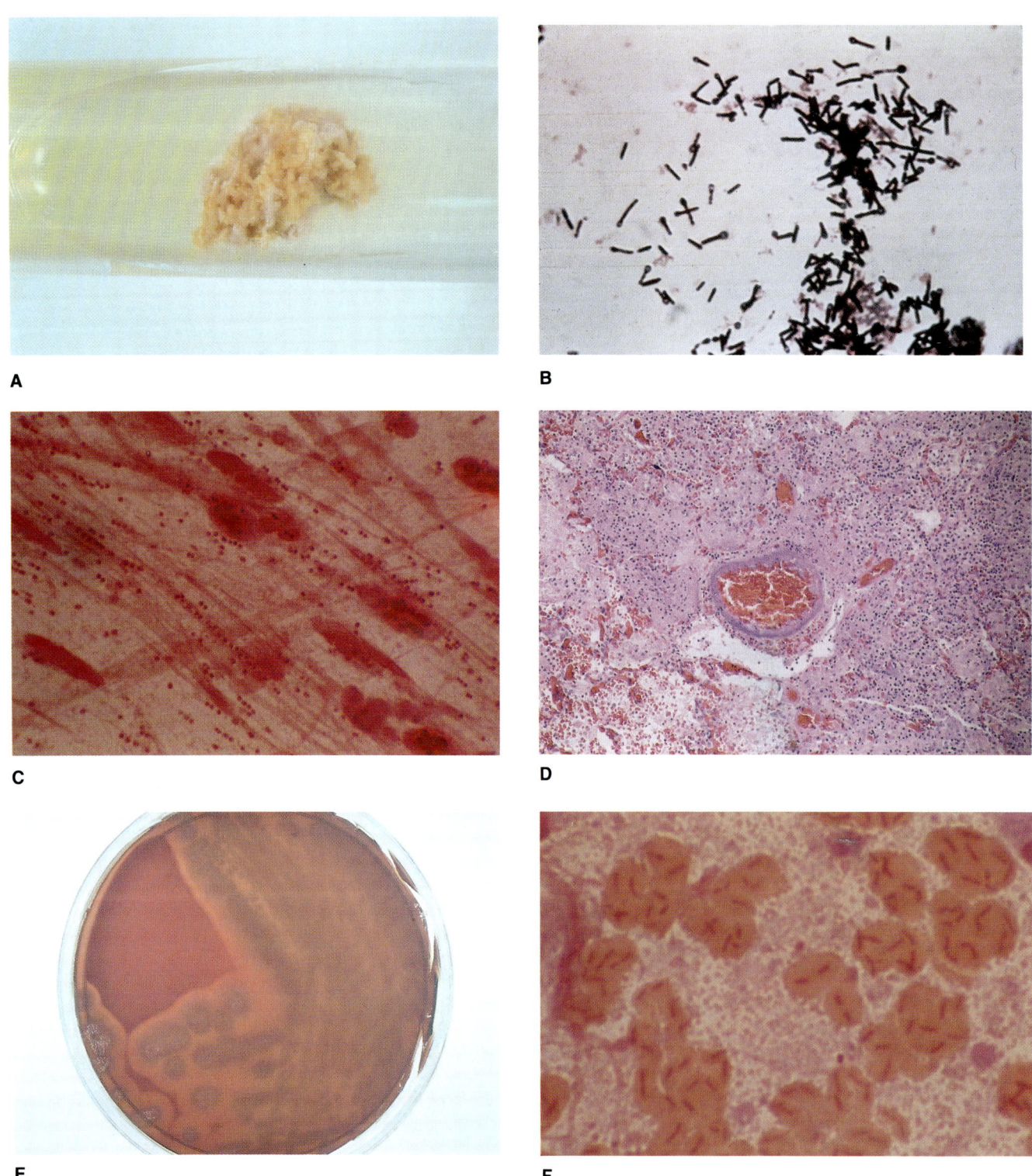

Plate IV. *A,* Colonies of Nocardia asteroides on Sabouraud's dextrose agar. *B,* Cells of Clostridium tetani (Gram stain, ×400). *C,* Smear of sputum shows many extracellular and intracellular gram-negative diplococci (Branhamella catarrhalis; Gram stain, ×400). *D,* Section of lung from a patient with necrotizing Pseudomonas aeruginosa pneumonia shows characteristic vessel involvement (hematoxylin and eosin, ×157.5). *E,* Colonies of Pseudomonas aeruginosa on sheep blood agar. *F,* Smear of sputum shows gram-negative bacilli with thick capsules (Pseudomonas aeruginosa; Gram stain, ×512).

Plate V

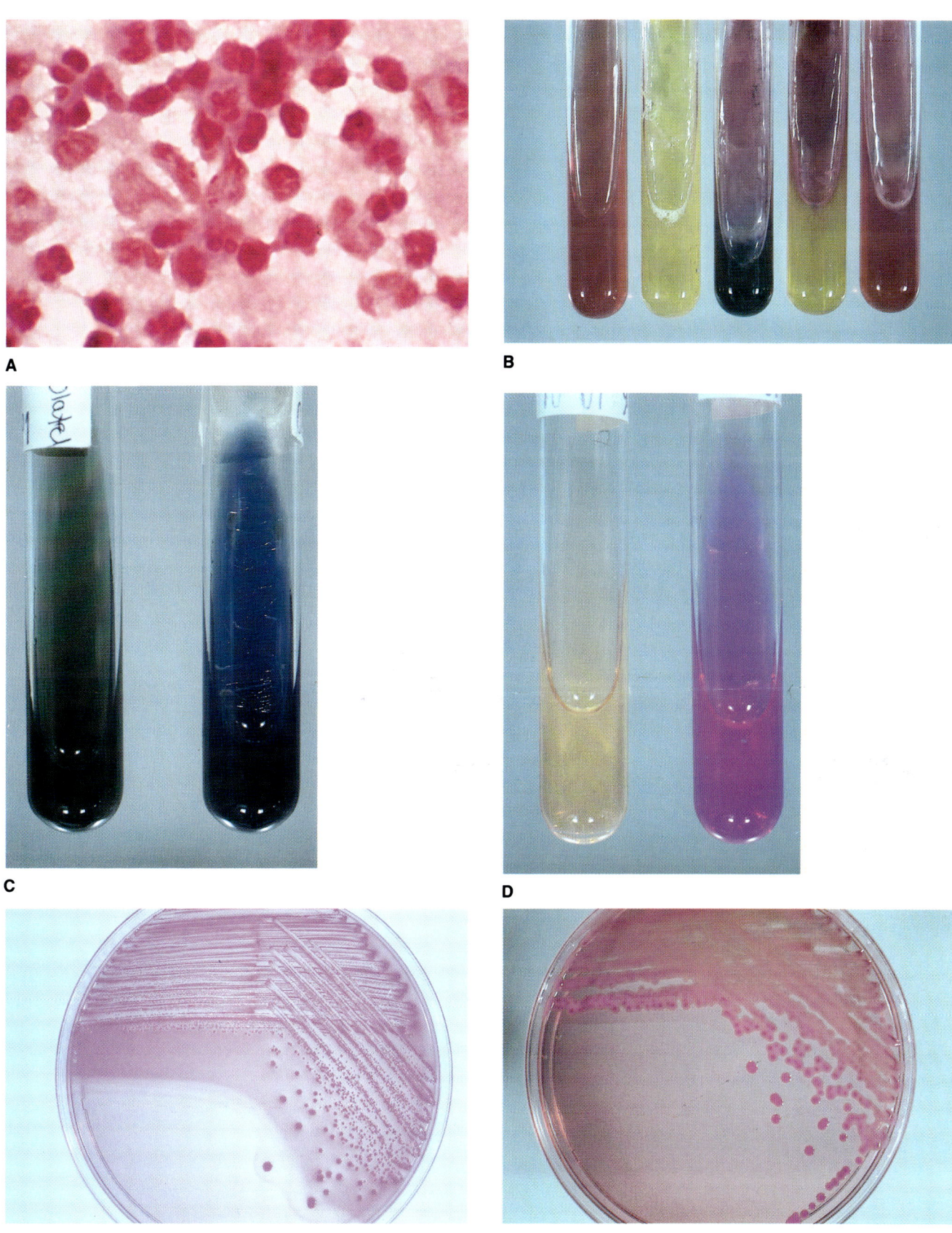

Plate V. *A*, Smear of cerebrospinal fluid shows gram-negative bacilli (Gram stain, ×400) Culture grew Enterobacter cloacae. *B*, Kligler's iron agar: uninoculated, *left,* and *left to right,* reactions when inoculated with Escherichia coli (A/A), Salmonella (K/A, H$_2$S), Shigella (K/A), and Pseudomonas aeruginosa (K/K). *C*, Citrate agar uninoculated, left, and inoculated with Klebsiella pneumoniae, right. *D*, Christensen's urea agar uninoculated, left, and inoculated with Proteus mirabilis, right. *E*, Colonies of Escherichia coli on MacConkey agar. *F*, Colonies of Klebsiella pneumoniae on MacConkey agar.

Plate VI

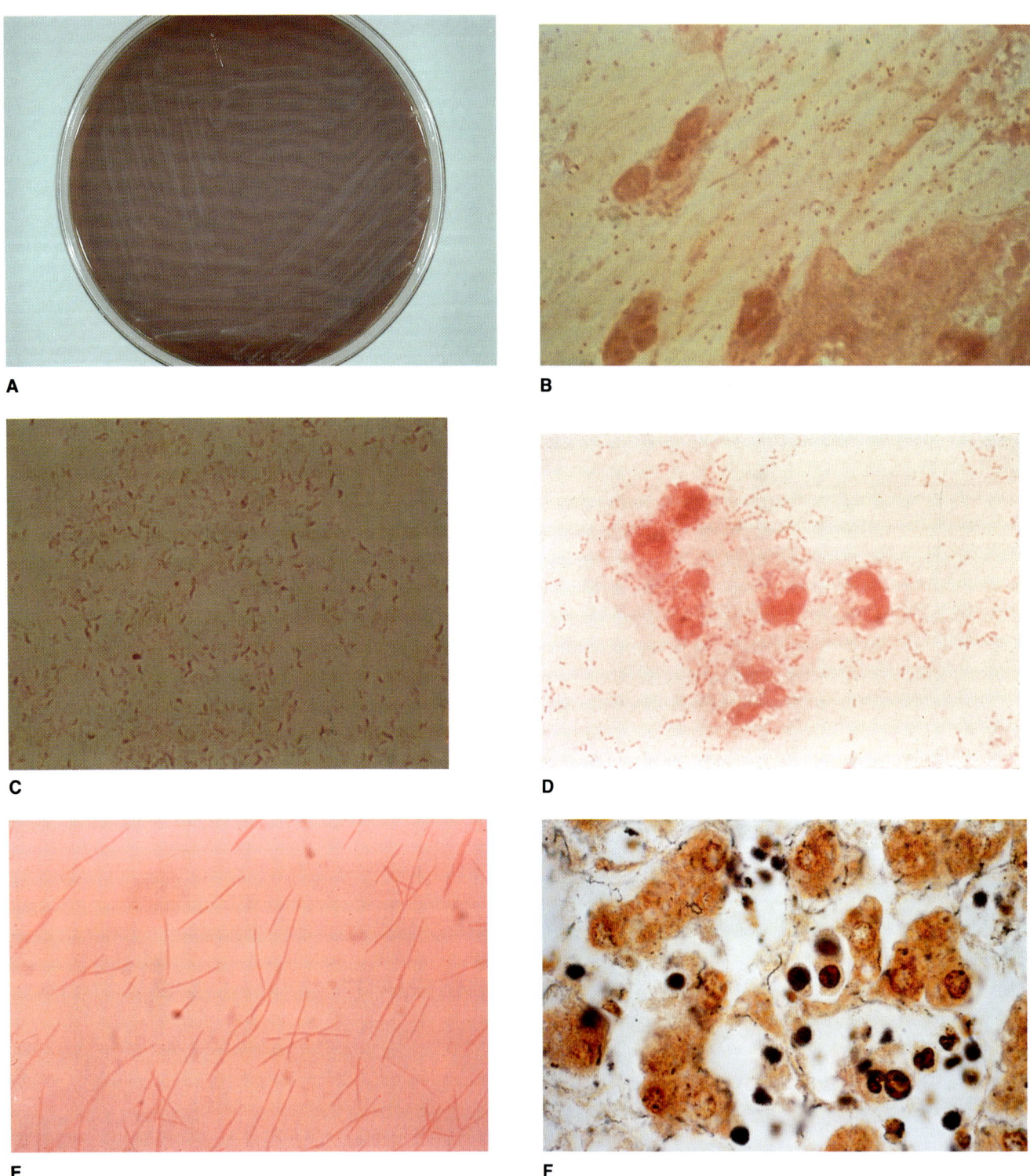

Plate VI. *A*, Swarming of Proteus mirabilis on sheep blood agar. *B*, Smear of sputum shows many tiny gram-negative bacilli (Haemophilus influenzae; Gram stain, ×400). *C*, Cells of Campylobacter jejuni (Gram stain, ×400). *D*, Smear of cerebrospinal fluid shows gram-negative coccobacilli (Gram stain, ×400. Culture grew Bacteroides fragilis. (Courtesy of Gerri Hall, PhD, Cleveland Clinic Foundation.) *E*, Cells of Fusobacterium nucleatum (Gram stain, ×400). (Courtesy of Gerri Hall, PhD, Cleveland Clinic Foundation.) *F*, Section of liver from an infant with congenital syphilis (Warthin-Starry stain, ×320).

Plate VII

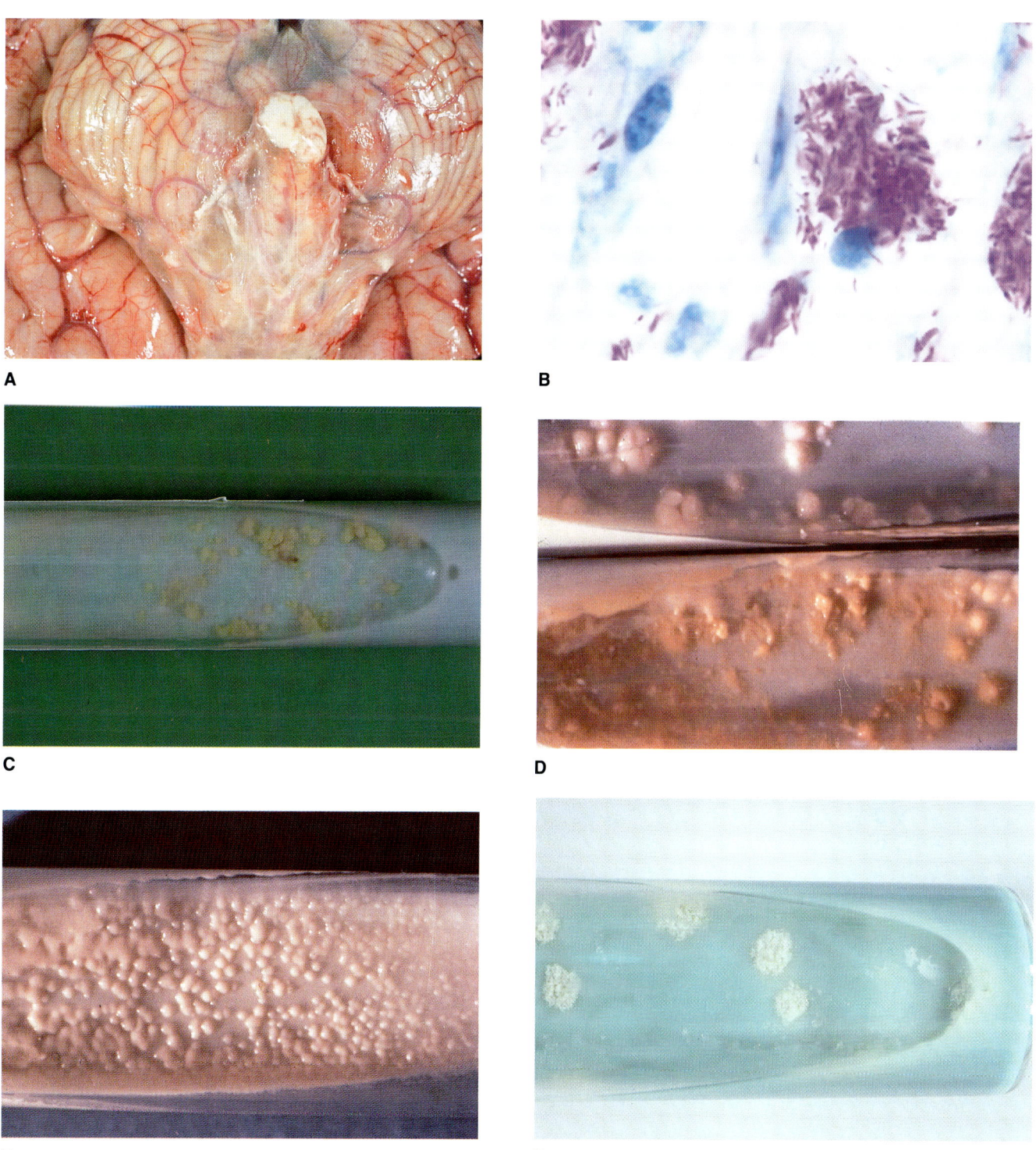

Plate VII. *A*, Brain from a patient with fatal tuberculous meningitis shows the characteristic exudate at the base. *B*, Imprint of a lymph node from a patient with AIDS shows intracellular acid-fast bacilli (Mycobacterium avium-intracellulare; Ziehl-Neelsen stain, ×400). *C*, Colonies of Mycobacterium tuberculosis on Lowenstein-Jensen medium. (Courtesy of Cathy Looby, MD, Medical College of Pennsylvania.) *D*, Colonies of Mycobacterium kansasii on Lowenstein-Jensen medium before, top, and after, bottom, exposure to light. (Courtesy of Gerri Hall, PhD, Cleveland Clinic Foundation.) *E*, Colonies of Mycobacterium avium-intracellulare on Lowenstein-Jensen medium. (Courtesy of Gerri Hall, PhD, Cleveland Clinic Foundation.) *F*, Colonies of Mycobacterium fortuitum on Lowenstein-Jensen medium.

Plate VIII

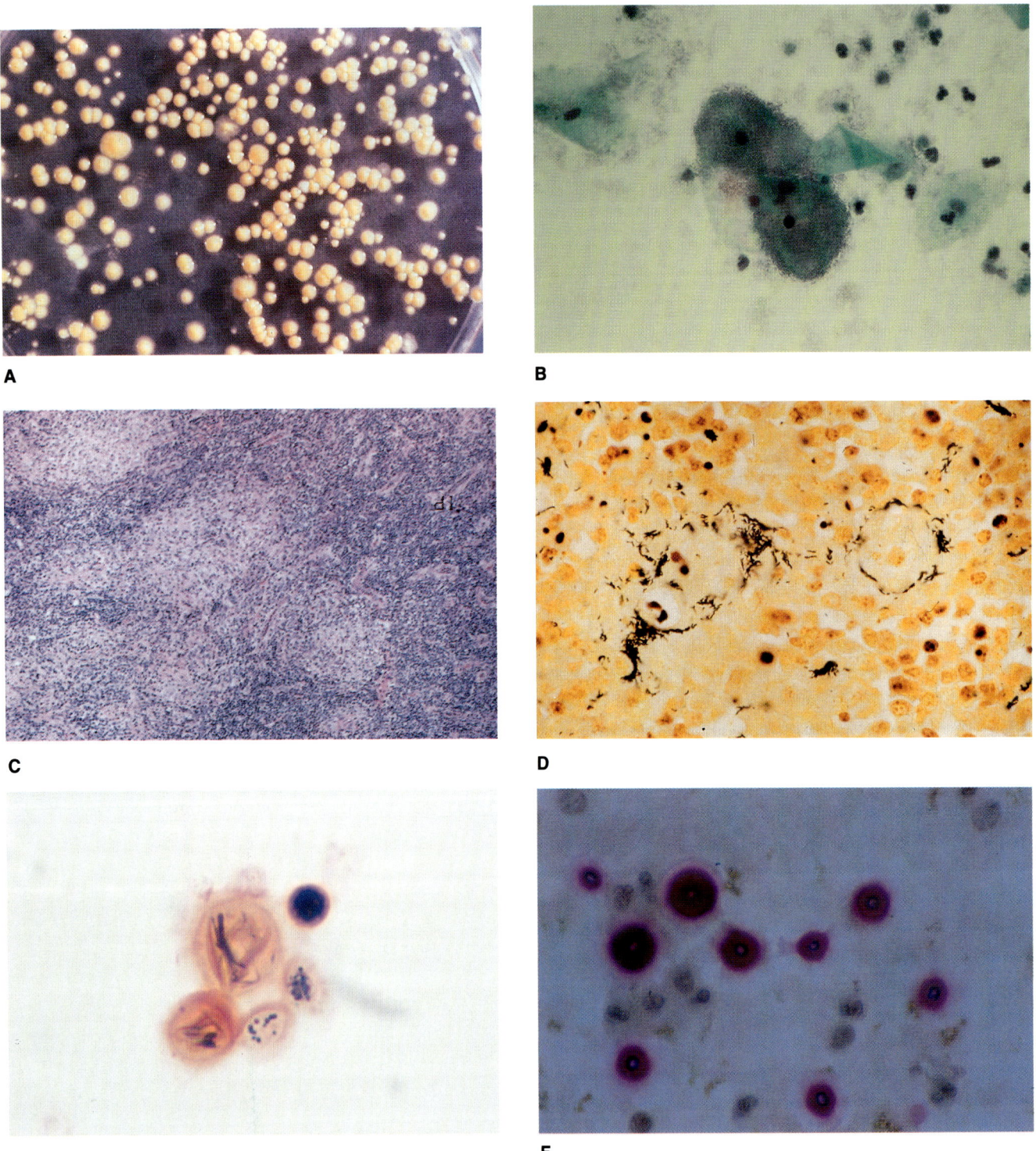

Plate VIII. *A*, Colonies of Mycobacterium gordonae on Middlebrook agar. (Courtesy of Gerri Hall, PhD, Cleveland Clinic Foundation.) *B*, Smear of endocervical cells shows "clue cells" (Papanicolaou stain, ×157.5). *C*, Section of lymph node demonstrates typical abscesses of cat scratch disease (hematoxylin and eosin, ×40). *D*, Section of lymph node shows the bacilli of cat scratch disease (Warthin-Starry stain, ×320). *E*, Smear of cerebrospinal fluid with budding yeast (Cryptococcus neoformans; Gram stain, ×256). *F*, Cells of Cryptococcus neoformans in smear of cerebrospinal fluid (mucicarmine, ×256). (Courtesy of Cathy Soldo, MD, Medical College of Pennsylvania.)

Plate IX

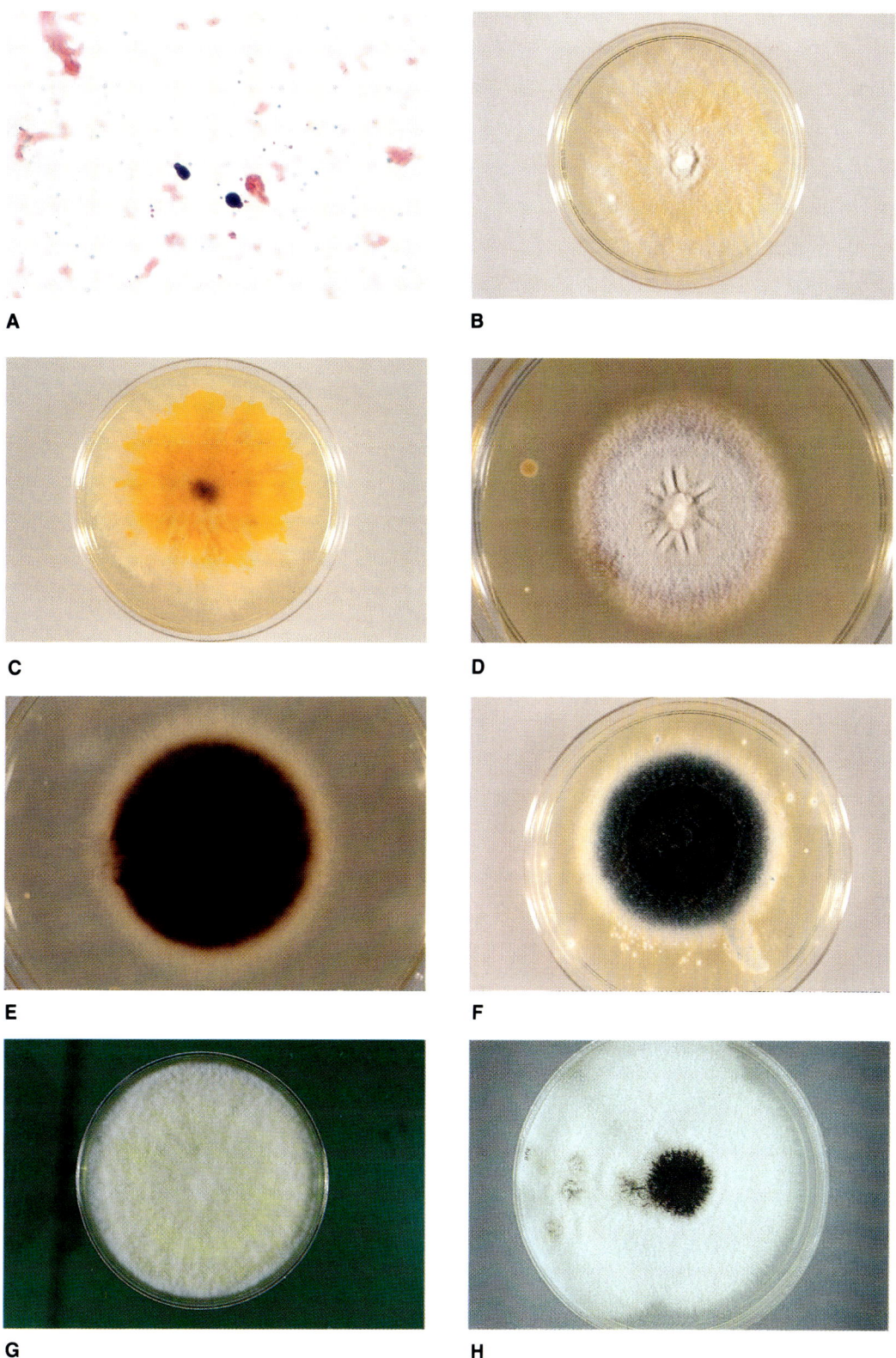

Plate IX. *A,* Yeast cells of Malassezia furfur in a smear of growth from a blood culture broth (Gram stain, ×320). *B,C,* Colony of Microsporum canis on Sabouraud's dextrose agar: *B,* front; *C,* reverse. *D,E,* Colony of Trichophyton mentagrophytes on Sabouraud's dextrose agar: *D,* front; *E,* reverse. *F,* Colony of Aspergillus fumigatus on Sabouraud's dextrose agar. *G,* Colony of Aspergillus flavus on Sabouraud's dextrose agar. *H,* Colony of Aspergillus niger on Sabouraud's dextrose agar.

Plate X

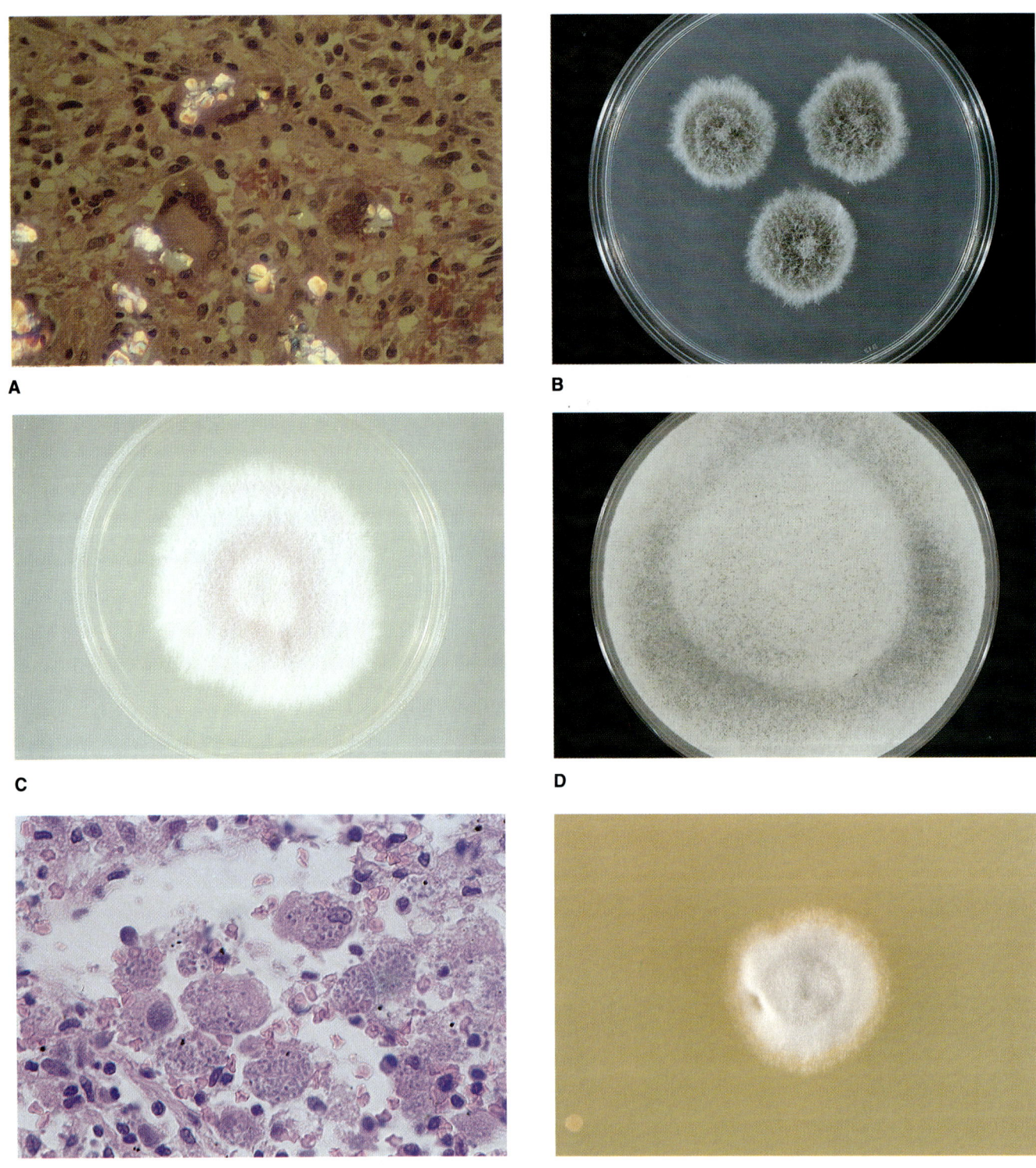

Plate X. *A*, Section of lung from a patient with Aspergillus niger pneumonia shows oxalate crystals. *B*, Colonies of Pseudallescheria boydii on Sabouraud's dextrose agar. *C*, Colony of Fusarium on Sabouraud's dextrose agar. *D*, Colony of Rhizopus on Sabouraud's dextrose agar. *E*, Section of liver from a patient with disseminated histoplasmosis shows Kupffer cells filled with yeast (hematoxylin and eosin, ×320). *F*, Colony of Blastomyces dermatitidis on Sabouraud's dextrose agar.

Plate XI

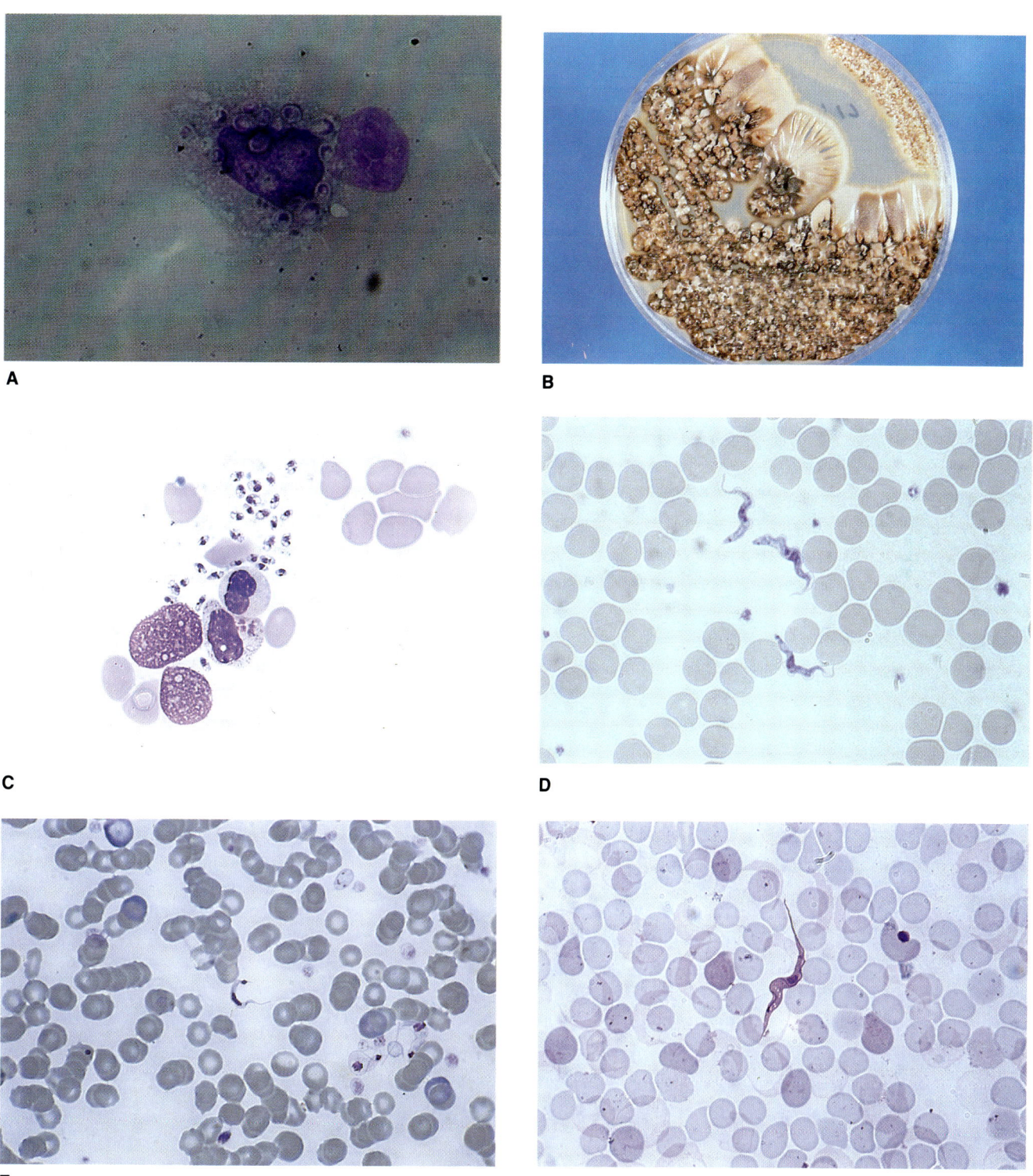

Plate XI. *A*, Smear of bone marrow from a patient with disseminated histoplasmosis shows a mononuclear cell filled with yeast (Wright stain, ×400). *B*, Colonies of Sporothrix schenckii on Sabouraud's dextrose agar. *C*, Leishmania donovani in a bone marrow smear (Giemsa ×320). *D*, Trypanosoma brucei in peripheral blood (Giemsa stain, ×320). *E*, Trypanosoma cruzi in peripheral blood (Giemsa stain, ×320). *F*, Trypanosoma rangeli in peripheral blood of mouse (Giemsa stain, ×320).

Plate XII

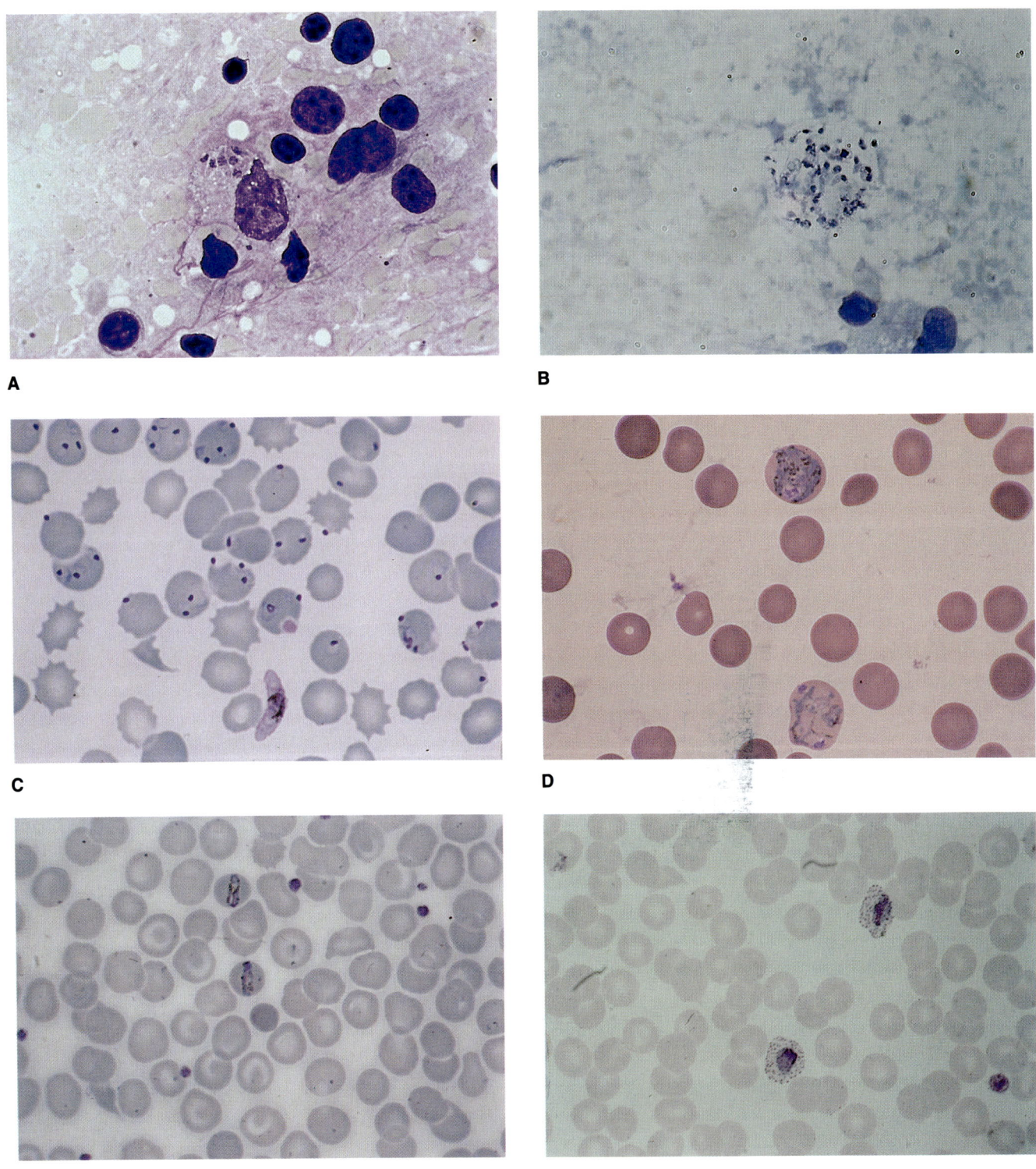

Plate XII. *A*, Toxoplasma gondii imprint of brain (Giemsa stain ×320). Note the tachyzoites in the cytoplasm of the cell. *B*, Toxoplasma gondii imprint of brain. Note the tachyzoites freed from the cell, an artifact of preparation of the smear, (Wright stain, ×320). *C*, Plasmodium falciparum in peripheral blood from person with a fatal infection (Giemsa stain, ×320). Note the number of parasitized red blood cells in normal-sized red blood cells. A gametocyte is also seen, indicating that infection has been present at least 3 weeks. *D*, P. vivax in human blood (Wright stain, ×320). Note a gametocyte, seen as a solid body almost filling the enlarged and deformed red blood cell, and a schizont (three nuclei) with numerous pseudopods. *E*, P. malariae in human blood (Giemsa stain, ×320). Two band forms are shown; note that the red blood cells are not deformed or enlarged. *F*, P. ovale in human blood (Giemsa stain, ×320). Note two trophozoites with little movement (no pseudopods). The stain shows the stippling of enlarged and deformed red blood cells.

Chapter 11

ORTHOMYXOVIRUSES

The orthomyxoviruses influenza A and influenza B have been responsible for recurrent epidemics of febrile respiratory tract disease every 1 to 3 years for at least four centuries (1). The illness typically is acute and self-limited, but it may be associated with significant morbidity and mortality, especially among elders and persons who have cardiac or pulmonary disease.

CLASSIFICATION

The orthomyxoviruses are classified in the family Orthomyxoviridae, which contains one genus, Influenzavirus, with two official members: influenza virus type A, first isolated in 1933, and influenza virus type B, first isolated in 1939 (2). Influenza A and B viruses are subtyped according to the hemagglutinin and neuraminidase glycoproteins (described later). Three hemagglutinins (H1, H2, and H3) and two neuraminidases (N1 and N2) are known. Within a subtype, each strain is identified by the site and year of virus isolation. For example, influenza A/Texas/77/H3N2 indicates influenza A virus of subtype H3N2 isolated in Texas in 1977. Influenza virus type C probably should be classified in another genus, but this is not official. Influenza A virus infects humans, swine, horses, seals, and birds; influenza B virus infects only humans; and influenza C virus infects primarily humans but in China has been isolated from swine (3). Only human viruses are discussed in this chapter.

STRUCTURE

With minor exceptions, all influenza viruses are morphologically similar. Virions, 80 to 120 nm in diameter, are pleomorphic spheres or filaments up to 400 nm long surrounded by a host cell membrane–derived lipid envelope from which surface glycoprotein spikes project (Fig. 11–1). A unique feature of influenza C virus is the organization of its surface glycoprotein molecules into orderly hexagonal arrays rather than the spikes of influenza A and B virus.

The influenza virus nucleocapsid exists as discrete segments, each containing one molecule of single-stranded, negative-sense RNA, multiple copies of the nucleoprotein (NP) polypeptides, and one or more polymerase polypeptides. The genomes of influenza A and B viruses contain 10 genes apportioned among eight segments, whereas the genome of influenza C virus, which codes for a single surface glycoprotein, has seven segments specifying eight known proteins (Table 11–1). Genome segments probably are randomly incorporated into mature virions, a process that would account for the high frequency of reassortment of RNA segments that occurs between two influenza viruses when both simultaneously infect one cell and that might be an important mechanism of antigenic variation (discussed later). The 60,000–molecular weight NP protein subunit of the helical nucleocapsid possesses the type-specific antigenicity upon which is based the classification of influenza virus into A, B, and C types.

Closely associated with the inner surface of the influenza virus envelope is the 26,000–molecular weight type-specific matrix or membrane (M) protein, an important structural component involved in the early assembly and budding stages of viral replication. Attached to and projecting from the outer layer of the lipid envelope are the neuraminidase (NA) and hemagglutinin (HA) peplomers of influenza A and B viruses and the single glycoprotein of influenza C virus. The rod-shaped HA molecule contains the site for attachment to host cells and to erythrocytes, and HA-specific antibodies prevent infection and hemagglutination. The mushroom-shaped NA spike enzymatically cleaves the sialic acid residue from any glycoconjugate that possesses that terminal sugar, including its own structural oligosaccharide chains and those of hemagglutinin. Potential roles of NA during infection include direction of protein transport to apical cell surfaces, removal of neuraminic acid from mucins in the respiratory tract that might interfere with viral attachment to host cell receptors, release of mature virions from an infected cell, prevention of virus aggregation, or a combination of these functions.

A unique feature of influenza A virus is its ability to undergo antigenic variation, or change in antigenicity, yielding a variant of the virus to which humans have minimal resistance. The change usually involves the hemagglutinin glycoprotein, but the neuraminidase glycoprotein and, less commonly, virion structural and nonstructural proteins may vary. Antigenic variation occurs less frequently with influenza B virus and has not been reported with influenza C virus. Minor antigenic variation ("antigenic drift") results from mutations in the RNA segments that code for hemagglutinin, or less often neuraminidase, and the subsequent alteration of a few amino acids in the protein structure. This occurs every year or every few years for any influenza subtype. Genetic reassortment causes major antigenic variation, called antigenic shift, yielding "new" viruses with hemagglutinin and neuraminidase antigens that show little or no cross-reaction with those of the "old" virus and to which the population has no immunity.

REPLICATION

Infection with an influenza virus is initiated by attachment of the hemagglutinin glycoprotein spike to a sialic

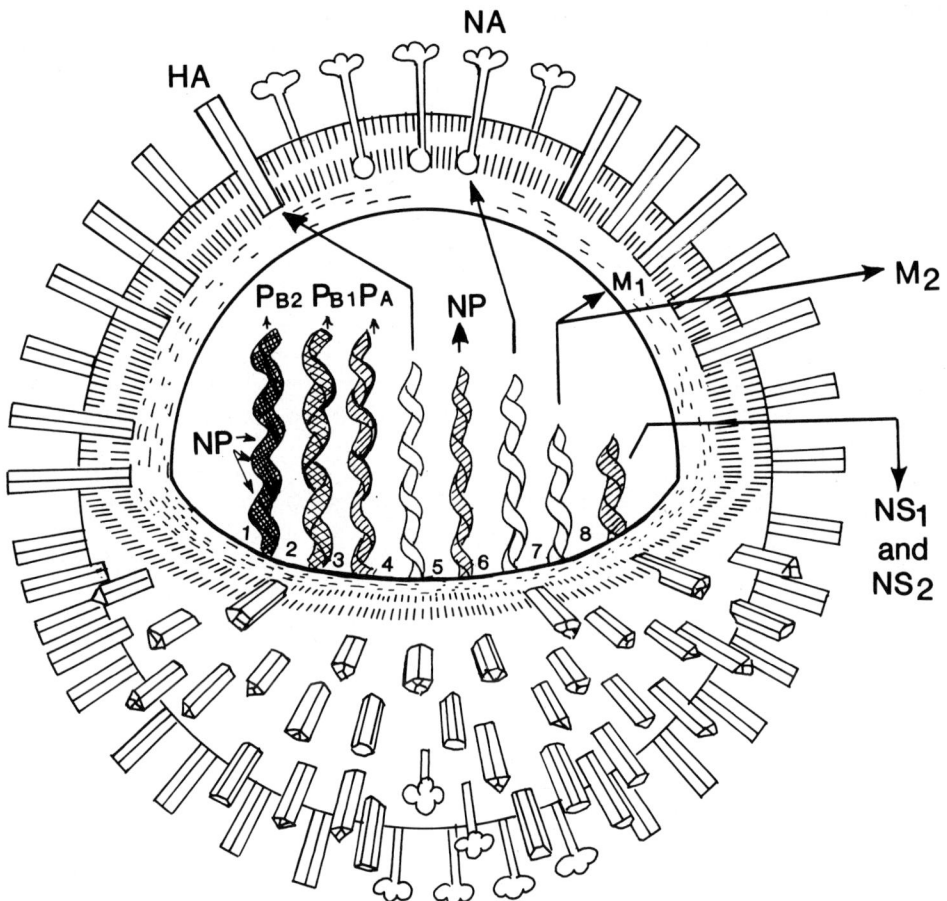

Fig. 11–1. Diagram of influenza virus structure. Inside the membrane and matrix shell are the eight segments of genomic RNA (1–8). Each codes for one or more proteins (see Table 11–1). Projecting from the lipid envelope are rod-shaped hemagglutinin (HA) and mushroom-shaped neuraminidase (NA) glycoproteins. (From Murphy BR, and Webster RG. Orthomyxoviruses. In Fields' Virology. 2nd ed. Edited by BN Fields, and DM Knipe. New York, Raven Press, 1990.)

acid residue on the host cell membrane. The viral envelope and host cell membrane fuse, and the virus enters the cell in an endosome. The pH in the endosome decreases, releasing the nucleocapsid. Cellular RNA polymerase II initiates the synthesis of viral messenger RNA; the viral genome then is transcribed. The nucleocapsid is assembled in the host cell nucleus, and the envelope is assembled at the cell surface membrane.

EPIDEMIOLOGY

Localized epidemics of influenza typically begin abruptly, peak in 2 to 3 weeks, and last 5 to 6 weeks (4).

Children usually are affected first. Hospital admissions for patients with pneumonia, exacerbation of chronic obstructive lung disease, croup, and congestive heart failure; school and work absenteeism; and the number of deaths due to pneumonia and influenza then increase. The average overall attack rate is 10 to 20%, but it can reach 40 to 50% in selected populations or age groups (5).

Epidemics typically occur in winter in the Northern Hemisphere, but they may begin as early as October if a strain with significantly different antigenicity is introduced. In the Southern Hemisphere epidemics occur from May to September and often predict the type of virus that

Table 11–1. Genes of Influenza Viruses and Their Protein Products

RNA Segment Number*	Protein Encoded In Influenza Virus			Protein Name	Protein Function
	A	B	C		
1	PB1	PB1	P1[†]	Polymerase	RNA transcriptase
2	PB2	PB2	P2[†]	Polymerase	RNA transcriptase
3	PA	PA	P3[†]	Polymerase	RNA transcriptase
4	HA	HA	HE[‡]	Hemagglutinin	Viral attachment to host cell
5	NP	NP	NP	Nucleoprotein	Encapsidates RNA
6	NA	NA, NB	M	Neuraminidase	Release of virus from membranes, prevents aggregation
7	M_1, M_2	M_1, M_2	NS_1, NS_2	Matrix	Virion assembly and budding
8	NS_1, NS_2	NS_1, NS_2	—	Nonstructural	Unknown

* Numbered in order of decreasing molecular weight.
[†] Nomenclature is arbitrary since genes have not been sequenced and their functions are unknown.
[‡] Hemagglutinin-esterase.

will appear in the Northern Hemisphere that winter. In temperate climates influenza viruses rarely are recovered between epidemics; in the tropics influenza virus can be isolated year-round, but epidemics often follow changes in weather patterns such as monsoons. Factors other than antigenic variation involved in the development of an influenza epidemic, factors involved in halting an epidemic after several weeks when only a portion of susceptible persons has been infected, and the location of the virus between epidemics are unknown.

Worldwide epidemics—pandemics—follow antigenic shift and introduction of a "new" virus, an event that occurs at variable and unpredictable intervals. Since the first influenza pandemic in 1580, thirty-one have been described. The recent pandemics of 1957, 1968, and 1977 began in mainland China and spread to the Soviet Union and Western Europe, and then to the North American continent. Generally, pandemics are most severe when the hemagglutinin and neuraminidase undergo major alterations; however, the severity also is influenced by the intrinsic virulence of the virus and its transmissibility.

PATHOGENESIS

Influenza virus is transmitted from person to person by small-particle (less than 10 μm diameter) aerosols created by sneezing, coughing, and talking. Virions deposited on the respiratory tract epithelium attach to and penetrate columnar epithelial cells, initiating the replication cycle, which ends in cell death and the release of many newly assembled virions capable of infecting epithelial cells in the vicinity. The mucosa of the larynx, trachea, and bronchi soon becomes hyperemic and edematous, and the ciliated and mucus-producing cells are sloughed.

Viral shedding in respiratory tract secretions begins just before the onset of illness, peaks in 24 to 48 hours, then rapidly declines until it is indetectable after 5 to 10 days. Approximately 1 day after viral shedding begins interferon is detected in nasal secretions and serum; it reaches peak levels about 1 day after the virus titer peaks (6,7). The appearance of interferon coincident with decreasing virus titers and improvement of symptoms suggests that it may play a role in recovery from the infection.

Specific antibodies to HA and NA antigens are detected in the serum in about 80% of cases of primary influenza during the second week after exposure to the virus and the titer peaks about 2 weeks later (8). Hemagglutination-inhibiting and neutralizing antibodies (directed primarily against the HA glycoprotein) persist for months to years then gradually decline. Type-specific complement-fixing antibodies (predominantly immunoglobulin [Ig] M), directed against the ribonucleoprotein, disappear in weeks to months. Secretory IgA antibodies reach peak titers in the respiratory secretions by day 14 after the illness begins and disappear several months later. In sufficient quantity, these antibodies protect against infection; serum hemagglutination-inhibiting titers of 1:40 or greater, serum neutralizing titers of 1:8 or greater, and nasal neutralizing titers of 1:4 or greater appear to provide protection (9,10). Lower titers or antibodies specific for a heterologous strain may not prevent infection but may modify its severity. Antibodies directed against NA appear to inhibit infection and shorten the duration of the illness.

CLINICAL MANIFESTATIONS

After an incubation period of 1 to 2 days, persons infected with influenza A or B virus experience abrupt onset of fever, chills, headache, myalgia, malaise, anorexia, cough, nasal discharge, and sore throat. Fever generally resolves in 3 to 4 days, respiratory symptoms persist for an additional 3 to 4 days, and cough, lassitude, and malaise for 1 to 2 more weeks. In a recent study the most common manifestations of infection with influenza C virus were fever and cough (11).

Pulmonary complications of influenza—primary influenza viral pneumonia and secondary bacterial pneumonia—most often develop in elders and in persons who have chronic cardiovascular or pulmonary disease. Influenza pneumonia, characterized by rapid progression of fever, cough, dyspnea, and cyanosis after typical onset of influenza, is associated with a high mortality rate. At autopsy, lung tissue shows diffuse intra-alveolar hemorrhage with hyaline membranes and minimal inflammation. Secondary bacterial pneumonia follows classic influenza by 4 to 14 days and is manifest by fever recrudescence, cough, and sputum production. The infection, most often caused by Streptococcus pneumoniae, Staphylococcus aureus, or Haemophilus influenzae, generally resolves with appropriate antimicrobial therapy (see Chapters 28 and 36).

Nonpulmonary complications of influenza include myositis, myocarditis, toxic shock–like syndrome, encephalitis, and Reye's syndrome (12–21).

LABORATORY DIAGNOSIS

The most desirable specimen for diagnosing infections with the influenza viruses is a nasopharyngeal wash. A combination of nose and throat swabs is an acceptable alternative; and if bronchoalveolar lavage is planned the collected fluid may be submitted for virus isolation. Specimen collection, transport, and processing are discussed in Part III.

Conventional methods of detecting influenza viruses are (1) inoculation of embryonated hens' eggs, (2) testing fluids from the allantoic and amniotic cavities for viral hemagglutinin after 3 days, and (3) cell culture (preferred in most clinical virology laboratories). Primary monkey (rhesus or cynomolgus) kidney cells are used most often for isolation of influenza viruses; however, data from one study suggest that the continuous Madin-Darby canine kidney cell line with trypsin added to the medium is an acceptable alternative (22).

Inoculated cell cultures are maintained in minimum essential medium without serum (which may have viral inhibitory factors) at 33° to 35° C for at least 14 days, although cytopathic effect (CPE) frequently is recognized after about 4 to 6 days. Monkey kidney cells infected with influenza A or B virus are granular, swollen, and round (Fig. 11–2); become pyknotic and fragmented; and eventually degenerate and detach from the glass. Identification is confirmed by staining smears of infected cells with

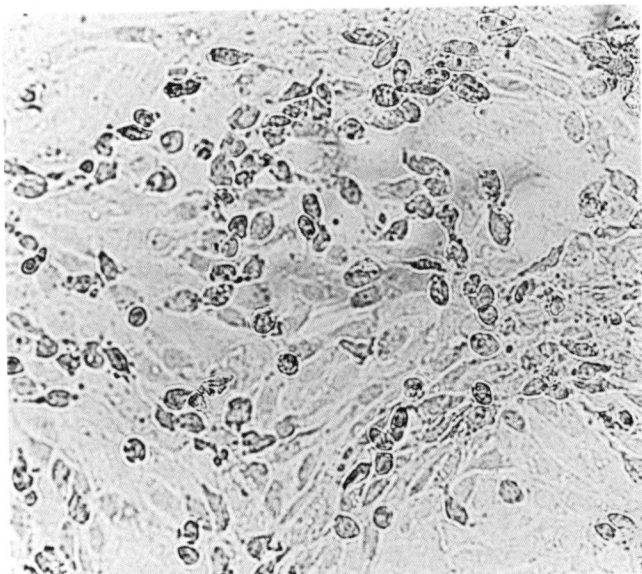

Fig. 11–2. Cytopathic effect produced by influenza A virus in primary monkey kidney cells (×100).

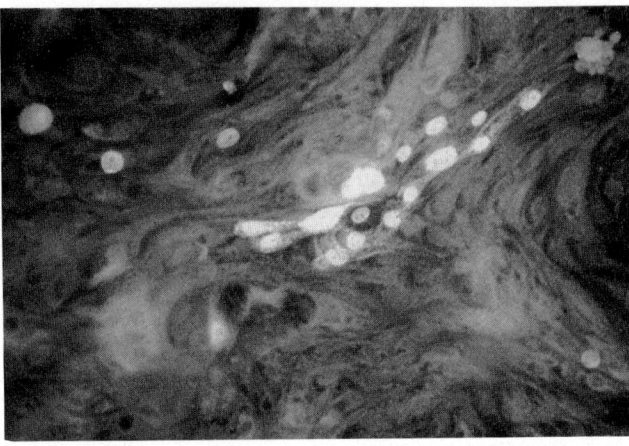

Fig. 11–3. Madin-Darby canine kidney cells stained with monoclonal antibodies to influenza A virus in the centrifugation-culture assay show fluorescence of intracytoplasmic and intranuclear inclusions, a positive reaction (×400).

monoclonal antibodies specific for influenza A and influenza B viruses. Some influenza virus isolates produce little or no recognizable CPE and are detected only by hemadsorption (see Appendix, Procedure 1) or by staining with monoclonal antibodies. Hemadsorption may be performed as early as day 3 after inoculation; but if the result is negative on day 3, monolayers should be washed with phosphate-buffered saline, reincubated, and tested for hemadsorption again on day 9 to 10 (23). For monolayers that demonstrate hemadsorption the virus is identified by staining the cells with monoclonal antibodies against influenza A and B and parainfluenza virus.

Centrifugation-culture, similar to that described for cytomegalovirus (see Chapter 5 and Appendix, Procedure 2), is a valuable adjunct to conventional cell culture for detection of influenza A and B viruses, eliminating the need for early (day 3) hemadsorption (23–25). Shell vials (purchased or prepared in house) or 24-well plates (prepared in house) containing coverslips seeded with Madin-Darby canine kidney cells or primary monkey kidney cells are inoculated with the specimen (two vials or wells per sample), centrifuged, and incubated at 35° C. After 40 hours one coverslip each is stained with monoclonal antibodies directed against influenza A virus and against influenza B virus. The presence of one or more cells demonstrating fluorescence in the cytoplasm, the nucleus, or both (Fig. 11–3) indicates that virus is present. The sensitivity of centrifugation-culture is about 85%, so it should supplement, not replace, conventional cell culture (25).

Influenza A and B viruses may be detected directly in clinical specimens by staining smears of nasal epithelial cells with fluorescein-conjugated monoclonal antibodies. This has the potential advantage of providing a diagnosis within a few hours of receiving the specimen. Disadvantages of this test are low sensitivity and problems with interpretation caused by interfering background fluorescence (25–27). In addition, a recently available 15-minute enzyme immunoassay membrane test specific for influenza A virus appears to be a good screening test for influenza A, but if results are negative it should be supported by cell culture (28).

Influenza also may be diagnosed by testing both acute- and convalescent-phase serum samples (collected early in the illness and 2 to 4 weeks later) for type-specific or strain-specific antibodies. A fourfold or greater rise or fall in titer is diagnostic of infection. Complement fixation and immunofluorescence tests detect antibodies to the influenza virus type (A or B), whereas the infecting strain is identified by hemagglutination inhibition. Because the latter requires using the correct antigen and is technically labor intensive, it generally is performed only in reference laboratories. All serologic methods, however, have limited clinical usefulness because a convalescent serum sample is required.

TREATMENT AND PREVENTION

Most cases of influenza require only symptomatic treatment. In the United States, amantadine is approved for treating infections with influenza A virus. Amantadine reduces the duration of signs and symptoms by about 50%, but it is associated with central nervous system side effects: insomnia, dizziness, and difficulty concentrating (29–31). Rimantadine, an agent structurally related to amantadine, has been used for several years in the former Soviet Union to treat infection with influenza A virus, but currently it is not approved for use in the United States. It is as effective as amantadine in uncomplicated influenza and is associated with fewer side effects. Resistance to rimantadine has emerged during therapy in young children who shed virus in high concentrations; however, treatment with amantadine probably would induce similar resistance (32). No antiviral agent effective against influenza B virus is approved for use.

The mainstay for preventing infection with influenza virus is the inactivated virus vaccine, which has an efficacy of approximately 70%. In general, the vaccine contains both influenza A and B viruses, usually the types isolated during the previous winter's influenza season. Yearly vaccination is recommended for persons in certain risk groups: Adults and children who undergo regular medical care or were hospitalized in the past year for chronic pulmonary or cardiac conditions and residents of nursing homes and other chronic care facilities are given the highest priority for vaccination. Healthy persons older than 65 years, those with chronic underlying diseases (diabetes mellitus, renal dysfunction, anemia, immunosuppression, asthma), and children and teenagers receiving chronic aspirin therapy are in the second risk category. Hospital personnel who have extensive contact with patients at high risk and those who provide home care to such patients also should be vaccinated. The only contraindication to vaccination is hypersensitivity to hens' eggs, because the vaccines are prepared from allantoic fluid harvested from embryonated hens' eggs infected with influenza A or B virus. For persons who were not vaccinated, amantadine is recommended for short-term (5 to 7 weeks) prophylaxis during a presumed outbreak of influenza A (33).

To prevent nosocomial spread of influenza, patients should be isolated in single rooms or "cohorted," staff should be cohorted to care for only ill or only well patients, and the use of gowns and masks and appropriate hand washing technique should be enforced.

REFERENCES

1. Noble GR: Epidemiological and clinical aspects of influenza. In Basic and Applied Influenza Research. Edited by AS Beare. Boca Raton, FL, CRC Press, 1982.
2. Murphy BR, and Webster RG: Orthomyxoviruses. In Fields' Virology. 2nd ed. Edited by BN Fields and DM Knipe. New York, Raven Press, 1990.
3. Guo Y, et al: Isolation of influenza C virus from pigs and experimental infection of pigs with influenza C virus. J Gen Virol, 64:177, 1983.
4. Glezen WP, and Couch RB: Interpandemic influenza in the Houston area, 1974–76. N Engl J Med, 298:587, 1978.
5. Monto AS, and Kioumehr F: The Techumseh study of respiratory illness. IX. Occurrence of influenza in the community, 1966–1971. Am J Epidemiol, 102:553, 1975.
6. Murphy BR, et al: Temperature sensitive mutants of influenza virus. IV. Induction of interferon in the nasopharynx by wild type and temperature-sensitive recombinant virus. J Infect Dis 128:488, 1973.
7. Jao RL, Wheelock EF, and Jackson GG: Production of interferon in volunteers infected with Asian influenza. J Infect Dis, 121:419, 1970.
8. Fox JP, Cooney MK, Hall CE, and Foy HM: Influenza virus infections in Seattle families, 1975–1979. II. Pattern of infection in invaded households and relation of age and prior antibody to occurrence of infection and related illness. Am J Epidemiol, 116:228, 1982.
9. Wenzel RP, Hendley JO, Sande MA, and Gwaltney JM Jr: Revised (1972–1973) bivalent influenza vaccine: Serum and nasal antibody responses to parenteral vaccination. JAMA, 226:435, 1973.
10. Kilbourne ED, Butler WT, and Rossen RD: Specific immunity in influenza—summary of influenza workshop III. J Infect Dis 127:220, 1973.
11. Morinchi H, et al: Community-acquired influenza C virus infection in children. J Pediatr, 118:235, 1991.
12. Dietzman DE, Schaller JG, Ray CG, and Reed ME: Acute myositis associated with influenza B infection. Pediatrics, 57:255, 1976.
13. Minow RA, Gorbach S, Johnson BL, and Dornfeld L: Myoglobinuria associated with influenza A infection. Ann Intern Med, 80:359, 1974.
14. Adams CW: Postviral myopericarditis associated with influenza virus: Report of eight cases. Am J Cardiol, 4:56, 1959.
15. Finland M, Parker F Jr, Barnes MW, and Joliffe LS: Acute myocarditis in influenza A infections. Two cases of nonbacterial myocarditis, with isolation of virus from the lungs. Am J Med Sci, 209:455, 1945.
16. MacDonald KL, et al: Toxic shock syndrome: A newly recognized complication of influenza and influenza-like illness. JAMA, 257:1053, 1987.
17. Hoult JG, and Flewett TH: Influenzal encephalopathy and postinfluenzal encephalitis. Histological and other observations. Br Med J, i:1847, 1958.
18. Flewett TH, and Hoult JG: Influenzal encephalopathy and postinfluenzal encephalitis. Lancet, ii:11, 1958.
19. Hurwitz ES, et al: National surveillance for Reye syndrome: A five-year review. Pediatrics, 70:895, 1982.
20. Corey L, et al: A nationwide outbreak of Reye's syndrome: Its epidemiologic relationship to influenza B. Am J Med, 61:615, 1976.
21. Corey L, Rubin RJ, Bregman D, and Gregg MB: Diagnostic criteria for influenza B–associated Reye's syndrome: Clinical vs pathologic criteria. Pediatrics, 60:702, 1977.
22. Frank AL, Couch RB, Griffis CA, and Baxter BD: Comparison of different tissue cultures for isolation and quantitation of influenza and parainfluenza viruses. J Clin Microbiol, 10:32, 1979.
23. Minnich LL, and Ray, GG: Early testing of cell cultures for detection of hemadsorbing viruses. J Clin Microbiol, 25:421, 1987.
24. Woods GL, and Johnson AM: Rapid 24-well plate centrifugation assay for detection of influenza A virus in clinical specimens. J Virol Methods, 24:35, 1989.
25. Mills RD, Cain KJ, and Woods GL: Detection of influenza virus by centrifugal inoculation of MDCK cells and staining with monoclonal antibodies. J Clin Microbiol, 27:2505, 1989.
26. Shalit I, McKee PA, Beauchamp H, and Waner JL: Comparison of polyclonal antiserum versus monoclonal antibodies for the rapid diagnosis of influenza A virus infections by immunofluorescence in clinical specimens. J Clin Microbiol, 22:877, 1985.
27. Stokes CE, Bernstein JM, Kyger SA, and Hayden FG: Rapid diagnosis of influenza A and B by 24-h fluorescent focus assay. J Clin Microbiol, 26:1263, 1988.
28. Waner JL, et al: Comparison of Directigen FLU-A with viral isolation and direct immunofluorescence for the rapid detection and identification of influenza A virus. J Clin Microbiol, 29:479, 1991.
29. Wingfield WL, Pollac D, and Grunert RR: Therapeutic efficacy of amantadine HCl and rimantadine HCl in naturally occurring influenza A2 respiratory illness in man. N Engl J Med, 281:579, 1969.
30. Van Voris LP, et al: Successful treatment of naturally occurring influenza A/USSR/77 H1N1. JAMA, 245:1128, 1981.
31. Younkin SW, Betts RF, Roth FK, and Douglas RG: Reduction in fever and symptoms in young adults with aspirin or amantadine. Antimicrob Agents Chemother, 23:577, 1983.
32. Hall CB, et al: Children with influenza A infection: Treatment with rimantadine. Pediatrics, 80:275, 1987.
33. Arden NH, et al: The role of vaccination and amantadine prophylaxis controlling an outbreak of influenza A (H3N2) in a nursing home. Arch Intern Med, 148:865, 1988.

Chapter 12

CORONAVIRUSES

In 1965 an agent, now called coronavirus, that could not be grown in cell culture, was ether sensitive, was not related to known ortho- or paramyxoviruses, and by electron microscopy resembled infectious bronchitis virus of chickens, was identified in nasal wash fluids from an adult with coldlike symptoms (1). Soon thereafter, several agents with similar morphologic and physiologic features were identified in the human respiratory tract and were recognized as pathogens in many animals (2–4). Subsequently, an international ad hoc committee recommended that this group of viruses be classified separately as a new genus: Coronavirus (5). Since then, coronaviruses have been detected in human feces as well as respiratory tract specimens. Human coronaviruses are discussed in this chapter.

CLASSIFICATION

Coronavirus, the only genus in the family Coronaviridae, contains four antigenic groups (I through IV). The five known strains of coronavirus that infect humans—229E, OC43, B814, OC16, and OC37—are members of groups I and II (1,2,6). Strains 229E and OC43 have been adapted to growth in cell culture and, therefore, are the best-studied. Most respiratory coronavirus isolates are antigenically related to one of these two strains. Enteric coronaviruses, difficult to cultivate, are detected only by electron microscopic examination of stool specimens. By immune electron microscopy some of these enteric coronaviruses appear to be antigenically related to the respiratory strain OC43 (7). Less well-studied enteric strains will be called "coronavirus-like particles" until evidence that affords definitive identification is available.

STRUCTURE AND REPLICATION

Coronavirus virions, 80 to 160 nm in diameter, consist of a single-stranded, positive-sense, 27- to 30-kilobase RNA genome with a molecular weight of about 6 million. The flexible, helical nucleocapsid is surrounded by a lipid envelope from which club-shaped glycoproteins project, giving virions a crown shape ("corona"; Fig. 12–1 and 12–2) (8).

Coronaviruses attach to target cell membrane receptors and penetrate by fusion of the viral envelope with the cell membrane. Replication occurs in the cell cytoplasm, and virions assemble by budding initially at the membranes between the rough endoplasmic reticulum and the Golgi apparatus. Virus-filled vesicles then are extruded from intact cells by reverse pinocytosis or are released by lysis of dying cells.

EPIDEMIOLOGY

Coronaviruses occur worldwide and in temperate climates more often cause disease in winter and spring. In the United States, strains 229E and OC43 have been responsible for large epidemics of respiratory tract illness at 2- to 3-year intervals (9). Respiratory tract disease is most common in children but affects all age groups. Reinfection may occur. Enteric coronaviruses are detected year-round, most frequently in neonates and infants younger than 1 year, and they have been found in adults with the acquired immunodeficiency syndrome (10). Asymptomatic shedding of virus in the feces for prolonged periods appears common.

CLINICAL MANIFESTATIONS

The human coronaviruses are an important cause of colds in adults and have been associated with pneumonia and pleuritis in military recruits, episodes of wheezing in asthmatic children, and exacerbations of bronchitis in adults with chronic obstructive respiratory disease (11–13). Coronaviruses have been implicated as a cause of pneumonia in infants, but their role in the disease has not been documented unequivocally (14,15). Gastrointestinal tract infections caused by coronaviruses have resulted in mild, self-limited bloody diarrhea, and in a more severe illness resembling necrotizing enterocolitis marked by abdominal distention, bloody stools, and pneumatosis intestinalis (16–18).

LABORATORY DIAGNOSIS

Because the coronaviruses are extremely difficult to grow in conventional cell culture most respiratory infections have been diagnosed retrospectively by testing acute and convalescent sera for antibodies to coronavirus antigens. Currently, antigens associated with strains 229E and OC43 are used for serologic testing in research laboratories; test systems are not commercially available.

Coronavirus strain 229E grows in human diploid cell lines, but recovering it from clinical specimens is difficult and often requires several blind passages. The cytopathic effect is nonspecific, resembling the natural degeneration of a cell monolayer. All other respiratory tract coronaviruses have been recovered from clinical specimens (such as nasal washes) only in organ cultures from human em-

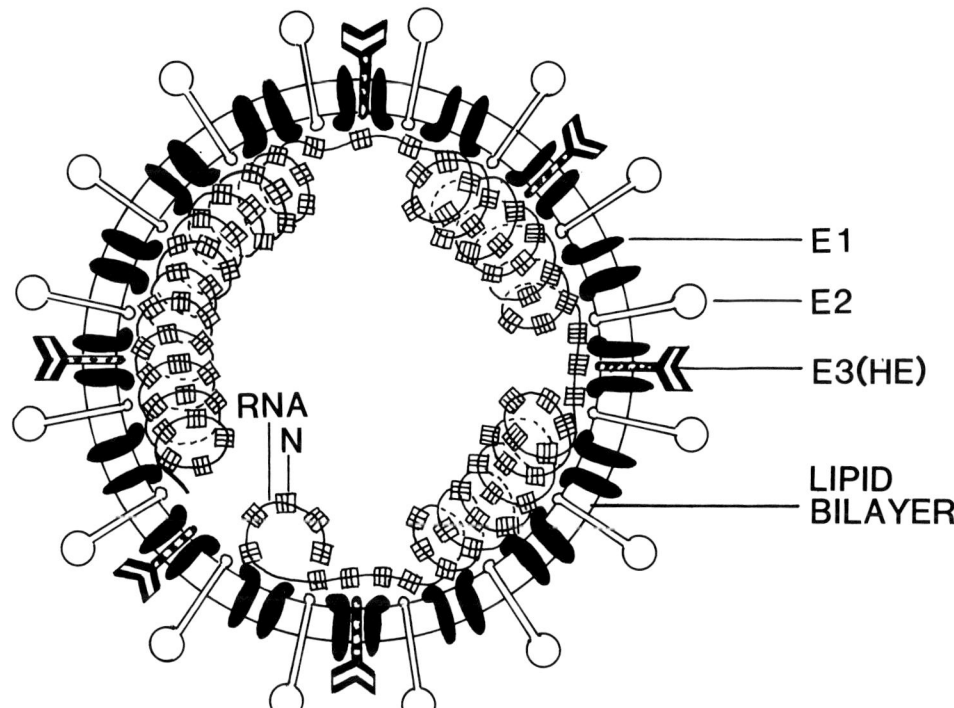

Fig. 12–1. Diagram of coronavirus structure. The nucleocapsid is a long, flexible helix composed of genomic RNA and many molecules of the nucleocapsid protein N. Surrounding the nucleocapsid is a host cell membrane–derived lipid envelope containing the viral glycoproteins E1 (now called M), E2 (now called S), and, on some coronaviruses, E3 (now HE). (From Holmes KV: Coronaviridae and their replication. In Fields' Virology. 2nd ed. Edited by BN Fields and DM Knipe. New York, Raven, 1990.)

bryonic trachea or nasal epithelium, which are not readily available.

Enteric disease caused by a coronavirus is diagnosed by identifying characteristic virus particles (see Fig. 12–2) in stool specimens by electron microscopy.

TREATMENT

Disease caused by coronaviruses is treated symptomatically. No specific antiviral agent is available.

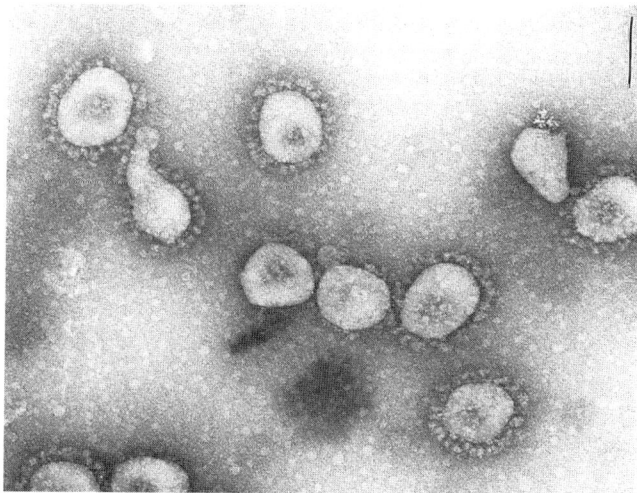

Fig. 12–2. Electron photomicrograph of coronavirus virions (×112,750). (Courtesy of the Division of Viral and Rickettsial Diseases, Centers for Disease Control, Atlanta, GA.)

REFERENCES

1. Tyrrell DAJ, and Bynoe ML: Cultivation of a novel type of common-cold virus in organ cultures. Br Med J, 1:1467, 1965.
2. McIntosh K, et al: Recovery in tracheal organ cultures of novel viruses from patients with respiratory disease. Proc Natl Acad Sci USA, 57:933, 1967.
3. McIntosh K, Becker WB, and Chanock RM: Growth in suckling mouse brain of "IBV-like" viruses from patients with upper respiratory tract disease. Proc Natl Acad Sci USA, 58:2268, 1967.
4. Witte KH, Tajima M, and Easterday BD: Morphologic characteristics and nucleic acid type of transmissible gastroenteritis virus of pigs. Arch Ges Virusforsch, 23:53, 1968.
5. Tyrrell DAJ, et al: Coronaviruses. Nature, 220:650, 1968.
6. Hamre D, and Procknow JJ: A new virus isolated from the human respiratory tract. Proc Soc Exp Biol, 121:190, 1966.
7. Gerna G, et al: Human enteric coronaviruses: Antigenic relatedness to human coronavirus OC43 and possible etiologic role in viral gastroenteritis. J Infect Dis, 151:796, 1985.
8. Holmes KV: Coronaviridae and their replication. In Fields' Virology. 2nd ed. Edited by BN Fields and DM Knipe. New York, Raven Press, 1990.
9. Monto AS: Medical reviews, coronaviruses. Yale J Biol Med, 47:234, 1974.
10. Kern P, et al: Detection of coronavirus-like particles in homosexual men with acquired immunodeficiency and related lymphadenopathy syndrome. Klin Wochenschr, 63:68, 1985.
11. Wenzel RP, et al: Coronavirus infections in military recruits: Three-year study with coronavirus strains OC43 and 229E. Am Rev Respir Dis, 109:621, 1976.
12. McIntosh K, et al: The association of viral and bacterial respiratory infections with exacerbations of wheezing in young asthmatic children. J Pediatr, 82:578, 1973.

13. Smith CB, et al: Association of viral and Mycoplasma pneumoniae infections with acute respiratory illness in patients with chronic obstructive pulmonary diseases. Am Rev Respir Dis, *121*:225, 1980.
14. McIntosh K, et al: Coronavirus infections in acute lower respiratory tract disease in infants. J Infect Dis, *130*:502, 1974.
15. McIntosh K, et al: Diagnosis of human coronavirus infection by immune fluorescence: Method and application to respiratory disease in hospitalized children. J Med Virol *2*:341, 1978.
16. Mortensen ML, et al: Coronavirus-like particles in human gastrointestinal disease. Epidemiologic, clinical, and laboratory observations. Am J Dis Child, *139*:928, 1985.
17. Chany C, et al: Association of coronavirus infection with neonatal necrotizing enterocolitis. Pediatrics, *69*:209, 1982.
18. Resta S, et al: Isolation and propagation of a human enteric coronavirus. Science, *229*:978, 1985.

Chapter 13

PICORNAVIRUSES

The picornaviruses are classified in the family Picornaviridae, so named because the viruses are very small (*pico*) and have an *RNA* genome. This family has more than 200 members that infect humans, other mammals, birds, fish, and possibly insects.

CLASSIFICATION

The Picornaviridae are divided into four genera: Enterovirus, Rhinovirus, Aphthovirus, and Cardiovirus. The latter two genera primarily infect cloven-footed animals and mice and will not be discussed here. Classification of the human picornaviruses is shown in Table 13–1.

STRUCTURE

The nonenveloped picornaviruses, 20 to 30 nm in diameter, have an icosahedral capsid composed of 60 protomers, and by electron microscopic examination appear similar to aggregates of glycogen (Fig. 13–1). The linear, single-stranded, positive-sense RNA genome has a molecular weight of about 2.6 million (about 7.5 kilobase pairs), and attached to the 5' end is a small protein called VPg, which apparently is important in packaging the genome into the capsid and initiating RNA synthesis. The viral protomers are composed of one molecule of each of the four major structural polypeptides (designated VP1 through VP4), which are formed by cleavage of one molecule of the structural protein precursor. Virions are resistant to ether, chloroform, and alcohol but readily inactivated by ionizing radiation, formaldehyde, and phenol.

REPLICATION

Infection with a picornavirus is initiated by attachment of the viral polypeptide VP1 to a specific host cell membrane receptor. The polypeptide VP4 then is released, which weakens the virion and allows it to be internalized by receptor-mediated endocytosis. In the acidic environment of the endosome, the virion dissociates, releasing the genome into the cytoplasm to bind to ribosomes and initiate transcription and translation. The RNA serves as a template for synthesis of additional RNA or as a messenger coding for a polyprotein that undergoes specific cleavages to form the four structural polypeptides, a virus-coded RNA replicase, proteases, and other polypeptides required for replication. As the viral genome is being replicated and translated, the structural proteins VP0, VP1, and VP3 are assembled into protomers. The latter associate into pentamers, 12 of which form the procapsid. Virions are assembled in the cell cytoplasm; viral RNA is inserted into the procapsid, after which VP0 is cleaved into VP2 and VP4. Virions are released by cell lysis, yielding about 10^5 particles per cell.

ENTEROVIRUSES

Historically, the enteroviruses were subdivided into polioviruses, coxsackievirus groups A and B, and echoviruses, based on antigenic relationships and differences in host range. Some enteroviruses, however, have biologic properties that bridge these major groups, making definitive categorization difficult; therefore, newly recognized enteroviruses are classified as enteroviruses numbered sequentially from type 68 on. The epidemiology and pathogenesis of infections caused by enteroviruses in general are discussed in the following paragraphs, and features unique to the individual species or serotypes are discussed separately later.

Epidemiology

Infections caused by enteroviruses occur worldwide throughout the year, but in temperate climates in the Northern Hemisphere they predominate in summer and fall. Infection is most common in infants and young children and, probably owing to crowding and poor hygiene, among lower socioeconomic classes.

The prevalence of a given serotype of enterovirus in the community varies. In the United States between 1970 and 1983 echoviruses and group B coxsackieviruses comprised approximately 50 and 25% of clinical isolates, respectively; however, group A coxsackieviruses probably were under-represented because most cannot be cultivated in the clinical laboratory (1,2). Echovirus types, 3, 4, 6, 7, 9 and 11 and coxsackievirus B5 occurred in seasonal epidemics, whereas the rest caused sporadic illness. Explanations for the appearance and disappearance of certain serotypes and their epidemic or endemic conditions are not known.

Enteroviruses are transmitted from person to person, predominantly via the fecal-oral route. Exceptions include some coxsackieviruses, especially A21, which probably is transmitted by the respiratory-oral route, and enterovirus 70, the agent of acute hemorrhagic conjunctivitis, which is spread by fomites, fingers, and contaminated ophthalmic instruments. Once the virus is introduced into a household, secondary attack rates for susceptible persons are 90 to 100% for wild polioviruses, 76% for coxsackieviruses, and less than 50% for echoviruses (3,4). The lower attack rates probably are related to a shorter period of fecal shedding of the virus. Infected persons generally excrete the virus in oral secretions or feces for several days before the onset of symptoms and in the feces for

Table 13–1. Classification of the Picornaviridae

Genus	Species (Serotype)	Comments
Enterovirus	Polioviruses 1–3	
	Coxsackieviruses A 1–22, 24	A 23 = echovirus 9
	Coxsackieviruses B 1–6	
	Echoviruses 1–9, 11–27, 29–34	Echovirus 10 = reovirus type 1
		Echovirus 28 = rhinovirus 1A
	Enteroviruses 68–72	Enterovirus 72 = hepatitis A virus
Rhinovirus	1 A, 1 B, 2–100	

several weeks thereafter; however, maximal contagion occurs early in the illness, when fecal excretion of the virus is greatest. Reinfection with the same serotype is rare and generally is not associated with illness.

The risk of certain enteroviral illnesses varies with sex and age. Aseptic meningitis is most common in young infants, pleurodynia and myopericarditis predominantly affect adolescents and young adults, and enteroviral infections in elders rarely are symptomatic. Among young children, enteroviral infection has no sex predilection, but boys develop aseptic meningitis and poliomyelitis nearly twice as often as girls. Symptomatic enteroviral infections are more severe in pregnant women and in persons who exercise vigorously before the onset of symptoms (5,6).

Pathogenesis

The pathogenesis of enteroviral infections is best understood for the polioviruses. After the virus is ingested, it replicates in susceptible cells of the pharynx or distal small intestine, although the specific cell is unknown. Further replication in the lymphoid tissue of the tonsils and Peyer's patches in the distal ileum occurs 1 to 3 days later, after which virions travel to the regional lymph nodes, enter the blood, and eventually reach the monocyte/macrophage cells of the liver, spleen, bone marrow, and deep lymph nodes. In subclinical infections, viral replication then stops or is contained by the host defenses. In a minority of infected persons further replication in the monocyte/macrophage system results in sustained viremia, clinically manifest as the "minor illness" of poliomyelitis or as nonspecific fever. Virions then disseminate to target organs, such as the meninges, heart, and skin, where tissue necrosis and inflammation ensue.

After natural infection with an enterovirus, type-specific immunity to infection with that enterovirus develops and persists for the life of the individual. Secretory immunoglobulins prevent enteroviruses from establishing infection in the gastrointestinal tract, and circulating neutralizing antibodies prevent hematogenous dissemination to target organs. Antibodies probably are involved in recovery from infection, because persons with isolated agammaglobulinemia may develop persistent infections with enteroviruses (7). Macrophages limit viral replication in target organs, and T lymphocytes may mediate the inflammatory component of coxsackievirus group B myocarditis.

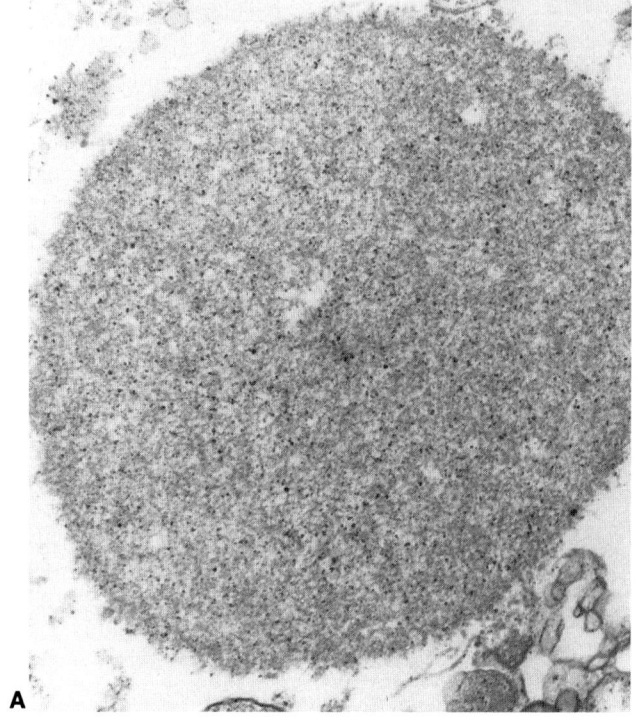
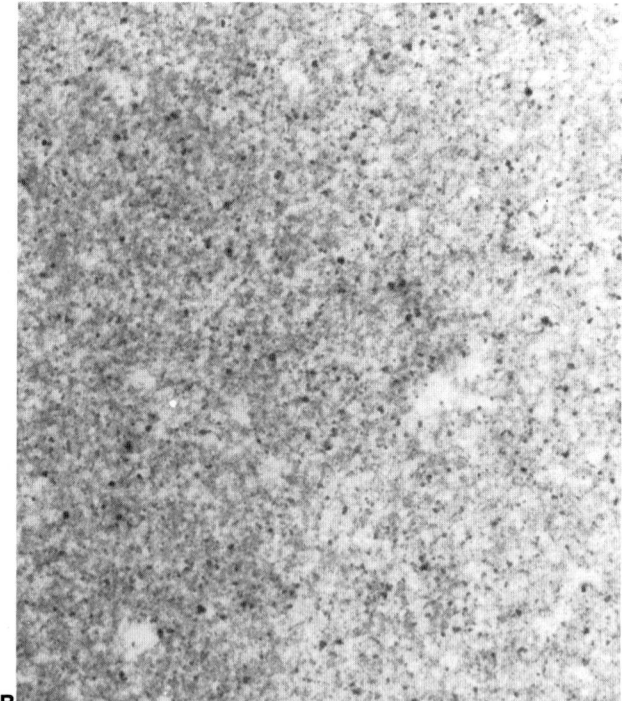

Fig. 13–1. Electron micrograph of a primary monkey kidney cell infected with an echovirus (A, ×94,500; B, ×150,000).

Polioviruses

The clinical features of poliomyelitis were described around 1840, but its epidemic nature was first recognized in Scandinavia and Western Europe around 1890 (8). Conclusive evidence of the infectious nature of the disease was demonstrated in 1908 by Landsteiner and Popper, who transmitted poliomyelitis to monkeys inoculated with human spinal cord homogenates. Poliovirus was propagated in vitro in 1949, and that same year three distinct serotypes (1, 2, and 3) were recognized (9,10). A formalin-inactivated poliovirus vaccine, developed by Salk in 1953, was licensed in the United States in 1955, and in 1962, the live attenuated polio vaccine developed by Sabin and colleagues was licensed (11).

Epidemiology

Humans are the only natural host and reservoir of polioviruses. Early in the twentieth century epidemics of polio in the United States primarily affected infants and children under the age of 5 years, but with improved hygiene the peak incidence shifted to the 5- to 9-year-old group by the late 1940s and early 1950s, when over one third of cases affected persons older than 15 years. With the introduction of poliovirus vaccines the incidence of paralytic poliomyelitis declined dramatically in developed countries. In the United States the attack rate fell from about 18 cases of poliomyelitis (paralytic and nonparalytic) per 100,000 population in 1955 to fewer than 1 case per 100,000 in 1962, and since 1972 fewer than 0.01 case per 100,000 has been reported, or 10 cases annually (12). In 1990 an estimated 116,000 cases of paralytic poliomyelitis occurred worldwide (13).

Owing to widespread use of the oral polio vaccine in the United States, wild poliovirus strains have disappeared, and epidemic polio no longer occurs, although outbreaks of disease in unvaccinated persons were described as recently as 1979 (14). Virtually all cases of poliomyelitis reported in the United States occur in recipients of the oral polio vaccine (usually after the first dose) and in their contacts (15). Cases in vaccine recipients occur 7 to 21 days after immunization, predominantly in children under 4 years of age, about 15% of whom have an immunodeficiency. Disease in contacts occurs principally in young adults, 20 to 29 days after vaccination. Oral polio vaccine virus types 3 and 2 most commonly cause vaccine-associated paralysis; however, more than one type may be involved (15). The estimated risk of oral polio vaccine–related disease is 1 case per 2.6 million doses of vaccine distributed. The overall mortality rate for vaccine-associated poliomyelitis is about 10%, and higher among persons with an immunodeficiency.

Several factors increase the risk of paralysis after infection with poliovirus: male gender (among preadolescents), pregnancy, fatigue, strenuous exercise, immune deficiency, especially isolated B-cell immunodeficiency or severe combined immunodeficiency syndrome, intramuscular injection or injury within 2 weeks before infection, tonsillectomy, and perhaps genetic factors (16,17).

Pathogenesis

The early events in the pathogenesis of poliomyelitis are similar to those described previously for the enteroviruses. Later, the virus reaches the central nervous system, probably via the hematogenous route, produces extensive necrosis of neurons in the gray matter of the brain and spinal cord, and elicits a local mixed inflammatory infiltrate (18). Destruction is maximal in the anterior horn of the spinal cord and in the motor nuclei of the pons and medulla, and less severe in the neurons of the mesencephalon, cerebellar roof nuclei, and precentral gyrus of the cerebral cortex. Virus titers in the spinal cord peak during the first few days after the onset of paralysis and cannot be detected by one week, but inflammation may persist for months.

Clinical Manifestations

Approximately 95% of infections caused by the polioviruses are asymptomatic or inapparent, and about 4 to 8% result in abortive poliomyelitis: fever, headache, sore throat, listlessness, anorexia, vomiting, and abdominal pain lasting a few hours to 3 days. Nonparalytic poliomyelitis is clinically indistinguishable from aseptic meningitis caused by other enteroviruses (described later). Frank paralysis (spinal or bulbar) occurs in about 0.1% of all polioviral infections. Encephalitis, manifested by confusion, altered consciousness, and seizures, and occasionally spastic paralysis, is an uncommon form of poliomyelitis that mainly affects infants.

Coxsackieviruses, Echoviruses, and Newer Enteroviruses

Over 90% of infections caused by the nonpolio enteroviruses are asymptomatic or are manifested as fever only. The epidemiology and pathogenesis of these infections are similar to those reviewed earlier for enteroviruses. Specific syndromes associated with these viruses (Table 13–2) are discussed.

Central Nervous System Infections. Enteroviruses account for more than 90% of cases of acute aseptic meningitis in which the pathogen is identified. Many nonpolio enteroviruses cause aseptic meningitis, but echoviruses, particularly types 4, 6, 9, 11, 16, and 30, most commonly are involved; and of the coxsackieviruses, B2, B3, B4, B5, A7, and A9 are implicated most frequently. Children younger than 1 year are at greatest risk of enteroviral aseptic meningitis, although the disease occurs in older children, young adults, and rarely in persons older than 40 years. The illness is characterized by fever, headache, stiff neck and back, nausea, and vomiting. In 5 to 10% of cases, seizures, lethargy, coma, sensory deficits, or movement disorders develop. Signs and symptoms generally subside in 1 week or less.

Enteroviruses account for 11 to 22% of cases of viral encephalitis, following the arthropod-borne viruses (Chapters 17–19), herpes simplex virus (Chapter 5), and lymphocytic choriomeningitis virus (Chapter 20) (19,20). Serotypes implicated most often are coxsackieviruses A9, B2, and B5 and echovirus types 6 and 9. Neonates, children, and young adults most frequently are affected. Clinical manifestations vary and include lethargy, drowsiness, personality changes, seizures, paresis, and coma. Most persons beyond the neonatal period recover completely, but neurologic sequelae and death may occur.

Coxsackievirus A7 and enterovirus 71 have caused outbreaks of paralytic disease, and sporadic cases have been

Table 13–2. Clinical Spectrum of Infections with Picornaviruses and Specimens for Diagnosis

Disease Manifestation	Responsible Viruses	Specimens
Aseptic meningitis	Cox A 1–11, 14, 16–18, 22, 24 Cox B 1–6 Echo (all but 24, 26, 29, 32) Enteroviruses 70, 71 Polioviruses	CSF, blood; throat swab or wash and feces
Encephalitis	Cox A 2, 5, 6, 7, 9 Cox B 1–3, 5, 6 Echo 2–4, 6, 7, 9, 11, 14, 17–19, 25 Enteroviruses 70, 71 Polioviruses	CSF, brain tissue, blood; throat swab or wash and feces
Paralysis	Cox A 4, 6, 7, 9, 11, 14, 21 Cox B 1–6 Echo 1–4, 6, 7, 9, 11, 14, 16, 18, 19, 30 Enteroviruses 70, 71 Polioviruses	CSF, brain or spinal cord tissue, blood; throat swab or wash and feces
Herpangina	Cox A 2–6, 8, 10, 22 Cox B 1–5 Echo 3, 6, 9, 16, 17, 25, 30	Scrapings of lesions; throat swab or wash and feces
Hand-foot-and-mouth disease	Cox A 5, 7, 9, 10, 16 Enterovirus 71	Scrapings of lesions, vesicle fluid; feces and throat swab or wash
Exanthems	Cox A 2, 4, 5, 9, 16 Cox B 1, 3, 4, 5 Echo 1–8, 11, 14, 18, 19, 25, 30, 32, 33 Enterovirus 71	Throat swab or wash and feces
Conjunctivitis hemorrhagic	Cox A 24 Enterovirus 70	Conjunctival scrapings; throat swab or wash and feces
Acute respiratory disease	Cox A 21, 24 Echo 4, 8, 9, 11, 20, 22, 25 Rhinoviruses	Throat swab or wash and feces Nasal swab or wash
Lymphonodular pharyngitis	Cox A10	Throat swab or wash and feces
Pleurodynia	Cox A 4, 6, 9, 10 Cox B 1–5 Echo 1, 6, 9, 16	Throat swab or wash and feces; ? serum
Myopericarditis	Cox A 4, 16 Cox B 1–6 Echo 9, 22	Pericardial fluid, myocardial biopsy; throat swab or wash and feces; ? serum
Generalized disease of newborn	Cox B 1–5 Echo 6, 9, 11, 14, 19, 31	Throat swab, urine, blood, CSF, tissue
Chronic meningoencephalitis*	Cox A 4, 11, 15 Cox B 2, 3 Echo 2, 3, 5, 9, 11, 19, 24, 25, 30, 33	CSF, brain tissue
Hepatitis	Enterovirus 72 (HAV)	Serum

* In persons with agammaglobulinemia.
Key: Cox A, coxsackievirus A; Cox B, coxsackievirus B; Echo, echovirus; CSF, cerebrospinal fluid; HAV, hepatitis A virus.

caused by coxsackieviruses A7, A9, B1, B2, B3, B4, and B5; echovirus types 6 and 9; and, less frequently, coxsackieviruses A4, A5, and A10 and other echoviruses (21,22). The disease is less severe than poliomyelitis. Muscle weakness is more common than paralysis, which generally resolves.

Exanthems. Echoviruses, especially type 9 but also types 2, 4, 11, 19, and 25 and coxsackievirus A9, cause summer epidemics of fever and maculopapular rashes resembling rubella (Chapter 17) in children under 10 years of age. Roseoliform exanthems in infants and young children, characterized by fever and nonpruritic, salmon-pink maculopapular rash, are caused most commonly by echovirus 16 but also by echoviruses 11 and 25 and coxsackieviruses B1 and B5.

Hand-foot-and-mouth disease, a vesicular eruption caused primarily by coxsackievirus A16 and less often by coxsackieviruses A5, A7, A9, A10, B2, and B5, occurs predominantly in children under the age of 10 years. Affected children present with fever, sore throat, and vesicles on the buccal mucosa, tongue, and in 75% of cases on the hands and feet, involving either the extensor surfaces or the palms and soles. Localized and generalized vesicular lesions caused by coxsackieviruses A9 and B1 and echovirus types 4, 33, and 11 have been reported (23–25).

Acute Respiratory Tract Disease. Fever and upper respiratory tract symptoms resembling the "common cold" may be caused by coxsackieviruses A21 and A24, echovirus 11, and possibly echovirus types 4, 8, 9, 20, 22, and 25 (26,27).

Herpangina. Herpangina, a painful, vesiculoulcerative enanthem of the fauces and soft palate accompanied by fever, sore throat, and pain on swallowing, affects children 3 to 10 years of age during the summer. Coxsackieviruses A1 through A10, A16, and A22 cause most cases, but occasionally coxsackieviruses B1 through B5 and echoviruses 3, 6, 9, 16, 17, 25, and 30 are implicated. Acute lymphonodular pharyngitis, caused by coxsackievirus A10, is similar to herpangina, but the lesions consist of small nodules of lymphocytes that resolve without becoming vesicular or ulcerated.

Pleurodynia. Pleurodynia (also called epidemic myalgia, devil's grippe, and Bornholm disease) was first described in 1872 in Norway, received worldwide attention in 1934 after Ejnar Sylvest's monograph describing his experiences with the disease on the island of Bornholm was translated, and was shown to be caused by the coxsackieviruses in 1949 (28). Group B coxsackieviruses are most commonly responsible, but echoviruses 1, 6, 9, 16, and 19 and coxsackieviruses A4, A6, A9, and A10, are implicated infrequently (29,30).

Pleurodynia generally affects adolescents and young adults. Major epidemics are reported at infrequent intervals, often 10 to 20 years apart, predominantly in Europe and North America, but the disease probably occurs worldwide. The illness begins abruptly with spasmodic pain, typically over the lower rib cage or upper abdomen, and fever, which peaks within 1 hour after the onset of each paroxysm and resolves as the pain subsides. Paroxysms, generally lessening in intensity, recur at varying intervals for 12 hours to 3 weeks (mean, 4 to 6 days).

Myopericarditis. Coxsackieviruses B2 through B5 are the most common causes of myopericarditis, and coxsackieviruses A4 and A16 and echoviruses 9 and 22 occasionally are implicated (31–35). Enteroviral myopericarditis usually occurs in adolescents and active young adults, although persons of any age may be affected. The male-female ratio is approximately 2:1. Fever, malaise, dyspnea, and pain in the precordial area are preceded by an upper respiratory tract illness in two thirds of cases. The most common electrocardiographic abnormalities are ST segment elevations or nonspecific ST and T-wave abnormalities. With severe disease, Q waves, ventricular tachyarrhythmias, and heart block may develop. Recovery is the rule, but recrudescence occurs in about 20% of persons during the first year or more after the initial infection, and the illness is fatal in as many as 4% of cases. Myocardial injury can be permanent, and idiopathic cardiomyopathy may be an occasional consequence of unrecognized infections caused by coxsackieviruses (31,32).

Neonatal Disease. Coxsackieviruses B2, B3, B4, and B5 and echovirus 11 are most commonly associated with overwhelming, systemic neonatal infections, and other echoviruses cause sporadic cases. Most infections are acquired perinatally from an infected mother but the virus may be transmitted nosocomially in nurseries on the hands of staff who care for an infected infant. Boys are affected more often than girls, and premature infants are at increased risk of infection.

Illness becomes apparent during the first week of life, as encephalomyocarditis, caused primarily by coxsackieviruses B1 through B5 and uncommonly by echovirus 11, or as the hemorrhage-hepatitis syndrome, caused by echovirus 11 in about 50% of cases and other echoviruses in the remainder (36–39). Infants with encephalomyocarditis present with respiratory distress, cyanosis, circulatory collapse, lethargy, and convulsions; about 50% die, usually within 1 week of onset. The hemorrhage-hepatitis syndrome, characterized by lethargy, poor feeding, jaundice, ecchymoses, bleeding from puncture sites, and metabolic acidosis, is fatal in 80 to 90% of cases.

Chronic Meningoencephalitis. Enteroviruses, primarily echoviruses, can cause persistent and sometimes fatal infections of the central nervous system in agammaglobulinemic and other immunocompromised persons (40,41). Chronic meningoencephalitis is manifested by nuchal rigidity, headache, lethargy, seizures, motor weakness, tremors, or ataxia, although neurologic signs and symptoms may be absent. Neurologic abnormalities fluctuate, progress, or disappear, and more than half of cases are accompanied by a dermatomyositis-like syndrome.

Acute Hemorrhagic Conjunctivitis. Enterovirus 70 and a variant of coxsackievirus A24 have caused epidemics and pandemics of acute hemorrhagic conjunctivitis since the disease emerged in 1969 in China and Indonesia, spreading throughout Asia, Africa, and some parts of Europe (42). In the Western Hemisphere, disease has been confined to seasonal outbreaks in Central America, Mexico, the Caribbean, and limited foci in Florida. Large epidemics occur predominantly in crowded, coastal areas of tropical countries during the hot, rainy season.

The disease begins abruptly with a burning, foreign body sensation, pain, photophobia, swelling of the eyelid, watery discharge, and pinpoint to diffuse subconjunctival hemorrhage in one eye, and within hours the other is involved. Subconjunctival hemorrhage occurs in 70 to 90% of infections caused by enterovirus 70, but is much less common in cases due to coxsackievirus A24. Fever, malaise, and headache develop in about 20% of affected persons. Symptoms subside by day 2 or 3, and recovery generally is complete by day 10. Possible complications include keratitis, which may persist for several weeks but rarely causes permanent damage, and motor paralysis. The latter is indistinguishable clinically from poliomyelitis, but it occurs 5 to 60 days (mean, 2 to 5 weeks) after an episode of acute hemorrhagic conjunctivitis due to enterovirus 70, almost always in persons older than 20 years.

Hepatitis A Virus (Enterovirus 72)

The existence of at least two agents that cause viral hepatitis syndrome was recognized during the 1950s and 1960s (43,44). In 1967, marmosets were infected with hepatitis A virus (HAV), and HAV virions were detected by immune electron microscopy in stool specimens of infected persons in 1973 (45,46). In 1979, HAV was propagated successfully and serially passaged in primary explant cultures of marmoset liver and in fetal rhesus monkey kidney cells (47).

Structure

The nonenveloped, spherical, 27- to 32-nm diameter virions of HAV are indistinguishable from other picornaviruses. Their RNA genome is surrounded by a capsid containing multiple copies of three or four viral proteins: VP1, (or 1D, the major surface protein), VP2, and VP3. A fourth protein VP4 or 1A) has not been documented with certainty; however, VP0, a presumptive uncleaved precursor of VP2 and VP4, and the structural protein VPg have been detected (48).

Similarities between HAV and the enteroviruses include the existence of a 22S double-stranded RNA replicative intermediate and a genome that can be divided into three parts: a 5' noncoding segment, a single open reading frame that appears to encode all of the viral proteins, and a short 3' noncoding region. However, HAV has unique features: the predicted lengths of its proteins and amino acid sequences differ from those of other enteroviruses; it is difficult to isolate and propagate in cell culture, replicates slowly, and generally is not cytopathic; it is resistant to temperatures and chemicals that inactivate other enteroviruses; and it has only one known serotype.

Epidemiology

HAV is found worldwide, often causing recurrent epidemics. The predominant mode of transmission is close personal contact, usually by the fecal-oral route. Communicability is highest during peak fecal shedding of the virus which occurs about 3 to 10 days before symptoms begin, although HAV has been detected in feces from 3 weeks before to 8 days after the onset of jaundice. Infrequently, HAV is transmitted by contact with body fluids other than feces, such as aerosolized respiratory secretions that contain infectious virus and by transfusion of contaminated blood or blood products (49–52). Hepatitis A virus also is spread via consumption of contaminated water, milk, and food, especially shellfish (53–56).

The reported incidence of hepatitis A in the United States is about 10 cases per 100,000 population; but because most primary infections are subclinical and only a small percentage of diagnosed cases are reported, the actual number of infections is probably much greater. Most reported cases are in adolescents and young adults, males and females in nearly equal numbers (57,58). Rates of infection with HAV, strongly influenced by the level of sanitation or hygiene in the environment, are high in populations where living conditions are crowded or sanitation is poor, such as institutions for developmentally disabled persons, military facilities and prisons (57). In the United States, homosexual men, and children and staff of day care centers also are at increased risk of infection (59,60).

Pathogenesis

Events involved in the pathogenesis of liver injury after natural infection with HAV are ill-understood. The port of entry after the virus is ingested is unknown, but early viral replication in the oropharynx or salivary glands is suspected. Later, HAV must penetrate the intestinal mucosa and spread to the liver. Immunoglobulin (IgA) coproantibodies are present in the feces of persons with acute hepatitis A, and although these antibodies lack neutralizing activity they may curtail communicability or prevent reinfection.

The histologic changes in the liver of persons with acute hepatitis A are minimal and include focal necrosis, acidophilic bodies, ballooning degeneration, and Kupffer cell proliferation; mild to moderate portal inflammation, slight disruption of the limiting plate, and cholestasis may be seen. Host immune cells such as natural killer cells or cytolytic T lymphocytes, rather than the virus, may mediate these alterations, because cellular injury is minimal during the early phase of maximal viral replication (61–63).

Clinical Manifestations

Infection with HAV may be inapparent, subclinical, or produce mild and transient to severe and prolonged symptoms. In general, the frequency of disease increases with age (64,65). Subclinical or anicteric hepatitis (meaning symptomatic disease without jaundice) develops in more than 90% of infected children younger than 5 years but in only 25 to 50% of adults.

Regardless of the route of transmission, the incubation period ranges from 10 to 50 days (mode, about 1 month) and generally is shorter when the viral inoculum is large. Fever, fatigue, malaise, myalgias, anorexia, nausea, and vomiting often begin abruptly and frequently are accompanied by epigastric or right upper quadrant pain, cough, coryza, sore throat, and, in children, diarrhea. Arthritis, vasculitis, and meningoencephalitis are rare (66,67). Just before the onset of jaundice, the urine becomes dark, and during the icteric phase, pruritus and acholic stools are common. Complete recovery is usual, but fatal fulminant hepatitis may occur.

The serum alanine aminotransferase (ALT) activity rises a few days after symptoms begin, peaks before the onset of jaundice, and generally returns to normal 2 to 3 weeks after the illness begins in children, and later in adults. Levels of ALT usually are higher than levels of aspartate aminotransferase (AST), and the ALT-AST ratio is less than 0.7 in almost all uncomplicated cases of acute hepatitis A.

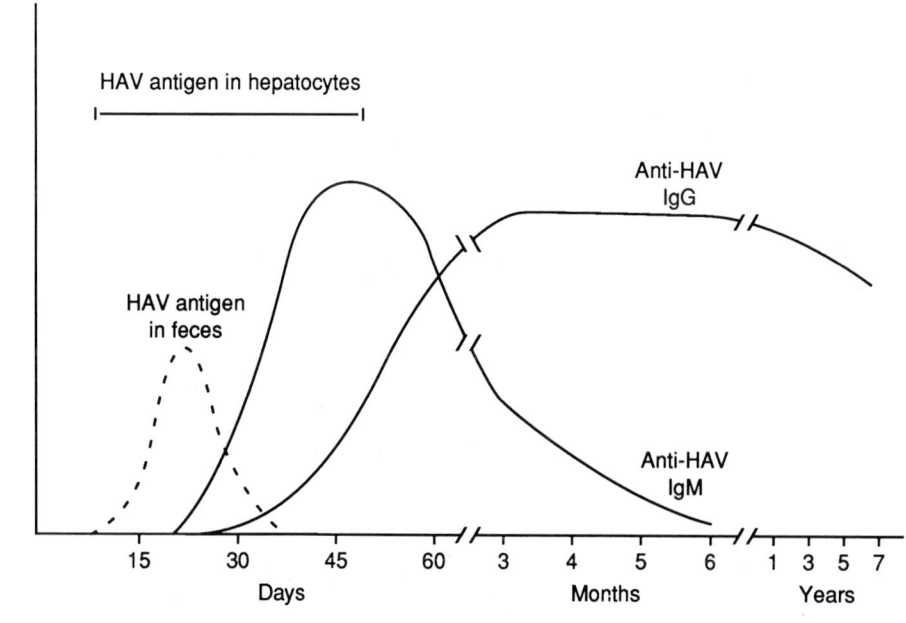

Fig. 13–2. Virologic and serologic events associated with hepatitis A.

The bilirubin level starts to rise 2 days to 2 weeks after the rise in ALT activity and returns to normal in about 1 month. Most persons have concurrent relative lymphocytosis.

The virologic and serologic events associated with hepatitis A are diagrammed in Figure 13–2 (68). After infection with HAV, high concentrations of virus are excreted in the feces and brief, low-grade viremia precedes the onset of symptoms. Specific IgM generally is present when symptoms begin and disappears 3 to 6 months later. Specific IgG rises shortly after IgM is detected and persists for years.

RHINOVIRUS

The first rhinovirus, later designated rhinovirus 1A, was isolated in 1956, and by 1986 100 immunotypes, numbered 1 to 100 and subtype 1A, were identified (69).

Structure

Rhinovirus virions, 20 to 27 nm in diameter, have four structural proteins (VP1, VP2, VP3, and VP4), forming an icosahedrally symmetric capsid, and an RNA genome containing approximately 7000 nucleotides. The nonenveloped viral shell consists of 60 repeated subunits containing the four viral proteins. The five VP1 subunits on the viral surface are separated by a deep cleft, which is the proposed site of viral attachment to the host cell receptor. Virions are ether resistant but are destroyed in an acidic environment (pH 3 to 5).

Epidemiology

Human rhinoviruses infect only humans and higher primates. They are distributed worldwide and are associated with fall and spring peaks of infection in temperate climates. Rhinoviruses also cause a large proportion of summer colds but they rarely cause illness during winter. In tropics and arctic areas outbreaks of rhinoviral infections occur during the rainy season and cold weather, respectively.

Rhinoviral colds, one of the most common human infections, occur throughout life, but rates are highest among infants and children and decrease with age. Rhinovirus is spread from person to person by close contact with infectious respiratory tract secretions. The hands of an infected person are contaminated with nasal secretions containing rhinovirus; hand-to-hand transmission then is followed by autoinoculation of the nasal and conjunctival mucosa. Alternatively, rhinovirus may be transmitted by inhalation of small or large airborne particles.

Pathogenesis

Infection with rhinovirus can be initiated in the laboratory by instilling less than one tissue culture mean infective dose ($TCID_{50}$) in the nose. After an incubation period of 1 to 4 days, shedding of the virus in nasal secretions begins; it peaks on day 2 or 3, then falls to lower levels, though the virus may be detected for 3 weeks. Symptoms begin on day 2 and peak on days 3 and 4.

The mechanisms by which rhinoviruses produce disease are not yet fully elucidated. Histologic examination of nasal mucosal biopsy specimens from symptomatic persons has shown marked submucosal edema with minimal inflammation; however these changes have not been consistent (70,71). Given that damage to the epithelium is minimal, the virus may trigger the release of chemical mediators, which ultimately are responsible for the clinical illness. The presence of high concentrations of bradykinin and lysylbradykinin and enzymes with arginine esterase activity, but not histamine, in nasal wash specimens of persons with experimental rhinoviral colds supports this hypothesis (72).

Natural infection with rhinovirus stimulates production of neutralizing antibodies, which are detected in serum and nasal secretions of about 80% of persons. Although most rhinoviral colds confer long-lasting type-specific immunity, protection by pre-existing antibodies can be overcome with a large inoculum.

Clinical Manifestations

The most common clinical manifestations of infection with rhinovirus are rhinorrhea, nasal obstruction, a sore or scratchy throat, headache, and malaise; cough and hoarseness occur in one third or fewer cases; fever is uncommon. The median duration of illness is 7 days, but in about 25% of persons symptoms persist up to 2 weeks. Complications of the infection include sinusitis and otitis media, and rhinoviruses may cause acute infectious exacerbations in persons with chronic bronchitis and attacks of asthma in children (73,74).

Laboratory Diagnosis

Specimens required for diagnosis of infections caused by the picornaviruses are listed in Table 13–2. Specimen collection, transport, and processing are discussed in Part III. Virus identification is reviewed here.

Enteroviruses. Detection of most enteroviruses requires conventional cell culture. At a minimum, primary monkey (rhesus, African green, or cynomolgus) kidney cells and a human diploid fibroblast cell line such as MRC-5 or WI-38 cells should be inoculated. Adding a continuous cell line such as HEp-2 or A-549 cells helps distinguish the different species, and inoculating the continuous BGM African green monkey kidney cell line and RD cells (a rhabdomyosarcoma cell line) may enhance recovery of group B coxsackieviruses and decrease the time to detection of cytopathic effect (CPE) (75–77). Many coxsackieviruses of group A, however, cannot be cultivated and are identified by their pathogenicity in suckling mice infected in the laboratory. Group A coxsackieviruses cause progressive flaccid paralysis without signs of encephalitis, whereas group B coxsackieviruses cause spastic paralysis with encephalitis. Moreover, only tissues of mice infected with group A coxsackieviruses show myositis.

Inoculated cell cultures are maintained a minimum of 2 weeks at 35° C. Typically, by day 5 to 7, cells of a monolayer infected with an enterovirus round up, become refractile, shrink, degenerate, and then detach from the surface of the culture tube (Fig. 13–3), although CPE may develop as early as day 2 or as late as day 21. The genus

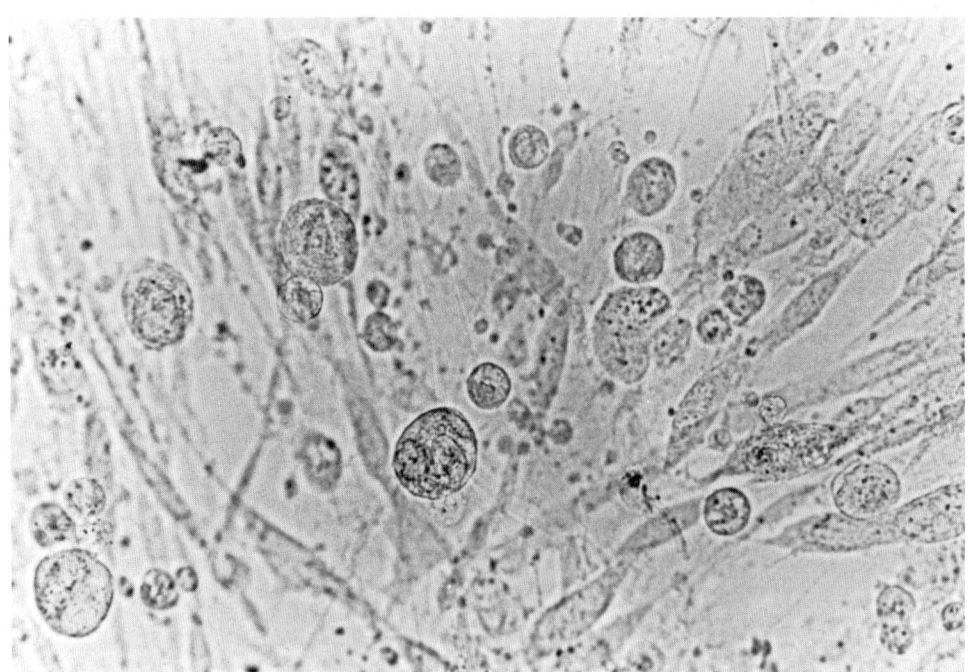

Fig. 13–3. Cytopathic effect produced by echovirus in MRC-5 cells (×100).

of enterovirus present often is suggested by the pattern of growth in different cell lines (Table 13–3) (75). Final identification requires neutralization using antiserum pools, performed in conventional cell culture tubes or microtiter plates seeded with a cell line sensitive to the viral isolate (78).

Serologic testing has limited value in diagnosis of infections with enteroviruses other than poliovirus and HAV because testing for antibodies to the many enterovirus serotypes that could cause a disease manifestation such as aseptic meningitis is not feasible. Moreover, the standard neutralization test often is difficult to interpret because cross-reactions occur between serotypes within a genus and occasionally between isolates of different genera. Serologic tests, however, might be useful for diagnosis of enteroviral syndromes caused by only a few serotypes such as hand-foot-and-mouth disease, myopericarditis, or pleurodynia. Paired acute- and convalescent-phase sera collected as early in the illness as possible and 2 to 4 weeks later should be tested concurrently because a high stable titer does not exclude past infection. A fourfold rise in titer indicates acute infection.

Given that enteroviruses may not be detected by conventional cell culture for 1 week or longer, a more rapid detection method would be valuable. Nucleic acid hybridization and gene amplification by polymerase chain reaction have been evaluated in research laboratories and in the future may be useful in the clinical virology laboratory (79,80).

Acute hepatitis A is diagnosed by testing serum or plasma for specific IgM, which is detected in almost all infected persons at the onset of symptoms. Although IgM generally becomes indetectable in 3 to 6 months, it persists more than 6 months in 10 to 15% of cases.

Rhinoviruses. Rhinoviruses are detected by conventional cell culture using human diploid fibroblasts, maintained at 33° to 35° C for a minimum of 2 weeks. Typical CPE becomes apparent after about 7 to 10 days as individual foci of rounded, refractile cells (Fig. 13–4) that may gradually spread, remain stable, or even disappear. Rhinoviruses are differentiated from the enteroviruses, which may cause a similar CPE, by demonstrating lability to pH 3 (enteroviruses are acid stable) (81).

Treatment

No antiviral agent effective against the picornaviruses is available currently. Management of infections is supportive.

Prevention

Poliovirus. Paralytic poliomyelitis is effectively prevented by an inactivated poliovirus vaccine or a live, attenuated oral poliovirus vaccine. The oral vaccine has

Table 13–3. Susceptibility of Tissue Culture Cells for the Enteroviruses

	Cell Line		
Genus	PMK	HDF	HEp-2/A-549
Poliovirus	++*	++	++
Coxsackie B	++	±	+
Coxsackie A[†]	0 to ++	0 to ++	0 to ++
Echovirus	++	++	0

* Degree of sensitivity: 0, not suitable for isolation; ±, some strains may be recovered; +, many strains may be recovered; ++, most strains will be recovered.
[†] Many strains detected only by suckling mouse inoculation (see text). Key: PMK, primary monkey kidney; HDF, human diploid fibroblasts (MRC-5, WI-38, foreskin); HEp-2/A-549, human heteroploid continuous cell line (squamous cell carcinoma).

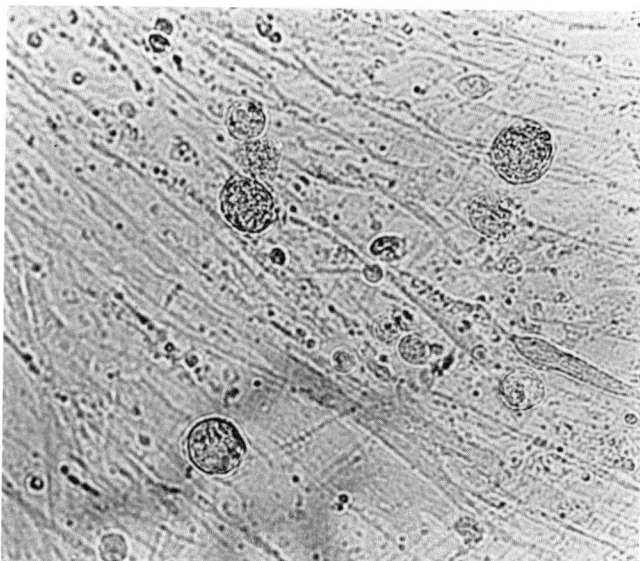

Fig. 13–4. Cytopathic effect produced by rhinovirus in MRC-5 cells (×100).

Table 13–4. Recommendations for Immune Globulin (Ig) Prophylaxis for Hepatitis A (HAV)

Pre-exposure prophylaxis
  Travelers to foreign countries where the risk of acquiring hepatitis A is enhanced owing to living conditions, the prevalence of HAV in the area, and the length of stay.
Postexposure prophylaxis
  Close personal contact: all household and sexual contacts of persons with hepatitis A.
  Day care centers: staff, attendees, and all members of households whose diapered children attend.
  Schools, preschools, and institutions for custodial care: not generally warranted unless an institutional- or classroom-centered outbreak is identified.
  Hospitals: not routinely indicated for hospital personnel. Instead, sound hygienic practices should be emphasized.
  Offices and factories: not indicated under usual working conditions for persons exposed to a fellow worker with hepatitis A.
  Common-source exposure: not warranted once cases have begun to appear. When a food handler with hepatitis A is identified, Ig should be given to other kitchen employees and may be considered for patrons if (a) the infected person is directly involved in handling foods that are not to be cooked, or handling cooked foods before they are eaten; (b) the hygienic practices of the worker are deficient; and (c) consumers can be identified and treated within 2 weeks of exposure.

(From Hollinger FB, and Glombicki AP: Hepatitis A virus. *In* Principles and Practice of Infectious Disease. 3rd ed. Edited by GL Mandell, RG Douglas, Jr, and JE Bennett. New York, Churchill Livingstone, 1990.)

been used almost exclusively in the United States since 1969 because of several perceived advantages: superior immunogenicity, lower cost, ease of administration, spread of vaccine virus to unimmunized, susceptible persons, and the induction of gastrointestinal immunity. The litigation resulting from vaccine-related paralytic disease, however, has caused a significant increase in the cost of the oral vaccine. Because the social and legal costs of the oral polio vaccine have increased and because a more potent inactivated poliovirus vaccine has been licensed, the polio vaccine policy in the United States currently is being reviewed (82–84).

Complete immunization using the trivalent oral polio vaccine requires a primary series of three doses administered at 2, 4, and 12 to 18 months of age and a booster at 4 to 6 years. The recommended primary series is identical for the enhanced inactivated polio vaccine, which is the preferred vaccine for immunocompromised persons and previously unvaccinated adults. In developing countries where poliomyelitis is still a problem, an immunization policy combining five doses of the oral polio vaccine with two doses of the inactivated vaccine appears to effectively control the disease and may make possible its eradication (85).

Hepatitis A Virus. General measures to prevent hepatitis A include careful hand washing by medical personnel who have contact with patients and laboratory workers who handle infective specimens, preventing close contact of infected young children with susceptible playmates during the first 2 weeks of illness or for 2 weeks after the onset of jaundice, and not sharing personal objects.

Passive immunization with immune globulin effectively modifies or prevents hepatitis A when given up to 6 days before the onset of illness. Indications for pre- and postexposure immune globulin prophylaxis are shown in Table 13–4. Research to develop a safe and efficacious attenuated vaccine and an effective molecularly engineered subunit vaccine is ongoing (86–88).

REFERENCES

1. Moore M: From the Centers for Disease Control: Enteroviral disease in the United States, 1970–1979. J Infect Dis, *146*: 103, 1982.
2. Strikas RA, Anderson LJ, and Parker RA: Temporal and geographic patterns of isolates of nonpolio enteroviruses in the United States. J Infect Dis, *153*:346, 1986.
3. Fox JP: Epidemiology of poliomyelitis in populations before and after vaccination with inactivated viruses. *In* Poliomyelitis. Papers and Discussions Presented at the Fourth International Poliomyelitis Conference. Philadelphia, JB Lippincott, 1958.
4. Kogon A, et al: The virus watch program. A continuing surveillance of viral infections in metropolitan New York families. VII. Observations on viral excretion, seroimmunity, intrafamilial spread and illness association in coxsackievirus and echovirus infections. Am J Epidemiol, *89*:51, 1969.
5. Baron RC, Hatch MHH, Kleeman K, and MacCormack JN: Aseptic meningitis among members of a high school football team. An outbreak associated with echovirus 16 infection. JAMA, *248*:1724, 1982.
6. Josselson J, Pula T, and Sadler JH: Acute rhabdomyolysis associated with an echovirus 9 infection. Arch Intern Med, *140*:1671, 1980.
7. McKinney RE Jr, Katz SL, and Wilfert CM: Chronic enteroviral meningoencephalitis in agammaglobulinemic patients. Rev Infect Dis, *9*:334, 1987.
8. Paul JR: A History of Poliomyelitis. New Haven, Yale University Press, 1971.
9. Enders JF, Weller TH, and Robbins FC: Cultivation of the Lansing strain of poliomyelitis virus in cultures of various human embryonic tissues. Science, *109*:85, 1949.

10. Bodian D, Morgan IM, and Howe HA: Differentiation of types of poliomyelitis viruses: III. The grouping of fourteen strains into three basic immunological types. Am J Hyg, 49:234, 1949.
11. Salk JE, et al: Studies in human subjects on active immunization against poliomyelitis. I. A preliminary report of experiments in progress. JAMA, 151:1081, 1953.
12. Centers for Disease Control: Summary of notifiable diseases, United States 1989. MMWR, 38(54):1, 1989.
13. Wright PF, et al: Strategies for the global eradication of poliomyelitis by the year 2000. N Engl J Med, 325:1774, 1991.
14. Schonberger LB, et al: Control of paralytic poliomyelitis in the United States. Rev Infect Dis, 6:S424, 1984.
15. Nkowane BM, et al: Vaccine-associated paralytic poliomyelitis: United States: 1973 through 1984. JAMA, 257:1335, 1987.
16. Greenberg M, Abramson H, Cooper HM, and Solomon HE: The relation between recent injections and paralytic poliomyelitis in children. Am J Public Health, 42:142, 1952.
17. van Eden W, et al: Differential resistance to paralytic poliomyelitis controlled by histocompatibility leukocyte antigens. J Infect Dis, 147:422, 1983.
18. Bodian D: Emerging concept of poliomyelitis infection. Science, 122:105, 1955.
19. Meyer HM, et al: Central nervous system syndromes of viral etiology. A study of 713 cases. Am J Med, 29:334, 1960.
20. Lennette EH, Magoflin RL, and Knouf EG: Viral central nervous system disease. JAMA, 179:687, 1962.
21. Voroshilova MK and Chumakov MP: Poliomyelitis-like properties of AB-IV-coxsackie A7 group of viruses. Progr Med Virol, 2:106, 1959.
22. Shindarov LM, et al: Epidemiological, clinical, and pathomorphological characteristics of epidemic poliomyelitis-like disease caused by enterovirus 71. J Hyg Epidemiol Microbiol Immunol, 23:284, 1979.
23. Cherry JD, Lerner AM, Klein JO, and Finland M: Coxsackie A9 infections with exanthems with particular reference to urticaria. Pediatrics, 31:819, 1963.
24. DeChamps C, et al: Four cases of vesicular lesions in adults caused by enterovirus infections. J Clin Microbiol, 26:2182, 1988.
25. Deseda-Tous J, Byatt PH, and Cherry JD: Vesicular lesions in adults due to echovirus 11 infections. Arch Dermatol, 113:1705, 1977.
26. Johnson KM, et al: The role of enteroviruses in respiratory disease. Am Rev Respir Dis, 88:240, 1963.
27. Jackson GG and Muidoon RL: Viruses causing common respiratory infections in man: II. Enteroviruses and paramyxoviruses. J Infect Dis, 128:387, 1973.
28. Sylvest E: Epidemic Myalgia: Bornholm Disease. London, Oxford University Press, 1934.
29. Assaad F and Cockburn WC: Four-year study of WHO virus reports on enteroviruses other than poliovirus. Bull WHO, 36:329, 1972.
30. Bell EJ and Grist NR: ECHO viruses, carditis, and acute pleurodynia. Am Heart J, 82:133, 1971.
31. Sainani GS, Krompotic E, and Slodki SJ: Adult heart disease due to the coxsackievirus B infection. Medicine, 47:133, 1968.
32. Koontz CH and Ray CG: The role of coxsackie group B virus infections in sporadic myopericarditis. Am Heart J, 82:750, 1971.
33. Ayuthya PSN, Jayavasu JJ, and Pongpanich B: Coxsackie group B virus and primary myocardial disease in infants and children. Am Heart J, 88:311, 1974.
34. Woodruff JF: Viral myocarditis. A review. Am J Pathol, 101:427, 1980.
35. Grist NR and Bell EJ: Coxsackieviruses and the heart. Am Heart J, 77:295, 1969.
36. Gear JHS and Measroch V: Coxsackievirus infections of the newborn. Progr Med Virol, 15:42, 1973.
37. Drew JH: Echo 11 virus outbreak in a nursery associated with myocarditis. Aust J Pediatr, 9:90, 1973.
38. Modlin JF: Perinatal echovirus infection: Insights from a literature review of 61 cases of serious infection and 16 outbreaks in nurseries. Rev Infect Dis, 8:918, 1986.
39. Spector SA and Straube RC: Protean manifestations of perinatal enterovirus infections. West J Med, 138:847, 1983.
40. McKinney RE, Katz SL, and Wilfert CM: Chronic enteroviral meningoencephalitis in agammaglobulinemic patients. Rev Infect Dis, 9:334, 1987.
41. O'Neill KM, et al: Chronic group A coxsackievirus infection in agammaglobulinemia: Demonstration of genomic variation or serotypically identical isolates persistently excreted from the same patient. J Infect Dis, 157:183, 1988.
42. Kono R: Apollo 11 disease or acute hemorrhagic conjunctivitis: A pandemic of a new enterovirus infection of the eyes. Am J Epidemiol, 101:383, 1975.
43. Murray R: Viral hepatitis. Bull NY Acad Med, 31:341, 1955.
44. Krugman S, Giles JP, and Hammond J: Infectious hepatitis: Evidence for two distinctive clinical, epidemiological, and immunological types of infection. JAMA, 200:365, 1967.
45. Deinhardt F, et al: Studies on the transmission of human viral hepatitis to marmoset monkeys. I. Transmission of disease, serial passages, and description of liver lesions. J Exp Med, 125:673, 1967.
46. Feinstone SM, Kapikian AZ, and Purcell RH: Hepatitis A: Detection by immune electron microscopy of a viruslike antigen associated with acute illness. Science, 182:1026, 1973.
47. Provost PJ, and Hilleman MR: Propagation of human hepatitis A virus in cell culture in vitro. Proc Soc Exp Biol Med, 160:213, 1979.
48. Gauss-Müller V, Lottspeich E, and Deinhardt F: Characterization of hepatitis A virus structural proteins. Virology, 155:732, 1986.
49. Dienstag JL, Szmuness W, and Stevens CE: Hepatitis A virus infection: New insights from seroepidemiologic studies. J Infect Dis, 137:328, 1978.
50. Centers for Disease Control: Hepatitis Surveillance Report Number 48. Atlanta, Centers for Disease Control, 1982.
51. Corey L, and Holmes KK: Sexual transmission of hepatitis A in homosexual men: Incidence and mechanism. N Engl J Med, 302:435, 1980.
52. Hadler SC, et al: Hepatitis A in day-care centers: A community-wide assessment. N Engl J Med, 302:1222, 1980.
53. Neefe JR and Stokes J Jr: An epidemic of infectious hepatitis possibly due to a water-borne agent. JAMA, 128:1063, 1945.
54. Aach RD, Evans J, and Losoc J: An epidemic of infectious hepatitis possibly due to airborne transmission. Am J Epidemiol, 87:99, 1968.
55. Barbara JAJ, et al: Post-transfusion hepatitis A. Lancet i:738, 1982.
56. Seeberg S, et al: Hospital outbreak of hepatitis A secondary to blood exchange in a baby. Lancet, i:1155, 1981.
57. Raska K: A milk-borne infectious hepatitis epidemic. J Hyg Epidemiol Microb Immunol, 10:413, 1966.
58. Rindge ME, Mason JO, and Elsea WR: Infectious hepatitis: Report of an outbreak in a small Connecticut school due to water-borne transmission. JAMA, 180:33, 1962.
59. Mason JO and McLean WR. Infectious hepatitis traced to the consumption of raw oysters: An epidemiologic study. Am J Hyg, 75:90, 1962.
60. Portnoy BL, et al: Oyster-associated hepatitis: Failure of

61. Kurane I, et al: Human lymphocyte responses to hepatitis A virus–infected cells: Interferon production and lysis of infected cells. J Immunol, 135:2140, 1985.
62. Vallbracht A, et al: Persistent infection of human fibroblasts by hepatitis A virus. J Gen Virol, 65:609, 1984.
63. Karron RA, et al: Studies of prototype live hepatitis A virus vaccines in primate models. J Infect Dis, 157:338, 1988.
64. Benenson MW, et al: A military community outbreak of hepatitis type A related to transmission in a child care facility. Am J Epidemiol, 112:471, 1980.
65. Lednar WM, et al: Frequency of illness associated with epidemic hepatitis A virus infection in adults. Am J Epidemiol, 122:226, 1985.
66. Inman RD, et al: Arthritis, vasculitis and cryoglobulinemia associated with relapsing hepatitis A virus infection. Ann Intern Med, 105:700, 1986.
67. Bromberg K, Newhall N, and Peter G: Hepatitis A and meningoencephalitis. JAMA, 247:815, 1982.
68. Hollinger FB and Glombicki AP: Heptatitis A virus. In Principles and Practice of Infectious Diseases. 3rd ed. Edited by GL Mandell, RG Douglas Jr, and JE Bennett. New York, Churchill Livingstone, 1990.
69. Price WH: The isolation of a new virus associated with respiratory clinical disease in humans. Proc Natl Acad Sci USA, 42:892, 1956.
70. Douglas RG Jr, Alford BR, and Couch RB: Atraumatic nasal biopsy for studies of respiratory virus infection in volunteers. Antimicrob Agents Chemother, 8:340, 1968.
71. Winther B, et al: Histopathologic examination and enumeration of polymorphonuclear leukocytes in the nasal mucosa during experimental rhinovirus colds. Acta Otolaryngol (Suppl) (Stockh), 413:19, 1984.
72. Naclerio RM, et al: Kinins are generated during experimental rhinovirus colds. J Infect Dis, 157:133, 1988.
73. Stenhouse AC: Rhinovirus infection in acute exacerbations of chronic bronchitis: A controlled prospective study. Br Med J, 3:461, 1967.
74. Minor TE, et al: Greater frequency of viral respiratory infection in asthmatic children as compared with their nonasthmatic siblings. Pediatrics, 85:472, 1974.
75. Johnston SG and Siegel CS: Presumptive identification of enteroviruses with RD, HEp-2, and RMK cell lines. J Clin Microbiol, 28:1049, 1990.
76. Menegus MA and Hollick GE: Increased efficiency of group B coxsackievirus isolation from clinical specimens by use of BGM cells. J Clin Microbiol, 15:945, 1982.
77. Woods GL and Young A: Use of A-549 cells in a clinical virology laboratory. J Clin Microbiol, 26:1026, 1988.
78. Egbertson SH and Mayo DR: A microneutralization test for the identification of enterovirus isolates. J Virol Methods, 14:305, 1986.
79. Chapman NH, Tracey S, Gaunt CJ, and Fortmueller U: Molecular detection and identification of enteroviruses using enzymatic amplification and nucleic acid hybridization. J Clin Microbiol, 28:843, 1990.
80. Rotbart HA, Kinsella JP, and Wasserman RL: Persistent enterovirus infection in culture-negative meningoencephalitis: Demonstration by enzymatic RNA amplification. J Infect Dis, 161:787, 1990.
81. Drew WL: Laboratory methods in basic virology. In Bailey and Scott's Diagnostic Microbiology. 8th ed. Edited by EJ Baron and SM Finegold. St. Louis, CV Mosby, 1990.
82. Centers for Disease Control: Poliomyelitis prevention: Enhanced-potency inactivated poliomyelitis vaccine—supplementary statement. MMWR, 36:795, 1987.
83. Institute of Medicine, National Academy of Sciences: An evaluation of poliomyelitis vaccine of enhanced potency. J Biol Stand, 14:127, 1986.
84. Faden H, et al: Comparative evaluation of immunization with live attenuated and enhanced-potency inactivated trivalent poliovirus vaccines in childhood: systemic and local responses. J Infect Dis, 162:1291, 1990.
85. Tulchinsky T, et al: A ten-year experience in control of poliomyelitis through a combination of live and killed vaccines in two developing areas. Am J Public Health, 79:1648, 1989.
86. Binn LN, et al: Preparation of a prototype inactivated hepatitis A-virus vaccine from infected cell cultures. J Infect Dis, 153:749, 1986.
87. Emini EA, et al: Induction of hepatitis A virus–neutralizing antibody by a virus-specific synthetic peptide. J Virol, 55:836, 1985.
88. Midthun K, et al: Safety and immunogenicity of a live attenuated hepatitis A virus vaccine in seronegative volunteers. J Infect Dis, 163:735, 1991.

Chapter 14

REOVIRUSES

Reoviruses are nonenveloped, segmented double-stranded RNA viruses, approximately 70 nm in diameter, that possess a double layer of icosahedral shells. These viruses are classified in the family Reoviridae, and those of medical importance are in the genera Orthoreovirus, Orbivirus, and Rotavirus.

ORTHOREOVIRUS

The ubiquitous orthoreoviruses cause infections in many vertebrates. Serotypes 1, 2, and 3 are associated with mammalian infections. Antibody surveys indicate that infections with orthoreoviruses are common in humans, though disease is rare. Enteritis of infants and children and upper respiratory tract infections have been reported (1,2). Reovirus type 1 has been implicated in an outbreak of fever, rhinorrhea, and pharyngitis in a nursery, and type 3 may cause neonatal hepatitis and extrahepatic biliary atresia (1,3).

ORBIVIRUS

Orbiviruses, divided into 13 antigenically distinct serogroups, are distinguished from orthoreoviruses by protein structure, arthropod transmission, and acid susceptibility. Of the seven orbiviruses that cause human disease, only Colorado tick fever virus, the orbivirus of importance in the United States, is discussed; features of the others are reviewed in Table 14–1 (4–6).

Colorado Tick Fever Virus

Colorado tick fever ("mountain fever") was described as early as 1850 but was not distinguished from Rocky Mountain spotted fever (Chapter 26) and tularemia (Chapter 33) until the 1930s. The responsible virus, which measures 50 to 60 nm in diameter and has an RNA genome of 12 segments, was isolated from Dermacentor andersoni ticks and transmitted to human volunteers in 1944 (7).

Epidemiology and Pathogenesis

Colorado tick fever occurs in mountainous areas where Dermacentor andersoni ticks are found: Colorado, Wyoming, Montana, Idaho, Utah, and parts of South Dakota, New Mexico, California, Oregon, Washington, Alberta, and British Columbia. In nature, the virus is amplified during the spring and summer in a cycle involving larval and nymphal ticks and ground squirrels and chipmunks. The virus is carried through the winter in hibernating nymphal and adult ticks, and the cycle begins again the next spring when infected nymphs feed on rodents. Humans acquire the virus via the bite of an adult D. andersoni tick, often between late May and early July. About 90% of persons diagnosed with the disease recall tick exposure. Young adult men exposed outdoors are at greatest risk of infection.

After the virus enters a susceptible host it circulates in erythrocytes for a long period. Viremia peaks during the second and third weeks after disease onset, and about half of infected persons are viremic 1 month after the illness begins.

Clinical Manifestations

After an incubation period of 3 to 6 days illness begins abruptly, with fever, chills, lethargy, prostration, headache, myalgia, ocular pain, photophobia, abdominal pain, nausea, and vomiting, and it lasts 7 to 10 days. Fever is biphasic in about half the cases, and a macular or maculopapular rash develops in 5 to 12%. Unusual complications in children include meningoencephalitis and a hemorrhagic syndrome. Complete recovery is usual, although adults older than 30 years may experience prolonged convalescence with asthenia. Infection induces long-lasting immunity, and reinfection is extremely rare.

ROTAVIRUS

Human rotaviruses were discovered in 1973 by electron microscopic examination of duodenal biopsy specimens from hospitalized children with nonbacterial gastroenteritis in Australia and of stool specimens from gastroenteritis patients in the United Kingdom, and shortly thereafter were found in persons with gastroenteritis in many parts of the world (8–14). In 1974, the virus was named rotavirus to describe the wheel-like appearance of intact virions in specimens stained with a negative stain and viewed under the electron microscope (Fig. 14–1) (15).

Structure

Rotavirus particles are about 70 nm in diameter, although incomplete, single-shelled 55-nm diameter particles also occur. The RNA genome has 11 segments, each with a molecular weight ranging from 400,000 to 2 million. The segments can be separated by polyacrylamide gel electrophoresis, a technique used predominantly for epidemiologic studies (16,17). The genes and major proteins of rotavirus are shown in Table 14–2.

Rotaviruses are divided into groups, subgroups, and serotypes. Until recently, all human and animal rotavirus strains were believed to possess a common group antigen.

Table 14-1. Orbiviruses Implicated in Human Disease Outside the United States

Agent	Clinical Manifestation	Vector	Geographic Location
Changuinola virus	Fever	Phlebotomus flies	Panama
Lebomo virus	Fever	Mosquitoes	Nigeria, South Africa
Kemerova, Lipounik, and Tribec viruses	Meningoencephalitis, polyradiculitis	Ticks	Soviet Republics, eastern Europe
Orungo virus	Fever, encephalitis	Mosquitoes	Sub-Saharan Africa

Table 14-2. Rotavirus Genes and Major Proteins

Gene Segment	Protein Product		
	Designation	Location	Biologic Function
1	VP1	Core	
2	VP2	Core	
3	VP3	Core	
4	VP4	Outer capsid	Hemagglutination; protease-enhanced plaque formation; growth restriction in cell culture
5	NS53		
6	VP6	Inner capsid	Major inner core structural protein; major subgroup antigen
7	NS34		
8 or 9	VP7	Major outer protein (glycosylated)	Serotype specificity; major neutralization determinant
10	NS28		
11	VP9		

Key: VP, viral protein; NS, nonstructural protein.
(Modified from Christensen ML: Human viral gastroenteritis. Clin Microbiol Rev, 2:51, 1989.)

However, morphologically indistinguishable rotaviruses that lack the common group antigen and possess different RNA electrophoretic patterns have been isolated from humans, many animals, and birds. These have various names: rotavirus-like organisms, antigenically distinct rotaviruses, pararotaviruses, atypical rotaviruses, and novel rotaviruses (18–30). The group designation of rotaviruses was introduced in 1983 (28): group A includes the original conventional rotaviruses that have the common group antigen; groups B, C, D, and E possess other group antigens and are genetically differentiated by electrophoresis and one-dimensional terminal fingerprinting analysis of the RNA segments. Most human rotaviruses belong to group A; group B rotaviruses cause severe epidemics of human diarrhea in China; and group C rotaviruses have been reported sporadically in humans (18,24,30,31).

The major rotavirus subgroup antigen, VP6, specifies one of two subgroups (I and II), which are differentiated by the electrophoretic migration patterns of gene segments 10 and 11, complement fixation, immune electron microscopy, radioimmunoassay, or enzyme-linked immunosorbent assay (ELISA). Serotype specificity is determined by VP7. Four human serotypes are known: serotype 2 is in subgroup I, and serotypes 1, 3, and 4 are in subgroup II. Possible serotypes 5 and 6 also have been described (32,33).

Epidemiology

Rotaviruses are a major cause of diarrhea in infants and young children, and are responsible for about half the cases of gastroenteritis in hospitalized pediatric patients. In developing countries the infant mortality rate for diarrheal diseases (many of which are caused by rotavirus) is high, whereas in developed parts of the world fatal infection by rotavirus is infrequent (34). Rotavirus is transmitted by the fecal-oral route, and in temperate climates disease occurs predominantly during the dry winter months.

Pathogenesis

Rotavirus selectively infects and replicates in the mature villus enterocytes of the small intestine, especially the duodenum. Although the mechanism of diarrhea is not completely understood, infection of the absorptive intestinal cells appears to inhibit absorption of salt and

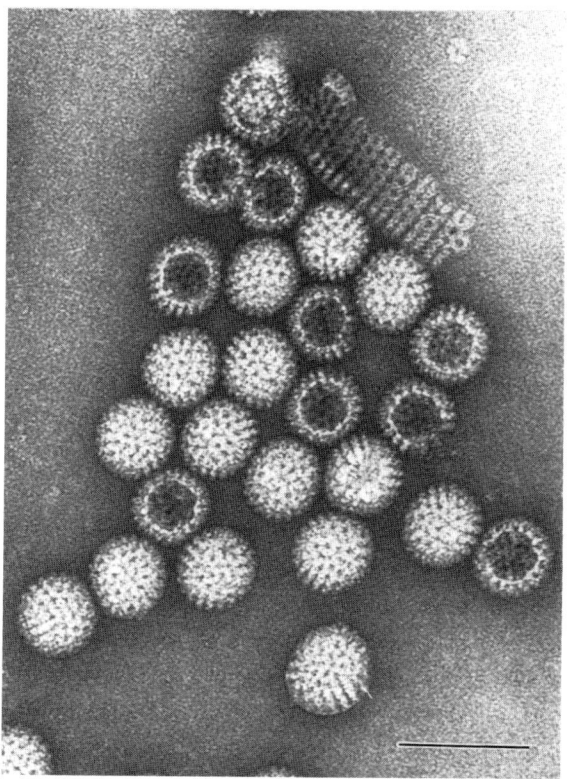

Fig. 14-1. Electron micrograph of rotavirus particles in a stool sample (X178,525). (Courtesy of the Division of Viral and Rickettsial Diseases, Centers for Disease Control, Atlanta, GA.)

water, resulting in net fluid secretion. Duodenal biopsy tissue from persons with rotaviral gastroenteritis shows mild to severe mucosal changes, including shortening and blunting of villi, mononuclear cell infiltration of the lamina propria, and cuboidal and irregular epithelial cells. By electron microscopic examination of the tissue rotavirus virions are seen in the endoplasmic reticulum of vacuolated epithelial cells.

Infection with rotavirus elicits the production of circulating and intestinal immunoglobulins, but their role in preventing infection is unclear because infections with rotavirus may be repetitive. Specific serum immunoglobulin (Ig) M appears during acute infection and declines during convalescence, when specific IgG appears and persists for 6 to 12 months. Neutralizing IgG, produced during convalescence, provides short-lived (less than 1 year) protection (35). Serum IgA appears within the first 2 weeks after illness and is indetectable 6 to 12 months later (36,37). It does not protect against infection but may lessen the severity of the disease (38). Fecal IgM, IgG, and IgA are detected by day 7 to 9 after the illness begins and gradually decline thereafter (39). Fecal IgA may limit the duration of diarrhea, but its role in resistance to reinfection is uncertain (40).

The role of the cellular immune response in recovery from and prevention of infection with rotavirus has not been evaluated extensively. In one study, the lymphoproliferative response to rotavirus antigens in vitro of lymphocytes from elderly and immunosuppressed adults was significantly lower than that of lymphocytes from healthy adults; however, acute natural infection in elderly persons, and in one adult organ transplant recipient, elicited good lymphoproliferative and antibody responses (41). In an animal model of rotaviral infection, neonatal T cell–deficient (athymic) mice developed self-limited infection similar to that in immunocompetent control animals, but they did not produce serum or intestinal antibodies, suggesting that in mice recovery from rotaviral infection is mediated by nonimmune mechanisms or by macrophages rather than by functional T lymphocytes or antibodies (42).

Clinical Manifestations

Symptomatic rotaviral infection typically begins suddenly, after a 1- to 2-day incubation period, with mild fever, vomiting, and then diarrhea, which usually lasts 4 to 5 days. Susceptibility to disease depends on age. In neonates infection often is asymptomatic, and in infants and children the likelihood of disease increases with age (43,44). In one study, fecal shedding of rotavirus was associated with diarrhea in 29% of neonates, 50% of infants aged 1 to 6 months, and 74% of 7- to 24-month-old children (43). Rotaviral infections are more serious before age 2 years, and more likely to cause moderate to severe dehydration than diarrhea caused by other infectious agents. Infection with rotavirus in adults often is asymptomatic, but it can result in disease, and in elders infection commonly causes severe, potentially fatal gastroenteritis (44–47).

Laboratory Diagnosis

Methods useful for diagnosis of infection with Colorado tick fever virus and with rotavirus are discussed.

Colorado Tick Fever Virus. Persons with Colorado tick fever frequently are leukopenic early in the illness, which may be useful diagnostically. However, a specific diagnosis requires the recovery of the virus from blood clot or washed erythrocytes by inoculating suckling mice or cell cultures or by demonstrating viral antigens in erythrocytes by immunofluorescence (48). Alternatively, specific IgM may be detected in serum, but usually it appears late in the illness. Culture of Colorado tick fever virus generally is not performed in the clinical virology laboratory, and reagents for the direct immunofluorescent and antibody tests are not commercially available; therefore, specimens must be shipped to special reference laboratories for testing.

Rotavirus. To diagnose infection with rotavirus, a fresh, undiluted stool sample should be collected early in the illness. If ELISA is used for virus detection, a rectal swab may be submitted, but stool is the best sample.

Electron microscopy is the reference method for detection of rotaviruses, and if an electron microscope is readily available this method is cost effective and provides rapid results. However, for laboratories without access to an electron microscope, other methods of detection must be used.

Rotavirus is very fastidious and, therefore, difficult to cultivate in the clinical virology laboratory. To isolate the virus from stool, the sample is pretreated with trypsin and inoculated into roller tube cultures of primary African green monkey kidney cells or MA-104 cells. Cultures are maintained in medium containing trypsin at 37° C for a minimum of 10 days and observed daily (49). When cytopathic effect is apparent cultures are frozen for further analysis. Drawbacks to culture are the long turn-around time, the need for supplemental tests, and the low sensitivity (about half of rotavirus-positive samples are detected).

In the clinical laboratory most rotaviral infections are diagnosed by an antigen detection test, usually ELISA (commercially available). ELISA for detection of group A rotaviruses provides results within 3 to 4 hours of receiving the specimen. In general, the sensitivities and specificities of these assays range from 88 to 100% and 84 to 98%, respectively (50–54). One problem identified in early evaluations of these kits was that ELISA produced false-positive results with specimens from neonates, a problem that can be eliminated in most cases by heat treatment of positive samples (55–57). Recently, a modified ELISA technique with a turn-around time of approximately 30 minutes, became commercially available. In preliminary evaluations its sensitivity ranged from 89 to 100% and its specificity from 90 to 99%; its major drawback is cost if large numbers of samples are tested (58–60).

Latex agglutination kits (commercially available) for detection of rotavirus antigens in stool specimens are easy to perform and provide results in less than 30 minutes. In general, the specificities of latex agglutination and ELISA are equivalent, but the sensitivity of latex agglutination is lower—from 61 to 86% (61–65).

Research techniques not used routinely in the clinical laboratory to detect rotaviruses include immune adherence hemagglutination, reverse passive hemagglutination, polyacrylamide gel electrophoresis, radioimmunofocusing, and nucleic acid hybridization (66–72).

Treatment and Prevention

No specific antiviral agents effective against Colorado tick fever virus or rotavirus are available currently. Therapy for both of these illnesses is supportive.

Because rotaviral gastroenteritis is a significant cause of infant morbidity and mortality in many areas of the world, much effort has been directed toward preventing rotaviral infection via active immunization. Orally administered animal strains of rotavirus have been evaluated as vaccine candidates because cross-protection occurs among animals infected with homotypic and heterotypic animal rotaviruses and with human rotaviruses (73,74). The Nebraska calf diarrhea virus strain of bovine rotavirus (designated RIT 4237) and the rhesus monkey rotavirus strain RRV-1 (designated MMU 18006), both of which are attenuated by passaging many times in cell culture, have been used most extensively in field trials. In several clinical trials in developing countries the RIT 4237 vaccine failed to protect against rotaviral disease; therefore, clinical studies with this vaccine are no longer being conducted (75–77). Results of clinical trials evaluating the MMU 18006 vaccine have varied. In two studies no significant differences in the development of gastroenteritis between vaccine and control groups occurred, but in another study vaccinated infants had significantly fewer episodes of rotaviral diarrhea (76–80).

Other rotavirus vaccines have been proposed. The WC3 vaccine, an attenuated bovine rotavirus vaccine, appears to provide protection against moderate to severe rotaviral diarrhea; however, few clinical trials have been conducted. Reassortant rotavirus vaccines derived from rhesus rotavirus and containing gene segments that code for neutralization proteins of serotypes 1, 2, or 4 or a combination of serotypes have been administered in human trials to determine safety and immunogenicity, but they have not yet been evaluated for protection against disease (81).

REFERENCES

1. Rosen L, et al: An outbreak of infection with a type 1 reovirus among children in an institution. Am J Hyg, 71:266, 1960.
2. Rosen L: Reovirus infection in human volunteers. Am J Hyg, 77:29, 1963.
3. Glaser JH, and Morecki R: Reovirus type 3 and neonatal cholestasis. Semin Liver Dis, 7:100, 1987.
4. Chumakov MP, et al: Report on the isolation from Ixodes persulcatus ticks and from patients in Western Siberia of a virus differing from the agent of tick-borne encephalitis. Acta Virol, 7:82, 1963.
5. Saluzzo JF: Etude ecologique du virus Orungo en Afrique Centrale. Ann Virol (Paris), 134:327, 1983.
6. Familusi JB, et al: Virus isolates from children with febrile convulsions in Nigeria. Clin Pediatr (Phila), 11:272, 1972.
7. Florio L, Steward MO, and Mugrage ER: The experimental transmission of Colorado tick fever. J Exp Med, 80:165, 1944.
8. Bishop RF, Davidson GP, Holmes IH, and Ruck BJ: Virus particles in epithelial cells of duodenal mucosa from children with acute gastroenteritis. Lancet, ii:1281, 1973.
9. Flewett TH, Bryden AS, and Davies H: Virus particles in gastroenteritis. Lancet, ii:1497, 1973.
10. Tan GS, et al: Virus in faecal extracts from children with gastroenteritis. Lancet, i:1109, 1974.
11. Middleton PJ, et al: Orbivirus acute gastroenteritis of infancy. Lancet, i:1241, 1974.
12. Cruickshank JG, Axton JHM, and Webster OF: Viruses in gastroenteritis. Lancet, i:1353, 1974.
13. Holmes IH, et al: Orbiviruses and gastroenteritis. Lancet, ii:658, 1974.
14. Kapikian AZ, et al: Reovirus-like agent in stools: Association with infantile diarrhea and development of serologic tests. Science, 185:1049, 1974.
15. Flewett TH, et al: Relation between viruses from acute gastroenteritis of children and newborn calves. Lancet, ii:61, 1974.
16. Flores J, et al: Genetic relatedness among human rotaviruses as determined by RNA hybridization. Infect Immun, 37:648, 1982.
17. Chanock SJ, Wenske EA, and Fields BN: Human rotaviruses and genome RNA. J Infect Dis, 148:49, 1983.
18. Bridger JC, Pedley S, and McCrae MA: Group C rotaviruses in humans. J Clin Microbiol, 23:760, 1986.
19. Dai G-Z, et al: First report of an epidemic of diarrhoea in human neonates involving the new rotavirus and biological characteristics of the epidemic virus strain (KMB/R85). J Med Virol, 22:365, 1987.
20. Dimitrov DH, et al: Detection of antigenically distinct rotaviruses from infants. Infect Immun, 41:523, 1983.
21. Espejo RT, Puerto F, Soler C, and Gonzalez N: Characterization of human pararotavirus. Infect Immun, 44:112, 1984.
22. Gerna G, Passarani N, Sarasini A, and Battaglia M: Characterization of serotypes of human rotavirus strains by solid-phase immune electron microscopy. J Infect Dis, 152:1143, 1985.
23. Nicolas JC, et al: Isolation of an human pararotavirus. Virology, 124:181, 1983.
24. Hung T, et al: Rotavirus-like agent in adult nonbacterial diarrhea in China. Lancet, ii:1078, 1983.
25. Rodger SM, Bishop RF, and Holmes IH: Detection of a rotavirus-like agent associated with diarrhea in infants. J Clin Microbiol, 16:724, 1982.
26. Eiden J, et al: Genetic and antigenic relatedness of human and animal strains of antigenically distinct rotaviruses. J Infect Dis, 154:972, 1986.
27. Bohl EH, et al: Porcine pararotaviruses: Detection, differentiation from rotavirus, and pathogenesis in gnotobiotic pigs. J Clin Microbiol, 15:312, 1982.
28. Pedley S, Bridger JC, Brown JF, and McCrae MA: Molecular characterization of rotaviruses with distinct group antigens. J Gen Virol, 64:2093, 1983.
29. Pedley S, Bridger JC, Chasey D, and McCrae MA: Definition of two new groups of atypical rotaviruses. J Gen Virol, 67:131, 1986.
30. Hung T, et al: Waterborne outbreak of rotavirus diarrhoea in adults in China caused by a novel rotavirus. Lancet, i:1139, 1984.

31. Chen GM, Hung T, Bridger JC, and McCrae MA: Chinese adult rotavirus is a group B rotavirus. Lancet, *ii*:1123, 1985.
32. Matsumo S, Hasegawa A, Mukoyama A, and Inouye S: A candidate for a new serotype of human rotavirus. J Virol, *54*:623, 1985.
33. Clark HF, et al: Rotavirus isolate W161 representing a presumptive new human serotype. J Clin Microbiol, *25*:1757, 1987.
34. Hieber JP, et al: Comparison of human rotavirus disease in tropical and temperate settings. Am J Dis Child, *132*:853, 1978.
35. Chiba S, et al: Protective effect of naturally acquired homotypic and heterotypic rotavirus antibodies. Lancet, *ii*:417, 1986.
36. Hjelt K, et al: Antibody response in serum and intestine in children up to six months after a naturally acquired rotavirus gastroenteritis. J Pediatr Gastroenterol Nutr, *5*:74, 1986.
37. Hjelt K, et al: Intestinal and serum immune response to a naturally acquired rotavirus gastroenteritis in children. J Pediatr Gastroenterol Nutr, *4*:60, 1986.
38. Hjelt K, et al: Protective effect of pre-existing rotavirus-specific immunoglobulin A against naturally acquired rotavirus infection in children. J Med Virol, *21*:39, 1987.
39. Sonza S, and Holmes IH: Coproantibody response to rotavirus infection. Med J Aust, *2*:496, 1980.
40. Stals F, Walther FJ, and Bruggeman CA: Faecal and pharyngeal shedding of rotavirus and rotavirus IgA in children with diarrhea. J Med Virol, *14*:333, 1984.
41. Totterdell BM, et al: Systemic lymphoproliferative responses to rotavirus. J Med Virol, *25*:37, 1988.
42. Eiden J, Lederman HM, Vonderfecht S, and Yolken R: T cell–deficient mice display normal recovery from experimental rotavirus infection. J Virol, *58*:706, 1986.
43. Champsaur H, et al: Rotavirus carriage, asymptomatic infection, and disease in the first years of life. I. Virus shedding. J Infect Dis, *149*:667, 1984.
44. Champsaur H, et al: Rotavirus carriage, asymptomatic infection, and disease in the first two years of life. II. Serological response. J Infect Dis, *149*:675, 1984.
45. Wenman WM, et al: Rotavirus infection in adults: Result of a prospective family study. N Engl J Med, *301*:303, 1979.
46. Echeverria P, et al: Rotavirus as a cause of severe gastroenteritis in adults. J Clin Microbiol, *18*:663, 1983.
47. Marrie TJ, et al: Rotavirus infection in a geriatric population. Arch Intern Med, *142*:313, 1982.
48. Emmons RW, and Lennett EH: Immunofluorescent staining in the laboratory diagnosis of Colorado tick fever. J Lab Clin Med, *68*:923, 1966.
49. Kutsuzawa T, et al: Isolation of human rotavirus subgroups 1 and 2 in cell culture. J Clin Microbiol, *16*:727, 1982.
50. Yolken RH, and Leister FJ: Evaluation of enzyme immunoassays for the detection of human rotavirus. J Infect Dis, *144*:379, 1981.
51. Cheung EY, Hnatko SI, Gunning H, and Wilson J: Comparison of Rotazyme and direct electron microscopy for detection of rotavirus in human stools. J Clin Microbiol, *16*:562, 1982.
52. Rubenstein AS, and Miller MF: Comparison of an enzyme immunoassay with electron microscopic procedures for detecting rotavirus. J Clin Microbiol, *15*:938, 1982.
53. Christensen ML: Human viral gastroenteritis. Clin Microbiol Rev, *2*:51, 1989.
54. Chernesky M, Castriciano S, Mahony J, and DeLong D: Examination of the Rotazyme II enzyme immunoassay for the diagnosis of rotavirus gastroenteritis. J Clin Microbiol, *22*:462, 1985.
55. Krause PJ, et al: Unreliability of Rotazyme ELISA test in neonates. J Pediatr, *103*:259, 1983.
56. Pai CH, and Mayock D: Rotazyme test in neonates. J Pediatr, *106*:343, 1985.
57. Rand KH, Houck HJ, and Swingle HM: Rotazyme assay in neonates with diarrhea. Am J Clin Pathol, *84*:748, 1985.
58. Marchlewicz B, Spiewak M, and Lampinen J: Evaluation of Abbott TESTPACK ROTAVIRUS with clinical specimens. J Clin Microbiol, *26*:2456, 1988.
59. Chernesky M, et al: Ability of TESTPACK ROTAVIRUS enzyme immunoassay to diagnose rotavirus gastroenteritis. J Clin Microbiol, *26*:2459, 1988.
60. Brooks RG, Brown L, and Franklin RB: Comparison of a new rapid test (TestPack Rotavirus) with standard enzyme immunoassay and electron microscopy for the detection of rotavirus in symptomatic hospitalized children. J Clin Microbiol, *27*:775, 1989.
61. Cevenini R, et al: Evaluation of a new latex agglutination test for detecting human rotavirus in faeces. J Infect, *7*:130, 1983.
62. Sambourg MA, et al: Direct appraisal of latex agglutination testing, a convenient alternative to enzyme immunoassay for the detection of rotavirus in childhood gastroenteritis, by comparison of two enzyme immunoassays and two latex tests. J Clin Microbiol, *21*:622, 1985.
63. Brandt CD, et al: Evaluation of a latex test for rotavirus detection. J Clin Microbiol, *25*:1800, 1987.
64. Pai CH, Shahrabadi MS, and Ince B: Rapid diagnosis of rotavirus gastroenteritis by a commercial latex agglutination test. J Clin Microbiol, *22*:846, 1985.
65. Shinozaki T, et al: Comparison of five methods for detecting human rotavirus in stool specimens. Eur J Pediatr, *144*:513, 1986.
66. Nagayoski SH, et al: Changes of the rotavirus concentration in faeces during the course of acute gastroenteritis as determined by the immune adherence hemagglutination test. Eur J Pediatr, *134*:99, 1980.
67. Sanekata T, and Okada H: Human rotavirus detection by agglutination of antibody-coated erythrocytes. J Clin Microbiol, *17*:1141, 1983.
68. Moosai RB, et al: Detection of rotavirus by a latex agglutination test Rotalex: Comparison with electron microscopy, immunofluorescence, polyacrylamide gel electrophoresis, and enzyme-linked immunosorbent assay. J Clin Pathol, *38*:694, 1985.
69. Liu S, Birch C, Coulepis A, and Gust I: Radioimmunofocus assay for detection and quantitation of human rotavirus. J Clin Microbiol, *20*:347, 1984.
70. Dimitrov DH, Graham DY, and Estes MK: Detection of rotaviruses by nucleic acid hybridization with cloned DNA of simian rotavirus SA11 genes. J Infect Dis, *152*:293, 1985.
71. Eiden J, Sato S, and Yolken R: Specificity of dot hybridization assay in the presence of rRNA for detection of rotaviruses in clinical specimens. J Clin Microbiol, *25*:1809, 1987.
72. Lin M, et al: Diagnosis of rotavirus infection with cloned cDNA copies of viral genome segments. J Virol, *55*:509, 1985.
73. Zissis G, et al: Protection studies in colostrum-deprived piglets of a bovine rotavirus vaccine candidate using human rotavirus strains for challenge. J Infect Dis, *148*:1061, 1983.
74. Wyatt RG, et al: Rotaviral immunity in gnotobiotic calves: Heterologous resistance to human virus induced by bovine virus. Science, *203*:548, 1979.
75. DeMol P, et al: Failure of live, attenuated oral rotavirus vaccine. Lancet, *ii*:108, 1986.

76. Hanlon P, et al: Trial of an attenuated bovine rotavirus vaccine (RIT 4237) in Gambian infants. Lancet, i:1342, 1986.
77. Albert MJ: Failure of live, oral vaccine in developing countries. J Infect Dis, 155:1350, 1987.
78. Wright PF, et al: Candidate rotavirus vaccine (rhesus rotavirus strain) in children: An evaluation. Pediatrics, 80:473, 1987.
79. Flores J, et al: Protection against severe rotavirus diarrhea by rhesus rotavirus vaccine in Venezuelan infants. Lancet, i: 882, 1987.
80. Rennels MB, et al: Preliminary evaluation of rhesus rotavirus vaccine strain MMU 18006 in young children. Pediatr Infect Dis J, 5:587, 1986.
81. Perez-Schael I, et al: Clinical studies of a quadrivalent rotavirus vaccine in Venezuelan infants. J Clin Microbiol, 28:553, 1990.

Chapter 15

CALICIVIRUSES

Caliciviruses were first recognized in humans in 1976, by electron microscopic examination of stool of infants with diarrhea (1). Initially considered picornaviruses, they are now classified in a separate family, Caliciviridae.

STRUCTURE

Caliciviruses, 30 to 35 nm in diameter, have a single-stranded RNA genome coding for one known structural protein. By electron microscopy virions have a scalloped border with 32 cup-shaped depressions on their surface (Fig. 15–1), giving a spiky appearance to their periphery and a Star of David configuration at certain rotations.

EPIDEMIOLOGY

Infections with caliciviruses occur worldwide throughout the year but peak in winter. Most individuals are infected with caliciviruses at an early age. Antibodies, generally acquired between age 6 and 24 months, are present in about 90% of older children and adults. Caliciviruses are responsible for about 1 to 6% of cases of gastroenteritis in hospitalized patients and have caused outbreaks of diarrhea in infants and young children, school children, and elders (2–5).

CLINICAL MANIFESTATIONS

Disease caused by caliciviruses is indistinguishable from rotaviral illness: mild, self-limited diarrhea and low-grade fever, with or without vomiting, lasting 1 to 3 days.

LABORATORY DIAGNOSIS

Infections with caliciviruses are diagnosed by electron microscopic examination of a diarrheic stool sample.

TREATMENT

No available antiviral agent is effective against the caliciviruses. Supportive treatment includes maintaining fluid and electrolyte balance.

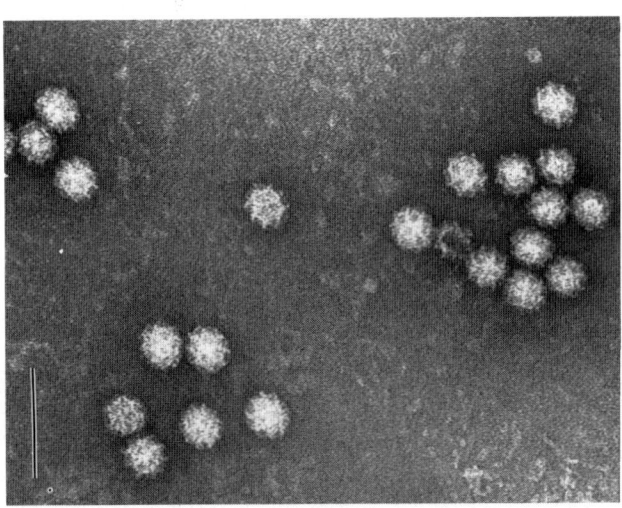

Fig. 15–1. Electron photomicrograph of calicivirus particles in a stool sample (X167,980). (Courtesy of the Division of Viral and Rickettsial Diseases, Centers for Disease Control, Atlanta, GA.)

REFERENCES

1. Madeley CR, and Cosgrove BP: Caliciviruses in man. Lancet, i:199, 1976.
2. McSwiggan DA, Cubitt D, and Moore W: Calicivirus associated with winter vomiting disease. Lancet, i:1215, 1978.
3. Cubitt WD, and McSwiggan DA: Calicivirus gastroenteritis in North West London. Lancet, ii:975, 1981.
4. Cubitt WD, Pead PJ, and Saeed AA: A new serotype of calicivirus associated with an outbreak of gastroenteritis in a residential home for the elderly. J Clin Pathol, 34:924, 1981.
5. Grohmann G, et al: Outbreak of human calicivirus gastroenteritis in a day-care center in Sydney, Australia. J Clin Microbiol, 29:544, 1991.

Chapter 16

RHABDOVIRUSES

More than 100 rhabdoviruses infect and cause disease in vertebrates and invertebrates, including many plants. In general, rhabdoviruses have a wide host range, although many have been adapted to grow in specific hosts. In this chapter, an overview of the classification, structure, and replication of rhabdoviruses is presented, vesiculoviruses are reviewed briefly, and rabies virus is discussed in detail.

CLASSIFICATION

Rhabdoviruses are classified in the family Rhabdoviridae, which contains two named genera: Vesiculovirus and Lyssavirus, designated on the basis of distinct antigenic and biologic characteristics, and two proposed but currently unnamed genera: one for bovine ephemeral fever–like viruses and one for the many ungrouped rhabdoviruses of mammals, birds, fish, arthropods, and plants. Vesiculoviruses commonly infect wild and domestic animals and occasionally are transmitted to humans. The lyssaviruses include rabies virus and five rabies-related viruses (Table 16–1), of which two, Duvenhage and Mokola, infect humans.

STRUCTURE AND REPLICATION

Bullet-shaped rhabdovirus virions (Fig. 16–1), 70 to 85 nm in diameter and 130 to 180 nm long, consist of a helical nucleocapsid surrounded by a bilayered lipid envelope derived primarily from host cell membranes (1). The negative-sense, single-stranded RNA genome of molecular weight 4.6 million codes for four or five major proteins. Rhabdoviruses initiate infection by attaching to a host cell receptor, after which virions penetrate into the cell and are uncoated, releasing their genome into the cytoplasm, where transcription and translation occur. Nucleocapsid RNA and proteins are assembled in the cytoplasm, and virions are released from the cell by budding upon plasma or intracytoplasmic membranes.

VESICULOVIRUS

Seven vesiculoviruses infect humans (Table 16–2) (2). Vesicular stomatitis virus (VSV)-New Jersey and VSV-Indiana, which are responsible for most cases of clinically apparent disease, are discussed.

Epidemiology

Vesicular stomatitis viruses are transmitted among wild and domestic animals in the respective geographic areas of endemicity via insect vectors. In the United States, most human infections due to VSV result from direct contact with oral secretions of infected animals, during which virions enter through skin abrasions or directly through the oral mucosa (3–5). Disease occurs during summer and fall epidemics of vesicular stomatitis in horses and cattle, principally in states bordering the Gulf of Mexico, in the Upper Mississippi River valley, and in the Rocky Mountains. The other five vesiculoviruses probably are transmitted similarly.

Clinical Manifestations

In horses and cattle infection caused by vesicular stomatitis virus is characterized by a vesicular eruption of the mouth, tongue, and teats, and in humans by an influenza-like illness (fever, chills, malaise, myalgias, nausea, vomiting, and pharyngitis) occasionally accompanied by oral vesicular lesions. Chandipura virus has been recovered from the blood of three persons with a febrile illness, and Piry virus has been associated with influenza-like symptoms (5–7). Serologic studies suggest that infection with the other vesiculoviruses is common in their respective endemic areas, but the associated clinical manifestations are unknown.

Laboratory Diagnosis

Infections caused by vesiculoviruses are diagnosed by demonstrating seroconversion. Complement-fixing and neutralizing antibodies are detected 10 to 14 days after the onset of symptoms. The titer of complement-fixing antibodies falls in several months, but neutralizing antibodies persist for about 1 year. These serologic tests, however, are performed only in specialized research laboratories. The virus can be recovered from vesicular lesions of animals, but it has not been isolated from vesicles of humans.

Treatment

Human infections caused by vesiculoviruses are self-limited and require only symptomatic therapy.

LYSSAVIRUS

Rabies Virus

Rabies, described in Middle Eastern civilizations before 2300 B.C., is one of the oldest known human diseases (8). It appears to have been introduced to North and South America by dogs accompanying conquistadors in the early 1800s (8). The disease was transmitted in the laboratory by inoculating a normal dog with saliva from a rabid dog in 1809, establishing its infectious nature (9). In 1885

Table 16-1. Rabies-related Viruses

Virus	Source in Nature
Lagos bat	Bats
Mokola	Shrews, humans, dogs, cats
Duvenhage	Humans, bats
Obodhiang	Mosquitoes
Kotonkan	Mosquitoes

Table 16-2. Vesiculoviruses That May Infect Humans

Virus	Areas of Endemicity
Vesicular stomatitis virus	
VSV-New Jersey	Southeastern United States, Central America, northern South America
VSV-Indiana	Central America, northern South America
VSV-Alagoas	Colombia, Brazil
Calchaqui	Argentina
Piry	Brazil
Chandipura	India
Isfahan	Iran

Pasteur vaccinated a boy who was bitten by a rabid dog with an extract of serially passaged fixed virus, and the boy survived (10). The viral etiology of rabies was demonstrated in 1903, and that same year Negri described intracytoplasmic inclusions (now called Negri bodies) in neural tissue infected with the virus (11,12).

Structure

Enveloped rabies virions, 180 by 75 nm, enclose a nucleocapsid, 50 by 165 nm, consisting of 30 to 35 coils. Five viral proteins have been identified. The primary structural component of the surface spikes is a glycoprotein (G) that induces specific neutralizing antibodies and is the postulated site for attachment of rabies virus to the host cell membrane, possibly by interacting with host acetylcholine receptors. The nucleocapsid (N) protein contains the group-specific antigen common to all lyssaviruses, the M protein is associated with the lipoprotein viral envelope, the NS(P) protein is associated with the nucleocapsid, and the viral polymerase (large [L]) is involved in replication.

Epidemiology

Rabies is predominantly a disease of wild and domestic animals, among which susceptibility to infection with the

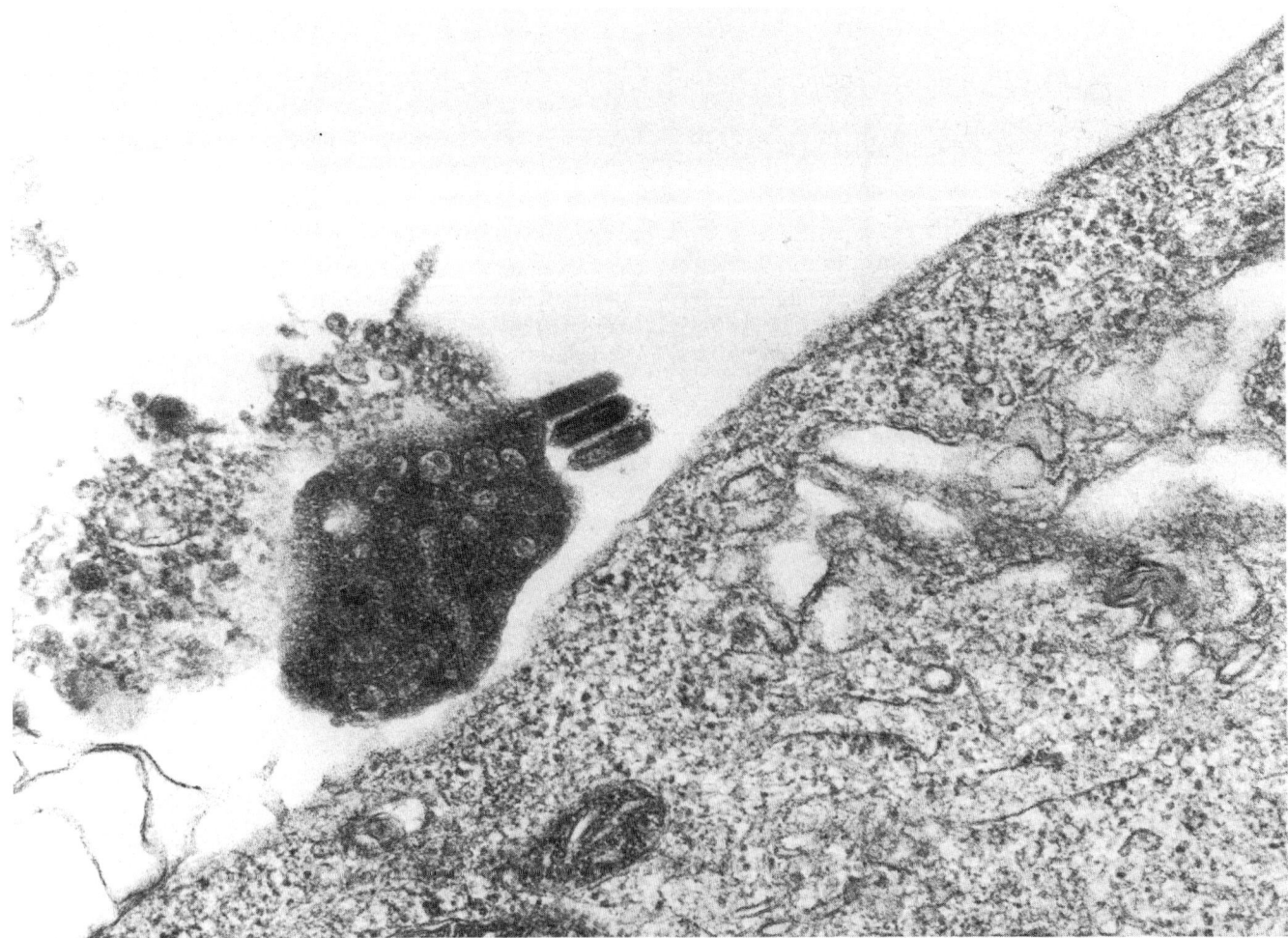

Fig. 16-1. Electron micrograph of rabies virus in BHK-21 cells (×82,900). (Courtesy of C.E. Rupprecht, J. Weibel, and G. Maul, The Wistar Institute, Philadelphia, PA.)

Table 16–3. Principal Wildlife Vectors of Rabies

Location	Vector
Africa	Mongoose, jackal
Europe	Fox
Arctic, sub-Arctic	Fox
Western Asia	Wolf
Latin America	Vampire bat
United States	Striped skunk, raccoon, Insectivorous bat

virus varies: foxes, coyotes, jackals, and wolves are highly susceptible; dogs, cats, raccoons, and skunks are moderately susceptible; and opossums are among the least susceptible. Most cases of rabies in humans result from direct or indirect exposure to a rabid animal. Dogs account for at least 90% of reported cases in areas where domestic rabies has not been controlled and for fewer than 5% where domestic rabies is well controlled, such as the United States, Canada, and many western European countries. Domestic animals other than dogs (primarily cats and cattle) are responsible for 5 to 10% of reported animal rabies worldwide. The principal wildlife vectors of rabies vary in different areas of the world (Table 16–3). Human-to-human transmission of rabies rarely has been documented in recipients of corneal transplants, and occasionally no source of infection is found (13–17).

Human rabies has been reported on all continents except Australia and the Antarctic, and the largest numbers of cases occur in countries where domestic animal rabies is not adequately controlled. In countries where rabies is endemic the estimated annual rates of human disease vary, depending on control of domestic animal rabies, from less than 0.01 per million population per year in the United States to nearly 30 per million in India (18). About 60 countries, including the United Kingdom, Japan, Finland, Sweden, Norway, Portugal, many Caribbean Islands, and most of Pacific Oceania reportedly are free of rabies, owing to geographic isolation, animal control programs, and quarantine regulations (2,19).

In the United States the prevalence of rabies in domestic animals and in humans (Fig. 16–2) has decreased dramatically since the 1950s, when canine vaccination and programs on stray-dog control were introduced. Each year during the 1950s, 4 to 20 persons died of rabies, which was acquired via contact with infected native animals; whereas between 1980 and 1988, no more than 3 persons died of rabies each year, and 73% of cases were acquired by contact with animals outside the United States (20). Moreover, as the prevalence of human rabies in the United States has decreased, the proportion of affected persons who have no known exposure to rabid animals has increased. Between 1960 and 1979 no source of infection could be identified in 6 of 38 (16%) cases, and since 1980 no source was identified in 6 of 10 (60%) cases (21–26).

Pathogenesis and Pathology

Rabies virus initially replicates in muscle tissue at the wound site and then enters an eclipse phase during which neither viral antigens nor the virus can be identified in any organ (27). After a lengthy dormancy at the bite site, virions travel in the peripheral nerves to the spinal ganglia and then through the spinal cord to the brain, where they replicate (27). From the brain, virions spread centrifugally down efferent nerves to many tissues and organs, including the salivary glands and the cornea.

The histologic findings of human rabies, which are limited to the central nervous system, include the pathognomonic intracytoplasmic inclusions termed Negri bodies (Fig. 16–3), minimal perivascular inflammation, some neuronophagia, and minimal neuronal necrosis.

Clinical Manifestations

Exposure to rabies virus is followed by an incubation period that ranges from 4 days to 9 years (20 to 90 days is usual) and often is shorter after a bite on the head than on an extremity (28,29). Not all persons bitten by rabid animals develop rabies. Factors that influence the out-

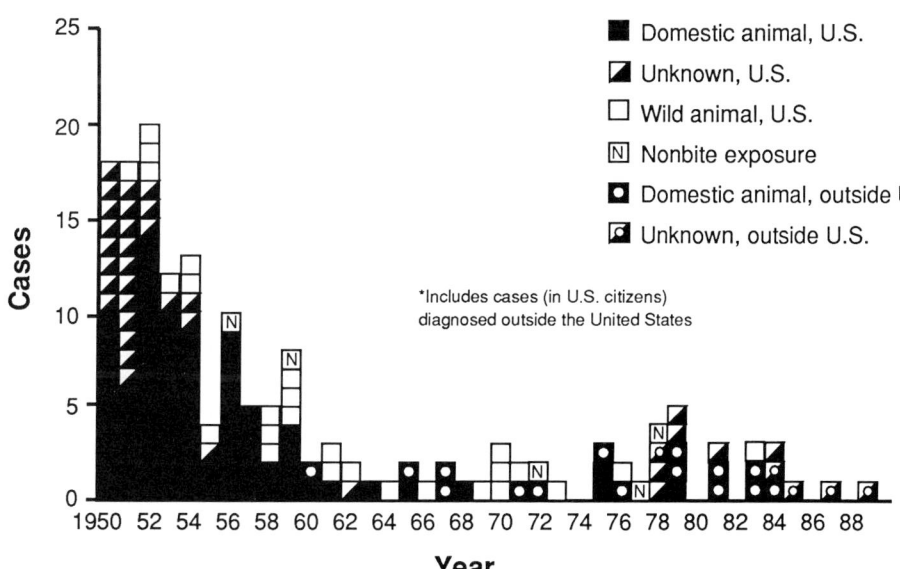

Fig. 16–2. Cases of human rabies in the United States by year and exposure category, including cases in U. S. citizens diagnosed outside the United States, 1950–1988. (From Centers for Disease Control: Rabies surveillance, United States, 1988. MMWR, *38*(SS-1):1, 1989.)

come of an exposure include the location and the severity of the bite, the animal involved, genetic differences in individuals bitten, and possibly the virulence of the virus (30–33).

Rabies begins with a 2- to 10-day prodrome of nonspecific symptoms: malaise, fatigue, fever, headache, anorexia, cough, chills, sore throat, abdominal pain, nausea, vomiting, or diarrhea, accompanied by apprehension, anxiety, agitation, nervousness, insomnia, or depression. In about 50% of cases pain or paresthesia is felt at the site of inoculation. The prodrome merges with the acute neurologic period, characterized by episodes of hyperactivity, disorientation, hallucinations, or bizarre behavior. Other symptoms and signs include fever, muscle fasciculations, hyperventilation, hypersalivation, seizures, nuchal rigidity, and rarely priapism. Moreover, attempts at drinking result in severe spasms of the pharynx and larynx. Paralysis develops, and within 4 to 10 days the patient becomes confused, disoriented, stuporous, and finally comatose. Untreated persons experience respiratory arrest shortly thereafter, whereas survival may be prolonged weeks by respiratory assistance. The mortality rate approaches 100%. Only three persons presumed to have rabies have survived: each received either post- or pre-exposure prophylaxis before symptoms began (34–36).

Rabies-Related Viruses

The rabies-related viruses occur naturally only in sub-Saharan Africa, and very little is known about their epidemiology and clinical significance. Duvenhage virus was recovered from a person in South Africa with fatal rabies-like encephalitis, and Mokola was associated with a case of fatal paralytic encephalitis (37,38).

Laboratory Diagnosis

Specimens useful for diagnosing rabies include cerebrospinal fluid (CSF), biopsy specimens of brain and skin, corneal impression smears, saliva, urine, tracheal secretions, and serum. None of the available tests, however, can diagnose rabies before symptoms begin. Examination of the CSF is abnormal in about two thirds of persons during the first week of illness and in 90% thereafter. The CSF white blood cell count generally is 75 to 300/µl; the protein content is normal early but elevated (100 to 200 mg/dl) in the later stages of illness.

Detection of rabies viral antigens, Negri bodies, rabies virus, or neutralizing antibodies is diagnostic of disease; however, none of these tests is positive in all cases, so evaluation of serial specimens may be necessary. Direct detection of rabies viral antigens in brain or skin biopsy or corneal impression smears by immunofluorescent antibody staining provides rapid diagnosis, but antigens may not be detectable after neutralizing antibodies develop (39,40). When using direct immunofluorescence the most reliable and reproducible results are obtained by examining a skin biopsy of the neck: a 6- to 8-mm full-thickness wedge or punch biopsy specimen containing as many hair follicles as possible should be collected from the posterior neck above the hair line, placed fresh in a small vial with a small piece of moist gauze, frozen at −70° C, and shipped to a reference laboratory familiar with the technique. Negri bodies: eosinophilic, 2- to 10-µm diameter, round to oblong intracytoplasmic inclusions (see Fig. 16–3), most commonly are found in the hippocampus, the horn of Ammon, and Purkinje cells of the cerebellum, and less often in the motor area of the cerebral cortex or spinal cord, but they are absent in 20 to 30% of cases.

In about 60% of cases rabies virus may be isolated intermittently from saliva as early as 2 days after the onset of symptoms; however, the viral titer declines when neutralizing antibodies appear. The virus also may be recovered from brain tissue, CSF, urine sediment, and tracheal secretions. Postmortem, tissue from the thalamus, midbrain, and upper spinal cord are the preferred specimens for virus isolation. Rabies viral culture, however, is available only in specialized reference laboratories.

Specific neutralizing antibodies, detected by the rapid fluorescent focus inhibition test, appear in the serum early in the second week after the onset of symptoms and usually are detected in the CSF 4 to 7 days later. Antibody titers in CSF may be useful in differentiating antibodies induced by vaccination from those induced by infection, because a high titer in CSF (2 to 25% of that in serum) occurs only with clinical disease.

Treatment

No antiviral agent effective against rabies virus is available. Treatment includes supportive care, especially respiratory and cardiovascular support. Patients are placed in isolation to prevent secondary bacterial infection and exposure of the hospital staff to rabies virus, which may be present in the saliva, tears, urine, other body fluids, and tissues of an infected person. Staff should wear face masks, gloves, and gowns; and if a staff member sustains a bite or mucous membrane contamination with an infected patient's body fluids, post- or pre-exposure rabies prophylaxis should be administered (described in the next section).

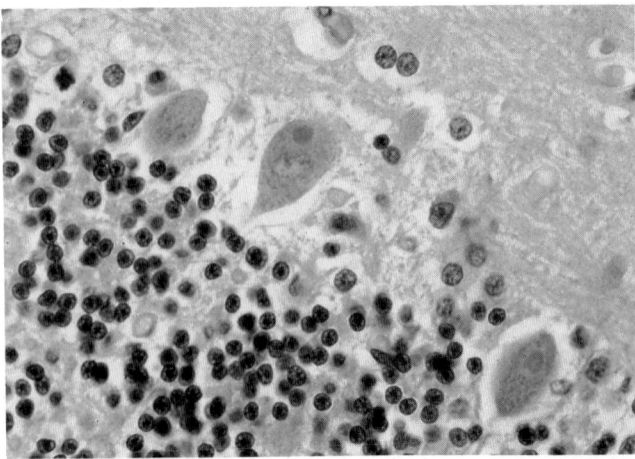

Fig. 16–3. Negri body in cytoplasm of a Purkinje cell in the cerebellum of a person who died of rabies (hematoxylin and eosin, ×400).

Table 16-4. Recommendations for Rabies Prophylaxis, Centers for Disease Control, 1991

Animal Vector	Evaluation and Disposition of Animal	Recommendations
Dogs, cats	Healthy, available for 10-day observation	No prophylaxis unless animal develops symptoms of rabies*
	Rabid or suspected rabid	Vaccinate immediately
	Unknown (escaped)	Consult public health officials
Skunks, raccoons, bats, foxes, most other carnivores; woodchucks	Considered rabid unless geographic area is known to be free of rabies or until animal is proven negative by laboratory tests†	Vaccinate immediately
Livestock, rodents, rabbits, hares	Consider individually	Consult public health officials; rodent bites almost never require antirabies treatment.

* At the first sign of rabies in the animal, begin treatment with human rabies immune globulin and the rabies vaccine. The animal should be killed and tested.
† The animal should be killed and tested as soon as possible. Holding for observation is not recommended. If the test results for rabies are negative, the vaccine should be discontinued.
(Modified from Centers for Disease Control: Rabies prevention—United States, 1991. MMWR, 40(RR-3):1, 1991.)

Prevention

Control of rabies in animals, especially domestic animals, is key to preventing human rabies. However, if exposure to a rabid animal occurs, human rabies almost always can be prevented by administering appropriate postexposure prophylaxis (Table 16-4) (41).

Bat exposure routinely requires postexposure prophylaxis; but because rodents such as squirrels, hamsters, guinea pigs, gerbils, chipmunks, rats, mice, and rabbits rarely are infected with rabies virus and have not been known to cause human rabies, postexposure prophylaxis following a bite by one of these animals generally is unnecessary. A bite from a cat or dog that is unavailable for quarantine in an area where rabies is present in wild terrestrial animals justifies prophylaxis. Only domestic dogs and cats need to be quarantined and observed. Because the median duration of illness in cats and dogs is 5 and 3 days, respectively, 10 days' observation adequately determines whether the animal had rabies virus in its saliva at the time of the exposure.

Postexposure Prophylaxis. Postexposure prophylaxis includes local wound treatment, passive antibody administration, and vaccination. The wound should be cleaned with nitric acid or a quaternary ammonium compound, and human rabies immune globulin is given in a single dose of 20 IU/kg body weight. Half the calculated dose is infiltrated around the wound site, and the remainder is given intramuscularly in a buttock or thigh.

The duck embryo vaccine used in the United States between 1958 and 1980 had low potency, failing to elicit antibodies after the recommended 23 subcutaneous abdominal injections in 10 to 20% of recipients, and it was associated with a 35% incidence of minor local reactions, a 30% incidence of transient systemic reactions, and a rate of neurologic complications around 1 in 24,000 (42). An inactivated human diploid cell rabies vaccine, administered as five intramuscular doses, started as soon as is reasonable after exposure and on each of days 3, 7, 14, and 28 after the first dose, has been used worldwide since 1974 and in the United States since 1980. In addition, an inactivated adsorbed rabies vaccine (prepared from the Kissling strain of Challenge Virus Standard rabies virus adapted to fetal rhesus lung diploid cell culture), which is considered as efficacious and as safe as the human diploid cell rabies vaccine, currently is available in the United States (41).

Pre-exposure Prophylaxis. Three intramuscular doses of human diploid cell rabies vaccine given on days 0, 7, and 21 or 28, is recommended for persons at high risk of exposure to rabies virus such as veterinarians, veterinary students, some laboratory workers, spelunkers, and persons who for longer than 30 days live in or visit countries where rabies is a constant threat. Persons at continuing risk of exposure should have their antibody titer determined every 2 years, and should receive a booster dose if levels are inadequate. Persons who work with live rabies virus should have their antibody titer determined every 6 months.

REFERENCES

1. Wagner RR: Rhabdovirus biology and infection: An overview. *In* Rhabdoviruses. Edited by RR Wagner. New York, Plenum Press, 1987.
2. Stoeckle M: Vesicular stomatitis virus and related viruses. *In* Principles and Practice of Infectious Diseases. 3rd ed. Edited by GL Mandell, RG Douglas, Jr, and JE Bennett. New York, Churchill Livingstone, 1990.
3. Hanson RP, Rasmussen AF, Brandly CA, and Brown JW: Human infection with the virus of vesicular stomatitis. J Lab Clin Med, 36:754, 1955.
4. Fellowes ON, Dimopoullos GT, and Callis JJ: Isolation of vesicular stomatitis virus from an infected laboratory worker. Am J Vet Res, 16:623, 1955.
5. Fields BN, and Hawkins K: Human infection with the virus of vesicular stomatitis during an epizootic. N Engl J Med, 277:989, 1967.
6. Rodrigues JJ, et al: Isolation of Chandipura virus from the blood in acute encephalopathy syndrome. Indian J Med Res, 77:303, 1983.
7. Karabatsos N (ed): International Catalogue of Arboviruses Including Certain other Viruses of Vertebrates. San Antonio, American Society of Tropical Medicine and Hygiene, 1985.
8. Steele JH: History of rabies. *In* The Natural History of Rabies. Edited by G Baer. New York, Academic Press, 1975.
9. Zinke G: Neue Ansichten der Hundswuth, ihrer Ursachen und Folgen nebst einer sicheren Behandlungsart der von tollen Thieren gebissenen Menschen. Gabler Jena, 16:212, 1908.

10. Pasteur L: Methode pour prevenir la rage apres morsure. C R Acad Sci [D], *101*:765, 1885.
11. Remlinger P: Isolement de virus rabique par filtration. C R Soc Biol, *55*:1433, 1903.
12. Negri A: Beitrag zum Studium der Aetiologie der Tollwuth. Zeit Hyg Infekionskr, *43*:507, 1903.
13. Smith JS, Fishbein DB, Rupprecht CE, and Clark K: Unexplained rabies in three immigrants in the United States. N Engl J Med, *324*:205, 1991.
14. Houff SA, et al: Human-to-human transmission of rabies virus by corneal transplant. N Engl J Med, *300*:603, 1979.
15. Centers for Disease Control: Human-to-human transmission of rabies via a corneal transplant—France. MMWR, *29*:25, 1980.
16. Centers for Disease Control: Human-to-human transmission of rabies via corneal transplant—Thailand. MMWR, *30*:473, 1981.
17. Gode GR, and Bhide NK: Two rabies deaths after corneal grafts from one donor [letter]. Lancet, *ii*:791, 1988.
18. Bogel K, and Motschwiller E: Incidence of rabies and postexposure treatment in developing countries. Bull WHO, *64*:883, 1986.
19. World Health Organization: World Survey of Rabies XXII (for Years 1984/85). Geneva, World Health Organization, 1987.
20. Centers for Disease Control: Rabies surveillance, United States, 1988. MMWR, *38*(SS-1):1, 1989.
21. Centers for Disease Control: Rabies surveillance, United States, 1987. MMWR, *37*(SS-4):1, 1988.
22. Centers for Disease Control: Human rabies—California, 1987. MMWR, *37*:305, 1987.
23. Centers for Disease Control: Human rabies diagnosed 2 months postmortem—Texas. MMWR, *34*:700, 1985.
24. Centers for Disease Control: Human rabies—Pennsylvania. MMWR, *33*:633, 1984.
25. Centers for Disease Control: Human rabies—Texas. MMWR, *33*:469, 1984.
26. Centers for Disease Control: Human rabies—Michigan. MMWR, *32*:159, 1983.
27. Murphy FA: The pathogenesis of rabies virus infection. *In* World's Debt to Pasteur. Edited by H Kaprowski and S Plotkin. New York, Alan R Liss, 1985.
28. Kaplan C, Turner GS, and Warrell DA: Rabies: The Facts. Oxford, Oxford University Press, 1986.
29. Held JR, Tierkel ES, and Steele JH: Rabies in man and animals in the United States, 1946–1965. Public Health Rep, *82*:1009, 1967.
30. Veeraraghavan N: Phenolized vaccine treatment of people exposed to rabies in Southern India. Bull WHO, *10*:789, 1954.
31. Nikolic M: The results of rabies inoculations in man after injuries inflicted by wolves. Trop Dis Bull, *49*:946, 1952.
32. Templeton JW, Holmberg G, Garber T, and Sharp RM: Genetic control of serum neutralizing–antibody response to rabies vaccination and survival after a challenge infection in mice. J Virol, *59*:98, 1986.
33. Sikes RK: Pathogenesis of rabies in wildlife. I. Comparative effect of varying doses of rabies virus inoculated into foxes and skunks. Am J Vet Res, *23*:1041, 1962.
34. Hattwick MAW, et al: Recovery from rabies: A case report. Ann Intern Med, 76:931, 1972.
35. Porras C, et al: Recovery from rabies in man. Ann Intern Med, *85*:44, 1976.
36. Centers for Disease Control: Rabies in a laboratory worker—New York. MMWR, *26*:183, 1977.
37. Meredith CD, Rossouw AP, and Van Praag Koch H: An unusual case of human rabies thought to be of Chiropteran origin. S Afr Med J, *45*:767, 1971.
38. Familusi JB, and Moore DL: Isolation of a rabies-related virus from the cerebrospinal fluid. Afr J Med Sci, *3*:93, 1972.
39. Emmons RW, et al: A case of human rabies with prolonged survival. Intervirology, *1*:60, 1973.
40. Rubin RH, et al: A case of human rabies in Kansas: Epidemiologic, clinical and laboratory consideration. J Infect Dis, *122*:318, 1970.
41. Centers for Disease Control: Rabies prevention—United States, 1991. MMWR, *40*(RR-3):1, 1991.
42. Rubin RH, et al: Adverse reactions to duck embryo rabies vaccine: Range and incidence. Ann Intern Med, *78*:643, 1973.

Chapter 17

TOGAVIRUSES

Togaviruses, which cause infection and disease in animals and humans, are classified in the family Togaviridae on the basis of size, type of genome, and mechanism of transmission. Flaviviruses originally were included in this family but were reclassified when differences in their genome structure and replication cycle were recognized (see Chapter 18). In this chapter an overview of the classification, structure, and replication of togaviruses is presented, and the most commonly encountered members of medical importance—eastern equine encephalitis virus, western equine encephalitis virus, Venezuelan equine encephalitis virus, and rubella virus—are discussed.

CLASSIFICATION

In the Togaviridae family are three genera: Alphavirus, Rubivirus, and Pestivirus. Many alphaviruses infect, and may cause disease in, animals and humans. The most important alphavirus agents of human disease are those associated with encephalitis. Rubella virus, the only member of the genus Rubivirus, causes disease in humans. The pestiviruses cause disease in animals but not in humans and are not discussed here.

STRUCTURE

Togaviruses are enveloped, spherical, 60- to 70-nm diameter particles with a single-stranded, positive-sense RNA genome encapsidated by a single species of protein with an icosahedral configuration. Projecting from and embedded in the lipid envelope are the virus-encoded glycoproteins, designated E1 and E2.

REPLICATION

The replication cycle is initiated by attachment of viral glycoprotein spikes to the host cell receptors. Virions then localize to coated pits and are endocytosed, forming coated vesicles. Subsequent pH changes trigger fusion between virion and vesicle membranes, releasing the nucleocapsid into the cytoplasm and uncoating the genome. Translation, transcription, and replication of the genomic RNA ensue. Virions assemble at the plasma membrane of the infected cell and are released by budding.

ALPHAVIRUSES

The mosquito-transmitted alphaviruses are maintained in nature by passage from mosquito to vertebrate to mosquito. Humans may be infected accidentally but are not involved in further propagation of the virus. Most human infections caused by alphaviruses are asymptomatic and detectable only by seroconversion, though sometimes they produce a transient, febrile illness. Infection with the virus of eastern or western equine encephalitis, or Venezuelan equine encephalitis may result in encephalitis, and infection with other alphaviruses may cause acute febrile arthropathy (described briefly in Table 17–1).

Eastern, Western, and Venezuelan Equine Encephalitis Viruses

Epidemiology

Infections caused by eastern, western, and Venezuelan equine encephalitis viruses, transmitted by mosquitoes, occur in the summer and early fall in temperate climates. Western and Venezuelan equine encephalitis viruses also may be transmitted transplacentally, producing encephalitis in the newborn, and Venezuelan equine encephalitis virus has been transmitted via aerosol inhalation to persons working with the virus in the laboratory (1,2).

Eastern equine encephalitis virus is endemic along the eastern coast of the United States from southern Canada to northern South America. In North America, the natural cycle of infection involves the Culiseta mosquito vector and wild and sentinel avian amplifying hosts, and infection is transmitted to humans by Culex and Aedes mosquitoes. In the United States, small outbreaks of eastern equine encephalitis (five or fewer cases in humans and more in horses) occur annually, and occasionally outbreaks resulting in hundreds of horses' death have been reported in northeastern states and Florida (3).

Western equine encephalitis viruses are distributed throughout the Americas, and subtypes are found in the former Soviet Union, Europe, Scandinavia, and New Zealand. The natural cycle of infection involves the Culex mosquito vector and avian amplifying hosts. Transmission to humans by Culex mosquitoes is uncommon, but western equine encephalitis virus causes human morbidity and mortality each year (4). Recent equine vaccination programs and improved vector control have significantly reduced the prevalence of western equine encephalitis in the United States, but the disease remains a problem in South America.

Six subtypes (I through VI) of Venezuelan equine encephalitis virus are known. Subtypes IA, IB, and IC, referred to as "epizootic" strains, require an amplification cycle in horses for transmission during an epidemic. Although during epidemics these strains have been detected in many different species of mosquitoes, their natural cycle remains unknown. The remaining subtypes, termed "enzootic" strains, are maintained in nature by cycling between Culex mosquito vectors living in tropical and subtropical swamps and forests throughout the Americas

Table 17-1. Alphaviruses That Cause Acute Arthropathy

Virus	Vector/Reservoir	Geographic Location	Clinical Manifestations
Chikungunya (CHIK) virus	Aedes mosquito/nonhuman primates	Sub-Saharan Africa; temperate and tropical Asia	Adults: fever, chills, headache, anorexia; migratory, polyarticular arthralgias (small joints); maculopapular rash Children: high fever, headache, injected pharynx, rash; no joint involvement
O'nyong-nyong (ONN) virus	Anopheles mosquito/none known	East African epidemic 1959–mid-1960s	Low-grade fever, arthropathy, rash
Mayaro (MAY) virus	Haemagogous mosquito/marmosets, ? humans, ? birds	Brazil, Bolivia, Central America	Fever, chills, headache, myalgias, arthralgias, rash
Ross River virus (RRV)	Aedes and Culex mosquitoes/marsupials, domestic animals, rodents	Australia, Pacific Islands	Severe joint pain, rash, myalgia, headache; no fever
Sinbis	Culex mosquito/birds	Europe (60°–65° north latitude), Asia, Australia	Rash, low-grade fever, headache, fatigue, migratory arthralgias

and rodent (and possibly avian) amplifying hosts. In the United States an endemic focus of the virus exists in Florida; however, human disease is rare. Epizootics of Venezuelan equine encephalitis occurred in South and Central America, Mexico, and southern Texas at intervals of 10 years or less from the 1930s to 1972, when the last major focus of epizootic virus activity was recognized. Clinical attack rates in humans during these epizootics ranged from 10 to 60% and were higher in males, possibly because they more frequently experience occupational and recreational exposure (5–7).

Pathogenesis.

Transmission of eastern, western, and Venezuelan equine encephalitis viruses to a susceptible host is followed by viremia, often accompanied by fever, during which the virions localize and replicate in extraneural tissues. The infection may be terminated by the host immune response at this time, or the virus may invade the central nervous system, producing encephalitis with neuronal destruction, neutrophilic and microglial cell infiltrates, vasculitis, and perivascular mononuclear cell infiltrates throughout the brain and spinal cord (Fig. 17–1).

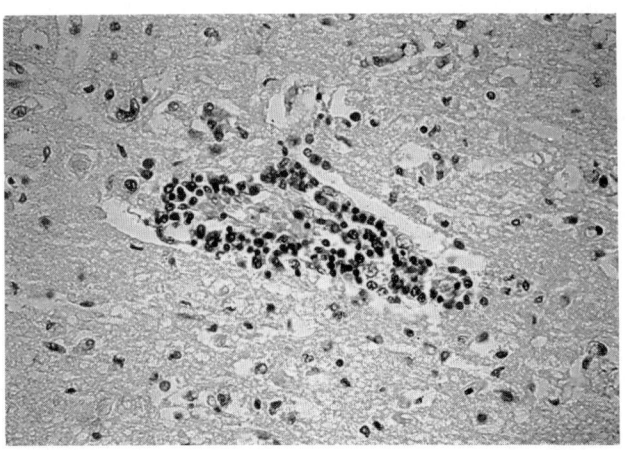

Fig. 17–1. Micrograph of brain tissue from a patient with Eastern equine encephalitis (hematoxylin and eosin, ×100).

Clinical Manifestations.

Children and elders are most susceptible to severe illness following infection with eastern, western, and Venezuelan equine encephalitis viruses. Western and eastern equine encephalitis begin with fever, headache, chills, nausea, and vomiting, followed in 24 to 48 hours by confusion, somnolence, variable neurologic findings (stiff neck, altered reflexes, tremors, spastic paralysis, and bulging fontanelles in infants), seizures in infants and children, and possibly coma. The cerebrospinal fluid protein concentration and white blood cell count are elevated (50 to 2000 cells/µl with a lymphocyte predominance, although neutrophils may predominate early in the illness). The case-fatality rate is 3 to 7% for western and 50 to 75% for eastern equine encephalitis. Neurologic sequelae—mental retardation, behavioral changes, seizure disorders, and paralysis—occur in 30 to 70%, respectively, of infants recovering from western and eastern equine encephalitis and are less common in adults.

Infection with Venezuelan equine encephalitis virus most commonly produces a febrile illness with myalgia, lethargy, somnolence, vomiting, diarrhea, and pharyngitis. Encephalitis occurs in less than 1% (in adults) to 4% (in children) of cases. The overall case fatality rate is under 1%, increasing to 10 to 20% with encephalitis.

RUBIVIRUS

The single Rubivirus organism, rubella virus, produces an acute exanthematous illness resembling a mild case of measles in children and adults. If acquired during the first trimester of pregnancy, it can infect the fetus, causing its demise or inducing various congenital defects. Although the exanthematous illness had been recognized as a distinct illness since the late nineteenth century, maternal rubella was not associated with birth defects until 1941 (8). Rubella virus was first isolated in 1962 and subsequently classified in a separate genus in the Togaviridae (9).

Structure

The spherical, 60-nm diameter, enveloped rubella virus virions have three distinct structural proteins: E1, an envelope glycoprotein with domains independently involved in attachment of the virion to the surface of erythrocytes and initiation of infection; E2, an envelope glycoprotein of unknown function; and the capsid or C protein.

Epidemiology

Humans are the only known host for rubella virus. Before a vaccine was available, minor epidemics of rubella occurred every 6 to 9 years, with peaks in the spring, and disease was recognized most often in children 5 to 9 years of age (10). In countries where the vaccine is widely used epidemics have stopped and the prevalence of the illness among older persons has increased (11). A live attenuated vaccine was licensed for use in the United States in 1969, and by 1986, when about 550 cases of postnatal rubella were reported to the Centers for Disease Control (CDC), the incidence of reported cases had declined by 99% compared with the prevaccine era (12). In 1988, an all-time low 225 cases of rubella were reported, but the number of reported cases almost doubled in 1989, and increased threefold more in 1990 (Fig. 17-2) (13,14).

In the United States from 1988 through 1990 the incidence of rubella increased principally in the West and Midwest. In 1990, half of the reported cases were in California, and outbreaks in Amish communities accounted for increases in cases from Minnesota, New York, and Ohio. The greatest increase in incidence occurred in persons aged 15 to 29 years (from 0.1 to 0.6 per 100,000) and in those 30 years of age and older (from 0.02 to 0.2 per 100,000). The 26 distinguished outbreaks in 1990 could be classified into two categories: those in which all cases occurred in or were linked to settings in which unvaccinated adults congregate (such as prisons, colleges, and workplaces) and those occurring among children and adults in religious communities with low levels of rubella vaccination coverage. Data on the vaccination status of persons with rubella indicate that almost 90% of affected persons had no history of rubella vaccination.

The prevalence of congenital rubella depends on the number of susceptible individuals, the circulation of the virus in the community, and the use of the vaccine. During the 1964 rubella epidemic approximately 30,000 affected infants were born. In the United States, between 1969 and 1979 an average of about 40 cases of congenital rubella were reported annually to the CDC. Since then, fewer than 10 cases per year were reported until 1990, when 10 cases of congenital rubella syndrome were confirmed (12,13).

Rubella virus is transmitted by aerosolization of respiratory secretions of infected persons. They are most contagious at the onset of the rash, but may shed the virus in respiratory secretions from 10 days before to 15 days after the appearance of the rash.

Pathogenesis

Virions enter via the upper respiratory tract mucosa, replicate in the nasopharyngeal lymphoid tissue, spread via the lymphatics or a transient viremia to regional (posterior cervical and occipital) lymph nodes, and replicate again, producing the lymphadenopathy that characteristically appears 5 to 10 days before the onset of the rash. Secondary viremia and shedding of the virus in the nasopharyngeal secretions and feces follow in about 1 week. The maculopapular rash appears 2 to 3 weeks after exposure, which coincides with the production of specific antibodies and the cessation of cell-free viremia, suggesting that the rash is immune mediated. Circulating immune complexes are detected frequently, but no evidence of their involvement in the development of the rash or other potential manifestations of the illness has been observed. During the rash the virus can be isolated from the skin and throat and has been recovered from the conjunctiva, urine, synovial fluid, lung, and cerebrospinal fluid.

Reinfection with rubella virus can occur following naturally acquired infection or vaccination, despite the presence of specific immunity, though in most cases of reinfection virion replication is limited to the nasopharynx; viremia is rare. Most reinfections in persons who had natural disease are asymptomatic, recognized only by a fourfold or greater rise in the pre-existing antibody titer; however, arthritis and rash have been described (15). Asymptomatic reinfection following immunization is more common, especially in persons with hemagglutination inhibition antibody titers of 1:64 or less (16,17). Reinfection during pregnancy rarely results in spread of the virus to the fetus (18,19).

Congenital rubella, transmitted to the fetus during maternal viremia, has the most serious effects on the fetus when the maternal infection is acquired early in gestation. Infection during the first 8 weeks of gestation results in fetal demise and spontaneous abortion or multiple congenital defects in 40 to 60% of cases; whereas if infection is acquired during the third or fourth month of gestation the chances of developing a single congenital defect such as deafness or congenital heart disease are 30 to 35% and 10%, respectively. Thereafter, the fetus is infected with rubella virus but fetal damage is rare.

Early in gestation infection of the placenta with rubella virus causes vasculitis and focal necrosis of syncytiotrophoblasts and cytotrophoblasts; and later, placental hypo-

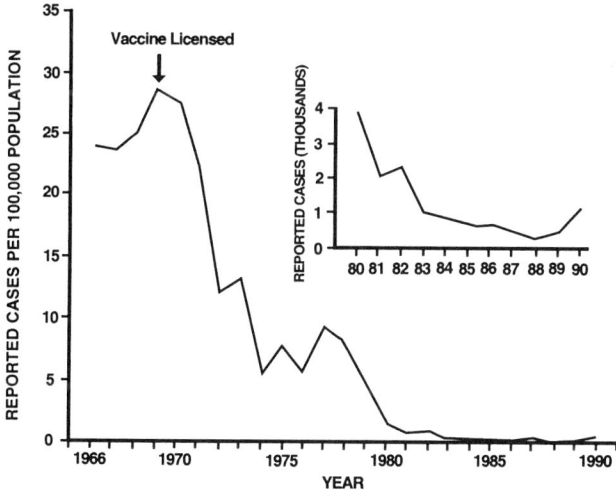

Fig. 17-2. Cases of rubella in the United States, 1966-1990. (From Centers for Disease Control: Summary of notifiable diseases, United States, 1990. MMWR, 39:1, 1990.)

plasia with vasculitis and mononuclear cell infiltrates in the placental membranes, umbilical cord, and decidua are seen. Following infection of the placenta the virus may spread to the developing fetus and infect almost any organ, causing spontaneous abortion, premature delivery, stillbirth, or any of a range of congenital malformations. At birth rubella virus can be recovered from nasopharyngeal secretions and urine of over 80% of congenitally infected newborns, and about 3% continue to shed virus as long as 20 months thereafter.

The pathogenesis of the congenital rubella syndrome is unknown, but several hypotheses have been suggested. Virion replication may damage clones of cells during critical stages of organ development, giving rise to the congenital abnormalities (20). Persistent infection with rubella virus may arrest cellular mitoses, inhibiting cellular and organ growth (21). Virus-induced angiopathy and subsequent vasculitis of the placenta and fetus may compromise fetal growth (22). Finally, lymphocyte abnormalities may predispose to organ-specific autoimmunity (23).

Clinical Manifestations

Many cases of postnatal rubella are subclinical. In persons who develop symptoms the predominant manifestations are enlargement of the posterior auricular, posterior cervical, and suboccipital lymph nodes and a maculopapular rash beginning on the face, spreading down the body, and often desquamating during convalescence. Typically, the rash lasts 3 to 5 days (hence the name "3-day measles") and may be accompanied by mild coryza, conjunctivitis, and fever. Arthritis or arthralgia has been reported in up to a third of women but is less common in children and men (24–26). Uncommon complications of rubella are immune-mediated thrombocytopenia (primarily in children) and encephalitis, which complicates about 1 in 5000 cases, is more frequent in adults, and is associated with a 20 to 50% fatality rate.

The symptoms of congenital rubella, which occasionally are inapparent until weeks or months after birth, may be classified as temporary, permanent, and developmental (Table 17–2). The most common manifestations are deafness, cataract or glaucoma, congenital heart disease, and mental retardation. In the first 18 months of life the mortality rate associated with congenital rubella ranges from 13 to 20%.

Table 17–2. Common Manifestations of Congenital Rubella

Classification	Manifestations
Transient	Low birth weight, thrombocytopenic purpura, hepatosplenomegaly, bone lesions, large anterior fontanelle, meningoencephalitis
Permanent	Cataracts, microphthalmia, retinopathy, patent ductus arteriosus, cryptorchidism, inguinal hernia, spastic diplegia, microcephaly
Developmental and Permanent	Pulmonic stenosis, mental retardation, behavior disorders, central language disorders, hearing loss

Laboratory Diagnosis

Alphaviruses. Most commonly, encephalitis and arthropathy caused by the alphaviruses are diagnosed serologically. To diagnose encephalitis, cerebrospinal fluid and serum should be tested for specific immunoglobulin (Ig) M, whose presence indicates recent infection. A presumptive diagnosis can be made if a fourfold or greater rise in IgG titer is observed between acute- and convalescent-phase serum. Interpretation of IgG titers may be difficult, however, because antibodies may be heterologous (related to a virus of the same group), and the diagnosis is delayed due to the requirement for a convalescent-phase serum sample. Currently, cerebrospinal fluid and serum samples should be sent to an experienced reference laboratory for testing.

Western, eastern, and Venezuelan equine encephalitis viruses may be isolated from brain tissue obtained by biopsy or at autopsy, and Venezuelan equine encephalitis virus may be recovered from blood and pharyngeal swab specimens. The preferred isolation method is intracerebral inoculation of mice, which generally die within 2 days if one of these viruses is present in the inoculum. Alternatively, Vero cells, mosquito cells, and primary chicken and duck embryo cells may be inoculated. Isolation usually is not performed in clinical virology laboratories, and specimens must be sent to a special reference laboratory such as the Vector-Borne Virus Diseases Division of the CDC (Fort Collins, CO) in the United States.

Rubella Virus. To diagnose recent infection with rubella virus, serum should be tested for specific IgM, which is detectable a few days after the onset of symptoms, peaks 8 to 21 days later, and then declines over the next 4 to 5 weeks, becoming indetectable. Detection of specific IgG, which is present at the onset of symptoms, rises for the next 7 to 21 days, levels off, and remains detectable indefinitely, is used primarily to determine immune status.

Rubella virus isolation is indicated in few situations: suspected rubella with severe complications, fatal cases for which serologic confirmation of the pathogen is not possible, and cases in which characterization of the infecting strain (vaccine-like versus wild-type) may be required for epidemiologic purposes. The virus is present in most body fluids and tissues of congenitally infected infants. For primary isolation of rubella virus from clinical specimens, inoculating African green monkey kidney, Vero, or RK-13 cell cultures is recommended (27). To detect rubella virus in cultures of African green monkey kidney cells (which is the standard method for isolating rubella virus), a challenge enterovirus such as echovirus 11 or coxsackievirus A9 is added to the culture 10 days postinoculation (9). Failure of the challenge virus to induce cytopathic effect (CPE) is presumptive evidence that rubella virus is present. Definitive identification requires neutralizing the interference with antibodies to rubella virus. In Vero and RK-13 cell systems, rubella virus produces CPE, but the latter often becomes apparent only after several passages of cell culture fluids. Once cytopathic effect is present the virus is identified by direct neutralization or indirect immunofluorescent staining. Because most clinical virology laboratories are unfamiliar with rubella virus detection techniques, specimens for rubella virus isolation probably should be sent to a reference laboratory.

Treatment and Prevention

No specific therapy for infections caused by togaviruses is known. For encephalitis caused by the alphaviruses, supportive measures, relief of symptoms, and intensive nursing care are indicated. Preventing human eastern and western equine encephalitis depends on controlling the mosquito vectors. Human infection with Venezuelan equine encephalitis virus is prevented by equine immunization because transmission of epidemic virus strains requires amplification in horses. Commercial vaccines against western, eastern, and Venezuelan equine encephalitis viruses are used in horses, and experimental vaccines are used to protect laboratorians working with these viruses.

Most cases of postnatal rubella do not require therapy, and its complications are treated symptomatically. Infection with rubella virus can be prevented by immunization. The Wistar RA27/3 vaccine, currently used in the United States, induces immunity in 95% or more of vaccine recipients. Potential side effects—fever, rash, lymphadenopathy, and arthritis—are most common in women older than 25 years. Routine vaccination of all children with the combination measles-mumps-rubella vaccine is recommended at 15 months of age. Immunization is contraindicated for women who are pregnant; however, because the currently recognized risk to the fetus following inadvertent vaccination during early pregnancy is minimal automatic termination of such a pregnancy is not mandated (28).

REFERENCES

1. Copps SC, and Giddings LE: Transplacental transmission of western equine encephalitis. Pediatrics, 24:31, 1959.
2. Shinefield HR, and Townsend TE: Transplacental transmission of western equine encephalomyelitis. J Pediatr, 43:21, 1953.
3. Monath TP: Arthropod-borne encephalitides in the Americas. Bull WHO, 57:513, 1979.
4. Centers for Disease Control: Arboviral infections of the central nervous system—United States, 1987. MMWR, 37:506, 1988.
5. Hinman AR, McGown JE, Jr, and Henderson BE: Venezuelan equine encephalomyelitis: Surveys of human illness during an epizootic in Guatemala and El Salvador. Am J Epidemiol 93:130, 1971.
6. Martin DH, et al: An epidemiologic study of Venezuelan equine enccphalomyclitis in Costa Rica, 1970. Am J Epidemiol, 95:565, 1972.
7. Sanmartin C: Diseased hosts: Man. *In* Proceedings of the Workshop Symposium on Venezuelan Encephalitis Virus. Sci Publ. 243. Washington, DC, Pan American Health Organization, 1972.
8. Gregg NM: Congenital cataract following German measles in the mother. Trans Ophthalmol Soc Aust, 3:35, 1941.
9. Parkman PD, Buescher EC, and Artenstein MS: Recovery of rubella virus from army recruits. Proc Soc Exp Biol Med, 111:225, 1962.
10. Witte JJ, et al: Epidemiology of rubella. Am J Dis Child, 118:107, 1969.
11. Krugman S: Present status of measles and rubella immunization in the United States: A medical progress report. J Pediatr, 90:1, 1977.
12. Centers for Disease Control: Rubella and congenital rubella—United States, 1984–1986. MMWR, 36:664, 1987.
13. Centers for Disease Control: Increase in rubella and congenital rubella syndrome—United States, 1988–1990. MMWR, 40:93, 1991.
14. Centers for Disease Control: Summary of notifiable diseases—United States, 1990. MMWR, 39(53):1, 1990.
15. Wilkins J, Leedom JM, Salvatore MA, and Portney B: Clinical rubella with arthritis resulting from reinfection. Ann Intern Med, 77:930, 1972.
16. Horstmann DM, et al: Rubella: Reinfection of vaccinated and naturally immune persons exposed in an epidemic. N Engl J Med, 283:771, 1970.
17. Chang T-W, Des Rosiers S, and Weinstein L: Clinical and serologic studies of an outbreak of rubella in a vaccinated population. N Engl J Med, 283:246, 1970.
18. Fosgren M, Carlson G, and Strongert K: Case of congenital rubella after maternal reinfection. Scand J Infect Dis, 11:81, 1979.
19. Bott LM, and Eizenberg DH: Congenital rubella after successful vaccination. Med J Aust, 1:514, 1982.
20. Rawls WE: Viral persistence in congenital rubella. Prog Med Virol, 18:273, 1974.
21. Naeye RL, and Blanc W: Pathogenesis of congenital rubella. JAMA, 194:1277, 1965.
22. Driscoll SG: Histopathology of gestational rubella. Am J Dis Child, 118:44, 1969.
23. Rabinowe SL, et al: Congenital rubella. Monoclonal antibody–defined T-cell abnormalities in young adults. Am J Med, 81:779, 1986.
24. Grahame R, Armstrong R, and Simon N. Chronic arthritis associated with the presence of intrasynovial rubella virus. Ann Rheum Dis, 42:2, 1983.
25. Heggie AD, and Robbins FC: Natural rubella acquired after birth: Clinical features and complications. Am J Dis Child, 118:12, 1969.
26. Chantler JK, Ford DK, and Tingle AJ: Persistent rubella infection and rubella-associated arthritis. Lancet, i:1323, 1982.
27. Chernesky MA, and Mahony JB: Rubella virus. *In* Manual of Clinical Microbiology. 5th ed. Edited by A Balows, et al. Washington, DC, American Society for Microbiology, 1991.
28. Centers for Disease Control: Rubella vaccination during pregnancy, 1971–1986. MMWR, 36:457, 1987.

Chapter 18

FLAVIVIRUSES

The flaviviruses (previously called group B togaviruses) infect domestic and wild animals and humans. In this chapter, an overview of the classification, structure, and replication of flaviviruses is presented, and four of the most important arthropod-borne afflictions of humans are discussed: dengue, yellow fever, St. Louis encephalitis, and Japanese encephalitis. The epidemiology and clinical manifestations associated with the flaviviruses that most frequently cause human disease are outlined in Table 18–1 (1).

CLASSIFICATION

The 66 known flaviviruses in the family Flaviviridae are grouped according to their mode of transmission: mosquito-borne, tick-borne, or vector unknown. Forty-nine flaviviruses have been placed into eight antigenic subgroups based on cross-neutralization using polyclonal, hyperimmune antisera; 17 additional viruses remain unassigned (discussed in detail in references 2 and 3).

STRUCTURE AND REPLICATION

The enveloped flavivirus virions, 37 to 50 nm in diameter, contain a nucleocapsid core composed of a single-stranded positive-sense RNA genome, approximately 11 kilobases long, complexed with a single species of capsid protein. The membrane surrounding the nucleocapsid consists of a lipid bilayer and two proteins: E (envelope), which defines the type specificity of the virus, and M (membrane).

The specific steps in flavivirus replication have not been described in detail. The initial steps of attachment and entry have not been defined. After uptake of the virion and uncoating of the nucleocapsid, transcription and translation ensue in the cytoplasm. Virions mature by budding from the membrane of the endoplasmic reticulum and Golgi apparatus, after which virus particles are released by exocytosis or cell lysis.

DENGUE VIRUS

Epidemics of dengue, first described in Philadelphia in the 1780s, were common in North America, the Caribbean, Asia, and Australia during the eighteenth and nineteenth century (4,5). Mosquito transmission and the viral etiology of the disease were demonstrated in the early 1900s (5). The dengue virus was isolated in mice in 1944, after which four serotypes were identified (6). Hemorrhagic dengue fever was described in 1954 in Asia, where it remains an important epidemic disease, and was recognized in Cuba in 1981. Between 1977 and 1987 345 cases of imported dengue were reported in the United States, and because the mosquito vector Aedes aegypti is found in the southeastern United States, indigenous transmission of the virus in those areas is possible (7).

Epidemiology

Dengue is endemic and epidemic in tropical areas of Asia, Oceania, Africa, Australia, and the Americas where Aedes aegypti, the principal vector, is found. The virus is maintained in a cycle involving humans and mosquitoes and, in Malaysia and Africa, in cycles involving monkeys and mosquitoes. Transmission to humans most often occurs by a bite, but mechanical spread by A. aegypti and other species of Aedes is possible. Where and how dengue viruses are maintained between epidemics are not clearly defined. Individuals of all ages and both sexes are susceptible to infection, but in endemic areas outbreaks are more common in children because most adults are immune. In tropical areas epidemics predominate during the monsoon or rainy season.

Pathogenesis

In nonhuman primates infected in the laboratory, dengue virus replicates primarily in monocytes. Classic dengue fever in humans is a self-limited infection; biopsy of involved skin shows endothelial cell swelling and a perivascular mononuclear cell infiltrate. Dengue hemorrhagic fever, characterized by increased vascular permeability, bleeding, and occasionally intravascular coagulation, typically occurs during second infections with dengue virus in persons with pre-existing antibodies to a heterologous dengue virus serotype. These changes may be mediated by circulating virus-antibody complexes, complement activation, and release of proteases and lymphokines; moreover, some strains of dengue viruses may be more virulent than others.

Clinical Manifestations

Classic dengue begins abruptly after an incubation period of 2 to 8 days with high fever, headache, retro-orbital pain, and backache, followed by myalgia or bone pain, anorexia, nausea, vomiting, and weakness. A transient macular rash may appear on the first or second day. Fever usually lasts 5 to 7 days, and coincident with defervescence, a secondary maculopapular or morbilliform rash appears on the trunk, spreads to the face and extremities sparing the palms and soles, and may desquamate. Fever may reappear, producing a "saddle-back" fever curve. Lymphadenopathy and mild hemorrhagic phenomena (petechiae, epistaxis, intestinal bleeding) may occur; complications such as encephalitis and myocarditis are

Table 18–1. Flaviviruses Associated With Human Disease

Virus	Disease	Primary Transmission Cycle		
		Principal Vector(s)	Host(s)	Geographic Location
Mosquito-borne				
Yellow fever	Hepatitis, gastrointestinal hemorrhage	Aedes aegypti (urban); Aedes spp. (sylvan)	Humans Simian spp.	South America, Africa South America, Africa
Dengue	Fever with rash, hemorrhagic fever (HF)	Aedes aegypti	Humans	Worldwide; HF in SE Asia, Caribbean
West Nile	Fever with rash, encephalitis	Culex spp.	Birds	Africa, Asia, Middle East, Europe
St. Louis encephalitis	Encephalitis	Culex spp.	Birds	Western Hemisphere
Rocio	Encephalitis	? Aedes spp.	? Birds	São Paulo State, Brazil
Japanese encephalitis	Encephalitis	Culex spp.	Pigs, birds	Japan, Korea, China, SE Asia, India
Murray Valley encephalitis	Encephalitis	Culex spp.	Birds	Australia
Tick-borne				
Tick-borne encephalitis*	Encephalitis	Ixodes persulcactus, Ixodes ricinus	Rodents, birds, goats, cattle	Former USSR, Central Europe, Scandinavia
Kyasanur Forest disease	Hemorrhagic fever	Haemaphysalis spp.	Rodents, monkeys	Karnataka State, India
Omsk hemorrhagic fever	Hemorrhagic fever	Dermacentor, Ixodes spp.	Rodents	Siberia

* Also transmitted to humans by ingestion of contaminated unpasteurized goat's milk.

rare. Manifestations of dengue hemorrhagic fever are fever, hemorrhagic manifestations (see above), thrombocytopenia, and hemoconcentration, often accompanied by hypotension and circulatory failure. The 50% mortality rate for untreated dengue hemorrhagic fever can be reduced to 1 to 3% with appropriate therapy (discussed later).

YELLOW FEVER VIRUS

Yellow fever, recognized as a distinct illness during the seventeenth century, was shown in 1900 to be a mosquito-transmitted viral disease (8). The yellow fever virus was first isolated by inoculating a rhesus monkey with the blood of a patient in Ghana in 1927, and 10 years later the strain was attenuated for use as the 17D yellow fever vaccine. Yellow fever remains a major public health problem in South America and Africa.

Epidemiology

In nature, yellow fever virus cycles between nonhuman primates and tree hole–breeding aedine mosquitoes (urban yellow fever, Aedes aegypti; sylvan yellow fever, Aedes species in Africa and Haemogogous species in South America). Humans are exposed when they encroach on this cycle ("jungle yellow fever"), after which epidemic spread is continued by sylvatic vectors. Alternatively, A. aegypti mosquitoes, living in proximity to humans, may transmit the virus only from human to human ("urban yellow fever").

Yellow fever occurs throughout tropical South America and sub-Saharan Africa (Fig. 18–1) (2). Approximately 1000 cases of yellow fever are reported in humans each year; however, the actual number probably is several times greater. In tropical America the prevalence of jungle yellow fever is highest in young males during hot, humid, rainy months (January to March). In Africa, where virus transmission peaks during the late rainy and early dry season, the age distribution is determined primarily by background immunity.

Pathogenesis

Yellow fever virus is viscerotropic, damaging the liver, kidneys, heart, and gastrointestinal tract. The histologic changes in the liver are characteristic: midzonal necrosis with little or no inflammation, fatty change, and intracellular hyaline deposits (Councilman bodies). Subsequent decreased synthesis of vitamin K–dependent coagulation factors by the damaged liver is the major factor responsible for the bleeding diathesis associated with yellow fever, although disseminated intravascular coagulation may occur. Renal changes include acute tubular necrosis and fatty metamorphosis. The myocardium is pale and flabby, and the myocardial fibers show cloudy swelling, degeneration, and fatty change. Petechial hemorrhages are seen in the stomach and duodenum and may develop in the brain.

Clinical Manifestation

Classic yellow fever begins abruptly after an incubation period of 3 to 6 days with chills, fever, headache, backache, generalized pain, nausea, and vomiting. This period of infection, which coincides with viremia, is followed by a period of remission, during which symptoms resolve. The period of intoxication—fever, vomiting, prostration, jaundice, oliguria, and bleeding diathesis—ensues within 24 hours. Abnormal laboratory findings include leukopenia, thrombocytopenia, elevated bilirubin and transaminase values, prolonged prothrombin time, and albuminuria. Death occurs in 20 to 50% of persons who develop jaundice 7 to 10 days after the onset of symptoms.

ST. LOUIS ENCEPHALITIS VIRUS

St. Louis encephalitis was first recognized in 1932, when an outbreak occurred in Illinois (9). The responsi-

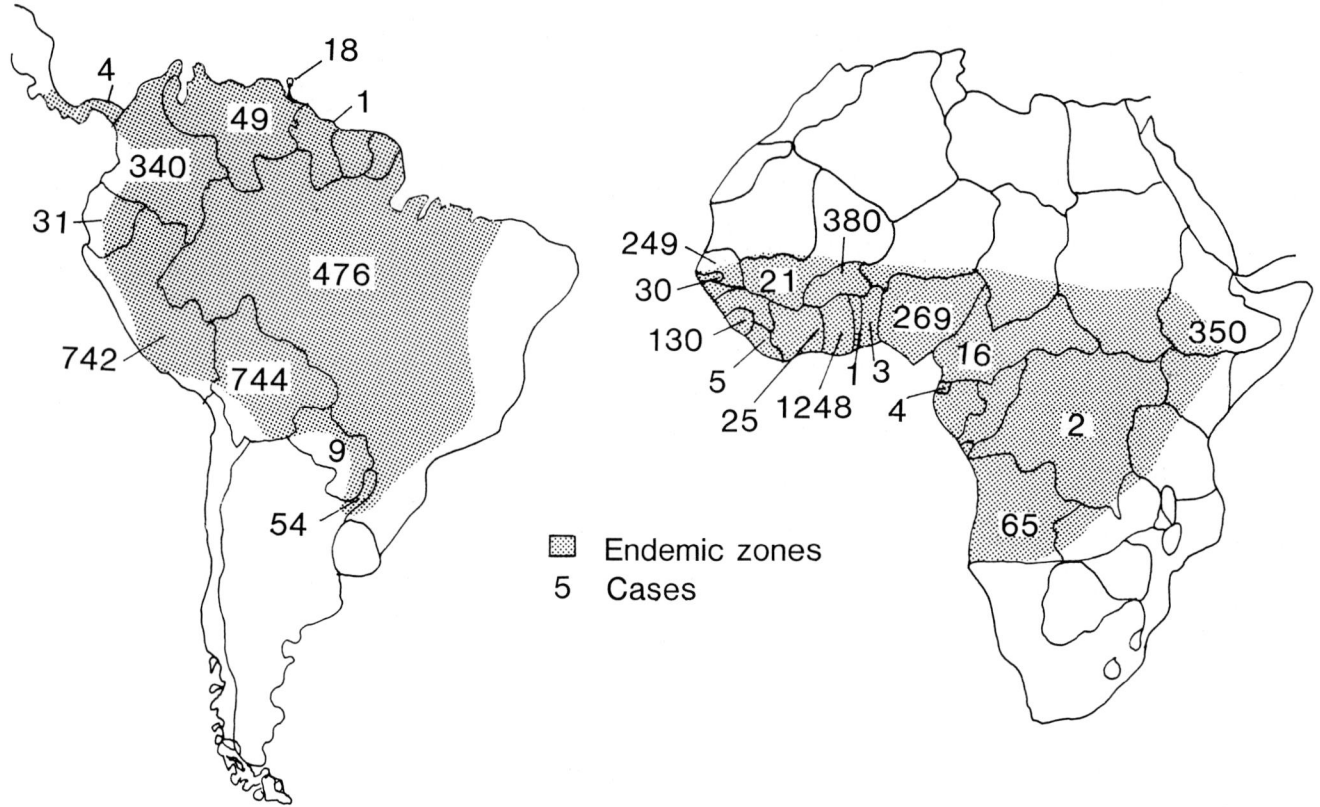

Fig. 18–1. Areas of endemic yellow fever (shaded) are labelled with the number of cases officially reported to the World Health Organization, by country, 1965–1985. (From Monath TP: Flaviviruses. In Fields' Virology. 2nd ed. Edited by BN Fields, and DM Knipe. New York, Raven Press, 1990.)

ble virus was isolated from human brain tissue during a large epidemic in St. Louis the following year, and mosquito transmission was documented in the 1940s. Since its recognition St. Louis encephalitis virus has caused several outbreaks, affecting as many as 2000 persons during a single outbreak in the United States, Canada, and Mexico (10).

Epidemiology

St. Louis encephalitis virus is responsible for summer epidemics about every 10 years, predominantly in the Ohio–Mississippi Valley, eastern Texas, Florida, Kansas, Colorado, and California, and for sporadic cases between epidemics. In nature, the virus cycles between wild birds, which develop viremia without becoming ill, and Culex mosquitoes, the vector that transmits the virus to humans. Most infections in humans are asymptomatic; the disease is most prevalent and severe in elders.

Pathogenesis

After entry into a susceptible host, virions replicate in lymphoid tissue, muscle, or endothelial cells, initiating sustained viremia, and then penetrate into the central nervous system, most likely via the blood. The pathologic findings in the brain of fatal cases of St. Louis encephalitis include mononuclear cell infiltration of the leptomeninges and parenchymal lesions, most prevalent in the substantia nigra and thalamus, characterized by neuronal degeneration and perivascular aggregates of reactive microglial cells and lymphocytes.

Clinical Manifestations

Symptomatic infections caused by St. Louis encephalitis virus are manifest after an incubation period of 4 to 21 days as fever and headache, aseptic meningitis, or encephalitis. Fever, headache, chills, malaise, myalgia, and drowsiness are followed in 1 to 4 days by acute meningeal signs, neuroparenchymal signs, or both. In persons who develop encephalitis, a decreased level of consciousness (confusion, disorientation, lethargy, stupor, coma) is the most frequent finding; abnormal reflexes and tremors also are common. The cerebrospinal fluid protein concentration and white blood cell count are elevated (up to 500 cells/μl with early predominance of neutrophils and later, of lymphocytes). The case-fatality rate varies from 2% in young adults to almost 25% in persons older than 60 years, and of the fatalities 50% occur within 1 week and 80% within 2 weeks of disease onset.

JAPANESE ENCEPHALITIS VIRUS

In the late 1800s an illness resembling Japanese encephalitis was recognized in horses and humans. The responsible virus was recovered from a human brain in 1924, during a severe epidemic in Japan, and from the brain tissue of a sick horse in 1937. Mosquito transmission was proven in 1938.

Epidemiology

Japanese encephalitis virus is widely distributed in Japan, China, Taiwan, Korea, the Philippines, the far eastern part of the former Soviet Union, Southeast Asia, and India. In nature the virus cycles between bird and pig amplifying hosts and Culex mosquito vectors, which transmit it to humans and to horses. In tropical climates sporadic cases occur throughout the year; in temperate areas summer outbreaks are common. In endemic areas children most often acquire disease, as a high rate of immunity exists in older age groups. In epidemic and nonendemic regions, disease predominates in young children and elders, who are at highest risk of fatal infection. The ratio of inapparent to apparent infections, 200:1 to 300:1, is influenced by age, strain of the infecting virus, and cross-protective immunity to other flaviviruses.

Pathogenesis

The pathologic findings in fatal cases of Japanese encephalitis are similar to those described earlier for St. Louis encephalitis.

Clinical Manifestations

After an incubation period of 6 to 16 days, symptomatic infection with Japanese encephalitis virus may manifest as fever and headache, aseptic meningitis, or encephalitis. The latter begins abruptly with headache, fever, chills, nausea, vomiting, dizziness, and drowsiness, followed by nuchal rigidity, decreased consciousness, hyperexcitability, mask-like facies, tremors, and pathologic reflexes. Findings of cerebrospinal fluid examination are similar to those in St. Louis encephalitis (described earlier). During epidemics, death occurs 5 to 9 days after disease onset in 20 to 70% of cases. Up to 70% of survivors experience neuropsychiatric sequelae—parkinsonism, seizures, motor abnormalities, mental retardation, and emotional disorders—all of which are more severe in children.

Laboratory Diagnosis

Because the tests required to diagnose infections caused by the viruses discussed in this chapter are not available in clinical virology laboratories, specimens must be sent to a specialized reference laboratory, which should be contacted for specimen requirements.

Dengue Virus. Dengue is diagnosed serologically or by isolating the virus from blood. The latter requires inoculation of mosquito cells or adult mosquitoes.

Yellow Fever Virus. A specific diagnosis of yellow fever can be made serologically, by detecting the virus, or by observing typical histologic changes in liver biopsy or autopsy tissue (described earlier). Yellow fever virus can be isolated from blood during the first 4 days of illness, or viral antigens may be detected in blood or liver tissue by enzyme-linked immunosorbent assay. A serologic diagnosis is made by detecting specific immunoglobulin (Ig) M, which appears within 5 days after the onset of symptoms. Specific IgG also may be measured; however, acute- and convalescent-phase serum samples must be tested, and cross-reacting antibodies to other flaviviruses may complicate interpretation of the results.

St. Louis and Japanese Encephalitis Viruses. St. Louis and Japanese encephalitis most often are diagnosed serologically. Detecting specific IgM in serum, cerebrospinal fluid, or both is most useful, although specific IgG may be measured in acute- and convalescent-phase serum samples. These viruses rarely are recovered from blood or cerebrospinal fluid, but they may be isolated from brain biopsy or autopsy tissue, and viral antigens can be detected in frozen sections of brain tissue by immunofluorescent staining.

Treatment and Prevention

Treatment of dengue, yellow fever, and St. Louis and Japanese encephalitis is supportive; no specific antiviral agents are currently available.

To prevent yellow fever, persons should be protected from mosquito bites, mosquito vectors should be eliminated, and the live 17D yellow fever vaccine should be given to persons living in or traveling to endemic areas, except pregnant women and immunocompromised persons. The vaccine provides long-lasting immunity, and severe adverse reactions are rare.

Prevention of dengue and St. Louis and Japanese encephalitis requires reducing mosquito vector populations. Live attenuated vaccines against the four dengue virus serotypes are being developed, and a formalin-inactivated vaccine against Japanese encephalitis virus (BIKEN JE) has been evaluated in humans and is recommended for United States citizens who may be at risk of exposure to the virus (11).

REFERENCES

1. Monath TP: Flavivirus (yellow fever, dengue, and St. Louis encephalitis). *In* Principles and Practice of Infectious Diseases. 3rd ed. Edited by GL Mandell, RG Douglas, Jr, and JE Bennett. New York, Churchill Livingstone, 1990.
2. Calisher CH, et al: Antigenic relationships among flaviviruses as determined by cross-neutralization tests with polyclonal antisera. J Gen Virol, *70*:37, 1989.
3. Monath TP: Flaviviruses. *In* Fields' Virology. 2nd ed. Edited by BN Fields and DM Knipe. New York, Raven Press, 1990.
4. Carey ED: Chikungunya and dengue: A case of mistaken identity? J Hist Med, *26*:243, 1971.
5. Siler JF, Hall MW, and Kitchens AP: Dengue: Its history, epidemiology, mechanisms of transmission, etiology, clinical manifestations, immunity and prevention. Philippine J Sci, *29*:1, 1926.
6. Sabin AB, and Schlesinger RW: Production of immunity to dengue with virus modified by propagation in mice. Science, *101*:640, 1945.
7. Centers for Disease Control: Imported dengue—United States, 1987. MMWR, *38*:463, 1989.
8. Strode GK: Yellow Fever. New York, McGraw-Hill, 1951.
9. Chamberlain RW: History. *In* St. Louis Encephalitis. Edited by TP Monath. Washington, DC, American Public Health Association, 1980.
10. Monath TP, and Tsai TF: St. Louis encephalitis: Lessons from the last decade. Am J Trop Med Hyg, *37*:40S, 1987.
11. Poland JD, Cropp CB, Craven RB, and Monath TP: Evaluation of the potency and safety of inactivated Japanese encephalitis vaccine in US inhabitants. J Infect Dis, *161*:878, 1990.

Chapter 19

BUNYAVIRUSES

The bunyaviruses are classified in the family Bunyaviridae, which is the largest family of RNA animal viruses, having more than 250 serologically distinct members that share certain common structural, genetic, replicative, and morphogenic properties. Most viruses in the family are transmitted by or have been recovered from arthropods, except the rodent-borne hantaviruses, which are transmitted via aerosolized rodent excreta. In this chapter, an overview of the classification, structure, and replication of members of the Bunyaviridae is presented, and those viruses that cause serious human disease—California viruses, Rift Valley fever virus, hantaviruses, and Crimean-Congo hemorrhagic fever virus—are discussed.

CLASSIFICATION

In the family Bunyaviridae, five genera—Bunyavirus, Phlebovirus, Hantavirus, Nairovirus, and Uukuvirus—and several unassigned viruses are recognized. Included in the genus Bunyavirus are approximately 160 virus serotypes, subtypes, and varieties divided into 16 serogroups. The genus Hantavirus includes one serologic group of at least eight viruses, and 32 viruses assigned to six serogroups comprise the tick-borne nairoviruses. Thirty-nine viruses divided among nine serogroups are in the genus Phlebovirus, and one serogroup of 13 viruses comprises the genus Uukuvirus.

STRUCTURE

The spherical bunyavirus virions, 80 to 120 nm in diameter, contain three internal nucleocapsids, each consisting of a unique negative-sense single-stranded RNA genome, many copies of a nucleocapsid protein, and a few copies of a large protein, presumably a transcriptase component. Surrounding the nucleocapsids is an envelope composed of a lipid bilayer containing glycoprotein spikes designated G1 and G2. The RNA genome is divided into three segments: Large (L) codes for the large protein, presumed to be a polymerase. Medium (M) codes for the two envelope glycoproteins, and in some genera for one or more nonstructural proteins. Small (S) codes for a nucleocapsid protein (N).

REPLICATION

One or both of the viral envelope glycoproteins mediate attachment to host cell receptors, which have not been defined for any member of the family. Viral entry and uncoating probably occur by endocytosis, forming an endosome which becomes acidified, triggering fusion of the viral and endosomal membranes and subsequent release of the nucleocapsid into the cytoplasm, where transcription, translation, and genome replication occur. Virions assemble by budding into the Golgi cisternae, forming cytoplasmic vesicles which fuse with the plasma membrane, releasing mature virions from the cell.

BUNYAVIRUS

California Serogroup Viruses

California encephalitis virus was first isolated in 1943, and subsequent serologic studies of persons with acute encephalitis identified three cases due to this "new" virus (1). Since then, California encephalitis virus has not been associated with encephalitis in California but has been isolated sporadically from mosquitoes. Moreover, other arthropod-borne viruses related to California encephalitis virus, designated the California serogroup (features of those causing human disease are shown in Table 19–1), have been identified (2). Medically, the LaCrosse virus (discussed below), isolated from a fatal case of encephalitis in 1960, is the most significant of the California serogroup of viruses in the United States. The Jamestown Canyon virus, recently recognized as a potential human pathogen, produces an illness resembling LaCrosse encephalitis, except that adults rather than children predominantly are affected (3,4).

Epidemiology

In nature, the LaCrosse virus cycles between chipmunk, squirrel, fox, and woodchuck amplifying hosts during the summer, and the vector Aedes triseriatus, a forest-dwelling, tree hole–breeding mosquito of the north central and northeastern United States, in which the virus is maintained by transovarial and venereal transmission. Transmission to humans occurs by a bite of a female mosquito.

LaCrosse virus and human encephalitis are concentrated in the upper Mississippi and Ohio River valleys: more than 90% of cases are reported from Minnesota, Wisconsin, Iowa, Illinois, Indiana, and Ohio. Between 1963 and 1981, on average about 75 cases were reported annually in the United States, most in children and young adults (1 to 19 years of age) who participated in activities such as hiking and camping in forested areas in the summer and early fall, when the risk of exposure to the vector is greatest (5).

Clinical Manifestations

Infection with the California viruses most often is asymptomatic. Illness due to infection with LaCrosse virus manifests after an incubation period of 3 to 7 days as a nonspecific fever, meningoencephalitis, or encephalitis,

Table 19–1. Features of California Serogroup Viruses Associated With Human Disease

Virus	Geographic Location	Vertebrate Host	Disease
California encephalitis	Western US, Canada	Rodents	Encephalitis
La Crosse	Midwestern US	Chipmunk, squirrels	Encephalitis
Tahyna	Europe	Domestic animals, rabbits	Influenza-like illness
Jamestown Canyon	North America	White-tailed deer	Encephalitis

which cannot be distinguished clinically or pathologically from acute encephalitis caused by alphaviruses or flaviviruses (see Chapters 17 and 18). The mortality rate of LaCrosse encephalitis is less than 1%; but 75% of the survivors have electroencephalographic abnormalities 1 to 5 years later, 10% experience persistent emotional lability, and 6 to 10% have chronic epilepsy.

PHLEBOVIRUS

Rift Valley Fever Virus

Rift Valley fever virus was first isolated in 1930 from ill ewes and lambs in the Rift Valley in East Africa, and in 1980 its classification as a phlebovirus was confirmed (6,7). During the first large epizootic-epidemic of Rift Valley fever in Egypt in 1977 to 1978, 25 to 50% of all sheep and cattle were infected and as many as 200,000 persons became ill; about 600 died (8).

Epidemiology

Rift Valley fever virus, transmitted by mosquitoes (Culex in Egypt and South Africa and Aedes in East Africa are the major vectors), can produce severe disease in several domestic animals: sheep are more suscpetible than cattle, and goats are least susceptible. Sporadic outbreaks frequently are associated with a rainy season, and interepizootic intervals may be many years. During an epizootic the virus is transmitted to humans by contact with tissues or blood of infected animals, and possibly by transcutaneous or aerosol exposure. Sporadic cases (not associated with an outbreak) are transmitted by mosquitoes and laboratory personnel working with Rift Valley fever virus have acquired infection, probably by aerosol inhalation.

Pathogenesis

The pathogenesis of infection with Rift Valley fever virus has been studied in animals infected in the laboratory (9–11). Inoculated virions probably spread from the skin to local lymph nodes, where they replicate, and then enter the circulation, travel to the liver and replicate again, damaging hepatocytes and yielding high titers of virus, which again enter the circulation. Virions may cross the blood-brain barrier and infect neurons and glia, but the meningoencephalitis and retinitis that develop 2 to 3 weeks after natural infection most likely are immune mediated.

Clinical Manifestations

After an incubation period of 2 to 6 days, most persons with Rift Valley fever experience a febrile, influenza-like illness (see Chapter 11) lasting 2 to 5 days. In 10 to 20% of cases, retinitis develops, which may cause permanent loss of vision. Fulminant hepatitis with hemorrhage or encephalitis complicates up to 1% of infections, and both are frequently fatal.

HANTAVIRUS

Four ecologically and antigenically distinct virus complexes in the Hantavirus are recognized: Hantaan, Puumala, Seoul, and Prospect Hill. These viruses infect rodents and insectivores and are the only bunyaviruses not transmitted by arthropods. Hantaan, Puumala, and Seoul viruses cause human disease and are reviewed briefly. Prospect Hill virus, which is found in the United States, infects humans but is not associated with any known disease and will not be discussed further.

Epidemiology

In nature, Hantaan virus is found in field mice in eastern Asia and eastern Europe; Puumala virus infects bank voles in Scandinavia, Europe, and the western part of the former Soviet Union; and Seoul virus is found worldwide in rats, especially in seaports, but human disease occurs predominantly in eastern Asia. The hantaviruses probably are transmitted primarily via inhalation of dusty aerosols contaminated by infectious rodent urine, although transmission by the bite of an infected rodent can occur. Persons visiting or working in forests and on farms in fall and early winter are at greatest risk of acquiring infection with Hantaan or Puumala virus. Infections caused by Seoul virus peak in winter and spring in China.

Pathogenesis

The pathogenesis of hemorrhagic fever is poorly understood. The major findings in fatal cases are disseminated hemorrhages and acute interstitial nephritis. The latter may be mediated by immune complex deposition (12).

Clinical Manifestations

Infection with Hantaan virus causes severe Asian hemorrhagic fever with renal syndrome, characterized by fever, thrombocytopenia, and acute renal failure, which develop after an incubation period of 9 to 35 days. Survivors progress through toxic (fever, headache, abdominal and back pain), hypotensive, oliguric, and polyuric stages. A mucosal bleeding diathesis, pneumonitis, and pulmonary edema frequently complicate the oliguric stage. The fatality rate ranges from 5 to 10%. Seoul virus causes a similar but milder illness associated with a lower mortality rate.

Infection caused by Puumala virus usually is asymptomatic but may result in nephropathia epidemica, an acute febrile illness marked by abdominal and back pain, polyuria, and mild hemorrhagic manifestations without shock, associated with a mortality rate of less than 1%.

NAIROVIRUS

Crimean-Congo Hemorrhagic Fever Virus

This virus was first isolated independently from farmers with an illness characterized by fever and hemorrhages in the Crimean peninsula and from patients with a severe febrile illness in Zaire (Congo). In 1969, the two agents were shown to be identical (13,14).

Epidemiology

Crimean-Congo hemorrhagic fever virus is widely distributed in the former southwestern Soviet Republics, the Balkans, the Middle East, and Africa, where Hyalomma ticks, the principal vectors, are found. In nature the virus is passed during molting from immature ticks, infected by feeding on viremic small mammals, to mature ticks, which parasitize larger wild and domestic animals. The virus usually is transmitted to humans by a tick bite, and nosocomial outbreaks, during which infection is transmitted via direct exposure to blood and secretion of infected patients, have been reported (15,16).

Clinical Manifestations

After an incubation period of 3 to 6 days Crimean-Congo hemorrhagic fever begins abruptly with influenza-like symptoms, followed in several days by hemorrhagic manifestations—petechiae, ecchymoses, hematemesis, and melena—accompanied by icteric hepatitis. Laboratory abnormalities include thrombocytopenia, elevated levels of fibrin split products, and prolonged prothrombin and partial thromboplastin times. Death occurs in 20 to 50% of cases, usually during the second week of illness.

Laboratory Diagnosis

Infections caused by the bunyaviruses discussed are diagnosed serologically. To diagnose infection with the California encephalitis viruses, specific immunoglobulin (Ig) M, often present at the onset of symptoms, is measured in serum and cerebrospinal fluid; attempting to isolate the virus is not useful because it is not present in blood or secretions when central nervous system disease is apparent. In persons with Asian hemorrhagic fever with renal syndrome specific IgM and IgG are detected in serum shortly after the onset of symptoms, and the virus is present in circulating monocytes but is difficult to recover in the laboratory. Antibodies to Rift Valley fever virus and Crimean-Congo hemorrhagic fever virus generally appear within 10 to 14 days of disease onset. Both of these viruses are readily recovered from the blood of acutely ill persons; however, owing to the aerosol hazard to laboratory personnel, isolation attempts should be performed in maximum-containment facilities. Approximately two thirds of persons with nephropathia epidemica develop specific antibodies within 10 days of disease onset, and in some cases the diagnosis is based on clinical and epidemiologic features alone.

Treatment and Prevention

All severe infections caused by bunyaviruses require supportive therapy. Clinical trials to evaluate the antiviral agent ribavirin for treating hemorrhagic fever with renal syndrome are in progress in China, and studies in laboratory animals suggest that ribavirin may be effective treatment for severe Rift Valley fever (17). No antiviral agents effective against the California encephalitis viruses or Crimean-Congo hemorrhagic fever virus are available.

Infections with these viruses may be prevented by using mosquito and tick repellents, and for the California encephalitis viruses, aerial spraying of slow-release insecticides over forested areas known to have a large vector population may be effective.

REFERENCES

1. Hammon W McD, and Reeves WC: California encephalitis virus—a newly described agent. I. Evidence of natural infection in man and other animals. Calif Med 77:303, 1952.
2. Gonzalez-Scarano F, and Nathanson N: Bunyaviruses. *In* Fields' Virology. 2nd ed. Edited by BN Fields and DM Knipe. New York, Raven Press, 1990.
3. Deibel R, et al: Jamestown Canyon virus: The etiologic agent of an emerging human disease? *In* California Serogroup Viruses. New York, Alan R Liss, 1983.
4. Srihongse S, Grayson MA, and Deibel R: California serogroup viruses in New York State: The role of subtypes in human infections. Am J Trop Med Hyg, *33*:1218, 1984.
5. Kappus KD, et al: Reported encephalitis associated with California serogroup virus infections in the United States. 1963–1981. *In* California Serogroup viruses. Edited by CH Calisher and WH Thompson. New York, Alan R Liss, 1983.
6. Daubney R, and Hudson JR: Enzootic hepatitis or Rift Valley fever: An undescribed virus disease of sheep, cattle and man from East Africa. J Pathol Bacteriol, *34*:545, 1931.
7. Rice RM, et al: Biochemical characterization of Rift Valley fever virus. Virology, *105*:256, 1980.
8. Meegan JM: The Rift Valley fever epizootic in Egypt 1977–78. I. Description of the epizootic and virological studies. Trans R Soc Trop Med Hyg, *73*:618, 1979.
9. Mims CA: Rift Valley fever virus in mice. I. General features of the infection. Br J Exp Pathol, *37*:99, 1956.
10. Mims CA: Rift Valley fever virus in mice. II. Adsorption and multiplication of virus. Br J Exp Pathol, *37*:110, 1956.
11. Mims CA: Rift Valley fever virus in mice. III. Further quantitative features of the infective process. Br J Exp Pathol, *37*: 120, 1956.
12. Penttinen K, et al: Circulating immune complexes, immunoagglutinins, and rheumatoid factors in nephropathia epidemica. J Infect Dis, *143*:15, 1981.
13. Casals J: Antigenic similarity between the virus causing Crimean hemorrhagic fever and Congo virus. Proc Soc Exp Biol Med, *131*:233, 1969.
14. Chumakov MP, Smirnova SE, and Tkaschenko EA: Relationship between strains of Crimean hemorrhagic fever and Congo viruses. Acta Virol, *14*:82, 1970.
15. Shepherd AJ, et al: A nosocomial outbreak of Crimean-Congo hemorrhagic fever at Tygerberg Hospital. Part V. Virological and serological observations. S Afr Med J, *68*:733, 1985.
16. Van Eeden PJ, et al: A nosocomial outbreak of Crimean-Congo hemorrhagic fever at Tygerberg Hospital. Part I. Clinical features. S Afr Med J, *68*:711, 1985.
17. Peters CJ, et al: Prophylaxis of Rift Valley fever with antiviral drugs, immune serum, an interferon inducer, and a macrophage activator. Antiviral Res, *6*:285, 1986.

Chapter 20

ARENAVIRUSES

The arenaviruses were named to describe the "sandy" appearance (Latin *arena, arensos*; sand, sandy) of the virus particles when viewed by electron microscopy. These viruses have a predilection for rodents or bats as normal hosts and vectors, and many establish persistent infections in cell culture and in neonatal rodents via transmission in utero or within a few days of birth (1,2). Most persistently infected animals have viremia and virurias throughout life, despite an immune response to the virus.

CLASSIFICATION

The 14 known arenaviruses are classified in the family Arenaviridae, which is divided into Old World and New World species. Only the four viruses that cause human disease—lymphocytic choriomeningitis virus, Lassa virus, Junin virus, and Machupo virus—are discussed here.

STRUCTURE

Round, oval, or pleomorphic arenavirus virions, 50 to 300 nm in diameter (average, 100 to 130 nm), are surrounded by a host cell membrane–derived envelope from which club-shaped viral glycoproteins project (Fig. 20–1) (3). Within the virion's interior are a variable number of host cell ribosomes, which are responsible for the sandy appearance. The internal viral nucleocapsid consists of a helical nucleocapsid protein (N or NP) and a linear, single-stranded, negative-sense RNA genome composed of two segments: large (L, molecular weight 2.6×10^6) and small (S, molecular weight 1×10^6). The small segment codes for three viral proteins: the nucleocapsid core protein and a glycoprotein precursor polypeptide (GP-C) that is cleaved and glycosylated, forming the structural proteins G1, which most likely represents viral surface projections, and G2, probably a membrane-embedded protein with partial surface expression. The G1 protein is important in arenavirus neutralization, and GP-C is a target of T cell–mediated cytolysis of virus-infected cells (4,5). The large segment codes for a viral polymerase and is associated with virulence in guinea pigs.

REPLICATION

Arenaviruses produce high titers of progeny virus with minimal disturbance of host cell processes, yet the replication cycle is slow compared to that of other negative-sense RNA viruses. A viral envelope glycoprotein probably attaches to a host cell membrane receptor; however, neither the glycoprotein nor the receptor involved has been identified. The exact mechanism of viral entry and uncoating is likewise unknown. Once inside the cell, transcription, translation, and replication of the RNA genome ensue in the cytoplasm. After assembly, mature virions are released by budding from the host plasma membrane. Alternatively, the virus may establish a persistent infection, during which infected cells express little, if any, glycoprotein and yield few infectious virus particles.

LYMPHOCYTIC CHORIOMENINGITIS VIRUS

Epidemiology and Epizootology

Lymphocytic choriomeningitis virus, identified in focal areas of Europe and the Americas, may be transmitted to humans from the mouse reservoir via aerosols, direct contact, or a bite; however, the exact mechanism of transmission is unknown. Most human infections occur during the fall, winter, and spring among young adults, especially laboratory workers who handle mice or hamsters. Sporadic cases usually are related to contact with infected mice, but outbreaks have been associated with Syrian hamsters infected via exposure to virus-contaminated tumor cell lines and with exposure to pet hamsters (6–9).

Pathogenesis

Few descriptions of the histologic appearance of infection due to lymphocytic choriomeningitis virus in humans have been published. In one reported fatal case with predominant neurologic manifestations, multiple foci of perivascular macrophage infiltrates were distributed throughout the brain, and viral antigen was detected in the meninges and cortical cells (10).

Clinical Manifestations

Human infection with lymphocytic choriomeningitis virus may be asymptomatic or cause mild to moderate fever or central nervous system manifestations. After an incubation period of 1 to 3 weeks, the illness begins with the insidious onset of fever accompanied by headache, myalgia and malaise, often with relative bradycardia and dysesthesia. Anorexia, nausea, and dizziness are common, and as many as 50% of persons develop sore throat, vomiting, and arthralgias. Frank meningitis occurs in a minority of persons. Signs of encephalopathy—psychosis, paraplegia, or disturbances of cranial, sensory, or autonomic nerve function—develop in about a third of those with central nervous system manifestations. Convalescence is prolonged, but neurologic sequelae are unusual and the illness rarely is fatal.

LASSA VIRUS

Epidemiology and Epizootology

Lassa virus, endemic in West Africa, may be transmitted from rats, the natural reservoir, to humans via aerosol in-

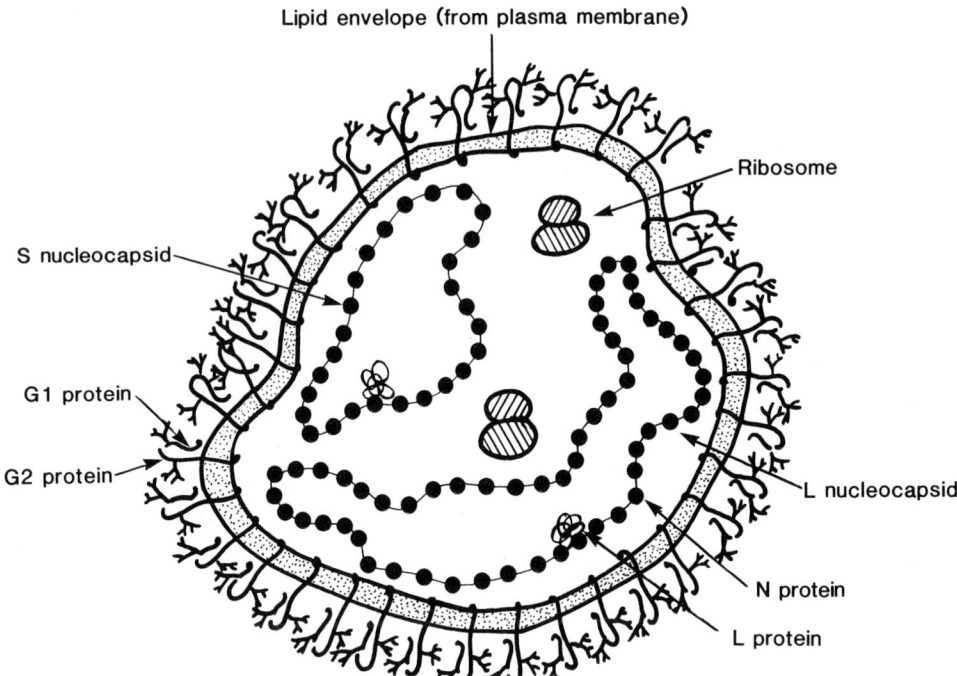

Fig. 20–1. Schematic diagram of an arenavirus particle. (From Bishop, DHL: Arenaviridae and their replication. In Fields' Virology. 2nd ed. Edited by BN Fields and DM Knipe. New York, Raven Press, 1990.)

halation and direct contact, and person-to-person spread has been documented (11). Endemic transmission occurs year-round, but more cases and most nosocomial outbreaks have been reported during the dry season (January to April). No age or sex preference for infection is apparent.

Pathogenesis

The most consistent findings in fatal human Lassa fever are foci of necrosis, accompanied by little or no inflammation, in the liver and spleen, and less frequently the adrenal glands. The liver necrosis, however, is insufficient to cause death. Data from studies in monkeys infected with Lassa virus suggest that platelet or endothelial cell dysfunction, mediated directly or indirectly by the virus, may be responsible for shock and death (12,13).

Clinical Manifestations

Most infections caused by Lassa virus are mild or subclinical, but 5 to 10% of patients develop severe multisystem disease (14–16). After an incubation period of 7 to 18 days the illness begins as described earlier for lymphocytic choriomeningitis virus infections, followed by cough, severe headache, sore throat, retrosternal or epigastric pain, vomiting, diarrhea, and in fewer than 20% of cases, mucosal bleeding. Clinical manifestations predictive of a fatal outcome—hypovolemic hypotension, vasoconstriction, oliguria, and facial and pulmonary edema—occur during the second week of illness. Case fatality rates in hospitalized patients range from 15 to 25%. Complications among survivors include transient alopecia, eighth nerve deafness, pericarditis, orchitis, and uveitis.

JUNIN AND MACHUPO VIRUSES

Epidemiology and Epizootology

Junin and Machupo viruses, endemic in Argentina and Bolivia, respectively, most likely are transmitted to humans via infectious aerosols or direct contact with infected rodent tissue, or food contaminated with infectious rodent urine. Argentine hemorrhagic fever occurs principally among adult males who harvest corn in the agricultural areas of northern Buenos Aires province between February and May. Bolivian hemorrhagic fever is a house-acquired infection of northern Bolivia (Beni province) with peak prevalence from April to July.

Pathogenesis

Autopsy findings in fatal cases of Argentine and Bolivian hemorrhagic fever include petechiae on organ surfaces, lymphadenopathy, mucosal hemorrhages of the gastrointestinal tract, hepatocyte necrosis, pericardial hemorrhage, and primary viral or secondary bacterial bronchopneumonia. In all involved organs the inflammatory response is minimal. During Argentine hemorrhagic fever interferon α levels are elevated, and they are highest in those who die, suggesting a detrimental rather than beneficial role for the cytokine (17).

Clinical Manifestations

Argentine and Bolivian hemorrhagic fever have a similar clinical presentation. The illness begins as described earlier for lymphocytic choriomeningitis virus. A few days after the onset of symptoms, nausea, vomiting, conjunctivitis, erythema of the face, neck, and thorax, generalized lymphadenopathy, cutaneous petechiae, and a pharyngeal enanthem develop. The disease may subside after about 1 week; or the second stage of the illness—vascular disease characterized by epistaxis, hematemesis, bleeding from mucosal surfaces or into the skin, pulmonary edema, and shock, or neurologic disease, hyporeflexia, tremors, clonic seizures, delirium, and coma—may begin (18). The rate of death, most often a result of neurologic disease, ranges from 10 to 20%.

Laboratory Diagnosis

Specimens useful for diagnosis of infections caused by arenaviruses are listed in Table 20–1. Acute infection may be diagnosed by demonstrating a fourfold or greater rise in the specific immunoglobulin (Ig) G titer or, in the case of Lassa virus, the presence of specific IgM in association with a compatible illness. Virus isolation in cell culture or laboratory animals provides the diagnosis during acute disease, but manipulation of these viruses requires laboratory biosafety level 4 or, for lymphocytic choriomeningitis virus, level 3.

Treatment and Prevention

Infections caused by the arenaviruses require supportive care. Convalescent-phase human plasma given before day 9 of illness is effective treatment for Argentine hemorrhagic fever (19). Ribavirin significantly reduces the mortality rate of Lassa fever if first given before day 7 of the disease (20).

Rodent control has been successful in curtailing outbreaks of Bolivian hemorrhagic fever and lymphocytic choriomeningitis (6,21). To prevent the spread of Lassa virus in hospitals, meticulous barrier nursing procedures and universal precautions to prevent contact with contaminated blood and other body fluids should be followed (22). To prevent laboratory-acquired infection (via infectious aerosols), work with the arenaviruses (except lymphocytic choriomeningitis) must be conducted in laboratories equipped for maximum biologic containment.

No licensed arenavirus vaccines are available; however, field trials to test the efficacy of an attenuated vaccine against Junin virus are in progress, and a genetically engineered Lassa virus vaccine is being evaluated in animals.

Table 20–1. Specimens Useful for Diagnosing Infections With Arenaviruses

Virus	Specimen Type	Time of Collection (Days)*
Lymphocytic choriomeningitis virus	Blood, CSF, ± throat	7
	Urine	≤67
Lassa virus	Blood, ± throat	7 to 10
	Urine	≤67
	Biopsy or autopsy tissue, especially liver	
Junin/Machupo viruses	Blood, ± throat	12
	Biopsy or autopsy tissue	

* Days after onset of disease.
Key: CSF, cerebrospinal fluid; ±, may or may not be useful.

REFERENCES

1. Rawls WE, Chan MA, and Gee SR: Mechanisms of persistence in arenavirus infections: A brief review. Can J Microbiol, 27:568, 1981.
2. McCormick JB; Arenaviruses. In Fields' Virology. 2nd ed. Edited by BN Fields and DM Knipe. New York, Raven Press, 1990.
3. Bishop DHL: Arenaviridae and their replication. In Fields' Virology. 2nd ed. Edited by BN Fields and DM Knipe. New York, Raven Press, 1990.
4. Parekh BS, and Buchmeier MJ: Proteins of lymphocytic choriomeningitis virus: Antigenic topography of the viral glycoprotein. Virology, 153:168, 1986.
5. Whitton JL, Southern PJ, and Oldstone MBA: Analyses of the cytotoxic lymphocyte responses to glycoprotein and nucleoprotein components of lymphocytic choriomeningitis virus. Virology, 162:321, 1988.
6. Hinman AR, et al: Outbreak of lymphocytic choriomeningitis virus infections in medical center personnel. Am J Epidemiol, 101:103, 1975.
7. Bowen GS, et al: Laboratory studies of a lymphocytic choriomeningitis virus outbreak in man and laboratory animals. Am J Epidemiol, 102:233, 1975.
8. Baum SG, Lewis AM, Jr, Rowe WP, and Huebner BJ: Epidemic nonmeningitic lymphocytic choriomeningitis virus infection. N Engl J Med, 274:934, 1966.
9. Biggar RJ, Woodall JP, Walter PD, and Haughie GE: Lymphocytic choriomeningitis outbreak associated with pet hamsters: Fifty-seven cases from New York state. JAMA, 232:494, 1975.
10. Warkel RL, et al: Fatal acute meningoencephalitis due to lymphocytic choriomeningitis virus. Neurology, 23:198, 1973.
11. Frame JD, Baldwin JM, Jr, Gocke DJ, and Troup JM: Lassa fever, a new virus disease of man from West Africa. I. Clinical description and pathological findings. Am J Trop Med Hyg 19:670, 1970.
12. Fisher-Hoch SP, et al: Physiologic and immunologic disturbances associated with shock in Lassa fever in a primate model. J Infect Dis, 155:465, 1987.
13. Fisher-Hoch SP, and McCormick JB. Pathophysiology and treatment of Lassa fever. Curr Topics Microbiol Immunol, 134:231, 1987.
14. McCormick JB, et al: Lassa fever: A case-control study of the clinical diagnosis and course. J Infect Dis, 155:445, 1987.
15. Monson MH, et al: Pediatric Lassa fever: A review of 33 Liberian cases. Am J Trop Med Hyg, 36:408, 1987.
16. McCormick JB: Epidemiology and control of Lassa fever. Curr Topics Microbiol Immunol, 134:69, 1987.
17. Lewis SC, et al: Endogenous interferons in Argentine hemorrhagic fever. J Infect Dis, 149:428, 1984.
18. Maiztegui JI: Clinical and epidemiological patterns of Argentine haemorrhagic fever. Bull WHO, 52:567, 1975.
19. Maiztegui JI, Fernandez NJ, and de Damilano AJ: Efficacy of immune plasma in treatment of Argentine haemorrhagic fever and association between treatment and a late neurological syndrome. Lancet, ii:1216, 1979.
20. McCormick JB, et al: Lassa fever: Effective therapy with ribavirin. N Engl J Med, 314:20, 1986.
21. Mackenzie RB: Epidemiology of Machupo virus infection. I. Pattern of human infection, San Joaquin, Bolivia, 1962–1964. Am J Trop Med Hyg, 14:808, 1965.
22. Holmes GP: Lassa fever in the United States. Investigation of a case and new guidelines for management. N Engl J Med, 323:1120, 1990.

Chapter 21

FILOVIRUSES

Filoviruses—Marburg virus, two named subtypes of Ebola virus (Sudan and Zaire), and an antigenically and genetically distinct filovirus that has some cross-reactivity with strains of Ebola virus—belong to the family Filoviridae, which has one genus, Filovirus. Marburg virus was first recognized in 1967 in Marburg, Germany (for which it was named) and in Yugoslavia, when 25 persons became ill after handling tissues from infected African green monkeys imported from Uganda (1). The mortality rate was 23% for primary cases, but no deaths occurred among the six secondary cases. The next cases of Marburg virus disease were reported in 1975 from South Africa (2). An Australian traveler, who acquired the infection in Zimbabwe, died, but neither of the two secondary cases was fatal. The third recognized outbreak of Marburg virus disease occurred in Kenya in 1980, another case occurred in South Africa in 1982, and the most recent case was reported from Kenya in 1987 (3–5).

Ebola virus (named after a river in Zaire) was first recognized in 1976 when two epidemics, the first in southern Sudan and the second in northwest Zaire, occurred within a short time (6,7). In the Sudan outbreak the index case, a worker in a cotton factory, was the source of a noscomial outbreak, and of the almost 300 recognized patients, 53% died. In the Zaire epidemic, 88% of more than 300 affected persons died. Another small outbreak occurred in 1979 in Sudan in the same area as the 1976 outbreak, and the index case was a worker in the same cotton factory (8). The case fatality rate was 65%.

Between November 1989 and March 1990, several shipments of cynomolgus monkeys imported from the Philippines were found to be actively infected with a filovirus (9–11). The virus was transmitted among monkeys in quarantine facilities, and many animals died. Four animal handlers who had much daily exposure to these animals demonstrated serologic evidence of a recent infection with a filovirus, but none developed an unexplained febrile illness.

Structure

Marburg and Ebola virus virions are pleomorphic, filamentous, U-shaped, 6-shaped, or circular forms with a uniform diameter of 80 nm. Virions are composed of a helical nucleocapsid, consisting of a linear, negative-sense, single-stranded RNA genome of molecular weight 4.2×10^6, and a host cell–derived envelope from which 10-nm peplomers project.

Replication

The mode of entry of filoviruses into cells is unknown. Uncoating, translation, and transcription are believed to occur in a manner similar to that of other negative-sense RNA viruses. Virion assembly involves budding of nucleocapsids from plasma membranes. Nucleocapsids also accumulate in the cytoplasm, forming prominent inclusion bodies.

Epidemiology

The geographic distribution of Marburg virus is ill-defined, but Central and East Africa should be considered endemic areas. Data from serologic studies indicate that Ebola virus may be endemic in certain parts of Sudan and Zaire and in other areas of East and Central Africa (12). The natural reservoir host for these two viruses and the mode of acquiring natural infection are unknown. Secondary transmission results from close personal contact with an infected person or close contact with infected blood, tissues, or body fluids.

For the animal handlers who became infected with the filovirus recently recognized in monkeys imported into the United States from the Philippines in one case the mode of transmission was presumed to be a laceration acquired during performance of necropsy on an infected animal, but it could not be determined for the other three cases.

Pathogenesis and Pathology

The pathophysiologic changes responsible for the morbidity and mortality of infections with Marburg and Ebola viruses are not fully understood. Visceral organ necrosis is due to viral replication in parenchymal cells, but the basis for the hemorrhagic shock syndrome is not clearly defined. Increased endothelial cell permeability, possibly due to decreased ability of these cells to secrete prostacyclin; platelet dysfunction, and thrombocytopenia are responsible for the dominant clinical manifestations (described later), but the mechanisms underlying these changes are unknown.

Autopsy studies of fatal cases of Marburg hemorrhagic fever have shown hemorrhage into the skin, mucous membranes, gastrointestinal tract, and visceral organs. Histologically, foci of necrosis associated with minimal inflammation are most prominent in the liver but also may be found in lymph nodes, spleen, kidneys, ovaries, and testes. Infected hepatocytes often contain large eosinophilic intracytoplasmic inclusions.

Clinical Manifestations

The clinical features of infection caused by Marburg and Ebola viruses—severe hemorrhagic fever—are similar. The illness begins abruptly after an incubation period of about 7 days (range, 2 to 21 days for Ebola, 3 to 10 days for Marburg virus) with fever, headache, malaise, joint pain, myalgia and sore throat, commonly followed by diarrhea and abdominal pain. A transient morbilliform rash that subsequently desquamates is common at the end of the first week of illness; and pharyngitis, conjunctivitis, jaundice, and edema may develop. Hemorrhagic manifestations—petechiae or frank bleeding from the gastrointestinal tract and other mucocutaneous sites—occur after the third day of illness. Infection with the recently recognized filovirus does not appear to cause disease in humans, though data are limited.

Laboratory Diagnosis

Filovirus infections are diagnosed serologically or by detection of the virus in blood or liver specimens, tests performed only in maximum-containment reference laboratories (Centers for Disease Control, Atlanta, GA; Central Public Health Laboratory, London, England; and the National Institute for Virology, Sandringham, South Africa).

A serologic diagnosis is made by demonstrating specific immunoglobulin (Ig) M or a fourfold or greater rise in IgG titer using indirect immunofluorescence and confirming positive results by radioimmunoprecipitation or Western blot assay. Antibodies may not appear in the blood until the second week of illness. Virus detection methods include isolation using Vero cells, electron microscopic examination of infected tissue, and direct or indirect immunofluorescence staining for detection of viral antigens in impression smears prepared from liver specimens.

Treatment and Prevention

Currently no antiviral agent effective against the filoviruses is available. Treatment is supportive and may require intensive care. Prevention of nosocomial transmission requires patient isolation and enforcement of strict barrier nursing techniques and universal precautions (outlined in detail in reference 5). To minimize the health hazard from filoviruses imported into the United States, a special permit must be obtained from the Director of the Centers for Disease Control for importation of individual shipments of cynomolgus, rhesus, or African green monkeys. Moreover, registered importers of nonhuman primates must submit a detailed written plan outlining steps that will be taken to prevent exposure of persons and animals to filoviruses during the importation and quarantine process (13).

REFERENCES

1. Siegert R, et al: Zur Atiologie einer unbekannten, von Affen ausgegangen menschlichen Infektionskrankheit. Dtsch Med Wochenschr, 92:2341, 1967.
2. Gear JSS, et al: Outbreak of Marburg virus disease in Johannesburg. Br Med J., 4:489, 1975.
3. Conrad JL, et al: Epidemiologic investigation of Marburg virus disease, southern Africa, 1975. Am J Trop Med Hyg, 27:1210, 1978.
4. van der Walls FJ, et al: Hemorrhagic fever virus infections in an isolated rainforest area of central Liberia. Limitations of the indirect immunofluorescence slide test for antibody screening in Africa. Trop Geogr Med, 38:209, 1986.
5. Centers for Disease Control: Management of patients with suspected viral hemorrhagic fever. MMWR, 37(S-3):1, 1988.
6. Bowen ETW, et al: Viral haemorrhagic fever in southern Sudan and northern Zaire. Lancet, i:571, 1977.
7. Johnson KM, Webb PA, Lange JV, and Murphy FA: Isolation and partial characterization of a new virus causing acute haemorrhagic fever in Zaire. Lancet, i:569, 1977.
8. Baron RC, McCormick JB, and Zubeir OA: Ebola hemorrhagic fever in southern Sudan: Hospital dissemination and intrafamilial spread. Bull WHO, 6:997, 1983.
9. Centers for Disease Control: Ebola virus infection in imported primates—Virginia, 1989. MMWR, 38:831, 1989.
10. Centers for Disease Control: Update: Filovirus infection in animal handlers. MMWR, 39:221, 1990.
11. Jahrling PB, et al: Preliminary report: Isolation of Ebola virus from monkeys imported to USA. Lancet, 335:502, 1990.
12. Emond RTD, Evans, B, Bowen ETW, and Lloyd G: A case of Ebola virus infection. Br Med J, 2:541, 1977.
13. Centers for Disease Control: Update: Filovirus infections among persons with occupational exposure to nonhuman primates. MMWR, 39:266, 1990.

Chapter 22

RETROVIRUSES

The retroviruses primarily infect vertebrates, causing viremia with no obvious ill effects or any of a spectrum of diseases: malignancies, wasting diseases, neurologic disorders, and immunodeficiencies. In this chapter an overview of retrovirus classification, structure, and replication is presented, and features unique to the retroviruses of medical importance—human T-cell leukemia virus types I and II (HTLV-I and HTLV-II) and human immunodeficiency virus types 1 and 2 (HIV-1 and HIV-2)—are discussed.

CLASSIFICATION

Retroviruses are classified in the family Retroviridae, which is divided on the basis of pathogenicity into three subfamilies, Oncovirinae, Lentivirinae, and Spumavirinae. They are further described according to virion structure (A through D, Table 22–1); utilization of specific cell receptors; whether the virus is endogenous (passed from parent to offspring as a provirus integrated into the germline) or exogenous; and the presence or absence of an oncogene (discussed in detail in reference 1). This classification, however, is not current with the more recently described retroviruses. For example, HTLV and HIV bud as C-type viruses do, but the envelope proteins of HTLV have a different appearance, and HIV has a distinctive bar-shaped nucleocapsid.

HTLV and HIV, respectively, belong to the subfamilies Oncovirinae and Lentivirinae. The Spumavirinae contains "foamy" viruses that may infect humans but are not associated with any known disease and, therefore, are not discussed further here.

STRUCTURE

The enveloped, spherical, 100-nm diameter retrovirus virions consist of a core of structural proteins (nucleocapsid, capsid, and matrix) that surround two molecules of single-stranded RNA and polymerase (1). Inserted into the lipid envelope, which is derived by budding from the cell membrane, are viral proteins composed of two different polypeptide chains. The larger polypeptide contains the receptor-binding function and is the predominant antigen to which neutralizing antibodies are directed. The smaller transmembrane protein anchors the complex to the envelope. Also included in the core are proteins essential for replication: protease; reverse transcriptase, an enzyme involved in converting the genomic single-stranded RNA to double-stranded DNA; and integrase, which is essential for provirus formation, covalently joining viral to cellular DNA.

The retrovirus genome, composed of two RNA molecules, is 7 to 10 kilobases long. The order of the genes encoding structural proteins is constant in all retroviruses: *gag-pro-pol-env*. The *gag*, the "5'-most" gene, encodes the matrix, capsid, and nucleic acid–binding proteins. The *pro* encodes the protease that cleaves *gag* and *pol* polyproteins. The *pol* encodes the reverse transcriptase and integrase proteins, and *env* encodes the two envelope glycoproteins. Other genes involved in regulating virus expression in HTLV and HIV are discussed later in the respective sections.

REPLICATION

The replication cycle of all retroviruses includes several common steps. First, the virion envelope glycoprotein attaches to a specific host cell surface receptor. The viral envelope and the cell membrane fuse, releasing the virion core into the cytoplasm. Reverse transcription of the viral genomic RNA into double-stranded DNA occurs within the core structure. The viral DNA then leaves the core, enters the nucleus, and integrates into random sites in host cell DNA, forming the provirus. Using the integrated provirus as a template, viral RNA is synthesized by cellular RNA polymerase II. Viral proteins then are synthesized, and virions assemble and are released from the cell by budding from the plasma membrane.

HUMAN T-CELL LEUKEMIA VIRUS TYPES I AND II

HTLV-I was first isolated in the United States in 1980 from T lymphocytes of a 28-year-old male who had cutaneous T-cell lymphoma (2). In 1981, Japanese investigators found retrovirus particles, tentatively named adult T-cell leukemia virus (ATLV), in cell lines from patients with adult T-cell leukemia, a malignancy first described in 1977 in southern Japan (3,4). Subsequently, HTLV-I and ATLV were shown to be the same virus, HTLV-I was identified as the agent of adult T-cell leukemia, and infection with HTLV-I was recognized worldwide in specific populations (5). In 1985, a high titer of antibody to HTLV-I was found in many persons with tropical spastic paraparesis in Martinique, an area where HTLV-I is endemic (6).

In 1982, an antigenically distinct retrovirus that shares 65 to 70% nucleotide sequence homology with HTLV-I was isolated from a person with a T-cell variant of hairy cell leukemia (7). A second isolate of this virus, HTLV-II, was recovered from an individual with a similar variant of hairy cell leukemia in 1986, suggesting a potential etiologic role for HTLV-II in this disease (8).

Structure and Replication

The 100-nm diameter, spherical HTLV virions are composed of an internal core of structural (*gag*) nucleocapsid (p15), capsid (p24), and matrix (p19) proteins that surround the RNA genome and polymerase enzyme, and an outer envelope consisting of the viral surface glycoprotein (gp46) and transmembrane protein (gp21), anchored in

Table 22-1. Classification of Retroviruses

Group	Description	Comments
A	Hollow, 60- to 90-nm, spherical, intracellular structures with double-walled appearance	First used to describe immature intracellular forms of mouse mammary tumor virus
B	Enveloped with surface spikes	Extracellular form of mouse mammary tumor virus
C	Progress from crescent-shaped patches at site of budding to immature hollow nucleocapsids to mature particles with an electron-dense core with barely visible surface projections	
D	Complete intracellular nucleocapsid with eccentric core, resembling B-type viruses but with less prominent surface projections	Occur only in retroviruses that infect primates

a lipid membrane. In addition to the universal retrovirus genes *gag* (group antigen), *pol* (reverse transcriptase), and *env* (envelope), HTLV-I and HTLV-II have unique genes: *tax* enhances viral replication by increasing viral RNA transcription, and *rex* regulates the levels of expression of genes encoding virion components, thus determining whether infectious virions are produced.

The replication cycle of HTLV is the same as that described earlier for retroviruses. The cellular receptor for these viruses has not been identified.

Epidemiology

Infection with HTLV-I is endemic in southwestern Japan, where about 20% of the adult population are seropositive; in the Caribbean basin, including the West Indies, northern South America, and the southeastern United States, where 2 to 5% of black adults are seropositive; and in parts of Central America and Africa (5,9–17). In the United States and Europe, serologic evidence of infection with HTLV-I is rare in the general population but is present in certain groups: homosexual males, female prostitutes, and intravenous drug users (especially blacks) (18–25). HTLV-I is transmitted from mother to child, principally via breast milk; by sexual contact from male to female, male to male, and occasionally from female to male; by transfusion of whole blood, packed cells, or platelet concentrates collected from HTLV-I–seropositive donors; and by contaminated needles (26–31).

The geographic distribution of HTLV-II is unknown. Only four cases of infection have been documented by virus isolation: two persons with T-cell hairy cell leukemia (described earlier), one individual with the acquired immunodeficiency syndrome (AIDS; described later), and one person with hemophilia A and pancytopenia (32,33). Seroprevalence studies have shown elevated rates of infection among intravenous drug users in New York City and in England; however serologic test results are difficult to interpret because antigens of HTLV-I and HTLV-II cross-react (21,25). Endemic foci of infection with HTLV-II recently have been identified in Changuinola, Panama, among the Guaymi Indians, who do not practice ritual scarification or tattooing, do not use intravenous drugs, and rarely receive blood transfusions; and in New Mexico among native Americans and Hispanics (34,35).

Pathogenesis

HTLV-I is believed to be the pathogen of adult T-cell leukemia/lymphoma because nearly all persons who have the disease have serologic evidence of infection with the virus. Moreover, in these persons HTLV-I provirus is monoclonally integrated into the genome of leukemic cells, indicating that infection antedated the malignancy. The mechanism of oncogenesis of HTLV-I is not understood, but the *tax* protein, which activates cellular genes and is responsible for oncogenesis in animals, may be important (36). The pathogenesis of HTLV-I–associated myelopathy is unknown.

Clinical Manifestations

Adult T-cell leukemia/lymphoma develops after a latent period of 20 to 30 years in only a small percentage of persons infected with HTLV-I and progresses through several stages: the asymptomatic carrier state, the preleukemic state, chronic or smoldering leukemia/lymphoma, and acute leukemia/lymphoma (37,38). The mean age at disease onset is 34 years in the United States and 55 years in Japan. The most common physical findings are diffuse peripheral lymphadenopathy without mediastinal involvement, hepatosplenomegaly, and skin lesions (localized or diffuse nodules and papules, localized erythema and plaques, and generalized erythroderma). Abnormal laboratory test results include leukocytosis (10,000 to 100,000 cells/μl) with circulating CD4-positive leukemic T cells in two thirds of cases, peripheral eosinophilia, and elevated serum calcium levels. The latter often is accompanied by diffuse lytic bone lesions. Opportunistic infections with organisms such as Pneumocystis carinii, Cryptococcus neoformans, or cytomegalovirus are common because cell-mediated immunity often is impaired, and recurrent infections with dermatophytes are frequent in persons with chronic disease.

HTLV-I also has been implicated as one cause of the similar, if not identical, neurologic diseases tropical spastic paraparesis, HTLV-I–associated myelopathy, and chronic progressive myelopathy, entities that are recognized only in areas where the virus is endemic. Sixty to eighty percent of affected persons have a high titer of antibody to HTLV-I in serum and cerebrospinal fluid (CSF), and in many affected persons viral DNA, viral proteins, and the virus are detected in CSF (39,40). Symptoms of bilateral lower extremity weakness and stiffness, peripheral numbness or dysesthesia, back pain, and urinary frequency, urgency, and incontinence begin at a mean age of 40 to 50 years. Physical examination reveals spastic paraparesis and hyperactive deep tendon reflexes with or without mild sensory changes. The CSF may be normal or slight elevations in protein levels and mononuclear cell counts and oligoclonal banding may be observed. Abnormal lymphocytes may be seen in the CSF or peripheral blood smears.

HUMAN IMMUNODEFICIENCY VIRUS TYPES 1 AND 2

A syndrome, now called AIDS, characterized by T-cell dysfunction, was first described in June, 1981, predominantly among homosexual men and intravenous drug users (41–43). A retrospective review of the medical literature disclosed several probable cases of AIDS during the 1960s and 1970s (44). By February, 1983, 1000 cases of AIDS had been reported in the United States (45). Though 32 states and the District of Columbia reported cases, almost 83% were from New York, California, New Jersey, and Florida, predominantly from major metropolitan areas. In addition to homosexual or bisexual men and intravenous drug users, other risk groups were recognized: Haitian natives, persons with hemophilia, recipients of blood transfusions, heterosexual partners of risk group members, and children born to mothers at risk. Persons with no identifiable risk factor accounted for a small percentage of cases.

A "presumptive" retrovirus, initially called lymphadenopathy-associated virus (LAV), was first isolated in Paris in 1983 from a person at risk for AIDS (46). In 1984 isolation of this virus was confirmed and the evidence linking it to AIDS was strengthened by investigators in the United States who named the virus human T-lymphotropic virus III (HTLV-III) (47,48). The virus since has been renamed human immunodeficiency virus type 1 (HIV-1). A related virus, HIV-2, was described in 1985 in asymptomatic West African prostitutes and, in 1986, was reported in two West Africans with AIDS (49,50). The variant subsequently was recovered from persons in Europe and North America, most of whom originally resided in West Africa (51–54).

Structure

The morphology of HIV virions, shown schematically in Figure 22–1, is similar to that of other members of the Lentivirinae. The particles are 90 to 130 nm in diameter with a double-membraned envelope surrounding an electron-dense cylindrical core. The HIV genome contains *gag, pol,* and *env* genes, common to all retroviruses, plus additional genes and open reading frames that code for regulatory proteins (55). The *gag* gene codes for a precursor protein (p55) that is cleaved, yielding the proteins p17, located outside the core just below the viral membrane; p24, the major constituent of the virion core structure; and p15, p9, and p7, whose functions are unknown. The *pol* gene codes for three viral proteins involved in replication: a proteinase (p10), a reverse transcriptase (p66/p51), and an integrase/endonuclease (p31). The *env* gene codes for a cell-associated glycosylated precursor protein (gp160) that is cleaved, yielding an external glycoprotein (gp120) and a transmembrane glycoprotein (gp41). Nucleotide sequence diversity in the *env* gene of HIV isolates is responsible for variable susceptibility of the virus to serum neutralization, a process mediated by an interaction between HIV and antibodies directed against gp120.

Four genes of HIV code for proteins that regulate viral gene expression: *vif* (virion infectivity factor), *nef* (negative factor), *tat* (transactivator of transcription), and *rev* (regulator of expression of virion proteins). The protein coded by *vif* (p23) probably influences viral infectivity, because virions with mutations in *vif* have reduced infectivity; however the mechanism has not been determined (56,57). The gene product of *nef* (p27) may down-regulate virus production, because virions with mutations in the *nef* gene replicate to higher titers than wild-type virus (58,59). The p27 product of different HIV isolates shows substantial sequence diversity, which supports its role in modulating the replicative properties of different HIV

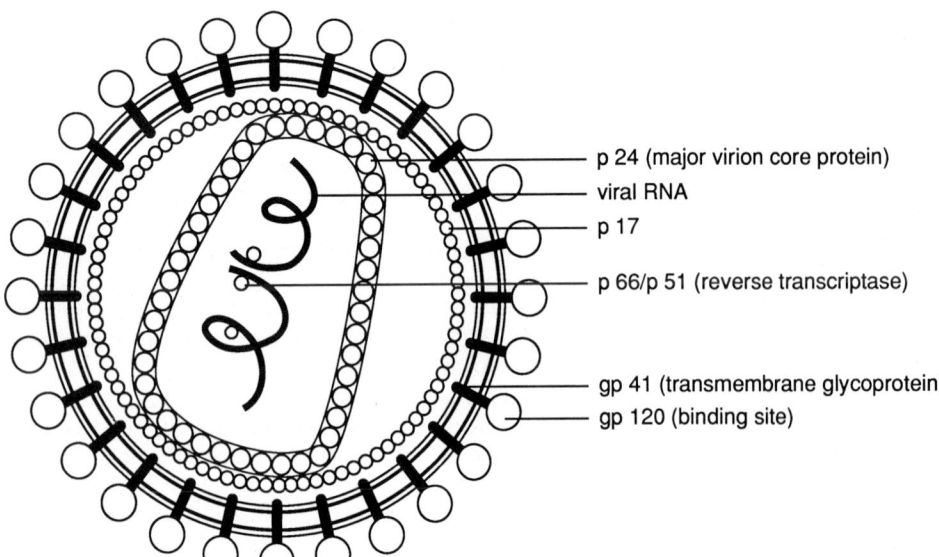

Fig. 22–1. Diagram of an HIV virion.

strains. The mechanism by which the *tat* gene product (p14) affects virus replication is not completely understood, although it appears to interact specifically with a region of the long terminal repeat (LTR) portion of the genome called the transacting responsive element (TAR) to enhance virus production (60,61). The *rev* regulatory protein (p20) is essential for viral replication and may control the level of processed viral messenger RNA (62). The functions of *vpr* and *vpu* gene products of HIV-1 and *vpx* gene products of HIV-2 are unknown.

Replication

The steps in the replication cycle of HIV (Fig. 22–2) are similar to those described earlier for retroviruses. The cycle begins with attachment of the viral gp120 surface glycoprotein to the cellular receptor—the CD4 antigen—found primarily on helper T lymphocytes and cells of the monocyte/macrophage lineage, although recent evidence suggests that alternate modes of HIV entry, as yet undefined, exist (63). After binding to target cells the viral envelope probably fuses directly with the cellular plasma membrane, a process that requires sequences located in gp41. The remainder of the cycle proceeds as outlined earlier for retroviruses.

Infection with HIV may induce a productive replication cycle, or the virus may establish a latent infection. The exact mechanism by which HIV is rendered latent is unknown; however, the *nef* gene product may down-regulate HIV replication from low levels of virus production to complete latency (64).

Different isolates of HIV have distinct biologic and molecular characteristics. For example, isolates of HIV-1 and HIV-2 vary in their ability to productively infect T lymphocytes, macrophages, glial cells, and fibroblasts, a trait apparently determined at least in part by the *env* region of the genome. Certain biologic characteristics of strains of HIV isolated from brain tissue differ from those of blood-derived strains. Brain isolates of HIV replicate well in primary macrophages, do not replicate in T-cell lines, are not cytopathic for CD4-positive cells, and are only minimally sensitive to serum neutralization. Blood isolates replicate poorly in primary macrophages but well in T-cell lines, are cytopathic for CD4-positive cells, and are much more sensitive to serum neutralization. The growth kinetics of isolates of HIV differ: some replicate rapidly, producing high titers of virus, whereas others replicate slowly and produce low levels of virus. Moreover, nucleotide sequences and biologic characteristics of HIV isolates obtained from the same person may change in vivo over time (64,65).

Epidemiology

In 1981, before HIV was discovered and a specific diagnostic test was available, investigators at the Centers for Disease Control (CDC) developed a specific, uniformly interpreted surveillance case definition of AIDS that included certain opportunistic diseases diagnosed by reliable methods in persons with no other known cause of immunodeficiency (67). This definition, used by all 50 states for the purpose of reporting cases of AIDS and adopted worldwide for surveillance of AIDS in all industrialized nations, was modified in 1985 and again in 1987 (68,69). The latter revision broadened the range of AIDS-indicative diseases (for example, by including HIV-induced encephalopathy and wasting syndrome), permitted inclusion of persons whose indicator disease was diagnosed presumptively, and improved the sensitivity and specificity of the definition by incorporating results of HIV diagnostic tests (Table 22–2) (70). Effective April 1, 1992, the CDC proposed a new AIDS case definition that includes those persons who meet the 1987 definition, and all adults and adolescents infected with HIV and with CD4 lymphocyte counts of less than 200 per microliter (70a).

As of December 31, 1991, 206,392 cases of AIDS, about

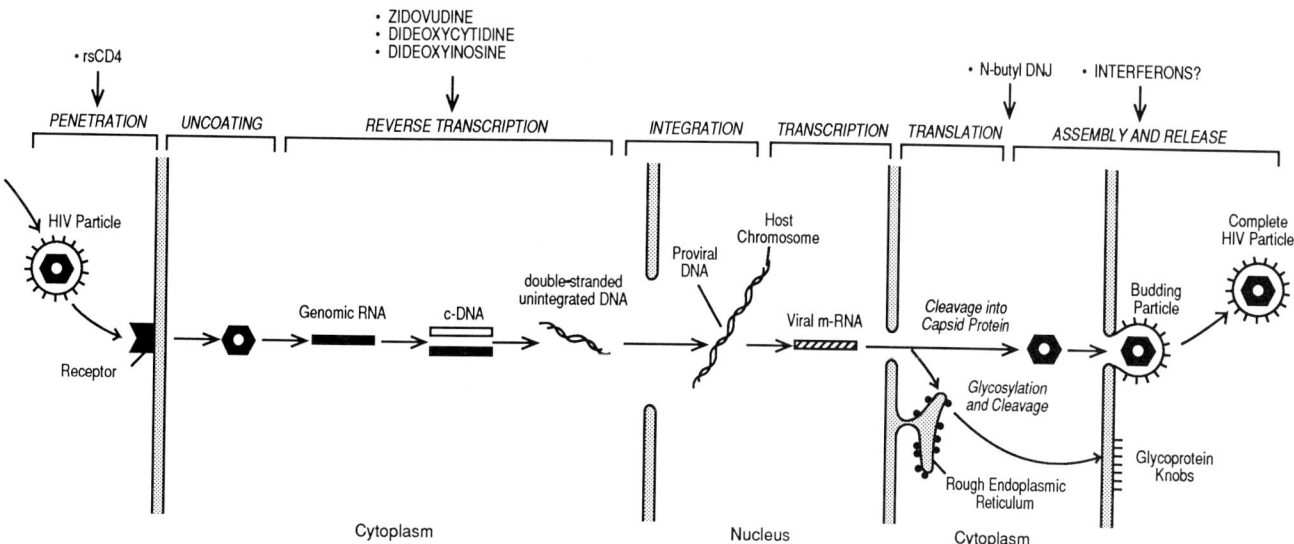

Fig. 22–2. Diagram of the replication cycle of HIV shows possible sites of attack for antiviral agents and examples of agents that act at specific targets. (From Hirsch, M.S.: Chemotherapy of human immunodeficiency virus infections: Current practice and future prospects. J. Infect. Dis., *161*:845, 1990.)

Table 22-2. 1987 Revised Surveillance Case Definition for AIDS

Laboratory Evidence of HIV Infection	Other Cause of Immunodeficiency	Diagnosis of Indicator Diseases	Indicator Diseases
Not performed or inconclusive	Absent	Definitive	Candidiasis of esophagus, trachea, bronchi, or lungs; extrapulmonary Cryptococcus neoformans; cryptosporidiosis (diarrhea >1 mo); CMV (excluding liver, spleen, lymph nodes) in person over age 1 mo; HSV mucocutaneous ulcer for >1 mo or bronchitis, pneumonitis, or esophagitis in person over age 1 mo; Kaposi's sarcoma in person under age 60 yr; primary CNS lymphoma in person under age 60 yr; LIP/PLH in child under age 13 yr; disseminated MAI or Mycobacterium kansasii; Pneumocystis carinii pneumonia; PML; CNS toxoplasmosis in person over age 1 mo.
Present	Absent or present	Definitive	All diseases listed above; multiple or recurrent serious bacterial infections* in child less than age 13 yr; disseminated coccidioidomycosis or histoplasmosis; isosporiasis (diarrhea >1 mo); Kaposi's sarcoma (any age); primary CNS lymphoma (any age); non-Hodgkin's lymphoma (B-cell or unknown phenotype); disseminated mycobacterial disease (not Mycobacterium tuberculosis); recurrent Salmonella septicemia; extrapulmonary M. tuberculosis; HIV wasting syndrome
Present	Absent or present	Presumptive	Esophageal candidiasis; CMV retinitis with vision loss; Kaposi's sarcoma; LIP/PLH in child under age 13 yr; disseminated mycobacterial disease (+ AFS; species not identified by culture); Pneumocystis carinii pneumonia; CNS toxoplasmosis in person over age 1 mo
Negative	Absent	Definitive	Pneumocystis carinii pneumonia; disease listed in first category above plus CD4 count <400/μl

* Caused by Haemophilus, Streptococcus, or other pyogenic bacteria.
Key: AIDS, acquired immunodeficiency syndrome; CMV, cytomegalovirus; HSV, herpes simplex virus; CNS, central nervous system; LIP/LPH, lymphoid interstitial pneumonia/pulmonary lymphoid hyperplasia; MAI, Mycobacterium avium-intracellulare; PML, progressive multifocal leukoencephalopathy; HIV, human immunodeficiency virus; AFS, acid-fast stain; +, positive.
(Data from Centers for Disease Control: Revision of the CDC surveillance case definition for acquired immunodeficiency syndrome. MMWR, 36 [suppl 1]: 1, 1987.)

98% in adults and adolescents, were reported in the United States (70,71). The first 100,000 cases were reported between June, 1981 and August, 1989; the second 100,000 between September, 1989 and November, 1991. The number of reported cases increased each year during the 1980s, and most patients were homosexual or bisexual males or intravenous drug users (72). The total number of AIDS cases and the number in these two risk groups increased most rapidly during the middle 1980s and more slowly in the late 1980s (Fig. 22-3). Cases associated with heterosexual transmission of HIV (predominantly to women) and those associated with perinatal transmission has increased steadily, whereas cases associated with transfusion of blood or blood products have stabilized (Figs. 22-4 through 22-6).

As a result of the 1987 revision of the case definition of AIDS, changes in the epidemiology of the disease in adults have been observed. The proportion of cases in whites decreased (63% in 1987; 56% in 1990) and increased in blacks and Hispanics (36% in 1987; 44% in 1990), reflecting the change in the proportion of cases among homosexual and bisexual males, which declined from 70% in 1987 to 60% in 1990, and among intravenous drug users, which increased from 14% in 1987 to 21% in 1990. Men have accounted for about 90% of all persons with AIDS reported in the United States, though the proportion of women with AIDS increased from 9% of the first 100,000 reported cases to 12% of the second 100,000 cases. In addition, the geographic distribution of AIDS cases in the United States has shifted. Cases reported from the mid-Atlantic region accounted for 54% of the total before 1984 and for only 32% of those reported in 1988 (69). During this same period the proportion of cases from all other regions increased, except the Pacific region, where it remained constant. The proportion of AIDS cases reported from standard metropolitan statistical areas with fewer than 500,000 population also has increased (from 12% before 1986 to 19% in 1988) (69).

The racial distribution of children with AIDS is similar to that of women with AIDS. As of December 31, 1988,

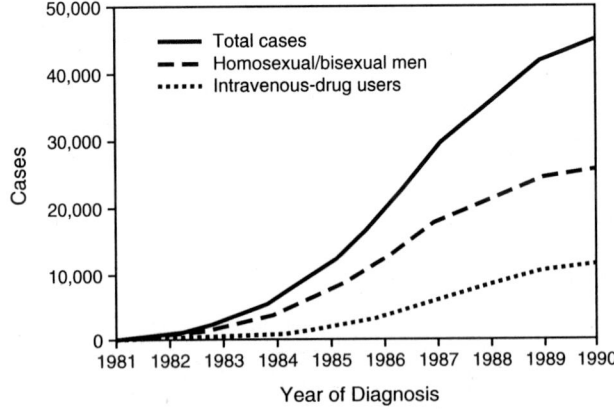

Fig. 22-3. Total cases of AIDS among homosexual or bisexual men (excluding intravenous drug users) and among women and heterosexual men who report intravenous drug use, by year of diagnosis in the United States, 1981-1990. Data are based on cases reported through March 1991 and adjusted for reporting delays. (From Centers for Disease Control: Update: Acquired immunodeficiency syndrome—United States, 1981-1990. MMWR, 40:358, 1991.)

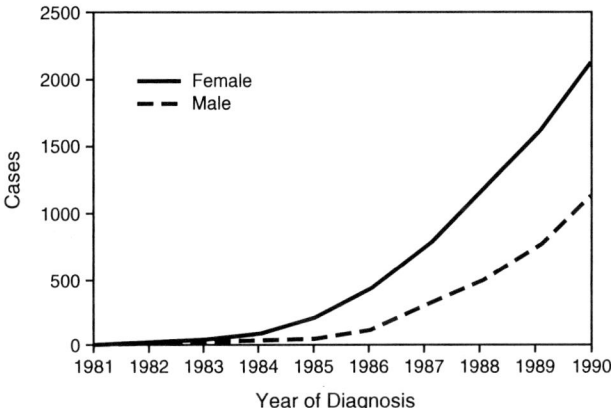

Fig. 22-4. AIDS cases among persons who report heterosexual contact with persons infected or at high risk of infection with HIV, by year of diagnosis in the United States, 1981–1990. Data are based on cases reported through March 1991 and adjusted for reporting delays. (From Centers for Disease Control: Update: Acquired immunodeficiency syndrome—United States, 1981–1990. MMWR, 40:358, 1991.)

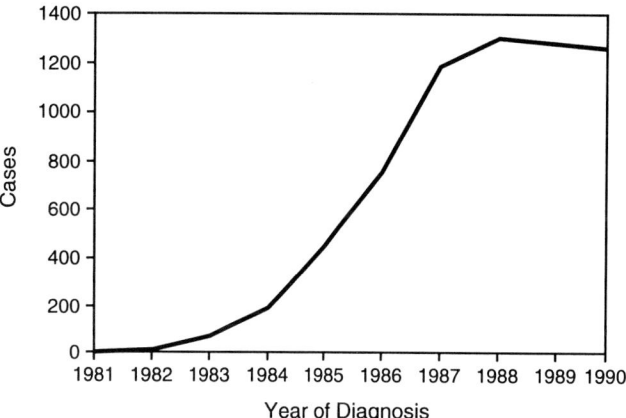

Fig. 22-5. Perinatally acquired pediatric AIDS cases, by year of diagnosis in the United States, 1981–1990. Data are based on cases reported through March 1991 and adjusted for reporting delays. (From Centers for Disease Control: Update: Acquired immunodeficiency syndrome—United States, 1981–1990. MMWR, 40:358, 1991.)

53% of children were black; 24%, white; 23%, Hispanic; and fewer than 1% each, Asian/Pacific Islander or American Indian/Alaskan Native (73). Risk factors for affected mothers of affected children included intravenous drug use (54%), sex with an intravenous drug user (19%) or with a man otherwise at increased risk of or infected with HIV (7%), birth in a country where heterosexual transmission of HIV predominates (11%), transfusion (2%), and undetermined (7%). The proportion of mothers whose sex partners were at increased risk of or infected with HIV increased from 11% before 1985 to 21% in 1988, whereas the proportion born in countries where heterosexual transmission predominates concurrently decreased from 22 to 7%. Black and Hispanic children with AIDS were more likely than white children to have mothers who reported intravenous drug use or sex with an intravenous drug user.

From 1981 through 1991, 133,232 deaths among persons with AIDS in the United States were reported to the CDC, nearly one third of them in 1990 (70,74). By 1988, AIDS had become the third leading cause of death among men 25 to 44 years of age and was second by the end of 1991 (72). Since 1984, AIDS has been the leading cause of premature death for single males aged 25 to 44 years in New York City and San Francisco, and by 1986, it had become the eighth leading cause of premature mortality in the United States (75,76). In women 25 to 44 years of age AIDS was the eighth leading cause of death in 1988, is estimated at fifth in 1991, and is the leading cause of death among black women in this age group in New York State and New Jersey (74,77,78). In certain parts of the country AIDS has become a leading cause of death among children. For example, in 1988 in New York State, AIDS was the leading cause of death among Hispanic children 1 to 4 years of age and the second leading cause among black children in the same age group (74). In all age groups death rates are highest among blacks and Hispanics. In 1990 the number of reported AIDS-related deaths per 100,000 population was about 29 for blacks, 22 for Hispanics, 9 for whites, and 3 each for Asian/Pacific Islanders and American Indians/Alaskan Natives.

Soon after the initial descriptions of AIDS in the United States, persons (primarily homosexual and bisexual men) with similar clinical, immune system, and epidemiologic features were reported from Europe; and by 1983, cases were recognized in natives of the Caribbean and Central Africa who resided in Europe (79,80). The epidemiology of the disease in the Caribbean and Central Africa was different. An equal proportion of cases among men and women suggested heterosexual transmission, and homosexuality and intravenous drug use were uncommon risk factors (81–84). Subsequent studies of the origin and global dissemination of infection with HIV showed that antibodies to HIV were present in stored serum speci-

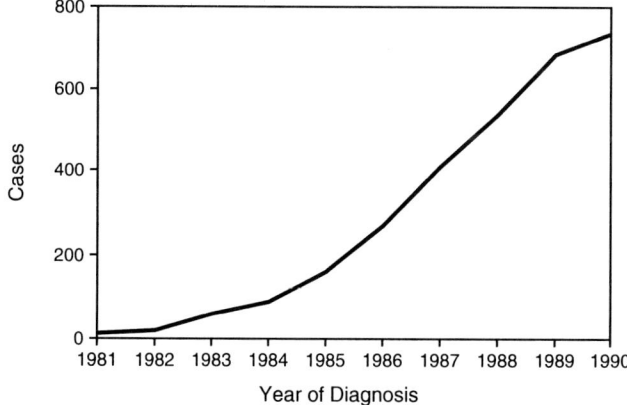

Fig. 22-6. Cases of AIDS associated with transfusion of blood or blood products, by year of diagnosis in the United States, 1981–1990. Data are based on cases reported through March 1991 and adjusted for reporting delays. (From Centers for Disease Control: Update: Acquired immunodeficiency syndrome—United States, 1981–1990. MMWR, 40:358, 1991.)

mens obtained in 1959 in Zaire and in 1963 in Burkina Faso, indicating that infection with HIV occurred sporadically before the recognized epidemic in the United States and Africa (85,86).

Today, infection with HIV is considered a pandemic. Cases of AIDS have been reported to the World Health Organization (WHO) from 163 countries, and infections with HIV have been documented in almost all countries (87). The WHO estimates that currently about 10 million adults (6 million in Africa, 1 million each in North America, South America, and Asia, and 500,000 in Europe) and 1 million children are infected with HIV and that 40 million persons may be infected by the year 2000 (71,87). By that time, more than 90% will reside in developing countries in sub-Saharan Africa, South and Southeast Asia, Latin America, and the Caribbean. Moreover, mothers or both parents of more than 10 million children will have died from HIV infection or AIDS during the 1990s.

HIV is transmitted during sexual contact; via artificial insemination; from mother to child in utero, by exposure to maternal blood at birth, or post partum in breast milk; via sharing of needles or other drug paraphernalia among intravenous drug users; and via transfusion of blood or blood products and transplantation of organs from HIV-seropositive donors, though the latter is unlikely when the donor's HIV immune status has been determined (88–96). A small but definite occupational risk of infection with HIV exists for health care workers exposed to HIV-infected blood via needlestick injury, contamination of skin lesions, or direct mucous membrane contact and for laboratory personnel who work with HIV (97–99). Moreover, HIV has been transmitted to persons receiving dental care from a dentist with AIDS (100–102).

In the United States sexual transmission has occurred predominantly between homosexual males, whose risk of infection increases with the number of sexual partners and with the frequency of receptive anal intercourse. However, heterosexual transmission, primarily male-to-female, is increasing in the United States, and it is the predominant mode of sexual transmission in Africa, where the level of sexual activity with multiple partners is the major risk factor, and the presence of genital ulcers in both males and females, and the lack of circumcision of males are important cofactors (83,103–105). In Western countries and in Africa, the most profoundly immunosuppressed persons are most likely to transmit the virus (93,106–108).

Pathogenesis

Infection with HIV results in a spectrum of immune system, neurologic, and enteropathic abnormalities. Profound immunosuppression results from depletion of the CD4-positive helper/inducer subset of T lymphocytes, which have many direct and indirect immune functions: they activate macrophages, secrete factors that stimulate hematopoiesis and the growth and differentiation of lymphocytes, and act as effector cells for B lymphocytes, cytotoxic and suppressor T lymphocytes, and natural killer cells. The mechanisms of this depletion, however, are not completely understood. HIV is cytopathic for CD4-positive lymphocytes in vitro, yet a direct viral cytopathic effect probably is not the only factor responsible for the dramatic decrease in CD4-positive lymphocytes, because a very small percentage of peripheral blood lymphocytes of HIV-infected persons express the virus at any given time (109). The mechanisms of direct cell killing by HIV are not known, but different hypotheses have been suggested (109–111). For example, infection of a cell with HIV may alter the membrane integrity, causing enhanced permeability to calcium, sodium, and potassium ions, subsequent increased intracellular volume, and, eventually, cell rupture. In HIV-infected cells, a reduction in phosphatidylcholine (an important structural component of the cell membrane) and diacylglycerol (an intermediate in phospholipid synthesis) may be involved in cell death. The accumulation of unintegrated viral DNA may interrupt cellular functions. Moreover, host immune responses such as antibody-dependent cellular cytotoxicity or cell-mediated cytotoxicity may kill infected cells.

In addition to direct killing of CD4-positive lymphocytes by HIV, cell death also may occur by indirect mechanisms (109–111). In vitro, HIV-infected CD4-positive cells with high levels of gp120 on their surface fuse with uninfected CD4-positive cells, forming nonviable multinucleate giant cells (syncytia), a phenomenon that could occur in vivo. Antilymphocyte antibodies linked to an 18-kd antigen on HIV-infected CD4-positive cells, which are detected in some persons with AIDS, may play a role in depleting CD4-positive cells. Attachment of circulating gp120 to uninfected CD4-positive cells may mediate autoimmune attack by gp120-specific antibody-dependent cellular cytotoxicity or cytotoxic T lymphocytes. Moreover, autoimmunization with class II–like antigens (see Chapter 2) may develop as follows: The CD4 molecule of the T lymphocyte recognizes a portion of the class II major histocompatibility complex (MHC) molecule and gp120 of HIV; therefore, if gp120 could mimic the configuration of a portion of the class II MHC antigen, antibodies and cytotoxic lymphocytes directed against gp120 could cross-react with class II MHC antigens.

Although quantitative depletion of CD4-positive lymphocytes is the predominant immune system abnormality in HIV infection, qualitative or functional defects occur in the subset of CD4-positive lymphocytes that recognize and respond to soluble antigens and in other immune cells (110,111). Circulating gp120 released from HIV-infected cells may suppress blastogenic activity, antigen presentation, allogeneic responses, and interleukin-2 activity. Natural killer cells have diminished cytotoxicity, and monocytes have defective chemotaxis and killing of certain organisms. Abnormalities of B lymphocytes include the inability to mount an adequate immunoglobulin (Ig) M response to antigenic challenge, the development of hypergammaglobulinemia with circulating immune complexes, and the formation of autoantibodies. Nonspecific deposition of immune complexes on platelet, neutrophil, and erythrocyte membranes may result in premature lysis or removal from the circulation. Autoantibodies in HIV-infected persons have been associated with thrombocytopenic purpura and depletion of CD4-positive lymphocytes (113,114).

The monocyte/macrophage, the predominant cell infected with HIV in the brain, may be essential in the pathogenesis of central nervous system disease in HIV-infected persons. Monocyte-derived cytokines are chemotactic for neutrophils and may be toxic to neuronal tissue (110). Moreover, partial sequence homology exists between HIV gp120 and the neurotropic factor neuroleukin, and competition between the two for neuroleukin receptors in the brain may inhibit neuroleukin-induced neuronal growth (115).

The monocyte/macrophage also may be involved in the pathogenesis of the diarrhea and intestinal malabsorption frequently associated with HIV infection (111). Aberrant macrophage function may allow infection with intestinal parasites such as cryptosporidia, Isospora belli, and Strongyloides stercoralis. Moreover, cytokines secreted by HIV-infected macrophages in the lamina propria or direct infection by HIV of enterochromaffin cells regulating motility and digestive function may contribute to the enteropathy, particularly when no intestinal pathogen is detected.

Clinical Manifestations

The clinical manifestations of infection with HIV range from no symptoms to severe immunosuppression and life-threatening infectious diseases or malignancies. In an attempt to improve reporting and surveillance of infection with HIV, epidemiologic studies, prevention and control activities, and public health policies and planning, investigators at the CDC established a hierarchical system by which adults who are infected with HIV are classified into four mutually exclusive groups (Table 22–3), defined below (116).

Group I includes persons who develop a mononucleosis-like syndrome (fever, arthralgias, malaise, diarrhea, sore throat, rash), with or without aseptic meningitis, associated with seroconversion to HIV. The interval between exposure to HIV and onset of the acute illness ranges from a few days to 3 months (117). HIV can be isolated from peripheral mononuclear cells and plasma during the acute illness, and frequently for several years thereafter (94,117). The serologic response to the infection is diagrammed in Figure 22–7. The core antigen (p24) of HIV is detected within 1 to 4 weeks. Specific IgM appears as early as 5 days after the onset of illness, peaks at about day 24, and disappears by about day 80. Immunoglobulin G to the core and envelope (gp41) antigens develops 3 to 12 weeks after infection and usually persists for life. In one study of 1000 HIV-seropositive homosexual males without AIDS four (0.4%) reverted to HIV seronegativity, yet provirus was detected by gene amplification in all four (118). All persons in group I are reclassified after the acute illness resolves.

Persons in group II have neither signs nor symptoms of infection and may be subclassified, based on the presence or absence of lymphopenia, thrombocytopenia, decreased number of CD4-positive lymphocytes, and cutaneous anergy. Group III exhibit lymph node enlargement of 1 cm or greater at at least two extrainguinal sites that persists more than 3 months in the absence of a concurrent illness

Table 22–3. Centers for Disease Control Classification Systems for Infection With Human Immunodeficiency Virus

I. Classification system for HIV infection in adults
   Group I   Acute infection
   Group II   Asymptomatic infection
   Group III Persistent generalized lymphadenopathy
   Group IV Other diseases
     Subgroup A Constitutional disease including HIV wasting syndrome in the CDC surveillance definition for AIDS (see Table 22–2)
     Subgroup B Neurologic disease including HIV encephalopathy in the CDC surveillance definition for AIDS
     Subgroup C Secondary infectious diseases
       Category C-1 Specified secondary infectious diseases in the CDC surveillance definition for AIDS
       Category C-2 Other specified secondary infectious diseases
     Subgroup D Secondary cancers in the CDC surveillance definition for AIDS
     Subgroup E Other conditions
II. Classification system for HIV infection in children under age 13 yr
   Class P-0 Indeterminate infection
   Class P-1 Asymptomatic infection
     Subclass A Normal immune function
     Subclass B Abnormal immune function
     Subclass C Immune function not tested
   Class P-2 Symptomatic infection
     Subclass A Nonspecific findings
     Subclass B Progressive neurologic disease, including HIV encephalopathy in the CDC surveillance definition for AIDS
     Subclass C Lymphoid interstitial pneumonitis in the CDC surveillance definition for AIDS
     Subclass D Secondary infectious diseases
       Category D-1 Specified secondary infectious diseases in the CDC surveillance definition for AIDS
       Category D-2 Recurrent serious bacterial infections in the CDC surveillance definition for AIDS
       Category D-3 Other specified secondary infectious diseases
     Subclass E Secondary cancers
       Category E-1 Specified secondary cancers in the CDC surveillance definition for AIDS
       Category E-2 Other cancers possibly secondary to HIV infection
     Subclass F Other diseases possibly due to HIV infection

(From Centers for Disease Control: Classification system for human T-lymphotropic virus type III/Lymphadenopathy-associated virus infection. MMWR, 35:334, 1986; and Centers for Disease Control: Classification system for human immunodeficiency virus [HIV] infection in children under 13 years of age. MMWR, 36:225, 1987.)

or condition other than infection with HIV to explain the lymphadenopathy.

The duration of the asymptomatic carrier state in adults varies but usually is prolonged, and the risk of disease progression, low in the first several years, increases with time. In one study of homosexual and bisexual men with known dates of seroconversion, 5% developed AIDS after 3 years and 48% after 10 years (119). In a similar study of adults with hemophilia, none developed AIDS within 2 years and 22% developed AIDS within 7 years; however, the rate of progression to AIDS in children and young adults with hemophilia who seroconverted before age 22 years appears to be lower: in one study only 11% had developed AIDS after 7 years (120,121). In contrast, the rate of disease progression in recipients of blood transfu-

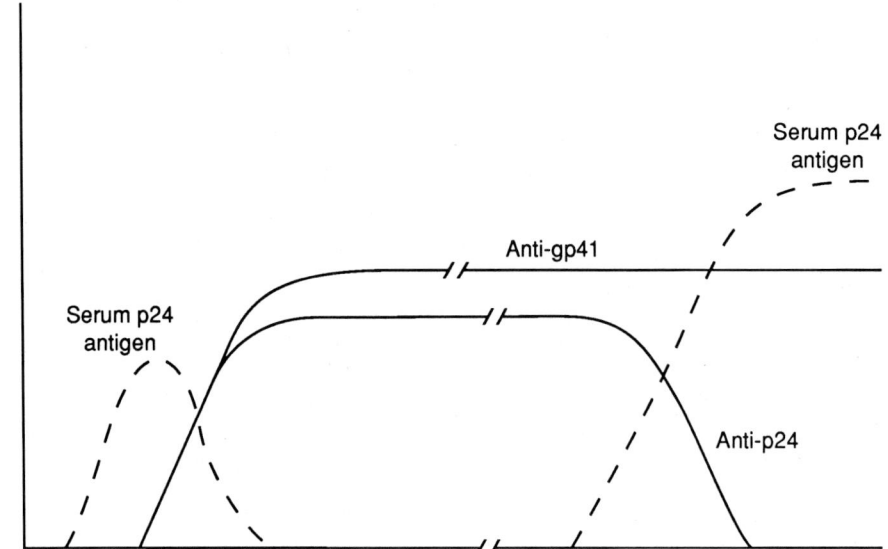

Fig. 22–7. Typical serologic response to HIV infection.

sions may be more rapid. In one analysis, 36 and 55% of persons with transfusion-acquired infection developed AIDS within 5 and 7 years, respectively (122). The rate of disease progression in intravenous drug users has not been firmly established.

Signs and symptoms that correlate with increased likelihood of developing AIDS include fever, night sweats, weight loss, oral candidiasis, hairy leukoplakia, and zoster; and once generalized lymphadenopathy is present its resolution or shrinking of lymph nodes may be associated with progression to AIDS (119). Laboratory predictors of disease progression are persistent HIV p24 antigenemia and a low absolute number of CD4-positive lymphocytes (fewer than 200 cells/μl) or a low CD4-CD8 (helper-suppressor) ratio (121,123). The rate of progression to AIDS or advanced AIDS-related complex in asymptomatic adults infected with HIV who have fewer than 500 CD4-positive lymphocytes per microliter, however, can be reduced significantly by zidovudine treatment (124).

Group IV includes persons with clinical signs and symptoms of infection with HIV other than or in addition to lymphadenopathy, further classified into one or more subgroups based on clinical findings. Subgroup A includes persons with one or more of the following: fever, diarrhea persisting more than 1 month, or involuntary weight loss of greater than 10% of baseline in the absence of a concurrent illness or condition other than infection with HIV to explain the findings. Subgroup B includes those with dementia, myelopathy, or peripheral neuropathy in the absence of a concurrent illness or condition other than infection with HIV to explain the findings.

Persons in subgroup C, secondary infectious diseases (indicative of a defect in cell-mediated immunity), are subdivided into two categories. Those in category C-1 have one of 12 specified secondary diseases included in the surveillance definition of AIDS: chronic cryptosporidiosis, toxoplasmosis, extraintestinal strongyloidiasis, isosporiasis, candidiasis of the esophagus, bronchi, or lung, cryptococcosis, histoplasmosis, infection with Mycobacterium avium-intracellulare or Mycobacterium kansasii, chronic cutaneous or disseminated infection with herpes simplex virus (HSV), and progressive multifocal leukoencephalopathy. Category C-2 includes those with one of six other specified secondary infectious diseases: oral hairy leukoplakia, multidermal herpes zoster, recurrent bacteremia caused by Salmonella, nocardiosis, tuberculosis, and oral candidiasis. Subgroup D includes persons with an HIV-associated malignancy indicative of a defect in cell-mediated immunity: Kaposi's sarcoma, non-Hodgkin's lymphoma (small, noncleaved lymphoma or immunoblastic sarcoma), or primary central nervous system lymphoma. In subgroup E are persons with other clinical findings or diseases that may be attributed to infection with HIV, are indicative of a defect in cell-mediated immunity, or both.

Once AIDS is diagnosed, the patient frequently survives less than 1 year, although the interval varies considerably. Among adults, survival is shorter for women, ethnic minorities, intravenous drug users, and elders (125,126). Data from early studies indicated that an initial presentation with pneumonia caused by Pneumocystis carinii was associated with decreased survival time, but more recently, survival among this group has improved significantly (125–129). Persons with Kaposi's sarcoma survive longer, and for them, younger age at diagnosis, absence of opportunistic infections, and earlier stages of clinical illness correlate with a more favorable prognosis (125–128). Moreover, persons with AIDS who are treated with zidovudine have less severe opportunistic infections and live longer (see Treatment) (129–131).

A separate system has been proposed to classify the manifestations of HIV infection in children (see Table 22–3). Class P-0 includes infants and children up to 15 months of age who have antibodies to HIV, indicating perinatal exposure to the virus, but who cannot be classified as definitely infected according to the definition outlined in Table 22–4 (132). Infants in class P-0 who become seronegative, whose blood and tissues are virus-culture negative (if cultured), and who have no clinical or laboratory-confirmed abnormalities associated with HIV probably are not infected. Class P-1 includes children who fulfill the criteria for infection with HIV (see Table 22–4) and have no signs or symptoms allowing classification in Class P-2. These children may be subclassified based on immune function.

Children in Class P-2 are subclassified based on signs and symptoms. Subclass A includes children who exhibit persistence of two or more of the following unexplained findings for more than 2 months: fever, failure to thrive or weight loss greater than 10% of baseline, hepatomegaly, splenomegaly, generalized lymphadenopathy, parotitis, and persistent or recurrent diarrhea. Subclass B includes children with at least one of the following progressive findings: regression beyond developmental milestones or loss of intellectual ability, impaired brain growth, or progressive symmetric motor deficits manifested by two or more of these findings: paresis, abnormal tone, pathologic reflexes, ataxia, or gait disturbances. Subclass C includes those with histologically confirmed pneumonitis (diffuse interstitial and peribronchial infiltrates of lymphocytes and plasma cells without identifiable pathogens) or, in the absence of a tissue and microbiologic diagnosis, radiographically diagnosed chronic pneumonitis that is unresponsive to appropriate antimicrobial therapy for at least 2 months.

Children in subclass D are subcategorized into D-1 (pneumonia caused by Pneumocystis carinii; chronic cryptosporidiosis; disseminated toxoplasmosis; infection with HSV with onset after 1 month of age; esophageal, bronchial, or pulmonary candidiasis; extrapulmonary cryptococcosis; disseminated histoplasmosis; noncutaneous, extrapulmonary, or disseminated infection with a Mycobacterium species other than Mycobacterium leprae; extrapulmonary or disseminated coccidioidomycosis; nocardiosis; and progressive multifocal leukoencephalopathy), D-2 (two or more serious bacterial infections—sepsis, meningitis, pneumonia, visceral abscess, osteomyelitis, arthritis—in 2 years), and D-3 (persistent oral candidiasis, two or more episodes of stomatitis caused by HSV in 1 year or multidermal or disseminated zoster). Children in subclass E are categorized as E-1 (those with Kaposi's sarcoma, B-cell non-Hodgkin's lymphoma, or primary central nervous system lymphoma) or E-2 (those with other malignancies possibly related to infection with HIV). Included in subclass F are children with other conditions possibly due to infection with HIV—hepatitis, cardiomyopathy, nephropathy, anemia, thrombocytopenia, and dermatologic diseases.

In children, the length of survival appears to be influenced by age at diagnosis and type of opportunistic disease at initial presentation. In one study, infants had a shorter median survival time than children over age 1 year (4 months versus 11 months). Those with pneumonia caused by Pneumocystis carinii had the worst prognosis (median survival, 1 month), and those developing encephalopathy, renal disease, or candidal esophagitis had a median survival under one year. Children with lymphocytic interstitial pneumonitis and recurrent bacterial infections had a better prognosis (median survival after diagnosis, 72 and 50 months, respectively) (133).

Many clinical manifestations of AIDS reflect a secondary infectious disease and so are discussed with the specific organisms elsewhere in the text. The opportunistic pathogens that most often cause disease in persons with AIDS are Pneumocystis carinii, cytomegalovirus, Cryptococcus neoformans, Mycobacterium avium-intracellulare, Mycobacterium tuberculosis, HSV, Candida species, Toxoplasma gondii, JC virus, Cryptosporidium, and Isospora belli. In geographic areas where Histoplasma capsulatum or Coccidioides immitis is endemic, histoplasmosis or coccidioidomycosis is common. Pyogenic bacteria such as Streptococcus pneumoniae, Haemophilus influenzae, and Salmonella species may cause recurrent infections, especially in children. Infections with Nocardia and Aspergillus are less frequent.

Manifestations of AIDS specifically related to infection with HIV include a wasting syndrome, chronic diarrhea, nephropathy (proteinuria and a mildly elevated serum creatinine value) and various neurologic complications (134–136). Aseptic meningitis, characterized by headache, fever, nuchal rigidity, and cranial nerve palsies, occurs early in the disease in 10 to 20% of cases. Vacuolar myelopathy, manifested by gait ataxia, progressive spastic paraparesis, posterior column deficits, and incontinence, develops in about 10 to 20%. Peripheral neuropathies—chronic distal symmetric polyneuropathy and chronic inflammatory demyelinating polyneuropathy—occur in 10 to 50% of persons with AIDS. Subacute encephalitis (or AIDS dementia complex), characterized by cognitive deficits, memory loss, depression, organic psychosis, psychomotor slowing, pryamidal tract signs, seizures, and incontinence, eventually develops in 70 to 90% of cases.

In addition to the opportunistic infections and manifes-

Table 22–4. Summary of the Definition of Infection With Human Immunodeficiency Virus in Children

Infants and children under 15 months of age with perinatal infection
1. Virus in blood or tissues
   or
2. HIV antibody
   and
      evidence of both cellular and humoral immune deficiency
   and
      one or more categories in Class P-2 (see Table 22–3)
   or
3. Symptoms meeting CDC case definitions for AIDS (Table 22–2)

Older children with perinatal infection and children with HIV infection acquired through other modes of transmission
1. Virus in blood or tissues
   or
2. HIV antibodies
   or
3. Symptoms meeting CDC case definition for AIDS

(From Centers for Disease Control: Classification system for human immunodeficiency virus [HIV] infection in children under 13 years of age. MMWR, 36:225, 1987.)

tations directly attributable to infection with HIV, malignancies, particularly Kaposi's sarcoma and non-Hodgkin's lymphoma, frequently cause morbidity and mortality in persons with AIDS. Kaposi's sarcoma in persons with AIDS differs from "classic" Kaposi's sarcoma, which is an uncommon, relatively indolent cutaneous neoplasm of elderly men in the United States, an endemic malignancy in central Africa, and a complication of corticosteroid administration in recipients of organ transplants (137–141). In persons with AIDS, predominantly homosexual males, Kaposi's sarcoma occurs at an earlier age; is more aggressive, rarely limited to a single anatomic region; and commonly involves the head and neck area and visceral organs (142,143). In early studies Kaposi's sarcoma was present at diagnosis in about 35% of persons with AIDS; whereas recently, fewer than 10% have the malignancy, and when present, it appears to be associated with a more rapid progression to death (144,145). Explanations for the predominance of Kaposi's sarcoma in male homosexuals, its declining prevalence, and its more rapid course still elude investigators. Recreational drug use, an as yet unidentified sexually transmitted virus, and HIV-induced endothelial growth factors have been suggested but not proven (146–148).

Non-Hodgkin's lymphoma, the second most common malignancy associated with AIDS, develops in fewer than 1% of persons with AIDS in the United States and has no preference for any specific group. This high-grade B-cell neoplasm (large-cell, undifferentiated, or immunoblastic types) involves the central nervous system, peripheral lymph nodes, and virtually any organ outside the central nervous system. Although its pathogenesis is unknown, a relationship to Epstein-Barr virus (EBV) has been proposed, because EBV DNA is found in tissue from some tumors (see Chapter 5) (149).

Laboratory Diagnosis

Human T-cell leukemia viruses. Infection with HTLV-1 should be suspected when an adult from an endemic area (discussed earlier) presents with a cutaneous T-cell malignancy such as mycosis fungoides, Sezary syndrome, or cutaneous T-cell lymphoma or with a progressive degenerative neurologic disease. The diagnosis of adult T-cell leukemia/lymphoma is confirmed by demonstrating antibodies to HTLV-I in serum and monoclonal integration of proviral DNA in the malignant cells. Neurologic disease caused by HTLV-I is diagnosed by demonstrating antibodies to the virus in serum, CSF (or both), detecting viral DNA or viral proteins in CSF, or isolating the virus from CSF (150). Serum specimens are first screened for antibodies to HTLV-I by an enzyme-linked immunoassay (EIA), and positive results are confirmed by Western blot assay, demonstrating antibodies to products of the *gag* (p24) and the *env* (gp46 or gp61/68) genes. With currently available EIA tests, antibodies to HTLV-I and to HTLV-II cannot be distinguished. Definitive characterization of the infecting virus requires its isolation from peripheral blood mononuclear cells or lymphoma tissue and gene amplification.

Human immunodeficiency viruses. Infection with HIV is diagnosed by detecting specific antibodies or viral antigens in serum or plasma; isolating HIV from peripheral blood mononuclear cells, plasma, or CSF; or detecting proviral DNA in peripheral blood mononuclear cells, nucleated cells from the CSF, or tissues. Of the serologic assays that detect antibodies to HIV-1, the EIA is used most frequently, principally as a screening test for blood donors and for persons at risk of infection with HIV (150). Sera that repeatably test positive for HIV-1 by EIA are confirmed with a supplemental test, most commonly the Western blot (Fig. 22–8).

The sensitivity and specificity of the Western blot for detection of antibodies to the different proteins of HIV is high; however currently the criteria for a positive Western blot test are not uniform (see Table 22–5). The criteria proposed by the Association of State and Territorial Public Health Laboratory Directors provide the highest percentage of positive and the lowest percentage of indeterminate results and, therefore, are recommended by the CDC (151). All groups agree on the definition of negative (absence of all bands) and indeterminate (the presence of any band or bands not meeting the positive criteria) Western blot results. Persons with repeatedly indeterminate Western blot results for at least 6 months may be considered negative for antibodies to HIV-1 if they have no known risk factors, clinical symptoms, or other findings.

Other supplemental tests used to confirm a repeatably positive HIV-1 EIA result are the indirect immunofluorescent assay and radioimmunoprecipitation. To perform the indirect immunofluorescent assay, a mixture of HIV-infected and uninfected lymphocytes is fixed on a slide, test serum is added, and the slide is incubated and stained with fluorescein isothiocyanate-labeled antihuman IgG. Results of this assay correlate well with those of the Western blot; a kit for commercial use recently was licensed by the Food and Drug Administration. Radioimmunoprecipitation requires actively growing HIV-1–infected cells to prepare radiolabeled viral proteins, so it is not practical for routine clinical use.

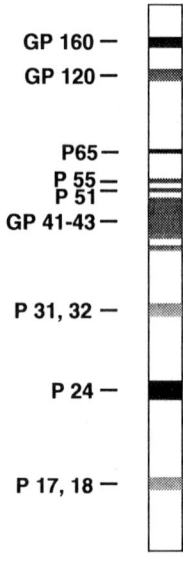

Fig. 22–8. Example of a positive Western blot assay result.

Table 22-5. Criteria for Positive Interpretation of Western Blot Tests

Organization	Criteria
Association of State and Territorial Public Health Laboratory Directors/CDC	Any two of: p24 gp41 gp120/gp160*
FDA-licensed DuPont test	p24 and p31 *and* gp41 or gp120/gp160
American Red Cross	≥3 bands −1 from each gene-product group: GAG *and* POL *and* ENV
Consortium for Retrovirus Serology Standardization	≥2 bands: p24 *or* p31, plus gp41 *or* gp120/gp160

* Distinguishing the gp120 band from the gp160 band often is very difficult. These two glycoproteins can be considered as one reactant for purposes of interpreting Western blot test results.
(From Centers for Disease Control: Interpretation and use of the Western blot assay for serodiagnosis of human immunodeficiency virus type 1 infections. MMWR, *38*[S-7]:1, 1989.)

Rapid screening assays for detection of antibodies to HIV-1 are based on hemagglutination, latex particle agglutination, or a form of immunoblotting (152-154). Results, however, are falsely positive in persons with various medical conditions, and because the end point of the assays is subjective, the reliability of the results depends on the skill of the individual performing the test. EIA tests to detect HIV-1 core antigen (p24) in body fluids are useful for monitoring the efficacy of antiviral therapy (discussed later) and for determining the prognosis for disease progression in asymptomatic persons infected with HIV-1 (150). A practical limitation of the test is its inability to detect the p24 antigen in the presence of high anti-p24 antibody titers; however, acid pretreatment of samples to dissociate immune complexes improves the detection and quantitation of p24 antigen (155).

Currently, the reference method for identifying infection with HIV is culture, performed by coculturing lymphocytes with an indicator cell line (for example, transformed T-cell lines: H9 or HUT-78 or monocyte/macrophage cells) or with peripheral blood mononuclear cells from a healthy, HIV-seronegative adult. Cultures are maintained for a minimum of 4 weeks and assayed weekly for evidence of virus-specific markers: reverse transcriptase or p24 antigen. Recently, the CDC published a standardized coculture procedure (155a). The rate of recovery of HIV-1 is greatest from blood (mononuclear cells or plasma), but virus has been cultured from cervical secretions, CSF, semen, saliva, human milk, and tears. Virus culture requires a maximum-containment facility and, so, cannot be performed in a routine clinical virology laboratory. Moreover, it is costly, time consuming, labor intensive, and creates the potential for exposure of laboratory personnel to high concentrations of the virus.

Enzymatic gene amplification using the polymerase chain reaction is an extremely sensitive method of detecting HIV, especially in situations where the viral RNA or proviral DNA is present in too few cells or in numbers too small for detection by other methods, such as identifying infection with HIV in infants (150,156,157). Because maternal IgG crosses the placenta and is present in the neonate's blood in approximately the same concentration as in the mother's blood, the neonate's HIV-1 (IgG) immune status cannot be used as a marker of viral infection, and reliable serum tests for HIV-1 IgM currently are not available. Usually, HIV-1 is present in a small proportion of the infant's peripheral blood mononuclear cells, so it is more likely to be detected by a very sensitive technique such as nucleic acid amplification than by culture.

Infection with HIV-2 is diagnosed serologically by detecting specific antibodies in serum or plasma or by recovering the virus from peripheral blood. Moreover, gene amplification has been used successfully to differentiate between infections with HIV-1 and HIV-2 (158).

Treatment

Human T-cell leukemia viruses. No agents that significantly prolong survival of individuals with adult T-cell leukemia/lymphoma are available currently. Treatment of HTLV-I–associated myelopathy with oral corticosteroids has had variable clinical efficacy (159).

Human immunodeficiency viruses. As the replication cycle and pathogenic mechanisms of HIV have become better understood, many approaches to therapy acting at virus-specific sites have been developed (see Fig. 22-2). Recombinant soluble preparations of the CD4 receptor molecule lacking the transmembrane and cytoplasmic domains should inhibit viral attachment to susceptible host cells; however, initial phase I clinical trials with various recombinant soluble CD4 preparations showed no significant changes in immune function or CD4 cell counts (160,161). Approaches to improve current preparations are under evaluation; but because certain cells may become infected by other mechanisms recombinant soluble CD4 preparations as single agents probably will not be sufficient for virus control (162-165).

The HIV DNA polymerase, a component of the reverse transcriptase, has been the major target for the antiviral agents developed to date. Antivirals that inhibit this step in the replicative cycle are the dideoxynucleoside analogues: zidovudine (AZT), dideoxycytidine, and dideoxyinosine (ddI), which become incorporated into the growing proviral DNA chain and terminate its elongation. Zidovudine, licensed in the United States in 1987 for treatment of symptomatic adults infected with HIV, is the mainstay of drugs active against HIV. It significantly prolongs survival of persons with advanced infection and delays progression of asymptomatic or early symptomatic infection in persons with 500 CD4 cells per microliter or fewer in the peripheral blood (129-131). However, clinical failures following AZT therapy occur, related to the emergence of HIV strains that are resistant to the drug (166,167).

Dideoxycytidine and ddI currently are in late stages of clinical evaluation (168-171). Results of phase I trials to evaluate the toxicity of ddI in persons with AIDS or AIDS-related complex indicate that the agent has antiretroviral activity. Its administration is associated with significant decreases in serum levels of p24 antigen, increases in numbers of CD4-positive lymphocytes, and clinical improvement or weight gain (170,171). Moreover, because the toxicity of both ddI and dideoxycytidine differs from that of AZT, combination therapy is being assessed and findings from an early study appear encouraging (172).

Late events in the viral replicative cycle may be blocked by inhibiting glycosylation of the envelope protein (gp120) and by preventing release from the cell of formed virus particles. Inhibitors of the enzyme α-glucosidase 1, such as castanospermine, which has antiviral activity in a murine leukemia virus model system, and N-butyl deoxynojirimycin inhibit glycosylation and interfere with the replication of HIV in vitro (173–176). Toxicity studies of N-butyl deoxynojirimycin in animals are completed, and phase 1 clinical trials are in progress (161). Interferon α (IFN-α) inhibits acute and chronic HIV infection in vitro. The mechanism is incompletely understood, but in chronic infection it appears to act late in the replication cycle, possibly during the release phase (177,178). In clinical studies, IFN-α appears to be most beneficial during early stages of infection (161). The combination of AZT, recombinant soluble CD4, and recombinant IFN-α synergistically inhibits replication of HIV-1 in vitro but has not yet been evaluated in vivo (179).

Prevention

The risk of sexual transmission of HIV can be eliminated completely by abstinence or participating in a mutually monogamous relationship with an uninfected person, and it can be reduced by limiting the number of sexual partners and by using condoms (180). Transmission of HIV in blood and blood products can be prevented by excluding blood and plasma donation by persons at risk of infection with HIV, testing donated blood and plasma for HIV antibodies, and heat-treating clotting factor concentrates (181–183). Approaches to preventing spread of HIV among intravenous drug users have included expanded methadone programs and experimental needle exchange programs; however, evidence suggests that altering the behavior is more difficult in this population than among homosexual and bisexual men (184). Perinatally acquired infection with HIV can be prevented by counseling and by testing women of childbearing age for antibodies to HIV where the prevalence of the virus is 0.5% or higher and if they are at risk of infection. Women infected with HIV should be advised to avoid pregnancy, and those who become pregnant and carry the pregnancy to term should not breast feed.

Research is under way to develop a safe and effective vaccine against HIV, but progress has been impeded by limited knowledge of the protective responses in humans, mutations of the viral envelope glycoprotein, lack of a readily available animal model, and the logistics of conducting clinical trials (185). An effective vaccine must induce an immune response that protects against free virus and deals with the infected cells that serve as viral reservoirs, possibly via neutralizing antibodies and antibody-dependent cell-mediated cytotoxicity, respectively. Vaccines being evaluated are inactivated virus, recombinant viruses such as vaccinia virus carrying relevant HIV proteins, genetically engineered subunit HIV proteins, and anti-idiotype preparations. Chimpanzees vaccinated with native HIV-1 gp120 or a vaccinia vaccine bearing the HIV envelope protein have not been resistant to challenge with homologous HIV, despite the presence of HIV-specific cytotoxic lymphocytes in animals immunized with the vaccinia vaccine (186,187). In a recent phase 1 trial in human volunteers of a genetically engineered HIV-1 vaccine (a nonglycosylated polypeptide representing the gp120 region of the *env* gene), induced antibody titers were low and had no neutralizing activity (188).

REFERENCES

1. Coffin JM: Retroviridae and their replication. *In* Fields' Virology. 2nd ed. Edited by BN Fields and DM Knipe. New York, Raven Press, 1990.
2. Poiesz BJ, et al: Detection and isolation of type C retrovirus particles from fresh and cultured lymphocytes of a patient with cutaneous T-cell lymphoma. Proc Natl Acad Sci USA, 77:7415, 1980.
3. Hinuma Y, et al: Adult T-cell leukemia: Antigen in an ATL cell line and detection of antibodies to the antigen in human sera. Proc Natl Acad Sci USA, 78:6474, 1981.
4. Uchiyama T, et al: Adult T-cell leukemia: Clinical and hematologic features of 16 cases. Blood, 50:481, 1977.
5. Wong-Staal F, and Gallo RC: Human T-lymphotropic retroviruses. Nature, 317:395, 1985.
6. Gessain A, et al: Antibodies to human T-lymphotropic virus type I in patients with tropical spastic paralysis. Lancet, ii: 407, 1985.
7. Kalyanaraman VS, et al: A new subtype of human T-cell leukemia virus (HTLV-II) associated with a T-cell variant of hairy cell leukemia. Science, 218:571, 1982.
8. Rosenblatt JD, et al: A second isolate of HTLV-II associated with atypical hairy cell leukemia. N Engl J Med, 315:372, 1986.
9. Hinuma Y, et al: Antibodies to adult T-cell leukemia virus–associated antigen (ATLA) in sera from patients with ATL and controls in Japan: A nationwide seroepidemiologic study. Int J Cancer, 29:631, 1982.
10. Schupbach J, et al: Antibodies against three purified proteins of the human type C retrovirus, human T-cell leukemia/lymphoma virus, in adult T-cell leukemia/lymphoma patients and healthy blacks from the Caribbean. Cancer Res, 43:886, 1983.
11. Schaffar-DesHayes L, et al: Antibodies to HTLV-I p24 in sera of blood donors, elderly people and patients with hemopoietic diseases in France and in French West Indies. Int J Cancer, 34:667, 1984.
12. Miller GJ, et al: Ethnic composition, age and sex, together with location and standard of housing as determinants of HTLV-I infection in an urban Trinidadian community. Int J Cancer, 38:801, 1986.
13. Wiktor SZ, et al: Human T-cell lymphotropic virus type I (HTLV-I) among female prostitutes in Kinshasa, Zaire. J Infect Dis, 161:1073, 1990.
14. Bunn PA, Jr, et al: Clinical course of retrovirus-associated adult T-cell lymphoma in the United States. N Engl J Med, 309:257, 1983.
15. Blayney DW, et al: The human T-cell leukemia/lymphoma virus in the southeastern United States. JAMA, 250:1048, 1983.
16. Catovsky D, et al: Adult T-cell lymphoma/leukaemia in blacks from West Indies. Lancet, i:639, 1982.

17. Hunsmann G, et al: Detection of serum antibodies to adult T-cell leukemia virus in nonhuman primates and in people from Africa. Int J Cancer, 32:329, 1983.
18. Minamoto GY, et al: Infection with human T-cell leukemia virus type I in patients with leukemia. N Engl J Med, 318:219, 1988.
19. Williams AE, et al: Seroprevalence and epidemiological correlates of HTLV-I infection in U.S. blood donors. Science, 240:643, 1988.
20. Manzari V, et al: HTLV-I is endemic in southern Italy: Detection of the first infectious cluster in a white population. Int J Cancer, 36:557, 1985.
21. Tedder RS, et al: Low prevalence in the UK of HTLV-I and HTLV-II infection in subjects with AIDS, with extended lymphadenopathy, and at risk of AIDS. Lancet, ii:125, 1984.
22. Robert-Guroff M, et al: HTLV-1 specific antibody in AIDS patients and others at risk. Lancet, ii:128, 1984.
23. Khabbaz RF, et al: Seroprevalence and risk factors for HTLV-I/II infection among female prostitutes in the United States. JAMA, 263:60, 1990.
24. Gradilone A, et al: HTLV-I and HIV infection in drug addicts in Italy. Lancet, ii:753, 1986.
25. Robert-Guroff M, et al: Prevalence of antibodies to HTLV-I, -II and -III in intravenous drug abusers from an AIDS endemic region. JAMA, 255:3133, 1986.
26. Ando Y, et al: Transmission of adult T-cell leukemia retrovirus (HTLV-I) from mother to child: Comparison of bottle-fed with breast-fed babies. Jpn J Cancer Res, 78:322, 1987.
27. Kinoshita K, et al: Milk-borne transmission of HTLV-I from carrier mothers to their children. Jpn J Cancer Res, 78:674, 1987.
28. Kajiyama W, et al: Intrafamilial transmission of adult T-cell leukemia virus. J Infect Dis, 154:851, 1986.
29. Murphy EL, et al: Sexual transmission of human T-lymphotropic virus type I (HTLV-I). Ann Intern Med, 111:555, 1989.
30. Ocochi K, Sato H, and Hinuma Y: A retrospective study on transmission of adult T-cell leukemia virus by blood transfusion: Seroconversion in recipients. Vox Sang, 46:245, 1984.
31. Jason JM, et al: Human T-cell leukemia virus (HTLV-I) p24 antibody in New York City blood product recipients. Am J Hematol, 20:129, 1985.
32. Hahn BH, et al: Detection and characterization of an HTLV-II provirus in a patient with AIDS. In Acquired Immune Deficiency Syndrome. Edited by MS Gottlieb and JE Groopman. New York, Alan R Liss, 1984.
33. Kalyanaraman VS, et al: Isolation and characterization of a human T-cell leukemia virus type II from a hemophilia-A patient with pancytopenia. EMBO J, 4:1455, 1985.
34. Heneine W, et al: HTLV-II endemicity among Guaymi Indians in Panama [letter]. N Engl J Med, 324:565, 1991.
35. Hjelle B, et al: Incidence of hairy cell leukemia, mycosis fungoides, and chronic lymphocytic leukemia in first known HTLV-II- endemic population. J Infect Dis, 163:435, 1991.
36. Nerenberg M, et al: The tat gene of human T-lymphotropic virus type 1 induces mesenchymal tumors in transgenic mice. Science, 237:1324, 1987.
37. Kawano F, et al: Variation in the clinical courses of adult T-cell leukemia. Cancer, 55:851, 1985.
38. Kondo T, et al: Risk of adult T-cell leukemia/lymphoma in HTLV-I carriers. Lancet, ii:159, 1987.
39. Bhagavati S, et al: Detection of human T-cell lymphoma/leukemia virus type I DNA and antigen in spinal fluid and blood of patients with chronic progressive myelopathy. N Engl J Med, 318:1141, 1988.
40. Jacobson S, et al: Isolation of an HTLV-I-like retrovirus from patients with tropical spastic paraparesis. Nature, 331:540, 1988.
41. Centers for Disease Control. Pneumocystis pneumonia—Los Angeles. MMWR, 30:250, 1981.
42. Gottlieb MS, et al: Pneumocystis carinii pneumonia and mucosal candidiasis in previously healthy homosexual men: Evidence of a new acquired cellular immunodeficiency. N Engl J Med, 305:1425, 1981.
43. Masur H, et al: An outbreak of community-acquired Pneumocystis carinii pneumonia: Initial manifestation of cellular immune dysfunction. N Engl J Med, 305:1431, 1981.
44. Huminer D, Rosenfeld JB, and Pitlik SD: AIDS in the pre-AIDS era. Rev Infect Dis, 9:1102, 1987.
45. Jaffe HW, Bregman DJ, and Selik RM: Acquired immune deficiency syndrome in the United States: The first 1000 cases. J Infect Dis, 148:339, 1983.
46. Barre-Sinoussi F, et al: Isolation of a T-lymphotropic retrovirus from a patient at risk for AIDS. Science, 220:868, 1983.
47. Gallo RC, et al: Frequent detection and isolation of cytopathic retroviruses (HTLV-III) from patients with AIDS and at risk for AIDS. Science, 224:500, 1984.
48. Popovic M, Sarngadharan MG, Read E, and Gallo RC: Detection, isolation, and continuous production of cytopathic retroviruses (HTLV-III) from patients with AIDS and pre-AIDS. Science, 224:497, 1984.
49. Barin F, et al: Serological evidence for virus related to simian T-lymphotropic retrovirus III in residents of West Africa. Lancet, ii:1387, 1985.
50. Clavel F, et al: Isolation of a new human retrovirus from West African patients with AIDS. Science, 233:343, 1986.
51. Centers for Disease Control: AIDS due to HIV-2 infection—New Jersey. MMWR, 37:33, 1987.
52. Popovsky MA, et al: Infection with HIV-2 in a resident of the United States [letter]. N Engl J Med, 322:1887, 1990.
53. Clavel F, et al: Human immunodeficiency virus type 2 infection associated with AIDS in West Africa. N Engl J Med, 316:1180, 1987.
54. Centers for Disease Control: Update: HIV-2 infection—United States. MMWR, 38:572, 1989.
55. Wong-Staal F: Human immunodeficiency viruses and their replication. In Fields' Virology. 2nd ed. Edited by BN Fields and DM Knipe. New York, Raven Press, 1990.
56. Fisher AG, et al: The sor gene of HIV-1 is required for efficient virus transmission in vitro. Science, 237:888, 1987.
57. Strebel K, et al: The HIV "A" (sor) gene product is essential for virus infectivity. Nature, 328:728, 1987.
58. Luciw PA, Cheng-Mayer C, and Levy JA: Mutational analysis of the human immunodeficiency virus: The orf-B region down-regulates virus replication. Proc Natl Acad Sci USA, 84:1434, 1987.
59. Fisher AG, et al: Infectious mutants of HTLV-III with changes in the 3' region and markedly reduced cytopathic effects. Science, 223:655, 1986.
60. Cullen BR: Trans-activation of human immunodeficiency virus occurs via a bimodal mechanism. Cell, 46:973, 1986.
61. Okamoto T, and Wong-Staal F: Demonstration of virus-specific transcriptional activator(s) in cells infected with HTLV-III by an in vitro cell-free system. Cell, 47:29, 1986.
62. Haseltine W, and Wong-Staal F: The molecular biology of the AIDS virus. Sci Am, 259:52, 1988.
63. Clapham PR, et al: Soluble CD4 blocks the infectivity of diverse strains of HIV and SIV for T cells and monocytes but not for brain and muscle cells. Nature, 337:368, 1989.
64. Cheng-Mayer C, Seto D, Tateno M, and Levy JA: Biologic

features of HIV-1 that correlate with virulence in the host. Science, 240:80, 1988.
65. Saag MS, et al: Extensive variation of human immunodeficiency virus type-1 in vivo. Nature, 344:440, 1988.
66. Levy JA: Mysteries of HIV: Challenges for therapy and prevention. Nature, 333:519, 1988.
67. Centers for Disease Control: Update on acquired immune deficiency syndrome (AIDS)—United States. MMWR, 31:507, 1982.
68. Centers for Disease Control: Revision of the case definition of acquired immunodeficiency syndrome for national reporting—United States. MMWR, 34:373, 1985.
69. Centers for Disease Control: Revision of the CDC surveillance case definition for acquired immunodeficiency syndrome. MMWR, 36(suppl 1):1, 1987.
70. Centers for Disease Control: The second 100,000 cases of acquired immunodeficiency syndrome—United States, June 1981–December 1991. MMWR, 41:28, 1992.
70a. Chang SW, Katz MH, and Hernandez SR: The new AIDS case definition. Implications for San Francisco. JAMA, 267:973, 1992.
71. Centers for Disease Control: The HIV/AIDS epidemic: The first 10 years. MMWR, 40:357, 1991.
72. Centers for Disease Control: Update: Acquired immunodeficiency syndrome—United States, 1981–1990. MMWR, 40:358, 1991.
73. Centers for Disease Control. Update: Acquired immunodeficiency syndrome—United States, 1981–1988. MMWR, 38:229, 1989.
74. Centers for Disease Control: Mortality attributed to HIV infection/AIDS—United States, 1981–1990. MMWR, 40:41, 1991.
75. Curran JW, et al: The epidemiology of AIDS: Current status and future prospects. Science, 229:1352, 1985.
76. Centers for Disease Control: Changes in premature mortality—United States, 1979–1986. MMWR, 327:47, 1986.
77. Kristal AR: The impact of the acquired immunodeficiency syndrome on patterns of premature death in New York City. JAMA, 255:2306, 1986.
78. Chu SY, Buehler JW, and Berkelman RL: Impact of the human immunodeficiency virus epidemic on mortality in women of reproductive age, United States. JAMA, 264:225, 1990.
79. Centers for Disease Control: Update: Acquired immunodeficiency syndrome—Europe. MMWR, 33:607, 1984.
80. Clumeck N, et al: Acquired immunodeficiency syndrome in African patients. N Engl J Med, 310:492, 1984.
81. Mann JM, et al: Surveillance for AIDS in a central African city, Kinshasa, Zaire. JAMA, 255:3255, 1986.
82. Quinn TC, et al: AIDS in Africa: An epidemiologic paradigm. Science, 234:955, 1986.
83. Piot P, et al: Acquired immunodeficiency syndrome in a heterosexual population in Zaire. Lancet, ii:65, 1984.
84. Clumeck N, et al: Heterosexual promiscuity among African patients with AIDS [letter]. N Engl J Med, 313:182, 1985.
85. Nahmias AJ, et al: Evidence for human infection with an HTLV-III/LAV-like virus in central Africa, 1959 [letter]. Lancet, i:1279, 1986.
86. Epstein JS, et al: Antibodies reactive with HTLV-III found in freezer-banked sera from children in West Africa (Abstract). In Proceedings and Abstracts of the 25th Interscience Conference on Antimicrobial Agents and Chemotherapy. Washington, DC, American Society for Microbiology, 1985.
87. Mann JM: AIDS—The second decade: A global perspective. J Infect Dis, 165:245, 1992.
88. Centers for Disease Control: HIV-1 infection and artificial insemination with processed semen. MMWR, 39:249, 1990.
89. Jovaisas E, et al: LAV/HTLV-III in 20-week fetus [letter]. Lancet, ii:1129, 1985.
90. Lapointe N, et al: Transplacental transmission of HTLV-III virus [letter]. N Engl J Med, 312:1325, 1985.
91. Colebunders R, et al: Breastfeeding and transmission of HIV [letter]. Lancet, ii:1487, 1988.
92. Weinbreck F, et al: Postnatal transmission of HIV infection. Lancet, i:482, 1988.
93. Curran JW, et al: Acquired immunodeficiency syndrome (AIDS) associated with transfusions. N Engl J Med, 310:69, 1984.
94. Feorino PM, et al: Transfusion-associated acquired immunodeficiency syndrome. Evidence for persistent infection in blood donors. N Engl J Med, 312:1293, 1985.
95. L'age-Stehr J, et al: HTLV-III infection in kidney transplant recipients [letter]. Lancet, ii:1361, 1985.
96. Centers for Disease Control: Human immunodeficiency virus infection transmitted from an organ donor screened for HIV antibody—North Carolina. MMWR, 36:306, 1987.
97. Centers for Disease Control: Update: Acquired immunodeficiency syndrome and human immunodeficiency virus infection among health-care workers. MMWR, 37:229, 1988.
98. Marcus R, and the CDC Cooperative Needlestick Surveillance Group: Surveillance of health care workers exposed to blood from patients infected with the human immunodeficiency virus. N Engl J Med, 319:118, 1988.
99. Gerberding JL, et al: Risk of transmitting the human immunodeficiency virus, cytomegalovirus, and hepatitis B virus to health care workers exposed to patients with AIDS and AIDS-related conditions. J Infect Dis, 156:1, 1987.
100. Centers for Disease Control: Possible transmission of human immunodeficiency virus to a patient during an invasive dental procedure. MMWR, 39:489, 1990.
101. Centers for Disease Control: Update: Transmission of HIV infection during an invasive dental procedure—Florida. MMWR, 40:21, 1991.
102. Centers for Disease Control: Update: Transmission of HIV infection during invasive dental procedures—Florida. MMWR, 40:377, 1991.
103. Piot P, et al: AIDS: An international perspective. Science, 239:573, 1988.
104. Kreiss JK, et al: AIDS virus infection in Nairobi prostitutes. Spread of the epidemic to East Africa. N Engl J Med, 314:414, 1986.
105. Greenblatt RM, et al: Genital ulceration as a risk factor for human immunodeficiency virus infection in Kenya [abstract]. In Proceedings of the Third International Conference on AIDS. Washington, DC, The U.S. Department of Health and Human Services and the WHO, 1987.
106. Curran JW, Jaffe HW, and Hardy AM: Epidemiology of HIV infection and AIDS in the United States. Science, 239:610, 1988.
107. Goedert JJ, Eyster ME, and Biggar RJ: Heterosexual transmission of human immunodeficiency virus (HIV): Association with severe T4-cell depletion in male hemophiliacs [Abstract]. In Proceedings of the Third International Conference on AIDS. Washington, DC, The U.S. Department of Health and Human Services and the WHO, 1987.
108. Redfield RR, et al: Correlation of HIV isolation rate and stage of infection [abstract]. In Proceedings of the Third International Conference on AIDS. Washington, DC, The U.S. Department of Health and Human Services and the WHO, 1987.

109. Rosenberg ZF, and Fauci AS: Immunopathogenic mechanisms of HIV infection. Clin Immunol Immunopathol, 50: S149, 1989.
110. Fauci AS: The human immunodeficiency virus: Infectivity and mechanisms of pathogenesis. Science, 239:617, 1988.
111. Evans LA, and Levy JA: Characteristics of HIV infection and pathogenesis. Biochimica Biophysica Acta, 989:237, 1989.
112. Stricker RB, et al: An AIDS-related cytotoxic antibody reacts with specific antigen on stimulated $CD4^+$ T cells. Nature, 327:710, 1987.
113. Stricker RB, Abrams DI, Corash L, and Shuman MA: Target platelet antigen in homosexual men with immune thrombocytopenia. N Engl J Med, 313:1375, 1985.
114. Morris L, Distenfeld A, Amorosi E, and Karpatkin S: Autoimmune thrombocytopenic purpura in homosexual men. Ann Intern Med, 86:714, 1982.
115. Lee MR, Ho DD, and Gurney ME: Functional interaction and partial homology between human immunodeficiency virus and neuroleukin. Science, 237:1047, 1987.
116. Centers for Disease Control: Classification system for human T-lymphotropic virus type III/lymphadenopathy–associated virus infections. MMWR, 35:334, 1986.
117. Cooper DA, Imrie AA, and Penny R: Antibody response to human immunodeficiency virus after primary infection. J Infect Dis, 155:1113, 1987.
118. Farzadegan H, et al: Loss of human immunodeficiency virus type 1 (HIV-1) antibodies with evidence of viral infection in asymptomatic homosexual men. A report from the Multicenter AIDS Cohort Study. Ann Intern Med, 108:785, 1988.
119. Lifson AR, Rutherford GW, and Jaffe HW: The natural history of human immunodeficiency virus infection. J Infect Dis, 158:1360, 1988.
120. Eyster ME, et al: Natural history of human immunodeficiency virus infections in hemophiliacs: Effects of T-cell subsets, platelet counts, and age. Ann Intern Med, 107:1, 1987.
121. Eyster ME, and Goedert JJ: The predictive value of T4-cell count and HIV antigen in antibody positive hemophiliacs [abstract 7764]. In Program and Abstracts of the Fourth International Conference on AIDS. Stockholm, Swedish Ministry of Health and Social Affairs, 1988.
122. Ward J, et al: Variable progression to ARC/AIDS in HIV-infected blood recipients [abstract 342]. In Program and Abstracts of the 28th Interscience Conference on Antimicrobial Agents and Chemotherapy. Washington, DC, American Society for Microbiology, 1988.
123. Kaplan JE, Spira T, Fishbein D, and Pinsky P: Natural history of HIV infection in homosexual men with lymphadenopathy syndrome: Relationship with T-helper cell count [abstract 4095]. In Program and Abstracts of the Fourth International Conference on AIDS. Stockholm, Swedish Ministry of Health and Social Affairs, 1988.
124. Volberding PA, et al: Zidovudine in asymptomatic human immunodeficiency virus infection: A controlled trial in persons with fewer than 500 CD4-positive cells per cubic millimeter. N Engl J Med, 322:941, 1990.
125. Rothenberg R, et al: Survival with the acquired immunodeficiency syndrome: Experience with 5833 cases in New York City. N Engl J Med, 317:1297, 1987.
126. Bacchetti P, et al: Survival patterns of the first 500 AIDS cases in San Francisco. J Infect Dis, 157:1044, 1988.
127. Moss AR, et al: Mortality associated with mode of presentation in the acquired immunodeficiency syndrome. J Natl Cancer Inst, 73:1281, 1984.
128. Marasca G, and McEvoy M: Length of survival of patients with acquired immunodeficiency syndrome in the United Kingdom. Br Med J, 292:1727, 1986.
129. Lemp GF, et al: Survival trends for patients with AIDS. JAMA, 263:402, 1990.
130. Fischl MA, et al: The efficacy of azidothymidine (AZT) in the treatment of patients with AIDS and AIDS-related complex. N Engl Med, 317:185, 1987.
131. Moore RD, Hidalgo J, Sugland BW, and Chaisson RE: Zidovudine and the natural history of the acquired immunodeficiency syndrome. N Engl J Med, 324:1412, 1991.
132. Centers for Disease Control: Classification system for human immunodeficiency virus (HIV) infection in children under 13 years of age. MMWR, 36:225, 1987.
133. Scott GB, et al: Survival in children with perinatally acquired human immunodeficiency virus type 1 infection. N Engl J Med, 321:1791, 1989.
134. Pardo V, et al: AIDS-related glomerulopathy: Occurrence in specific risk groups. Kidney Int, 31:1167, 1987.
135. Rao TKS, Friedman EA, and Nicastri AD: The types of renal disease in the acquired immunodeficiency syndrome. N Engl J Med, 316:1062, 1987.
136. Hirsch MS, and Curran J: Human immunodeficiency virus. In Fields' Virology. 2nd ed. Edited by BN Fields and DM Knipe. New York, Raven Press, 1990.
137. Safai B, and Good RA: Kaposi's sarcoma: A review and recent developments. Clin Bull, 10:62, 1980.
138. Templeton AC: Kaposi's sarcoma. Pathol Annu, 16:315, 1981.
139. Hutt MSR: The epidemiology of Kaposi's sarcoma. Antibiot Chemother, 29:3, 1981.
140. Myers BD, et al: Kaposi's sarcoma in kidney transplant recipients. Arch Intern Med, 133:307, 1974.
141. Penn I: Kaposi's sarcoma in immunosuppressed patients. J Clin Lab Immunol, 12:1, 1983.
142. Levine AM: Non-Hodgkin's lymphomas and other malignancies in the acquired immune deficiency syndrome. Semin Oncol, 14:34, 1987.
143. Rogers MF, et al: National case-control study of Kaposi's sarcoma and Pneumocystis carinii pneumonia in homosexual men: Part 2, laboratory results. Ann Intern Med, 99: 151, 1983.
144. Des Jarlais DC, et al: Kaposi's sarcoma among four different AIDS risk groups. Lancet, i:1119, 1988.
145. Des Jarlais DC, Stoneburner R, Thomas P, and Friedman SR: Declines in proportion of Kaposi's sarcoma among cases of AIDS in multiple risk groups in New York City. Lancet, ii: 1024, 1987.
146. Marmor M, et al: Risk factors for Kaposi's sarcoma in homosexual men. Lancet, i:1083, 1987.
147. Haverkos HW: Factors associated with the pathogenesis of AIDS. J Infect Dis, 156:251, 1987.
148. Chaisson RE, and Volberding PA: Clinical manifestations of HIV infection. In Principles and Practice of Infectious Diseases. 3rd ed. Edited by GL Mandell, RG Douglas, Jr, JE Bennett. New York, Churchill Livingstone, 1990.
149. Subar M, et al: Frequent c-*myc* oncogene activation and infrequent presence of Epstein-Barr virus genome in AIDS-associated lymphoma. Blood, 72:667, 1988.
150. Schochetman G, Epstein JS, and Zuck TF: Serodiagnosis of infection with the AIDS virus and other human retroviruses. Ann Rev Microbiol, 43:629, 1989.
151. Centers for Disease Control: Interpretation and use of the western blot assay for serodiagnosis of human immunodeficiency virus type 1 infections. MMWR, 38(S-7):1, 1989.
152. Suarez A, Hodges S, Petruska J, and Scheffel J: Passive hemagglutination assay for HIV antibody screening. In Program

and Abstracts of the Fourth International Conference on AIDS. Stockholm, Swedish Ministry of Health and Social Affairs, 1988.
153. Quinn TC, et al: Rapid latex agglutination assay using recombinant envelope polypeptide for the detection of antibody to the HIV. JAMA, 260:510, 1988.
154. Santos JI, et al: Dot enzyme immunoassay: A simple, cheap, and stable test for antibody to human immunodeficiency virus (HIV). J Immunol Methods, 99:191, 1987.
155. Nishanian P, et al: A simple method for improved assay demonstrates that HIV p24 antigen is present as immune complexes in most sera from HIV-infected individuals. J Infect Dis, 162:21, 1990.
155a. Hollinger FB, et al: Standardization of sensitive human immunodeficiency virus coculture procedures and establishment of a multicenter quality assurance program for the AIDS Clinical Trials Group. J Clin Microbiol, 30:1787, 1992.
156. Guatelli JC, Gingeras TR, and Richman DD: Nucleic acid amplification in vitro: Detection of sequences with low copy numbers and application to diagnosis of human immunodeficiency virus type 1 infection. Clin Microbiol Rev, 2:217, 1989.
157. Laure F, et al: Detection of HIV-1 DNA in infants and children by means of the polymerase chain reaction. Lancet, i:538, 1988.
158. Rayfield M, et al: Mixed human immunodeficiency virus (HIV) infection of an individual: Demonstration of both HIV type 1 and HIV type 2 proviral sequences by polymerase chain reaction. J Infect Dis, 158:1170, 1988.
159. Vernant JC, et al: Endemic tropical spastic paraparesis associated with human T-lymphotropic virus type I: A clinical and seroepidemiological study of 25 cases. Ann Neurol, 21:123, 1987.
160. Schooley RT, et al: A phase I/II escalating dose trial of recombinant soluble CD4 therapy in patients with AIDS-related complex. Ann Intern Med, 112:247, 1990.
161. Hirsch MS: Chemotherapy of human immunodeficiency virus infections: Current practice and future prospects. J Infect Dis, 161:845, 1990.
162. Traunecker A, Luke W, and Karjalainen K: Soluble CD4 molecules neutralize human immunodeficiency virus type 1. Nature, 331:84, 1988.
163. Lifson JD, et al: Synthetic CD4 peptide derivatives that inhibit HIV infection and cytopathicity. Science, 241:712, 1988.
164. Capon DJ, et al: Designing CD4 immunoadhesins for AIDS therapy. Nature, 337:525, 1989.
165. Fischl MA, et al: Prolonged zidovudine therapy in patients with AIDS and advanced AIDS-related complex. JAMA, 262:2405, 1989.
166. Larder BA, Darby G, and Richman DD: HIV with reduced sensitivity to zidovudine (AZT) isolated during prolonged therapy. Science, 243:1731, 1989.
167. Larder BA, and Kemp SD: Multiple mutations in the HIV reverse transcriptase confer high-level resistance to zidovudine (AZT). Science, 246:1155, 1989.
168. Yarchoan R, et al: Phase I studies of 2', 3'-dideoxycytidine in severe human immunodeficiency virus infection as a single agent and alternating with zidovudine (AZT). Lancet, i:76, 1988.
169. Merigan TC, et al: Circulating p24 antigen levels and responses to dideoxycytidine in human immunodeficiency virus (HIV) infections. Ann Intern Med, 110:189, 1989.
170. Lambert JS, et al: 2',3'-Dideoxyinosine (ddI) in patients with the acquired immunodeficiency syndrome or AIDS-related complex. N Engl J Med, 322:1333, 1990.
171. Cooley TP, et al: Once daily administration of 2',3'-dideoxyinosine (ddI) in patients with the acquired immunodeficiency syndrome or AIDS-related complex. N Engl J Med, 322:1340, 1990.
172. Meng T-C, et al: Combination therapy with zidovudine and dideoxycytidine in patients with advanced human immunodeficiency virus infection. A phase I/II study. Ann Intern Med, 116:13, 1992.
173. Ruprecht RM, Mullaney S, Andersen J, and Bronson R: In vivo analysis of castanospermine, a candidate antiretroviral agent. J AIDS, 2:149, 1989.
174. Walker BD, et al: Inhibition of human immunodeficiency virus syncytium formation and virus replication by castanospermine. Proc Natl Acad Sci USA, 84:8120, 1987.
175. Gruters RA, et al: Interference with HIV-induced syncytium formation and viral infectivity by inhibitors of trimming glucosidase. Nature, 330:74, 1987.
176. Karpas A, et al: Aminosugar derivatives as potential anti–human immunodeficiency virus agents. Proc Natl Acad Sci USA, 85:9229, 1988.
177. Ho DD, et al: Recombinant human interferon α-A suppresses HTLV-III replication in vitro. Lancet, i:602, 1985.
178. Poli G, et al: Interferon-α but not AZT suppresses HIV expression in chronically infected cell lines. Science, 224:575, 1989.
179. Johnson VA, et al: Three-drug synergistic inhibition of HIV-1 replication in vitro by zidovudine, recombinant soluble CD4 and recombinant interferon-α A. J Infect Dis, 161:1059, 1990.
180. Centers for Disease Control: Condoms for prevention of sexually transmitted diseases. MMWR, 37:133, 1988.
181. Centers for Disease Control: Prevention of acquired immune deficiency syndrome (AIDS); report of interagency recommendations. MMWR, 32:101, 1983.
182. Centers for Disease Control: Provisional Public Health Service interagency recommendations for screening donated blood and plasma for antibody to the virus causing acquired immunodeficiency syndrome. MMWR, 34:1, 1985.
183. Stehr-Green JK, et al: Hemophilia-associated AIDS in the United States, 1981 to September 1987. Am J Public Health, 78:439, 1988.
184. Centers for Disease Control: Human immunodeficiency virus infection in the United States: A review of current knowledge. MMWR, 36(suppl 6):1, 1987.
185. Bolognesi DP: Prospects for prevention of and early intervention against HIV. JAMA, 261:3007, 1989.
186. Fauci AS, and Fischinger PJ: The development of an AIDS vaccine: Progress and promise. Public Health Rep, 103:230, 1988.
187. Hu S-L, et al: Effect of immunization with a vaccinia-HIV env recombinant on HIV infection of chimpanzees. Nature, 328:721, 1987.
188. Wintsch J, et al: Safety and immunogenicity of a genetically engineered human immunodeficiency virus vaccine. J Infect Dis, 163:219, 1991.

Chapter 23

UNCLASSIFIED AND UNCONVENTIONAL VIRUSES

ASTROVIRUSES

Astroviruses were discovered by electron microscopic examination of stools of human infants with diarrhea in 1975 (1,2). Since then, five distinct serotypes of astrovirus have been identified, and the virus has been recognized as a cause of diarrhea in the young of various animals (3–5).

Structure

Astroviruses, 28 to 30 nm in diameter, have a single-stranded RNA genome that codes for two to four structural proteins. By electron microscopic examination the round virions have a five- or six-pointed star-shape on their surface (Fig. 23–1).

Epidemiology

Astroviruses, recognized in Europe, the United Kingdom, Australia, Japan, and North America, account for about 5% of cases of gastroenteritis in infants and have caused nosocomial infections (5–7). Infants and young children typically are symptomatic but may be asymptomatic; adults become ill less frequently, although virus has been responsible for outbreaks of diarrhea in elders (8–12).

Clinical Manifestations

The illness begins after an incubation period of 24 to 36 hours with diarrhea, vomiting, or both. Symptoms last 12 hours to 4 days and generally are less severe than those caused by rotavirus (see Chapter 14).

NORWALK VIRUS AND NORWALK-LIKE VIRUSES

The Norwalk virus (Fig. 23–2) is the representative agent of a heterogeneous group of viruses, 24 to 40 nm in diameter, called small, round-structured viruses or Norwalk-like agents. The latter usually are named according to the geographic location of an outbreak: Norwalk, Hawaii, Snow Mountain, Montgomery County, Taunton, Amulree, Sapporo, and Otofuke. The Norwalk virus has a single structural protein and an RNA genome (13). Its protein and nucleic acid properties are typical of caliciviruses, but as yet its classification is uncertain.

Epidemiology

In the United States, illness resulting from infection with the Norwalk virus is most common among persons of school age and older. Antibodies to Norwalk virus, uncommon in young children, are present in about 50% of adults (14). In developing countries illness occurs among younger persons, and antibodies are acquired during childhood (15).

Outbreaks of gastroenteritis caused by Norwalk-like agents usually last 1 to 2 weeks and affect adults and older children. They have been reported in many settings: banquets, cruise ships, geriatric facilities, psychiatric wards, emergency rooms, cafeterias, recreational lakes, swimming pools, campgrounds, football teams, hotels, schools, dormitories, and fast food restaurants (6,16). Infection is transmitted by ingestion of contaminated water or food (especially shellfish and salads), by aerosols, by fomites, and by person-to-person contact. Viral shedding may continue up to 2 days after symptoms have resolved (17).

Antibody titers to the Norwalk virus peak by the third week after infection and begin to decline after the sixth week. Persons who have the highest pre-existing antibody titer are at greatest risk of developing symptoms, but an abrupt elevation of the titer appears to correlate with resistance to infection (14). The nature of resistance and susceptibility to the Norwalk-like agents are poorly understood.

Clinical Manifestations

The illness begins after an incubation period of 1 to 2 days with vomiting, nonbloody diarrhea, and abdominal cramps and generally resolves in 12 to 60 hours.

Laboratory Diagnosis

A diarrheic stool sample is necessary for diagnosis of infection with astroviruses, the Norwalk virus, and Norwalk-like agents. All of these viruses are detected by electron microscopy. Astroviruses can be isolated and propagated in human embryonic kidney cells; but because these cells are not easily obtained, culture is not performed in most clinical virology laboratories.

Treatment

No specific therapy is available for disease caused by astroviruses, the Norwalk virus, or Norwalk-like agents. Supportive treatment consists of maintaining fluid and electrolyte balance.

NON-A, NON-B HEPATITIS

Non-A, non-B hepatitis was recognized after sensitive serologic tests for diagnosis of hepatitis B and hepatitis A were developed and used to determine why testing serum from blood donors for hepatitis B surface antigen did not eliminate transfusion-associated hepatitis, as was expected, and to retrospectively investigate outbreaks of hepatitis related to contamination of the water supply with raw sewage in Delhi, India, in Ahmedabad, and in Kashmir (18–22). The pathogens of non-A, non-B hepatitis were unknown until hepatitis C virus was identified

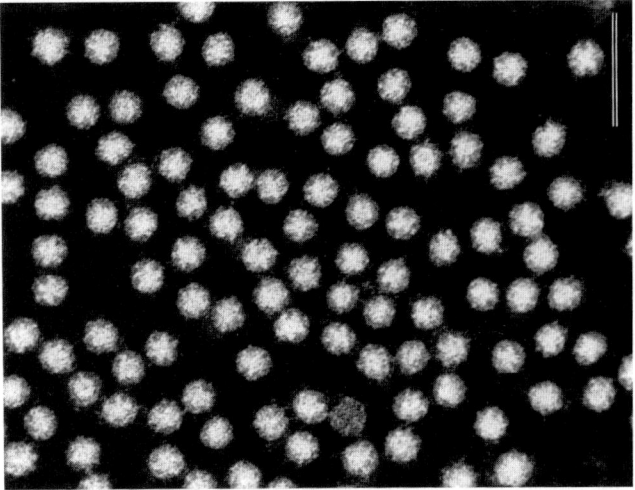

Fig. 23–1. Electron micrograph of astrovirus particles in a stool specimen (×180,049). (Courtesy of Dr. Charles Humphrey, Ultrastructure Activity, Division of Viral and Rickettsial Diseases, Centers for Disease Control, Atlanta, GA.)

by molecular studies as the pathogen of most cases of parenterally transmitted disease and hepatitis E virus was identified by studies in primates as one agent of enterically transmitted non-A, non-B hepatitis.

Hepatitis C Virus

Hepatitis C virus (HCV) is the major cause of transfusion-associated non-A, non-B hepatitis in the United States, Japan, and Europe, and is the leading cause of all cases of non-A, non-B hepatitis in the United States (23). The morphologic characteristics of HCV particles are still unknown, but its genome has been cloned from plasma of a chimpanzee infected in the laboratory with a blood product known to transmit non-A, non-B hepatitis (24). Clones synthesizing nonstructural HCV proteins have been identified, allowing production of large quantities of viral protein (termed C100-3) for detection of specific antibodies by radioimmunoassay and enzyme immunoassay (25).

Structure and Replication

The 30- to 60-nm diameter enveloped HCV virions consist of a positive-sense, single-stranded RNA genome of approximately 10,000 nucleotides, one or two envelope proteins (E1, E2), and four or five nonstructural (NS) proteins. NS1 may be E2, NS3 encodes a helicase, NS5 is an RNA-dependent polymerase, and the function of NS4 is not determined (24). Known antigenic proteins of HCV are c100-3 in the NS4 region, 5-1-1 and c33c in the NS region, and c22-3 in the core region. The specific events in the replication cycle are unknown. The organizational pattern of the HCV genome has characteristics similar to those of the flavivirus genome (see Chapter 18); but definitive classification requires further study.

Epidemiology

According to data from investigations in the United States, Europe, and Taiwan the prevalence of antibodies to HCV ranges from 0.4 to 1.5% among blood donors, from 48 to 96% among intravenous drug users, from 66 to 90% among hemophiliacs, and from 1 to 23% among persons receiving hemodialysis (25–31). Among household or sexual contacts of persons with non-A, non-B hepatitis who also develop non-A, non-B hepatitis, the prevalence of antibodies to HCV is 75%.

Hepatitis C virus is transmitted via the percutaneous route and via close personal contact. Data from one study conducted before HCV was recognized and a serologic assay was available suggested maternal-infant transmission of non-A, non-B hepatitis; however, this is not confirmed (32). In many cases the route of transmission of HCV is unknown. For example, in the United States almost 60% of persons with non-A, non-B hepatitis and no known source of infection have antibodies to HCV.

Pathogenesis

HCV-associated antigen has been demonstrated by immunohistochemical staining in the cytoplasm of hepatocytes in chimpanzees with acute and chronic hepatitis C and in humans with chronic non-A, non-B hepatitis who are seropositive for HCV (27). The mechanisms of hepatocyte damage, however, are unknown.

Clinical Manifestations

The incubation period of transfusion-associated hepatitis ranges from less than 2 weeks to 6 months (mean, 7 to 8 weeks). Acute infection usually is mild, but fulminant hepatitis can occur (33). Following recovery from the acute illness clinical or biochemical relapses are typical and they commonly lead to chronic persistent or chronic active hepatitis, or possibly to cirrhosis. The presence of antibodies to HCV in sera of 65 to 75% of persons with hepatocellular carcinoma in Italy and Spain, respectively,

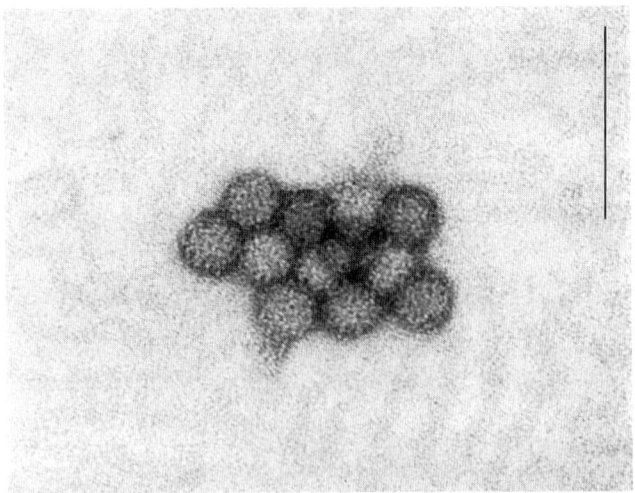

Fig. 23–2. Electron micrograph of Norwalk virus particles in a stool specimen (×303,760). (Courtesy of the Division of Viral and Rickettsial Diseases, Centers for Disease Control, Atlanta, GA.)

suggests that this malignancy is a potential complication of infection with HCV (26).

The natural history of hepatitis C has been studied prospectively in chimpanzees and retrospectively in humans who developed non-A, non-B hepatitis following blood transfusion. In chimpanzees inoculated with HCV in the laboratory the alanine transferase level peaks 50 to 70 days after inoculation, and of the animals followed longer than 12 months 60% have biochemical evidence of ongoing liver dysfunction (27). Serum of persistently infected, HCV-seropositive animals is highly infective, suggesting that the antibodies measured are non-neutralizing and that the development and maintenance of circulating antibodies may reflect ongoing viral replication.

Using stored serum samples from prospective studies of transfusion-associated non-A, non-B hepatitis in persons who underwent open heart surgery, Alter and his colleagues evaluated the frequency with which HCV caused the hepatitis and followed the natural history of the infection (34). All persons who had chronic non-A, non-B hepatitis proven by liver biopsy were seronegative for HCV before transfusion and developed antibodies to HCV 10 to 39 weeks (mean, 22 weeks) after transfusion or 4 to 32 weeks (mean, 15 weeks) after the onset of hepatitis. Antibodies persisted throughout follow-up (mean, 7 years; range, 14 months to 12 years) in all but one of these persons. Of five persons who developed acute, resolving non-A, non-B hepatitis, three developed antibodies to HCV, which then disappeared after an average of 4 years (range, less than 1½ to more than 9 years).

In another study of five persons who developed post-transfusion non-A, non-B hepatitis and were followed for 10 to 14 years after transfusion, HCV RNA was first detected by polymerase chain reaction within 3 weeks of transfusion in all five persons and within 1 week in three of them (35). The viremia lasted less than 4 months in the person with acute, self-limited hepatitis but persisted 10 to 14 years in the four who developed chronic disease. Antibodies to HCV were first detected 12 to 14 weeks after transfusion and became indetectable after 9 years in the person with self-limited disease and borderline after 5 years in one who had chronic hepatitis.

Hepatitis E Virus

Hepatitis E virus (HEV) is a leading cause of acute viral hepatitis in young to middle-aged adults in developing countries. The virus was transmitted successfully first in 1983 by Balayan, who self-administered an extract of fecal material collected from a person with hepatitis (acquired during an outbreak in Soviet Asia) and 5 weeks later developed non-A hepatitis (he was seropositive for hepatitis A virus) (36). A 27- to 30-nm particle was identified in an acute-phase stool sample by immune electron microscopy, and specific antibodies were detected in serum. The particle was transmitted to monkeys, which subsequently demonstrated evidence of liver disease and shed the virus in their stools. The existence of the particle has been confirmed by others, and its antigenic similarity to particles identified during outbreaks in different parts of the world has been established (37,38).

Structure

HEV virions have not been fully characterized because the virus has not been grown in cell culture. The spherical, unenveloped 27- to 34-nm diameter virus particles have a surface structure similar to that of caliciviruses (see Chapter 15) and a single-stranded RNA genome of approximately 7.6 kilobases.

Epidemiology

HEV is the major cause of sporadic hepatitis in parts of India where it is endemic (39). Outbreaks of hepatitis caused by HEV have been reported in India, Pakistan, Nepal, Burma, Soviet Asia, North Africa, and Mexico; and although no outbreaks have been documented in the United States, imported cases have been described (34,40,41). Most epidemics have been related to consumption of contaminated water, but the mode of spread in sporadic cases is unknown. The highest attack rates during epidemics are among persons 15 to 40 years of age.

Clinical Manifestations

Like hepatitis A, hepatitis E has a short incubation period (mean, 6 weeks; range, 2 to 9 weeks), frequently is accompanied by cholestasis, and does not progress to chronic disease. Hepatitis E is more often fulminant, predominantly in pregnant women who acquire the infection during the third trimester. The fatality rate of hepatitis E is 10 to 20% for pregnant women and 1 to 2% for other hospitalized patients. In contrast, the mortality rate of hepatitis A is about 0.1% for hospitalized patients, and no difference for pregnant women (42).

Laboratory Diagnosis

Persons infected with HCV are identified by detection of specific antibodies in serum. The first-generation enzyme-linked immunosorbent assays (ELISA) approved by the United States Food and Drug Administration were associated with a significant number of false positive and some false negative results. Second-generation ELISA tests, which detect antibodies to three antigens rather than one, identify infection earlier. For a definitive diagnosis of HCV infection, however, serum samples that test positive by ELISA should be evaluated by a confirmatory test (immunoblot or Matrix) (43). Detection of hepatitis C viral sequences in blood by polymerase chain reaction may be a good predictor of infectivity; however, in its present form this test is not suitable for mass screening of blood donors (35,44). Diagnosis of infection with HEV currently requires identifying viral particles in stool specimens by electron microscopy.

Treatment and Prevention

No specific therapy effective against HCV or HEV is available currently; treatment is supportive. Screening blood donors for antibodies to HCV should reduce the risk of transfusion-associated hepatitis C (30).

UNCONVENTIONAL VIRUSES ("PRIONS")

The progressive dementing illness now called Creutzfeldt-Jakob disease first was described by Creutzfeldt in a 22-year-old woman in 1920, and in 1921, Jakob reported four persons with a similar clinical presentation and course (45). In 1959, neuropathologic similarities were observed between Creutzfeldt-Jakob disease and kuru, a degenerative disease of the cerebellum occurring in New Guinea natives, and between kuru and scrapie, a central nervous system disease of sheep and goats; and within a decade kuru and Creutzfeldt-Jakob disease were transmitted to nonhuman primates (46–49).

The transmissible neurodegenerative disorders (also called spongiform encephalopathies)—kuru, Creutzfeldt-Jakob disease, and Gerstmann-Straussler syndrome in humans (discussed later) and the animal diseases scrapie, transmissible mink encephalopathy, chronic wasting disease of elk and deer, and bovine spongiform encephalopathy—have several common features. After prolonged incubation, each disease progresses steadily, ending in death of the infected person or animal. The associated pathologic findings are confined almost exclusively to the central nervous system, and the histologic appearance of the lesions is similar (described later). The responsible pathogen or pathogens have unique properties that distinguish them from other known organisms (50,51). They resist inactivation by boiling, by ultraviolet irradiation, and by 70% alcohol and formaldehyde vapor, and they may remain active in tissues fixed in 10% formalin. Failure to destroy the infectious agent by methods that disrupt nucleic acids suggests that they do not contain a nucleic acid; that the nucleic acid is very small, consisting of fewer than 50 nucleotides; or that the nucleic acid is surrounded by a densely packed protein shell that prevents penetration of enzymes, psoralens, nucleophiles, or divalent cations that disrupt nucleic acids. The sensitivity of the infectious agent to substances that digest, denature, or chemically modify proteins indicates that protein is an integral component of the agent and is essential for infectivity. Moreover, infection with the agent does not induce a humoral or cellular immune response in the host. Given these unusual properties, various terms have been proposed for this infectious agent: unconventional virus, virino, and prion (52,53). The term prion ("small proteinaceous infectious particle that resists inactivation by procedures that modify nucleic acids") accurately describes the agent; however, until its nature is established unequivocally, kuru agent, Creutzfeldt-Jakob disease agent, and scrapie agent, respectively, may be more appropriate terms (52).

Structure and Replication

Much of what is known about the biologic, structural, and molecular properties of the agents responsible for the transmissible neurodegenerative disorders has been learned by studying the scrapie agent in different animal models. In 1981 Merz and coworkers identified filaments, which they termed scrapie-associated fibrils, 4 to 6 nm in diameter and 50 to 400 nm in length, appearing as helically intertwined doublets or tetramers in electron micrographs of extracts of scrapie-infected mouse brains (54,55). Scrapie-associated fibrils also have been observed in brain tissue from individuals with Creutzfeldt-Jakob disease (56). In 1982 Prusiner and his colleagues purified from brain homogenates of scrapie-infected hamsters a sialoglycoprotein with an apparent molecular weight of 27,000 to 30,000, designated PrP 27-30 (prion protein; molecular weight 27,000 to 30,000), which they believe represents the major component of the scrapie agent (57–59). This protein polymerizes into rodlike structures 25 nm wide and 50 to 200 nm long with characteristics of amyloid. Similar rod-shaped particles have been isolated from persons who died of Creutzfeldt-Jakob disease (Fig. 23–3) (60). The molecular weight of the major protein component of scrapie-associated fibrils is similar to that of PrP 27-30, its N-terminal amino acid sequence is identical to that of PrP 27-30, and antisera to PrP 27-30 react with scrapie-associated fibrils, suggesting that the two structures are closely related, if not identical (61–63).

Once PrP 27-30 was purified, the sequence of the last seven N-terminal amino acids was determined and oligonucleotide probes containing nucleotide sequences that might possibly code for the identified heptapeptide were synthesized and used to identify a PrP complementary DNA (cDNA) (51,64). Chromosomal DNA analysis of

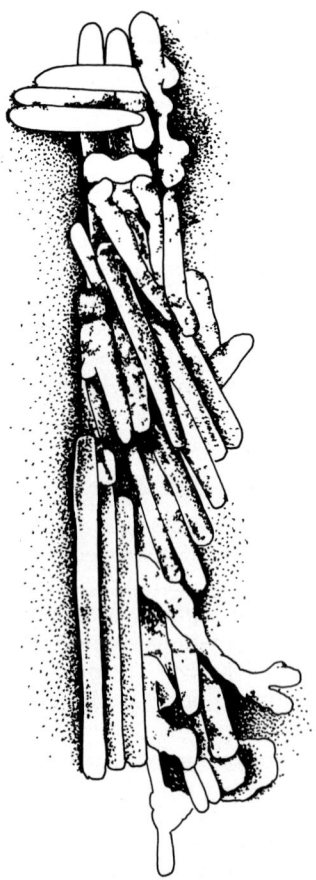

Fig. 23–3. Diagram of prion rods from brain tissue of a patient with Creutzfeldt-Jakob disease.

normal uninfected and scrapie-infected hamster brains by Southern blotting using this PrP cDNA as a probe identified a single gene with the same restriction pattern in uninfected and infected tissues; subsequently, related genes were found in DNA from humans and many other organisms, indicating that PrP is encoded by a host cell gene (65,66). Levels of PrP messenger RNA in normal and scrapie-infected hamster brains are similar, suggesting that differences in gene transcription are not responsible for disease induction (64). Prusiner and his colleagues believe that in healthy cells the product of the PrP gene is a protein designated PrP^c, which is susceptible to digestion by proteases and solubilizes when exposed to detergents; whereas in scrapie-infected cells the product of the PrP gene is the precursor of PrP 27-30, termed PrP^{sc}, which is resistant to proteases, polymerizes into amyloid rods and filaments when exposed to detergents, and upon proteinase K digestion yields PrP 27-30 (64). The differences in the properties of these two proteins may arise from a post-translational event (67). Moreover, the presence of PrP^c in normal tissues may render the host tolerant to the abnormal isoform PrP^{sc}, accounting for the lack of an immune response to infection with these agents.

The agents responsible for the transmissible neurodegenerative diseases are capable of replication, though the process by which this occurs is unknown.

Epidemiology

Creutzfeldt-Jakob disease occurs worldwide, affecting both sexes equally, with a peak occurrence between the ages of 40 and 60 years. It is associated with an annual mortality rate of about 1 case per million in metropolitan areas and a lower rate in rural areas. The disease has a higher prevalence among Libyan Jews and is familial in about 10 to 15% of cases. The natural mode of transmission is unknown; however, iatrogenic transmission via corneal transplantation, the use of depth electrodes for electroencephalogram monitoring, and administration of growth hormone prepared from pooled pituitary glands has been reported (50,68–70).

Approximately 80% of all cases of kuru occur among the Fore peoples of the eastern highlands of New Guinea, and the remainder in other groups of people in that same region. Mortality from kuru steadily declined from about 200 deaths per year during the 1960s to fewer than 15 deaths per year since 1985, a trend associated with the cessation of endocannibalism, a ritual in which the body of the deceased is consumed (50). Endocannibalism was practiced almost exclusively by women, although children of both sexes helped prepare the brain, which explains the previous female predominance of kuru among adults and the equal sex ratio among preadolescents. Kuru probably is transmitted from infected tissues of the deceased to another individual by self-inoculation while preparing the body for consumption. Potential ports of entry are the conjunctivae, oropharynx, and breaks in the skin.

The Gerstmann-Straussler syndrome is a rare familial transmissible neurodegenerative disease with clinical and pathologic features distinct from those of Creutzfeldt-Jakob disease (described later).

Pathogenesis and Pathology

The present understanding of the pathogenesis of the transmissible neurodegenerative diseases is based on studies of scrapie-infected animals and animals inoculated in the laboratory with tissues from persons with kuru and Creutzfeldt-Jakob disease. The incubation period for kuru in animals inoculated in the laboratory with brain suspensions from persons with the disease ranges from 8 months for smaller animals to 8 years for monkeys. Creutzfeldt-Jakob disease has been transmitted by inoculation to monkeys, goats, cats, guinea pigs, mice, and hamsters; and recently agents responsible for both diseases have been transmitted by feeding infected tissues to squirrel monkeys (71).

After animals are inoculated in the laboratory, agents of Creutzfeldt-Jakob disease and kuru multiply in cells of the monocyte/macrophage system, particularly the spleen but also the liver and lymph nodes, and then travel by an unknown pathway to the brain, where they replicate to very high titers. These agents also are found in lungs, kidney, cornea, vitreous, lenses, cerebrospinal fluid, and leukocytes of infected animals. The mechanism by which they cause neurologic disease is unknown; however, because prion protein levels are higher in infected brains, the accumulation of this protein may be toxic (51).

Studies of the scrapie agent in different strains of inbred mice have shown that host factors influence the nature and outcome of the infection and the interval between inoculation of the agent and disease (51,64). In mice, the genes *Pid-1* and *Prn-i* influence susceptibility to infection with the scrapie agent and the incubation time, respectively. The *Prn-i* gene appears closely linked to the structural gene, *Prn-p,* that encodes the prion protein (72,73). Variations in the nature of the agent itself also can influence the incubation period. The sequences of proteins coded by the prion protein genes (*Prn-p*) from strains of inbred mice that exhibit long and short incubation times differ in two amino acids (64,73).

The histopathologic findings that characterized the central nervous system lesions of the transmissible neurodegenerative diseases are similar: neuronal cell loss; diffuse astrocytosis; and vacuolization of the cytoplasm of neurons and astrocytes (termed spongiosus), appearing as empty vacuoles with redundant membranes by electron microscopic examination. In a variable percentage of cases (kuru, 70%; Creutzfeldt-Jakob disease, 10%), plaques resembling amyloid are found. The location of the lesions in each disease, however, differs. In kuru the cerebellum is predominantly involved, whereas in Creutzfeldt-Jakob disease neuronal loss and diffuse spongiosus are most prominent in all cortical layers of the frontal lobes. Unlike kuru and Creutzfeldt-Jakob disease, the spongiform change in the Gerstmann-Straussler syndrome principally involves the white matter.

Clinical Manifestations

Kuru, a rapidly progressive cerebellar degenerative disease with features of cortical and brain stem dysfunction, begins insidiously with cerebellar ataxia (a shivering tremor involving the head, trunk, and legs), dysarthria, strabismus, and mood changes. With disease progression, inability to walk, involuntary movements, dementia, and dysphagia develop. Death due to inanition, pneumonia, or respiratory failure occurs 3 to 12 months after onset of disease. The Gerstmann-Straussler syndrome likewise is characterized by cerebellar ataxia and dementia.

The hallmarks of Creutzfeldt-Jakob disease include rapidly progressive dementia, focal neurologic changes, and myoclonus. Changes in behavior, emotional responses, memory, and reasoning and visual disturbances occur early. Dementia becomes prominent within 6 months, and later in the disease myoclonic contractions develop. Ataxia, dysarthria, and delirium progress to stupor and coma. Death from an intercurrent infection usually occurs in less than 1 year, although 6 to 10% of persons survive 2 years or longer.

Laboratory Diagnosis

Kuru and the Gerstmann-Straussler syndrome usually are diagnosed on the basis of appropriate clinical findings in the correct epidemiologic setting. The electroencephalogram, cerebrospinal fluid and serum electrolytes and other chemistry tests usually are normal. The diagnosis is confirmed by histologic examination of brain biopsy or autopsy tissue (described earlier).

Laboratory tests may be useful for diagnosis of Creutzfeldt-Jakob disease. More than half of affected persons have characteristic electroencephalographic findings sometime during their illness: periodic, biphasic or triphasic high-amplitude sharp waves, often appearing time locked to myoclonic jerks. The cerebrospinal fluid is normal except for a slightly elevated protein concentration. A 27-kd protein has been identified in Western blots of infected brain tissue preparations from persons with Creutzfeldt-Jakob disease and kuru by using antibodies specific for a purified fraction of scrapie-infected brain; however, further evaluations are needed to establish the sensitivity and specificity of this test (74). The diagnosis is confirmed by observing the characteristic histologic features in brain biopsy or autopsy tissue (described earlier).

Treatment and Prevention

No effective treatment for the transmissible neurodegenerative disorders is known.

The prevalence of kuru has decreased dramatically with the abandonment of endocannibalism, and cases no longer occur among children or adolescents (50). How Creutzfeldt-Jakob disease is transmitted in nature is not known, so natural transmission cannot be effectively prevented. Iatrogenic transmission of the disease can be prevented, however, by observing certain precautions when caring for infected patients and when handling infected materials (75). Neither demented patients nor patients with an unexplained, possibly infectious illness should donate blood, blood products, or organs or serve as sources of tissue for preparation of biologic products for use in humans: corneal transplants, dura mater, pituitary hormone, interferon. Needles, needle electrodes, scalpels, ophthalmic tonometers, surgical instruments, and all other potentially contaminated materials should be autoclaved for 4 to 5 hours at 15 lb/in^2 or sterilized by three successive 30-minute immersions in 1 N sodium hydroxide at 25°C.

Special isolation of patients with Creutzfeldt-Jakob disease is not necessary. Exposure to oral secretions, urine, or feces of infected patients and simple contamination of the skin by blood should be followed by thorough washing of the hands or other exposed body parts with hospital detergent or ordinary soap. In case of accidental percutaneous exposure to blood, cerebrospinal fluid, or tissue of infected patients, the wound should be cleaned with an iodine or phenolic antiseptic or 0.5% sodium hypochlorite or swabbed with a 1:3000 potassium permanganate solution.

Special decontamination procedures should be followed when performing an autopsy on a person who might have had Creutzfeldt-Jakob disease. Autopsy room personnel should wear long-sleeved gowns, gloves, and masks. When opening the skull and spinal canal care should be taken not to cut the brain and cord. All tissues should be considered potentially infectious. All instruments should be autoclaved before being cleaned for reuse, and containers used to collect autopsy tissues should be externally disinfected (as discussed earlier). The sink in which water from the autopsy table collects should be plugged and the wash water collected and autoclaved; alternatively, four volumes or more of 5% sodium hypochlorite bleach should be added to the water and left for at least 2 hours before it is discarded. The body should be sponged with 5% sodium hypochlorite before it leaves the autopsy room.

All tissues from a patient with Creutzfeldt-Jakob disease should be considered fully infectious, even after prolonged fixation in formalin and histologic processing. Tissues processed for histologic examination should be washed in several changes of water, on a shaker rather than in running tap water. Wash water, formalin, and subsequent aqueous or alcoholic washes should be pooled and decontaminated, by autoclaving or chemically (as described). Glassware, forceps, and tissue carriers, likewise should be decontaminated. Xylene, toluene, or other organic solvents should be autoclaved and discarded. The microtome blade used to cut potentially infected tissue may be decontaminated by flaming, autoclaving, or soaking in disinfectant.

REFERENCES

1. Madeley CR, and Cosgrove BP: Viruses in infantile gastroenteritis. Lancet, ii:124, 1975.
2. Madeley CR, and Cosgrove BP: 28-nm particles in faeces in infantile gastroenteritis. Lancet, ii:451, 1975.
3. Kurtz JB, and Lee TW: Human astrovirus serotypes. Lancet, ii:1405, 1984.
4. Lee TW, and Kurtz JB: Human astrovirus serotypes. J Hyg, 89:539, 1982.
5. Christensen ML: Human viral gastroenteritis. Clin Microbiol Rev, 2:51, 1989.
6. Centers for Disease Control: Viral agents of gastroenteritis: Public health importance and outbreak management. MMWR, 39(RR-5):1, 1990.
7. Ellis ME, et al: Micro-organism in gastroenteritis. Arch Dis Child, 59:848, 1984.

8. Konno T, et al: Astrovirus-associated epidemic gastroenteritis in Japan. J Med Virol, 9:11, 1982.
9. Oshiro LS, et al: A 27-mm virus isolated during an outbreak of acute infectious nonbacterial gastroenteritis in a convalescent hospital: A possible new serotype. J Infect Dis, 143:791, 1981.
10. Ashley CR, Caul EO, and Paver WK: Astrovirus-associated gastroenteritis in children. J Clin Pathol, 31:939, 1978.
11. Kurtz JB, Lee TW, and Pickering D: Astrovirus associated gastroenteritis in a children's ward. J Clin Pathol, 30:948, 1977.
12. Gary JJ, Wreghitt TG, Cubitt WD, and Elliot PR: An outbreak of gastroenteritis in a home for the elderly associated with astrovirus type 1 and human calicivirus. J Med Virol, 23:377, 1987.
13. Jiang X, Graham DY, Wang K, and Estes MK: Norwalk virus genome cloning and characterization. Science, 250:1580, 1990.
14. Blacklow NR, et al: Immune response and prevalence of antibody to Norwalk enteritis virus as determined by radio-immunoassay. J Clin Microbiol, 10:903, 1979.
15. Greenberg HB, et al: Prevalence of antibody to the Norwalk virus in various countries. Infect Immun, 25:270, 1979.
16. Kaplan JE, et al: Epidemiology of Norwalk gastroenteritis and the role of Norwalk virus in outbreaks of acute nonbacterial gastroenteritis. Ann Intern Med, 96:756, 1982.
17. White KE, et al: A foodborne outbreak of Norwalk virus gastroenteritis: evidence for post-recovery transmission. Am J Epidemiol, 124:120, 1986.
18. Feinstone SM, et al: Transfusion associated hepatitis not due to viral hepatitis type A or B. N Engl J Med, 292:767, 1975.
19. Mosley JW, et al: Multiple hepatitis viruses in multiple attacks of acute viral hepatitis. N Engl J Med, 296:75, 1977.
20. Viswanathan R: Infectious hepatitis in Delhi (1955–1956): A critical study; epidemiology. Indian J Med Res, 45(suppl):1, 1957.
21. Wong DC, et al: Epidemic and endemic hepatitis in India: Evidence for a non-A, non-B hepatitis virus aetiology. Lancet, ii:876, 1980.
22. Khuroo MS: Study of an epidemic of non-A, non-B hepatitis. Possibility of another human hepatitis virus distinct from post-transfusion non-A, non-B type. Am J Med, 68:818, 1980.
23. Alter MJ, et al: Risk factors for acute non-A, non-B hepatitis in the United States and association with hepatitis C virus infection. JAMA, 264:2231, 1990.
24. Choo Q-L, et al: Isolation of a cDNA clone derived from a blood-borne non-A, non-B viral hepatitis genome. Science, 244:359, 1989.
25. Kuo G, et al: An assay for circulating antibodies to a major etiologic virus of human non-A, non-B hepatitis. Science, 244:362, 1989.
26. Stevens CE, et al: Epidemiology of hepatitis C virus: A preliminary study in volunteer blood donors. JAMA, 263:49, 1990.
27. Krawczynski K: Newer hepatitis viruses: Hepatitis E virus and Hepatitis C virus. Sixth Annual Clinical Virology Symposium and Annual Meeting—Pan American Group for Rapid Viral Diagnosis. Clearwater Beach, Florida, 1990.
28. van den Hoek JAR, et al: Prevalence, incidence, and risk factors of hepatitis C virus infection among drug users in Amsterdam. J Infect Dis, 162:823, 1990.
29. Chen D-S, et al: Hepatitis C virus infection in an area hyperendemic for hepatitis B and chronic liver disease: The Taiwan experience. J Infect Dis, 162:817, 1990.
30. Esteban II, et al: Evaluation of antibodies to hepatitis C virus in a study of transfusion-associated hepatitis. N Engl J Med, 323:1107, 1990.
31. Dawson GJ, et al: Detection of antibodies to hepatitis C virus in U.S. blood donors. J Clin Microbiol, 29:551, 1991.
32. Tong MJ, et al: Studies on the maternal infant transmission of the viruses which cause acute hepatitis. Gastroenterology, 80:999, 1981.
33. Feinstone SM: Non-A, non-B hepatitis. In Principles and Practice of Infectious Diseases. 3rd ed. Edited by GL Mandell, RG Douglas, Jr, JE Bennett. New York, Churchill Livingstone, 1990.
34. Alter HJ, et al: Detection of antibody to hepatitis C virus in prospectively followed transfusion recipients with acute and chronic non-A, non-B hepatitis. N Engl J Med, 321:1494, 1989.
35. Farci P, et al: A long-term study of hepatitis C virus replication in non-A, non-B hepatitis. N Engl J Med, 325:98, 1991.
36. Balayan MS, et al: Evidence for a virus in non-A, non-B hepatitis transmitted via the fecal-oral route. Intervirology, 20:23, 1983.
37. Bradley DW, et al: Enterically transmitted non-A, non-B hepatitis: Serial passage of disease in cynomolgus macaques and tamarins and recovery of disease-associated 27- to 34-nm viruslike particles. Proc Natl Acad Sci USA, 84:6277, 1987.
38. Arankalle VA, et al: Aetiological association of a virus-like particle with enterically transmitted non-A, non-B hepatitis. Lancet, i:550, 1988.
39. Khuroo MS, et al: Failure to detect chronic liver disease after epidemic non-A, non-B hepatitis [letter]. Lancet, ii:97, 1980.
40. Khuroo MS, et al: Acute sporadic non-A, non-B hepatitis in India. Am J Epidemiol, 118:360, 1983.
41. Bradley DW, et al: Enterically transmitted non-A, non-B hepatitis: Etiology of disease and laboratory studies in nonhuman primates. In Viral Hepatitis and Liver Disease. Edited by AJ Zuckerman, New York, Alan R Liss, 1988.
42. Khuroo MS: Incidence and severity of viral hepatitis in pregnancy. Am J Med, 70:252, 1981.
43. Chaudhary RK, and MacLean C: Evaluation of first and second-generation RIBA kits for detection of antibody to hepatitis C virus. J Clin Microbiol, 29:2329, 1991.
44. Garson JA, et al: Detection of hepatitis C viral sequences in blood donations by "nested" polymerase chain reaction and prediction of infectivity. Lancet, 335:1419, 1990.
45. Jakob A: Uber eigenartige Erkrankungen des zentral nerven Systems mit bemerkenswertem anatomischen Befunde (spatische pseudosklerose—Encephalomyelopathie mit disseminierten Degenerationsherden). Z Gasamte Neurol Psych, 64:147, 1921.
46. Klatzo I, Gajdusek DC, and Zigas V: Pathology of kuru. Lab Invest, 8:799, 1959.
47. Hadlow WJ: Scrapie and kuru. Lancet, ii:289, 1959.
48. Gajdusek DC, Gibbs CJ, Jr, and Alpers M: Experimental transmission of a kuru-like syndrome to chimpanzees. Nature, 209:794, 1966.
49. Gibbs CJ Jr, et al: Creutzfeldt-Jakob disease (spongiform encephalopathy): Transmission to the chimpanzee. Science, 161:388, 1968.
50. Lehrich JR and Tyler KL: Slow infections of the central nervous system. In Principles and Practice of Infectious Diseases. 3rd ed. Edited by GL Mandell, RG Douglas, Jr, and JE Bennett. New York, Churchill Livingstone, 1990.
51. Tyler KL: Prions. In Principles and Practice of Infectious Diseases. 3rd ed. Edited by GL Mandell, RG Douglas, Jr, and JE Bennett. New York, Churchill Livingstone, 1990.
52. Prusiner SB: Novel proteinaceous infectious particles cause scrapie. Science, 216:136, 1982.
53. Gajdusek DC: Unconventional viruses and the origin and disappearance of kuru. Science, 197:943, 1977.

54. Merz PA, et al: Abnormal fibrils from scrapie-infected brains. Acta Neuropathol (Berl), 54:63, 1981.
55. Merz PA, et al: Infection specific particle from the unconventional slow virus diseases. Science, 225:437, 1984.
56. Merz PA, et al: Scrapie-associated fibrils in Creutzfeldt-Jakob disease. Nature, 305:474, 1983.
57. McKinley MP, Bolton DC, and Prusiner SB: A protease-resistant protein is a structural component of the scrapie prion. Cell, 35:57, 1983.
58. Bolton DC, McKinley MP, and Prusiner SB: Molecular characteristics of the major scrapie prion protein. Biochemistry, 23:5898, 1984.
59. Bolton DC, Meyer RK, and Prusiner SB: Scrapie PrP 27-30 is a sialoglycoprotein. J Virol, 53:596, 1985.
60. Bockman JM, et al: Creutzfeldt-Jakob disease prion proteins in human brain. N Engl J Med, 312:73, 1985.
61. Diringer H, et al: Scrapie infectivity, fibrils, and low molecular weight protein. Nature, 306:476, 1983.
62. Hope J, et al: The major polypeptide of scrapie-associated fibrils (SAF) has the same size, charge distribution and N-terminal protein sequence as predicted for the normal brain protein (PrP). EMBO J, 5:2591, 1986.
63. Merz PA, et al: Antisera to scrapie-associated fibril protein and prion protein decorate scrapie-associated fibrils. J Virol, 61:42, 1987.
64. Prusiner SB: Prions and neurodegenerative diseases. N Engl J Med, 317:1571, 1987.
65. Oesch B, et al: A cellular gene encodes scrapie PrP 27-30 protein. Cell, 40:735, 1985.
66. Westaway D, and Prusiner SB: Conservation of the cellular gene encoding the scrapie prion protein. Nucleic Acids Res, 14:2035, 1986.
67. Basler K, et al: Scrapie and cellular PrP isoforms are encoded by the same chromosomal gene. Cell, 46:417, 1986.
68. Brown P, Gajdusek C, Gibbs CJ, and Asher DM: Potential epidemic of Creutzfeldt-Jakob disease from human growth hormone therapy. N Engl J Med, 313:728, 1985.
69. Koch TK, Berg BO, DeArmond SJ, and Gravina RF: Creutzfeldt-Jakob disease in a young adult with idiopathic hypopituitarism: Possible relation to the administration of cadaveric human growth hormone. N Engl J Med, 313:731, 1985.
70. Gibbs CJ, et al: Clinical and pathological features and laboratory confirmation of Creutzfeldt-Jakob disease in a recipient of pituitary-derived human growth hormone. N Engl J Med, 313:734, 1985.
71. Gibbs CJ, Jr, et al: Oral transmission of kuru, Creutzfeldt-Jakob disease and scrapie to nonhuman primates. J Infect Dis, 142:205, 1980.
72. Carlson GA, et al: Linkage of prion protein and scrapie incubation time genes. Cell, 46:503, 1986.
73. Westaway D, et al: Distinct prion proteins in short and long scrapie incubation period mice. Cell, 51:651, 1987.
74. Brown P, et al: Diagnosis of Creutzfeldt-Jakob disease by western blot identification of marker protein in human brain tissue. N Engl J Med, 314:547, 1986.
75. Gajdusek DC, et al: Precautions in medical care of, and in handling materials from, patients with transmissible virus dementia (Creutzfeldt-Jakob disease). N Engl J Med, 297:1253, 1977.

Section II

BACTERIA

Chapter 24

INTRODUCTION TO BACTERIA

Bacteria are single-celled prokaryotes, most of which reproduce by binary fission. Most are free-living and possess the genetic information and energy-producing and biosynthetic systems required for growth and reproduction; however, a few—chlamydiae (Chapter 25) and rickettsiae (Chapter 26)—are obligate intracellular parasites that lack one or more of these properties. Almost all bacteria have a layered cell envelope composed of the plasma membrane, cell wall, and associated proteins; some produce an external polysaccharide covering, termed a capsule or slime; and some have filamentous surface appendages, called flagella or pili (Fig. 24–1) (1). Internal to the cell wall is the central fibrillar chromatin network or nucleoid, surrounded by an amorphous cytoplasm containing ribosomes, energy storage granules, and in a few bacteria, endospores. Bacteria lack the membrane-bound organelles present in eucaryotic cells—a nucleus, lysosomes, endoplasmic reticulum, Golgi bodies. In this chapter, bacterial classification, structure, laboratory diagnosis (methods of detection and identification), and susceptibility testing are discussed.

CLASSIFICATION

Bacteria are classified functionally in this book—by their ability to grow outside cells, the presence or absence of a cell wall, Gram-stain reaction, shape (cocci, rods, spirochetes), oxygen requirement (aerobic, facultative, microaerophilic, anaerobic), need for special growth factors, and ability to resist decolorization by acid after staining. In each group, bacteria are further divided to the species level, based on genome size, guanine-plus-cytosine content, deoxyribonucleic acid (DNA) relatedness under optimal and supraoptimal conditions for DNA reassociation, and the thermal stability of related DNA sequences (2). Members of a species should have a similar-sized genome and guanine-plus-cytosine content, and the DNA relatedness should be 70% or more at an optimal reassociation temperature (25° to 30°C below the temperature at which native double-stranded DNA is denatured into single strands) with 0 to 4% divergence in related sequences, and 60% or more at a supraoptimal reassociation temperature (10° to 14°C below the temperature at which native double-stranded DNA is denatured). However, using these genetic parameters to identify bacterial isolates currently is not practical in the clinical laboratory. Identification usually is based on biochemical tests or the recognition of specific bacterial antigens, and nucleic acid probes specific for a few bacteria are commercially available.

STRUCTURE

The bacterial cell envelope, which accounts for about 20% of the cell's dry weight, is a multilayered structure that includes the plasma membrane, the cell wall, specialized proteins or polysaccharides, and any outer adherent materials. It contains transport sites for nutrients and components that are potentially toxic to the host and is the site of interaction with host antibodies and complement (see Chapter 2). The plasma (or cytoplasmic) membrane, a delicate, trilaminar unit-membrane composed of 60 to 70% protein, 30 to 40% lipid, and a small amount of carbohydrate (sterols also are present in the plasma membranes of the mycoplasmas), serves as an osmotic barrier for the cell, contains the energy-producing cytochrome and oxidative phosphorylation system and transport systems for solutes, and regulates transport of cell products to the extracellular environment.

The cell wall, present in all free-living pathogenic bacteria except the mycoplasmas, protects the cell from rupture in low osmotic pressure environments and maintains the cell's shape. The basic cell wall structure of gram-positive and gram-negative bacteria is different (see Fig. 24–1), which in large part is responsible for the differential staining properties. The thick (15 to 80 nm) cell wall of gram-positive bacteria consists of a peptidoglycan layer composed of chains of alternating subunits of N-acetylglucosamine and N-acetylmuramic acid cross-linked through carboxyl groups of terminal D-alanine residues on tetrapeptides. All gram-positive cell walls contain teichoic acid bound to the plasma membrane and, in most gram-positive cells, also covalently linked to the peptidoglycan layer. The cell wall of streptococci contains the specific group carbohydrates; and some gram-positive bacteria have important proteins on their surface, such as the M protein of group A Streptococcus and protein A of Staphylococcus aureus (Chapter 28).

Structurally, the gram-negative cell wall is more complex. External to the plasma membrane is a thin (1 to 2 nm) peptidoglycan layer, outside of which is the phospholipid outer membrane (not present in gram-positive cells); and between the outer membrane and the plasma membrane is an area called the periplasmic space. The outer membrane, which prevents the loss of periplasmic proteins and provides protection against hydrolytic enzymes and toxic substances such as bile in the gastrointestinal tract, consists of a lipid bilayer composed of proteins, a lipoprotein layer, and lipopolysaccharide (LPS). The outer membrane proteins have several functions. They are involved in the functional integrity of the membrane, in cell division, and in conjugation. They function as nonspecific diffusion pores, allowing the passage of low–molecular weight nutrients, and protect against the loss of hydrolytic enzymes and nutrient-binding proteins residing in the periplasmic space. Porin proteins form grating channels in the membrane that regulate transport, which in part is responsible for antimicrobial resistance. Moreover, outer

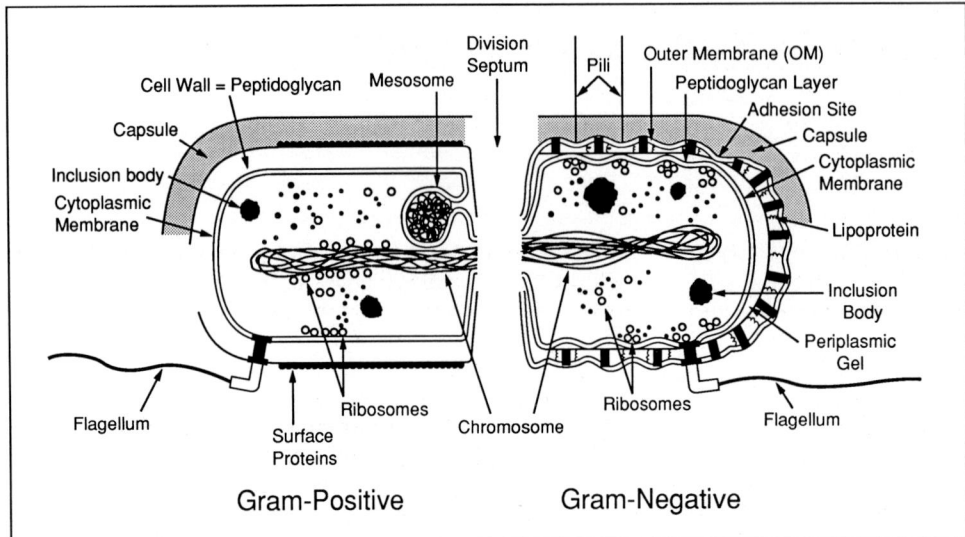

Fig. 24–1. Diagram of typical gram-positive and gram-negative cells, showing similarities and cell wall differences. (From Wheat, R. W.: Bacterial morphology and ultrastructure. In Zinsser Microbiology. 19th ed. Edited by W. K. Joklik, H. P. Willett, D. B. Lange, and C. M. Wilfert. Norwalk, Appleton & Lange, 1988.)

membrane proteins of some organisms appear to be associated with virulence and to play a role in immunity to infection by inducing antibody production. The lipoprotein layer gives stability to the outer membrane and crosslinks it to diaminopimelic acids in the peptidoglycan layer.

The LPS (or endotoxin), the major component of the outer membrane of gram-negative bacteria, consists of lipid A, the endotoxin moiety, which anchors the LPS to the membrane, and polysaccharide or oligosaccharide chains (O, or somatic, antigens), major immunodeterminants of the organism, which extend outward from lipid A. Lipid A plays a primary role in the structural integrity of the membrane and is the toxic portion of LPS, associated with fever, hypothermia, local Schwartzman reaction, leukopenia and leukocytosis, induction of prostaglandin synthesis by macrophages, mitogenesis for lymphocytes, lethal toxicity in animals in the laboratory, enhancement of monocyte migration, interferon induction, adjuvant activity, and production of interleukin-1 and tumor necrosis factor (see Chapter 2) (3–6).

Surrounding the cell wall of many invasive gram-positive and gram-negative bacteria is a capsular polysaccharide, or slime layer, that serves an antiphagocytic function, allowing the organism to evade normal host defense mechanisms (see Chapter 2) (5). Capsular polysaccharides may be useful diagnostically, because the capsule often is sloughed into the surrounding fluids as the organism grows and may be detected in soluble form as free antigens in the cerebrospinal fluid, serum, and urine of infected persons (discussed later). The capsular antigen corresponds to the K antigens of the Enterobacteriaceae (and the Vi antigens of some serotypes of Salmonella) (see Chapter 34).

Extending from the surface of many pathogenic bacteria are helical protein filaments of uniform length and diameter, called flagella, that are responsible for motility. Bacteria with a single polar flagellum are termed monotrichous; those with a tuft of several polar flagella, lophotrichous; those with flagella at both poles, amphitrichous; and those with many flagella distributed over the entire cell surface, peritrichous. Located on the flagella are heat-labile H antigens, which can undergo phase variation, the property by which a bacterium alternates the expression of one type of flagellar antigen with an unrelated type, thus preventing its immobilization by antibodies directed against the first type. In place of flagella, spirochetes (see Chapter 39) are motile by means of flagellum-like axial filaments located in the periplasmic space between the inner and outer membranes of the cell, around which the cell is coiled.

Fimbriae, or pili, which are hairlike microfibrils 0.004 to 0.008 μm long, composed of about 1000 subunits of an identical protein arranged in a helix, are located on the surface of many bacteria, predominantly gram-negative organisms. These structures serve as adhesins, promoting adherence of the bacteria to mucosal surfaces, an essential first step in their colonization of the host. In addition, fimbriae may prevent phagocytosis, acting as evasins; they may be leukocidal; and they may act as sex pili, functioning in cell-to-cell adhesion during bacterial conjugation.

Cytoplasmic structures found in all bacterial cells include the nuclear body, ribosomes, and cytoplasmic granules. The bacterial genome, representing 2 to 3% of the cell's weight, is a single circular chromosome composed of double-stranded DNA that replicates amitotically. The molecular weight of DNA in most bacteria is between 1 and 8 billion; it specifies 1500 to 6000 average-sized genes. Polyribosome-membrane aggregates, composed of chains of 70S ribosomes which dissociate into 30S and 50S subunits, attached to messenger RNA, are the sites of protein synthesis. Various granules represent accumulations of food reserves, predominantly glycogen but also lipids and polyphosphates.

In addition to these structures, species of Bacillus and Clostridium (Chapters 29 and 30, respectively) may produce endospores, highly refractile bodies formed within the vegetative bacterial cell that allow them to survive adverse environmental conditions of dryness, heat, and poor nutrient supply. The spore coat includes a peptidoglycan layer and surface antigens, both of a different composition from that of the parent vegetative cell.

LABORATORY DIAGNOSIS

Detection of bacteria in clinical samples first involves the collection of an appropriate specimen and timely transport to the laboratory (discussed in Part III). The specimen then is processed to allow the detection of bacteria by several methods: microscopic examination, culture, antigen detection, and nucleic acid hybridization. In addition, infections with certain bacteria are diagnosed most easily by serologic tests or by histologic examination of involved tissue. Each of these methods, and techniques that may be used in the future, are discussed.

Microscopic Examination. Microscopic examination of unstained fresh material or smears prepared from clinical specimens or bacterial colonies and variously stained is valuable for several reasons. The type and degree of the inflammatory response can be assessed, the quality of the specimen can be determined, and visualization of micro-organisms may provide sufficient information to allow initiation of empiric antimicrobial therapy. Unstained specimens are evaluated by examining *wet mount preparations* by darkfield or phase-contrast microscopy, an approach used principally to diagnose infections caused by spirochetes (Chapter 39) that also may provide a presumptive diagnosis of diarrhea caused by Campylobacter jejuni if characteristic short, curved bacilli showing darting motility are seen in stool samples (Chapter 37).

Of the various stains available, the *Gram stain,* first devised by Hans Christian Gram in the late nineteenth century, remains the most efficient and cost-effective test for rapid diagnosis of bacterial infections. With the Gram stain (see Appendix, Procedure 3), bacteria are divided into two groups, gram-positive (Plate IB) and gram-negative (Plate IC)—based on the difference in their cell wall composition. The extensive teichoic acid cross-links of gram-positive cell walls presumably contribute to the organisms' ability to resist decolorization and retain the crystal violet. In addition to determining the Gram reaction and cellular structure of bacteria forming individual colonies, a direct Gram stain of clinical material may be used to assess the suitability of sputum for culture (see Chapter 57), to determine the numbers and structure of bacteria present, and to determine the presence of significant bacteriuria (see Chapter 61).

Acridine orange, a fluorochrome that binds to native or denatured nucleic acid, has been used as an alternative to blind subculturing of blood cultures (see Chapter 58) and to detect bacteria in smears prepared from fluids such as cerebrospinal fluid and exudates in which organisms are expected to be present in low concentrations or may be difficult to visualize by Gram staining because of the large amount of background debris (7). To perform the staining, an air-dried, methanol-fixed smear of the material to be examined is flooded with acridine orange for 2 minutes, rinsed with tap water, air dried, and examined with a fluorescence microscope. The stain detects living bacteria but does not distinguish gram-positive from gram-negative organisms; therefore, specimens that demonstrate bacteria with the acridine orange stain should be stained with Gram stain to determine the differential staining characteristics of the organisms.

Mycobacteria (Chapter 40) have long-chain (50 to 90 carbon atoms) fatty acids, termed mycolic acids, in their cell walls, which property is responsible for their ability to resist decolorizing by strong organic solvents such as a mixture of ethanol and hydrochloric acid. These organisms, characterized as acid fast, may be distinguished from other bacteria by staining with *acid-fast stains*: Ziehl-Neelson, Kinyoun, and the fluorochrome dyes auramine and rhodamine (see Appendix, Procedures 4–6, and Plates ID, IE). Acid-fast stains also may be used to identify nonbacterial micro-organisms, such as the oocysts of Cryptosporidium and Isospora belli (see Chapter 49). The Nocardia (see Chapter 29), decolorized by the acid-alcohol step of a standard acid-fast stain but not by a mild decolorizer such as 0.5 to 1% sulfuric acid, are partially or weakly acid fast bacteria and may be differentiated from other filamentous, branching, gram-positive rods by staining with a modified acid-fast stain (see Appendix, Procedure 7, and Plate IF).

The Warthin-Starry silver stain is used to detect spirochetes in formalin-fixed tissue sections, and modified Dieterle stain is useful in demonstrating spirochetes of Borrelia burgdorferi in tissue sections from persons with Lyme disease. The Giemsa stain may be used to visualize inclusions of Chlamydia trachomatis in corneal scrapings from a person with conjunctivitis, but because this method lacks sensitivity and specificity it has been replaced by a stain utilizing fluorescein isothiocyanate–labeled monoclonal antibodies (see Chapter 25).

Polyclonal and monoclonal antibodies bound to the fluorochrome fluorescein isothiocyanate are used to directly visualize certain bacteria by fluorescence microscopy. Commercially available antibodies specific for Chlamydia trachomatis (Chapter 25), Bordetella pertussis (Chapter 33), and species of Legionella (Chapter 33) are used to detect these organisms directly in clinical specimens and for culture confirmation. In addition, other fluorescein-conjugated antibodies are used to identify isolates of group A Streptococcus (Chapter 28) and Neisseria gonorrhoeae (Chapter 31).

Culture. Different types of media are used for primary recovery of bacteria from clinical specimens. The chlamydiae and rickettsiae (except Rochalimaea quintana) cannot be recovered on artificial media but may be isolated in cell culture, a technique reviewed in Chapter 3 and discussed in more detail in Chapters 25 and 26. Media may be *nonselective*—free of inhibitors and able to support the growth of most organisms encountered in the clinical laboratory—or *selective*—containing one or more agents, such as dyes or antimicrobial agents, that inhibit all organisms except the organism or group of organisms being sought. *Enrichment media* are used to recover a limited number of bacteria from a specimen containing large numbers of commensal organisms, such as stool. *Differential media* contain a factor or factors that allow differentiation of colonies of bacteria based on specific metabolic or cultural characteristics of those organisms. Inoculating broth media for primary recovery of bacteria is recommended only for specimens in which detection of a few organisms in low concentration may be significant (body fluids, needle biopsy specimens, or aspirates from deep tissue infections). Listed in Table 24–1 are the primary planting media used routinely in the clinical laboratory, the ingredients that afford them selective, enrichment, or differential capability, and their main purpose. Media used less frequently, and generally for the purpose of recovering a specific pathogen, are discussed in Part III (see Table 54-4).

The appearance of individual colonies growing on the agar medium (size, form, elevation, margin, color, surface, density, and consistency) and the reactions on the agar (hemolysis of blood, pigment production, and changes in differential media) are useful identifying features. Preliminary impressions derived from these observations are confirmed by examining smears of the colonies stained with Gram stain. Isolates then are identified by performing biochemical tests (discussed in detail in the following chapters) selected on the basis of colony characteristics and Gram reaction, by detecting specific antigens, or by nucleic acid hybridization.

Antigen Detection. The ability to detect bacterial antigens, for example cell wall components, capsular material, and bacterial products such as toxins, by one or more techniques—counterimmunoelectrophoresis (CIE), particle agglutination, and enzyme-linked immunosorbent assay (ELISA)—allows rapid detection of several organisms. With CIE, an electrical current is placed across a double-diffusion system to accelerate the reaction of any negatively charged antigens and uncharged antibodies, recognized as a visible precipitin band in agarose gel. It has been used to detect polysaccharide antigens of Streptococcus pneumoniae, Haemophilus influenzae type b, and Neisseria meningitidis in cerebrospinal fluid (CSF); however, because the test is labor intensive and costly, the bands often are difficult to interpret, results are not available for several hours, and the sensitivity is only 0.01 to 0.05 mg/ml antigen (or about 1000 organisms per milliliter of fluid), CIE has been replaced in most laboratories by the more sensitive and more rapid particle agglutination tests.

Particle agglutination tests include latex agglutination, in which antibodies bound to the surface of latex beads bind to antigens present in the solution being tested, forming visible cross-linked aggregates, and coagglutination, which is similar in principle to latex agglutination but utilizes antibodies bound to protein A of Staphylococcus aureus (8). Kits for detection of antigens of Streptococcus pneumoniae, group B Streptococcus, Haemophilus influenzae type b and several capsular types of Neisseria meningitidis (N. meningitidis type b and Escherichia coli cross-react) in body fluids (primarily CSF but also urine and serum); for detection of antigens of group A Streptococcus in throat swabs; and for colony confirmation of Streptococcus groups A, B, C, D, F, and G, Streptococcus pneumoniae, Neisseria meningitidis, Neisseria gonorrhoeae, Staphylococcus aureus and Haemophilus influenzae types a through f are commercially available. These tests are technically simple and provide rapid results.

Table 24–1. Primary Planting Media Commonly Used in the Clinical Laboratory

Medium	Ingredients	Primary Use
Blood agar	Trypticase soy agar, Brucella agar, or beef heart infusion base with 5% sheep blood	Cultivation of most unfastidious bacteria; determining hemolytic reactions
Chocolate agar	Peptone base agar enriched with 2% hemoglobin or IsoVitaleX	Cultivating Haemophilus and Neisseria
MacConkey agar	Peptone base agar, crystal violet and bile salts (inhibit gram-positive organisms), lactose, neutral red indicator	Isolate gram-negative bacteria and differentiate lactose fermenters from lactose nonfermenters
Eosin methylene blue (EMB) agar	Peptone base; lactose, sucrose; eosin and methylene blue as indicators and inhibitors of gram-positive bacteria	As for MacConkey
Hektoen enteric agar	Peptone base agar; bile salts (inhibit gram-positive organisms); lactose, sucrose, salicin; ammonium sulfate to detect H_2S production; bromthymol blue and acid fuchsin indicators	Differential and selective medium for isolating Salmonella and Shigella from stool and differentiating them from gram-negative bacteria of the normal fecal flora
CDC anaerobic blood agar	Trypticase soy agar with 5% sheep blood, hemin, L-cysteine, vitamin K	Isolation of anaerobes
Columbia colistin–nalidixic acid (CNA) agar	Columbia agar base; 5% sheep blood; colistin, nalidixic acid	Selective recovery of gram-positive bacteria
Thayer-Martin agar	Blood agar base; hemoglobin, supplement B; colistin, vancomycin, nystatin, trimethoprim	Selective isolation of Neisseria gonorrhoeae
Xylose lysine deoxycholate (XLD) agar	Yeast extract agar; sodium deoxycholate inhibits gram-positive bacteria; lysine, xylose, lactose, sucrose; ferric ammonium citrate to detect H_2S production; phenol red indicator	As for Hektoen enteric agar
Campy-blood agar	Brucella agar base; sheep blood; trimethoprim, polymyxin B, amphotericin B, cephalothin	Selective recovery of Campylobacter from stool
Gram-negative (GN) broth	Peptone base broth; glucose, mannitol; sodium citrate and sodium deoxycholate as inhibitory agents	Enrichment broth medium for Salmonella and Shigella
Thioglycolate broth	Pancreatic digest of casein, soy broth and glucose; thioglycolate and low concentration of agar	Supports growth of most aerobes, anaerobes, and microaerophilic and fastidious bacteria

However, the kits used to detect bacterial antigens in CSF are expensive (about 100 times the cost of the Gram stain) and their sensitivity for diagnosing bacterial meningitis is similar to that of the Gram stain. Therefore, particle agglutination is recommended only to confirm a Gram stain result and for diagnosis of partially treated meningitis. Moreover, the sensitivity of the kits for detection of group A Streptococcus organisms in throat swabs is only about 70%; consequently, a negative result does not exclude the diagnosis and should be followed by culture (9,10).

Different types of ELISA systems, consisting of antibodies bonded to enzymes that catalyze a reaction yielding a visible end product while attached to the antibodies, are available commercially. In solid-phase immunosorbent assays antibodies are firmly fixed to a solid matrix—wells of a microtiter tray or plastic or metal beads; in membrane-bound solid-phase immunosorbent assays antibodies are mobilized on a membrane such as nitrocellulose or nylon. ELISA is simple, rapid, and in some cases able to detect antigen in concentrations as weak as 1 ng/ml. Kits for detection of Chlamydia trachomatis in cervical or urethral swab specimens or in urine of males, group A Streptococcus in throat swabs, and Clostridium difficile toxin in stool are commercially available. Their sensitivity ranges from about 70% for group A Streptococcus to over 90% for C. difficile toxin (see Chapters 25, 28, and 30) (11–13).

Nucleic Acid Probes. Nucleic acid probes—discrete sequences of DNA or RNA forming strong covalently bonded hybrids with the specific complementary strand of nucleic acid—may be used to detect bacteria in clinical specimens or for culture confirmation. Radiolabeled, biotin-labeled, or chemiluminescent probes are commercially available to detect Chlamydia trachomatis, Neisseria gonorrhoeae, and species of Legionella directly in clinical specimens and for culture confirmation of Staphylococcus aureus, group B Streptococcus, Enterococcus, Neisseria gonorrhoeae, Haemophilus influenzae type b, thermophilic campylobacters, and several species of Mycobacterium (14–18).

Serologic Tests. Infections with certain fastidious or uncultivable bacteria—Rickettsia organisms, Mycoplasma pneumoniae, Francisella tularensis, species of Brucella, Treponema pallidum, Borrelia burgdorferi, Leptospira interrogans, and perhaps Helicobacter pylori—are diagnosed most easily by detecting specific antibodies in serum. Tests that detect immunoglobulin (Ig) M specific for Mycoplasma pneumoniae are commercially available, providing early diagnosis; but for most of the other organisms mentioned above, only tests for detection of specific IgG, which usually is not present early in the acute phase of infection, are available. To diagnose infection with these organisms, therefore, acute- and convalescent-phase serum samples must be tested, which delays the diagnosis a few weeks.

Future Technology. Gene amplification via the polymerase chain reaction is a very sensitive and specific tool for detecting micro-organisms and in the future may be used in the clinical laboratory (19). In addition, flow cytometry, in which organisms stained with fluorescent dyes pass through a detector module in a thin stream of liquid and are recognized by the size, charge, and staining characteristics of the particles, has been suggested as a possible means to detect bacteria in body fluids such as blood and urine (20).

SUSCEPTIBILITY TESTING

Antimicrobial susceptibility testing should be performed on all clinically significant isolates of rapidly growing, unfastidious aerobic and facultative bacteria except the β-hemolytic species of Streptococcus, which have a consistently predictable susceptibility pattern (see Chapter 28). The basic principles of the susceptibility testing methods used most often in the clinical laboratory—broth dilution, disk diffusion, and β-lactamase detection—are described; more comprehensive discussions are available elsewhere (7,21–26). Special situations pertaining to specific organisms are discussed separately in the appropriate chapters. Additional topics briefly reviewed here are susceptibility testing of anaerobes, selection and reporting of antimicrobial agents, tests to evaluate bactericidal activity, and therapeutic drug monitoring.

Broth Dilution. In general, broth dilution testing—macrotube or, commonly in the clinical laboratory, microdilution using commercially available multiwell plates (Fig. 24–2)—determines the lowest or minimum concentration of an antimicrobial agent that inhibits the growth of an organism. These techniques have been standardized by the National Committee for Clinical Laboratory Standards (NCCLS), and published guidelines should be followed (24). A standard inoculum of the isolate is prepared as follows: Several similar-looking colonies are inoculated to a broth medium such as brain-heart infusion or Mueller-Hinton broth. The broth is incubated 4 to 6 hours (until growth is considered to be in the logarithmic phase), and the density of the suspension is adjusted to equal about 10^8 colony-forming units (cfu) per milliliter by visually comparing its turbidity to that of a 0.5 McFarland standard (commercially available or prepared in

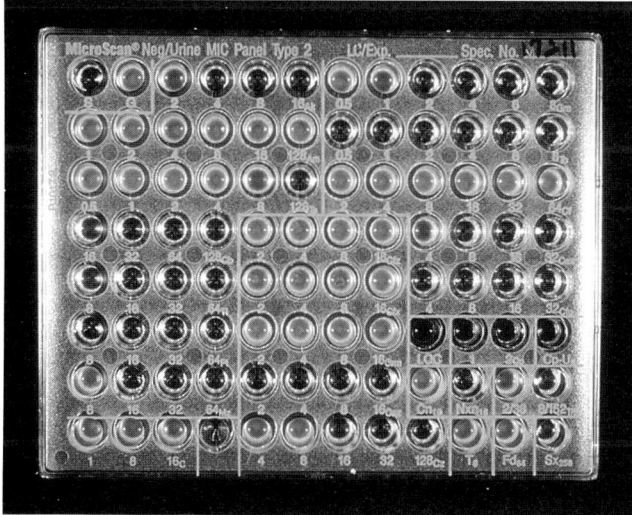

Fig. 24–2. Microdilution susceptibility testing of an isolate of Pseudomonas aeruginosa.

house by adding 0.5 ml of 0.048 M barium chloride to 99.5 ml 0.36 N sulfuric acid) against a white background on which black lines are drawn. Alternatively, the broth is inoculated directly with young colonies (representing overnight growth), and the turbidity is adjusted to the appropriate density. This suspension is diluted to yield a final inoculum of about 5×10^5 cfu/ml and inoculated into a series of tubes, each containing one concentration of the antimicrobial agent prepared in Mueller-Hinton broth supplemented with calcium, 20 to 25 mg/L, and magnesium, 12.5 mg/L, or to a microdilution tray containing a series of dilutions of several agents (final inoculum about 5×10^4 cfu per well). Cation supplementation is necessary to ensure acceptable results when evaluating the activity of aminoglycosides against isolates of Pseudomonas aeruginosa, which may appear (falsely) susceptible if cation concentrations are insufficient (22).

Tubes or plates are incubated at 35°C in ambient air overnight (16 to 18 hours) and examined for bacterial growth, which is best determined by comparison with the growth control. In general, growth is indicated by turbidity, one sedimented button 2 mm or more in diameter, or several smaller buttons. The lowest concentration that inhibits growth of the organism is called the minimum inhibitory concentration (MIC). Trailing end points may occur with trimethoprim or the sulfonamides, in which case the concentration of drug associated with 80 to 90% diminution of growth (compared with the growth control) should be considered the MIC. The "skipped" tube or well—growth is absent at one drug concentration but present at lower and higher concentrations—presents another potential interpretation problem. In this situation the skipped tube or well is ignored, and the concentration that inhibits growth with no growth occurring at higher concentrations is the MIC. If more than one tube or well is skipped, or if growth occurs at higher but not at lower concentrations of drug, results should not be reported and the test should be repeated.

The concentration of an antimicrobial agent that can be achieved in the serum with optimal therapy is called the breakpoint, and organisms with an MIC at or below that level are considered susceptible to that agent. If the MIC is above the achievable level or within a range that is toxic to the host, the organism is resistant to that agent. For certain organism–antimicrobial agent combinations other categories exist: "intermediate" indicates that the susceptibility of that particular organism cannot be predicted at that particular MIC, and "moderately susceptible" indicates that the organism may be inhibited by the antimicrobial agent if larger doses are used or in body sites where the drug is physiologically concentrated, such as urine. The MIC interpretive standards are published by the NCCLS (see reference 24).

Quality control of macrotube or microtiter dilution testing must be performed to evaluate the precision and accuracy of the dilutions and test procedures used, to monitor reliability of reagents, and to evaluate the performance of personnel who perform the tests. Reference strains should be genetically stable and give MICs in the midrange of each antimicrobial agent tested. Organisms recommended for quality control—Escherichia coli ATCC 25922 and ATCC 35218, Pseudomonas aeruginosa ATCC 27853, Enterococcus faecalis ATCC 29212, and Staphylococcus aureus ATCC 29213—may be purchased from the American Type Culture Collection or another commercial source. Testing Enterococcus faecalis ATCC 29212 against trimethoprim-sulfamethoxazole is useful in detecting inappropriate concentrations of substances such as thymidine that interfere with the activity of antifolate drugs in vitro; MICs greater than 0.5/9.5 µg/ml indicate that interfering substances are present. Working stock cultures of control organisms may be maintained on soybean-casein digest agar with weekly subcultures, and they must be replaced at least once a month (or sooner if results are questionable) from commercial cultures, lyophilized cultures, or cultures that have been frozen at $-20°$ C or lower in a stabilizer such as a broth medium with 15% glycerol, defibrinated sheep or rabbit blood, or 50% fetal calf serum in broth.

Quality control of each new lot of microtiter plates, panels, or trays prepared in house or purchased should be performed to determine accuracy (see references 22 and 24 for acceptable ranges) and sterility. Lots that fail to pass accuracy or sterility checks should be rejected. Quality control also should be performed daily, or at least every day that the panels are used to test clinical isolates. Two or more consecutive out-of-control MICs or more than two nonconsecutive out-of-control results in 20 consecutive tests indicate problems in the procedure that must be identified and solved. Daily testing may be abandoned for weekly testing if accuracy is documented by these criteria: When each drug–reference strain combination is tested for 30 consecutive days to obtain 30 MICs for each combination, three or fewer MICs per combination are outside the accuracy range. If during weekly testing a single MIC is outside the accuracy range, testing must be performed daily for 5 days. If all five MICs for the problem drug–organism combination are within the accuracy range, weekly testing may be resumed, but if one or more MICs fall outside the accuracy range, daily testing must be performed until for 30 consecutive days no more than three MICs are outside the accuracy range.

Disk Diffusion. To perform disk diffusion testing, filter paper disks, each impregnated with a specific concentration of an antimicrobial agent, are placed on the surface of a Mueller-Hinton agar plate (which may be supplemented with 5% defibrinated sheep blood to enhance bacterial growth, if necessary) that has been inoculated with a lawn of a standardized inoculum (prepared as described earlier for dilution testing) of the test isolate. Disks should be stored in the refrigerator or frozen at $-20°$ C or lower, and those containing β-lactam compounds must be frozen to ensure preservation of their potency. Plates are incubated overnight (16 to 18 hours) at 35°C in ambient air, and the zone of inhibition of growth surrounding the disk is measured (Fig. 24–3). Zone size is interpreted as susceptible, resistant, intermediate, or moderately susceptible (defined earlier) according to standards provided by NCCLS, guidelines based on results of regression analyses performed by plotting the zone sizes and MIC values of many strains of rapidly growing bacteria (Fig. 24–4) (25). Break point zone diameters

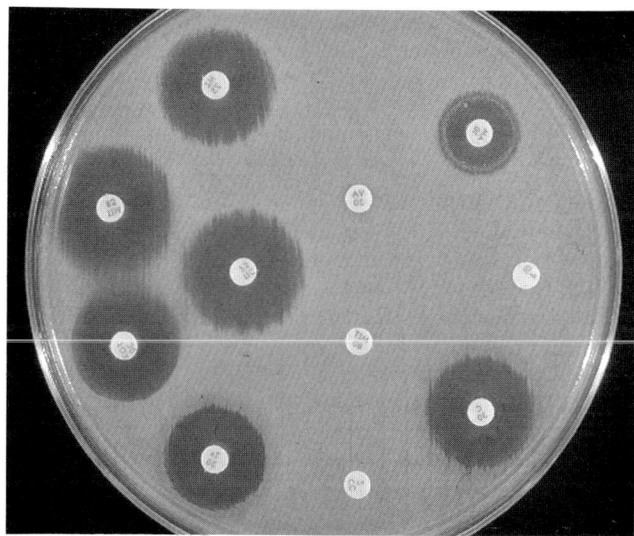

Fig. 24–3. The disk diffusion susceptibility test is interpreted by measuring the zone of inhibition (across its center, including the diameter of the disk) with a millimeter rule or calipers.

corresponding to MICs in the susceptible and resistant ranges, based on achievable serum levels, are selected. Disk diffusion testing should be used only to test isolates of bacteria that have been thoroughly evaluated by this method and should not be used to test bacteria that grow slowly, need special nutrients, or require carbon dioxide or anaerobic conditions to grow, although the test may be modified to evaluate isolates of Streptococcus pneumoniae (Chapter 28), Neisseria gonorrhoeae (Chapter 31), or Haemophilus influenzae (Chapter 36).

Quality control of disk diffusion testing, similar to that described above for dilution testing, must be performed. Recommended control strains are Escherichia coli ATCC 25922, Staphylococcus aureus ATCC 25923, Pseudomonas aeruginosa ATCC 27853, and Enterococcus faecalis ATCC 29212 or 33186 (see references 23 and 25 for acceptable zone diameters). One E. faecalis strain is included to detect trace amounts of thymidine, thymine, or p-aminobenzoic acid, which interfere with trimethoprim and trimethoprim-sulfamethoxazole testing. Quality control must be performed on each new lot of Mueller-Hinton agar received and every day that clinical isolates are tested. In laboratories where satisfactory performance has been documented for 30 consecutive days, quality control testing may be reduced to once a week.

β-Lactamase Detection. Some bacteria are resistant to certain penicillins and cephalosporins because they produce β-lactamases, plasmid-mediated enzymes that bind to antimicrobial agents that possess a β-lactam ring (Fig. 24–5) and open the ring, inactivating the drug. Of the methods that may be used to detect β-lactamase production, only the most sensitive, the chromagenic cephalosporin method, is discussed here. (A more extensive review may be found in references 21 and 26.) Nitrocefin, a cephalosporin compound that is yellow when intact and red if the β-lactam ring is broken, is impregnated into disks (commercially available) onto which growth of the test organism (preferably from the primary isolation plate) is rubbed. Development of a red color within 30 minutes indicates the presence of β-lactamase. This test is most useful for testing Neisseria gonorrhoeae, Haemophilus influenzae, Branhamella catarrhalis, and all anaerobes, but also may be used to test species of Staphylococcus and Enterococcus.

Susceptibility Testing of Anaerobes. Susceptibility testing of anaerobes is indicated in few situations (28): to determine patterns of susceptibility to new antimicrobial agents, to monitor susceptibility patterns in various centers (reference laboratories) and periodically in local communities and hospitals, and at times, to assist in managing individual infections. Testing isolates that cause

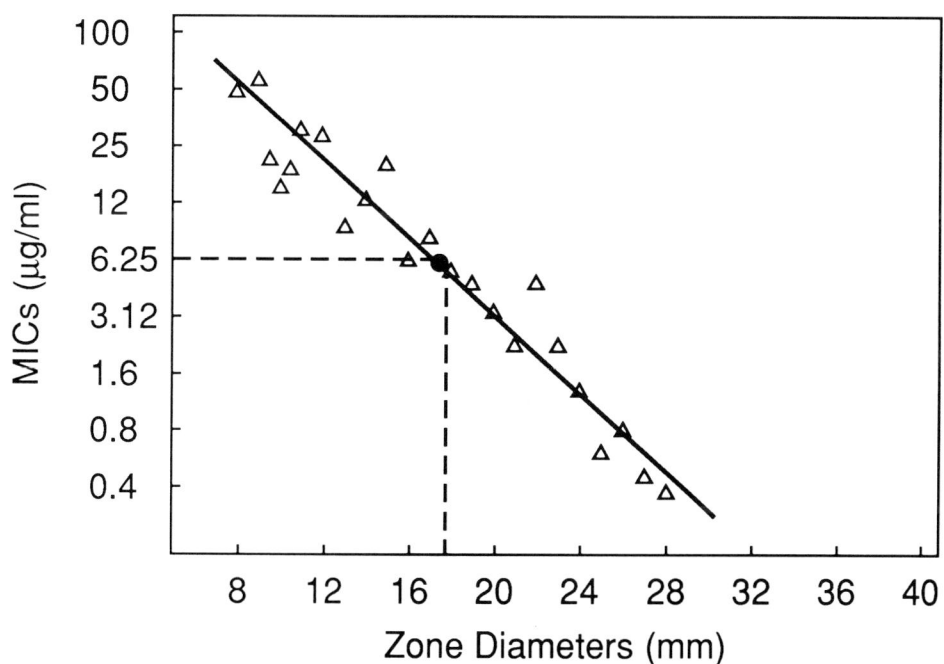

Fig. 24–4. Typical regression curve compares MICs (in micrograms per milliliter) with zone sizes (in millimeters). Each triangle represents the MIC and inhibitory zone for a single isolate. (From Koneman, EW, et al. (eds.): Color Atlas and Textbook of Diagnostic Microbiology. 3rd ed. Philadelphia, J.B. Lippincott, 1988.)

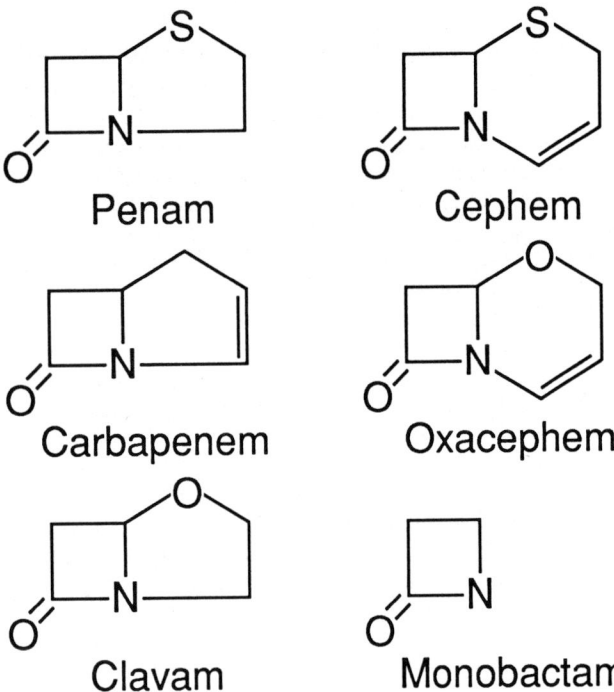

Fig. 24–5. Structural nuclei of the major β-lactam agents. Penicillin is a penem; cephalosporins and cephamycins are cephems; imipenem is a carbapenem; moxalactam is an oxacephem; clavulanic acid has a clavam nucleus; and aztreonam is a monobactam. (From Willett, H. P.: Antimicrobial agents. *In* Zinsser Microbiology. 19th ed. Edited by W. K. Joklik, H. P. Willett, D. B. Amos, and C. M. Wilfert. Norwalk, Appleton & Lange, 1988.)

brain abscesses, endocarditis, osteomyelitis, joint infections, infections of prosthetic devices or vascular grafts, and refractory or recurrent bacteremia is recommended. If multiple anaerobes are recovered, testing virulent or commonly resistant organisms should be considered—members of the Bacteroides fragilis group, species of Prevotella and Porphyromonas (formerly Bacteroides), some Fusobacterium, and some species of Clostridium (Clostridium perfringenes, Clostridium tertium, and Clostridium ramosum).

Several methods for determining the susceptibility of anaerobes to antimicrobial agents have been described: broth disk elution, β-lactamase, agar dilution, and broth micro- and macrodilution. Broth disk elution is not recommended owing to problems in performance, especially with newer cephalosporins; clustering about the break point of MICs to many drugs; and the lack of established quality control procedures. Beta-lactamase testing using a chromogenic cephalosporin (described earlier) rapidly detects β-lactamases produced by species of Prevotella, Porphyromonas, Bacteroides, and other anaerobes and accurately predicts resistance to penicillin G and ampicillin. However, because resistance of some organisms—Bilophila wadsworthia, Bacteroides gracilis, and some isolates of Bacteroides distasonis and Bacteroides fragilis—to β-lactam agents is not always mediated by β-lactamase production, and because the hydrolysis of drugs such as imipenem and cefoxitin may not be predictable by conventional β-lactamase testing the β-lactamase test result is limited in its clinical application.

Agar dilution is the established reference method for determining the activity of antimicrobial agents against anaerobes, but no "gold standard" has been accepted (28). A series of Wilkins-Chalgren agar plates (plain or supplemented with 5% defibrinated sheep blood or lysed sheep blood to allow growth of fastidious anaerobes), each containing a specific concentration of the antimicrobial agent to be tested, are spot inoculated with a standardized inoculum (1×10^4 cfu) of the test isolate, incubated anaerobically for 48 hours, and examined for growth. The lowest concentration of an agent that allows no more than one or two colonies or only a slight haze of growth is the MIC. Broth dilution is performed as described earlier for aerobic and facultative organisms, except that a different broth medium (Schaedler's, West-Wilkins, brain-heart infusion, or Wilkins-Chalgren) is used and tubes or microtiter trays (available commercially) are incubated anaerobically for 48 hours. Quantitative breakpoints indicating "susceptible" and "resistant" categories for the anaerobes have been established for some antimicrobial agents (see reference 28).

Selection and Reporting of Antimicrobial Agents. The antimicrobial agents commonly used, their mechanisms of action, and the organisms against which they usually are active are listed in Table 24–2. Agents that are tested in the clinical laboratory and reported should be determined jointly by the members of the hospital medical staff and the pharmacy, taking into consideration agents on the hospital formulary. The NCCLS has published guidelines based on proven clinical efficacy for the organism group and acceptable test performance in vitro for selection of antimicrobial agents to test against the rapidly growing aerobic and facultative bacteria (24). Recommendations based on these guidelines and personal experience are listed in Table 24–3. However, certain NCCLS guidelines pertaining to reporting or testing of antimicrobial agents must be followed to ensure a high standard of care. For example, cephalosporins and clindamycin should not be tested or reported against species of Enterococcus because the results may be misleading. Isolates of Staphylococcus that are resistant to the penicillinase-resistant penicillins (oxacillin, nafcillin, methicillin) should be considered resistant to the cephalosporins, amoxicillin-clavulanate, ticarcillin-clavulanate, ampicillin-sulbactam, and imipenem and reported as such, regardless of results of susceptibility testing. Moreover, cephalothin, not cefazolin, should be used to predict the susceptibility of isolates of Enterobacteriaceae, especially isolates of Escherichia coli, to other first-generation cephalosporins, because a significant number of false-susceptible errors would result if cefazolin were used.

For anaerobes susceptibility to penicillin G, one or more broad-spectrum antipseudomonal penicillin (carbenicillin, ticarcillin), clindamycin, cefoxitin, and certain other cephalosporins active against anaerobes (cefmetazole, cefoperazone, cefotaxime, cefotetan, ceftizoxime) should be evaluated (28). Metronidazole, chloramphenicol, imipenem, ampicillin-sulbactam, amoxicillin-clavulanate, and ticarcillin-clavulanate almost always are active

Table 24–2. Commonly Used Antimicrobial Agents, Their Mechanism of Action, and Usual Spectrum of Activity

Antimicrobial Agent	Mechanism of Action	Spectrum of Activity
Penicillins	Bind to penicillin-binding proteins in the cell wall, inhibiting cell wall synthesis	

Natural penicillins
    Penicillin G
    Penicillin V
		Streptococcus pneumoniae, β-hemolytic streptococci, viridans streptococci, Streptococcus bovis, Neisseria meningitidis, β-lactamase–negative staphylococci and Neisseria gonorrhoeae, gram-positive anaerobes

Penicillinase-resistant penicillins
    Oxacillin
    Nafcillin
    Methicillin
		β-lactamase–positive staphylococci

Aminopenicillins
    Ampicillin
    Amoxicillin
		Proteus mirabilis, many Escherichia coli, β-lactamase–negative Haemophilus and Neisseria gonorrhoeae, Enterococcus (plus an aminoglycoside for serious infections), Listeria

Anti-Pseudomonas penicillins
    Azlocillin
    Carbenicillin
    Ticarcillin
		Pseudomonas

Extended-spectrum penicillins
    Mezlocillin
    Piperacillin
		Pseudomonas

Cephalosporins	As for penicillins	

First generation
    Cefazolin
    Cephalothin
		Gram-positive cocci (except methicillin-resistant staphylococci), Escherichia coli, Klebsiella pneumoniae, Proteus mirabilis

Second generation
    Cefamandole
    Cefuroxime
    Cefotetan
    Cefoxitin
		Active against many Enterobacteriaceae and Haemophilus; cefoxitin active against many anaerobes (including many Bacteroides)

Third generation
    Cefotaxime
    Ceftizoxime
    Ceftriaxone
		β-lactamase–positive Neisseria gonorrhoeae, many Enterobacteriaceae; meningitis due to β-lactamase–positive Haemophilus influenzae

Third generation with anti-Pseudomonas activity
    Ceftazidime
    Cefoperazone
		Pseudomonas

Other β-lactams	As for penicillins	
Carbapenems Imipenem		Enterobacteriaceae, Pseudomonas, anaerobes
Monobactams Aztreonam	Binds to penicillin-binding proteins only in gram-negative aerobic bacteria	Enterobacteriaceae, some Pseudomonas spp.
β-lactamase inhibitors Amoxicillin-clavulanate		Otitis media due to β-lactamase–positive Haemophilus influenzae and Branhamella
Ticarcillin-clavulanate		Aerobic gram-negative bacilli
Ampicillin-sulbactam		Mixed aerobic and anaerobic intra-abdominal and pelvic infections

Aminoglycosides
  Gentamicin
  Tobramycin
  Amikacin
	Inhibit bacterial proteins synthesis	Enterobacteriaceae, Pseudomonas, Acinetobacter

Streptomycin		Brucella, Francisella, Yersinia pestis
Tetracyclines	Inhibit bacterial protein synthesis (reversibly bind to 30S ribosome)	Brucella, Rickettsia
Chloramphenicol	Inhibits bacterial protein synthesis (reversibly binds 50S subunit of ribosome)	Haemophilus, Salmonella, anaerobes, many Enterobacteriaceae
Metronidazole	Bactericidal by damaging DNA	Anaerobes (except gram-positive cocci), Clostridium difficile colitis
Erythromycin	Inhibits RNA-dependent bacterial protein synthesis	Aerobic gram-positive cocci, Legionella, Campylobacter, Mycoplasma pneumoniae, Chlamydia, Branhamella
Clindamycin	Inhibits bacterial protein synthesis	Anaerobes, gram-positive cocci
Vancomycin	Inhibits synthesis and assembly of cell wall peptidoglycan polymers by complexing with D-alanyl-D-alanine precursor	Methicillin-resistant staphylococci, Clostridium difficile colitis, ampicillin-resistant Enterococcus (plus an aminoglycoside)
Trimethoprim-sulfamethoxazole	Sulfonamides: bacteriostatic by interfering with microbial folic acid synthesis; Trimethoprim: inhibits bacterial dihydrofolate reductase	Shigella, Branhamella, Haemophilus, some Enterobacteriaceae (especially urine isolates)

Quinolones
  Ciprofloxacin
  Norfloxacin
	Inhibit DNA gyrase	Active against aerobic gram-positive and gram-negative bacteria (recommended primarily for complicated urinary tract infections, bacterial gastroenteritis, osteomyelitis with gram-negative bacilli, and exacerbations of pneumonia in persons with cystic fibrosis)

Table 24-3. Antimicrobial Agents to Consider for Routine Testing and Reporting

Organisms	Antimicrobial Agents*
Enterobacteriaceae and Acinetobacter†	amikacin, ampicillin, cefazolin, cephalothin, cefotaxime (or ceftizoxime or ceftriaxone), gentamicin, mezlocillin, tobramycin, trimethoprim-sulfamethoxazole, [norfloxacin, trimethoprim]
Pseudomonas and Acinetobacter†	amikacin, ceftazidime (or cefoperazone), gentamicin, mezlocillin (or piperacillin), tobramycin, trimethoprim-sulfamethoxazole [norfloxacin]
Staphylococcus spp	ampicillin, cephalothin, clindamycin, erythromycin, gentamicin, oxacillin, penicillin G, rifampin, trimethoprim-sulfamethoxazole, vancomycin [norfloxacin, trimethoprim]
Enterococcus spp	penicillin G (or ampicillin), vancomycin [erythromycin, norfloxacin, tetracycline], streptomycin and gentamicin synergy
Streptococcus spp	penicillin G, cephalothin, chloramphenicol, erythromycin, vancomycin [norfloxacin]
Haemophilus spp	ampicillin, ceftriaxone (or cefotaxime or ceftizoxime), cefuroxime, chloramphenicol, trimethoprim-sulfamethoxazole

* Agents in brackets [ ] could be included for isolates from urine.
† For very resistant organisms only, ciprofloxacin and imipenem should be reported.

(Data from National Committee for Clinical Laboratory Standards: Dilution procedures for susceptibility testing of aerobic bacteria. Approved Standard NCCLS Publication M7-A2. 2nd ed. Villanova, PA, NCCLS, 1990.)

against anaerobes and currently do not need to be tested for clinical purposes (28). When reporting susceptibility test results for anaerobes, the following footnote should be added: "Metronidazole, chloramphenicol, imipenem, ampicillin-sulbactam, amoxicillin-clavulanate, and ticarcillin-clavulanate are not tested against anaerobes because, currently, almost all isolates are susceptible (except most non–spore-forming anaerobic gram-positive rods and some isolates of Peptostreptococcus are resistant to metronidazole, and many isolates of Bilophila wadsworthia are resistant to imipenem and the β-lactam–β-lactamase inhibitors)."

If microdilution testing was performed, both the minimum inhibitory concentration and the interpretation should be included in reports of susceptibility test results. In addition, reporting only selected agents, noting the cost of different drugs, or both may limit the utilization of expensive cephalosporins and aminoglycosides in situations when a less costly agent would be equally effective. For example, if a gram-negative bacillus is susceptible to a first-generation cephalosporin, the results for second- and third-generation cephalosporins are not reported; likewise, tobramycin and amikacin results are not reported for a gentamicin-susceptible gram-negative bacillus.

Tests of Bactericidal Activity. Tests that measure bactericidal activity are the minimum bactericidal concentration (MBC) and the serum bactericidal test. The MBC, the lowest concentration of an antimicrobial agent that kills more than 99.9% of the bacteria being tested, is performed by first determining the MIC of the organism to a specific drug by broth macrodilution and then subculturing to agar plates a known volume (0.1 ml is recommended) of inoculum from tubes of broth that show no visible growth. Plates are incubated 24 to 48 hours, and the colonies are counted and compared to the number of cfu per milliliter in the original inoculum. The clinical value of the MBC is questionable, especially because the test is associated with technical problems and interpretation of results is ill-defined (29,30).

The serum bactericidal test (also known as the Schlichter test) measures the activity of the host's own serum against the pathogen in question (reviewed in reference 31). The test format is similar to that of the MBC. Current recommendations include testing an inoculum of 10^5 cfu/ml from an actively growing suspension of organisms in peak and trough serum samples (obtained 30 minutes after and immediately before delivery of an antimicrobial agent, respectively) serially diluted in a diluent containing at least 50% normal, noninhibitory, pooled human serum. From tubes that show no growth 0.1 ml of broth is subcultured to agar plates, which are incubated overnight and examined for growth. The serum bactericidal test most often is used to guide therapy for infective endocarditis. Data from one study of patients with bacterial endocarditis showed that a peak serum bactericidal titer of 1:64 or greater and a trough titer of 1:32 or greater were 100% predictive of bacteriologic cure, although lower titers did not predict treatment failure, because many patients with endocarditis caused by viridans streptococci (Chapter 28) were cured despite low serum bactericidal titers (32). The serum bactericidal test also has been recommended as a means to assess and monitor the adequacy of therapy of osteomyelitis and suppurative arthritis, and it may be useful for assessing combinations of antimicrobial agents for immunocompromised patients with bacterial infections (31).

Therapeutic Drug Monitoring. The amount of antimicrobial agent in the serum or body fluid of a patient is measured to determine whether an effective level is being achieved and, for agents that are therapeutically effective at concentrations very close to those that may be toxic to the host, levels are monitored to prevent toxicity while maintaining adequate therapeutic concentrations. Serum specimens most often are obtained immediately before administering a dose (trough) or 30 minutes after completing an intravenous infusion, 60 minutes after an intramuscular dose, or 1 to 2 hours after an oral dose (peak). Both the time of specimen collection and the time that the antimicrobial agent was given must be indicated to appropriately interpret results. For many years drug levels were measured by a microbiologic assay, but this method has been replaced by more sensitive, precise, and accurate methods such as gas-liquid chromatography, high-pressure liquid chromatography, enzyme assays, and various immunoassays, which often are performed in clinical chemistry rather than microbiology laboratories.

REFERENCES

1. Wheat RW: Bacterial morphology and ultrastructure. *In* Zinsser Microbiology. 19th ed. Edited by WK Joklik, HP Willett, DB Amos, and CM Wilfert. Norwalk, CT, Appleton & Lange, 1988.
2. Brenner DJ: Taxonomy, classification, and nomenclature of bacteria. *In* Manual of Clinical Microbiology. 5th ed. Edited by A Balows, et al. Washington, DC, American Society for Microbiology, 1991.
3. Michie HR, et al: Detection of circulatory tumor necrosis factor after endotoxin administration. N Engl J Med, *318*:1481, 1988.
4. Dinarello CA, and Mier JW: Lymphokines. N Engl J Med, *317*:940, 1987.
5. Kasper DL: Bacterial capsule—old dogmas and new tricks. J Infect Dis, *153*:407, 1986.
6. Morrison DC, and Alving CR (eds): Molecular concepts of lipid A. Rev Infect Dis, *6*:427, 1984.
7. Koneman EW, et al (eds): Color Atlas and Textbook of Diagnostic Microbiology. 3rd ed. Philadelphia, JB Lippincott, 1988.
8. Tinghitella TJ, and Edberg SC: Agglutination tests and Limulum assay for diagnosis of infectious diseases. *In* Manual of Clinical Microbiology. 5th ed. Edited by A Balows, et al. Washington, DC, American Society for Microbiology, 1991.
9. Radetsky M, Solomon JK, and Todd JR: Identification of streptococcal pharyngitis in the office laboratory: reassessment of new technology. Pediatr Infect Dis J, *6*:556, 1987.
10. Campos JM: Noncultural diagnosis of group A streptococcal pharyngitis. Clin Microbiol Newslett, *9*:152, 1987.
11. Gilligan P, et al: Evaluation of the PREMIER Clostridium difficile toxin A enzyme immunoassay. *In* Abstracts of the 1990 Interscience Conference on Antimicrobial Agents and Chemotherapy. Washington, DC, American Society for Microbiology, 1990.
12. Kraft J, et al: Detection of C. difficile toxin A by EIA in patient stools. *In* Abstracts of the 1990 Interscience Conference on Antimicrobial Agents and Chemotherapy. Washington, DC, American Society for Microbiology, 1990.
13. Barnes RC: Laboratory diagnosis of human chlamydial infections. Clin Microbiol Rev, *2*:119, 1989.
14. Pfaller MA: Laboratory diagnosis of infections due to Legionella species: Practical application of DNA probes in the clinical microbiology laboratory. Lab Med, *19*:301, 1988.
15. Kleemold SRM, Karjalainen JE, and Raty RKH: Rapid diagnosis of Mycoplasma pneumoniae infection: Clinical evaluation of a commercial probe test. J Infect Dis, *162*:70, 1990.
16. Woods GL, et al: Evaluation of a nonisotopic probe for detection of Chlamydia trachomatis in endocervical specimens. J Clin Microbiol, *28*:370, 1990.
17. Ellner PD, Kiehn TE, Cammarata R, and Hosmer M: Rapid detection and identification of pathogenic mycobacteria by combining radiometric and nucleic acid probe methods. J Clin Microbiol, *26*:1349, 1988.
18. Daly JA, Clifton NL, Seskin KC, and Gooch WM III: Use of rapid, nonradioactive DNA probes in culture confirmation tests to detect Streptococcus agalactiae, Haemophilus influenzae, and Enterococcus spp from pediatric patients with significant infections. J Clin Microbiol, *29*:80, 1991.
19. Desforges JF: The polymerase chain reaction. N Engl J Med, *322*:178, 1990.
20. Shapiro HM: Flow cytometry in laboratory microbiology: new directions. ASM News, *56*:584, 1990.
21. Baron EJ, and Finegold SM (eds): Bailey and Scott's Diagnostic Microbiology. 8th ed. St. Louis, CV Mosby Company, 1990.
22. Sahm DF, and Washington JA II: Antibacterial susceptibility tests: Dilution methods. *In* Manual of Clinical Microbiology. 5th ed. Edited by A Balows, et al. Washington, DC, American Society for Microbiology, 1991.
23. Barry AL, and Thornsberry C: Susceptibility tests: Diffusion test procedures. *In* Manual of Clinical Microbiology. 5th ed. Edited by A Balows, et al. Washington, DC, American Society for Microbiology, 1991.
24. National Committee for Clinical Laboratory Standards: Dilution procedures for susceptibility testing of aerobic bacteria. Approved Standard NCCLS Publication M7-A2. Villanova, PA, NCCLS, 1990.
25. National Committee for Clinical Laboratory Standards: Performance standards for antimicrobial disk susceptibility tests. Approved Standard NCCLS Publication M2-T4. Villanova, PA, NCCLS, 1990.
26. Stratton CW, and Cooksey RC: Susceptibility tests: Special tests. *In* Manual of Clinical Microbiology. 5th ed. Edited by A Balows, et al. Washington, DC, American Society for Microbiology, 1991.
27. Willett HP: Antimicrobial agents. *In* Zinsser Microbiology. 19th ed. Edited by WK Joklik, HP Willett, DB Amos, and CM Wilfert. Norwalk, CT, Appleton & Lange, 1988.
28. National Committee for Clinical Laboratory Standards: Methods for antimicrobial susceptibility testing of anaerobic bacteria. 2nd ed. Approved Standard NCCLS Document M11-A2. Villanova, PA, NCCLS, 1990.
29. Pearson RD, et al: Method for reliable determination of minimal lethal concentrations. Antimicrob Agents Chemother, *18*:699, 1980.
30. National Committee for Clinical Laboratory Standards: Methods for determining bactericidal activity of antimicrobial agents. Proposed Guideline. NCCLS Document M26-P. Villanova, PA, NCCLS, 1987.
31. Stratton CW: Serum bactericidal test. Clin Microbiol Rev, *1*:19, 1988.
32. Weinstein MP, et al: Multicenter collaborative evaluation of a standardized serum bactericidal test as a prognostic indicator in infective endocarditis. Am J Med, *83*:218, 1987.

Chapter 25

CHLAMYDIAS

The chlamydiae, for many years considered viruses because of their strict intracellular parasitism, are obligate intracellular bacteria with a tropism for columnar epithelial cells. Unlike viruses, the chlamydiae have a cell wall similar to that of gram-negative bacteria (see Chapter 24); they contain both DNA and RNA, have prokaryotic ribosomes, and synthesize their own proteins, nucleic acids, and lipids; they divide by binary fission and are susceptible to antibiotics. Unlike most bacteria, the chlamydiae cannot replicate outside cells or synthesize high-energy adenosine triphosphate metabolites: they are "energy parasites."

CLASSIFICATION

The chlamydiae have a unique developmental cycle and, therefore, are classified in a separate order, Chlamydiales, with one family, Chlamydiaceae, containing one genus, Chlamydia, in which three species are recognized: Chlamydia trachomatis, Chlamydia psittaci, and Chlamydia pneumoniae (formerly called the TWAR agent). Chlamydia trachomatis is susceptible to sulfonamides and produces a single glycogen-containing (and therefore iodine-positive) inclusion that displaces the nucleus. Chlamydia psittaci is resistant to sulfonamides and produces glycogen-negative (and iodine-negative) inclusions that rupture early and are distributed around the nucleus without displacing it. The DNA homology between these two species is only about 10%. Chlamydia pneumoniae, initially considered to be a strain of Chlamydia psittaci, represents a separate species because it lacks appreciable DNA homology with either Chlamydia trachomatis or Chlamydia psittaci; it has different restriction endonuclease patterns; and it lacks extrachromosomal DNA, which both Chlamydia trachomatis and Chlamydia psittaci have.

STRUCTURE

Two morphologically distinct forms of chlamydiae are recognized. The dense, spherical, 0.2- to 0.4-μm diameter elementary body, which contains prokaryotic ribosomal RNA and has a rigid cell wall, is the infectious form of the organism, capable of limited extracellular survival. The osmotically fragile reticulate body, 0.6 to 1.0 μm in diameter, is the intracellular, metabolically active form, and is incapable of existing outside cells. The closed circular DNA of both forms, compactly organized in a central nucleoid, has a molecular weight of 660 million, and codes for about 600 proteins.

The nonmotile chlamydiae lack flagella and pili but have about 20 cylindrical surface projections, anchored in the cytoplasmic membrane and protruding through holes in the cell wall. In developing chlamydiae these projections penetrate the cellular endosomal membrane surrounding the chlamydial microcolony, recognized histologically as a cytoplasmic inclusion, permitting uptake of nutrients from the host cell cytoplasm.

The outer membrane of the chlamydial elementary body, like that of many gram-negative bacteria, has several components, the most prominent being the major outer membrane protein (MOMP), a transmembrane protein with type-, subspecies-, species-, and genus-reactive epitopes defined by monoclonal antibodies (1). Infection with chlamydiae induces MOMP-specific antibodies, but their role in protective immunity and in diagnosis is unclear. The chlamydial outer membrane also contains a lipopolysaccharide (LPS) antigen that is structurally similar to that of Salmonella minnesota Re strains (2,3). The LPS of Chlamydia trachomatis and of Chlamydia psittaci has antigens shared by other members of the Enterobacteriaceae and structurally different genus-specific antigens (2). The extractable chlamydial LPS is the major antigen detected in genus-specific serologic tests for chlamydiae, and monoclonal antibodies and monospecific polyvalent antisera to the LPS are used in enzyme immunoassays to detect chlamydial antigen in clinical specimens (4).

REPLICATION

Chlamydiae replicate in the cytoplasm of infected host cells. Their developmental cycle (Fig. 25–1) has five phases: (1) attachment and penetration of the elementary body, (2) transition of the metabolically inert elementary body into the metabolically active reticulate body, (3) growth and division of the reticulate body, producing many progeny, (4) maturation of the noninfectious reticulate body into infectious elementary bodies, and (5) release of the elementary bodies from the host cell.

The infectious process begins with attachment of the elementary body to a microvillus of a susceptible columnar cell; specific receptors have not been identified. The elementary body travels down the microvillus and localizes in indentations of the host cell plasma membrane that resemble coated pits, forming an endosome, where both Chlamydia psittaci and Chlamydia trachomatis remain throughout their intracellular development. Endosomes containing elementary bodies of Chlamydia psittaci do not interact with cellular lysosomes and proceed to the nuclear hoff area, whereas endosomes containing Chlamydia trachomatis elementary bodies fuse with one another, and perhaps with lysosomes. Within 6 to 8 hours after entering the host cell, changes in the elementary body cell wall result in a transition to the reticulate body and subsequent initiation of DNA, RNA, and protein synthesis, permitting growth of the reticulate body and its division by binary fission. Host cell mitochondria migrate to and are positioned against the enlarging endosome, allowing the reticulate body to utilize host cell adenosine

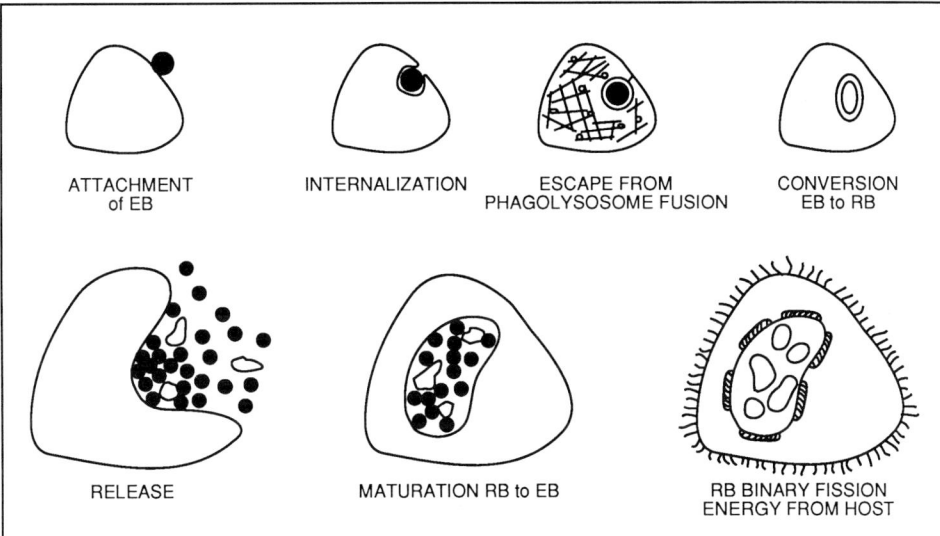

Fig. 25–1. Diagram of the developmental cycle of chlamydiae. Key: EB, elementary body; RB, reticulate body. (From Wyrick, P. B., Gutman, L. T., and Hodinka, R. L.: Chlamydiae. In Zinsser Microbiology. 19th ed. Edited by W. K. Joklik, J. P. Willett, D. B. Amos, and C. M. Wilfert. Norwalk, Appleton & Lange, 1988.)

triphosphate. During reticulate body growth, chlamydia-specific lipopolysaccharide is exported to the surface of the infected cell, possibly protecting the organism from cytotoxic T cells by reducing plasma membrane fluidity and perpetuating chlamydial disease by prolonging the inflammatory response (5). By 18 to 24 hours after infection, reticulate bodies begin to reorganize, and presumably when nutrients are depleted they mature into elementary bodies, which are released from the host cell. Cells infected with Chlamydia psittaci usually are severely damaged, and the organisms are released by cell lysis within 48 hours, whereas the inclusion of Chlamydia trachomatis appears to be extruded 72 to 96 hours after infection, leaving a scar in the surviving host cell.

CHLAMYDIA TRACHOMATIS

Chlamydia trachomatis is the most common cause of sexually transmitted disease in the United States and an important cause of blindness in trachoma-endemic regions of the Middle East, North Africa, and northern India (6,7). The organism was first isolated in the yolk sac of embryonated eggs in 1938 and in cell culture in 1965. In 1970 the microimmunofluorescent method for detecting antibodies to C. trachomatis and for immunotyping was introduced. These culture and serologic techniques confirmed the etiologic role of C. trachomatis in nongonococcal urethritis and cervicitis, and the development within the past decade of methods to detect C. trachomatis antigens immunochemically has allowed rapid diagnosis of infection with the organism.

Classification

Fifteen serotypes of Chlamydia trachomatis are distinguishable by microimmunofluorescence (Table 25–1), and recently, three new serovars, Da, Ia, and L_{2a}, have been proposed (9). Types A, B, Ba, and C are associated with endemic trachoma; types D through K are isolated principally from persons with genital and neonatal infections but may cause ocular infections in adults in developed countries; types L_1, L_2, and L_3 are associated with lymphogranuloma venereum (LGV). Types D, E, F, and G are responsible for most non-LGV infections. These 15 immunotypes may be grouped into two subspecies serogroups: the B complex includes B, Ba, D, E, L_1, L_2; the C complex includes C, J, H, I, and A. Types G and F are related to the B complex, and types K and L_3, related to the C complex, bridge both C and B complexes.

Pathology

The histologic findings of cervical and ocular infections with non-LGV strains of Chlamydia trachomatis include shallow mucosal erosions, epithelial cell metaplasia, intracytoplasmic inclusions in mucosal epithelial cells, a patchy mononuclear cell inflammatory infiltrate, and submucosal lymphoid hyperplasia with germinal centers. Lymph nodes involved with LGV contain granulomas with stellate abscesses, indicating the greater importance of the cellular immune response to C. trachomatis serotypes L_1, L_2, and L_3.

Epidemiology and Clinical Manifestations

Humans are the only known natural host for all strains of Chlamydia trachomatis except that responsible for mouse pneumonitis. The clinical spectrum and organ specificity of human infections with C. trachomatis are determined by the method of transmission and by the properties of

Table 25–1. Chlamydia Trachomatis Serotypes

Serotypes*	Associated Infections
A, B, Ba, C	Endemic trachoma
D, E, F, G, H, I, J, K	Non-LGV genital infections in adults, inclusion conjunctivitis in neonates and adults, pneumonitis in infants
L_1, L_2, L_3	LGV

*Da, Ia, and L_2a have been proposed as a new serotypes.
Key: LGV, lymphogranuloma venereum.

the infecting strain. C. trachomatis infections are divided epidemiologically into three categories: classic trachoma, sexually transmitted infections of adults, and perinatal eye and respiratory tract infections. Each is discussed in this section.

Classic trachoma is an important cause of blindness in areas where public sanitation is inadequate and personal hygiene poor, and it is the most common cause of preventable blindness worldwide (10). Typically, the infection is transmitted among children via fingers, fomites, and probably flies. In endemic areas, acute conjunctivitis of adults or infants is uncommon, but most children become chronically infected within a few years of birth. Repeated exposure to Chlamydia trachomatis eventually results in chronic follicular keratoconjunctivitis, conjunctival scarring, and pannus formation (invasion of vessels into the cornea).

The sexually transmitted infections of adults include lymphogranuloma venereum and infections produced by non-LGV serotypes of Chlamydia trachomatis. LGV, the only infection caused by Chlamydia trachomatis that produces multisystem involvement and constitutional manifestations, has three phases. During the primary phase, a small, painless vesicle or a nonindurated papule or ulcer develops 3 days to 3 weeks after exposure and heals quickly without scarring. This transient lesion occurs on the penis of about one third of men with inguinal LGV, less frequently on the labia, fourchette, or posterior vagina of women, and in homosexual men (and occasionally in women), may involve the anus or rectosigmoid colon. The secondary stage, beginning 2 to 6 weeks after exposure, is characterized by suppurative regional lymphadenopathy accompanied by fever, chills, anorexia, headache, myalgias, and arthralgias. Involved lymph nodes become matted, with fixed and inflamed overlying skin, and eventually suppurate, producing multiple draining fistulas that heal with scarring over a period of several months. The fibrosis and resultant abnormal lymphatic drainage are responsible for the urethral or rectal strictures or induration and lymphedema of the genitalia that develop during the third stage.

LGV is endemic in Asia, Africa, and South America, and approximately 500 cases are reported in the United States each year. In the United States LGV affects males three times as frequently as females and is most common in persons of low socioeconomic status living in the Southeast, in homosexual men, and in persons returned from LGV-endemic areas outside the United States. LGV is transmitted sexually, although transmission by fomites and by aerosolization produced during laboratory accidents has caused pneumonitis, pleural effusions, and mediastinal or hilar lymphadenopathy (11). The reservoirs of infection probably have asymptomatic or ignored symptomatic urethral, cervical, or anorectal infection, but this has not been proven.

The clinical spectrum of sexually transmitted infections due to non-LGV strains of Chlamydia trachomatis is similar to the spectrum of infections caused by Neisseria gonorrhoeae (see Chapter 31). In men, Chlamydia trachomatis (serotypes D to K) is responsible for 30 to 50% of cases of nongonococcal urethritis, which is manifested by urethral discharge, itching, or dysuria; although as many as a third of men who harbor C. trachomatis in the urethra are asymptomatic (12–14). Of cases of urethritis caused by C. trachomatis, 1 to 2% progress to epididymitis, and C. trachomatis is the most common agent of epididymitis in young heterosexual men who have no structural abnormality of the genitourinary tract (15). Among homosexual males, non-LGV strains of C. trachomatis have been associated with proctitis. The organism also has been recovered from the urethra of as many as 70% of men with untreated Reiter's syndrome associated with urethritis (16).

Genital infection with Chlamydia trachomatis probably is more prevalent in women than in men. In the United States, C. trachomatis has been recovered from the cervix of 30 to 60% of women who have gonorrhea or whose partner has gonorrhea or nongonococcal urethritis, from 10 to 20% of women attending sexually transmitted disease clinics who have not had a partner with urethritis, and from 5 to 10% of college students or young women attending gynecology, family planning, or prenatal clinics (6). The prevalence of cervical infection with C. trachomatis is greater among women who are young, single or divorced, black, of low socioeconomic status, and have multiple sexual partners (6,17). Infection of the endocervix with C. trachomatis may cause mucopurulent cervicitis, which can spread to the urethra and urinary bladder, resulting in the "acute urethral syndrome" of abacteriuric pyuria, or to the endometrium and fallopian tubes, producing endometritis or salpingitis (10,18–20). Infections of the upper reproductive tract may progress to overt or subclinical pelvic inflammatory disease or cause scarring and dysfunction of the oviduct transport system, which could result in infertility or ectopic pregnancy. Intraperitoneal spread of the infection may cause acute peritonitis, perihepatitis (Fitz-Hugh-Curtis syndrome), periappendicitis, or perisplenitis (11).

A small percentage of adults with chlamydial genital infections develop inclusion conjunctivitis, which begins abruptly with a foreign body sensation, photophobia, mucopurulent discharge, and follicular conjunctivitis, often accompanied by keratitis. If reinfection does not occur, lesions usually heal in several months to a few years.

In developed countries where sexually transmitted infection with Chlamydia trachomatis is epidemic, the organism may be transmitted from infected mother to infant during passage through the birth canal. Data from studies in North America indicate that 60 to 70% of infants exposed to C. trachomatis during vaginal delivery become infected with the organism, and infection has been documented after cesarean section, although with much lower frequency (11). C. trachomatis is recovered from the conjunctiva of infected infants after 1 to 2 weeks and from the nasopharynx shortly thereafter. The rate of isolation from the conjunctiva falls by 5 to 6 weeks, but C. trachomatis can be recovered from the nasopharynx, conjunctiva, rectum, and vagina (usually without producing symptoms) for many months.

In infants the most common manifestation of infection with Chlamydia trachomatis is inclusion conjunctivitis, which develops in nearly 80% of infants whose conjunctival cultures or cytologic examination demonstrate the organism (11). Two to 25 days after birth a mucopurulent discharge appears, and the conjunctiva becomes inflamed and edematous. Without therapy the manifestations usually resolve in several months with no sequelae, although in one study nearly half of infected infants developed mild trachoma (21).

Approximately 20% of infants who acquire infection with Chlamydia trachomatis at birth develop interstitial pneumonitis between 2 weeks and 3 months of age (peak, 3 to 6 weeks), approximately half of whom have, or have had, conjunctivitis. Infants initially present with nasal congestion and gradually develop a distinctive staccato cough with tachypnea and rales; fever is absent. Clinical illness lasts several weeks, but inspiratory rales and chest roentgenographic changes may persist for months.

CHLAMYDIA PSITTACI

Pneumonia associated with exposure to birds was described in Switzerland in 1879, and in 1894 parrots were determined to be the source of an outbreak of a similar respiratory tract illness, named *psittakos*, after the Greek word for parrot. The disease was rare in the United States and Europe until pet tropical birds became fashionable in the late 1920s, and many outbreaks were described in 1929 and 1930 following large-scale importation of infected South American birds. The pathogen was isolated from human and avian tissue in 1930 by Bedson, who was investigating an outbreak at the London Zoo.

Epidemiology

Infection caused by Chlamydia psittaci (termed psittacosis) occurs worldwide. Psittacine birds are considered the major reservoir, but most species of birds can serve as a host for the organism. Birds infected with C. psittaci may be obviously ill and die of the disease, but they often have minimal symptoms such as anorexia, diarrhea, lethargy, and ruffled feathers. Human illness occurs sporadically and has been associated with exposure to parrots, canaries, pigeons, sparrows, ducks, cockatiels, fowl (especially turkeys), and occasionally mammals. Owners of pet birds account for about half of the 40 to 60 cases reported annually in the United States. Pet shop employees, pigeon fanciers, zoo workers, veterinarians, and others who work with birds are at increased risk of infection, and recent outbreaks have occurred in turkey-processing plants, principally among workers who killed the birds and plucked their feathers and those who eviscerated carcasses (22). Over the past two decades the number of cases of psittacosis in the United States has declined dramatically as a result of adding tetracycline to poultry feed, requiring that commercially imported psittacine birds be medicated for 30 days before entering the country, and breeding parakeets domestically.

Chlamydia psittaci is present in the blood, tissues, excreta, and feathers of infected birds and may be shed for months after acute infection. Most often, infection is transmitted to humans via inhalation of infectious aerosols derived from feces, fecal dust, and secretions of C. psittaci–infected birds, in which the organism can long survive. Human infection also has resulted from handling contaminated plumage or tissues, from bird bites, and from mouth-to-beak contact. Contact with birds does not have to be close or prolonged; infection has been acquired during a brief exposure in an environment in which an infected bird previously had been present. Person-to-person spread of C. psittaci is rare but may result in more severe disease.

Pathogenesis and Pathology

Chlamydia psittaci enters the body via the respiratory tract and is transported to the monocyte/macrophage cells of the liver and spleen, where the organisms replicate and then enter the blood, to be transported to the lung, the primary target of infection, and other organs. In the lung, lymphocytes are found in the alveolar and interstitial spaces; small hemorrhages account for the hemoptysis that occasionally develops; mucus plugging of the bronchioles is common; and macrophages with intracytoplasmic inclusions may be seen. The hilar lymph nodes, liver, and spleen may be enlarged and contain foci of necrosis, and in fatal cases the myocardium, pericardium, meninges, brain, and adrenals may be involved.

Clinical Manifestations

After an incubation period of 7 to 15 days or longer, psittacosis begins—abruptly, with chills and fever, or gradually, with increasing fever and malaise. The heart rate frequently is slow relative to body temperature; a diffuse, severe headache is usual; malaise, anorexia, painful myalgias, and arthralgias are common; and a macular rash (Horder spots) resembling the rose spots of typhoid fever (see Chapter 34) may occur. Persistent cough, often dry and hacking but occasionally productive of blood-streaked mucoid sputum, is prominent. Decreased mentation may develop at the end of the first week of illness, and a few persons have gastrointestinal complaints. Chlamydia psittaci is a rare cause of destructive endocarditis in persons who have a history of rheumatic heart disease, or congenital valvular abnormalities, and rarely in those who had no cardiac disease (23,24).

CHLAMYDIA PNEUMONIAE

Recently, a unique chlamydial organism has been associated with acute respiratory tract disease in humans (25). The organism, initially considered to be a strain of Chlamydia psittaci, was named TWAR for the laboratory identifying letters of the first two isolates: TW-183, isolated from the eye of a control child in a trachoma vaccine study in Taiwan in 1965, and AR-39, recovered from the throat of a student with pharyngitis at the University of Washington in 1965. Data from DNA homology and electron microscopy studies demonstrated that these organisms were a separate species, Chlamydia pneumoniae (26–29). Strains of C. pneumoniae and Chlamydia psittaci have 10% or less DNA sequence homology, and the elementary body of Chlamydia pneumoniae is pear shaped and has a large periplasmic space, different from the typically round elementary bodies of Chlamydia psittaci and Chlamydia trachomatis.

Epidemiology

The current concept of the epidemiology of infection with Chlamydia pneumoniae is based on serologic data collected by testing sera acquired during previous studies of respiratory tract illnesses. In adults, antibodies to C. pneumoniae have been found 5 to 10 times more frequently than antibodies to Chlamydia trachomatis (30). Immunoglobulin (Ig) G titers detected in about 50% of adults in seven countries ranged from approximately 40% in Nova Scotia, Canada, to over 60% in Taiwan and Panama. In Denmark and Seattle, Washington, antibody prevalence rates were low in children, increased sharply in teenagers, continued to increase until middle age, and remained high into old age. In the seven countries evaluated, seropositivity rates were 10 to 25% higher for males. The acquisition of antibodies after school age and the higher prevalence in males suggest that the source of infection may be outside the household more often than is usual with many respiratory tract infections. Data from retrospective and prospective serologic studies indicate that disease caused by Chlamydia pneumoniae is endemic in the United States and epidemic in Scandinavia and Finland and that infection does not occur with any consistent seasonal periodicity (31).

Though evidence indicates that Chlamydia pneumoniae is a primary human pathogen transmitted from human to human without an avian or animal reservoir, the mechanism and place of transmission, the incubation period, and the infectiousness of the organism are unknown. Retrospective serologic data from Finnish military trainees showed that epidemics of pneumonia caused by C. pneumoniae lasted 5 to 8 months, suggesting that the infection spreads slowly, even in a closed population, an environment that usually promotes transmission of respiratory tract infections (32).

Pathogenesis

The pathogenesis of infection by Chlamydia pneumoniae currently is unknown. No animal models of infection exist, and because the illness generally is mild and self-limited, autopsy studies are unavailable.

Clinical Manifestations

Approximately 10% of the community-acquired and nosocomial pneumonias have been associated with evidence of infection with Chlamydia pneumoniae (25). The pneumonia usually is mild with a single subsegmental infiltrate, but it may be severe, especially in elders and in persons with chronic disease. Frequently, illness begins with upper respiratory tract symptoms, particularly pharyngitis with hoarseness, followed by persistent cough and other symptoms of lower respiratory disease. Although pneumonia has been the most common syndrome associated with infection with C. pneumoniae, serologic studies during epidemics among military trainees showed that only about 10% of infections with C. pneumoniae resulted in pneumonia, suggesting that the infections frequently are mild or asymptomatic and go unrecognized (32).

In young adults about 4% of cases of bronchitis are caused by Chlamydia pneumoniae. Pharyngitis with hoarseness is a common manifestation of infection with C. pneumoniae; and although up to 80% of persons with pneumonia due to C. pneumoniae have a sore throat, fewer than 1% who have pharyngitis but do not develop lower respiratory tract disease have evidence of infection with C. pneumoniae. About 5% of cases of primary sinusitis in young adults are caused by C. pneumoniae, and at least 5% of persons with pneumonia due to C. pneumoniae have evidence of sinusitis (24). Infection with C. pneumoniae also has been associated with fever of undetermined origin, otitis, influenza-like illness, myocarditis, and endocarditis (33,34).

LABORATORY DIAGNOSIS

Specimens needed for diagnosis of infections with the chlamydiae are listed in Table 25-2. Specimen collection, transport, and processing are discussed in Part III and are briefly reviewed in the following discussion of organism identification.

Chlamydia trachomatis. Most infections with C. trachomatis involve mucous membranes, and specimens should be collected directly from the involved surface and must contain an adequate sample of infected epithelial cells. Purulent discharge is not an appropriate specimen for chlamydia detection and should be removed before collection of a swab or brush specimen. Of the different types of swabs available, those with wooden shafts should be avoided because wood is toxic to the organism. Calcium alginate swabs may be toxic to the chlamydiae or to the cells that support their growth; dacron-, rayon-, or cotton-tipped swabs are acceptable, though cotton swabs occasionally are toxic.

To collect ocular specimens, the eyelid should be everted and the swab rotated directly against the conjunctival surface. To diagnose urethritis caused by Chlamydia

Table 25–2. Diseases Caused by the Chlamydiae and Specimens Required for Diagnosis

Disease	Species	Specimen
Mucopurulent cervicitis	C. trachomatis	Endocervical swab
Acute urethral syndrome	C. trachomatis	Urethral swab
Acute endometritis	C. trachomatis	Endometrial aspirate
Acute salpingitis	C. trachomatis	Fallopian tube biopsy
Nongonococcal urethritis	C. trachomatis	Urethral swab, urine
Inclusion conjunctivitis	C. trachomatis	Conjunctival scrapings/swab
Trachoma	C. trachomatis	Conjunctival scrapings/swab
Lymphogranuloma venereum	C. trachomatis (L_1–L_3)	Lymph node aspirate, biopsy of ulcerated lesion, serum
Pneumonia	C. trachomatis	Tracheobronchial aspirate, nasopharyngeal swab, serum
	C. psittaci	Serum
	C. pneumoniae	Serum, nasopharyngeal swab, throat swab

trachomatis, a urethral swab specimen or urine (when using an enzyme-linked immunosorbent assay [ELISA] to detect C. trachomatis antigen) is appropriate (35). In nonpregnant women, collection of endocervical specimens with a cytologic brush (rather than a swab) may increase the sensitivity of direct fluorescent antibody staining—and possibly of other diagnostic methods—for C. trachomatis (36). To diagnose LGV pus is aspirated by inserting a needle into an enlarged, fluctuant lymph node through healthy adjacent skin; if no material is obtained sterile saline may be injected into the node and then aspirated into the same syringe.

Of the techniques that may be used to detect Chlamydia trachomatis (Table 25–3), cell culture is the reference method and must be used when the diagnosis is disputed or in criminal cases, including sexual assault and abuse investigations. Swabs, aspirates, or tissues are placed in transport medium (2-sucrose phosphate and sucrose-glutamate-phosphate are used most commonly) and transported promptly to the laboratory (37,38). Adding 2 to 10% fetal bovine serum to the transport medium may preserve chlamydial viability when storage at $-70°$ C is necessary, but the optimal concentration of serum has not been determined. If $-70°$ C storage is not required, transport in tryptose phosphate broth is acceptable (39). To inhibit overgrowth of bacteria and fungi, vancomycin (100 µg/ml), gentamicin (10 to 50 µg/ml), and nystatin, (25 to 50 U/ml) or amphotericin B (2.5 to 4.0 µg/ml) frequently are added to the medium. However, media containing penicillin, which inhibits growth of chlamydiae in cell culture, cannot be used. Specimens submitted for isolation of chlamydiae should be processed as soon as possible after collection. If a delay in processing is unavoidable, specimens should be stored at 4° C if they can be processed within 48 hours or at $-70°$ C if a longer interval is anticipated, although freezing may decrease the isolation rate of C. trachomatis in cell culture by 20% (40,41).

Cell lines used to isolate Chlamydia trachomatis include HeLa-229, McCoy, BHK-21, and Buffalo green monkey kidney (42,43). Pretreatment of HeLa-229 cell monolayers with diethylaminoethyl-dextran increases the susceptibility of the monolayer to infection, and adding cycloheximide (0.5 to 1.5 µl/ml) to the growth medium of McCoy cells enhances sensitivity and eliminates the need for iododeoxyuridine pretreatment or irradiation of the cell monolayer (43,44). Cell monolayers usually are grown on glass coverslips in shell vials or 24-well plates or on the polystyrene surface of 96-well or 48-well cell culture dishes (45). Recovery of C. trachomatis in cell culture is enhanced by sonicating specimens or mixing them on a vortex mixer to release elementary bodies from host cells before inoculating cell monolayers and by centrifuging the inoculated shell vials or culture plates (43,44). In 96-well culture systems detection may be enhanced by passaging specimens that do not grow C. trachomatis at 48 hours; however, passaging does not significantly increase detection in shell vials or 24-well plates (46,47). After incubation for 48 to 72 hours, monolayers may be stained with Giemsa or iodine, but staining with fluorescein-conjugated monoclonal antibodies to C. trachomatis increases the sensitivity of cell culture (48). A sensitive, practical method for culturing C. trachomatis in the clinical laboratory is outlined in Procedure 8 in the Appendix.

Although cell culture is the reference method for diagnosing infection with Chlamydia trachomatis, its use is associated with several disadvantages: Culture of a single endocervical specimen has an estimated sensitivity of only 70 to 80%; it is costly; and results are not available for 48 to 96 hours (49,50). Therefore, various nonculture methods have been developed (see below).

Chlamydia trachomatis antigens may be detected by direct visualization of the organism in smears stained with fluorescein-conjugated monoclonal antibodies specific for C. trachomatis (DFA) or by immunochemical detection of solubilized chlamydial components using an ELISA. Direct immunofluorescence using monoclonal antibodies allows rapid detection of C. trachomatis elementary bodies (Plate IIA) in endocervical, urethral, rectal, conjunctival and nasopharyngeal smears and permits an assessment of the adequacy of the specimen (51–54). Genital or conjunctival specimens with columnar epithelial cells are acceptable, whereas samples that contain few columnar cells, excessive amounts of cervical mucus, or a predominance of squamous cells are inadequate. However, a high-performance fluorescent microscope is essential, interpretation is subjective, and the potential for operator fatigue limits the number of specimens that can be processed in a day.

Several different monoclonal antibody formulations for direct staining of specimens are available commercially. In general, antibodies directed against the species-specific major outer membrane protein of Chlamydia trachomatis, which stain only the morphologically homogenous elementary bodies, are superior to those directed against the chlamydial lipopolysaccharide, because the former produce more intense fluorescence and are more specific (55). Occasionally, even the species-specific monoclonal antibodies stain bacteria other than C. trachomatis, a reaction that may result from nonspecific immunoglobulin binding or monoclonal antibody cross-reactivity through

Table 25–3. Methods for Detection of Chlamydia Trachomatis

Method	Turn-around time (hr)	Comments
Cell culture	48–96	Reference method
Direct immunofluorescence	1	Allows assessment of specimen quality; interpretation subjective; recommended for use in high-prevalence populations
Enzyme-linked immunoassay	3–4	Objective interpretation; useful for processing large numbers of specimens; most reliable in high-prevalence populations
Membrane enzyme immunoassay	½	Variable sensitivity; high specificity (≥95%)
DNA probe	1	Sensitivity and specificity comparable to those of culture

epitope similarity (56). Staining organisms other than C. trachomatis is especially frequent with rectal specimens, owing to the high concentrations of bacteria, and possibly to the presence of Peptostreptococcus productus, which has cross-reactive antigens (55,57).

The sensitivity of direct immunofluorescence in women ranges from 70 to 100%, depending on the prevalence of infection in the population being evaluated and the number of elementary bodies that represent a positive result (49,58–62). In general, the sensitivity is greater in studies that have lower cutoff values for elementary bodies and in those that evaluate populations with a high prevalence of infection. The sensitivity of DFA staining of urethral specimens from men is about 70%. In most studies the specificity of DFA is greater than 95% for specimens from both males and females.

ELISA kits provide objective results in a few hours and are most useful and most cost effective in laboratories where large numbers of specimens are processed daily. The sensitivity of ELISA (range, 70 to 100% in women and 67 to 92% in men) is higher in populations with a high prevalence of infection, such as persons attending sexually transmitted disease clinics (58,59,63–71). In general, ELISA is associated with more false-positive results than direct immunofluorescence staining; however, this problem can be reduced significantly by improving the specimen collection technique (removing the cervical mucus and obtaining an endocervical sample) and by using blocking antibodies (72).

Monoclonal antibody–based membrane antigen capture enzyme immunoassays that detect Chlamydia trachomatis antigen in clinical specimens within 30 minutes only recently became commercially available, so data on their reliability are limited. Compared with culture, the specificity of the assays is 95% or greater, but the sensitivity varies in different situations: 59 to 88% and 65% for diagnosing urogenital infection in females and males, respectively, and 93% for diagnosing conjunctivitis in infants (73–75).

A chemiluminescence-labeled DNA probe, complementary to Chlamydia trachomatis ribosomal RNA (available commercially), provides results within a few hours of receiving the specimen. In early evaluations of the probe in different populations the sensitivity ranged from 60 to 94% and the specificity from 75 to 100% (76). The assay was modified subsequently; and in one study of women attending an emergency room the sensitivity and specificity of the modified probe compared with culture were 93 and 98%, respectively (77).

Serologic tests have limited value in diagnosing infections caused by Chlamydia trachomatis, for two reasons. First, antibodies to C. trachomatis persist after the infection resolves, so their presence in serum does not necessarily correlate with active disease. Second, many serologic tests are not specific for C. trachomatis because they detect genus-specific antibodies that may be produced during infection with C. trachomatis, Chlamydia psittaci, or Chlamydia pneumoniae. However, the complement-fixation test, which uses a group-reactive antigen, may be useful for diagnosis of LGV. Because LGV has a long latent period and clinical diagnosis often is delayed, antibodies usually are present when the acute-phase serum sample is obtained, and fourfold rises in titer between acute- and convalescent-phase serum samples often cannot be documented. Consequently, a single or a stable titer of 1:64 or greater is very suggestive of LGV. These titers have been detected in 80% of persons with LGV, in 77% with psittacosis, in 9% of adults with inclusion conjunctivitis, in 18% of women with uncomplicated cervical infection with Chlamydia trachomatis, and in none of 60 men with nongonococcal urethritis due to C. trachomatis (11). The serovar-specific microimmunofluorescence test is more sensitive than complement fixation and can be used to measure IgM and IgG in serum and tears. Detection of IgM by microimmunofluorescence indicates recent infection and may be the method of choice for diagnosis of C. trachomatis pneumonia in infants (a titer of 1:32 or greater is diagnostic) (78).

Chlamydia psittaci. C. psittaci grows well in L cells, but because the organism is especially virulent and has been responsible for laboratory-acquired infections, culture should be performed only in specially equipped laboratories. Specimens are suspended in sterile, balanced salt solution and inoculated onto a confluent monolayer of indicator cells. After incubation for 1 hour at 37° C, the monolayer is washed and chlamydial growth medium is added. If C. psittaci is present, cytopatholytic plaques form in 5 to 10 days. Monolayers then are fixed in methanol and stained with a commercially available genus-specific immunofluorescent culture-confirmation reagent. C. psittaci is distinguished from Chlamydia trachomatis by failure of its inclusions to stain with antibodies specific for C. trachomatis.

Infection with Chlamydia psittaci typically is diagnosed serologically: a fourfold or greater rise in complement-fixing antibody titers between acute- and convalescent-phase serum specimens is diagnostic, and a single titer of 1:32 or greater in an individual with a compatible illness constitutes presumptive evidence of psittacosis. Antibody titers usually begin to rise by the end of the second week of illness; however, early antibiotic therapy (discussed later) can delay the appearance of antibodies for several weeks. False-positive rises in antibody titer occur uncommonly in individuals with Legionnaires' disease.

Chlamydia pneumoniae. Laboratory diagnosis of infection with C. pneumoniae is based predominantly on serologic tests (25). The microimmunofluorescence test with the TWAR antigen, capable of distinguishing IgM and IgG, is specific for C. pneumoniae. IgM appears about 3 weeks after the onset of primary illness, usually declines over the next 2 to 6 months to a level that cannot be detected, and may not reappear with reinfection. IgG, detected 6 to 8 weeks after the onset of the primary illness, persists for life and may rise 1 to 2 weeks following reinfection. A fourfold rise in IgG titer between acute- and convalescent-phase serum samples, a single IgG titer of 1:512 or greater, or an IgM titer of 1:16 or greater is consistent with acute infection. C. pneumoniae can be isolated in cell culture; however, the organism is more difficult to grow than Chlamydia trachomatis, and currently monoclonal antibodies specific for Chlamydia pneumoniae, essential for identification, are not commercially available.

TREATMENT

Tetracyclines are the mainstay of treatment of infections with chlamydiae. For genital infections due to Chlamydia trachomatis doxycycline is the agent of choice. Other effective agents include erythromycin, sulfisoxazole, ofloxacin, and possibly high-dose amoxicillin (11). Ocular infections with C. trachomatis are treated systemically with tetracycline (for adults) or erythromycin or sulfisoxazole (for neonates), because topical therapy suppresses signs of infection but does not eradicate the organism. The tetracyclines are also considered the most effective antimicrobial agents against Chlamydia psittaci and Chlamydia pneumoniae. Erythromycin is an acceptable alternative agent for infections caused by C. pneumoniae; however, the sulfonamides are ineffective against both Chlamydia psittaci and Chlamydia pneumoniae.

REFERENCES

1. Stephens RS, Tam MR, Kuo C-C, and Nowinski RC: Monoclonal antibodies to Chlamydia trachomatis: Antibody specificities and antigen characterization. J Immunol, 128:1083, 1982.
2. Brade L, et al: Antigenic and immunogenic properties of recombinants from Salmonella typhimurium and Salmonella minnesota rough mutants expressing in their lipopolysaccharide and genus-specific chlamydial epitope. Infect Immun, 55:482, 1987.
3. Brade L, Schramek S, Schade U, and Brade H: Chemical, biological, and immunochemical properties of the Chlamydia psittaci lipopolysaccharide. Infect Immun, 54:568, 1986.
4. Pugh SF, et al: Enzyme amplified immunoassay: A novel technique applied to direct detection of Chlamydia trachomatis in clinical specimens. J Clin Pathol, 38:1139, 1985.
5. Wyrick PB, Gutman LT, and Hodinka RL: Chlamydiae. In Zinsser Microbiology. 19th ed. Edited by WK Joklik, HP Willett, DB Amos, and CM Wilfert. Norwalk, CT, Appleton & Lange, 1988.
6. Centers for Disease Control: Chlamydia trachomatis infections: Policy guidelines for prevention and control. MMWR, 34(suppl 3):53S, 1985.
7. Thompson SE, and Washington AE. Epidemiology of sexually transmitted Chlamydia trachomatis infections. Epidemiol Rev, 5:96, 1983.
8. Gordon FB, and Quan AL: Isolation of the trachoma agent in cell culture. Proc Soc Exp Biol Med, 354:354, 1965.
9. Wang SP, and Grayston JT: Three new serovars of Chlamydia trachomatis: Da, Ia, and L_{2a}. J Infect Dis, 163:403, 1991.
10. Schachter J: Chlamydial infections. N Engl J Med, 298:428; 540, 1978.
11. Bowie WR, and Holmes KK: Chlamydia trachomatis (Trachoma, perinatal infections, lymphogranuloma venereum, and other genital infections). In Principles and Practice of Infectious Diseases. 3rd ed. Edited by GL Mandell, RG Douglas, Jr, and JE Bennett. New York, Churchill Livingstone, 1990.
12. Bowie WR, et al: Etiology of nongonococcal urethritis: Evidence for Chlamydia trachomatis and Ureaplasma urealyticum. J Clin Invest, 59:735, 1977.
13. Holmes KK, et al: Etiology of nongonococcal urethritis. N Engl J Med, 292:1199, 1975.
14. Stamm WE, et al: Chlamydia trachomatis urethral infections in men. Prevalence, risk factors, and clinical manifestations. Ann Intern Med, 100:47, 1984.
15. Berger RE, et al: Chlamydia trachomatis as a cause of "idiopathic" epididymitis. N Engl J Med, 298:301, 1978.
16. Keat A, Thomas BJ, and Taylor-Robinson D. Chlamydial infection in the aetiology of arthritis. Br Med Bull, 39:168, 1983.
17. Handsfield HH, et al: Criteria for selective screening for Chlamydia trachomatis infection in women attending family planning clinics. JAMA, 255:1730, 1986.
18. Brunham RC, et al: Mucopurulent cervicitis—the ignored counterpart in women of urethritis in men. N Engl J Med, 311:1, 1984.
19. Stamm WE, Tam M, Koester M, and Cles L: Detection of Chlamydia trachomatis inclusions in McCoy cell cultures with fluorescein-conjugated monoclonal antibodies. J Clin Microbiol, 17:666, 1983.
20. Schachter J, and Grossman M: Chlamydial infections. Ann Rev Med, 32:45, 1981.
21. Mordhorst CH: Clinical epidemiology of oculogenital chlamydia infection. In Nongonococcal Urethritis and Related Infections. Edited by D Hobson and KK Holmes. Washington, DC, American Society for Microbiology, 1977.
22. Centers for Disease Control: Psittacosis at a turkey processing plant—North Carolina, 1989. MMWR, 39:460, 1990.
23. Jariwalla AG, Davies BH, and White J: Infective endocarditis complicating psittacosis: Response to rifampin. Br Med J, 280:155, 1980.
24. Jones RB, Priest JB, and Kuo C: Subacute chlamydial endocarditis. JAMA, 247:655, 1982.
25. Grayston JT, et al: A new respiratory pathogen: Chlamydia pneumoniae strain TWAR. J Infect Dis, 161:618, 1990.
26. Chi EY, Kuo CC, and Grayston JT: Unique ultrastructure in the elementary body of Chlamydia sp. strain TWAR. J Bacteriol, 169:3757, 1987.
27. Kuo CC, Chi EY, and Grayston JT: Ultrastructural study of entry of Chlamydia strain TWAR into HeLa cells. Infect Immun, 56:1668, 1988.
28. Campbell LA, Kuo CC, and Grayston JT: Characterization of the new Chlamydia agent, TWAR, as a unique organism by restriction endonuclease analysis and DNA-DNA hybridization. J Clin Microbiol, 25:1911, 1987.
29. Cox RL, Kuo CC, Grayston JT, and Campbell LA: Deoxyribonucleic acid relatedness of Chlamydia sp. strain TWAR to Chlamydia trachomatis and Chlamydia psittaci. Int J Syst Bacteriol, 38:265, 1988.
30. Wang SP, and Grayston JT: Microimmunofluorescence serological studies with the TWAR organism. In Chlamydial Infections. Edited by JD Oriel, et al. Cambridge, Cambridge University Press, 1986.
31. Grayston JT, Wang SP, Kuo CC, and Campbell LA: Current knowledge on Chlamydia pneumoniae, strain TWAR, an important cause of pneumonia and other acute respiratory diseases. Eur J Clin Microbiol Infect Dis, 8:191, 1989.
32. Kleemola M, et al: Epidemics of pneumonia caused by TWAR, a new Chlamydia organism, in military trainees in Finland. J Infect Dis, 157:230, 1988.
33. Marrie TJ, et al: Culture-negative endocarditis probably due to Chlamydia pneumoniae. J Infect Dis, 161:127, 1990.
34. Ogawa H, Fujisawa T, and Kazuyama Y: Isolation of Chlamydia pneumoniae from middle ear aspirates of otitis media with effusion: A case report. J Infect Dis, 162:1000, 1990.

35. Chernesky M, et al: Detection of Chlamydia trachomatis antigens in urine as an alternative to swabs and cultures. J Infect Dis, *161*:124, 1990.
36. Lindner LE, Nettum JA, Miller SL, and Altman KH: Comparison of scrape, swab, and cytobrush samples for the diagnosis of cervical chlamydial infection by immunofluorescence. Diagn Microbiol Infect Dis, *8*:179, 1987.
37. Bovarnick MR, Miller JC, and Syncer JC: The influence of certain salts, amino acids, sugars, and proteins on the stability of rickettsiae. J Bacteriol, *59*:509, 1950.
38. Gordon FB, et al: Detection of Chlamydia (Bedsonia) in certain infections of man. I. Laboratory procedures: Comparison of yolk sac and cell culture for detection and isolation. J Infect Dis, *120*:451, 1969.
39. Smith TF, Brown SD, and Weed LA: Diagnosis of Chlamydia trachomatis infections by cell cultures and serology. Lab Med, *13*:92, 1982.
40. Mahony JB, and Chernesky MA: Effect of swab type and storage temperature on the isolation of Chlamydia trachomatis from clinical specimens. J Clin Microbiol, *22*:865, 1985.
41. Reeve PJ, Owen J, and Oriel JD: Laboratory procedures for the isolation of Chlamydia trachomatis from the human genital tract. J Clin Pathol, *28*:910, 1975.
42. Croy TR, Kuo C-C, and Wang S-P: Comparative susceptibility of eleven mammalian cell lines to infection with trachoma organisms. J Clin Microbiol, *1*:434, 1975.
43. Barnes RC: Laboratory diagnosis of human chlamydial infections. Clin Microbiol Rev, *2*:119, 1989.
44. Rota TR, and Nichols RL: Chlamydia trachomatis in cell culture. I. Comparison of efficiencies of infection in several chemically defined media, at various pH and temperature values, and after exposure to diethylaminoethyl-dextran. Appl Microbiol, *26*:560, 1973.
45. McComb DE, and Puzniak CI: Micro cell culture method for isolation of Chlamydia trachomatis. Appl Microbiol, *28*:727, 1974.
46. Jones RB, et al: Effect of blind passage and multiple sampling on recovery of Chlamydia trachomatis from urogenital specimens. J Clin Microbiol, *24*:1029, 1986.
47. Schachter J, and Martin DH: Failure of multiple passages to increase chlamydial recovery. J Clin Microbiol, *25*:1851, 1987.
48. Zapata M, Chernesky M, and Mahony J: Indirect immunofluorescnece staining of Chlamydia trachomatis inclusions in microculture plates with monoclonal antibodies. J Clin Microbiol, *19*:937, 1984.
49. Lefebvre J, Laperiere H, Rousseau H, and Masse R: Comparison of three techniques for detection of Chlamydia trachomatis in endocervical specimens from asymptomatic women. J Clin Microbiol, *26*:726, 1988.
50. Schachter J: Biology of Chlamydia trachomatis. *In* Sexually Transmitted Diseases. Edited by KK Holmes, P-A Mardh, PF Sparling, and PJ Wiesner. New York, McGraw-Hill, 1984.
51. Friis B, et al: Rapid diagnosis of Chlamydia trachomatis pneumonia in infants. Acta Pathol Microbiol Immunol Scand Sect B, *92*:139, 1984.
52. Paisley JW, et al: Rapid diagnosis of Chlamydia trachomatis pneumonia in infants by direct immunofluorescence microscopy of nasopharyngeal secretions. J Pediatr, *109*:653, 1986.
53. Tam MR, et al: Culture-independent diagnosis of Chlamydia trachomatis using monoclonal antibodies. N Engl J Med, *310*:1146, 1984.
54. Taylor HR, Rapoza PA, Kiessling LA, and Quinn TC: Rapid detection of Chlamydia trachomatis with monoclonal antibodies. Lancet, *ii*:38, 1984.
55. Cles LD, Bruch K, and Stamm WE: Staining characteristics of six commerically available monoclonal immunofluorescence reagents for direct diagnosis of Chlamydia trachomatis infections. J Clin Microbiol, *26*:1735, 1988.
56. Stamm WE: Diagnosis of Chlamydia trachomatis genitourinary infections. Ann Intern Med, *108*:710, 1988.
57. Rompalo AM, Suchland RJ, Price CB, and Stamm WE: Rapid diagnosis of Chlamydia trachomatis rectal infection by direct fluorescence staining. J Infect Dis, *155*:1075, 1987.
58. Baselski VS, McNeeley SG, Ryan G, and Robinson MA: A comparison of nonculture-dependent methods for detection of Chlamydia trachomatis infections in pregnant women. Obstet Gynecol, *70*:47, 1987.
59. Chernesky MA, et al: Detection of Chlamydia trachomatis antigens by enzyme immunoassay and immunofluorescence in genital specimens from symptomatic and asymptomatic men and women. J Infect Dis, *154*:141, 1986.
60. Lipkin ES, et al: Comparison of monoclonal antibody staining and culture in diagnosing cervical chlamydial infection. J Clin Microbiol, *23*:114, 1986.
61. Phillips RS, Hanff PA, Hauffman RS, Aronson MD: Use of a direct fluorescent antibody test for detecting Chlamydia trachomatis cervical infection in women seeking routine gynecologic care. J Infect Dis, *156*:575, 1987.
62. Quinn TC, et al: Screening for Chlamydia trachomatis infection in an inner-city population: A comparison of diagnostic methods. J Infect Dis, *152*:419, 1985.
63. Amortegui AJ, and Meyer MP: Enzyme immunoassay for detection of Chlamydia trachomatis from the cervix. Obstet Gynecol, *65*:523, 1985.
64. Hipp SS, Yangsook H, and Murphy D: Assessment of enzyme immunoassay and immunofluorescence test for detection of Chlamydia trachomatis. J Clin Microbiol, *25*:1938, 1987.
65. Levy RA, and Warford AL: Evaluation of the modified Chlamydiazyme immunoassay for the detection of chlamydial antigen. Am J Clin Pathol, *86*:330, 1986.
66. Mumtaz G, Mellars BJ, Ridgway GL, and Oriel JD: Enzyme immunoassay for detection of Chlamydia trachomatis antigen in urethral and endocervical swabs. J Clin Pathol, *38*:740, 1985.
67. Moi H, and Danielsson D: Diagnosis of genital Chlamydia trachomatis infection in males by cell culture and antigen detection test. Eur J Clin Microbiol, *5*:563, 1986.
68. Ryan RW, et al: Rapid detection of Chlamydia trachomatis by an enzyme immunoassay method. Diagn Microbiol Infect Dis, *5*:225, 1986.
69. LeBar WD, Schubiner H, Jemal C, and Herschman BR: Comparison of IDEIA III and cell culture for the detection of Chlamydia trachomatis in endocervical specimens. J Clin Microbiol, *28*:1447, 1990.
70. Phillips LE, et al: Ortho enzyme immunoassay versus McCoy cell monolayers stained by iodine or fluorescent antibody for detection of Chlamydia trachomatis. J Clin Microbiol, *28*:1541, 1990.
71. Gaydos CA, et al: Evaluation of Syva enzyme immunoassay for detection of Chlamydia trachomatis in genital specimens. J Clin Microbiol, *28*:1541, 1990.
72. Kellogg JA, Sieple JW, Murray CL, and Levisky JS: Effect of endocervical specimen quality on detection of Chlamydia trachomatis and on the incidence of false-positive results with the Chlamydiazyme method. J Clin Microbiol, *28*:1108, 1990.
73. Hammerschlag MR, Gelling M, Roblin PM, and Worku M: Comparison of Kodak Surecell Chlamydia test kit with culture for the diagnosis of chlamydial conjunctivitis in infants. J Clin Microbiol, *28*:1441, 1990.
74. Schubiner H, et al: Comparison of two membrane enzyme

immunoassays for the detection of Chlamydia trachomatis in clinical samples. *In* Abstracts of the 90th Annual Meeting of the American Society for Microbiology. Washington, DC, American Society for Microbiology, 1990.

75. Arumainayagam JT, Matthews RS, Uthayakumar S, and Clay JC: Evaluation of a novel solid-phase immunoassay, Clearview Chlamydia, for the rapid detection of Chlamydia trachomatis. J Clin Microbiol, 28:2813, 1990.

76. Woods GL, et al: Evaluation of a nonisotopic probe for detection of Chlamydia trachomatis in endocervical specimens. J Clin Microbiol, 28:370, 1990.

77. Iwen PC, Blair TMH, and Woods GL: Comparison of the Gen-Probe PACE 2 system, direct fluorescent-antibody and cell culture for detecting Chlamydia trachomatis in cervical specimens. Am J Clin Pathol, 95:578, 1991.

78. Schachter J, Grossman M, and Azimi PH: Serology of Chlamydia trachomatis in infants. J Infect Dis, 146:530, 1982.

79. Kuo CC, and Grayston JT: Factors affecting viability and growth in HeLa 229 cells of Chlamydia sp. strain TWAR. J Clin Microbiol, 26:812, 1988.

Chapter 26

RICKETTSIAE

Rickettsiae are the agents of some of the most serious, difficult to diagnose, infectious diseases (Table 26–1) (1,2). The definition of a rickettsia is related to its host and its ecology: rickettsiae are small, obligate intracellular, gram-negative bacteria that have an arthropod host during at least a portion of their natural history.

Rickettsial diseases such as Rocky Mountain spotted fever (RMSF), Q fever, louse-borne epidemic typhus, flea-borne murine typhus, scrub typhus, ehrlichiosis, boutonneuse fever, Queensland tick typhus, and Israeli spotted fever have fatal potential. The rickettsial disease now known as scrub typhus was described in Chinese medical texts contemporary with the Roman empire (3). Epidemic typhus, first clearly described in Europe in the early 1500s, played a major role in determining the outcome of most of the important military campaigns there for the ensuing 400 years (4). During World War I, the Russian Revolution, and their aftermath, 25 million persons suffered from epidemic louse-borne typhus, and 3 million died. Scrub typhus affected 16,000 Allied troops in Asia and the Pacific during World War II. Despite the development of antimicrobial agents that make these diseases easily treatable in their early stages, clinical pathology has generally neglected the diagnosis of rickettsial diseases (2). Usually, the patient is dependent on a tentative clinical diagnosis and empiric treatment. Unfortunately, the clinical diagnosis is also difficult, as very suggestive clinical signs and epidemiologic clues are often absent, particularly early in the course of illness (5). Moreover, the antimicrobial drugs that are most effective against rickettsiae are not those most frequently used for empirical coverage of febrile patients.

Rickettsiae offer many challenges to the diagnostic pathologist who wishes to establish expeditiously the diagnosis of rickettsiosis. Scientifically, they pose interesting questions that range from their intracellular life style to their ecology (6,7). Rapid advances in diagnosis are being achieved by the molecular biology revolution, but these entrenched zoonoses are likely to remain diagnostic problems.

CLASSIFICATION

Because the definition of rickettsiae is based upon relationships of the organisms to their hosts (growth only within eukaryotic cells and ecologic niche involving arthropods) rather than properties of the bacteria themselves, rickettsial taxonomy has not been based on their evolutionary relationships. Recently, the use of nucleotide sequence data from 16S ribosomal RNA has permitted construction of a bacterial evolutionary tree that includes rickettsiae (8). Members of the spotted fever–typhus complex of the genus Rickettsia and species of Ehrlichia are relatively closely related in this system, and Rochalimaea is also a related member of the α lineage of the purple bacteria. Located relatively distant from this branch of the bacterial evolutionary tree in the γ subdivision of the purple bacteria, Coxiella is more closely related to Legionella, a genus of facultative intracellular bacteria. The available data regarding Rickettsia tsutsugamushi, including proteins, cell wall ultrastructure, DNA hybridization, and lack of lipopolysaccharides and peptidoglycan, indicate that it is not truly a member of the genus Rickettsia (9,10). Further studies are necessary to determine its taxonomic position, but the present data suggest that its obligate intracellular parasitism and vasculotropism with consequent clinical and pathologic similarities to spotted fevers and typhus fevers are an accident of apparent convergent evolution. The medically important rickettsiae are contrasted with the other genus of obligate intracellular bacteria, Chlamydia, which, according to the 16S ribosomal RNA scheme occupies a phylum of its own with no known close relatives (Table 26–2).

STRUCTURE AND PHYSIOLOGY

Rickettsiae are small coccobacilli with a gram-negative cell wall. Typical Rickettsia rickettsii are 0.3 μm wide and 1.0 μm long and are barely resolved by the ordinary brightfield microscope. Rickettsiae are poorly visualized by routine Gram stain methods but are stained bright red by carbol fuchsin in the Gimenez technique. Acridine orange stains the DNA and RNA of rickettsiae for visualization by ultraviolet microscopy. The Giemsa stain was used by Wolbach from 1916 through the years following World War I to demonstrate that the vascular endothelium of patients with RMSF and epidemic typhus fever contains bacteria-like forms (11–13). Lack of attention to details of fixation and differentiation have rendered the Giemsa stain virtually useless for the demonstration of rickettsiae in most histology laboratories today. Even the modified Brown-Hopps tissue Gram stain, which can be used to visualize Legionella in paraffin-embedded sections, stains only a small fraction of the rickettsial organisms actually present when compared with sensitive immunohistologic methods.

Electron microscopy reveals that spotted fever and typhus group rickettsiae have a cell wall with an outer leaflet 2 to 2.5 nm thick, an inner leaflet 5 to 7.7 nm thick, and a prominent electron-lucent zone that has been considered to be a carbohydrate-rich slime layer (Fig. 26–1) (9,14). The cell wall of Rickettsia tsutsugamushi has a thicker outer leaflet of 8.5 nm and a thinner inner leaflet of 2.5 nm and seems to lack the slime layer. The cell wall of Ehrlichia species has not been examined as carefully, but it differs appreciably from spotted fever and typhus rickettsiae ultrastructurally and lacks lipopolysaccharide (Fig. 26–2). Several morphologic forms of Coxiella bur-

Table 26-1. Rickettsial Diseases: Pathogens, Distribution, and Mode of Transmission

Disease	Etiologic Agent	Geographic Distribution	Mode of Transmission
Spotted fevers			
Rocky Mountain spotted fever	R. rickettsii	North, Central & South America	Bite of Dermacentor, Rhipicephalus, or Amblyomma ticks
Rickettsialpox	R. akari	USA, Ukraine, Korea	Bite of Lipnyssoides sanguineus mite
Boutonneuse fever	R. conorii	Southern Europe, Africa, Ukraine, Russia, Georgia, Middle East, Indian subcontinent	Bite of Rhipicephalus, Hyalomma, Amblyomma, or Haemaphysalis ticks
North Asian tick typhus	R. sibirica	Russia, China, Mongolia, Pakistan	Bite of Dermacentor, Haemaphysalis, or Hyalomma ticks
Queensland tick typhus	R. australis	Eastern Australia	Bite of Ixodes ticks
Oriental spotted fever	R. japonica	Japan	Suspected bite of Japanese tick
Israeli spotted fever	Rickettsia sp. unnamed	Israel	Bite of Rhipicephalus tick
Typhus fevers			
Epidemic typhus	R. prowazekii	Potentially worldwide; recent decades in Africa, South America, Central America, Mexico, Asia	Feces of Pediculus louse
Brill-Zinsser disease	R. prowazekii	Worldwide; wherever persons with past epidemic typhus now reside	Recrudescence of latent infection
Flying squirrel typhus	R. prowazekii	USA	Presumably feces of flea or louse of flying squirrel
Murine typhus	R. typhi	Worldwide in tropics & subtropics	Feces of Xenopsylla, Ctenocephalides & other fleas
Scrub typhus	R. tsutsugamushi	SE Asia, Japan, China, Sri Lanka, India, Russia, Indonesia, Western Pacific, Northern Australia	Bite of Leptotrombidium chiggers
Ehrlichioses			
Human ehrlichiosis	E. chaffeensis	USA	Bite of undetermined ticks
Sennetsu rickettsiosis	E. sennetsu	Japan	Not known
Q fever	C. burnetii	Worldwide	Inhalation of aerosols from infected animals, possibly ingestion of animal products or tick bite
Rochalimaea infections			
Trench fever	R. quintana	Europe, North America	Feces of Pediculus louse
Bacillary angiomatosis and peliosis	R. henselae	USA	Not known

netii have been described, including the small cell variant, large cell variant, and an endospore-like structure (15). Integration of these morphologic variants into a defined developmental cycle and proof that the endospore-like structure functions as such have not been established. Rochalimaea quintana, Rochalimaea henselae (an agent of septicemia, bacillary angiomatosis, and bacillary peliosis hepatitis) and Bartonella bacilliformis are typical gram-negative bacilli, and because they have been cultivated on cell-free medium they do not meet the definition of rickettsiae. Genetic relationship to Rickettsia prowazekii, the louse vector, and tradition explain the inclusion of Rochalimaea and Bartonella in this chapter.

It is important to understand that rickettsiae have evolved to a highly adapted state in their natural host. For example, Rickettsia rickettsii is so well-adapted to its tick hosts that rickettsiae are vertically transmitted from one generation to the next transovarially (16). Coxiella burnetii can proliferate to very large numbers in the placenta of ungulate hosts, which show no signs of illness and give birth to offspring that are free of associated morbidity. Ehrlichia species grow successfully in macrophages, lym-

Table 26-2. Properties of Rickettsiae and Chlamydiae

Genus	G + C content (%)	LPS	ATP Synthesis	Developmental Cycle	Axenic Cultivation	Major Target Cell	Intracellular Location
Rickettsia*	29–33	+	+	None	No	Endothelium	Cytosol
Rickettsia†	28.5–30	None	+	None	No	Presumably endothelium	Cytosol
Ehrlichia	Unknown	None	+	None	No	Various leukocytes	Phagosome
Coxiella	43	+	+	+	No	Macrophages	Phagolysosome
Rochalimaea	39	+	+	None	Yes	Not applicable	Extracellular
Chlamydia	41–44	+	No	+	No	Ophthalmic, respiratory, & genital mucosal epithelium & macrophages	Phagosome

* Spotted fever and typhus groups.
† Rickettsia tsutsugamushi is so clearly distinct from the other members of the genus Rickettsia that a separate genus name, Orientia, has been proposed.

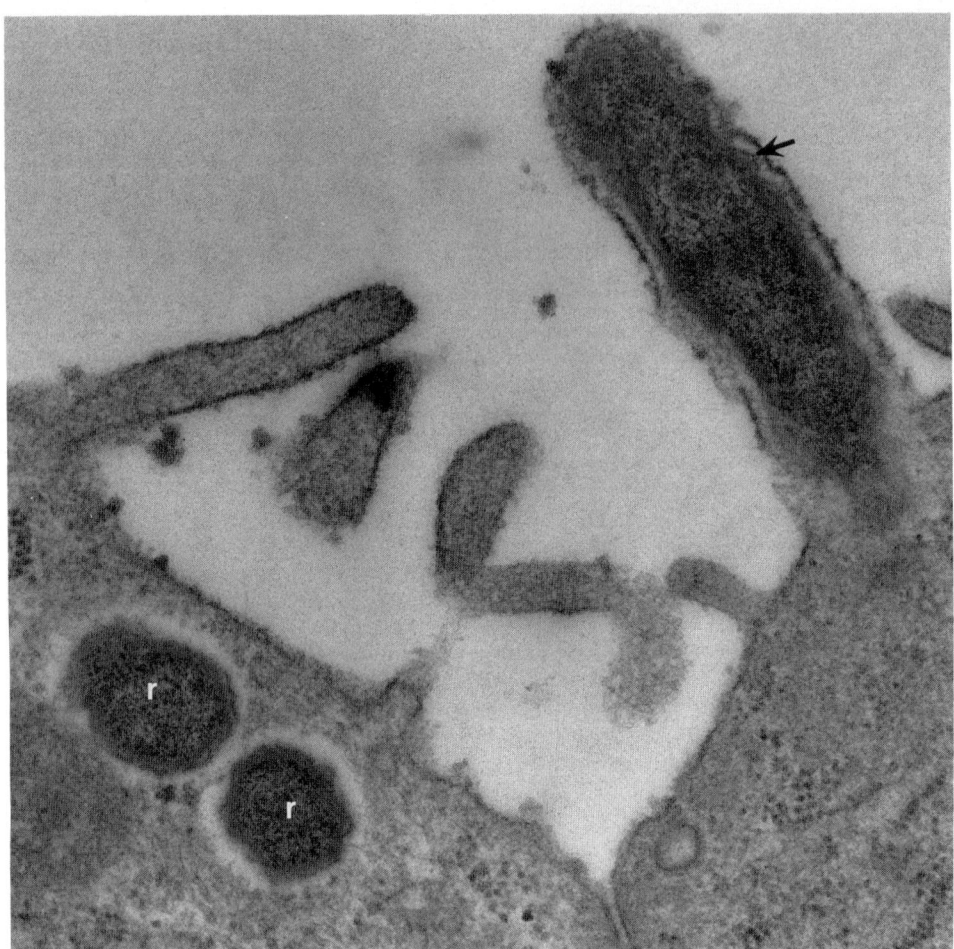

Fig. 26–1. Electron micrograph of intracellular spotted fever–group rickettsiae. A pair of organisms (*r*) cut in cross section have internal ribosomes, a plasma membrane, a cell wall, and an external electron-lucent zone. A longitudinally sectioned organism (*arrow*) is in the process of exit from the host cell via a filopodium.

phocytes, and polymorphonuclear leukocytes, all of which are important host defenses against most infectious diseases.

Further evidence for adaptation of rickettsiae to the intracellular niche includes a variety of specific transport mechanisms for acquiring amino acids, adenosine triphosphate (ATP), and other substances from the host cell (6). These adaptations, as well as possession of enzymes for biosynthetic pathways and generation of energy, indicate that rickettsiae are not defective life forms dependent on host cells but rather are highly evolved life forms that are particularly capable of exploiting the intracellular environment.

SPOTTED FEVERS

Rickettsia rickettsii contains 1.3×10^9 daltons of DNA, about the same as Neisseria meningitidis, less than Escherichia coli, and more than Mycoplasma pneumoniae. Organisms of the spotted fever and typhus groups are closely related genetically. DNA-DNA hybridizations demonstrate that Rickettsia rickettsii shares 91 to 94% DNA homology with Rickettsia conorii, 70 to 74% with Rickettsia sibirica, 53% with Rickettsia australis, 47% with Rickettsia prowazekii, 46% with Rickettsia akari, 42% with Rickettsia typhi, and 73% with the nonpathogenic spotted fever rickettsiae, Rickettsia montana. Spotted fever rickettsiae were grouped together on the basis of shared antigens, particularly the lipopolysaccharides of the cell wall. They are distinguished from typhus group rickettsiae by antigenic differences in the lipopolysaccharides. In practice the species of a spotted fever rickettsia is determined by species-specific heat-labile epitopes on a pair of surface-exposed major outer membrane proteins (17).

Rocky Mounted Spotted Fever

Epidemiology

RMSF occurs in the geographic distribution of ticks infected with Rickettsia rickettsii: Dermacentor variabilis in the eastern half of the United States, Dermacentor andersoni in the western United States and Canada, Rhipicephalus sanguineus in Mexico, and Amblyomma cajennense in Central and South America. Rickettsia rickettsii is maintained in nature principally by transovarian transmission from the adult female tick to infected ova, which hatch as infected larvae and maintain the infection as they molt from stage to stage (18). The tick-rickettsia relationship is not perfect, however, because on occasion rickettsial overgrowth occurs, resulting in increased mortality, decreased oviposition, and decreased egg development. Replenishment of the rickettsia-infected tick reservoir is apparently achieved by uninfected larval and nymphal ticks acquiring R. rickettsii in a blood meal from rodents during

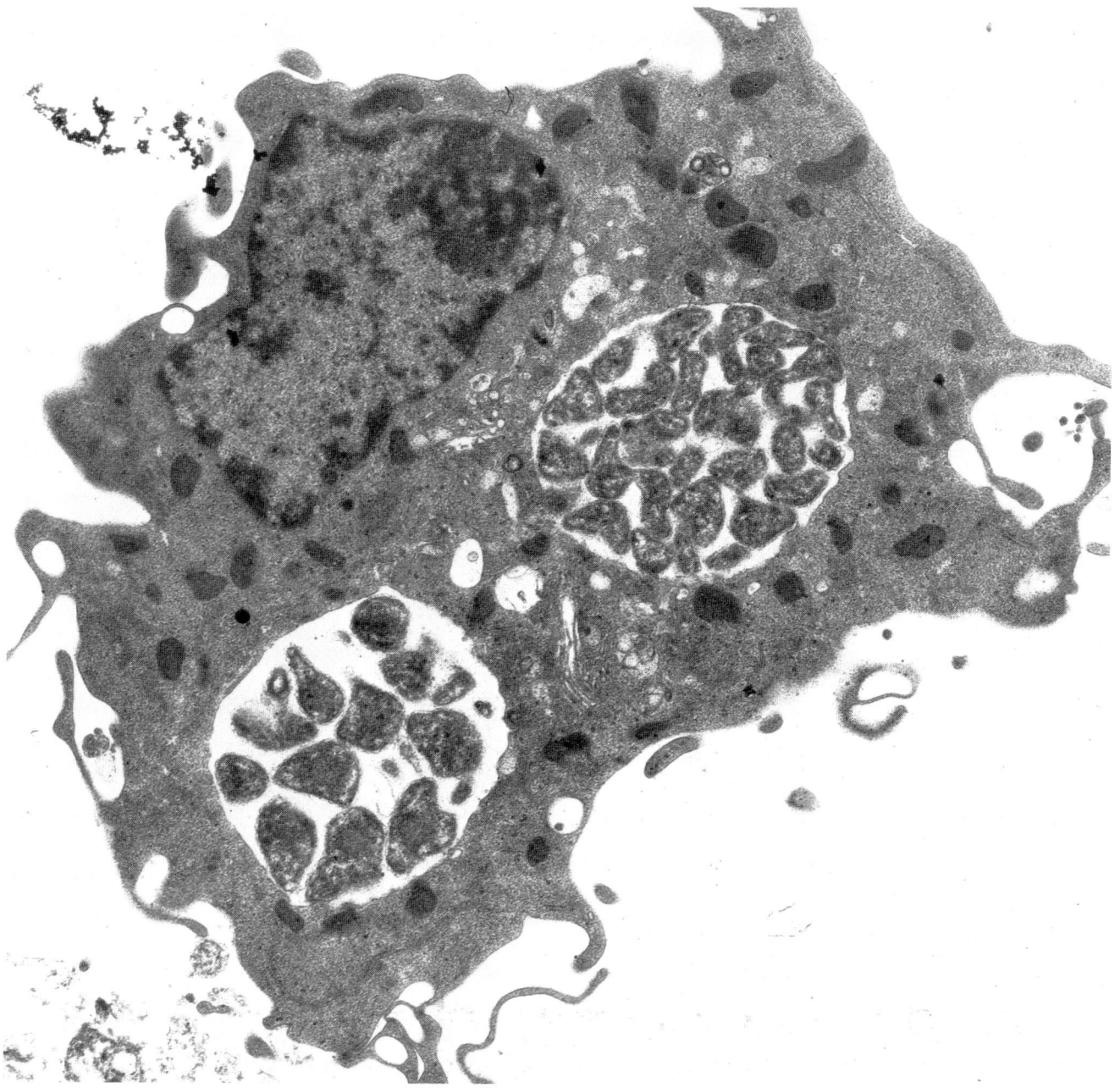

Fig. 26–2. Electron micrograph of ehrlichiae within membrane-bound cytoplasmic vacuoles (×15,200).

their relatively brief period of rickettsemia. This establishment of new lines for subsequent transovarial transmission does not appear to occur very efficiently. In fact, only a small portion of the ecologic niche is occupied by virulent R. rickettsii (fewer than 0.1% of individuals of the relevant tick species). Competition between some highly prevalent, nonpathogenic species of rickettsiae and R. rickettsii explains the absence of RMSF from particular geographic locations (19). However, in most endemic areas 96% of ticks contain no rickettsiae that would interfere with the establishment of R. rickettsii in them.

Dramatic fluctuations in the incidence of RMSF have been observed over the years and in various geographic locations (20). In the 1920s and 1930s, an incidence greater than 50 cases per 100,000 population in some regions of the Rocky Mountains gave the disease its name. A sharp fall in incidence in the Rocky Mountains in the mid-1940s and an increase in the South Atlantic states during the 1970s remain unexplained. From a low of 199 cases reported to the Centers for Disease Control (CDC) in 1959, there was a steady rise to 1192 cases in 1981, followed by a steady decline to approximately 600 cases annually since 1987. In the last decade the highest incidences have been reported in Oklahoma, North Carolina, South Carolina, Maryland, Virginia, Georgia, Tennessee, Ohio, Missouri, Arkansas, Texas, and Kansas. Asynchronous geographic fluctuations in incidence, recently including New Jersey, Pennsylvania, and the South Bronx in

New York, continue to defy explanation (21). Endemic areas at the fringes of the geographic distribution of the disease in Cape Cod and Long Island have persisted for many decades. Infected Dermacentor variabilis attached to dogs can be transported wherever the dog is taken or is allowed to go. When the infected eggs hatch, RMSF may become established if the ecology supports survival of the ticks. RMSF has been reported in nearly all of the 48 contiguous states.

Most cases occur between May and September, although wintertime cases are well-documented. The highest incidence is in children, particularly in the 5- to 9-year age group, who play outdoors and are exposed to the common American dog tick (22).

Pathogenesis

The sequence of pathogenic events leading to RMSF begins with attachment of the infected tick to human skin (2,12,16,18). Rickettsial virulence is reactivated by the warmth of the mammalian host's body and undefined components in the blood meal. Rickettsiae are inoculated from tick salivary glands into the human dermis, whence they spread throughout the body via the lymphohematogenous route. Rickettsiae attach to the endothelial cell membrane, induce phagocytosis, escape from the phagosome into the cytosol, divide by binary fission one or more times, and are released through the cell membrane at the end of long cellular projections (Fig. 26–1) (23). The released rickettsiae attach to and invade adjacent endothelial cells and vascular smooth muscle cells, exhibiting a capacity for invasiveness that no other rickettsial species possesses. Rickettsia rickettsii even invades the nucleus of some parasitized cells.

Cell injury is directly related to the quantity of intracellular rickettsiae (23). The ultrastructural cytopathology, dilated cisternae of rough endoplasmic reticulum, suggests that the cell membrane is injured by exiting and entering organisms. Reduction of cell injury by phospholipase A inhibitors and inhibitors of trypsin-like proteases is consistent with the cell membrane as a subcellular target (24,25). Another line of investigation suggests that membrane lipids are damaged by free radical–induced peroxidation. Rickettsia rickettsii destroys infected cells in vitro in the absence of host immune, inflammatory, and coagulation mechanisms (26). The organisms do not elaborate exotoxins or endotoxic lipopolysaccharides. Although host mediated mechanisms may play a role in some of the symptoms and signs of RMSF (e.g., interleukin [IL]-1 and tumor necrosis factor [TNF]-α may play a role in fever and other manifestations of the acute phase response), activation of the immune response, the kallikrein-kinin system, the intrinsic and extrinsic coagulation pathways, platelets, and the fibrinolytic system appear to confer more benefit than harm to the host (27,28). Disseminated intravascular coagulation occurs rarely, although thrombocytopenia, present in half of RMSF cases, is attributable to consumption of platelets in the numerous foci of damaged endothelium (5,29). The characteristic rickettsial lesion consists of swollen or necrotic, infected endothelial cells and perivascular hemorrhage, lymphocytes, and macrophages.

Clinical Manifestations

After an incubation period of 2 to 14 days (mean 7 days), onset of RMSF is marked by fever, severe headache, and myalgia (2,5,29). The fundamental pathophysiologic effects in all rickettsioses, including RMSF, stem from vascular injury leading to increased vascular permeability, edema, hypovolemia, hypoalbuminemia, and hypotension (30). Acute renal failure is observed in 14% of cases and is explained by hypovolemia leading to prerenal azotemia or hypotensive shock leading to acute tubular necrosis (5,29,31).

The cutaneous, gastrointestinal, neurologic, and respiratory tract signs and symptoms correlate well with the presence of rickettsial vascular lesions in these sites (Fig. 26–3). The diagnostically suggestive rash develops in 90% of patients with RMSF, but the onset of rash is after the third day of illness in slightly more than half the cases, and appears on days 5 or 6 in 18 to 20% of cases (5,29). The rash is initially macular, and the dilated blood vessels

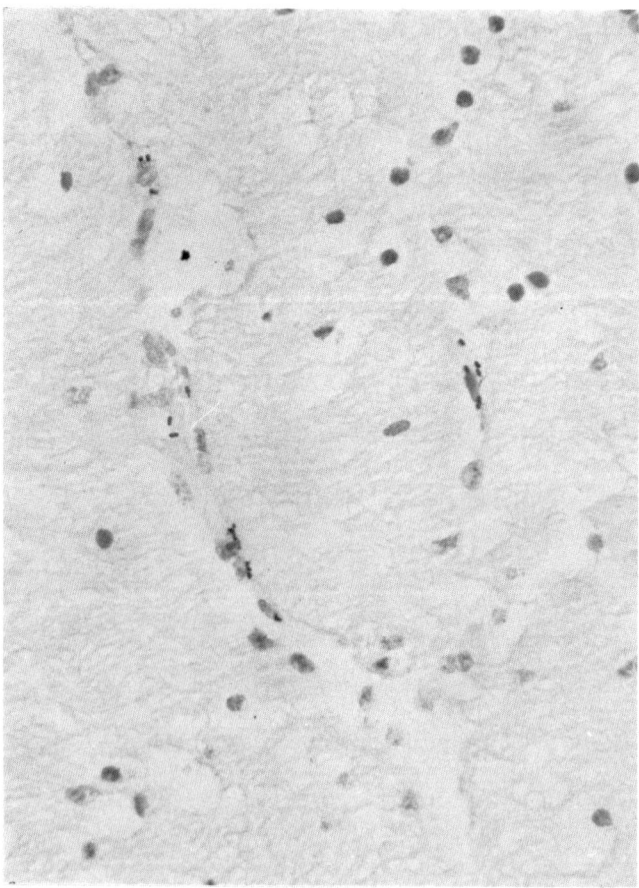

Fig. 26–3. Micrograph of brain tissue from a patient who died of Rocky Mountain spotted fever. Two longitudinally sectioned capillaries have endothelial cells infected with coccobacillary forms of Rickettsia rickettsii that were stained dark by immunoperoxidase.

blanch upon pressure. Eventually it becomes maculopapular, with central petechiae in 41 to 59% of patients. Nausea, vomiting, and abdominal pain occur early in the course and may suggest gastroenteritis or acute surgical abdomen (5,29,32). Central nervous system (CNS) involvement may mimic meningoencephalitis with mild to moderate cerebrospinal fluid (CSF) pleocytosis, confusion, and stupor or delirium (33). Coma and seizures affect the 8 to 10% of patients who are the most severely ill (5,29). Severe respiratory failure is seen in 12% of cases, the result of a rickettsial injury to the pulmonary microcirculation and consequent noncardiogenic pulmonary edema (29,34).

Immediately prior to the antimicrobial era, the case fatality rate for RMSF was 23%. Recently it has been approximately 3%, death being associated with delayed or inappropriate antimicrobial treatment, male sex, older age, and glucose-6-phosphate dehydrogenase (G6PD) deficiency.

Laboratory Diagnosis

During the first three days of illness when antimicrobial treatment is very effective, only 3% of patients with RMSF have the triad of fever, rash, and history of tick bite (5). Before the onset of the rash, the differential diagnosis is very large and includes influenza, nonspecific viral syndrome, infectious mononucleosis, dengue fever, typhoid fever, gastroenteritis, acute surgical abdomen, viral meningoencephalitis, leptospirosis, and bacterial sepis (2). Appearance of a rash suggests the possibility of meningococcemia, enteroviral exanthem, toxic shock syndrome, secondary syphilis, disseminated gonococcal infection, measles, rubella, thrombotic thrombocytopenic purpura, immune thrombocytopenic purpura, drug reaction, Kawasaki's syndrome, immune complex vasculitis including systemic lupus erythematosus, or another rickettsiosis.

The pathologist and microbiologist seldom offer diagnostic assistance to patients who may have RMSF during the acute phase of illness when antimicrobial therapeutic decisions are important. Some clinical laboratories offer the Weil-Felix serologic test for antibodies that agglutinate Proteus vulgaris strains OX-19 or OX-2. This archaic test, however, has poor sensitivity and specificity and should be relegated to medical history (35). During the acute phase of illness the Weil-Felix test produces more positive results for persons who do not have RMSF than for patients who do. Very seldom does even the most sensitive assay for antibodies to Rickettsia rickettsii yield positive results at the time of the patient's presentation. The serologic diagnosis of spotted fevers and typhus fevers is by nature retrospective. Confirmation of the diagnosis of RMSF is achieved, in decreasing order of sensitivity, by indirect hemagglutination assay, indirect immunofluorescence assay, latex agglutination, microagglutination, and complement fixation (Table 26–3) (36,37). Reagents are available commercially for indirect immunofluorescence assay and latex agglutination, either of which is preferable to the Weil-Felix reaction. Latex agglutination and indirect hemagglutination are based upon coating latex beads or erythrocytes with a heated alkaline extract of spotted fever group rickettsial proteins and lipopolysaccharide (38). All these assays contain antigens shared among the members of the group and, so, do not distinguish among the various spotted fevers. Enzyme immunoassays have been tailored to detect either spotted fever group-specific or species-specific antibodies. State and federal public health laboratories usually offer useful diagnostic serologic tests for RMSF, murine typhus, and Q fever. Convalescent-phase serologic confirmation is important to document long-lasting immunity, to sharpen the clinician's diagnostic acumen, and to provide a documented diagnosis for reporting to public health authorities.

Table 26–3. Comparison of Serologic Assays for the Diagnosis of Rocky Mountain Spotted Fever

Serologic Test	Sensitivity (%)	Specificity (%)	Antigen Detected
Indirect immunofluorescence	94–100	100	Group*
Indirect hemagglutination	91–100	99	Group
Latex agglutination	71–94	96–99	Group
Complement fixation	0–63	100	Group
Proteus OX-19 agglutination	70	78	X[†]
Proteus OX-2 agglutination	47	96	X

* Antigens shared among rickettsiae of the spotted fever group.
† Undefined cross-reactive antigens.

In the acute stage of the illness a timely diagnosis is afforded presently only by immunohistologic demonstration of Rickettsia rickettsii in 3-mm punch biopsy specimens of the skin rash that are processed as frozen sections of fresh tissue or paraffin-embedded sections of formalin-fixed tissue (35,39,40). The feasibility of detection of the DNA of R. rickettsii by polymerase chain reaction (PCR) amplification of DNA in blood samples has been demonstrated and may become generally available in the future (41).

The gold standard of infectious disease diagnosis is established by cultivation and identification of the etiologic agent (39). Cultivation of Rickettsia rickettsii has generally been considered to be cumbersome and hazardous. However, modern biohazard-containment laminar flow hoods, use of protective gloves, mask, and gown, safety procedures, and facilities such as those used for handling mycobacteria, fungi, and human immunodeficiency virus make cultivation and identification in shell vial centrifugation-enhanced cell cultures an attractive, less hazardous, relatively timely, diagnostic approach (42). Many cell lines, including human embryonic lung, L-929 cells, and Vero cells, support the growth of rickettsiae. The traditional approach of intraperitoneal inoculation of patient's blood or tissues into adult male guinea pigs, although effective, is rarely attempted.

Treatment

The drug of choice in most clinical situations is doxycycline (200 mg/day in two divided doses). Also effective are tetracycline (25 mg/kg per day in four doses) and chloramphenicol (50 mg/kg per day in four doses) (29). Antirickettsial activity in vitro has been reported for the quinolone antimicrobial agents (43). Many drugs used empirically in febrile patients, such as penicillins, cephalosporins, aminoglycosides, and erythromycin, have no benefit against RMSF.

Rickettsialpox

Rickettsialpox was first recognized in 1946 by a general practitioner in New York City (44). The etiology was rapidly elucidated to be Rickettsia akari, a new spotted fever–group rickettsia that is transmitted by the bite of Liponyssoides sanguineus, the mite of domestic mice, Mus musculus. The rickettsia is maintained in nature by transovarian transmission in mites. During the late 1940s and the 1950s more than 100 cases per year were frequently reported; today rickettsialpox is seldom diagnosed (45). Cases have been reported mainly in cities of the northeastern United States, but rickettsialpox has also occurred in Ohio, Utah, Arizona, and the Ukraine.

Rickettsia akari is introduced into the skin during a blood meal by an infected mite. A papule develops at the feeding site during the incubation period and progresses 2 to 7 days later to a 1- to 2.5-cm eschar. Histologic examination of the eschar shows coagulative necrosis of the epidermis and adjacent vascular injury and inflammation. Enlarged regional lymph nodes reflect lymphatic spread from the cutaneous inoculation site. Hematogenous spread results in a maculopapular rash, which typically becomes papular, then vesicular, forms a crust, and heals.

Onset of chills, fever, malaise, severe headache, and myalgia occurs approximately 10 days after the mite bite. Rash is noted 2 to 6 days later. Some patients also have nausea, vomiting, abdominal pain, anorexia, cough, conjunctivitis, pharyngitis, photophobia, nuchal rigidity, and splenomegaly.

The differential diagnosis is similar to that for RMSF, but the eschar adds to the list primary syphilis, cutaneous anthrax, and other rickettsioses. The vesicular rash may also suggest infection with varicella-zoster or herpes simplex virus. Laboratory diagnosis by rickettsial isolation has been achieved by inoculation of mice and guinea pigs, but it is rarely attempted. Serologic diagnosis of a spotted fever rickettsiosis is established by indirect immunofluorescence, but demonstration of species-specific antibodies to Rickettsia akari requires cumbersome cross-absorption with antigens of Rickettsia rickettsii and Rickettsia akari and indirect immunofluorescent antibody testing, as has been performed at the CDC. Neither acute- nor convalescent-phase serum reacts in the Weil-Felix test. Treatment with either tetracycline (15 to 30 mg/kg body weight per day, orally, in four doses) or chloramphenicol (50 mg/kg per day, orally, in four doses) is effective.

Tick-Borne Spotted Fever Rickettsioses of Europe, Africa, Asia, and Australia

At least five distinct species of tick-borne spotted fever rickettsiae cause human illness in the Eastern Hemisphere (see Table 26–1). The prototype of these spotted fevers, boutonneuse fever, is caused by Rickettsia conorii, which has greater antigenic and genetic diversity than the strains of Rickettsia rickettsii associated with RMSF. Each of these spotted fevers is transmitted by tick bite, and the rickettsiae are maintained in nature principally by transovarian transmission (46). The seasonal occurrence correlates with the period of activity of the vector tick. Often patients seek medical care in the United States and northern Europe upon returning home from Africa or southern Europe infected with Rickettsia conorii (47). In many areas of the Mediterranean basin, Africa, Asia, Japan, and Australia, numerous healthy persons have antibodies reactive with spotted fever group rickettsiae. It has yet to be determined whether these observations are due to prior undiagnosed illness, immune stimulation by nonpathogenic rickettsiae, or nonspecificity of the tests.

Disseminated endothelial infection by Rickettsia conorii results in multisystem injury manifest in biopsy and necropsy specimens as meningoencephalitis, vascular lesions in the skin, lungs, gastrointestinal tract, pancreas, liver, heart, kidneys, and spleen, and multifocal hepatocellular necrosis (48–50). The pathogenic basis for tissue injury is demonstrated well in the site of the tick bite inoculation of rickettsiae, where the eschar develops in 50% of patients diagnosed with boutonneuse fever, 77% with North Asian tick typhus, 50% with Queensland tick typhus, 48% with Oriental spotted fever, and fewer than 1% with Israeli spotted fever. In the eschar of boutonneuse fever, commonly also referred to as *tache noire* (French: black spot), immunofluorescent R. conorii are present along with dermal edema, moderate to severe lymphohistiocytic vasculitis, and cutaneous necrosis (51). The mechanism of tissue injury appears to be associated with endothelial damage but is not caused by vascular thrombosis. As in RMSF, the systemic pathophysiologic events result from increased vascular permeability with edema, arterial hypotension, and hypoalbuminemia (52). Vascular endothelial damage results in consumption of platelets, decreased concentrations of plasma fibrinogen, elevated concentrations of fibrin split products, and increased von Willebrand factor antigen (the latter presumably derived from injured endothelium) (53). Although hemostatic mechanisms are activated by the vascular lesions, normal levels of factors XII, XI, X, IX, VII, II, and antithrombin-III indicate that true disseminated intravascular coagulation does not occur.

After an average incubation period of one week onset is marked by fever, headache, and myalgia. An eschar may be noted by the patient prior to onset or upon examination at presentation. A maculopapular rash typically appears 3 to 5 days after onset of illness and may develop into papules. Abdominal symptoms of nausea, vomiting, and diarrhea and elevated serum hepatic transaminase values are common. Although these spotted fevers of the Eastern Hemisphere were often considered benign, boutonneuse fever can be a severe disease, particularly in patients who are elderly or alcoholic or have underlying disease or G6PD deficiency (54). These patients may have a purpuric rash, other hemorrhagic phenomena, thrombocytopenia, respiratory impairment, hypoxemia, acute renal failure, and mental status alterations. Approximately 2% of patients hospitalized with boutonneuse fever and Israeli spotted fever die.

Spotted fever is often missed because the physician fails to consider the diagnosis, the clinical features frequently do not conform to the classic textbook description (e.g., eschar or rash may not be present), and laboratory diagnostic tests may not be available in many parts of the world. The diagnosis can be established in the acute phase by immunohistologic demonstration of spotted fever rickettsiae in the eschar or rash. A clinically useful diagnosis can be achieved by culture of blood utilizing the centrifugation shell vial technique in which blood is inoculated into antibiotic-free cell culture (42). Spotted fever rickettsiae may be demonstrated in the monolayer after 48 hours of cultivation. A confirmatory diagnosis can be made by examination of acute- and convalescent-phase sera for a fourfold or greater rise in antibodies to spotted fever group antigens by indirect immunofluorescence assay, indirect immunoperoxidase, latex agglutination, line blot, Western immunoblot, or complement fixation.

Boutonneuse fever can be treated successfully with substantial decrease in the duration of fever and morbidity by administration of doxycycline (100 mg, orally every 12 hours), tetracycline (25 to 30 mg/kg body weight per day, orally, in four doses), chloramphenicol (50 to 60 mg/kg per day, orally, in four doses), ciprofloxacin (200 mg, intravenously, every 12 hours or 750 mg, orally, every 12 hours), or ofloxacin (200 mg, orally, every 12 hours) (55).

TYPHUS FEVERS

Rickettsia prowazekii and Rickettsia typhi have genetic relatedness of 73% as determined by DNA-DNA hybridization (56). The similarity of the typhus fevers was confusing to physicians for decades. Nicolle of the Pasteur Institute in Tunis was awarded the Nobel Prize for his 1909 demonstration that epidemic typhus was transmitted by the human body louse (57). Between 1898 and 1910 in New York, Brill described 221 cases of an illness that was not associated with lice and which he correctly considered to be a modified form of classic epidemic typhus fever. Rickettsia prowazekii was isolated from patients with the disease described by Brill. Zinsser concluded that these patients were suffering from recrudescence of latent infection with R. prowazekii years after the acute illness. By the early 1930s, it had been demonstrated that sporadic endemic typhus is caused by a rickettsial agent different from the agent of epidemic typhus, that rats are part of the natural cycle, and that fleas are the major vector (58-60). The clinical distinction between sporadic cases of endemic murine typhus and recrudescent typhus was impossible without elucidation of two distinct rickettsial species that have different epidemiology and ecology.

Murine Typhus

By far the most prevalent rickettsial disease in the United States during the 1940s—more than 5000 cases were reported some years—the incidence of murine typhus was curtailed sharply by the application of the insecticide DDT and by control of rat populations. In recent years fewer than 100 cases have been reported annually in the United States, mostly in Texas (61,62). Murine typhus is a very important, frequently misdiagnosed infection that is endemic in Africa, Asia, Australia, Europe, and South America.

In addition to the zoonotic cycle of Rickettsia typhi in rats and the rat flea (Xenopsylla cheopis), other mammals and arthropods have been indicted, including opossums and the cat flea (Ctenocephalides felis) (63). Rat fleas acquire Rickettsia typhi from rickettsemic rats, support rickettsial growth in the midgut epithelial cells, and shed organisms in their feces. Humans are thought to become infected by scratching the rickettsiae-laden feces into the skin, by the flea bite, or by inhaling dried flea feces in which the organisms are stable for a relatively long period. An apparently minor factor in maintaining R. typhi in nature is transovarian transmission by a small proportion of infected female fleas.

Rickettsiae, after entering the body via the skin or lungs, spread hematogenously throughout the body where endothelial infection and vascular lesions are produced in the skin, lungs, CNS, gastrointestinal tract, liver, heart, and kidneys (64). The most important pathologic consequences are diffuse alveolar damage and meningoencephalomyelitis. The pathophysiologic effects of increased vascular permeability and focal vascular lesions include hypoalbuminemia, hyponatremia, prerenal azotemia, elevated hepatic enzymes, and thrombocytopenia.

After an average incubation period of 11 days patients note onset of chills, fever, and severe headache (61). Usually they do not seek medical attention for several days, and the rash is seldom present when they do. Nausea, vomiting, diarrhea, abdominal pain, and cough are often prominent symptoms. Murine typhus is seldom the initial diagnosis, and antirickettsial treatment is initiated an average of 10 days after onset of illness. A rash is observed in varying proportions of patients, depending on the darkness of their skin pigmentation (in 80% of whites and 20% of blacks). The rash typically appears on day 5 to 6 of illness, involves the trunk most prominently, and is macular or maculopapular. A minority of patients develop chest roentgenographic abnormalities such as pneumonitis, pulmonary edema, atelectasis, or pleural effusion. Severely ill patients may suffer confusion, stupor, coma, hallucinations, ataxia, seizures, respiratory failure requiring intubation, or hematemesis. Severe illness is associated with increased age, prolonged interval before antirickettsial therapy, and treatment with a sulfonamide drug. Nearly 10% of hospitalized patients are admitted to the intensive care unit, and 1 to 2% of murine typhus cases are fatal.

Murine typhus can be diagnosed by immunohistologic demonstration of Rickettsia typhi in vascular lesions and by rickettsial isolation in animals or cell culture. In practice, confirmatory laboratory diagnosis is achieved by documenting seroconversion between negative acute-phase serum and a significant titer of antibodies in convalescent-phase serum. Although indirect immunofluorescent assay, latex agglutination, indirect hemagglutination, enzyme immunoassay, and complement fixation tests have been developed, only immunofluorescent antibody and latex agglutination are routinely available. Both methods are acceptably sensitive and specific.

Murine typhus responds well to treatment with doxycycline (100 mg, orally, every 12 hours), tetracycline (25 to 50 mg/kg per day, orally, in four doses), or chloramphenicol (50 to 75 mg/kg body weight per day, orally, in four doses). Body temperature returns to normal on average 3 days after initiation of appropriate antimicrobial therapy.

Rickettsia prowazekii Infection

Classic epidemics of typhus fever do not occur in louse-free populations. Thus, poverty, social disruption, and poor sanitation caused by war, flood, famine, and earthquakes are the usual setting for epidemics of louse-borne typhus. A single case of recrudescent typhus can ignite an epidemic in a louse-infested population. Although occasional cases of recrudescent typhus are diagnosed in the United States, person-to-louse-to-person transmission has not been observed in the United States in recent history. It came as a major surprise when Rickettsia prowazekii was discovered in eastern flying squirrels and their ectoparasites (65). Thirty-five human cases of typhus fever have been recognized to have originated from this enzootic cycle. Humans are not the only reservoir of R. prowazekii.

The human body louse lives in clothing, feeds on blood taken from the skin, and thereby acquires Rickettsia prowazekii from the rickettsemic typhus patient. When the louse leaves an ill or dead patient and feeds upon another person, rickettsiae are shed in the louse's feces and may enter the skin via scratching. It is noteworthy that the rickettsiae are pathogenic for the louse, which is killed by damage to its gastrointestinal epithelium. In humans rickettsiae spread through the bloodstream to skin, brain, heart, kidney, lungs, and other organs (13). Rickettsiae attach to endothelial cells, induce phagocytosis, escape from the phagosome, and divide by binary fission until the cell bulges with organisms and bursts (6). Infection and cellular damage are associated with phospholipase activity. Data from observations in vitro suggest that some portion of the cell injury may be mediated by cytokines such as interferon-γ and by cytotoxic T cells or natural killer cells (66–70). The lipopolysaccharide of R. prowazekii is relatively nontoxic (71).

The earliest pathologic lesion is swelling of infected endothelial cells, followed by infiltration of the vascular wall and perivascular space by lymphocytes and macrophages (13). The lymphohistiocytic vasculitis is present in the skin rash, brain, heart, lung, kidney, and liver.

Epidemic louse-borne typhus frequently affects persons who are undernourished and live in crowded, cold conditions. After a short prodrome of malaise, the patient develops chills, fever, severe headache, myalgias, vomiting, constipation, and insomnia (13). A rash appears 6 or more days later, along with conjunctivitis, rales, and cough. The rash usually appears first on the trunk as discrete, 2- to 6-mm, pink macules, and later on the extremities. After 1 to 2 days the blanchable vasodilatation gives way to focal dermal hemorrhage. Untreated patients may develop hypotension, delirium (48%), coma (6%), seizures (1%), rales (80%), and gangrene (3%) with fatality rates ranging from 7% to as high as 60%, presumably depending upon host factors. Recrudescent typhus is usually milder, possibly because of the anamnestic immune response.

Sylvatic typhus transmitted from flying squirrels causes fever (100%), headache (81%), centrifugal maculopapular rash (66%), myalgia (44%), confusion (44%), coma (28%), cough, and gastrointestinal symptoms (72). The fact that no fatalities have been reported may be attributed in part to antimicrobial treatment and in part to better underlying general health and nutrition.

The diagnosis of Rickettsia prowazekii infection presents the full set of problems faced by clinical rickettsiologists. In locations and situations where louse-borne typhus occurs, the other social, economic, and political problems are so enormous that the clinical diagnosis may be long delayed and laboratory diagnosis never even attempted. In the sporadic cases of flying squirrel–associated typhus in the United States, no physician or microbiologist has succeeded in considering the diagnosis during the acute illness, collecting a blood specimen before antirickettsial drugs are given, and sending it to a laboratory that subsequently isolated R. prowazekii. All diagnoses have been based on retrospective serologic, clinical, and epidemiologic data.

Demonstration of seroconversion with development of antibodies to typhus-group rickettsiae can be accomplished by indirect immunofluorescence assay, indirect hemagglutination, enzyme immunoassay, and complement fixation (73,74). Indirect immunofluorescence assay with Rickettsia typhi antigen is the most widely available of the tests in the United States. Detection of species-specific antibodies for Rickettsia prowazekii is cumbersome but can be achieved by indirect immunofluorescence after absorption with Rickettsia typhi and Rickettsia prowazekii.

Treatment consists of the usual regimen of doxycycline, tetracycline, or chloramphenicol. Under the dire conditions of epidemic typhus fever, treatment of patients with a single oral 200-mg dose of doxycycline has been used successfully.

SCRUB TYPHUS

Rickettsia tsutsugamushi differs so remarkably as an organism from other Rickettsia species (75) that a separate genus designation has been proposed. Within the species R. tsutsugamushi is a great mosaic of antigenic diversity (75,76). Variations in virulence for humans among the numerous strains have not been elucidated. Immunity to homologous strains lasts only a few years; immunity to heterologous strains, only months (77). Reinfection occurs frequently in some areas. Thus, differences in fatality rates from 0 to 35% reported in the preantibiotic era might plausibly be explained by undefined rickettsial virulence factors, immune status, and other host factors (78).

Scrub typhus occurs in Asia, islands of the western and southwestern Pacific Ocean, and northern Australia. Known mainly in Western countries for disease in soldiers during World War II and the Vietnam War, scrub typhus is an important ongoing problem for native populations. In rural Malaysia it is the most frequent diagnosis in febrile hospitalized patients (79). The actual incidence of scrub typhus in southeastern Asia or China could hardly even be guessed.

Rickettsia tsutsugamushi resides within the chigger (Leptotrombidium species), which transmits the bacteria transovarially. Infected ova hatch and the larval chiggers feed upon rodents and other mammals, including humans when they enter the infected areas. Areas of growth of scrub vegetation, such as along rivers or where forest has been cleared for farming and subsequently allowed to revert to forest, harbor the rat populations upon which the chiggers feed (80). These infected foci persist in parcels of land known as mite islands.

Rickettsiae are transmitted by the chigger during feeding upon tissue fluid (81). An eschar often forms at the feeding site. Organisms spread hematogenously and localize in the microcirculation, where they cause damage in the form of the skin rash, interstitial pneumonitis, cerebral glial nodules, and other vascular lesions.

After an incubation period of 6 to 21 days, the patient develops fever, headache, myalgia, cough, and gastrointestinal symptoms. The mite bite develops into a papule and then an eschar during the incubation period, but the eschar is generally absent in native patients and is observed in fewer than half of Westerners. Generalized lymphadenopathy or regional lymphadenopathy in the area that drains the eschar is often present. A rash is observed in approximately half of Westerners who have a primary infection. Discrete, pink to red, 3- to 8-mm macules or maculopapules appear 2 to 9 days after onset of fever. Untreated patients often develop hypotension, rales, meningoencephalitis, and sometimes renal failure and hemorrhage. The average fatality rate for untreated cases is 7%.

The laboratory diagnosis of scrub typhus can be established by recovery of Rickettsia tsutsugamushi in cell culture or by intraperitoneal inoculation of mice with the patient's blood. In practice, diagnosis by serologic demonstration of antibodies is more common. In primary infections the indirect immunofluorescence test demonstrates IgM antibody to R. tsutsugamushi on day 8 of illness and IgG antibody about day 12 (82). After reinfection, anamnestic IgG antibodies to scrub typhus rickettsiae are detected by day 6. These antibodies disappear within a year, the titer decreasing from greater than 50 to less than 50 in 61% of previously infected persons (83). In an endemic area, an indirect immunofluorescence titer of at least 400 is 96% specific and 48% sensitive, and a fourfold increase in titer to at least 200 is 98% specific and 54% sensitive (84). Newer methods include enzyme immunoassays.

The historic serologic test for scrub typhus is agglutination of Proteus mirabilis OX-K strain. The probability of a correct diagnosis of scrub typhus is 79% with a single titer of at least 320 (84). The sensitivity was rather low; however, a fourfold rise to a titer of at least 320 has 96% specificity but only 39% sensitivity. This test should not be used today to make the diagnosis of a rickettsial infection.

Scrub typhus is treated with the usual regimens of doxycycline, tetracycline, or chloramphenicol. For empiric treatment of an illness whose differential diagnosis includes scrub typhus, typhoid fever, and meningococcemia, chloramphenicol (2 g/day in four doses) is often chosen. Scrub typhus is the only human rickettsiosis for which an effective prophylactic regimen is established: 200 mg chloramphenicol, weekly during exposure and for 6 weeks thereafter (85).

EHRLICHIOSES

Ehrlichiae are obligate intracellular bacteria that grow within cytoplasmic phagosomes of macrophages, polymorphonuclear leukocytes, and lymphocytes (Fig. 26–2) (86). Ehrlichiae are known primarily as etiologic agents of veterinary diseases such as canine ehrlichiosis (Ehrlichia canis), canine granulocytic ehrlichiosis (Ehrlichia ewingii), infectious cyclic thrombocytopenia (Ehrlichia platys), equine monocytic ehrlichiosis (Ehrlichia risticii), equine ehrlichiosis (Ehrlichia equi), and tick-borne fever (Ehrlichia phagocytophilia). The first ehrlichial disease to be recognized, canine ehrlichiosis, was described in Algeria in 1935. Rhipicephalus sanguineus ticks transmit the agent to dogs, which develop a febrile illness with circulating monocytes containing clusters of small organisms demonstrable by Giemsa stain. German shepherd dogs are particularly susceptible to severe illness, and it occurred among military dogs during the Vietnam War.

Human Ehrlichiosis

The first case of human ehrlichiosis was diagnosed in 1986 as a severe febrile disease with hypotension, confusion, pancytopenia, coagulopathy, cutaneous and gastrointestinal hemorrhages, hepatocellular damage, and acute renal failure requiring hemodialysis (87). The diagnosis was made by observation of 2- to 5-μm morulae (cytoplasmic vacuoles containing mulberry-like clusters of organisms) in 1 or 2% of circulating white blood cells including lymphocytes, atypical lymphocytes, monocytes, polymorphonuclear leukocytes, and bands. Ultrastructurally the morula inclusions were membrane-bound vacuoles containing gram-negative bacteria 0.2 to 0.8 μm in diameter. The patient's serum contained a high titer of antibodies reactive with Ehrlichia canis.

A novel Ehrlichia species has been isolated from a patient at Fort Chaffee, Arkansas, who had human ehrlichiosis, and DNA sequences generated by polymerase chain reaction with primers corresponding to a portion of the gene for the 16S ribosomal RNA have been compared with sequences from known species of Ehrlichia (88,89). The new agent, Ehrlichia chaffeensis, is distinct from all the other ehrlichiae, having close sequence similarities with Ehrlichia canis and Ehrlichia ewingii, but only more distantly related to Ehrlichia risticii, Ehrlichia sennetsu and Ehrlichia equi. Nucleotide sequences corresponding to those of the novel isolate have also been generated by PCR from nucleic acids in the blood of other patients with human ehrlichiosis.

Epidemiology

Human ehrlichiosis apparently is a tick-borne zoonosis (90). The vast majority of patients with ehrlichiosis report exposure to ticks. There is a strong seasonality to the disease: 76% of cases occur between May and July. A large proportion of patients were exposed to rural areas. Most cases have been reported from the west south central, southeastern, and mid-Atlantic states; the highest incidences are in Oklahoma, Arkansas, Missouri, Virginia, and Tennessee. The Lone Star tick, Amblyomma americanum, and Dermacentor variabilis are the favorite candidate vectors because their geographic distribution is very similar to that of the reported cases, and the season of activity of the adults and nymphs of this species conforms to the seasonal onset of illness in most patients. The median age of patients is older than for RMSF, 42 years in one study, and there is strong male predominance.

Clues to the mechanisms of maintenance in nature and transmission of ehrlichiae are provided by Ehrlichia canis, for which Rhipicephalus sanguineus ticks are the vector (91). Larvae and nymphs of these ticks acquire ehrlichiae while feeding on infected dogs. Although ehrlichiae are transmitted from stage to stage as the tick molts, transovarian transmission does not occur. Ehrlichiae are present in the tick salivary glands and are transmitted to canine hosts during the blood meal by infected nymphal and adult ticks. The reservoir and vector of human ehrlichiosis remain to be determined.

Pathogenesis

The presumed pathogenic sequence of human ehrlichiosis is tick bite inoculation into the skin and lymphohematogenous spread of the bacteria to the lymph nodes, liver, spleen, lungs, brain, and bone marrow. Ehrlichia organisms apparently enter macrophages, lymphocytes, and polymorphonuclear leukocytes by phagocytosis and divide by binary fission in the phagosomal vacuole. The related species, Ehrlichia risticii, has the ability to inhibit phagosome-lysosome fusion (92). After extensive successful growth in vitro, ehrlichiae destroy the host cell by unknown mechanisms. The pathologic lesions in fatal human ehrlichiosis include perivascular mononuclear infiltrates in the kidneys, heart, and central nervous system, hepatocellular necrosis, pulmonary injury, and erythrophagocytosis in the liver and bone marrow (93). Ehrlichiae have been demonstrated in the spleen, liver, lymph nodes, lung, bone marrow, kidney, and epicardium (94). Bone marrow examination during the acute and convalescent phases of human ehrlichiosis has shown a bewildering variety of findings, including normal cellularity with normal maturation of all cell lines, erythroid or myeloid hypoplasia, erythroid or myeloid hyperplasia, and noncaseating granulomas. Leukopenia and thrombocytopenia occur during the first week of illness and seem more likely to be caused by peripheral sequestration and destruction than by pathologic events in the bone marrow.

Clinical Manifestations

After an average incubation period of 7 days, the typical ehrlichiosis patient develops fever, chills, headache, and malaise, often accompanied by myalgia, anorexia, nausea, vomiting, diarrhea, or cough (95). Later in the course patients are more likely to have a rash, pharyngitis, confusion, weight loss, lymphadenopathy, dyspnea, anemia, and abdominal pain. A rash is observed routinely in children, but in only 35% of adults. The median onset of rash is day 8 of illness, and it has been described as either maculopapular or petechial. Lymphadenopathy is unilateral. Nearly half of patients with chest radiographs have pulmonary infiltrates.

Severely ill patients often have respiratory failure requiring intubation and mechanical ventilation, acute renal failure, and CNS abnormalities including encephalopathy, coma, and CSF pleocytosis (90). Fatalities have been reported, including 5% of the cases that occurred in 1988. A mild form of the infection was recorded among Army reservists exposed to ticks in New Jersey (96). Among nine serologically diagnosed subjects, none was hospitalized, only a third missed work, and two remained asymptomatic although untreated. A woman treated prophylactically with tetracycline after a tick bite remained asymptomatic and exhibited seroconversion with production of antibodies reactive with Ehrlichia canis (97).

Laboratory Diagnosis

The laboratory diagnosis of human ehrlichiosis has been accomplished by a variety of methods, including visualization of morulae in peripheral blood leukocytes by Giemsa stain and electron microscopy, immunohistologic visualization of ehrlichial antigen in morulae in human tissues, cultivation of the pathogen in cell culture, detection of specific nucleotide sequences that had been amplified by PCR from peripheral blood, and demonstration of antibodies cross-reactive with Ehrlichia canis. Only the last method has been employed in a substantial number of cases with an acceptable level of sensitivity of the results. The major diagnostic criterion for human ehrlichiosis is based on indirect immunofluorescence assay utilizing E. canis–infected cells as the antigen, and it requires a fourfold or greater rise or fall in antibody titer with a minimum peak titer of 80 (98). Among 85 patients who tested positive by this assay at the CDC, only 22% were positive during the first week of illness. The majority seroconverted in the second week, and all by 4 weeks after onset. The peak geometric mean titer of 1280 occurred 6 weeks after onset and decreased to less than 80 by 17 to 31 weeks. Problems with this test include false-positive results in 5% of patients and unexplained concurrent presence of a significant titer of antibodies to Rickettsia rickettsii, Rickettsia typhi, or Coxiella burnetii in 36.5% of these patients. A greater proportion of patients make antibodies to the human isolate than to Ehrlichia canis. In the setting of a new infectious disease such as this, rapidly developing improvements in laboratory diagnosis can be expected.

Treatment

Human ehrlichiosis responds to treatment with tetracycline with defervescence after about 2 days. Although one human subject and an experimental study in canines (99) showed successful prophylaxis with tetracycline, prophylactic antimicrobial treatment has not been recommended for any population exposed to ticks.

Sennetsu Ehrlichiosis

The first organisms of the genus Ehrlichia isolated from a human were recovered in 1953 from the blood, bone marrow, and lymph node of a patient in Japan with an infectious mononucleosis–like syndrome including fever, severe headache, myalgia, lymphadenopathy, and a large quantity of circulating atypical lymphocytes (100). Human volunteers inoculated with the isolate developed a similar illness.

After an average incubation period of 2 weeks, there is sudden onset of chills, fever, headache, and myalgia (101). Enlargement of the postauricular and posterior cervical lymph nodes appears 5 to 7 days later. Hepatosplenomegaly and elevated serum transaminase values occur frequently, aseptic meningitis occasionally, and rash rarely. Leukopenia early in the course is followed by absolute lymphocytosis with more than 10% atypical lymphocytes. Specific laboratory diagnosis is made by isolation of ehrlichiae in mice or by demonstration of antibodies to Ehrlichia sennetsu by indirect immunofluorescence or complement fixation. Treatment with one of the tetracyclines produces defervescence after 1 to 2 days.

Q FEVER

Q fever was described in 1937 by Derrick in Australia as an occupational disease of abattoir workers and dairy farmers. The designation Q referred to *query*, because of the unknown cause of the disease. The pathogen, Coxiella burnetii, differs remarkably from other bacteria categorized as rickettsiae in its resistance to chemicals and desiccation, possession of a plasmid, morphologic variation suggesting a hypothetical life cycle, and stimulation of metabolic activity by acid pH of the phagolysosome where they reside (Fig. 26–4). A laboratory peculiarity of C. burnetii has obsessed rickettsiologists for decades and is important for understanding its diagnostic serology. Essentially as a phenomenon confined to the laboratory manipulation of C. burnetii, repeated cultivation of the bacteria in embryonated eggs or cell culture results in so-called phase variation (102). Phase I is the complete pathogenic organism as it occurs in nature and in human infections. Phase II is the laboratory-derived, avirulent form with truncated lipopolysaccharide in the cell wall, analogous to the conversion from smooth to rough phenotype by the Enterobacteriaceae. The Coxiella literature burgeons

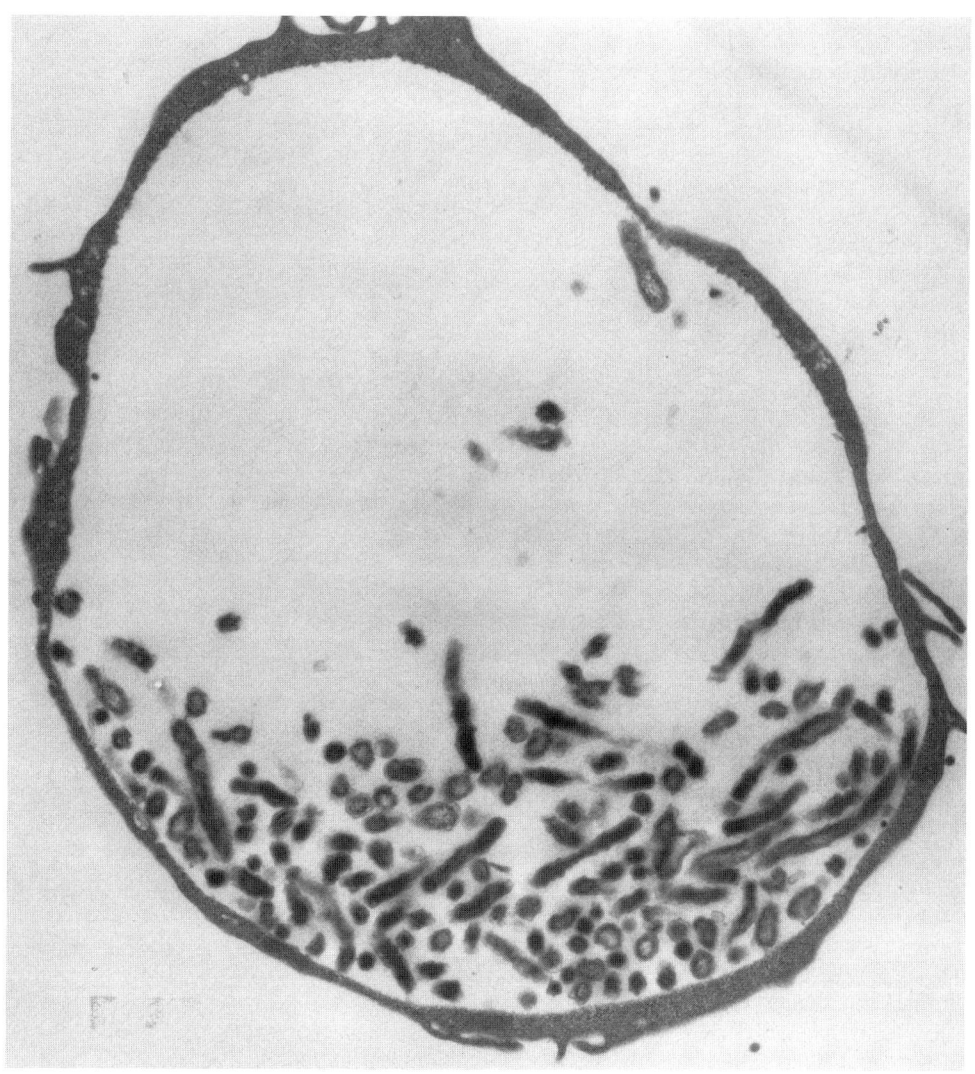

Fig. 26–4. Electron micrograph of a cell with a large phagolysosome containing a variety of morphologic forms of Coxiella burnetii (×19,250).

with arcane treatises on these phases, yet there are only two related facts of any importance: a vaccine composed of phase II organisms does not confer protection, and serologic responses to phase I and II distinguish acute and chronic Q fever.

Epidemiology

Coxiella burnetii has a worldwide distribution and is found in 40 species of ticks, domestic livestock, and many wild mammals and birds. Q fever occurs principally in humans exposed to aerosols of infected placenta and birth fluids of infected cattle, sheep, goats, camels, and other ungulates. Thus, cases are associated with farms, abattoirs, research laboratories that use sheep, and exposure to contaminated wool. Humans exposed to parturient infected cats and to wild rabbits also acquire the infection. Organisms are shed in milk, urine, and feces of infected animals. Ingestion of C. burnetii in raw milk is suspected to be a mode of infection. These bacteria have the ability to persist in the environment long after being shed from the animal reservoir.

Serosurveys support the concept that the infection is widespread. Large outbreaks demonstrate the wide spectrum of disease: 54% were asymptomatic and only 3.4% were hospitalized in a Swiss epidemic (103). A longitudinal, community-based study in Nova Scotia demonstrated a 2% annual rate of seroconversion; all appeared to lack symptoms of Q fever (104). The most serious form of Q fever, chronic endocarditis, has been diagnosed nearly everywhere acute Q fever has been seen. Hepatomegaly and splenomegaly vary in geographic incidence, affecting 11% and 4%, respectively, in California and 51% and 30%, respectively, in Australia. The pathogenic or microbial explanation for these differences in virulence and for the geographic variations in clinical manifestations has not been determined.

Pathogenesis

Q fever has both acute and chronic forms. The etiologic organism, Coxiella burnetii, has intrinsic differences in its lipopolysaccharides and plasmid genetic composition which correlate with the clinical form of the human disease (102,105,106). A single organism of one acute Q fever strain is capable of causing febrile disease in guinea pigs, while a million organisms of an equally infectious chronic endocarditis strain are required to stimulate a febrile response. The purified lipopolysaccharides of C. burnetii contain relatively little toxic lipid A and are nonendotoxic. It could be hypothesized that the pathogenic mechanisms of Q fever are host mediated and that the acute Q fever strains are more active in stimulating T lymphocytes to secrete lymphokines such as IL-2 and macrophages to secrete cytokines such as IL-1, IL-6, and TNF-α. These factors mediate the febrile acute-phase response and stimulate the formation of immune granulomas, which destroy the bacteria. In contrast, patients with chronic endocarditis have a remarkable lack of lymphocyte stimulation by antigens of Coxiella. Athymic nude mice develop massive infection without overt illness (107). The interaction of C. burnetii and host cells in culture is minimally cytopathic.

Experimental human infection by aerosol results in rickettsemia beginning late in the incubation period that is dose dependent and varies from 9 to 18 days (108). Granulomatous hepatic lesions also appear during the incubation period and even 36 days later remain, a sign of the successful immune struggle with Coxiella burnetii. The target cells in experimentally infected animals are macrophages.

In human Q fever granulomas have been observed in spleen, bone marrow, and liver where the characteristic, but not pathognomonic, form is that of a doughnut with a central lipid vacuole surrounded by a fibrin ring and epithelioid macrophages (109). Not all Q fever granulomas manifest this appearance, and other agents can stimulate doughnut granulomas. A pulmonary portal of entry causes a mixed interstitial-alveolar-bronchiolar pneumonia with a predominance of mononuclear inflammatory cells (Fig. 26–5).

Chronic Q fever endocarditis usually affects native mitral and aortic valves that were previously abnormal because of rheumatic, atherosclerotic, or congenital disease or prosthetic valves. In contrast with the lesions of acute Q fever, in which organisms are difficult to detect, there are numerous foamy macrophages filled with Coxiella

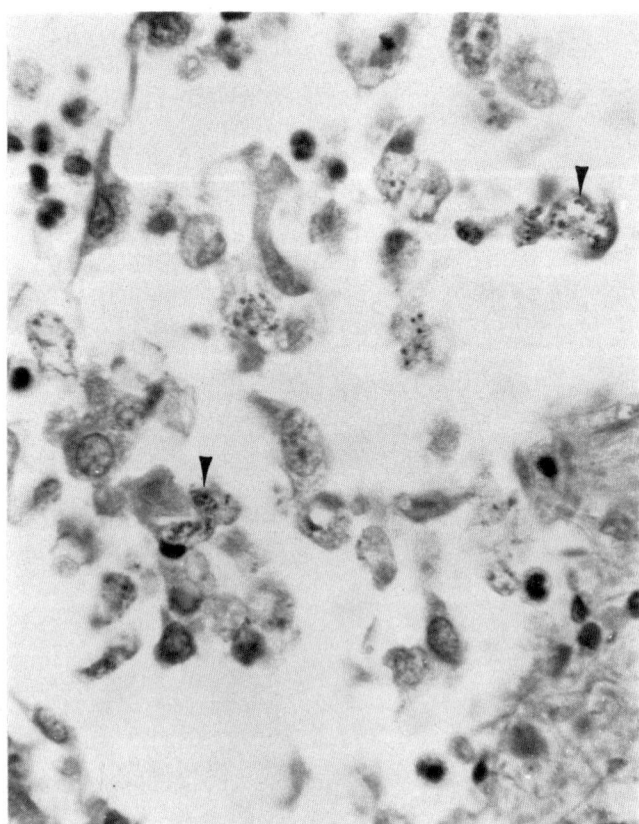

Fig. 26–5. Photomicrograph of lung from a patient with Q fever demonstrates numerous macrophages in the alveolar space. Coxiella burnetii in cytoplasmic vacuoles (*arrows*) in these macrophages are stained by immunoperoxidase.

burnetii in the valvular vegetations. Circulating immune complexes are usually detectable and may cause glomerulonephritis and vasculitis with a purpuric rash.

Clinical Manifestations

Acute Q fever is usually a self-limited illness marked by abrupt onset of chills, fever, and headache that is more pronounced than in other lower respiratory tract infections (110). Without effective treatment fever lasts 13 days or less in 67% of patients. Cough affects as many as 70 to 90% of patients, but the prevalence is usually 25 to 30%. It is the dry, nonproductive cough of atypical pneumonia. The characteristic chest radiograph shows multiple, rounded, segmental consolidations. Pneumonia occurs more frequently in the United States than in Australia. Nausea, vomiting, and diarrhea occur often, but with no greater frequency than in pneumonia of other causes. Rash and meningoencephalitis are reported rarely.

Chronic Q fever is virtually synonymous with chronic Coxiella endocarditis affecting previously damaged valves or valvular or vascular prostheses (111). Some patients may have concurrent chronic, nonspecific, reactive hepatitis. Rarely, chronic Q fever manifests as chronic osteomyelitis. Chronic Coxiella burnetii infection is afebrile in 33% of cases. Frequent symptoms are weakness, malaise, weight loss, anorexia, and night sweats. Most patients develop cardiac failure, often requiring valve replacement. Echocardiography frequently does not demonstrate vegetations. An illustration of the often remarkably long clinical course is the presence of digital clubbing in 37% of cases. Patients may have a purpuric rash or peripheral emboli. Clinical laboratory abnormalities often include microscopic hematuria, anemia that may be hemolytic, thrombocytopenia, and hypergammaglobulinemia.

Q fever occurs as an opportunistic infection in compromised hosts (e.g., with malignancy, corticosteroid therapy, acquired immunodeficiency syndrome, and ethanol abuse). The potential for reactivation of latent Coxiella burnetii infection has been demonstrated in guinea pigs after corticosteroid or cytotoxic drug treatment, irradiation, or pregnancy.

Laboratory Diagnosis

The diagnosis of acute Q fever is seldom considered by most physicians. Thus, despite the high prevalence of Coxiella burnetii infection indicated by the presence of antibodies in some populations, the diagnosis of acute Q fever is seldom established except in the setting of an epidemiologically investigated common-source outbreak. Q fever hepatitis is evaluated and diagnosed usually in the patients with classic doughnut granulomas in hepatic biopsy specimens, and chronic Q fever endocarditis is considered in patients with culture-negative endocarditis.

Specific laboratory diagnosis is achieved most often by serologic methods, although cultivation of the organisms or visualization of them in infected tissues can also establish the diagnosis (112). The two serologic methods currently most used are complement fixation (CF) and indirect fluorescent antibody (IFA) assay. In acute Q fever, IgM IFA is diagnostic in 53% of cases in the first week and in 89% in the second week. The CF test is less sensitive; diagnostic titers begin to appear in the second week. Because antibodies to Coxiella burnetii phase II antigen appear earlier than antibodies to phase I antigen, the ratio of anti–phase II titer to anti–phase I titer is greater than 1 in acute Q fever. In contrast, in chronic Q fever, the antibody titers are higher and the ratio of anti–phase II titer to anti–phase I titer is no greater than 1. Chronic Q fever can be diagnosed with a single serum antibody titer to Coxiella burnetii phase I of at least 400 by IFA or at least 200 by CF. IgA antibodies to phase I antigen at titers of 50 or greater by IFA are also considered diagnostic of chronic Q fever.

Few laboratories undertake the cultivation of Coxiella burnetii, in part because of the biohazard of this highly infectious organism. As small an inoculum as one organism is capable of initiating infection. Although traditionally C. burnetii has been recovered by intraperitoneal inoculation of guinea pigs, mice, or hamsters, recently shell vial centrifugation-enhanced cell culture has been demonstrated to be an efficient means of recovering the pathogens from cardiac valves, and even peripheral blood (113). Among inoculated guinea pigs monitored by rectal temperatures for fever, one is sacrificed on day 10 for similar passage of harvested spleen. Serum collected from other guinea pigs or mice on day 21 after inoculation is evaluated for seroconversion, sufficient documentation of the diagnosis.

The shell vial centrifugation method for isolation of Coxiella burnetii could be utilized in laboratories with P-3 level biohazard containment facilities for cell culture. This approach is also considerably less cumbersome than animal inoculation. Replicate inoculated shell vials are monitored by immunofluorescence for the presence of proliferating C. burnetii. Cultivated organisms are usually detected and identified within 7 days (113).

Treatment

Because acute Q fever is seldom diagnosed, only 33% of patients receive optimal antimicrobial treatment. Either tetracycline or doxycycline reduces the duration of fever in acute Q fever; however, without a specific diagnosis it is considered wise to treat atypical pneumonia in which the differential diagnosis includes mycoplasma pneumonia, Legionnaires' disease, and Q fever with a combination of erythromycin and rifampin (110). Combinations of antimicrobial agents that are effective against chronic Q fever such as doxycycline-rifampin or tetracycline-trimethoprim-sulfamethoxazole are also very likely to be effective in acute infection.

Treatment of chronic Q fever is a matter of prolonged suppression of the infection without elimination of the organisms from the host (111). The combination of doxycycline or tetracycline with rifampin is preferred currently. Fluoroquinoline antimicrobials such as ciprofloxacin or ofloxacin are also useful for treatment of Q fever endocarditis. Organisms have been recovered from valves removed after various regimens of prolonged therapy, indicating this infection's proclivity to relapse. Recommendations include following antibody titers for the disappearance of IgA antibodies and reduction of IgG anti–phase I antibodies to less than 400 and treating the patient for at least 2 years, possibly for life. Valve replacement is frequently required for hemodynamic reasons, and the prosthetic valve is also subject to becoming infected.

ROCHALIMAEA INFECTIONS

Rochalimaea has been largely ignored since the end of World War I, when it was a major cause of infection among troops. This genus emphasizes the artificial nature of the classic definition of rickettsiae. Rochalimaea quintana, after years of study by rickettsiologists as a louse-borne agent, was finally propagated axenically, extracellularly, on blood agar (114). Suddenly, it was no longer an obligate intracellular bacterium and, by definition, not a rickettsia.

Recently Rochalimaea has entered the medical consciousness again when a new species, Rochalimaea henselae, was identified as the agent of bacillary angiomatosis and bacillary peliosis of the liver and spleen (115). This condition has been recognized to be a medically interesting and important infectious disease as a result of the epidemic of the acquired immune deficiency syndrome (AIDS).

Trench Fever

Rochalimaea quintana, despite its extracellular nature, is related to organisms in the genus Rickettsia. It shares 30% similarity to Rickettsia prowazekii as determined by DNA-DNA hybridization. Strangely, its 16S ribosomal RNA sequence is not as closely related to R. prowazekii as Ehrlichia risticii is.

The pathogens are excreted in the feces of infected lice and apparently enter the skin through excoriation (116). After an incubation period of approximately 8 days, an illness of host-determined severity occurs. The symptoms range from mild and afebrile to moderately severe with a long course and numerous relapses. The acute illness is usually characterized by fever, headache, myalgias, pretibial pain, and an evanescent macular rash. The duration of fever is generally less than 1 week; however, relapses often occur at 4- to 5-day intervals. Rochalimaea quintana organisms are present in the blood for weeks, months, and in some documented cases for more than a year, even in the presence of specific antibodies.

This organism was responsible for a large number of infections among troops engaged in trench warfare during World War I. Subsequently, Rochalimaea quintana was isolated on blood agar from patients in Mexico, and Koch's postulates were fulfilled in human volunteer studies (114). Growth of organisms on blood agar is often detected only after cultivation for weeks.

Rochalimaea henselae

Rochalimaea henselae recently has been identified as a cause of persistent fever and bacteremia, bacillary angiomatosis, and bacillary peliosis hepatis (117–126). Bacillary angiomatosis (also called epithelioid angiomatosis) is a distinct vascular proliferative disease that involves the skin, lymph nodes, and viscera of persons who are seropositive for human immunodeficiency virus (HIV), other immunocompromised persons, and rarely, immunocompetent hosts. A few cases of bacillary angiomatosis have been associated with a cat scratch; therefore, the entity may be difficult to distinguish from cat scratch disease (see Chapter 41) (120,121).

Pathology

Regardless of location, lesions of bacillary angiomatosis have in common a lobular pattern of vascular proliferation, and in most cases small capillaries are arranged in clusters around ectatic ones. Vascular lobules are composed of rounded vessels lined by protuberant endothelial cells and, typically, are separated by an edematous, mucinous, or fibrotic stroma. In all cases clusters of neutrophils, neutrophil debris, and granular material are found adjacent to the capillaries (Fig. 26–6). The granular material has been shown by staining with the Warthin-Starry stain and electron microscopic examination to be bacteria resembling those observed in cat scratch disease. These pleomorphic bacteria, 0.2 to 0.5 μm by 1 to 3 μm, have trilaminar walls and grow in clumps (Fig. 26–7). Occasionally, small areas of necrosis containing neutrophils and foamy macrophages also are present. The histologic

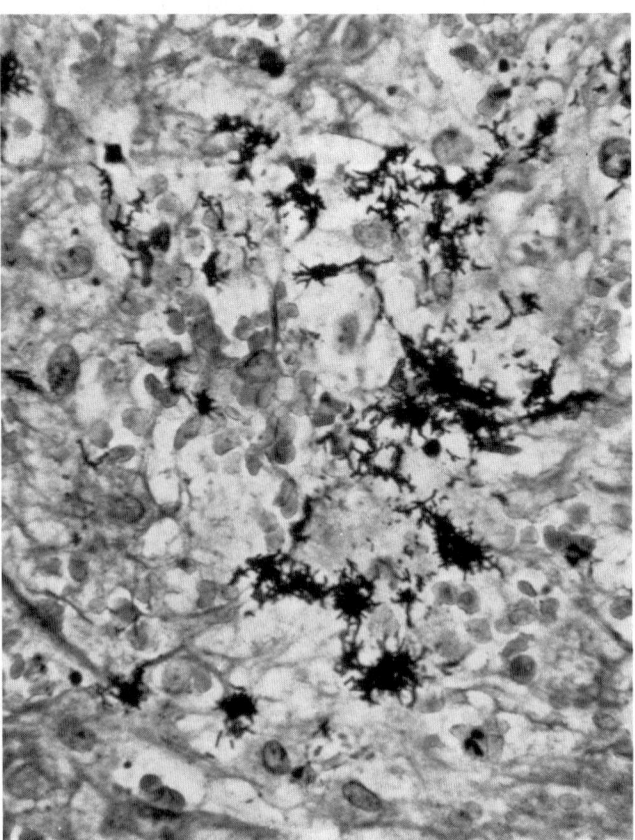

Fig. 26–6. Photomicrograph of a cutaneous vascular lesion of bacillary angiomatosis contains numerous bacteria stained by the Warthin-Starry silver impregnation method.

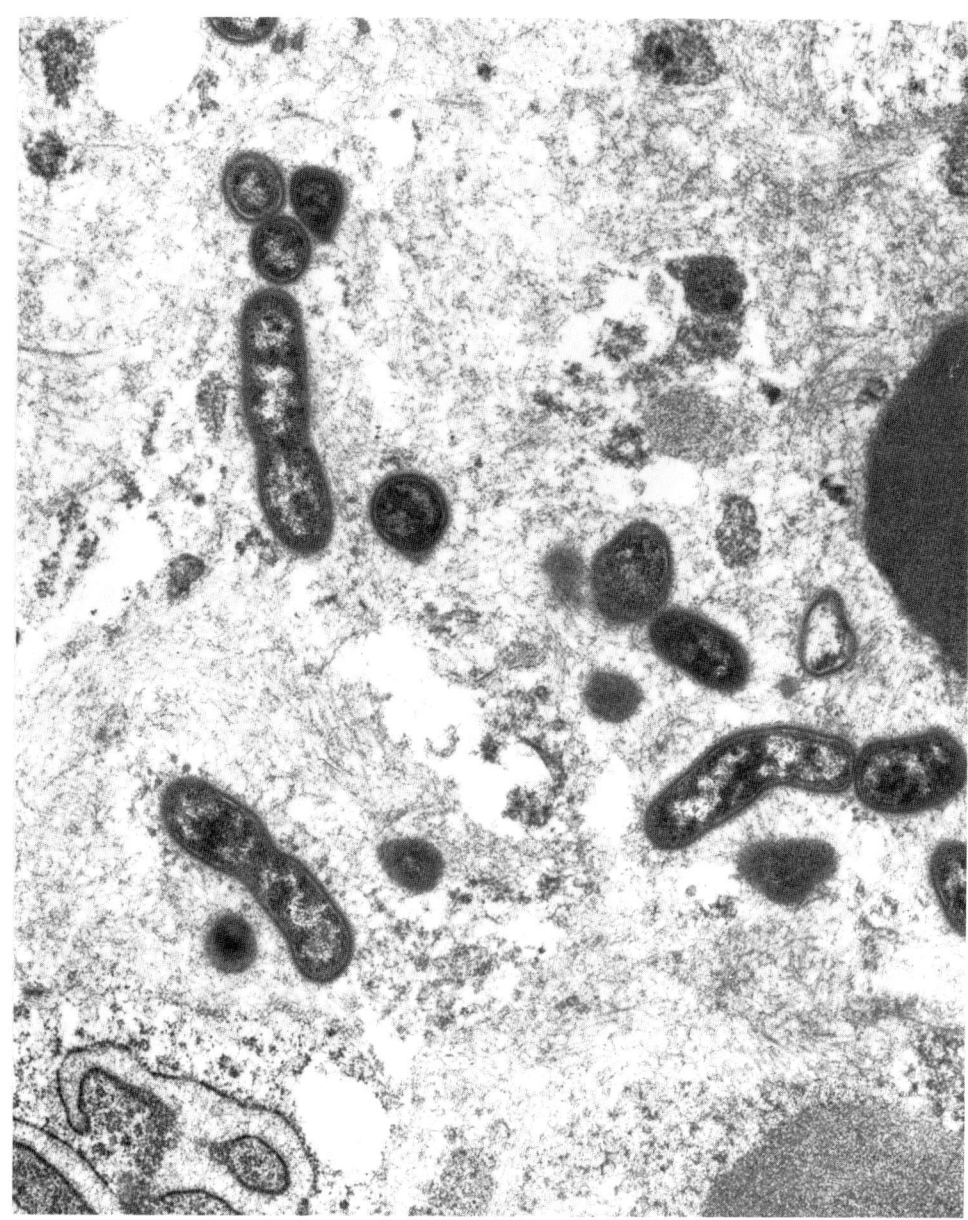

Fig. 26–7. Electron micrograph of typical extracellular bacteria in a lesion of bacillary angiomatosis (×27,500).

features resemble those of bacillary peliosis hepatis in HIV-seropositive persons (123).

Laboratory Diagnosis

Diagnosis of bacteremia caused by Rochalimaea henselae requires collection of blood. To date, the organism has been recovered only from blood specimens processed by lysis-centrifugation (see Chapter 58). Optimal growth occurs on enriched media supplemented with blood (sheep blood or chocolate agar) and on charcoal-yeast extract agar. Initial colonies, typically cauliflower-like and embedded in the agar, are visible after 9 to 15 days' incubation at 35° C in a humidified atmosphere of 5% carbon dioxide or at 30° C in air. Subsequent passages result in more rapid growth and a change in colony structure: smooth, shiny colonies that are not embedded in agar appear in 4 to 5 days.

Cells of Rochalimaea henselae are slightly curved gram-negative bacilli about 1 to 2 μm long and 0.5 to 0.6 μm wide that stain readily with the Gimenez stain. They are oxidase- and catalase-negative (or weakly catalase positive), do not utilize carbohydrates, and are urease negative. Definitive identification requires analysis of cellular fatty acid composition and nucleic acid hybridization, techniques usually unavailable in the clinical laboratory. Suspect isolates, therefore, should be sent to a reference laboratory for identification.

Bacillary angiomatosis and bacillary peliosis hepatis are diagnosed by histologic examination of involved tissue. Bacillary angiomatosis must be differentiated from other entities that may have a similar histologic appearance, such as pyogenic granuloma, histiocytoid hemangioma, verruga peruana (described later), angiosarcoma, and Kaposi's sarcoma (see reference 117 for a discussion of distinguishing features).

Treatment

Isolates of Rochalimaea henselae are susceptible in vitro to many antimicrobial agents, including cephalothin, aztreonam, trimethoprim-sulfamethoxazole, chloramphenicol, erythromycin, aminoglycosides, quinolones, and rifampin, and are resistant to nalidixic acid. Bacillary angiomatosis responds clinically to erythromycin and tetracycline and may be fatal if not treated.

BARTONELLA

Bartonella bacilliformis is the only species in the genus Bartonella, which is classified in the order Rickettsiales and in the family Bartonellaceae. It is a small, aerobic, slightly curved pleomorphic bacillus that causes bartonellosis or Carrion's disease, a biphasic illness limited to the remote mountainous regions at elevations between 2000 and 8000 feet in Colombia, Ecuador, Peru, Chile, Bolivia, and probably Guatemala (127). The cutaneous manifestations of bartonellosis (called verruga peruana) have been recognized since pre-Incan times in Peru, and the acute form (termed Oroya fever) was described in 1870, when an epidemic of fever and anemia developed among workmen building a railway between Lima and Oroya. Daniel Carrion, a medical student in Peru, established the common bacterial cause of the two forms of the disease in 1885, when he inoculated himself with blood from a skin lesion of an individual with verruga peruana and developed Oroya fever. The pathogen was described by Barton in 1909.

Epidemiology

Bartonellosis is transmitted by the bite of the Phlebotomus sand fly, which determines the geographic occurrence of the disease (discussed earlier). Asymptomatic persons and longterm carriers are the reservoirs of the infection.

Pathogenesis

Bartonella bacilliformis enters the blood during the bite of an infected sandfly. The bacteria then adhere to erythrocytes, inducing the formation of a vacuole in which they enter the erythrocyte and replicate without being released into the cytoplasm (128). The internal cytoskeleton of the erythrocyte is altered by the bacteria, causing deformation of the red cell and increasing its fragility. Infected erythrocytes are phagocytosed and destroyed by cells of the monocyte/macrophage system, and the erythropoietic response of the bone marrow is decreased, both of which contribute to the rapid development of anemia.

As the infection resolves, an event that appears to coincide with the development of immunity, erythropoiesis is enhanced and bacteria disappear from the blood or decline to a very low level. The chronic benign form of the disease becomes manifest after a variable latent period. Verruga peruana is characterized by cutaneous and subcutaneous hemangiomatous nodules consisting of many newly formed vessels with proliferating endothelial cells and occasionally containing the bacteria.

Clinical Manifestations

After an incubation period of about 3 weeks Oroya fever begins insidiously, with anorexia, headache, malaise, and low-grade fever, or acutely, with high fever, chills, headache, and change in mentation (129). Severe muscle and joint pain, dyspnea, chest pain, and insomnia may develop. If the patient survives, the convalescent phase follows. The organisms disappear from the blood, and the fever resolves. However, intercurrent infections (salmonellosis, amebiasis, malaria, tuberculosis, various enteric infections) are most common at this stage and account for up to 50% of deaths (127,130).

Verruga peruana may follow Oroya fever or occur without prior symptoms, especially in persons who had previous episodes of bartonellosis. Red to purple, nontender nodules that may resemble Kaposi's sarcoma develop in crops over 1 to 2 months, most frequently on the exposed parts of the body but occasionally involving mucous membranes or internal organs, and they may persist months to years (131,132). Lesions, reaching 1 to 2 cm in diameter, may be sessile, miliary, nodular, pedunculated, confluent, or, if they become secondarily infected pustular or ulcerated. Joint pains and low-grade fever are present initially but decrease after the cutaneous lesions appear.

Laboratory Diagnosis

During the acute illness, organisms are easily visualized in smears of peripheral blood stained with the Giemsa stain, appearing as cocci or bacilli with occasional curved or ring forms, and Bartonella bacilliformis may be cultured from blood. Verruga peruana is diagnosed by culturing the organism from cutaneous lesions, and occasionally from blood and bone marrow. Optimal growth occurs on brain-heart infusion agar, modified to contain 0.4% agar and 5% human, rabbit, or horse blood, and incubated at room temperature in ambient air.

Treatment

Acute bartonellosis responds to therapy with chloramphenicol, penicillin, and possibly tetracycline and streptomycin. Blood transfusion may be necessary in cases of severe anemia. Cutaneous lesions exhibit varying responses to antimicrobial therapy and may require surgical excision.

REFERENCES

1. Weiss E, and Moulder JW: The rickettsias and chlamydias. *In* Bergey's Manual of Systematic Bacteriology. Vol. 1. Edited by NR Kreig and JG Holt. Baltimore, Williams & Wilkins, 1984.
2. Walker DH: Rocky Mountain spotted fever: A disease in need of microbiologic concern. Clin Microbiol Rev, 2:227, 1989.
3. Fan MY, Walker DH, Yu SR, and Liu QH: Epidemiology and ecology of rickettsial diseases in the People's Republic of China. Rev Infect Dis, 9:823, 1987.
4. Zinsser H (ed): Rats, Lice, and History. New York, Little, Brown, 1935.
5. Helmick CG, Bernard KW, and D'Angelo LJ: Rocky Moun-

tain spotted fever: Clinical, laboratory and epidemiological features of 262 cases. J Infect Dis, 150:480, 1984.
6. Winkler HH: Rickettsia species (as organisms). Ann Rev Microbiol, 44:131, 1990.
7. Walker DH: The rickettsia-host interaction. In Intracellular Parasitism. Edited by JW Moulder. Boca Raton, CRC Press, 1989.
8. Weisburg WG: Polyphyletic origin of bacterial parasites. In Intracellular Parasitism. Edited by JW Moulder. Boca Raton, CRC Press, 1989.
9. Silverman D, and Wisseman CL, Jr: Comparative ultrastructural study on the cell envelopes of Rickettsia prowazekii, Rickettsia rickettsii, and Rickettsia tsutsugamushi. Infect Immun, 21:1020, 1978.
10. Amano K, Tamura A, Ohashi N, et al: Deficiency of peptidoglycan and lipopolysaccharide components in Rickettsia tsutsugamushi. Infect Immun, 55:2290, 1987.
11. Wolbach SB: Studies on Rocky Mountain spotted fever. J Med Res, 41:2, 1919.
12. Wolbach SB, Todd JL, and Palfrey FW: Clinical observations; Pathology of typhus in man. In The Etiology and Pathology of Typhus. Edited by The League of Red Cross Societies. Cambridge, Harvard University Press, 1922.
13. Harden VA: Rocky Mountain Spotted Fever. History of a Twentieth-Century Disease. Baltimore, The Johns Hopkins University Press, 1990.
14. Silverman DJ, Wisseman CL, Waddell AD, et al: External layers of Rickettsia prowazekii: Occurrence of a slime layer. Infect Immun, 22:233, 1978.
15. McCaul TF, and Williams JC: Developmental cycle of Coxiella burnetii: Structure and morphogenesis of vegetative and sporogenic differentiations. J Bacteriol, 147:1063, 1981.
16. Burgdorfer W: Ecological and epidemiological considerations of Rocky Mountain spotted fever and scrub typhus. In Biology of Rickettsial Diseases. Edited by DH Walker. Boca Raton, CRC Press, 1988.
17. Li H, Lenz B, and Walker DH: Protective monoclonal antibodies recognize heat-labile epitopes on surface proteins of spotted fever group rickettsiae. Infect Immun, 56:2587, 1988.
18. McDade JE, and Newhouse VF: Natural history of Rickettsia rickettsii. Ann Rev Microbiol, 40:287, 1986.
19. Burgdorfer W, Hayes SF, and Mavros AJ: Nonpathogenic rickettsia in Dermacentor andersoni: A limiting factor for the distribution of Rickettsia rickettsii. In Rickettsiae and Rickettsial Disease. Edited by W Burgdorfer and RL Anacker. New York, Academic Press, 1981.
20. Hattwick MAW, O'Brien RJ, and Hanson BF: Rocky Mountain spotted fever: Epidemiology of an increasing problem. Ann Intern Med, 84:732, 1976.
21. Salgo MP, Edward ET, Currie B, et al: A focus of Rocky Mountain spotted fever within New York City. N Engl J Med, 318:1345, 1988.
22. Wilfert CM, MacCormack JN, Kleeman K, et al: Epidemiology of Rocky Mountain spotted fever as determined by active surveillance. J Infect Dis, 150:469, 1984.
23. Walker DH, and Cain GB: The rickettsial plaque. Evidence for direct cytopathic effect of Rickettsia rickettsii. Lab Invest, 43:388, 1980.
24. Walker DH, Firth WT, Ballard JF, et al: Role of the phospholipase-associated penetration mechanism in cell injury by Rickettsia rickettsii. Infect Immun, 40:840, 1983.
25. Walker DH, Tidwell RR, Rector TM, et al: Effect of synthetic protease inhibitors of the amidine type on cell injury by Rickettsia rickettsii. Antimicrob Agents Chemother, 25:582, 1984.
26. Silverman DJ, and Santucci LA: A potential protective role for thiols against cell injury caused by Rickettsia rickettsii. Ann NY Acad Sci, 590:111, 1990.
27. Yamada T, Harber P, Pettit GW, et al: Activation of the kallikrein-kinin system in Rocky Mountain spotted fever. Ann Intern Med, 88:764, 1978.
28. Rao AK, Schapiro M, Clements ML, et al: A prospective study of platelets and plasma proteolytic systems during the early stages of Rocky Mountain spotted fever. N Engl J Med, 318:1021, 1988.
29. Kaplowitz LG, Fischer JJ, and Sparling PF: Rocky Mountain spotted fever: A clinical dilemma. Curr Clin Topics Infect Dis, 2:89, 1981.
30. Harrell GT, and Aikawa JK: Pathogenesis of circulatory failure in Rocky Mountain spotted fever. Arch Intern Med, 83:331, 1949.
31. Walker DH, and Mattern WD: Acute renal failure in Rocky Mountain spotted fever. Arch Intern Med, 139:443, 1979.
32. Randall MR, and Walker DH: Gastrointestinal and pancreatic lesions and rickettsial infection in Rocky Mountain spotted fever. Arch Pathol Lab Med, 108:963, 1984.
33. Horney LF, and Walker DH: Meningoencephalitis as a major manifestation of Rocky Mountain spotted fever. South Med J, 81:915, 1988.
34. Walker DH, Crawford CG, and Cain BG: Rickettsial infection of the pulmonary microcirculation: The basis of interstitial pneumonitis of Rocky Mountain spotted fever. Human Pathol, 11:263, 1980.
35. Walker DH, Burday MS, and Folds JD: Laboratory diagnosis of Rocky Mountain spotted fever. South Med J, 73:1443, 1980.
36. Philip RN, Casper EA, MacCormack JN, et al: A comparison of serologic methods for diagnosis of Rocky Mountain spotted fever. Am J Epidemiol, 105:56, 1977.
37. Kaplan JE, and Schonberger LB: The sensitivity of various serologic tests in the diagnosis of Rocky Mountain spotted fever. Am J Trop Med Hyg, 35:840, 1986.
38. Hechemy KE, Michaelson EE, Anacker RL, et al: Evaluation of latex–Rickettsia rickettsii test for Rocky Mountain spotted fever in 11 laboratories. J Clin Microbiol, 18:938, 1983.
39. Kaplowitz LG, Lange JV, Fischer JJ, et al: Correlation of rickettsial titers, circulating endotoxin, and clinical features in Rocky Mountain spotted fever. Arch Intern Med, 143:1149, 1983.
40. Dumler JS, Gage WR, Pettis GL, et al: Rapid immunoperoxidase demonstration of Rickettsia rickettsii in fixed cutaneous specimens from patients with Rocky Mountain spotted fever. Am J Clin Pathol, 93:410, 1990.
41. Tzianabos T, Anderson BE, and McDade JE: Detection of Rickettsia rickettsii DNA in clinical specimens by using polymerase chain reaction technology. J Clin Microbiol, 27:2866, 1989.
42. Marrero M, and Raoult D: Centrifugation–shell vial technique for rapid detection of Mediterranean spotted fever rickettsia in blood culture. Am J Trop Med, 40:197, 1989.
43. Raoult D, Roussellier P, Vestris G, et al: Susceptibility of Rickettsia conorii and R. rickettsii to pefloxacin, in vitro and in ovo. Br Assoc Antimicrob Chemother, 19:303, 1987.
44. Roueche B: The alerting of Mr. Pomerantz. The New Yorker, 38:1, 1947.
45. Brettman LR, Lewin S, Holzman RS, et al: Rickettsialpox: Report of an outbreak and a contemporary review. Medicine, 60:363, 1981.
46. Walker DH, and Fishbein DB: Epidemiology of rickettsial diseases. Eur J Epidemiol, 7:237, 1991.
47. Harris RL, Kaplan SL, Bradshaw MW, et al: Boutonneuse fever in American travelers. J Infect Dis, 153:126, 1986.

48. Walker DH, and Gear JHS: Correlation of the distribution of Rickettsia conorii, microscopic lesions, and clinical features in South African tick bite fever. Am J Trop Med Hyg, 34:361, 1985.
49. Walker DH, Herrero-Herrero JI, Ruiz-Beltran R, et al: The pathology of fatal Mediterranean spotted fever. Am J Clin Pathol, 87:669, 1987.
50. Walker DH, Staiti A, Mansueto S, et al: Frequent occurrence of hepatic lesions in boutonneuse fever. Acta Trop, 43:175, 1986.
51. Walker DH, Occhino C, Tringali GR, et al: Pathogenesis of rickettsial eschars: The *tache noire* of boutonneuse fever. Human Pathol, 19:1449, 1988.
52. Ruiz R, Herrero I, Martin AM, et al: Vascular permeability in boutonneuse fever. J Infect Dis, 149:1036, 1984.
53. Vicente V, Alberca I, Ruiz R, et al: Coagulation anomalies in Mediterranean spotted fever. J Infect Dis, 153:128, 1986.
54. Raoult D, Zuchelli P, Weiller PJ, et al: Incidence, clinical observations and risk factors in the severe form of Mediterranean spotted fever among patients admitted to hospital in Marseilles 1983–84. J Infect, 12:111, 1986.
55. Raoult D, Gallais H, DeMicco P, et al: Ciprofloxacin therapy for Mediterranean spotted fever. Antimicrob Agents Chemother, 30:606, 1986.
56. Myers WF, and Wisseman CL, Jr: Genetic relatedness among the typhus group of rickettsiae. Intl J Syst Bacteriol, 30:143, 1980.
57. Nicole C, Compte C, and Conseil E: Transmission experimentale du typhus exanthematique par le poudu corps. CR Acad Sci, 149:486, 1909.
58. Dyer RE, Rumreich A, and Badger LF: Typhus fever. A virus of the typhus type derived from fleas collected from wild rats. Public Health Rep, 46:334, 1931.
59. Maxcy KF: An epidemiological study of endemic typhus (Brill's disease) in the southeastern United States. Public Health Rep, 41:2967, 1926.
60. Traub R, Wisseman CL, and Farhang-Azad A: The ecology of murine typhus—a critical review. Trop Dis Bull, 75:237, 1978.
61. Dumler JS, Taylor JP, and Walker DH: Clinical and laboratory features of murine typhus in Texas, 1980–1987. JAMA, 266:1365, 1991.
62. Taylor JP, Betz TG, and Rawlings JA: Epidemiology of murine typhus in Texas (1980 through 1984). JAMA, 255:2173, 1986.
63. Azad AF: Relationship of vector biology and epidemiology of louse- and flea-borne rickettsioses. In Biology of Rickettsial Disease. Vol. I. Edited by DH Walker. Boca Raton, CRC Press, 1988.
64. Walker DH, Parks FM, Betz TG, et al: Histopathology and immunohistologic demonstration of the distribution of Rickettsia typhi in fatal murine typhus. Am J Clin Pathol, 91:720, 1989.
65. McDade JE, Shepard CC, Redus MA, et al: Evidence of Rickettsia prowazekii infections in the United States. Am J Trop Med Hyg, 29:277, 1980.
66. Wisseman CL, Jr, and Waddell A: Interferonlike factors from antigen- and mitogen-stimulated human leukocytes with antirickettsial and cytolytic actions on Rickettsia prowazekii. J Exp Med, 157:1780, 1983.
67. Rollwagen FM, Dasch GA, and Jerrells TR: Mechanisms of immunity to rickettsial infection: Characterization of a cytotoxic effector cell. J Immunol, 136:1418, 1986.
68. Rollwagen FM, Bakun AJ, Dorsey CH, et al: Mechanisms of immunity to infection with typhus rickettsiae: Infected fibroblasts bear rickettsial antigens on their surfaces. Infect Immun, 50:911, 1985.
69. Carl M, Ching W-M, and Dasch GA: Recognition of typhus group rickettsia–infected targets by human lymphokine–activated killer cells. Infect Immun, 56:2526, 1988.
70. Carl M, Robbins F-M, Hartzman RJ, et al: Lysis of cells infected with typhus group rickettsiae by a human cytotoxic T-cell clone. J Immunol, 139:4203, 1987.
71. Schramek S, Brezina R, and Kazar J: Some biological properties of an endotoxic lipopolysaccharide from the typhus group rickettsiae. Acta Virol, 21:439, 1977.
72. McDade JE, Shepard CC, Redus MA, et al: Evidence of Rickettsia prowazekii infections in the United States. Am J Trop Med Hyg, 29:277, 1980.
73. Philip RN, Casper EA, Ormsbee RA, et al: Microimmunofluorescence test for the serological study of Rocky Mountain spotted fever and typhus. J Clin Microbiol, 3:51, 1976.
74. Hechemy KE, Osterman JV, Eisemann CS, et al: Detection of typhus antibodies by latex agglutination. J Clin Microbiol, 13:214, 1981.
75. Amano KI, Tamura A, Ohashi N, et al: Deficiency of peptidoglycan and lipopolysaccharide components in Rickettsia tsutsugamushi. Infect Immun, 55:2290, 1987.
76. Elisberg BL, Campbell JM, and Bozeman FM: Antigenic diversity of Rickettsia tsutsugamushi: Epidemiologic and ecologic significance. J Hyg Epidemiol Microbiol, 12:18, 1968.
77. Hanson B: Role of the composition of Rickettsia tsutsugamushi in immunity to scrub typhus. In Biology of Rickettsial Diseases. Vol II. Edited by DH Walker. Boca Raton, CRC Press, 1988.
78. Maxcy KF: Scrub typhus (tsutsugamushi disease) in the U.S. Army during World War II. In Rickettsial Disease of Man. Edited by FR Moulton. Washington, DC, Thomas, Adams, and Davis, 1946.
79. Brown GW, Shirai A, Jegathesan M, et al: Febrile illness in Malaysia—an analysis of 1,629 hospitalized patients. Am J Trop Med Hyg, 33:311, 1984.
80. Audy JR: The red mites of Japan. In Red Mites and Typhus. Edited by JR Audy. New York, University Press, 1968.
81. Brown GW: Scrub typhus: Pathogenesis and clinical syndrome. In Biology of Rickettsial Diseases. Vol I. Edited by DH Walker. Boca Raton, CRC Press, 1988.
82. Bourgeois AL, Olson JG, Fang RCY, et al: Humoral and cellular responses in scrub typhus patients reflecting primary infection and reinfection with Rickettsia tsutsugamushi. Am J Trop Med Hyg, 31:532, 1982.
83. Saunders JP, Brown GW, Shirai A, et al: The longevity of antibody to Rickettsia tsutsugamushi in patients with confirmed scrub typhus. Trans R Soc Trop Med Hyg, 74:253, 1980.
84. Brown GW, Shirai A, Rogers C, et al: Diagnostic criteria for scrub typhus: Probability values for immunofluorescent antibody and Proteus OXK agglutinin titers. Am J Trop Med Hyg, 32:1101, 1983.
85. Twartz JC, Shirai A, Selvaraju G, et al: Doxycycline prophylaxis for human scrub typhus. J Infect Dis, 146:811, 1982.
86. Walker DH: Ehrlichiosis. In Principles and Practice of Infectious Diseases. Update 5. Edited by GL Mandell, RG Douglas, Jr, and J Bennett. Philadelphia, JB Lippincott, 1989.
87. Maeda K, Markowitz N, Hawley RC, et al: Human infection with Ehrlichia canis, a leukocytic rickettsia. N Engl J Med, 316:853, 1987.
88. Dawson J, Anderson B, Fishbein D, et al: Isolation and characterization of an Ehrlichia sp. from a patient diagnosed with human ehrlichiosis. J Clin Microbiol, 29:2741, 1991.
89. Anderson B, Dawson J, Jones DC, et al: Ehrlichia chaffeensis, a new species associated with human ehrlichiosis. J Clin Microbiol, 29:2838, 1991.
90. Eng TR, Harkess JR, Fishbein DB, et al: Epidemiologic, clini-

cal, and laboratory findings of human ehrlichiosis in the United States, 1988. JAMA, 264:2251, 1990.
91. Smith RD, Sells DM, Stephenson EH, et al: Development of Ehrlichia canis, causative agent of canine ehrlichiosis, in the tick Rhipicephalus sanguineus and its differentiation from a symbiotic rickettsia. Am J Vet Res, 37:119, 1976.
92. Wells MY, and Rikihisa Y: Lack of lysosomal fusion with phagosomes containing Ehrlichia risticii in P388D$_1$ cells: Abrogation of inhibition with oxytetracycline. Infect Immun, 56:3209, 1988.
93. Dumler JS, Aronson JF, and Walker DH: Human ehrlichiosis: Pathologic findings in three fatal cases. Lab Invest, 64:87A, 1991.
94. Dumler JS, Brouqui P, Aronson J, et al: Identification of ehrlichia in human tissue. N Engl J Med, 325:1109, 1991.
95. Fishbein DB, Kemp A, Dawson JE, et al: Human ehrlichiosis: Prospective active surveillance in febrile hospitalized patients. J Infect Dis, 160:803, 1989.
96. Petersen LR, Sawyer LA, Fishbein DB, et al: An outbreak of ehrlichiosis in members of an Army unit exposed to ticks. J Infect Dis, 159:562, 1989.
97. Taylor JP, Betz TG, Fishbein DB, et al: Serological evidence of possible human infection with Ehrlichia in Texas. J Infect Dis, 158:217, 1988.
98. Dawson JE, Fishbein DB, Eng TR, et al: Diagnosis of human ehrlichiosis with the indirect fluorescent antibody test: Kinetics and specificity. J Infect Dis, 162:91, 1990.
99. Amyx HL, Huxsoll DL, Zeiler DC, et al: Therapeutic and prophylactic value of tetracycline in dogs infected with agent of tropical canine pancytopenia. JAVMA, 159:1428, 1971.
100. Misao T, and Kobayashi Y: Studies on infectious mononucleosis (glandular fever) I. Isolation of etiologic agent from blood, bone marrow and lymph node of a patient with infectious mononucleosis by using mice. Kyushu J Med Sci, 6:145, 1955.
101. Tachibana N: Sennetsu fever: The disease, diagnosis, and treatment. *In* Microbiology—1986. Edited by L Leive. Washington, DC, American Society for Microbiology, 1986.
102. Hackstadt T: The role of lipopolysaccharides in the virulence of C. burnetii. Ann NY Acad Sci, 590:27, 1990.
103. Dupuis G, Peter O, Pedroni D, et al: Aspects cliniques observes lors d'une epidemie de 415 cas de fievre Q. Schweiz Med Wochenschr, 115:814, 1985.
104. Marrie TJ, and Yates L: Incidence of Q fever: Pilot studies in two areas in Nova Scotia. Ann NY Acad Sci, 590:275, 1990.
105. Samuel JE, Frazier ME, and Mallavia LP: Correlation of plasmid type and disease caused by Coxiella burnetii. Infect Immun, 49:775, 1985.
106. Hackstadt T: Antigenic variation in the phase I lipopolysaccharide of Coxiella burnetii isolates. Infect Immun, 52:337, 1986.
107. Kishimoto RA, Rozmiarek H, and Larson EW: Experimental Q fever infection in congenitally athymic nude mice. Infect Immun, 22:69, 1978.
108. Tigertt WD, and Benenson AD: Studies on Q fever in man. Trans Assoc Am Physicians, 69:98, 1956.
109. Walker DH: Pathology of Q fever. *In* Biology of Rickettsial Diseases. Vol II. Edited by DH Walker. Boca Raton, CRC Press, 1988.
110. Marrie TJ: Acute Q fever. *In* Q Fever. Vol I. Edited by TJ Marrie. Boca Raton, CRC Press, 1990.
111. Raoult D, Raza A, and Marrie TJ: Q fever endocarditis and other forms of chronic Q fever. *In* Q Fever. Vol I. Edited by TJ Marrie. Boca Raton, CRC Press, 1990.
112. Walker DH, and Peacock MG: Laboratory diagnosis of rickettsial diseases. *In* Biology of Rickettsial Diseases. Vol II. Edited by DH Walker. Boca Raton, CRC Press, 1988.
113. Raoult D, Vestris G, and Enea M: Isolation of 16 strains of Coxiella burnetii from patients by using a sensitive centrifugation cell culture system and establishment of the strains in HEL cells. J Clin Microbiol, 28:2482, 1990.
114. Vinson JW, Varela G, and Molina-Pasquel C: Trench fever. III. Induction of clinical disease in volunteers inoculated with Rickettsia quintana propagated on blood agar. Am J Trop Med Hyg, 18:713, 1969.
115. Relman DA, Loutit JS, Schmidt TM, et al: The agent of bacillary angiomatosis. An approach to the identification of uncultured pathogens. N Engl J Med, 323:1573, 1990.
116. Bruce D: Trench fever. Final report of the war office trench fever investigation committee. J Hyg, 20:258, 1921.
117. LeBoit PE, Berger TG, Egbert BM, et al: Bacillary angiomatosis. The histopathology and differential diagnosis of a pseudoneoplastic infection in patients with human immunodeficiency virus disease. Am J Surg Pathol, 13:909, 1989.
118. Stoler MH, Bonfiglio TA, Steigbigel RT, and Pereira M: An atypical subcutaneous infection associated with acquired immune deficiency syndrome. Am J Clin Pathol, 80:714, 1983.
119. Cockerell CJ, Whitlow MA, Webster GF, and Friedman-Kien AE: Epithelioid angiomatosis: A distinct vascular disorder in patients with the acquired immunodeficiency syndrome or AIDS-related complex. Lancet, ii:654, 1987.
120. Milam MW, et al: Epithelioid angiomatosis secondary to disseminated cat scratch disease involving the bone marrow and skin in a patient with acquired immune deficiency syndrome: A case report. Am J Med, 88:180, 1990.
121. Kemper CA, Lombard CM, Deresinski SC, and Tompkins LS: Visceral bacillary epithelioid angiomatosis: Possible manifestations of disssseminated cat scratch disease in the immunocompromised host: A report of two cases. Am J Med, 89:216, 1990.
122. Cockerell CJ, Bergstresser PR, Myrie-Williams C, and Tierno PM: Bacillary epithelioid angiomatosis occurring in an immunocompetent individual. Arch Dermatol, 126:787, 1990.
123. Perkocha LA, et al: Clinical and pathological features of bacillary peliosis hepatis in association with human immunodeficiency virus infection. N Engl J Med, 323:1581, 1990.
124. Slater LN, Welch DF, Hensel D, and Coody DW: A newly recognized fastidious gram-negative pathogen as a cause of fever and bacteremia. N Engl J Med, 323:1587, 1990.
125. Regnery RL, et al: Characterization of a novel Rochalimaea species, R. henselae sp. nov., isolated from blood of a febrile, human immunodeficiency virus–positive patient. J Clin Microbiol, 30:265, 1992.
126. Welch DF, et al: Rochalimaea henselae sp. nov., a cause of septicemia, bacillary angiomatosis, and parenchymal bacillary peliosis. J Clin Microbiol, 30:275, 1992.
127. Howe C: Carrion's disease. Immunologic studies. Arch Intern Med, 72:147, 1943.
128. Benson LA, et al: Entry of Bartonella bacilliformis into erythrocytes. Infection Immun, 54:347, 1986.
129. Schultz MG: Daniel Carrion's experiment. N Engl J Med, 278:1323, 1968.
130. Ureteaga BO, and Payne EH: Treatment of the acute febrile phase of Carrion's disease with chloramphenicol. Am J Trop Med, 4:507, 1955.
131. Arias-Stella J, et al: Verruga peruana mimicking malignant neoplasms. Am J Dermatopathol, 9:279, 1987.
132. Garcia FU: Tissue reaction in bartonellosis may suggest Kaposi's sarcoma. Arch Pathol Lab Mcd, 109:703, 1985.

Chapter 27

MYCOPLASMAS

The first mycoplasma was isolated in 1898 from cattle with contagious pleuropneumonia, and 2 years later the typical colony morphology of these organisms, which often required a dissecting microscope for visualization, was described: small, dome-shaped colonies with dense central cores and a light periphery, resembling fried eggs, that appeared after incubation for up to 3 weeks (1,2). Since then, mycoplasmas have been isolated from many animals and from the environment (3). In 1937 the first human isolate (recovered from a Bartholin's gland abscess) was reported, but mycoplasmas were not proven to be causally related to human disease until 1962, when a mycoplasma (subsequently named Mycoplasma pneumoniae) was identified as the pathogen of primary atypical pneumonia (4,5).

Mycoplasmas, the smallest free-living organisms, are pleomorphic, spherical, pear-shaped, or filamentous cells, 0.2 to 0.8 μm in diameter. Most are facultative anaerobes. They replicate by binary fission, like all bacteria except Chlamydia and Rickettsia, but mycoplasmas are unique among the bacteria because they have no cell wall, they cannot synthesize cell wall precursors, and they require cholesterol and related sterols for membrane synthesis. Mycoplasmas also lack the enzymatic pathways for purine and pyrimidine synthesis and, therefore, require complex media (such as beef heart infusion broth supplemented with horse serum, yeast extract, and nucleic acids) for growth in vitro.

Human mycoplasmas are classified in general as follows (6):

Order: Mycoplasmatales
Family: Mycoplasmataceae
Genus: Mycoplasma
Species: pneumoniae, salivarium, orale, buccale, faucium, lipophilum, primatum, fermentans, hominis, genitalium
Genus: Ureaplasma
Species: urealyticum
Family: Acholeplasmataceae
Genus: Acholeplasma
Species: laidlawaii

The potential pathogens, Mycoplasma pneumoniae, Mycoplasma hominis, and Ureaplasma urealyticum, are discussed; the remaining species are part of the normal human flora, primarily of the respiratory and genitourinary tracts.

MYCOPLASMA PNEUMONIAE

In 1938 the term primary atypical pneumonia was used to describe a type of pneumonia that differed clinically from the typical pneumonias caused by micro-organisms then known, and in 1943 high titers of cold agglutinins were detected in the serum of persons with the illness (7,8). In 1944 Eaton and associates produced pneumonia in rats and hamsters inoculated with filtered secretions from persons with "atypical pneumonia," and they prevented disease in animals by giving convalescent-phase antiserum before inoculation (9). The responsible organism, initially called Eaton's agent, was grown on agar and proven to be a mycoplasma in 1962, and that same year respiratory tract disease was reproduced in human volunteers (5,10).

Epidemiology

Mycoplasma pneumoniae is found worldwide and causes infections year-round. However, during epidemics, which typically occur at 4- to 8-year intervals among confined populations such as children in schools, families, and military recruits, disease is most prevalent in late summer and fall. Spread of the infection generally is slow, apparently requiring close contact with an ill person, and it occurs first among school-aged children, who subsequently introduce the infection into the family. Epidemics, however, may progress rapidly, and the occurrence of point-source outbreaks in which a close and prolonged exposure is not identified suggests that M. pneumoniae may be transmitted via small-particle aerosols (11–13). Rates of infection with M. pneumoniae are greatest in school-aged children and young adults, and pneumonia most frequently occurs in persons aged 5 to 20 years, especially those between the ages of 15 and 19 years. Infection with M. pneumoniae is common before age 5 years, but it usually is asymptomatic or produces a mild illness with coryza and wheezing but no fever or pneumonia (14).

Pathogenesis and Pathology

Organism- and host-related factors are involved in the pathogenesis of Mycoplasma pneumoniae disease. M. pneumoniae is a surface parasite that colonizes the mucosa of the respiratory tract, and its ability to attach to respiratory mucosal cells, evade phagocytosis, and modulate the immune system are essential to the initiation of disease. Its gliding motility may promote penetration through respiratory secretions, and its filamentous, flexible form with terminal attachment organelle may allow it to locate in crypts and folds of the host cell membrane and between microvilli and cilia, protected from phagocytosis. Attachment of M. pneumoniae to host cells is mediated by a protein designated P1, apparently contained in surface projections resembling viral peplomers (see Chapter 3), that interacts with glycoproteins containing neuraminic acid at the surface of the host cell membrane

(15–17). Hydrogen peroxide and superoxide produced by M. pneumoniae may injure mucosal cells, causing ciliostasis and sloughing of superficial cells (18).

The apparent high prevalence of infection with Mycoplasma pneumoniae in infants and young children, the mild nature of the disease in this age group, and the occurrence of a more severe illness during infection at a later age suggest that severe disease may result from host immune responses to reinfection; however, a precise mechanism for the host cell injury has not been identified. Moreover, the extrapulmonary manifestations of disease (discussed later) may be immune mediated, because the organism infrequently is recovered from these distant sites; however, this has not been proven. The interaction of M. pneumoniae with the I antigenic determinant of human erythrocytes, which contains the necessary 2,3-sialylated poly-N-acetylgalactosamine sequences, may render the I antigen antigenic, thus stimulating production of cold agglutinins. Other autoimmune antibodies produced during infection with M. pneumoniae (antibodies to lung, brain, smooth muscle, and lymphocytes) may have similar derivations.

During primary infection with Mycoplasma pneumoniae the first line of defense is activation of the alternate complement pathway and phagocytosis of the organism at the mucosal surface. Galactosyl and glycosyl derivatives on the surface membrane of the organism apparently stimulate production of antibodies, of which immunoglobulin (Ig) A, found predominantly in respiratory tract secretions, appears to be most important for recovery. Intracellular protein antigens of M. pneumoniae exposed during phagocytosis and degradation of the organism stimulate T-lymphocyte reactions, which apparently determine the severity of disease.

Few descriptions of the pathologic findings of Mycoplasma pneumoniae–induced disease are available because most infections are self-limited. In fatal cases the lungs have shown patchy areas of consolidation, characterized histologically by bronchitis, bronchiolitis, and interstitial and alveolar pneumonitis with peribronchiolar collections of lymphocytes and plasma cells, accompanied by macrophages and neutrophils if cellular necrosis is present.

Clinical Manifestations

The most common manifestation of disease caused by Mycoplasma pneumoniae is tracheobronchitis. About a third of infected persons develop pneumonia, which begins gradually 2 to 3 weeks after exposure, with fever, malaise, headache, pharyngitis, and persistent nonproductive hacking cough. Clinically inapparent sinusitis frequently occurs, and myringitis also may develop. Chest roentgenograms show unilateral lower lobe bronchopneumonia, or occasionally bilateral feathery infiltrates. The peripheral white blood cell count is normal early and becomes elevated as the disease progresses. Maculopapular or, less commonly, vesicular skin eruptions occur in about 15% of cases a few days after disease onset (19–21). If the illness is not treated, fever resolves in 2 to 14 days; malaise, cough, and radiographic abnormalities persist 2 to 6 weeks. In about 2% of children and about 10% of adults, pneumonia is severe enough to warrant hospitalization, and these patients may develop lung abscess, pleural effusions, secondary bacterial infections, bronchiectasis, or clinical relapse (22–24). Extrarespiratory manifestations are uncommon and include clinically apparent hemolytic anemia, typically in persons with very high titers of cold agglutinins; erythema multiforme, erythema nodosum, and urticaria; encephalitis, meningoencephalitis, mono- or polyneuritis, and meningitis; myocarditis and pericarditis; and arthralgias and rarely arthritis (19,25–30).

MYCOPLASMA HOMINIS AND UREAPLASMA UREALYTICUM (GENITAL MYCOPLASMAS)

Epidemiology

Infants may become colonized with genital mycoplasmas during passage through an infected birth canal, colonization that usually persists less than 2 years. Ureaplasma urealyticum and Mycoplasma hominis may be recovered from the genital tract of as many as about 30% of infant girls (less frequently from the genital tract of infant boys), and they may be isolated from the nose and throat of up to 15% of infant boys and girls (31,32). In one study 20% of prepubertal girls were colonized with ureaplasmas and 6% with M. hominis, but these organisms seldom were recovered from prepubertal boys (33). Colonization with genital mycoplasmas after puberty results from sexual contact (34,35). About 60% of apparently healthy sexually active women carry Ureaplasma urealyticum and about 20% carry Mycoplasma hominis in the vagina.

Clinical Manifestations

Ureaplasma urealyticum is one cause of nongonococcal urethritis; it has been associated with postpartum fever, chorioamnionitis, and low birth weight, although a causal relationship with the latter is not proven, and it is a rare cause of chronic urethrocystitis in immunosuppressed persons (36–40). Mycoplasma hominis probably is involved in acute pelvic inflammatory disease, but its specific role has not been defined. It is responsible for some cases of postabortal and postpartum fever, probably by causing endometritis in the latter cases; and it is an uncommon cause of bacteremia, arthritis, peritonitis, meningitis, osteomyelitis, and wound infections, principally in immunocompromised persons but also in some who have no apparent underlying immune system abnormality (36,41–47).

Laboratory Diagnosis

Mycoplasma pneumoniae. Specimens most commonly submitted for diagnosis of infections caused by M. pneumoniae are throat swabs, sputum, and serum, although bronchoalveolar lavage fluid and lung tissue also are acceptable. Collection, transport, and processing of specimens are discussed in Part III.

Cold agglutinins, which are IgM antibodies specific for the I antigen of human erythrocytes, are detected by the end of the first week or early in the second week of illness in 50% or more of infected persons, but their presence is not diagnostic of Mycoplasma pneumoniae–induced disease. A definitive diagnosis requires detection of the organism or specific antibodies. To isolate M. pneumoniae, biphasic cultures (prepared in house or purchased) are inoculated, incubated up to 3 weeks in ambient air at 35° to 37° C in a sealed container, and examined microscopically (40×) once or twice per week. Spherical colonies embedded in the agar with a thin outer layer (resembling a "fried egg") are consistent with M. pneumoniae and should be tested for β-hemolysis (M. pneumoniae is β-hemolytic by virtue of hydrogen peroxide production) as follows: 1% melted agar, prepared in 0.85% saline and cooled to 50° C, is mixed with sheep or guinea pig blood to give a 5% erythrocyte concentration. A thin layer of the suspension is poured on the agar plate, which is reincubated for 24 hours and examined microscopically (48).

Because culture of Mycoplasma pneumoniae may require several weeks, more rapid diagnostic tests are needed. Data from evaluations of a DNA probe are favorable, especially when sputum is tested (49,50). Detection of specific IgM in a single serum sample is diagnostic of acute infection; whereas if IgG is measured, acute- and convalescent-phase samples must be tested, and the diagnosis is based on a four-fold or greater rise in titer.

Genital Mycoplasmas. Ureaplasma urealyticum and Mycoplasma hominis may be recovered from urethral, vaginal, or endocervical swab specimens, blood, urine, abscess material, prostatic secretions, semen, and tissues. Specimen collection, transport, and processing are discussed in Part III.

Various culture systems may be used to isolate the genital mycoplasmas (48,51–54). Traditionally, separate systems are used for each organism (U agar and U broth for Ureaplasma urealyticum and H agar and H broth for Mycoplasma hominis), because the optimal pH for growth of the two organisms differs (pH 5.5 to 6.5 for Ureaplasma urealyticum and pH 6 to 8 for Mycoplasma hominis). However, data from several studies indicate that certain commercially available culture systems effectively detect both organisms (52–54). Broth cultures are incubated aerobically in sealed test tubes. Agar cultures are incubated anaerobically or in an atmosphere of 5 to 7% carbon dioxide and observed daily under the microscope (×40). M. hominis also grows on sheep blood agar, producing nonhemolytic pinpoint colonies, and in most broth blood culture media without showing visible evidence of growth.

Colonies of Mycoplasma hominis, 200 to 300 μm in diameter with the typical fried-egg appearance, usually are visible in 5 days or less. In broth containing phenol red and 0.1% arginine, M. hominis metabolizes arginine to ammonia, causing a color change from yellow to red. Colonies of Ureaplasma urealyticum, 15 to 16 μm in diameter, usually are apparent in 2 days, and are best visualized by applying a calcium chloride stain to the agar surface and observing for a distinct dark brown precipitate, which appears around colonies of U. urealyticum in 5 minutes. In U broth, U. urealyticum produces a shift in pH, changing the color from yellow to red. A loopful of broth then is transferred to agar plates and streaked for isolation.

Treatment and Prevention

Mycoplasma pneumoniae. Antimicrobial therapy is not recommended for M. pneumoniae–induced pharyngitis or tracheobronchitis. Tetracycline and its derivatives and erythromycin are effective treatment for M. pneumoniae–induced pneumonia, but therapy apparently does not alter transmission of the organism. No effective method for prevention of infection and disease caused by M. pneumoniae is established, but persons with disease probably should be placed in isolation.

Genital Mycoplasmas. The tetracyclines are active against most isolates of Ureaplasma urealyticum and Mycoplasma hominis. However, about 10% of ureaplasmas are resistant to tetracycline, and infections caused by resistant strains generally respond to erythromycin (55,56).

REFERENCES

1. Nocard E, and Roux ER: Le microbe de la peripneumoniae. Ann Inst Pasteur (Paris), 12:240, 1898.
2. Couch RB: Introduction to Mycoplasma Diseases. *In* Principles and Practice of Infectious Diseases. 3rd ed. Edited by GL Mandell, RG Douglas, Jr, and JE Bennett. New York, Churchill Livingstone, 1990.
3. Freundt EA: The Mycoplasmas. *In* Bergey's Manual of Determinative Bacteriology. Edited by RE Buchanan and NE Gibbons. 8th ed. Baltimore, Williams & Wilkins, 1974.
4. Dienes L, and Edsall G: Observations of L organisms of Klieneberger. Proc Soc Exp Biol Med, 36:740, 1937.
5. Chanock RM, Hayflick L, and Barile MF. Growth on artificial medium of an agent associated with atypical pneumonia and its identification as a PPLO. Proc Natl Acad Sci, 48:41, 1962.
6. Couch RB: Mycoplasma pneumoniae (primary atypical pneumonia). *In* Principles and Practice of Infectious Diseases. 3rd ed. Edited by GL Mandell, RG Douglas, Jr, and JE Bennett. New York, Churchill Livingstone, 1990.
7. Reimann HA: An acute infection of the respiratory tract with atypical pneumonia. A disease entity probably caused by a filterable virus. JAMA, 111:2377, 1938.
8. Peterson OL, Han TH, and Finland M: Cold agglutinins (autohemagglutinins) in primary atypical pneumonias. Science, 97:167, 1943.
9. Eaton MD, Meiklejohn G, and van Herick W: Studies on the etiology of primary atypical pneumonia. A filterable agent transmissible to cotton rats, hamsters, and chick embryos. J Exp Med, 79:649, 1944.
10. Rifkind D, et al: Ear involvement (myringitis) and primary atypical pneumonia following inoculation of volunteers with Eaton agent. Am Rev Respir Dis, 35:479, 1962.
11. Evatt BL, et al: Epidemic mycoplasma pneumonia. N Engl J Med, 285:374, 1971.
12. Sande MA, Gadot F, and Wenzel RP: Point source epidemic of Mycoplasma pneumoniae infection in a prosthodontics laboratory. Am Rev Respir Dis, 112:213, 1975.
13. Broome CV, et al: An explosive outbreak of Mycoplasma pneumoniae infection in a summer camp. Pediatrics, 66:884, 1980.
14. Fernald GW, Collier AM, and Clyde WA, Jr: Respiratory infections due to Mycoplasma pneumoniae in infants and children. Pediatrics, 55:327, 1975.
15. Manchee RJ, and Taylor-Robinson D: Studies on the nature of receptors involved in attachment of tissue culture cells to mycoplasmas. Br J Exp Pathol, 50:66, 1969.
16. Chandler DKF, Grabowski MW, and Barile MF: Mycoplasma pneumoniae attachment: Competitive inhibition by myco-

plasmal binding component and by sialic acid–containing glycoconjugates. Infect Immun, *38*:598, 1982.
17. Geary SJ, and Gabridge MG: Characterization of a human lung fibroblast receptor site for Mycoplasma pneumoniae. Isr J Med Sci, *23*:462, 1987.
18. Almagor M, Kahane I, and Yatziv S: Role of superoxide anion in host cell injury induced by Mycoplasma pneumoniae infection. J Clin Invest, *73*:842, 1984.
19. Fleming PC, et al: Febrile mucocutaneous syndrome with respiratory involvement, associated with isolation of Mycoplasma pneumoniae. Can Med Assoc J, *97*:1485, 1967.
20. Lascari AD, Garfunkel JM, and Mauro DG: Varicella-like rash associated with Mycoplasma infection. Am J Dis Child, *128*:254, 1974.
21. Cherry JD, Hurwitz ES, and Welliver RC: Mycoplasma pneumoniae infections and exanthems. J Pediatr, *87*:369, 1975.
22. Foy HM, et al: Long-term epidemiology of infections with Mycoplasma pneumoniae. J Infect Dis, *139*:681, 1979.
23. Ponka A: Clinical and laboratory manifestations in patients with serological evidence of Mycoplasma pneumoniae infection. Scand J Infect Dis, *10*:271, 1978.
24. Watson GI: Mycoplasma pneumoniae in general practice. J Coll Gen Pract, *13*:174, 1967.
25. Jacobson LB, Longstreth GF, and Edgington TS: Clinical and immunologic features of transient cold agglutinin hemolytic anemia. Am J Med, *54*:514, 1973.
26. Foy HM, Kenny GE, and Koler J: Mycoplasma pneumoniae in Stevens-Johnson syndrome. Lancet, *ii*:550, 1967.
27. Cassel GH, and Cole BC: Mycoplasmas as agents of human disease. N Engl J Med, *304*:80, 1981.
28. Ponka A: The occurrence and clinical picture of serologically verified Mycoplasma pneumoniae infections with emphasis on central nervous system, cardiac, and joint manifestations. Ann Clin Res, *24*:1, 1979.
29. Ponka A: Central nervous system manifestations associated with serologically verified Mycoplasma pneumoniae infection. Scand J Infect Dis, *12*:175, 1980.
30. Jones MC: Arthritis and arthralgia in infection with Mycoplasma pneumoniae. Thorax, *25*:748, 1970.
31. Klein JO, Buckland D, and Finland M: Colonization of newborn infants by mycoplasmas. N Engl J Med, *280*:1025, 1969.
32. Foy HM, et al: Acquisition of mycoplasmata and T strains during infancy. J Infect Dis, *121*:579, 1970.
33. Hammerschlag MR, et al: Microbiology of the vagina in children: Normal and potentially pathogenic organisms. Pediatrics, *62*:57, 1978.
34. McCormack WM, Lee Y-H, and Zinner SH: Sexual experience and urethral colonization with genital mycoplasmas. A study in normal men. Ann Intern Med, *78*:696, 1973.
35. McCormack WM, et al: Sexual activity and vaginal colonization with genital mycoplasmas. JAMA, *221*:1375, 1972.
36. Taylor-Robinson D, and McCormack WM: Medical progress: The genital mycoplasmas. N Engl J Med, *302*:1003, 1980.
37. Bowie WR, et al: Etiology of nongonococcal urethritis: Evidence for Chlamydia trachomatis and Ureaplasma urealyticum. J Clin Invest, *59*:735, 1977.
38. Taylor-Robinson D, Furr PM, and Webster ADB: Ureaplasma urealyticum causing persistent urethritis in a patient with hypogammaglobulinemia. Genitourin Med, *61*:404, 1985.
39. Cassell GW, et al: Role of Ureaplasma urealyticum in amnionitis. Pediatr Infect Dis, *5*:S247, 1986.
40. Kass EH, et al: Genital mycoplasmas as a cause of excess premature delivery. Trans Assoc Am Phys, *94*:261, 1981.
41. Platt R, et al: Infection with Mycoplasma hominis in postpartum fever. Lancet, *ii*:1217, 1980.
42. Wallace RJ, Jr, et al: Isolation of Mycoplasma hominis from blood cultures in patients with postpartum fever. Obstet Gynecol, *51*:181, 1978.
43. DeGirolami PC, and Madoff S: Mycoplasma hominis septicemia. J Clin Microbiol, *16*:566, 1982.
44. Mokhbat JE, et al: Peritonitis due to Mycoplasma hominis in a renal transplant recipient. J Infect Dis, *146*:713, 1982.
45. Taylor-Robinson D, et al: The association of Mycoplasma hominis with arthritis. Sex Transm Dis, *10*:341, 1983.
46. Gewitz M, et al: Mycoplasma hominis. A cause of neonatal meningitis. Arch Dis Child, *54*:231, 1979.
47. McMahon DK, Dummer JS, Pasculle AR, and Cassell G: Extragenital Mycoplasma hominis infections in adults. Am J Med, *89*:275, 1990.
48. Clyde WA, Jr, Kenny GE, and Schachter J: Laboratory diagnosis of chlamydial and mycoplasmal infections. In Cumitech 29. Edited by WL Drew. Washington, DC, American Society for Microbiology, 1984.
49. Dular R, Kajioka R, and Kasatiya S: Comparison of Gen-Probe commercial kit and culture technique for the diagnosis of Mycoplasma pneumoniae infection. J Clin Microbiol, *26*:1068, 1988.
50. Kleemold SRM, Karjalainen JE, and Raty RKH: Rapid diagnosis of Mycoplasma pneumoniae infection: Clinical evaluation of a commercial probe test. J Infect Dis, *162*:70, 1990.
51. Fiacco V, Miller MJ, Carney E, and Martin WJ: Comparison of media for isolation of Ureaplasma urealyticum and genital Mycoplasma species. J Clin Microbiol, *20*:862, 1984.
52. Yajko DM, et al: Evaluation of PPLO, A7B, E, and NYC agar media for the isolation of Ureaplasma urealyticum and Mycoplasma species from the genital tract. J Clin Microbiol, *19*:73, 1984.
53. Wood JC, Lu RM, Peterson EM, and de la Maza LM: Evaluation of Mycotrim-GU for isolation of Mycoplasma species and Ureaplasma urealyticum. J Clin Microbiol, *22*:789, 1985.
54. Phillips LE, Goodrich KH, Turner RM, and Faro S: Isolation of Mycoplasma species and Ureaplasma urealyticum from obstetrical and gynecological patients by using commercially available medium formulations. J Clin Microbiol, *24*:377, 1986.
55. Evans RT, and Taylor-Robinson D: The incidence of tetracycline-resistant strains of Ureaplasma urealyticum. J Antimicrob Chemother, *4*:57, 1978.
56. Taylor-Robinson D, and Furr PM: Clinical antibiotic resistance of Ureaplasma urealyticum. Pediatr Infect Dis, *5*:S335, 1986.

Chapter 28

AEROBIC AND FACULTATIVE GRAM-POSITIVE COCCI

Medically important aerobic and facultative gram-positive cocci are classified in two families, Micrococcaceae and Streptococcaceae. Members of these two families are distinguished by the presence or absence of cytochromes (iron-porphyrin components of the electron transport chain that carry electrons toward molecular oxygen), which are found in bacteria belonging to the Micrococcaceae but not in members of the Streptococcaceae. The catalase test (Appendix, Procedure 9, and Fig. 28–1) differentiates most Micrococcaceae, usually catalase positive, from most Streptococcaceae, which almost always are catalase negative. Occasionally, however, catalase-positive isolates of Streptococcaceae and catalase-negative isolates of Micrococcaceae must be identified by the benzidine test, which is positive with organisms containing cytochromes such as the Micrococcaceae.

The gram-positive cocci of medical importance are classified in general as follows:

Family: Micrococcaceae
Genus: Staphylococcus
Micrococcus
Stomatococcus
Family: Streptococcaceae
Genus: Streptococcus
Enterococcus
Aerococcus
Leuconostoc
Pedicoccus
Lactococcus

The commonly encountered species of these genera are discussed in this chapter.

MICROCOCCACEAE

The family Micrococcaceae has three genera of medical importance: Staphylococcus, Micrococcus, and Stomatococcus. Distinguishing features are listed in Table 28–1. Several species of Staphylococcus produce human disease. Species of Micrococcus are part of the normal flora of human skin and occasionally are recovered from clinical specimens, in which case they must be differentiated from Staphylococcus. These organisms are rare human pathogens and are not discussed further. One species of Stomatococcus, Stomatococcus mucilaginosus (previously Micrococcus mucilaginosus), recently has been recognized as a potential human pathogen.

Staphylococcus

Members of the genus Staphylococcus are immotile, non–spore-forming gram-positive cocci, 0.5 to 1.5 μm in diameter, that in broth cultures occur singly and in pairs, short chains, tetrads, and clusters. Of the 27 recognized species of Staphylococcus 14 are found on human skin and mucous membranes: Staphylococcus aureus, -epidermidis, -saprophyticus, -hominis, -haemolyticus, -warneri, -capitis, -saccharolyticus, -auricularis, -simulans, -cohnii, -xylosus, -lugdunensis, and -schleiferi. The remaining species colonize animals. The species that infect humans are facultative anaerobes and grow better aerobically, except Staphylococcus saccharolyticus which prefers anaerobic conditions. Staphylococci may be divided into two groups based on the presence or absence of the enzyme coagulase. Of the species that infect humans, only Staphylococcus aureus is coagulase positive; the remaining species often are referred to collectively as coagulase-negative staphylococci. Three species of Staphylococcus commonly associated with human infection are discussed: S. aureus, Staphylococcus epidermidis, and Staphylococcus saprophyticus.

Staphylococcus aureus

Epidemiology

Staphylococcus aureus is a component of the normal microflora of some humans, termed carriers; the organisms reside in the anterior nasal vestibule, perineum, or axilla without producing symptoms. The mechanisms by which S. aureus is acquired and maintained as a component of normal flora are not completely understood. Infants become colonized soon after birth, but the carrier rate falls during the first several months of life, at least partly owing to transplacental acquisition of maternal antibodies. About 15 to 30% of healthy, non–hospital-associated adults are colonized with S. aureus. Some are chronic or persistent carriers, but most harbor the organism intermittently, for a few weeks at a time. The carrier rate is higher among physicians, nurses, and hospital ward attendants, among persons with atopic dermatitis, and among persons who use needles regularly, such as diabetes patients who take insulin, persons who repeatedly undergo hemodialysis, those who receive allergy injections, and intravenous drug users (1).

Most infections caused by S. aureus are endogenous: the organism is transferred from a site of colonization such as the anterior nares, to the skin, where dermal breaks provide a portal of entry. Direct contact with the hands of carriers or others with mild staphylococcal skin lesions also is an important route of transmission.

Pathogenesis

A polysaccharide capsule, specific cell wall components, and various enzymes and toxins elaborated by Staphylococcus aureus are responsible for its pathogenicity (1). The capsule, if present, protects the organism from

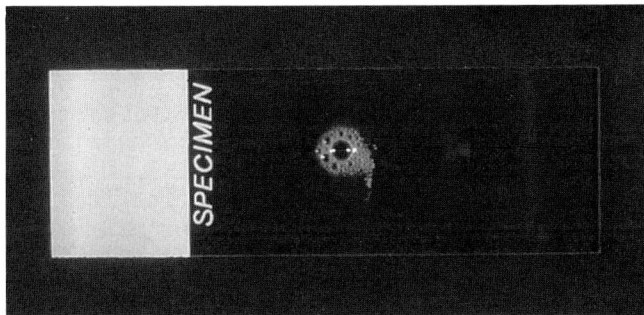

Fig. 28-1. Positive catalase test result.

complement-mediated attack by polymorphonuclear leukocytes, and it enhances spread of the organism through tissues. Cell wall components are these: The peptidoglycan (see Chapter 24) elicits interleukin 1 production by macrophages, activates complement, and is chemotactic for neutrophils. Teichoic acid interacts with components of the alternate complement pathway, activating the coagulation and kinin systems to produce septic shock, and perhaps potentiating bacterial adherence at sites of colonization. Protein A, an immunologically active substance with a high affinity for the Fc fragment of immunoglobulin (Ig) G, binds to and aggregates IgG molecules, fixing complement in the process, and it enhances natural killer cell activity.

Extracellular enzymes produced by Staphylococcus aureus include catalase, which promotes survival of the organism by interfering with the neutrophil oxygen–dependent bactericidal mechanisms; β-lactamase, a plasmid-mediated enzyme responsible for penicillin resistance; and lipases, which are essential for invasion of healthy cutaneous and subcutaneous tissues. Among the toxins elaborated are exfoliatin serotypes A and B, a toxin responsible for the scalded skin syndrome; toxic shock syndrome toxin 1 (TSST-1), responsible for toxic shock syndrome, perhaps by eliciting production of tumor necrosis factor (TNF); δ toxin, which inhibits water absorption and stimulates cyclic adenosine monophosphate (cAMP) production in rabbit and guinea pig ileum, suggesting a role in the pathogenesis of acute diarrhea in some staphylococcal infections; and enterotoxins (serotypes A–E), which are major causes of food poisoning (2). Enterotoxins B and C also have been identified in a few cases of toxic shock syndrome, principally those not associated with menstruation (3–5).

Clinical Manifestations

Infections caused by Staphylococcus aureus may affect multiple organ systems (1,6,7). Among the most common are those involving the skin and its appendages. Impetigo is a superficial cutaneous infection of children that affects primarily exposed areas such as the face and legs. It is characterized by vesicles that rupture, leaving yellow crusts. Most often impetigo is caused by S. aureus, but Streptococcus pyogenes (discussed later) or both organisms may be involved. Folliculitis is a localized cutaneous infection of hair follicles caused by Staphylococcus aureus, presenting as painful, red pustules. Local extension of folliculitis, especially on the face, neck, axillae, and buttocks, produces a furuncle, a red, painful dermal nodule with central necrosis. Coalescence of multiple furuncles in the subcutaneous tissue forms a carbuncle. S. aureus may cause mastitis, an inflammation of the mammary ducts of lactating women, and it is the major cause of infections of surgical wounds.

Staphylococcus aureus is among the leading causes of bacteremia (seeding of the blood) in hospitalized patients. The bacteremia commonly originates from an infected intravascular catheter, a postoperative wound, a skin infection, or pneumonia, but in about 20% of cases no focus is evident (8). Fewer than 10% of persons who are bacteremic with S. aureus develop endocarditis. At highest risk are those with left-sided organic valvular heart disease and intravenous drug users, who generally have right-sided lesions and a less rapidly progressive illness.

Infection with Staphylococcus aureus may result in a septic shock syndrome by one of four mechanisms: (1) In persons with a severe local infection, loss of large volumes of fluid into the interstitial spaces may cause hypovolemia. (2) In those with endocarditis, aortic valve rupture or myocardial abscess formation may impair cardiac function. (3) An unencapsulated strain of S. aureus in the blood may activate the coagulation and kinin systems via an interaction between the organisms' teichoic acid–peptidoglycan complex and the components of the alternate complement pathway. (4) Infection with a strain of S. aureus that produces TSST-1 may cause a septic shock syndrome by eliciting production of TNF (2).

Table 28-1. Characteristics of the Micrococcaceae

Characteristic	Staphylococcus	Micrococcus	Stomatococcus
Catalase	+	+	±
Capsule	∓	−	+
Growth in 5% NaCl	+	+	−
Anaerobic growth in glucose	+	−	+
Lysostaphin susceptibility	S	R	R
Aerobic acid production from glycerol in presence of erythromycin (0.4 μg/ml)	+	−	−
Modified oxidase	−	+	−
Bacitracin (0.04-U disk)	R	S	S*
Furazolidone (100-μg disk)	R	S	S*

* Data are limited; however some Stomatococcus mucilaginosus are susceptible.
Key: +, positive; −, negative; R, resistant; S, susceptible.

In the central nervous system Staphylococcus aureus is the most common cause of spinal epidural abscess and suppurative intracranial phlebitis. Organisms reach the epidural space by hematogenous spread from a distant focus of infection or by local extension, and septic intracranial thrombophlebitis usually follows infection of the paranasal sinuses, middle ear, mastoid, face, or oropharynx, spreading centrally along the emissary veins (see Chapter 55). S. aureus is recovered from 10 to 15% of brain abscesses and is the most common pathogen in brain abscesses following trauma. Acute pyogenic meningitis caused by S. aureus is an uncommon infection that generally follows head trauma or a neurosurgical procedure but may occur in conjunction with brain abscesses, paranasal sinusitis, or endocarditis.

Staphylococcus aureus, a major cause of musculoskeletal infection, is responsible for most cases of osteomyelitis (see Chapter 64). Clinically, acute osteomyelitis is characterized by the abrupt onset of fever and pain and erythema in the affected area, and chronic infection generally is manifested by local pain and draining sinuses. S. aureus is the most common cause of septic arthritis in prepubertal children, is occasionally responsible for septic arthritis in adults and in persons with rheumatoid arthritis, and is a major cause of infections in joints with prostheses. Persons with septic arthritis are febrile, and the affected joint is hot, swollen, and painful. Common symptoms of an infected prosthesis are protracted pain or instability of the involved joint. In the tropics, S. aureus may cause pyomyositis, spontaneous deep abscesses of muscles (usually in malnourished persons who have an intercurrent parasitic infection) (9).

Staphylococcus aureus is an infrequent cause of community-acquired pneumonia but the second most common cause of nosocomial pneumonia (after Pseudomonas aeruginosa) (10). Primary bronchopneumonia follows aspiration of endogenous nasopharyngeal organisms or, less commonly, inhalation of microbes from an exogenous source. Factors that predispose to pneumonia include infection with measles or influenza A virus, cystic fibrosis, hospitalization, and immune deficiency. The infection is most common in infants, young children, and adults in the fifth or sixth decade; in all age groups males are predominantly affected. Secondary pneumonia, due to hematogenous spread of Staphylococcus aureus from an extrapulmonary focus of infection, is most common in persons who have a chronic illness or receive immunosuppressive therapy and in intravenous drug users who have bacterial endocarditis. Complications of pneumonia caused by S. aureus include abscess formation, empyema, and pneumatoceles (thin-walled cystlike structures filled with air or partially filled with fluid that develop after an abscess drains into a bronchus). Although neither roentgenographic nor clinical features are diagnostic, rapid cavitation of bronchopneumonia, the appearance of multiple areas of pulmonary consolidation, and the development of pleural empyema in a person who has one of these risk factors suggest infection with S. aureus.

Urinary tract infections caused by Staphylococcus aureus are pyelonephritis, intrarenal abscess, and perinephric abscess. Pyelonephritis most often is a complication of bacteremia or endocarditis, intrarenal abscess is a complication of pyelonephritis, and perinephric abscess occurs secondary to obstruction of an infected kidney or calyx but may follow bacteremia. The classic manifestations of these infections are fever and flank pain, often with frequency, urgency, and dysuria. Intrarenal and perinephric abscesses, however, differ from pyelonephritis because symptoms do not respond to appropriate antimicrobial therapy or do so more slowly. With intrarenal and perinephric abscesses the urine sediment may be normal, and cultures of the urine and blood may not yield S. aureus. The diagnosis is suspected by the findings of intravenous pyelography, computed tomography, or ultrasonography, and it is confirmed by needle aspiration of the abscess and microscopic examination of the aspirate.

Toxin-mediated diseases caused by Staphylococcus aureus include scalded skin syndrome, toxic shock syndrome (TSS), and food poisoning. Scalded skin syndrome, an exfoliative dermatitis, occurs in infants infected with a strain of S. aureus that produces exfoliative toxin. The illness begins abruptly with erythema, followed in 2 to 3 days by the formation of flaccid bullae which slough, leaving moist denuded areas that eventually resolve completely.

TSS is a multisystem disease of persons who have no antibodies to TSST-1 and are colonized or infected with strains of Staphylococcus aureus that produce that toxin, or rarely enterotoxin B or C. The illness is most common in women 15 to 25 years of age who use tampons during menstruation, an association first recognized in 1980 (11). The syndrome also may be unrelated to menstruation, as in women in the postpartum period or persons who have surgical wounds or other focal infections or who have undergone a surgical procedure in the nose or sinuses (3–5,11,12). TSS begins abruptly with fever, myalgias, vomiting, and diarrhea, soon followed by hypotension, hypovolemic shock, and shortly by an erythematous rash that frequently involves the palms and soles and desquamates in 1 to 2 weeks. The diagnosis of TSS is confirmed if (1) all of the major criteria—fever (38.8° C or

Table 28–2. Minor Criteria for Toxic Shock Syndrome

Organ System	Clinical or Laboratory Findings
Gastrointestinal	Vomiting or diarrhea at onset
Musculoskeletal	Severe myalgias; >two fold increase in CPK
Mucous membranes	Hyperemia of vagina, pharynx, or conjunctiva
Renal	>Twofold increase in BUN and creatinine; >5 WBC per high-power field in urine sediment in the absence of a urinary tract infection
Hepatic	>Twofold increase in bilirubin and transaminases
Hematologic	Platelets <100,000/μl
Central nervous system	Disorientation, altered consciousness without focal neurologic signs

Key: CPK, creatinine phosphokinase; BUN, blood urea nitrogen; WBC, white blood cells.

greater), rash, skin desquamation, hypotension—and three or more of the minor criteria (Table 28–2) are present; (2) cultures of the throat (for group A Streptococcus), blood, and cerebrospinal fluid demonstrate no pathogens other than S. aureus; and (3) serologic tests fail to demonstrate Rocky Mountain spotted fever, leptospirosis, or measles (11). Isolation of S. aureus from any site is not required. Full recovery is the rule, although repeated episodes may occur.

Since May 1980 the total number of cases of TSS reported annually to the Centers for Disease Control has decreased substantially (Fig. 28–2), owing primarily to the decline in the number of cases associated with menstruation (13). Factors that contribute to the lower prevalence of menstruation-associated TSS include manufacturers reducing the absorbency of tampons, increased public awareness, and, possibly, a change in tampon composition.

Staphylococcal food poisoning follows ingestion of foods contaminated with preformed enterotoxin produced by Staphylococcus aureus. The illness—nausea, vomiting, abdominal cramps, and watery diarrhea—generally occurs in epidemics 2 to 6 hours after contaminated food is ingested, especially custard-filled bakery goods, canned foods, processed meats, potato salad, and ice cream. Symptoms usually abate without treatment in 24 hours or less.

Staphylococcus epidermidis

Epidemiology

Staphylococcus epidermidis is the most prevalent and persistent of the Staphylococcus species that colonize human glabrous skin and mucous membranes. Most S. epidermidis infections are hospital acquired, resulting from contamination of a surgical site by organisms that colonize the patient or hospital personnel, although community-acquired infections occur.

Pathogenesis

In immunocompetent persons, Staphylococcus epidermidis has low virulence, but in immunocompromised persons and those who have indwelling foreign devices such as prosthetic heart valves or joints, cerebrospinal fluid shunts, and peritoneal or vascular catheters, it may cause serious infections (14). Foreign bodies become contaminated with S. epidermidis during surgical implantation or during bacteremia following the surgical procedure. The organisms colonize foreign bodies by hydrophobic binding, and to facilitate adherence some isolates of S. epidermidis produce a viscous extracellular polysaccharide substance called slime, which appears to be associated with virulence (15). The slime layer eventually completely covers the bacteria, forming a biofilm on the surface of

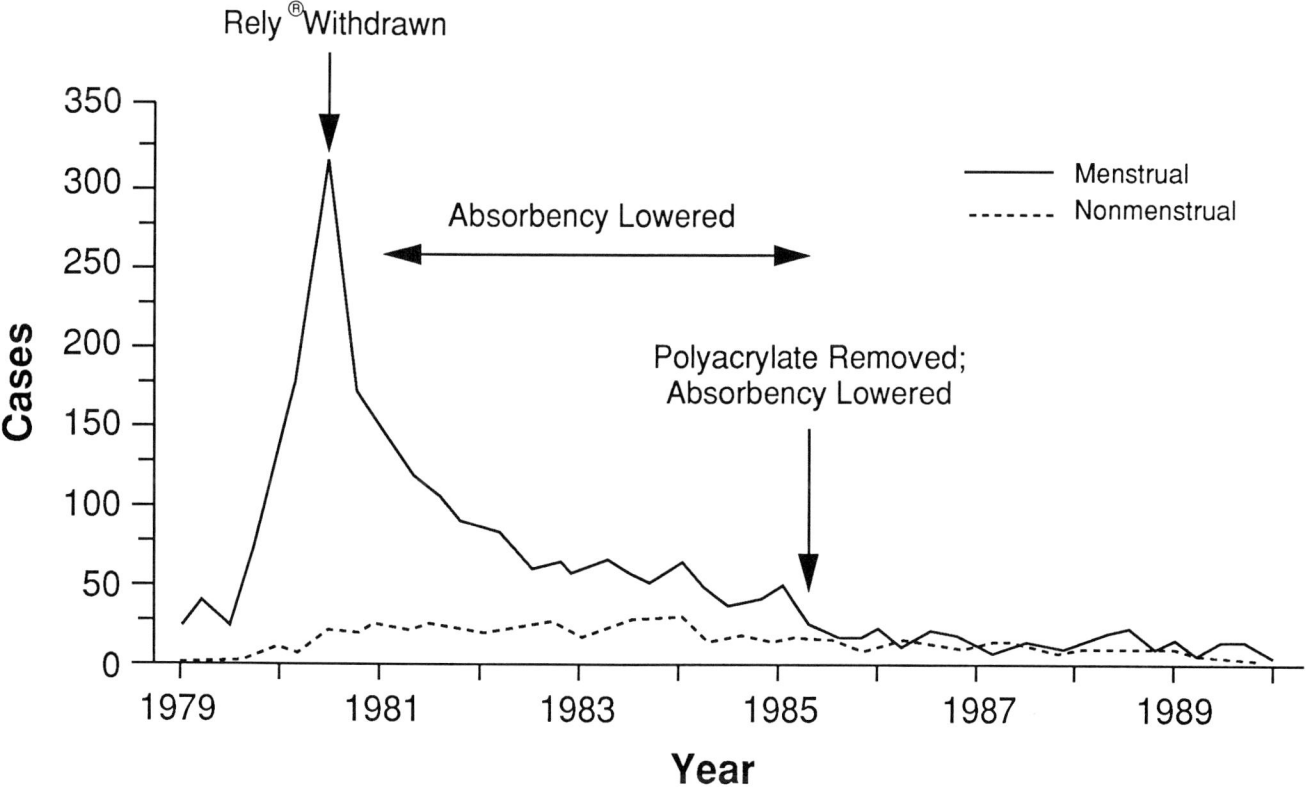

Fig. 28–2. Reported cases of toxic shock syndrome, by quarter, in the United States from January 1, 1979, to March 31, 1990. (From Centers for Disease Control: Reduced incidence of menstrual toxic shock syndrome—United States, 1980–1990. MMWR, 39:421, 1990).

the foreign material in which the organisms become embedded. This polysaccharide is believed to act as an ion-exchange resin for enhanced nutrition, to protect the bacteria from antimicrobial agents and host immune cells, to interfere with coagulation, neutrophil chemotaxis, and bactericidal activity, and to potentiate further adherence of bacteria (16–18).

Clinical Manifestations

Staphylococcus epidermidis is the most common cause of infections of foreign devices (intravascular catheters, cerebrospinal fluid shunts, prosthetic cardiac valves and joints, and vascular grafts) and of endophthalmitis after a surgical procedure involving the eye (14,19–24). It also is an important cause of bacteremia in immunocompromised persons and of sternal osteomyelitis following cardiothoracic surgery (25–27). Moreover, S. epidermidis may cause urinary tract infections, principally in hospitalized persons aged 50 years or older who have a history of urinary tract complications. Cerebrospinal fluid shunt infections usually are manifested within 2 weeks of implantation, revision, or manipulation, by low-grade fever, shunt malfunction, or wound infection without signs of meningeal irritation. Infection of a prosthetic valve caused by S. epidermidis typically develops during the first year after its placement, and because the infection may involve the sewing ring, complications of dehiscence, dysrhythmia from extension of the infection into the conducting system, or obstruction of the valve orifice from overgrowth of the vegetation are common. Manifestations of valve dysfunction and fever in the absence of peripheral emboli and of multiple positive blood cultures are common.

Infections of joints with prostheses due to Staphylococcus epidermidis commonly manifest more than 1 year after implantation by pain in the involved joint, and (in fewer than 50% of cases) fever, swelling, joint dislocation, and draining fistulae develop. Infections of vascular grafts caused by S. epidermidis typically develop in the late postoperative period and are characterized by anastomotic aneurysms and pseudoaneurysms, inguinal sinus tracts, and vasculoenteric fistulas.

Staphylococcus saprophyticus

Epidemiology and Pathogenesis

Staphylococcus saprophyticus transiently colonizes the skin of the periurethra and the mucosa of the urethra, colonization aided by specific oligosaccharide receptors on its cell membrane that allow selective adherence to urothelial cells. Moreover, some isolates of S. saprophyticus produce an extracellular enzyme complex that inhibits growth of other bacteria.

Clinical Manifestations

Staphylococcus saprophyticus is a common cause of cystitis, characterized by urinary frequency, urgency, and dysuria, in sexually active young women. The organism may cause pyelonephritis and is a rare cause of endocarditis (28).

Stomatococcus

The only species of Stomatococcus that causes human disease is Stomatococcus mucilaginosus, which is part of the normal flora of the oral cavity and upper respiratory tract. S. mucilaginosus is an uncommon human pathogen but has been recovered from the blood of persons who have endocarditis and septicemia (29,30).

Laboratory Diagnosis

Specimens for diagnosis of infections caused by staphylococci are listed in Table 28–3; Stomatococcus mucilaginosus typically is recovered from blood cultures. Specimen collection, transport, and processing are discussed in Part III. Identifying features of the different species, antimicrobial susceptibility testing, and epidemiologic typing are reviewed here.

Organism Identification

Staphylococcus aureus. After overnight incubation colonies of S. aureus typically are smooth, convex, about 1 to 3 mm in diameter, often yellow to orange, and on blood agar most are surrounded by a zone of complete hemolysis (Plate IIB). Fewer than 1% of isolates exhibit diminished growth on culture media not supplemented with essential nutrients (hemin, menadione, thiamine, pantothenate), producing "dwarf" or "G" colonies that often are nonhemolytic and may "satellite" around other bacteria in mixed culture (31,32).

Several tests differentiate Staphylococcus aureus from the remaining species of Staphylococcus (Table 28–4). S. aureus produces coagulase, an enzyme that binds plasma fibrinogen, causing the organisms to agglutinate or plasma to clot; almost all other species of Staphylococcus do not. More than 95% of isolates to S. aureus are identified by the slide coagulase test (Appendix, Procedure 10), which detects cell-bound enzyme (clumping factor), and almost all isolates are identified by the tube coagulase test (Appendix, Procedure 11), which detects free coagulase. The detection of thermostable DNase is especially useful for identifying S. aureus in blood culture broths containing gram-positive cocci in clusters (Plate IB) (33,34). Positive reactions with particle agglutination tests (latex beads or sensitized sheep red blood cells) that detect protein A, clumping factor, or both, rapidly identify S. aureus; however, these tests may yield false-positive results with isolates of Staphylococcus saprophyticus and species of Micrococcus and false-negative results with isolates of methicillin (oxacillin)-resistant Staphylococcus aureus, especially those that are also resistant to trimethoprim-sulfamethoxazole and rifampin (35–39). Staphylococcus intermedius, a rare cause of canine bite wounds in humans, also produces coagulase but is distinguished from Staphylococcus aureus by the fact that it produces the enzyme pyroglutamyl-β-naphthylamide aminopeptidase (detected by the PYR test, described later) and S. aureus does not (40).

A serum specimen for detection of antibodies to teichoic acid has questionable diagnostic value (41). The presence of these antibodies in the serum of persons who

Table 28–3. Infections Produced by Staphylococcus and Specimens Required for Diagnosis

Infection	Species	Specimens
Localized skin infection	S. aureus	Aspirated pus, vesicle fluid, swab of lesion
Wound infection	S. aureus	Aspirated pus, swab of lesion
Bacteremia	S. aureus S. epidermidis	Blood
Endocarditis	S. aureus S. epidermidis	Blood, vegetation, ? serum for teichoic acid antibodies (S. aureus)
Pneumonia	S. aureus	Sputum, transtracheal aspirate, bronchoalveolar lavage, blood, pleural fluid (if present)
Arthritis		
Native joint	S. aureus	Joint fluid
Prosthetic joint	S. epidermidis	Joint fluid, swab of prosthesis
Osteomyelitis	S. aureus	Needle aspiration, bone biopsy of radiographic lesion
Cerebrospinal fluid shunt infection*	S. epidermidis S. aureus	Blood, cerebrospinal fluid, peritoneal fluid
Intravascular catheter infection†	S. epidermidis S. aureus	Blood, catheter tip
Vascular graft infection	S. epidermidis S. aureus	Graft material, blood, abscess drainage
Peritoneal dialysis–associated peritonitis	S. epidermidis S. aureus	Peritoneal fluid
Ocular infections	S. epidermidis	Vitreous (needle aspiration)
Urinary tract infection	S. saprophyticus S. epidermidis S. aureus	Urine
Scalded skin syndrome	S. aureus	Swab of nasopharynx, skin
Toxic shock syndrome‡	S. aureus	?Swab of vagina, surgical site, wound, antibodies to TSST-1
Food poisoning	S. aureus	Potentially contaminated food, gastric contents, vomitus

* Cerebrospinal fluid should be collected through the shunt and via lumbar puncture; blood and peritoneal fluid are collected from ventriculoatrial and ventriculoperitoneal shunts, respectively.
† Blood should be collected through the potentially infected catheter and from a peripheral uncatheterized vein.
‡ Diagnosis is based on clinical criteria (see text) and the exclusion of infection with group A Streptococcus, Rocky Mountain spotted fever, leptospirosis, and measles.

Table 28–4. Tests to Differentiate Staphylococcus Aureus from Other Staphylococci

Test	Comments
Coagulase	
Slide test	Identifies >95% of S. aureus; detects cell-bound coagulase (clumping factor); results available in seconds
Tube test	Identifies almost all S. aureus; detects free coagulase; results available in 18 hours
Thermostable DNase	Useful for testing blood culture broths; results available in 2–4 hours
Particle agglutination	Detects protein A and/or clumping factor; results available in seconds; false-positive results may occur with S. saprophyticus and micrococci; false-negative results may occur with methicillin-resistant isolates

not required, detection of the toxin, and failure to detect antitoxin antibodies in serum, confirm the diagnosis. Currently, tests to detect TSST-1 and anti-TSST-1 antibodies are not commercially available, so specimens must be sent to a specialized reference laboratory.

Coagulase-Negative Species of Staphylococcus. Colonies of Staphylococcus epidermidis are white and nonhemolytic on blood agar; those of Staphylococcus saprophyticus are nonhemolytic and often become yellow to orange with age. To identify the coagulase-negative staphylococci, isolates first must be differentiated from species of Micrococcus (see Table 28–1), which produce nonhemolytic colonies that are bright yellow and smooth or white and sticky. Then, conventional biochemical tests such as those proposed by Kloos and Schleifer or by Herbert and coworkers (Fig. 28–3) or commercially available kit systems may be used (42–47). Isolates of coagulase-negative staphylococci from urine that are resistant to novobiocin (Appendix, Procedure 12) presumptively are called S. saprophyticus. Other novobiocin-resistant coagulase-negative species of Staphylococcus—Staphylococcus cohnii, Staphylococcus lentus, Staphylococcus sciuri, and Staphylococcus xylosus—rarely are isolated from humans.

Stomatococcus. Characteristics that distinguish Stomatococcus from Staphylococcus and Micrococcus are listed in Table 28–1. Colonies of Stomatococcus mucilaginosus are white, nonhemolytic on blood agar, and often mucoid and adherent to the agar surface. Isolates are differentiated from enterococci and from group D streptococci (described later) by their inability to grow in media containing 6.5% NaCl and by their failure to agglutinate with group D serologic typing reagents, respectively. Additional biochemical reactions useful for identifying Stomatococcus are described elsewhere (29,30).

Susceptibility Testing

Susceptibility testing (see Chapter 24) should be performed on all clinically significant isolates of Staphylococcus and Stomatococcus mucilaginosus. Most isolates of Staphylococcus aureus and many of the coagulase-negative species of Staphylococcus produce β-lactamase and therefore are resistant to penicillin, a characteristic usu-

have Staphylococcus aureus bacteremia has been used as a marker of deep-seated invasive disease, but as many as 20% of persons who have S. aureus–induced bacteremia and antiteichoic acid antibodies do not have deep-seated disease. Moreover, antiteichoic acid antibodies may not be detected in as many as half of persons who have complicated bacteremia or endocarditis caused by S. aureus, especially those who are immunosuppressed.

The diagnosis of TSS is based on clinical criteria (described earlier) after excluding infection with group A Streptococcus, Rocky Mountain spotted fever, leptospirosis, and measles. Although isolation of Staphylococcus aureus to determine whether it produces TSST-1 is

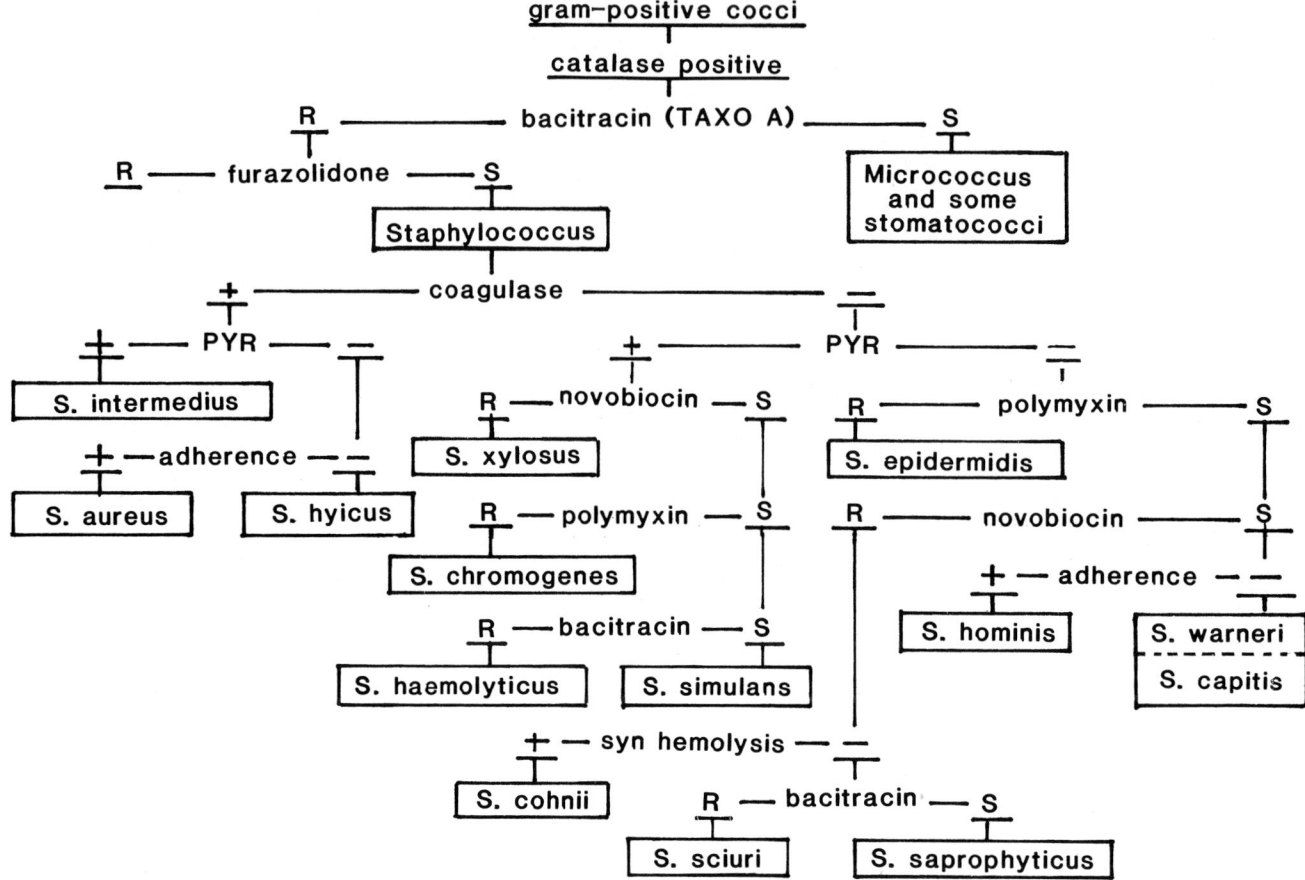

Fig. 28–3. Criteria for identification of coagulase-negative staphylococci and some other members of the Micrococcaceae. R and S indicate resistant and susceptible organisms, as defined by Herbert and coworkers, not by a standardized susceptibility test. (From Herbert, GA, et al.: Characteristics of coagulase-negative staphylococci that help differentiate these species and other members of the family Micrococcaceae. J. Clin. Microbiol., 26: 1939, 1988.)

ally detected by broth microdilution testing using an inoculum of 3 to 5 × 10^5 cfu/ml, or by disk diffusion testing. For occasional isolates, however, β-lactamase production must be induced by exposing the organism to a penicillin: a blood agar plate is inoculated with the organism and a 1-μg oxacillin disk is applied to the surface. After overnight incubation at 35° C, β-lactamase production is detected by rubbing growth from the edge of the zone of inhibition on a moistened nitrocefin filter paper disk (commercially available) and observing for the development of a red color within 30 minutes (discussed in more detail in Chapter 24). Testing for inducible β-lactamase is recommended for isolates whose penicillin minimum inhibitory concentration (MIC) is 0.06 to 0.25 μg/ml.

Resistance to the penicillinase-resistant penicillins (methicillin, oxacillin, nafcillin) was recognized in Great Britain in coagulase-negative species of Staphylococcus, and shortly thereafter—in the early 1960s—in Staphylococcus aureus, but it did not become a problem in the United States until the late 1970s (48,49). Because resistance to these agents typically is heterogenous, meaning that only rare cells (1 in 10^4 to 10^8) express the resistance trait, specific guidelines must be followed to detect resistant isolates (48): (1) An inoculum equal to the turbidity of a 0.5 McFarland standard should be prepared in 0.85% sterile saline directly from overnight growth on a blood agar plate for disk diffusion and microdilution testing. (2) Mueller-Hinton agar plates and a 1-μg oxacillin disk should be used for disk diffusion testing. (3) Oxacillin in cation (calcium and magnesium)-supplemented Mueller-Hinton broth containing 2% sodium chloride should be used for microdilution testing. (4) Agar plates and microtiter trays should be incubated a full 24 hours at 35° C. To screen for oxacillin resistance, Mueller-Hinton agar supplemented with 4% sodium chloride and containing 6 μg/ml oxacillin is spot inoculated with a cotton swab that has been dipped into the inoculum solution prepared as described above, and plates are incubated at 35° C for 24 hours, under which conditions only resistant isolates grow.

Epidemiologic Typing

Occasionally, epidemiologic typing of staphylococcal isolates is desirable. Bacteriophage typing and plasmid profiles are most useful for Staphylococcus aureus, and biotyping, antibiograms, and plasmid profiles are used to type Staphylococcus epidermidis.

Treatment

The treatment of infections caused by Staphylococcus organisms depends on the species and the location and severity of the infection. Superficial infections and uncomplicated urinary tract infections are adequately controlled with oral antimicrobial therapy, whereas serious, invasive infections require parenterally administered antimicrobial agents. Infected intravascular devices, shunts, and prostheses generally must be removed, and abscesses must be drained in addition to providing appropriate antimicrobial therapy.

Serious infections caused by Staphylococcus aureus initially are treated with a penicillinase-resistant penicillin such as oxacillin or nafcillin, because most isolates produce β-lactamase; however, if the organism is susceptible penicillin should be used. Patients infected with an isolate of S. aureus that is resistant to the penicillinase-resistant penicillins must be placed in strict isolation and treated with vancomycin. Isolates of Staphylococcus epidermidis generally are more resistant than Staphylococcus aureus to antimicrobial agents, including the penicillinase-resistant penicillins, so infections with these organisms often require vancomycin therapy, but spatial isolation of the patient is not necessary. Recently, vancomycin-resistant isolates of coagulase-negative staphylococci have been reported (50,51). Alternative therapy for such organisms is limited, but daptomycin may be effective (52). Staphylococcus saprophyticus generally responds to antimicrobial agents commonly used to treat urinary tract infections, such as ampicillin or trimethoprim-sulfamethoxazole, but it is resistant to nalidixic acid.

STREPTOCOCCACEAE

The family Streptococcaceae has seven genera. Streptococcus and Enterococcus are encountered frequently in the clinical microbiology laboratory and are discussed in detail. Aerococcus, Leuconostoc, Pediococcus, and Lactococcus, which rarely cause human disease, are reviewed briefly. Members of the genus Gemella are not known to be human pathogens and are not discussed further.

Streptococcus

Species of Streptococcus are facultative anaerobes, although some are microaerophilic and grow better anaerobically. The medially important species of Streptococcus ferment glucose to lactic acid (they are homofermentative). In smears prepared from broth cultures and stained with Gram stain, streptococci usually form chains (Plate IIC) and may elongate under certain conditions, appearing as gram-positive bacilli rather than cocci. Streptococci are classified according to the specific cell wall carbohydrates identified by Rebecca Lancefield, designated with capital letters, and the pattern of hemolysis on sheep blood agar (53,54). Complete hemolysis of blood around the colony (Plate IID) is referred to as β hemolysis; partial hemolysis or "greening of the agar" (Plate IIE) as α hemolysis, and no hemolysis as γ hemolysis.

Group A Streptococcus (Streptococcus pyogenes)

Epidemiology

Pharyngitis caused by group A streptococci is most common in children attending school, during winter months. Transmission occurs by aerosol droplets or intimate contact with secretions from persons who have the disease or from asymptomatic carriers, and correlates with the number of persons per room in a family's living quarters (55). Outbreaks of pharyngitis due to group A streptococci have been linked to contaminated food and milk (56). Streptococcal pyoderma (impetigo) occurs predominantly in children during the late summer and early fall in temperate climates. The exact mechanism of transmission is unknown, but insects such as mosquitoes and flies are suspected vectors.

Nonsuppurative sequelae may follow pharyngitis or pyoderma caused by group A streptoccci. Acute rheumatic fever occurs most commonly in children and young adults as a complication only of pharyngitis, although nearly a third of those affected give no history of recent sore throat. The prevalence of acute rheumatic fever peaked in northern Europe during the 1880s, when the major manifestations of the syndrome, which occurred predominantly among the lower socioeconomic groups, were first defined clearly, and after the turn of the century it began to decline slowly, suggesting that factors other than penicillin (such as improved living conditions) may have been responsible for modifying the disease before the discovery of antibiotics (57). The reappearance of acute rheumatic fever in the United States began in 1985 in several geographic areas. Outbreaks occurred in relatively affluent communities in Utah, Ohio, and Pennsylvania and among military recruits in California and Missouri (58–63). Acute poststreptococcal glomerulonephritis may follow cutaneous or pharyngeal infections with group A streptococci of specific M protein types (including 1–4,12,15,49,55,57,59–61), known as nephritogenic strains.

Pathogenesis

Streptococcal cell wall components and extracellular products (enzymes and toxins) and host responses are involved in the pathogenesis of infections caused by Streptococcus pyogenes. The most significant bacterial factor is the cell wall M protein, which prevents phagocytosis of the organism. Antibodies against the specific M protein confer lifelong type-specific immunity; however, because over 60 M protein types exist, infection with a group A Streptococcus that possesses a different M protein may occur. Another important cell wall component is lipoteichoic acid, which permits bacterial adherence to respiratory tract epithelium.

Streptococcus pyogenes elaborates about 20 extracellular products, including enzymes (streptolysins, hyaluronidase, streptokinase, deoxyribonucleases [DNases], and nicotinamide adenine dinucleotidase [NADase]) and erythrogenic toxins. Streptolysin O, an antigenic, oxygen-labile enzyme, produces subsurface β hemolysis on blood agar plates; and streptolysin S, a nonantigenic, oxygen-stable enzyme, produces surface β hemolysis. Neither streptolysin has a proven role in the pathogenesis of human disease. Streptokinase, an enzyme that promotes fibrinolytic activity by converting plasminogen to plasmin, and hyaluronidase may enhance the spread of the organism through connective tissue. The pathogenic significance of the DNases and of NADase is unknown. Serologic tests to detect antibodies to streptolysin O, streptokinase, and DNase B are useful in diagnosing nonsuppurative complications (described earlier) of group A streptococcal infections.

Pyrogenic (erythrogenic) toxins (serotypes A, B, C), produced by isolates of Streptococcus pyogenes infected with a specific temperate bacteriophage, are immunologically distinct proteins that share toxic properties, including pyrogenicity (due to direct action on the hypothalamus), enhancement of susceptibility to lethal shock, and in animal models of infection liver and myocardial damage (64). In the past these toxins were believed to be responsible for the rash of scarlet fever (described later), though more recently it has been proposed that the rash is a hypersensitivity response, depending on an interplay between host cellular and humoral factors (65). From the seventeenth century to the early 1900s, most strains of S. pyogenes associated with scarlet fever produced type A pyrogenic toxin, and epidemics caused by these organisms were accompanied by high mortality rates (5 to 25%). Between 1976 and 1986, strains of S. pyogenes that were tested produced either type B toxin or both types B and C, and the severity of nonbacteremic infections with group A Streptococcus was attenuated, possibly reflecting the virtual disappearance of type A pyrogenic toxin. Recently, however, severe soft-tissue infections associated with a toxic shock–like syndrome due to strains of S. pyogenes producing pyrogenic toxin A have been reported (66–68).

The pathogenesis of acute rheumatic fever is not fully understood (69). Certain M protein types of Streptococcus pyogenes may be rheumatogenic. A type 18 M protein strain was isolated during the recent outbreaks of acute rheumatic fever, during an outbreak in the United States in 1968, and from several cases in Great Britain in the early 1970s (70). The presence of complexes of immunoglobulin and the C3 component of complement along the sarcolemmal sheaths of cardiac myofibers from persons with rheumatic carditis suggests that myocarditis results from the production of antibodies directed against a streptococcal cell wall M protein that cross-reacts with myocardial tissue. Moreover, a heart- or tissue cross-reactive antigen of S. pyogenes that shares immunologic epitopes with but is distinct from the M protein recently was identified (71).

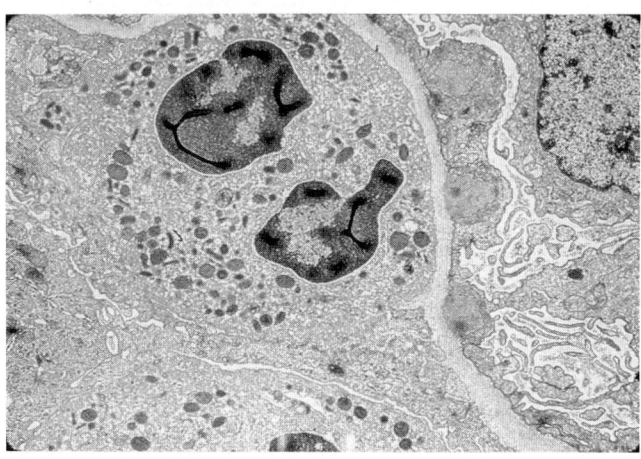

Fig. 28–5. Electron micrograph of the subepithelial immune deposits of poststreptococcal acute glomerulonephritis.

The renal damage in acute glomerulonephritis (Fig. 28–4) is caused by deposits of circulating streptococcal-antistreptococcal immune complexes in the glomeruli (Fig. 28–5) and the subsequent activation of complement. Cell-mediated reactions to an altered glomerular basement membrane or activation of the alternate complement pathway also may be involved.

Clinical Manifestations

Typically, pharyngitis caused by group A Streptococcus is manifested as fever, sore throat, exudative tonsillitis, and tender regional lymphadenopathy, but symptoms may be minimal. Pharyngitis may be accompanied by scarlet fever, a punctate exanthem overlying diffuse erythema that usually appears first on the neck or upper chest, becomes generalized, and then desquamates. Erythema of the tongue (strawberry tongue) and lymphadenopathy also may be present.

Skin infections due to group A Streptococcus include cellulitis, erysipelas, and pyoderma. Cellulitis is characterized by fever, with pain and erythema of the involved area. Erysipelas is an acute inflammation of the skin with prominent lymphangitis, accompanied by fever, chills, and systemic toxicity. It begins as a localized area of erythema and swelling and spreads rapidly with a raised, discrete red border that demarcates normal and affected skin. The infection generally affects the face of infants and persons over age 30 years, who frequently give a history

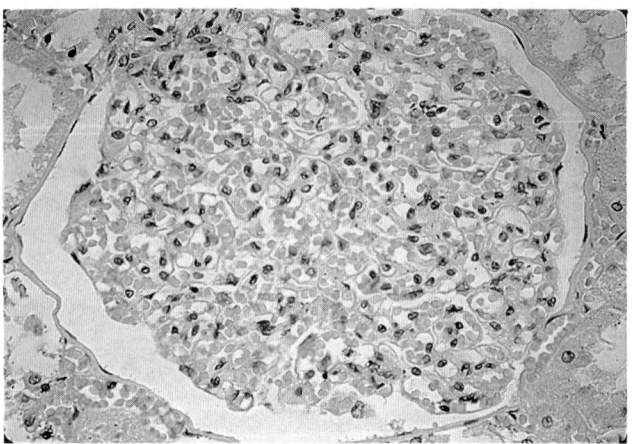

Fig. 28–4. Micrograph of hypercellular glomerulus of poststreptococcal acute glomerulonephritis (hematoxylin and eosin, ×100).

of a recent episode of streptococcal pharyngitis, but it may involve a surgical site or wound on the trunk or extremities. Pyoderma (impetigo) has a clinical presentation identical to that of Staphylococcus aureus impetigo (discussed earlier).

In the soft tissues, group A Streptococcus may cause type II necrotizing fasciitis, a rare, life-threatening form of gangrene. The infection, which usually occurs at a site of trauma on an extremity but occasionally develops without an obvious portal of entry, begins as a local painful area of erythema and edema. In a few days the skin becomes dusky; bullae containing yellow to red-black fluid rupture and become covered by necrotic debris. The infection may spread along fascial planes, and bacteremia and death may ensue if appropriate antimicrobial therapy is not administered promptly.

A toxic shock–like syndrome recently has been described in persons with soft tissue infections such as cellulitis and necrotizing fasciitis or bacteremia with group A Streptococcus (66–68). The mortality rate for this multisystem disease manifested by shock, renal impairment, and respiratory distress, with or without a rash, can be as high as 30%.

Acute rheumatic fever, characterized by carditis (Fig. 28–6 and 28–7), polyarthritis, chorea, erythema marginatum, subcutaneous nodules, or a combination of these, develops 1 to 5 weeks (average, 19 days) after group A streptococcal sore throat. To assist in diagnosis, guidelines known as the Jones Criteria have been established (Table 28–5). Given two major or one major and two minor criteria, plus evidence of a recent group A streptococcal infection (increased antistreptolysin O or anti-DNase B antibody titers, positive throat culture, or scarlet fever), acute rheumatic fever is highly probable.

Acute glomerulonephritis, manifested by fatigue, malaise, weakness, edema, hypertension, and smoky or rust-colored urine, generally without fever, develops 10 days to 3 weeks after group A streptococcal pharyngitis or pyoderma.

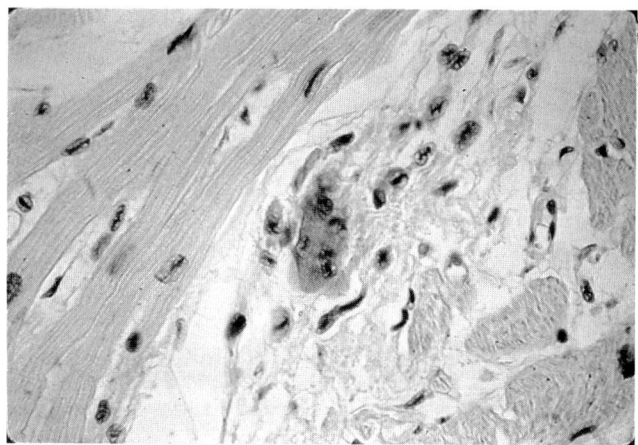

Fig. 28–7. Aschoff body characteristic of the myocarditis of acute rheumatic fever (hematoxylin and eosin, ×157.5).

Group B Streptococcus (Streptococcus agalactiae)

Epidemiology

Five serotypes of group B Streptococcus are recognized: Ia, Ib, Ic, II, and III. Serotypes Ia and III, which, respectively, have a predilection for the respiratory tract and central nervous system, most often are associated with neonatal disease. Group B Streptococcus is part of the normal flora of the pharynx, lower gastrointestinal tract, and vagina. It is present without producing symptoms in the vagina of 5 to 40% of pregnant women; however, the lower gastrointestinal tract most likely is the principal reservoir for the organism (72–74).

Vertical transmission of group B Streptococcus from mother to infant occurs in utero by the ascending route or during delivery, resulting in colonization of the newborn's mucous membranes. From 30 to 70% (average, 50%) of colonized women transmit the organism to their infants. Infants born to heavily colonized mothers are at increased risk of developing early-onset invasive disease (within the first 5 days of life), and infants who become heavily colonized are more likely to develop early-onset or late-onset disease (from age 6 days to 3 months). Factors that favor early-onset disease in infants born to colonized mothers are prolonged (over 24 hours) or premature rupture of membranes, multiple births, maternal fever, and amnionitis. Moreover, data from a recent study showed that blacks are at increased risk of disease (75). Less commonly, horizontal (nosocomial) transmission of group B Streptococcus to neonates occurs in the nursery, espe-

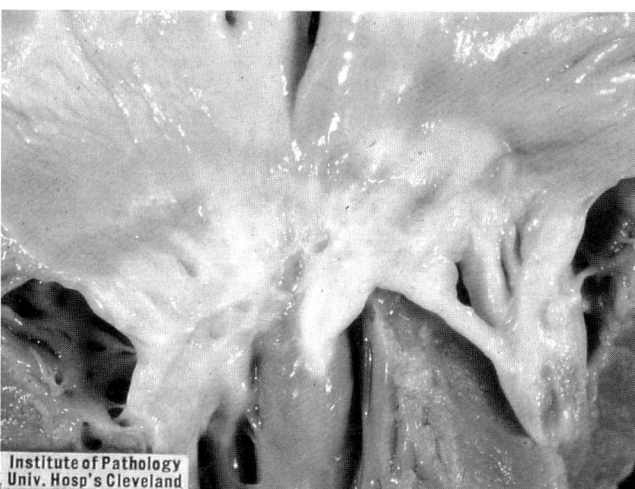

Fig. 28–6. "Old" rheumatic heart disease: Thickening of the leaflets of the mitral valve and the attached chordae tendineae.

Table 28–5. Modified Jones Criteria for Diagnosing Acute Rheumatic Fever

Criteria	Findings
Major	Polyarthritis, carditis, chorea, erythema marginatum, subcutaneous nodules
Minor	Clinical: History of rheumatic fever or rheumatic heart disease, arthralgias, fever
	Laboratory: Accelerated sedimentation rate, increased C-reactive protein, leukocytosis, prolonged PR interval

cially when maternal colonization rates are high, nursery conditions crowded, and hand-washing techniques poor.

The incidence of early-onset infection with group B Streptococcus ranges from 0.7 to 3.7 per 1000 live births (average, 2.0 per 1000) (76–78). Attack rates, inversely proportional to birth weight, may exceed 20 per 1000 live births among infants who weigh less than 1 kg. The incidence of late-onset neonatal infection with group B Streptococcus is about 1 per 1000 live births.

Pathogenesis

Neonatal factors that increase susceptibility to invasive group B streptococcal infection are a low level or no type-specific antibodies to group B Streptococcus and low levels of the complement components C1q and C4, which correlate with deficient bactericidal activity (79). Bacterial virulence factors that may contribute to the host-parasite interaction that determines the outcome of infections caused by group B Streptococcus are the amount of capsular material elaborated, the unique capsular structure, and the production of extracellular enzymes such as neuraminidase. Moreover, the presence of the γ antigen of the c protein (a protein associated with certain type-specific carbohydrates, principally type Ib but also Ia and II) appears to be a virulence factor in strains that cause early-onset sepsis (80).

Clinical Manifestations

Persons of all ages may develop infection with group B Streptococcus, but the majority are neonates (81). Approximately a third of neonates with early-onset infection have bacteremia but no identifiable focus of infection, another third have pneumonia, and the remainder have meningitis. Affected infants present with lethargy, anorexia, jaundice, abnormal temperature, and respiratory distress. About 50% of those who have meningitis develop seizures within 24 hours of onset. Mortality ranges from 13 to 37% (82). Neonates with late-onset infection most commonly have bacteremia with meningitis, although bacteremia may occur without a focus of infection. The mortality rate is less than 20%, and 25 to 50% of survivors have permanent neurologic sequelae (82).

In adults, most infections caused by group B Streptococcus occur postpartum and include endometritis, wound infections associated with cesarean section, and urinary tract infections. Bacteremia occurs in elderly persons with underlying diseases such as diabetes mellitus, peripheral vascular disease, liver disease, and malignancies. Group B Streptococcus also may cause skin and soft tissue infections, pneumonia, endocarditis, meningitis, arthritis, and osteomyelitis.

Streptococcus pneumoniae

Epidemiology

Streptococcus pneumoniae is the most common cause of acute community-acquired bacterial pneumonia. Approximately 2 cases per 1000 population (150,000 to 300,000 cases) of pneumococcal pneumonia occur annually in the United States, and the incidence is higher among closed populations such as the military, and in certain occupational groups such as painters and welders. Those most susceptible to pneumococcal pneumonia include infants and elders, owing to the weaker immune defenses at the extremes of age; persons who have an underlying disease such as chronic lung or heart disorders, diabetes mellitus, and chronic alcoholism; persons who lack a spleen; and those with impaired immunoglobulin production or defective opsonic factors, as occurs with multiple myeloma and sickle cell disease, respectively.

Streptococcus pneumoniae is normal flora of the upper respiratory tract of 25 to 50% of preschool children and nearly 20% of adults, who are termed carriers (83). Its spread is enhanced by upper respiratory tract infections and crowding, which explains the winter peak of pneumococcal infections. Pneumococcal pneumonia, however, is a disease of carriers, and cases occur sporadically throughout the year. Epidemics are uncommon but have been reported (84).

Pathogenesis

Pneumococcal pneumonia develops when the host immune defenses are impaired. Most cases are endogenous, following aspiration of oral secretions containing normal flora that includes Streptococcus pneumoniae. Person-to-person transmission during epidemics occurs by droplet aerosols. Impairment of the cough reflex or mucociliary action then predisposes the lower respiratory tract to invasion by aspirated or inhaled bacteria. In the alveolar spaces S. pneumoniae provokes an outpouring of edema fluid and neutrophil recruitment.

The major virulence factor of Streptococcus pneumoniae is its antiphagocytic polysaccharide capsule, and strains that have a thick, mucoid capsule, such as type 3, are especially virulent. Opsonization of cells of S. pneumoniae by complement and IgG promotes phagocytosis, and IgG provides lifelong type-specific immunity. In adults, pneumonia usually involves one or more complete lobes (lobar); but in infants, young children, and elders the process is often patchy and peribronchial (bronchopneumonia). Infection with an especially virulent strain such as type 3 may result in cavity formation (Fig. 28–8). From the primary (pulmonary) focus, S. pneumoniae may spread to the pleural cavity or pericardium or enter the blood and seed the meninges, heart valves, or joints.

Clinical Manifestations

Classically, pneumococcal pneumonia begins abruptly with fever, productive cough, and chest pain; but in elderly or debilitated persons the illness may have an insidious onset with low-grade or no fever, mental obtundation and signs of congestive heart failure.

In all age groups, Streptococcus pneumoniae is a major cause of acute pyogenic meningitis, beginning abruptly with fever, headache, nuchal rigidity, nausea, and vomiting. Vasculitis of meningeal vessels may result in altered consciousness. Mortality approaches 80% in infants and elders. S. pneumoniae may produce spontaneous bacteremia in persons who lack a spleen and in persons infected with human immunodeficiency virus, and the organism is

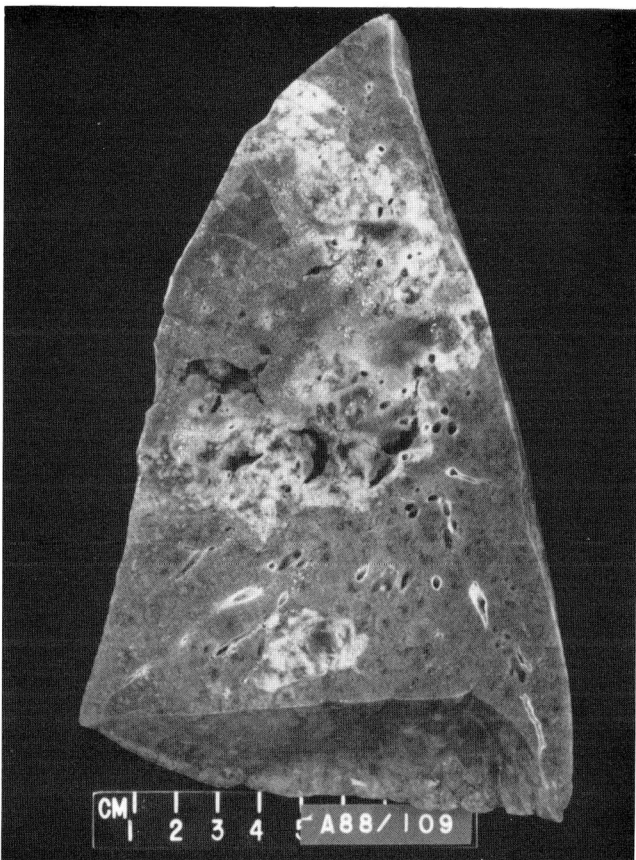

Fig. 28–8. Lung involved with cavitary pneumonia caused by Streptococcus pneumoniae type 3.

an important cause of otitis media, sinusitis, mastoiditis, endocarditis, and spontaneous peritonitis.

Nonhemolytic (Viridans) Streptococci

Epidemiology and Pathogenesis

The nonhemolytic streptococci are a heterogeneous group of organisms that do not produce clear zones on sheep blood agar (meaning they are not β hemolytic) (except some isolates of Streptococcus anginosus). Because many isolates produce greenish discoloration on blood agar, this group of organisms also is called the viridans streptococci. Most of these organisms do not react with Lancefield grouping sera, except the β-hemolytic strains of S. anginosus, which react with Lancefield A, C, F, or G antiserum, and Streptococcus bovis, which reacts with Lancefield D antiserum. The nonhemolytic streptococci are a major component of the normal oral and gastrointestinal flora but can cause disease and death, especially when they enter normally sterile sites. Characteristics of the most common nonhemolytic streptococci are shown in Table 28–6 (85).

Clinical Manifestations

Bacterial endocarditis is the most common serious infection caused by the viridans streptococci, which are the agents of nearly half of all valve infections (86). The infection, characterized by fever, fatigue, weight loss, sweats, arthralgias, and peripheral embolic phenomena involving the central nervous system, spleen, skin, and eye, affects persons with underlying valvular heart disease, follows an indolent and protracted course, and has a cure rate of over 90%. Cerebral emboli, most commonly involving the middle cerebral artery and its branches, occur in about one third of all cases. Infarcts of the spleen, reported in over 40% of cases of endocarditis seen at autopsy, rarely are detected clinically. Cutaneous or conjunctival petechiae develop in 20 to 40% of cases. Other peripheral cutaneous findings include Osler's nodes (characterized microscopically by intimal proliferation of dermal arterioles, venules, and capillaries, occasionally accompanied by immune complex deposition, thrombosis and necrosis, and a perivascular infiltrate of neutrophils and monocytes) and Janeway lesions (subcutaneous abscesses due to septic emboli). Roth spots in the nerve fiber layer of the retina consist of aggregates of lymphocytes surrounded by edema and hemorrhage. Cardiac murmurs are audible in more than 85% of cases, although changing murmurs are unusual, and congestive heart failure due to valvular dysfunction may develop. Typical abnormal laboratory test results include an elevated sedimentation rate, anemia, and microscopic hematuria.

Table 28–6. Characteristics of the Common Viridans Streptococci

Species of Streptococcus	Sites of Colonization	Associated Diseases	Virulence Factors	Comments
S. anginosus	Mouth, gastrointestinal tract, vagina	Abscesses (liver, brain, joints, other spaces), neonatal sepsis	Production of hydrolytic enzymes	Phenotypically heterogeneous,* three biotypes
S. bovis	Gastrointestinal	Bacteremia, endocarditis (esp. in adults with tumor in GIT)	?	Normal flora of 5–10% of normal adults and larger percentage of adults with colon cancer
S. mitis	Mouth	Endocarditis	Production of glucans	
S. sanguis	Mouth	Endocarditis	Production of glucans	
S. mutans	Mouth	Dental caries, endocarditis	Production of glucans	Group of seven species†
S. salivarius	Mouth	Rare	?	
S. vestibularis	Mouth	Rare	?	New species

* Includes S. constellatus, S. intermedius, Streptococcus MG, group F, S. milleri, and minute hemolytic strains.
† S. mutans, S. rattus, S. cricetus, S. sobrinus, S. ferus, S. macacae, S. downei.

The viridans streptococci, predominantly Streptococcus anginosus, are the micro-organisms most frequently recovered from brain abscesses, which cause symptoms of a space-occupying mass: headache, impaired mental status, focal neurologic findings, nausea, vomiting, and seizures. Moreover, they are frequently isolated from abscesses of the lung, liver, pancreas, and abdominal cavity.

Other Streptococcus Species

Group C and group G streptococci are normal flora of the upper respiratory and gastrointestinal tract of many animals and may be found in the human pharynx, gastrointestinal tract, and vagina, and on the skin. Human infections follow exposure to animals or animal products or are endogenous, originating from sites of colonization. Extracellular products such as hyaluronic acid, fibrinolysins, streptokinase, streptolysin O, and erythrogenic toxin may be involved in the pathogenesis of the infections caused by these organisms (Table 28–7) (86,87).

Nutritionally deficient streptococci (Streptococcus defectivus and Streptococcus adjacens), which require pyridoxal (vitamin B_6) for growth, are an uncommon cause of endocarditis and, therefore, may be encountered in blood culture specimens (88).

Enterococcus

Based on results of nucleic acid hybridization studies, Streptococcus faecalis and Streptococcus faecium (previously members of the group D streptococci) in 1984 were reassigned to a new genus, Enterococcus (89). Since then, several additional species of Streptococcus were shown to be sufficiently closely related to other enterococci to be transferred to that genus, and new species of Enterococcus have been recognized (90,91). Members of the genus Enterococcus are gram-positive, oval-shaped, facultative anaerobes that appear as single cells or in pairs or chains in smears prepared from both cultures and stained with the Gram stain. Most react with group D antisera, and some also react with group Q antisera. Enterococcus faecalis, followed by Enterococcus faecium and occasionally Enterococcus durans, are the species of Enterococcus most often encountered in the clinical microbiology laboratory (for a review of other species, see reference 91).

Epidemiology and Pathogenesis

Enterococcus faecalis is normal flora in the oral cavity and gastrointestinal and genitourinary tract of adults, and Enterococcus faecium is present in the gastrointestinal tract of about 25% of adults. Most infections with the enterococci are endogenous, resulting from invasion of the colonizing bacteria; however, nosocomial transmission of the enterococci occurs, and the risk of infection with enterococci is increased by much cephalosporin use in hospitals (92,93).

Clinical Manifestations

Enterococcus is a common cause of urinary tract infections in hospitalized persons with an indwelling catheter but an infrequent cause in otherwise healthy persons. About 10 to 20% of cases of bacterial endocarditis and 5% of bacteremias are caused by species of Enterococcus. Enterococcal endocarditis, most common in elders with

Table 28–7. Infections Produced by Streptococcaceae and Specimens Required for Diagnosis

Infection	Organism	Specimen
Pharyngitis	Groups A, C, G	Throat swab,* serum†
Skin, soft tissue, wound	Groups A, C, G Enterococci, viridans streptococci	Aspirated pus or fluid, swab of lesion
Puerperal infection	Groups B, C, G	Endometrial tissue or aspirate
Neonatal sepsis	Groups B, G	Blood
Bacteremia	Groups A, B, C, G, D, enterococci, S. pneumoniae, viridans streptococci, nutritionally deficient streptococci, Leuconostoc	Blood
Endocarditis	Viridans streptococci, groups B, C, G, D, enterococci, S. pneumoniae, nutritionally deficient streptococci, Leuconostoc	Blood, vegetation
Meningitis	S. pneumoniae Groups A, B, C, G; Leuconostoc	CSF
Arthritis	Group B, G S. pneumoniae	Joint fluid
Urinary tract infection	Enterococci Group B, aerococci	Urine
Pneumonia	S. pneumoniae groups A, B	Sputum, transtracheal aspirate, bronchoalveolar lavage, blood, pleural fluid (if present)
Sinusitis	S. pneumoniae group A	Sinus aspirate
Otitis media	S. pneumoniae	Tympanocentesis
Acute rheumatic fever	Group A	Throat swab, serum†
Acute glomerulonephritis	Group A, C	Throat swab, serum†
Localized tissue abscess (brain, liver, lung)	Viridans streptococci	Aspirated pus

* Collection of two swabs, one for direct antigen detection and one for culture, is recommended.
† Antistreptolysin O (ASO) and anti-DNase B titers.

underlying disease and in intravenous drug users, generally has a subacute onset and an indolent clinical course characterized by recurrent fever and valve destruction with resultant audible murmurs and congestive heart failure. Sources of enterococcal bacteremia include infections of the urinary tract and intra-abdominal abscesses, although in nearly 40% of cases no source is found.

Other Streptococcaceae

Species of Aerococcus most often are environmental contaminants, but they have been associated with urinary tract infections and endocarditis. Leuconostoc species, first recognized as potential human pathogens in 1985, have been isolated from blood of persons (primarily neonates and immunocompromised persons) with bacteremia, endocarditis, and pneumonia, and from the cerebrospinal fluid of those with meningitis (94–96). Pediococcus acidilactici has been recovered from wounds and from the blood of immunocompromised hosts; however, further information is needed to clarify its role in human disease (97,98). Of the members of Lactococcus, only Lactococcus garviae has been recovered from human specimens.

Laboratory Diagnosis

Specimens useful for diagnosis of infections caused by members of the Streptococcaceae are listed in Table 28–7. Specimen collection, transport, and processing are reviewed in Part III of the book. Colony characteristics, cell structure, an approach to organism identification (Table 28–8), and susceptibility testing are discussed here.

Colony Characteristics

After overnight incubation colonies of groups A, C, and G Streptococcus are about 0.5 mm in diameter, domed, translucent or gray with a smooth or "semimatte" surface, and surrounded by a wide zone of complete (β) hemolysis, usually two to four times the diameter of the colony (Plate IID). Occasional strains of Streptococcus pyogenes produce mucoid colonies. Colonies of group B Streptococcus are larger; most are surrounded by a narrow zone of complete hemolysis, but 5 to 15% of isolates are nonhemolytic.

Colonies of Streptococcus pneumoniae are about 1 mm in diameter, round, mucoid, or flattened with a depressed center, and surrounded by a zone of α hemolysis (Plate IIE). Colonies of Enterococcus are gray, 0.5 to 1 mm in diameter, and nonhemolytic or exhibit α-, or rarely β, hemolysis. Colonies of nonhemolytic (viridans) streptococci are smaller than those of enterococci and exhibit α- or γ hemolysis; some isolates of Streptococcus anginosus form small, pinpoint colonies (less than 0.5 mm diameter) surrounded by a narrow to wide zone of β hemolysis. Isolates of Aerococcus are α hemolytic, or occasionally nonhemolytic. Colonies of Leuconostoc resemble those of nonhemolytic enterococci, and colonies of Pediococcus are white to gray, smooth, and nonhemolytic on blood agar, although after prolonged incubation greenish discoloration of the agar surrounding the colonies may be visible.

Cellular Structure

Cells of streptococci are gram positive, round to oval, and form chains in broth cultures (Plate IIC). Occasionally cells are elongate, resembling corynebacteria or lactobacilli (see Chapter 29), and they may appear gram negative if cultures are old or if the individual from whom the specimen was obtained was receiving antimicrobial agents. To differentiate elongate gram-positive cells, a blood agar plate is inoculated with a lawn of the organism and a 10-U penicillin disk is placed on the surface. After overnight incubation a smear prepared from growth just outside the zone of inhibition is stained with Gram stain: cells of Lactobacillus appear as long bacilli and cells of Streptococcus are spherical. Moreover, staining a smear of growth in thioglycollate broth with Gram stain provides useful information: species of Streptococcus form long chains of cocci; Aerococcus and Pediococcus form large, spherical cocci arranged singly and in tetrads and pairs; Lactococcus grows as rods and filaments. Observing classic gram-positive lancet-shaped diplococci suggests Streptococcus pneumoniae (Plate IIF), and cells of Leuconostoc typically are coccobacillary.

Organism Identification

β-Hemolytic Streptococcus Species. Tests commonly used in the clinical microbiology laboratory to presumptively name the β-hemolytic species of Streptococcus are shown in Figure 28–9. Over 99% of isolates of group A Streptococcus are susceptible to bacitracin (Appendix, Procedure 13, Plate IID), but a very small percentage of isolates of group B Streptococcus, and 10 to 20% of isolates of groups C and G, also are susceptible. Therefore, results of the bacitracin susceptibility test provide presumptive identification. Alternatively, an isolate may be called group A Streptococcus presumptively based on the

Table 28–8. Laboratory Tests Commonly Used to Name Streptococci and Enterococci

Organism	Test (Expected Reaction)
Group A Streptococcus	PYR *(positive), bacitracin (growth inhibited), particle agglutination, fluorescence
Group B Streptococcus	Hippurate *(positive), CAMP* (positive), particle agglutination
Streptococcus pneumoniae	Optochin *(growth inhibited), particle agglutination
Viridans streptococci†	Optochin *(growth not inhibited), 6.5% NaCl *(no growth), biochemical tests
Groups C and G Streptococcus	Particle agglutination
Enterococcus species	PYR *(positive), 6.5% NaCl* (growth), biochemical tests

* Performing these tests names the organism presumptively.
† The viridans streptococci typically are named after excluding S. pneumoniae and Enterococcus by performing the tests indicated.

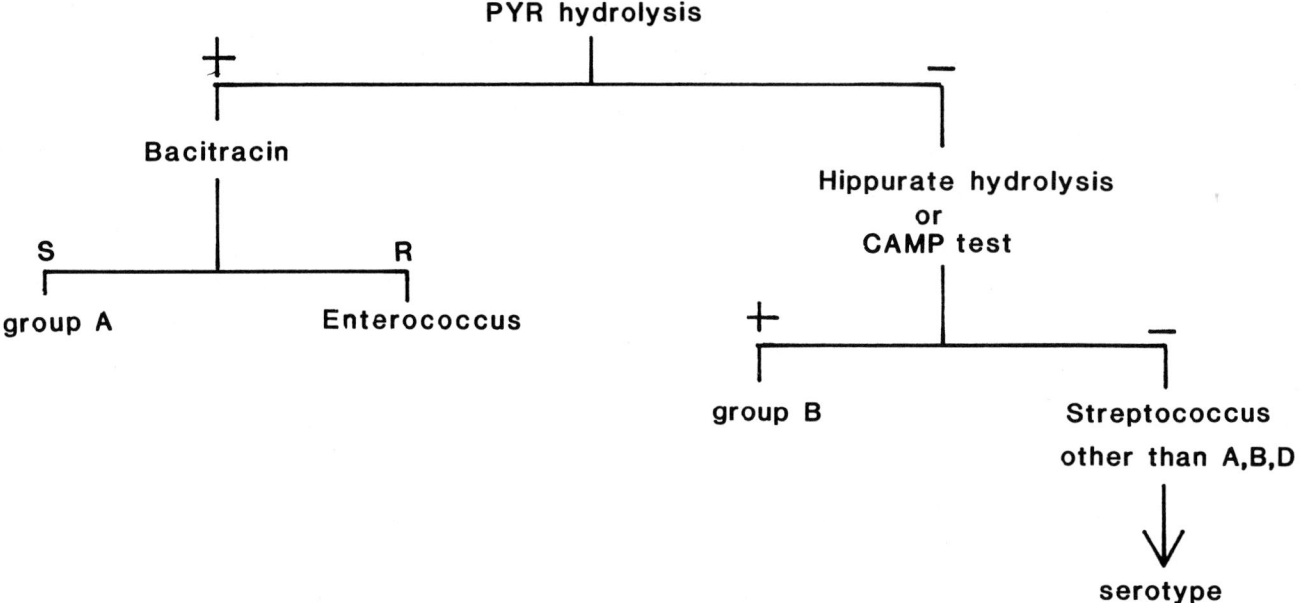

Fig. 28–9. Decision tree of tests to presumptively name the β-hemolytic species of Streptococcus. Key: +, positive result; −, negative result; S, susceptible; R, resistant.

hydrolysis of pyrrolidonyl-β-naphthylamide (PYR test) (99–101). The PYR test may be performed by one of several commercially available methods: agar requires overnight incubation, broth requires 4 hours' incubation, and disks impregnated with the reagent provide results within 5 minutes. All isolates of group A Streptococcus, and more than 99% of isolates of Enterococcus, are PYR positive. Identification of a β-hemolytic colony as group A Streptococcus is confirmed by serotyping using latex agglutination or coagglutination, or by staining a smear with fluorescent monoclonal antibodies.

Group A Streptococcus may be detected directly in throat swab specimens within 5 to 15 minutes by using commercially available kits. The group A antigen is extracted from the swab chemically or enzymatically and identified by latex agglutination, coagglutination, or enzyme-linked immunosorbent assay. These tests are very specific, but given their low sensitivity, a negative direct result should be followed by culture (102–106).

Serologic tests to detect antibodies to streptolysin O and DNase B are used primarily to diagnose acute rheumatic fever and acute glomerulonephritis following infection with group A Streptococcus, but they also may be used to distinguish persons who carry Streptococcus pyogenes in their pharynx from those who have active infection. Measuring titers of both antibodies is important because antistreptolysin O is not produced following group A streptococcal skin infections. A fourfold rise in antibody titer between acute- and convalescent-phase serum collected 3 to 4 weeks apart is evidence of recent infection with group A Streptococcus.

An isolate that hydrolyzes hippurate (Appendix, Procedure 14) or has a positive CAMP test reaction (Appendix, Procedure 15, Plate IIIA) presumptively is called group B Streptococcus. Isolates of presumed group B Streptococcus from sterile body sites such as blood and cerebrospinal fluid (CSF) should be identified by serotyping with commercially available latex agglutination or coagglutination tests, by staining a smear with fluorescent monoclonal antibodies, or by using a chemiluminescent DNA probe (107). Group B streptococcus may be detected directly in endocervical swab specimens using kits similar to those described earlier for group A streptococci. However, because these tests also have low sensitivity; specimens that produce a negative direct result should be cultured (108). Meningitis caused by group B Streptococcus may be diagnosed within 1 hour of receiving the specimen by latex particle agglutination (see Chapter 24) to detect specific capsular antigens, preferably in CSF, though urine is acceptable. When testing urine specimens from neonates, false-positive latex test results have been attributed to antibiotics administered to the mother during labor (109).

Isolates of β-hemolytic groups C, D, F, and G Streptococcus are identified by serotyping with latex agglutination or coagglutination reagents.

α- and γ-Hemolytic Streptococci and Enterococci. Tests used to presumptively name α- and γ-hemolytic streptococci and enterococci are shown in Figure 28–10. α-Hemolytic colonies that are mucoid or flattened with a depressed center are suggestive of Streptococcus pneumoniae and should be tested for susceptibility to ethylhydroxycupreine hydrochloride, more commonly called optochin (P disk; Appendix, Procedure 16); S. pneumoniae is susceptible (Plate IIE), whereas other α-hemolytic streptococci are resistant. Isolates from sterile body sites presumed to be S. pneumoniae should be identified by serotyping with commercially available latex agglutination or coagglutination reagents. Pneumococcal meningitis may be diagnosed by using commercially available latex particle agglutination tests to detect capsular antigens in CSF.

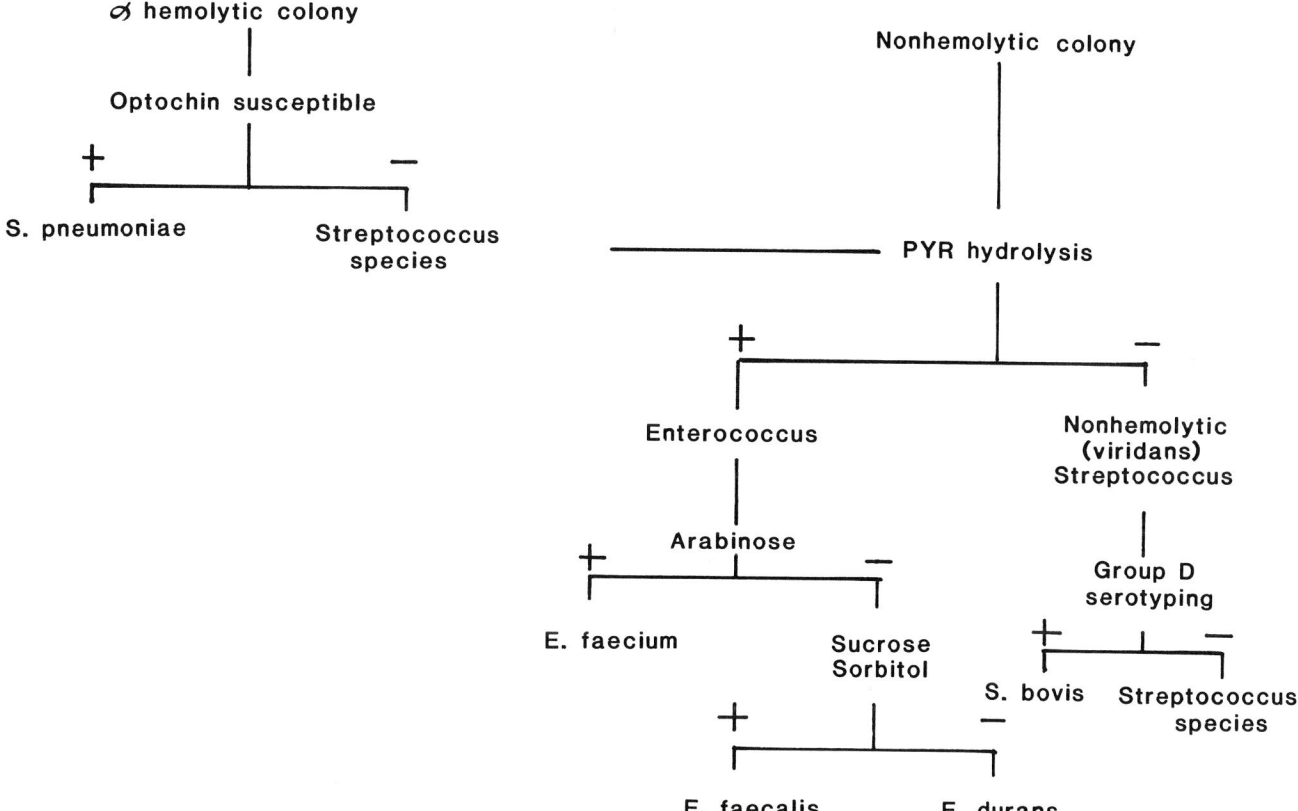

Fig. 28–10. Decision tree of tests to presumptively name the α-hemolytic and γ-hemolytic species of Streptococcus and Enterococcus. Key: +, positive result; −, negative result.

α-Hemolytic colonies determined not to be Streptococcus pneumoniae and γ-hemolytic colonies are tested for PYR hydrolysis: all enterococci are PYR positive; viridans streptococci are negative. Moreover, all species of Enterococcus grow in the presence of 6.5% sodium chloride in trypticase soy broth (incubated up to 3 days); viridans streptococci do not. A DNA probe to identify colonies of enterococci also is available (107). Isolates of Enterococcus hydrolyze esculin in the presence of bile (recognized by visible growth and blackening of the agar), but as many as 10% of the viridans streptococci also are bile-esculin positive. The three species of Enterococcus commonly encountered in the clinical laboratory may be identified by biochemical tests (Fig. 28–10) (see reference 110 for a comprehensive list of tests) or by using commercially available kit systems (111–113).

α-Hemolytic streptococci that are optochin resistant and PYR negative and γ-hemolytic streptococci that are PYR negative and do not grow in 6.5% sodium chloride are grouped as nonhemolytic (viridans) streptococci. Identification of the individual species of viridans streptococci requires conventional biochemical testing (described in reference 85). Kit systems to identify these organisms are commercially available, but because the taxonomy has changed these systems should be modified and evaluated again. Streptococcus bovis may be identified by serotyping (group D) with latex agglutination or coagglutination reagents.

Other Streptococcaceae. Aerococcus has a variable bile esculin reaction and grows in broth containing 6.5% sodium chloride, similar to Enterococcus; but Aerococcus does not grow at 10° C and most are susceptible to bacitracin, whereas Enterococcus grows at 10° C and is bacitracin resistant. Characteristics that help differentiate isolates of Leuconostoc and Pediococcus from those of Enterococcus are listed in Table 28–9 (reviewed in references 110 and 114). Pediococcus is differentiated from

Table 28–9. Characteristics that Differentiate Enterococcus, Leuconostoc, and Pediococcus

Characteristic	Enterococcus	Leuconostoc	Pediococcus
Gram stain from broth	Cocci in pairs, long chains	Cocci, coccobacilli, rods in pairs and chains	Large, spherical cocci in tetrads and pairs
Bile esculin	+	+	+
Growth in 6.5% NaCl	+	V	V
PYR test	+	−	−
Gas from glucose	−	+	−
Vancomycin resistance	S*	R	R

* Fewer than 1% of isolates are resistant.
Key: +, positive; −, negative; V, variable; S, susceptible; R, resistant.

Aerococcus by its ability to grow anaerobically; Aerococcus is a strict aerobe.

Typically, nutritionally deficient streptococci are detected in broth blood culture systems. Growth in the broth medium is recognized, a smear stained with the Gram stain reveals gram-positive cocci in chains, but subcultures to solid media are sterile when incubated in ambient air, in increased carbon dioxide, and in an anaerobic environment. Organisms are recovered by performing a "Staph streak": a lawn of the organism from the blood culture broth is spread over the surface of a sheep blood agar plate and then streaked with an isolate of Staphylococcus aureus, which provides the needed pyridoxal. The small colonies of catalase-negative gram-positive cocci that grow at the periphery of the S. aureus, called "satelliting" colonies, are the nutritionally deficient streptococci. Alternatively, pyridoxal may be added to the growth medium. Differential characteristics of Streptococcus defectivus and Streptococcus adjacens are reviewed elsewhere (115).

Susceptibility Testing

The antibiograms of groups A, B, C, and G Streptococcus are predictable (all are susceptible to penicillin); therefore, routine antimicrobial susceptibility testing of these organisms is unnecessary. Because strains of Streptococcus pneumoniae with intermediate (relative) or high-level resistance to penicillin (MIC, 0.1 to 1.0 mg/L and at least 2 mg/L, respectively) are found worldwide, isolates of S. pneumoniae recovered from sterile body sites such as blood or CSF should be screened for susceptibility to penicillin using the disk diffusion technique (see Appendix, Procedure 17) (116). The latter method, however, does not distinguish isolates with intermediate resistance from those with high-level resistance to penicillin, so isolates with a zone of 19 mm or less must be further evaluated by macrodilution or microdilution testing, using Mueller-Hinton broth supplemented with 5% sheep blood, lysed horse blood, or Haemophilus test medium, to determine the MIC of penicillin (117).

Susceptibility testing should be performed on isolates of nonhemolytic (viridans) streptococci from sterile body sites, because resistance to penicillin has been reported. Moreover, susceptibility testing may provide information on the organism's identity. The cellular and colony morphology of nonhemolytic streptococci may resemble those of species of Leuconostoc, Pediococcus, and often Lactobacillus; however, viridans streptococci are susceptible to vancomycin, whereas Leuconostoc, Pediococcus, and some Lactobacillus are resistant (114).

Susceptibility testing of isolates of Enterococcus should be performed, primarily to identify high-level resistance to penicillin or ampicillin, high-level resistance to streptomycin and gentamicin, and resistance to vancomycin (93,118,119). Susceptibility to penicillin, ampicillin, and vancomycin is determined by routine microdilution. To detect high-level aminoglycoside resistance, broth macrotube dilution, agar dilution, and disk diffusion using a 120-μg gentamicin disk and a 300-μg streptomycin disk provide valid results; however, the necessary disks are not commercially available (91). For agar dilution, Mueller-Hinton agar plates containing 2000 μg of streptomycin or gentamicin are spot-inoculated with a cotton swab that has been dipped into a suspension of the isolate with a turbidity equal to a 0.5 McFarland standard. Any growth by agar dilution or a zone of inhibition less than 10 mm by disk diffusion after incubation for 24 hours indicates resistance. Commercially available microtiter susceptibility systems provide tests that detect high-level aminoglycoside resistance, though currently some systems require 48 hours' incubation to identify such resistance reliably (120,121). Strains of Enterococcus that produce β-lactamase have been reported; but because these strains are uncommon, testing all isolates of Enterococcus for β-lactamase production probably is not cost effective (122).

Treatment

Most streptococci are susceptible to penicillin or ampicillin, erythromycin, and the first-generation cephalosporins. However, in Finland between 1988 and 1990, the prevalence of strains of group A Streptococcus resistant to erythromycin was 20 to 44%, depending on the site of infection and the geographic locale (123). Serious infections due to group B Streptococcus usually are treated with ampicillin plus either gentamicin or streptomycin. Large-dose penicillin alone is sufficient therapy for bacteremic or nonbacteremic pneumonia due to strains of Streptococcus pneumoniae with intermediate resistance to penicillin. Bacteremia and meningitis caused by highly resistant strains of S. pneumoniae and meningitis due to intermediate-resistance strains, however, should be treated with an agent other than penicillin, such as chloramphenicol (if the organism is susceptible), cefotaxime, ceftriaxone, or vancomycin, possibly with rifampin added (116).

Isolates of Enterococcus require higher concentrations of penicillin or ampicillin to inhibit growth and are resistant to achievable serum levels of cephalosporins. Although uncomplicated enterococcal urinary tract infections generally respond to ampicillin, serious Enterococcus infections require therapy with the synergistic combination of penicillin or ampicillin plus streptomycin or gentamicin. Recently, isolates of Enterococcus faecalis and E. faecium with high-level resistance to one or both of these aminoglycosides or high-level resistance to penicillin have been identified, and the infections they cause have been difficult to treat (91). Persons allergic to penicillin who have infections due to Enterococcus can be treated with vancomycin, although vancomycin-resistant isolates of Enterococcus have been reported (91).

Prevention

Group A Streptococcus (Nonsuppurative Complications). Treatment of pharyngitis caused by group A Streptococcus with penicillin or erythromycin within 1 week of the onset of symptoms will prevent acute rheumatic fever, and recent data suggest that delaying antimicrobial treatment for 48 hours may be more beneficial than immediate therapy. In one study children treated immediately with penicillin were more than twice as likely to experience reinfection with group A Streptococcus within the next 4 months, and delaying therapy 48 hours did not increase intrafamilial spread of the infection or the occurrence of nonsuppurative sequelae (124). Acute streptococcal glomerulonephritis cannot be prevented despite appropriate therapy.

Streptococcus pneumoniae. A vaccine for S. pneumoniae containing 14 different capsular polysaccharides representing serotypes that accounted for about 80% of bacteremic infections was licensed in the United States in 1978 and modified in 1983 to include 23 different capsular polysaccharides representing serotypes that account for more than 90% of bacteremic infections caused by S. pneumoniae in the United States and other countries. Vaccine-induced antibody levels start to decline about 1 year after immunization, and among healthy adults antibody levels decline to about three fourths of peak levels 5 years after vaccination, suggesting that booster immunization might be necessary to maintain adequate antibody levels and that a second dose of vaccine might be administered 5 to 10 years after initial immunization in adults (125). The Centers for Disease Control recommends reimmunizing persons who received the 14-valent vaccine and persons at high risk of developing serious infection with S. pneumoniae who were immunized with the 23-valent vaccine more than 6 years previously.

Pneumococcal vaccine currently is recommended for these persons: healthy adults over age 65 years; adults at high risk of serious pneumococcal infection because of splenic dysfunction, asplenia, or chronic illness such as Hodgkin's disease, multiple myeloma, alcoholism, cirrhosis, renal failure, CSF leaks, and any condition that causes immunosuppression; adults with chronic cardiovascular or pulmonary disease; children over age 2 years who have chronic illnesses associated with increased risk of serious pneumococcal infection (sickle cell disease, splenectomy, immunosuppression, CSF leaks, nephrotic syndrome); and anyone over 2 years of age infected with human immunodeficiency virus. The efficacy of immunizing high-risk populations, however, is controversial (126–130).

REFERENCES

1. Sheagren JN: Staphylococcus aureus—the persistent pathogen (first of two parts). N Engl J Med, *310*:1368, 1984.
2. Fast DJ, Schlievert PM, and Nelson RD: Toxic shock syndrome–associated staphylococcal and streptococcal pyrogenic toxins are potent inducers of tumor necrosis factor production. Infect Immun, *57*:291, 1989.
3. Garbe PL, et al: Staphylococcus aureus isolates from patients with nonmenstrual toxic shock syndrome. Evidence for additional toxins. JAMA, *253*:2538, 1985.
4. Schlievert PM: Staphylococcal enterotoxin B and toxic shock syndrome toxin-1 are significantly associated with nonmenstrual TSS. Lancet, *i*:1149, 1986.
5. Rizkallah MF, et al: Toxic shock syndrome caused by a strain of Staphylococcus aureus that produces enterotoxin C but not toxic shock syndrome toxin-1. Am J Dis Child, *143*:848, 1989.
6. Sheagren JN: Staphylococcus aureus—the persistent pathogen (second of two parts). N Engl J Med, *310*:1437, 1984.
7. Musher DM, and McKenzie SO: Infections due to Staphylococcus aureus. Medicine, *56*:383, 1977.
8. Mylotte JM, McDermott C, and Spooner JA: Prospective study of 114 consecutive episodes of Staphylococcus aureus bacteremia. Rev Infect Dis, *9*:891, 1987.
9. Chiedozi LC: Pyomyositis: Review of 205 cases in 112 patients. Am J Surg, *137*:255, 1979.
10. Craven DE, Steger KA, and Barber TW: Preventing nosocomial pneumonia: State of the art and perspectives for the 1990s. Am J Med, *91*(suppl 3B):44S, 1991.
11. Todd JK: Toxic shock syndrome. Clin Microbiol Rev, *1*:432, 1988.
12. Ferguson MA, and Todd JK: Toxic shock syndrome associated with Staphylococcus aureus sinusitis in children. J Infect Dis, *161*:953, 1990.
13. Centers for Disease Control: Reduced incidence of menstrual toxic shock syndrome—United States, 1980–1990. MMWR, *39*:421, 1990.
14. Pfaller MA, and Herwaldt LA: Laboratory, clinical, and epidemiological aspects of coagulase-negative staphylococci. Clin Microbiol Rev, *1*:281, 1988.
15. Younger JJ, et al: Coagulase-negative staphylococci isolated from cerebrospinal fluid shunts: Importance of slime production, species identification, and shunt removal to clinical outcome. J Infect Dis, *156*:548, 1987.
16. Gristina AG: Biomaterial-centered infection: Microbial adhesion versus tissue integration. Science, *237*:1588, 1987.
17. Bykowska K, et al: Anticoagulant properties of extracellular slime substance produced by Staphylococcus epidermidis. Thromb Haemostasis, *54*:853, 1985.
18. Johnson GM, et al: Interference with granulocyte function by Staphylococcus epidermidis slime. Infect Immun, *54*:13, 1986.
19. Archer G: Antimicrobial susceptibility and selection of resistance among Staphylococcus epidermidis isolates recovered from patients with infections of indwelling foreign devices. Antimicrob Agent Chemother, *14*:353, 1978.
20. Baddour LM, and Christensen GD: Prosthetic valve endocarditis due to small-colony staphylococcal variants. Rev Infect Dis, *9*:1168, 1987.
21. Karchmer AW, Archer GL, and Dismukes WE: Staphylococcus epidermidis causing prosthetic valve endocarditis: Microbiologic and clinical observations as guides to therapy. Ann Intern Med, *98*:447, 1983.
22. Baum JL: Ocular infections. N Engl J Med, *299*:28, 1978.
23. Burke JP: Infections of cardiac and vascular prostheses. *In* Hospital Infections. Edited by JV Bennett and PS Brachman. Boston, Little, Brown, 1986.
24. Goldstone J, and Moore WS: Infection in vascular prostheses: Clinical manifestations and surgical management. Am J Surg, *128*:225, 1974.
25. Winston DJ, et al: Coagulase-negative staphylococcal bacteremia in patients receiving immunosuppressive therapy. Arch Intern Med, *143*:32, 1983.
26. Wade JC, Schimpff SC, Newman KA, and Wiernik PH: Staphylococcus epidermidis: An increasing cause of infection in patients with granulocytopenia. Ann Intern Med, *97*:503, 1982.
27. Culliford AT, et al: Sternal and costochondral infections following open-heart surgery: A review of 2594 cases. J Thorac Cardiovasc Surg, *72*:714, 1976.
28. Singh VR, and Raad I: Fatal Staphylococcus saprophyticus native valve endocarditis in an intravenous drug addict. J Infect Dis, *162*:783, 1990.

29. Coudron PE, et al: Isolation of Stomatococcus mucilaginosus from drug user with endocarditis. J Clin Microbiol, 25:1359, 1987.
30. Pelman DA, Ruoff K, and Ferraro MJ: Stomatococcus mucilaginosus endocarditis in an intravenous drug abuser. J Infect Dis, 155:1080, 1987.
31. Koneman EW, et al (eds): Color Atlas and Textbook of Diagnostic Microbiology. 3rd ed. Philadelphia, JB Lippincott, 1988.
32. Gilligan PH, et al: Prevalence of thymidine-dependent Staphylococcus aureus in patients with cystic fibrosis. J Clin Microbiol, 25:1258, 1987.
33. Madison BM, and Baselski VS: Rapid identification of Staphylococcus aureus in blood cultures by thermonuclease testing. J Clin Microbiol, 18:722, 1983.
34. Faruki H, and Murray P: Medium dependence for rapid detection of thermonuclease activity in blood culture broths. J Clin Microbiol, 24:482, 1986.
35. Berke A, and Tilton RC: Evaluation of rapid coagulase methods for the identification of Staphylococcus aureus. J Clin Microbiol, 23:916, 1986.
36. Smith SM, and Berezny C: Comparative evaluation of identification systems for testing methicillin-resistant strains of Staphylococcus aureus. J Clin Microbiol, 24:173, 1986.
37. Ruane PJ, Morgan MA, Citron DM, and Mulligan ME: Failure of rapid agglutination methods to detect oxacillin-resistant Staphylococcus aureus. J Clin Microbiol, 24:490, 1986.
38. Lairscey R, and Buck GE: Performance of four slide agglutination methods for identification of Staphylococcus aureus when testing methicillin-resistant staphylococci. J Clin Microbiol, 25:181, 1987.
39. Gregson DB, Low DE, Skulnick M, and Simor AE: Problems with rapid agglutination methods for identification of Staphylococcus aureus when Staphylococcus saprophyticus is being tested. J Clin Microbiol, 26:1398, 1988.
40. Talan DA, et al: Staphylococcus intermedius in canine gingiva and canine-inflicted human wound infections: Laboratory characterization of a newly recognized zoonotic pathogen. J Clin Microbiol, 27:78, 1989.
41. Abramson C, Bergdoll MS, and Wheat LJ: Immunoserology of staphylococcal disease. In Cumitech 22. Edited by C Abramson. Washington, DC, American Society for Microbiology, 1987.
42. Kloos WE, and Schleifer KH: Simplified scheme for routine identification of human Staphylococcus species. J Clin Microbiol, 1:82, 1975.
43. Herbert GA, et al: Characteristics of coagulase-negative staphylococci that help differentiate these species and other members of the family Micrococcaceae. J Clin Microbiol, 26:1939, 1988.
44. Grasmick AE, Naito N, and Bruckner DA: Clinical comparison of the AutoMicrobic System Gram-Positive Identification Card, API Staph-Ident, and conventional methods in the identification of coagulase-negative Staphylococcus spp. J Clin Microbiol, 18:1323, 1983.
45. Hussain Z, et al: Comparison of the MicroScan system with the API Staph-Ident system for species identification of coagulase-negative staphylococci. J Clin Microbiol, 23:126, 1986.
46. Kloos WE, and Wolfshohl JF: Identification of Staphylococcus species with the API Staph-Ident system. J Clin Microbiol, 16:509, 1982.
47. Giger O, Charilaou CC, and Cundy KR: Comparison of the API Staph-Ident and DMS Staph-Trac systems with conventional methods used for the identification of coagulase-negative staphylococci. J Clin Microbiol, 19:68, 1984.
48. Chambers HF: Methicillin-resistant staphylococci. Clin Microbiol Rev, 1:173, 1988.
49. Brumfitt W, and Hamilton-Miller J: Methicillin-resistant Staphylococcus aureus. N Engl J Med, 320:1188, 1989.
50. Schwalbe RS, et al: Emergence of vancomycin resistance in coagulase-negative staphylococci. N Engl J Med, 316:927, 1987.
51. Veach LA, et al: Vancomycin resistance in Staphylococcus haemolyticus causing colonization and bloodstream infection. J Clin Microbiol, 28:2064, 1990.
52. Johnson AP: Resistance to vancomycin and teicoplanin: An emerging clinical problem. Clin Microbiol Rev, 3:280, 1990.
53. Lancefield RC: A serological differentiation of human and other groups of hemolytic streptococci. J Exp Med, 57:571, 1933.
54. Brown JH: The use of blood agar for the study of streptococci. New York, The Rockefeller Institute for Medical Research, 1919.
55. Ayoub EM, and Schiebler GL: Acute rheumatic fever: Practice of pediatrics. Philadelphia, Harper and Row, 1987.
56. Bisno AL: Streptococcus pyogenes. In Principles and Practice of Infectious Diseases. 3rd ed. Edited by GL Mandell, RG Douglas, Jr, and JE Bennett. New York, Churchill Livingstone, 1990.
57. Quinn RW: Comprehensive review of morbidity and mortality trends for rheumatic fever, streptococcal disease, and scarlet fever: The decline of rheumatic fever. Rev Infect Dis, 11:928, 1989.
58. Daly JA: Resurgence of group A streptococcal disease: rheumatic fever. Clin Microbiol Newslett, 11:161, 1989.
59. Veasy LG, et al: Resurgence of acute rheumatic fever in the Intermountain area of the United States. N Engl J Med, 316:421, 1987.
60. Hosier DM, et al: Resurgence of rheumatic fever. Am J Dis Child, 111:730, 1987.
61. Congeni B, et al: Outbreak of acute rheumatic fever in Northeast Ohio. J Pediatr, 111:176, 1987.
62. Centers for Disease Control: Acute rheumatic fever at a navy training center—San Diego, California. MMWR, 37:101, 1988.
63. Centers for Disease Control. Acute rheumatic fever among trainees—Fort Leonard Wood, Missouri, 1987–1988. MMWR, 37:519, 1988.
64. Kim YB, and Watson DW: Streptococcal exotoxins: Biological and pathological properties. In Streptococci and streptococcal diseases: recognition, understanding, and management. Edited by LW Wannamaker and JM Matsen. New York, Academic Press, 1972.
65. Gallis HA: Streptococcus. In Zinsser Microbiology. 19th ed. Edited by WK Joklik, HP Willett, DB Ames, and CM Wilfert. Norwalk, Appleton & Lange, 1988.
66. Cone LA, Woodard DR, Schlievert PM, and Tomory GS: Clinical and bacteriologic observations of a toxic shock–like syndrome due to Streptococcus pyogenes. N Engl J Med, 317:146, 1987.
67. Stevens DL, et al: Severe group A streptococcal infections associated with a toxic shock–like syndrome and scarlet fever toxin A. N Engl J Med, 321:1, 1989.
68. Bartter T, et al: 'Toxic strep syndrome'—a manifestation of group A streptococcal infection. Arch Intern Med, 148:1421, 1988.
69. Unny SK, and Middlebrooks BL: Streptococcal rheumatic carditis. Microbiol Rev, 47:97, 1983.
70. Marcon MJ, et al: Occurrence of mucoid M-18 Streptococcus pyogenes in a central Ohio pediatric population. J Clin Microbiol, 26:1539, 1988.

71. Barnett LA, and Cunningham MW: A new heart–cross-reactive antigen in Streptococcus pyogenes is not M protein. J Infect Dis, 162:875, 1990.
72. Gordon JS, and Sbarra AJ: Incidence, technique of isolation, and treatment of group B streptococci. Am J Obstet Gynecol, 126:1023, 1976.
73. Anthony BF, et al: Genital and intestinal carriage of group B streptococci during pregnancy. J Infect Dis, 143:761, 1981.
74. Dillon HC, Jr, Khare S, and Gray BM: Group B streptococcal carriage and disease: A 6-year prospective study. J Pediatr, 110:31, 1987.
75. Schuchat A, et al: Population-based risk factors for neonatal group B streptococcal disease: Results of a cohort study in metropolitan Atlanta. J Infect Dis, 162:672, 1990.
76. Pass MA, Gray BM, Khare S, and Dillon HC: Prospective studies of group B streptococcal infections in infants. J Pediatr, 95:437, 1979.
77. Stewardson-Krieger PB, and Gotoff SP: Risk factors in neonatal group B streptococcal infections. Infection, 6:50, 1978.
78. Opal SM, Cross A, Palmer M, and Almazan R: Group B streptococcal sepsis in adults and infants. Arch Intern Med, 148:641, 1988.
79. Stewardson-Krieger PB, et al: Perinatal immunity to group B β-hemolytic Streptococcus type Ia. J Infect Dis, 136:649, 1977.
80. Chun CSY, et al: Group B streptococcal c protein-associated antigens: Association with neonatal sepsis. J Infect Dis, 163:786, 1991.
81. Patterson MJ, and Hafeez AEB: Group B streptococci in human disease. Bacteriol Rev, 40:774, 1976.
82. Edwards MS, and Baker CJ: Streptococcus agalactiae (group B Streptococcus). In Principles and Practice of Infectious Diseases. 3rd ed. Edited by GL Mandell, RG Douglas, Jr, and JE Bennett. New York, Churchill Livingstone, 1990.
83. Hendley JO, et al: Spread of Streptococcus pneumoniae in families. Carriage rates and distribution of types. J Infect Dis, 132:55, 1975.
84. Centers for Disease Control: Outbreak of invasive pneumococcal disease in a jail—Texas, 1989. MMWR, 38:733, 1989.
85. Coykendall AL: Classification and identification of the viridans streptococci. Clin Microbiol Rev, 2:315, 1989.
86. Salata RA, et al: Infections due to Lancefield group C streptococci. Medicine, 68:225, 1989.
87. Venezio FR, et al: Group G streptococcal endocarditis and bacteremia. Am J Med, 81:29, 1986.
88. Roberts RB, Krieger AG, and Schiller NL: Viridans streptococcal endocarditis: The role of various species including pyridoxal-dependent streptococci. Rev Infect Dis, 1:955, 1979.
89. Schleifer KH, and Kilpper-Balz R: Transfer of Streptococcus faecalis and Streptococcus faecium to the genus Enterococcus nom. rev. as Enterococcus faecalis comb. nov. and Enterococcus faecium comb. nov. Int J Syst Bacteriol, 34:31, 1984.
90. Collins MD, et al: Enterococcus avium nom. rev., comb. nov.; E. casseliflavus nom. rev., comb. nov; E. durans nom. rev., comb. nov., E. gallinarum comb. nov.; and E. malodoratus sp. nov. Int J Syst Bacteriol, 34:220, 1984.
91. Murray BE: The life and times of the enterococcus. Clin Microbiol Rev, 3:46, 1990.
92. Morrison AJ, Jr, and Wenzel RP: Nosocomial urinary tract infections due to enterococcus: Ten years' experience at a University hospital. Arch Intern Med, 146:1549, 1986.
93. Zervos MJ, et al: Nosocomial infection by gentamicin-resistant Streptococcus fecalis: An epidemiologic study. Ann Intern Med, 106:687, 1987.
94. Rubin LG, Vellozzi E, Shapiro J, and Isenberg HB: Infection with vancomycin-resistant "streptococci" due to Leuconostoc species. J Infect Dis, 157:216, 1988.
95. Handwerger S, et al: Infection due to Leuconostoc species: Six cases and review. Rev Infect Dis, 12:602, 1990.
96. Friedland JR, Snipelisky M, and Khoosal M: Meningitis in a neonate caused by Leuconostoc sp. J Clin Microbiol, 28:2125, 1990.
97. Riebel WJ, and Washington JA II: Clinical and microbiologic characteristics of Pediococci. J Clin Microbiol, 28:1348, 1990.
98. Mastro TD, et al: Vancomycin-resistant Pediococcus acidilactici: Nine cases of bacteremia. J Infect Dis, 161:956, 1990.
99. Bosley GS, Facklam RR, and Grossman D: Rapid identification of enterococci. J Clin Microbiol, 18:1275, 1983.
100. Facklam RR, Thacker LG, Fox B, and Eriquez L: Presumptive identification of streptococci with a new test system. J Clin Microbiol, 15:987, 1982.
101. Wellstood SA: Rapid, cost-effective identification of group A streptococci and enterococci by pyrrolidonyl-β-naphthylamide hydrolysis. J Clin Microbiol, 25:1805, 1987.
102. Kellogg JA, and Manzella JP: Detection of group A streptococci in the laboratory or physician's office: Culture vs antibody methods. JAMA, 255:2638, 1986.
103. Gerber MA: Diagnosis of group A beta-hemolytic streptococcal pharyngitis—use of antigen detection tests. Diagn Microbiol Infect Dis, 4:55, 1986.
104. Centor RM, Meier FA, and Dalton HP: Throat cultures and rapid tests for diagnosis of group A streptococcal pharyngitis. Ann Intern Med, 105:892, 1986.
105. Facklam RR: Specificity study of kits for detection of group A streptococci directly from throat swabs. J Clin Microbiol, 25:504, 1987.
106. Radetsky M, Solomon JA, and Todd JK: Identification of streptococcal pharyngitis in the office laboratory: Reassessment of new technology. Pediatr Infect Dis J, 6:556, 1987.
107. Daly JA, Clifton NL, Seskin KC, and Gooch WM III: Use of rapid nonradioactive DNA probes in culture confirmation tests to detect Streptococcus agalactiae, Haemophilus influenzae, and Enterococcus spp. from pediatric patients with significant infections. J Clin Microbiol, 29:80, 1991.
108. Kotnick CM, and Edberg SC: Direct detection of group B streptococci from vaginal specimens compared with quantitative culture. J Clin Microbiol, 28:336, 1990.
109. Harris MC, Deuber C, Polin RA, and Nachamkin I: Investigation of apparent false-positive urine latex particle agglutination tests for the detection of group B Streptococcus antigen. J Clin Microbiol, 27:2214, 1989.
110. Facklam RR, and Collins MD: Identification of Enterococcus species isolated from human infections by a conventional test scheme. J Clin Microbiol, 27:731, 1989.
111. Tritz DM, Iwen PC, and Woods GL: Comparative evaluation of MicroScan and conventional media for species identification of enterococci. J Clin Microbiol, 28:1477, 1990.
112. Appelbaum PC, et al: Comparative evaluation of the API 20S system and the AutoMicrobic system Gram-Positive Identification card for species identification of streptococci. J Clin Microbiol, 19:164, 1984.
113. Appelbaum PC, et al: Accuracy and reproducibility of the IDS RapID STR system for species identification of streptococci. J Clin Microbiol, 23:843, 1986.
114. Facklam R, Hollis D, and Collins MD: Identification of gram-

positive coccal and coccobacillary vancomycin-resistant bacteria. J Clin Microbiol, 27:724, 1989.
115. Ruoff KL: Update on nutritionally variant streptococci (Streptococcus defectivus and Streptococcus adjacens). Clin Microbiol Newslett, 12:97, 1990.
116. Klugman KP: Pneumonococcal resistance to antibiotics. Clin Microbiol Rev, 3:171, 1990.
117. Jorgensen JH, Maher LA, and Howell AW: Use of Haemophilus test medium for broth microdilution antimicrobial susceptibility testing of Streptococcus pneumoniae. J Clin Microbiol, 28:430, 1990.
118. Bush LM, et al: High-level penicillin resistance among isolates of enterococci. Ann Intern Med, 110:515, 1989.
119. Uttley AHC, Collins CH, Naidoo J, and George RC. Vancomycin-resistant enterococci. Lancet, i:57, 1988.
120. Spiegel CA: Laboratory detection of high-level aminoglycoside-aminocyclitol resistance in Enterococcus spp. J Clin Microbiol, 26:2270, 1988.
121. Sahm DF, et al: Factors influencing determination of high-level aminoglycoside resistance in Enterococcus faecalis. J Clin Microbiol, 29:1934, 1991.
122. Rhinehart E, et al: Rapid dissemination of β-lactamase–producing, aminoglycoside-resistant Enterococcus faecalis among patients and staff on an infant-toddler surgical ward. N Engl J Med, 323:1814, 1990.
123. Seppälä H, et al: Resistance to erythromycin in group A streptococci. N Engl J Med, 326:292, 1992.
124. Pichichero ME, et al: Adverse and beneficial effects of immediate treatment of group A β-hemolytic streptococcal pharyngitis with penicillin. Pediatr Infect Dis J, 6:635, 1987.
125. Mufson MA, et al: Pneumococcal antibody levels one decade after immunization of healthy adults. Am J Med Sci, 30:279, 1987.
126. Bentley DW, et al: Pneumococcal vaccine in the institutionalized elderly: Design of a nonrandomized trial and preliminary results. Rev Infect Dis, 3(suppl):S71, 1981.
127. Austrian R: Some observations on the pneumococcus and on the current status of pneumococcal disease and its prevention. Rev Infect Dis, 3(suppl):S1, 1981.
128. Bolan G, et al: Pneumococcal vaccine efficacy in selected populations in the United States. Ann Intern Med, 104:1, 1986.
129. Schwartz JS: Pneumococcal vaccine: Clinical efficacy and effectiveness. Ann Intern Med, 96:208, 1982.
130. Williams JH, Jr, and Moser KM: Pneumococcal vaccine and patients with chronic lung disease. Ann Intern Med, 104:106, 1986.

Chapter 29

AEROBIC AND FACULTATIVE GRAM-POSITIVE BACILLI

The aerobic and facultative gram-positive bacilli are a heterogeneous group of organisms frequently found in the environment. Because the taxonomy of many of these bacteria has not been determined unequivocally, in this chapter they are discussed according to spore formation and microscopic appearance as follows: endospore-forming bacilli, Bacillus; regular non–spore-forming bacilli, Listeria, Erysipelothrix, Lactobacillus, Kurthia; irregular or coryneform non–spore-forming bacilli, Corynebacterium, Arcanobacterium, Rothia; nocardioforms and aerobic actinomycetes, Nocardia, Actinomadura, Streptomyces, Nocardiopsis, Dermatophilus, Rhodococcus, and Oerskovia. An approach to identification of these organisms is shown in Figure 29–1.

ENDOSPORE-FORMING BACILLI

Bacillus species are aerobic or facultative, endospore-forming, catalase-positive, gram-positive bacilli. Bacillus anthracis once was considered the only human pathogen of the genus, but other species now are recognized as potential pathogens, capable of causing food poisoning and serious infections in immunocompromised persons.

Bacillus anthracis

Epidemiology

Bacillus anthracis, principally a pathogen of herbivores, is the agent of anthrax. Cutaneous anthrax results from direct contact with animals that have the disease or from contact with anthrax spores contaminating raw materials such as hides, goat hair, wool, and bones used in a manufacturing process. Inhaling aerosols of anthrax spores generated during processing of goat hair causes pulmonary anthrax (woolsorters' disease); gastrointestinal and oropharyngeal anthrax follow ingestion of contaminated undercooked meat.

The reservoir of Bacillus anthracis is the soil, but its cycle in the environment is not fully understood. In the United States B. anthracis is found in the environment in focal areas of Louisiana, Oklahoma, and Colorado.

The actual incidence of anthrax worldwide is not known, but 20,000 to 100,000 cases are reported annually (1). Anthrax is rare in most developed countries. Fewer than 10 cases were reported in the United States during the past decade, the most recent being a case of cutaneous anthrax that occurred in 1987 in a 42-year-old male maintenance worker at a North Carolina textile mill who came in contact with cashmere contaminated with Bacillus anthracis from Western Asia (2).

Pathogenesis

After spores of Bacillus anthracis are inhaled, those larger than 5 μm are cleared from the lung by the mucociliary system, but smaller particles reach the alveoli, are phagocytosed by pulmonary macrophages, and are carried to the mediastinal lymph nodes. Hemorrhagic mediastinitis ensues followed by bacteremia and often meningitis. After they are ingested, bacilli travel to the mesenteric lymph nodes, where they multiply, causing hemorrhagic lymphadenitis and ascites, followed by septicemia. Bacilli also may pass from contaminated meat directly across the pharyngeal mucosa to local lymph nodes, causing edema and adenopathy, and eventually they enter the blood.

The virulence of Bacillus anthracis is due to an antiphagocytic polyglutamic acid capsule and plasmid-mediated production of a three-component exotoxin (protective antigen, edema factor, and lethal factor), responsible for brawny edema and tissue necrosis.

Clinical Manifestations

Cutaneous anthrax, which accounts for more than 95% of anthrax cases, begins 1 to 7 days after contact with an infected animal as a pruritic papule, most commonly on exposed parts of the body, that enlarges and progresses into a painless ulcer surrounded by vesicles and eventually covered by a characteristic black eschar. Edema is prominent, and lymphangitis and regional lymphadenopathy may occur. If untreated, cutaneous anthrax is fatal in about 20% of cases.

Pulmonary anthrax initially resembles influenza (see Chapter 11), and in 2 to 3 days severe hypoxia, dyspnea, and hypotension develop, accompanied by meningeal signs in about half the cases. The mortality rate approaches 100%. Features of gastrointestinal anthrax are abdominal pain, bleeding, and ascites.

Other Bacillus Species

Epidemiology

Bacillus species are found in decaying organic matter, dust, soil, vegetables, and water. Some are part of the normal human flora, and from sites of colonization can easily cause disease in immunocompromised or traumatized persons. Outbreaks of bacteremia related to contaminated dialysis equipment and wound and burn infections have been reported (3,4). Serious infections have occurred among drug users, possibly from contaminated heroin or paraphernalia (5). Outbreaks of food poisoning caused by Bacillus cereus have been reported from Asia, Australia, Europe, and North America (6).

Pathogenesis

Some species of Bacillus elaborate enzymes and toxins that may contribute to their virulence. Bacillus cereus produces two enterotoxins, diarrheal toxin, which causes

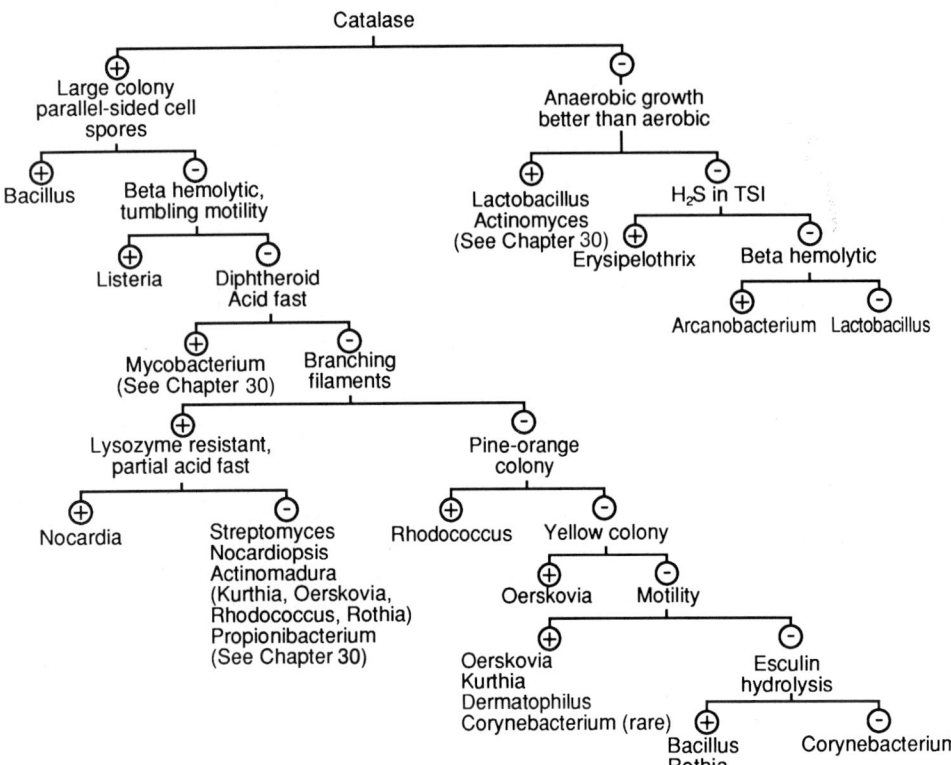

Fig. 29–1. Decision tree for preliminary identification of aerobic and facultative gram-positive bacilli. (From Baron, E. J., and Finegold, S. M. (eds.): Bailey and Scott's Diagnostic Microbiology. 8th ed. St. Louis, C.V. Mosby, 1990.)

fluid accumulation in rabbit ileal loops, increases vascular permeability in rabbits, and is lethal for mice when injected intravenously, and emetic toxin; and two lethal toxins, loop fluid-inducing/skin test/necrotic toxin and cereolysin. Phospholipase C, an enzyme produced by B. cereus, may play a role in ocular infections by disrupting host cell membrane phospholipids exposed by the action of other toxins.

Clinical Manifestations

Infections caused by Bacillus species are listed in Table 29–1 (7–12). Food poisoning due to Bacillus cereus, which follows the consumption of preformed toxin, begins abruptly with nausea and vomiting 1 to 6 hours after ingesting toxin-contaminated warmed foods such as fried or steamed rice (short-incubation disease) or with abdominal cramps and diarrhea 6 to 24 hours after ingesting meat or vegetables (long-incubation disease). Both syndromes are self-limited. B. cereus also is an important cause of endophthalmitis, especially following trauma or soil contamination (9).

Laboratory Diagnosis

Specimens for diagnosis of infection with species of Bacillus are listed in Table 29–1. Collection, transport, and processing of these specimens are discussed in Part III. Organism identification is reviewed here.

Bacillus anthracis. A smear prepared from an aspirate or swab collected from a cutaneous ulcer or vesicle and stained with Gram stain shows short chains of large, gram-positive bacilli (3 to 5 μm × 1 to 1.25 μm) with flattened ends; spores are rare. In smears prepared from a colony of B. anthracis, bacilli with non-swollen central to subterminal endospores are in long chains, resembling a jointed bamboo rod.

On sheep blood agar after overnight incubation, colonies of Bacillus anthracis are 2 to 5 mm in diameter, non-hemolytic, and with age develop a rough texture and curled peripheral projections, the classic Medusa head appearance. Typically, cells of B. anthracis lack a capsule, but when grown on medium containing 0.5% sodium bicarbonate and incubated in 5% carbon dioxide, virulent strains become encapsulated, producing mucoid colonies.

Colony appearance alone is not sufficient to identify Bacillus anthracis. Although most other species of Bacillus cause β hemolysis on sheep blood agar, this trait is variable among strains of Bacillus cereus and Bacillus thuringiensis. Moreover, Bacillus cereus, Bacillus mycoides, and Bacillus thuringiensis may exhibit the Medusa head colony. A motility test (described in reference 13) is a useful screen, because Bacillus anthracis is nonmotile and most other species of Bacillus are motile. In addition, testing for susceptibility to penicillin with a 10-U penicillin G disk on Mueller-Hinton agar will differentiate B. anthracis, which is highly susceptible, from Bacillus cereus, Bacillus mycoides, and Bacillus thuringiensis, which are resistant. Direct examination under oil immersion of a wet-mount preparation of cells of Bacillus anthracis growing at the leading edge of the zone of inhibition shows bulging cylinders, referred to as the "string of pearls" reaction. Additional tests for identification of B. anthracis are outlined in references 13 and 14.

Anthrax also may be diagnosed by demonstrating serum antibodies to Bacillus anthracis protective antigen and le-

Table 29-1. Infections Caused by Bacillus and Specimens for Diagnosis

Infection (reference)	Species	Specimen
Anthrax (1)	B. anthracis	Swabs of vesicle exudate,* blood, cerebrospinal fluid, serum (for serology)
Bacteremia, septicemia (7)	B. alvei, cereus, laterosporus, megaterium, pumilis, sphaericus, subtilis	Blood
Meningitis (8)	B. alvei, circulans, megaterium, pumilis, sphaericus, subtilis	Cerebrospinal fluid
Ocular infections† (8,9)	B. brevis, cereus, coagulans, subtilis, thuringiensis	Corneal scrapings, aspirate of vitreous
Pneumonia (10)	B. cereus, subtilis, sphaericus	Sputum, bronchoalveolar lavage fluid, transtracheal aspirate, lung tissue, pleural fluid (if present), blood
Endocarditis (11)	B. cereus, subtilis	Blood
Food poisoning (12)	B. cereus	Implicated food (25–50 g), stool, vomitus‡

* One for culture and one for preparing smears for staining with Gram and fluorescent antibody stains.
† Includes corneal ulcer, endophthalmitis, keratitis, iridocyclitis, panophthalmitis, and orbital abscess.
‡ Quantitative culture must be performed.

thal factor, but these tests are not available commercially (1).

Other Bacillus Species. After overnight incubation, colonies of most Bacillus species are β hemolytic, and many are large with a frosted-glass appearance (Color Plate IIIB), occasionally becoming opaque and variable in color. Colonies of Bacillus cereus, 3 to 8 mm in diameter, are raised and irregular, with a greenish frosted-glass appearance and undulate margins, and usually are surrounded by a wide zone of β hemolysis. Colonies of Bacillus mycoides (formerly Bacillus cereus var. mycoides) are larger with rootlike outgrowths from the colony margin. Some isolates of Bacillus grow poorly on MacConkey agar and may be mistaken for gram-negative bacilli, especially because some species are gram variable and may stain gram negative. A potassium hydroxide test may be useful for classifying isolates of indeterminate Gram reaction (Appendix, Procedure 18). More detailed descriptions of differential characteristics of the species of Bacillus are provided elsewhere (13,14).

Treatment and Prevention

Treatment of cutaneous anthrax includes local wound care and penicillin administration. Inhalation anthrax requires large intravenous doses of penicillin plus streptomycin and supportive care; however, the mortality rate is high despite therapy. Vaccinating workers involved in the industrial processing of imported animal products and the decline in the use of fibers of animal origin are responsible for the low incidence of human anthrax in the United States (2).

Treatment of infections with other species of Bacillus is based on the antibiogram of the infecting organism. β-Lactam antimicrobial agents rarely are effective against Bacillus cereus, but other species often are susceptible. Many species are susceptible to tetracycline, chloramphenicol, clindamycin, erythromycin, vancomycin, gentamicin, imipenem, and ciprofloxacin. Food poisoning caused by B. cereus is a self-limited illness that requires only supportive care.

REGULAR NONSPORE-FORMING BACILLI

Listeria

Eight species of Listeria, all found in the environment, are recognized. Only Listeria monocytogenes causes human disease; the others cause disease in animals or are nonpathogenic and are not discussed further. L. monocytogenes, a motile, catalase-positive, facultative anaerobe, has been recovered from soil, dust, water, animal feed, sewage, decaying vegetation, fish, insects, many animals, and asymptomatic humans. Isolates can be grouped according to five heat-labile flagellar antigens and 14 carbohydrate-containing heat-stable antigens into 16 serotypes (serovars), of which three (serotypes 4 b, 1/2 b, and 1/2 a) cause more than 90% of human infections.

Epidemiology

The prevalence of listeriosis in the United States is difficult to estimate because reporting is incomplete and bacterial isolation and identification procedures are not uniform. In 1986, when the Centers for Disease Control (CDC) initiated an active surveillance program, the estimated overall annual incidence was 7.1 per million, but it varied significantly among different populations. The attack rate was 12.4 per 100,000 for cases associated with pregnancy, 5.4 per million for cases not associated with pregnancy, and 21 per million for persons older than 70 years.

In the United States and Denmark, one third of cases of listeriosis are in pregnant women and neonates, groups that account for two-thirds of cases in Sweden and Germany (15). Adults older than 40 years are at increased risk of infection, possibly reflecting the decline in immunocompetence with increasing age (see Chapter 2). The fatality rate is 35% overall in nonperinatal cases, 11% for persons under 40 years, and 63% for those older than 60 years.

Transmission of the organism by foods such as cole slaw, pasteurized milk, and soft cheeses has resulted in major epidemics in North America and Europe during the past decade (16–19). Most cases of listeriosis, however, occur sporadically, and except with transplacental transmission, the source is unknown. Food-borne transmission is postulated but not proven. Listeria monocytogenes has been detected in 2 to 3% of processed dairy products tested by the Food and Drug Administration since 1986, resulting in recall of more than 40 commercial products (20). Moreover, the organism has been isolated from 4 to 8% of samples of shrimp and cooked crabmeat, and may be present in as many as 30% of raw, ready-to-eat meat products, 15 to 20% of ground meat samples, and 15 to 80% of retail poultry, although these products have not yet been implicated unequivocally in the transmission of listeriosis.

Pathogenesis

The port of entry of Listeria monocytogenes (excluding transplacental transmission during maternal bacteremia) to persons with sporadic bacteremia or meningitis is unknown, but it is presumed to be the gastrointestinal tract. Given that L. monocytogenes is present in the gastrointestinal tract of about 1% of adults without producing symptoms (carriers), some additional factor(s) must be necessary to produce disease. Defects in the immune system probably are involved because many persons with listeriosis are immunosuppressed. Macrophages and T lymphocytes are the most important host defenses against L. monocytogenes; immunoglobulins and complement, necessary for opsonization, play a less important role.

The virulence of Listeria monocytogenes probably is related to production of listeriolysin O, a 52-kd protein with hemolytic and cytotoxic properties that is secreted under conditions of low pH and low iron concentration, as would exist in a phagolysosome. The protein is postulated to act intracellularly by binding irreversibly to cholesterol in the lysosome membrane, thus disrupting the membrane and allowing unrestricted growth of the bacteria within the phagocyte cytoplasm.

Clinical Manifestations

Clinical manifestations of listeriosis differ in each of the high-risk groups: pregnant women, neonates, and immunocompromised persons. Listeriosis during pregnancy is most common in the third trimester. Women present with a flulike illness: fever, headache, and myalgias, occasionally with diarrhea and abdominal cramping. Bacteremia occurs concurrently, during which the uterine contents are infected. Progression to amnionitis may result in premature labor or septic abortion in 3 to 7 days. Infection in the mother is self-limited because the source of the infection is removed with delivery of the infected fetus and uterine contents.

Two forms of neonatal listeriosis occur, early- and late-onset, which clinically resemble neonatal infections caused by group B Streptococcus (see Chapter 28). Early-onset disease, manifested at birth or within the first few days of life, results from infection in utero. Infants present with signs and symptoms of bacterial sepsis: temperature instability, hemodynamic compromise, and respiratory distress; widely disseminated granulomas, particularly involving the placenta, posterior pharynx, and skin, are characteristic of the illness but are not always present (21). Late-onset disease, affecting full-term infants of mothers who have uncomplicated pregnancies, is assumed to be acquired postpartum, but in most cases the source is unknown. Clinical manifestations of meningitis become apparent several days to several weeks after birth (mean, 14 days).

Nonperinatal listeriosis occurs in persons who have a malignancy, are recipients of organ transplants or for another reason receive immunosuppressive agents, as well as in elders, diabetics, persons with alcoholic and nonalcoholic liver disease, chronic renal disease, and collagen-vascular diseases. For about one third of affected adults no risk factor can be identified. Approximately half of these infections are manifested as meningitis with nuchal rigidity and fever. The cerebrospinal fluid (CSF) contains 100 to 10,000 white blood cells (WBC) per microliter, with a predominance of neutrophils in 70% of cases, elevated protein levels, and a normal glucose concentration in more than 60% of cases; 60 to 75% of blood cultures yield Listeria monocytogenes. In other forms of central nervous system (CNS) listeriosis—cerebritis and brain stem and spinal cord abcesses—fever is common but nuchal rigidity is rare; CSF cultures are sterile in over half the cases (20). The diagnosis is based on positive blood cultures and the results of imaging tests.

In addition to CNS infections, listeriosis in adults may present as primary bacteremia or, rarely, focal infections: endocarditis, endophthalmitis, arthritis, osteomyelitis, liver abscess, cholecystitis, peritonitis, pleuropulmonary infections, and cutaneous infections (22–30).

Laboratory Diagnosis

Specimens necessary to diagnose Listeria monocytogenes infection vary with the clinical syndrome (Table 29–2). Collection, transport, and processing of these specimens are discussed in Part III. Organism identification is reviewed below.

On sheep blood agar, colonies of Listeria monocytogenes are round, translucent, and surrounded by a narrow zone of complete hemolysis, similar to colonies of group B Streptococcus (see Chapter 28). In smears of clinical specimens and broth cultures stained with the Gram stain, cells of L. monocytogenes vary in appearance: typical short, intra- and extracellular gram-positive bacilli, coccobacilli in short chains resembling streptococci, longer

Table 29–2. Clinical Syndromes Associated with Listeria Monocytogenes and Specimens for Diagnosis

Syndrome	Specimen
Listeriosis of pregnancy	Blood, amniotic fluid, genital tract secretions
Listeriosis in neonates	Placenta, blood, cerebrospinal fluid (CSF), fetal tissue* (if fatal)
Meningitis	CSF, blood
Bacteremia	Blood
Nonmeningitic infections of the central nervous system†	CSF, brain tissue, blood

* Lesions are most common in liver, but may involve brain, adrenal glands, spleen, kidneys, lung, and the gastrointestinal tract.
† Include meningoencephalitis, cerebritis, and brain stem and spinal cord abscesses.

gram-positive bacilli in a palisade formation characteristic of diphtheroids (discussed later), or unevenly stained pleomorphic organisms similar to Haemophilus (see Chapter 36) may be observed. Biochemical tests useful for identification are listed in Table 29–3.

Treatment

Although the optimal antimicrobial therapy for listeriosis has not been established, the synergistic combination of ampicillin and gentamicin usually is recommended. For persons allergic to penicillin the combination of sulfamethoxazole and trimethoprim has documented efficacy (20).

Erysipelothrix

Erysipelothrix rhusiopathiae is a nonmotile, nonencapsulated gram-positive bacillus, commensal in many animals, birds, and fish, but also found in dead and decaying organic matter. It is principally a pathogen of swine but can cause disease in horses, sheep, cows, other animals, and humans.

Epidemiology

Although no national data are available on the prevalence of human erysipeloid in the United States, approximately one case is reported to the CDC in any given year (31). Human infection, an occupational disease of fishermen, fish handlers, butchers, meat processing and poultry workers, farmers, veterinarians, abattoir workers, and housewives, generally follows skin trauma during contact with infected animals or animal products, though as many as 20% of infected persons have no known animal exposure.

Pathogenesis

A potential virulence factor of Erysipelothrix rhusiopathiae is its production of neuraminidase, an enzyme that cleaves sialic acid residues from host cell membranes, increasing the susceptibility of affected cells to lysis via activation of the alternate complement pathway.

Clinical Manifestations

A painful, pruritic, violaceous cutaneous lesion with sharply defined, irregular borders appears 2 to 7 days following trauma to the skin, most commonly involving the hands. Arthritis ensues in approximately 5% of cases. Bacteremia, usually associated with endocarditis, occurs infrequently, and about a third of affected persons have a concurrent cutaneous lesion.

Laboratory Diagnosis

The best specimen for recovery of Erysipelothrix rhusiopathiae from a cutaneous lesion is an aseptically collected full-thickness skin biopsy specimen (because organisms are found deep in the tissue) taken from the edge of a lesion. Alternatively, saline may be injected into the edge of the lesion, reaspirated without withdrawing the needle, and submitted for culture. Blood cultures are required to diagnose bacteremia and endocarditis.

Colonies of Erysipelothrix rhusiopathiae on sheep blood agar are smooth, convex, circular, and transparent, or rough with a matte surface and fimbriated edge. The blood underneath the colonies shows greenish discoloration. In a smear prepared from smooth colonies and stained with Gram stain, the bacilli are short, slender, and straight or slightly curved, and in smears from rough colonies, bacilli form long filaments and chains. E. rhusiopathiae is catalase- and oxidase-negative. In triple sugar iron agar (see Chapter 34) it produces an acid slant and butt and forms hydrogen sulfide, blackening the butt, a characteristic almost always indicating E. rhusiopathiae, because very few gram-positive bacilli form hydrogen sulfide. The "test tube brush" pattern of growth of E. rhusiopathiae in gelatin stab cultures incubated at 25° C is another unique identifying feature.

Treatment

Localized cutaneous disease generally is self-limited, resolving spontaneously in 3 to 4 weeks. The treatment of choice is a single intramuscular injection of benzathine penicillin, but oral erythromycin also is effective. Either penicillin or cefazolin is appropriate therapy for Erysipelothrix rhusiopathiae–induced endocarditis. Arthritis often requires drainage plus antimicrobial therapy.

Lactobacillus

Species of Lactobacillus, part of the normal flora of the human oral cavity and gastrointestinal and female genital tract, have been isolated from blood, CSF, abscess material, amniotic fluid, and pleural fluid, and rarely cause serious human infections such as endocarditis (32). Lactobacilli are facultative or strict anaerobes, but usually prefer microaerophilic conditions and demonstrate better growth when incubated anaerobically than when incubated in air. On blood agar colonies may be pinpoint, α hemolytic, resembling those of streptococci, or large, rough, and gray. Cells of lactobacilli may appear similar to those of Bacillus (described earlier), or they may be coccobacillary, spiral, or long and thin. Lactobacilli are nonmotile and give negative reactions for catalase, esculin hydrolysis, and hydrogen sulfide production. Differentiation of lactobacilli from streptococci (Chapter 28) may be difficult, but observing chains of bacilli in smears of growth in thioglycolate broth stained with Gram stain

Table 29–3. Characteristics of Listeria Monocytogenes

Test	Expected Reaction
Hanging-drop motility, 25° C	Tumbling
Motility medium, 25–30° C	Umbrella formation of growth
Catalase	+
Hydrogen sulfide production in triple sugar iron agar	−
Hippurate hydrolysis	+
Bile esculin hydrolysis	+
Growth in 6.5% sodium chloride	+
Glucose fermentation	+
Urease production	−

(Plate IIIC) and resistance to vancomycin help identify an isolate as a Lactobacillus. Features of the species of Lactobacillus most commonly isolated from clinical specimens are outlined in reference 33. Growth of lactobacilli is inhibited by penicillin, ampicillin, clindamycin, and cephalothin, but these agents are not bactericidal; therefore, the combination of penicillin plus an aminoglycoside, perhaps with rifampin, is recommended for treatment of endocarditis due to Lactobacillus.

Kurthia

Kurthia bessonii, a soil saprophyte, is a rare cause of endocarditis in humans. It is a nonsaccharolytic, strict aerobe that forms irregular colonies resembling those of Bacillus cereus (described earlier). The cells are large, straight-sided, and motile, similar to B. cereus but with no spores.

IRREGULAR OR CORYNEFORM NON–SPORE-FORMING BACILLI

Corynebacterium

Species of Corynebacterium are pleomorphic gram-positive bacilli that occur in angular arrangements and occasionally develop rudimentary branching and coccoid cells. Corynebacteria have mesodiaminopimelic acid, arabinogalactan, and short-chain (22 to 36 carbon atoms) mycolic acids, similar to those of mycobacteria (Chapter 40) and nocardiae (discussed later), in their cell wall, and a DNA guanine-plus-cytosine content of 51 to 65 mol% (34).

Pleomorphic gram-positive bacilli recovered in the clinical laboratory that stain irregularly and are arranged in palisades and V shapes (Plate IIID), commonly are called diphtheroids or coryneforms because they resemble the cuneiform configurations of cells of Corynebacterium diphtheriae and are presumed to be members of the genus Corynebacterium. However, in one study, only 59% of more than 1000 aerobic coryneform isolates from the skin of hospitalized patients and normal volunteers belonged to the genus Corynebacterium; 20% belonged to the genus Brevibacterium; the remainder could not be assigned to a genus (35). Most corynebacteria are nonmotile and catalase positive. These organisms are components of the normal skin flora and when recovered from clinical specimens often are regarded as contaminants. However, because the prevalence of opportunistic infections due to coryneform bacteria is increasing, they should be considered potential pathogens when isolated from sterile sites in immunocompromised persons. Corynebacterium diphtheriae, Corynebacterium jeikeium, and corynebacteria of group D2 are important human pathogens. Other species of Corynebacterium—Corynebacterium ulcerans, Corynebacterium minutissimum, Corynebacterium pseudotuberculosis, Corynebacterium pseudodiphtheriticum, Corynebacterium xerosis, and Corynebacterium bovis — infrequently cause disease in humans and are discussed briefly; a more detailed description of these organisms is provided in reference 34.

Corynebacterium diphtheriae

Epidemics of "throat distemper" were first recognized in New England in the early 1700s. The disease was named diphtheria by Bretonneau in 1821, from the Greek root for leather, to describe the pharyngeal membrane. In 1883, gram-positive bacilli were seen in histologic sections of the membrane, and the next year Loeffler isolated the organism in pure culture and reproduced the disease in guinea pigs, proving that the bacterium was the agent of diphtheria (36). Over the next 10 years toxin produced by Corynebacterium diphtheriae was proven to be responsible for death in guinea pigs, and antiserum directed against the toxin was shown to protect animals from death following infection and to significantly reduce the mortality rate of children from diphtheria. Clinical trials using "toxoid" (toxin made nontoxic by exposure to formalin and heat) to induce protection against diphtheria were initiated in 1924, and immunization programs were established in most western countries between 1930 and 1945.

Epidemiology

Humans are the only known reservoir for Corynebacterium diphtheriae, which is transmitted by airborne respiratory droplets, direct contact with infected respiratory secretions, or exudate from skin lesions, and fomites. Carriers (asymptomatic persons who harbor a toxigenic strain of C. diphtheriae in the nasopharynx or on the skin) and those in the incubation stage of the disease are the most important sources of infection (37–40).

Diphtheria occurs worldwide, causing nearly a million deaths annually in developing countries, where fewer than 10% of infants are fully immunized, but it is uncommon in Western Europe and the United States, where active immunization programs exist. In the United States only five cases of diphtheria were reported from 1980 to 1984, and between 1971 and 1981 the incidence was highest among American Indians (41). During these 10 years, outbreaks were most common in winter, when crowding and close interpersonal contact promote spread of the infection, among incompletely immunized school children of poor socioeconomic conditions. More recently, outbreaks of cutaneous diphtheria have been reported among adults who are longterm alcohol abusers (37,38).

Pathogenesis

At the initial site of infection on the tonsils and oropharynx, Corynebacterium diphtheriae multiplies on the epithelial cells and elaborates an exotoxin that causes local cell necrosis and subsequent inflammation. Exudative lesions coalesce, forming a grayish black adherent pseudomembrane composed of fibrin, necrotic epithelial cells, erythrocytes, leukocytes, and bacilli (Fig. 29–2). The organisms remain localized, and the toxin is absorbed into the circulation and distributed systemically, producing degenerative changes in the heart, nervous system, and kidneys.

Diphtheria toxin is produced only by strains of Corynebacterium diphtheriae infected with a temperate bacterio-

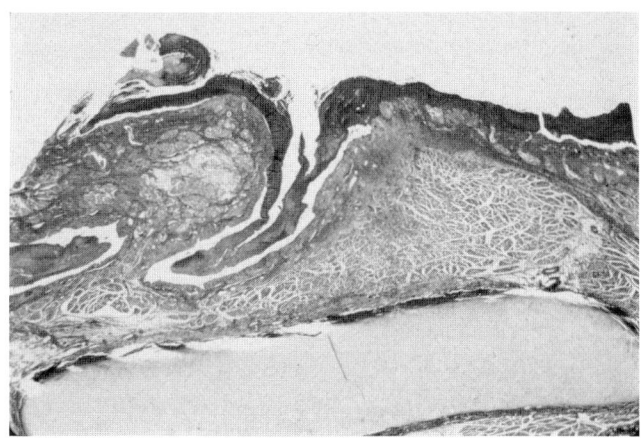

Fig. 29–2. Section of the larynx shows the pseudomembrane of diphtheria (hematoxylin and eosin, ×2.5).

phage carrying the gene for toxin production. The biologically active toxin molecule consists of two fragments: A, containing the enzymatically active site, and B, comprising the receptor-binding site, both of which are essential for cytotoxicity. Toxin molecules bound to host cells via fragment B are cleaved, and fragment A enters the cell by an incompletely understood process. In the cell, fragment A disrupts protein synthesis by catalyzing the inactivation of transfer RNA translocase, thus preventing the interaction of messenger RNA and transfer RNA and stopping further addition of amino acids to developing polypeptide chains (42). The toxin affects all cells in the body, but the heart, nerves, and kidneys are damaged most severely. Myocardial injury ranges from cloudy swelling of myocytes with loss of cross-striations to complete degeneration of muscle fibers with minute hemorrhages and mononuclear cell infiltration. Degenerative changes in the nervous system involve the ganglion cells of the anterior horns and posterior root ganglia of the spinal cord and the cranial nerves and their nuclei; sparing the cortex. Tubular necrosis occurs in the kidneys.

Clinical Manifestations

Pharyngeal diphtheria begins abruptly, with fever, malaise, sore throat, mild pharyngeal injection, and the development on one or both tonsils of a gray, necrotic, adherent pseudomembrane that may spread to involve the tonsillar pillars, uvula, soft palate, oropharynx, and nasopharynx. With extensive involvement, cervical adenopathy and swelling develop, creating a bull-necked appearance and respiratory stridor. Downward extension of the membrane into the larynx induces hoarseness, dyspnea, and cough. Involvement of the trachea and bronchi may cause respiratory embarrassment, requiring intubation.

Systemic manifestations produced by diphtheria toxin are most likely to develop with severe local disease. Myocardial damage occurs in 10 to 25% of cases after 1 to 2 weeks' illness, although up to two thirds of patients have subtle evidence of myocarditis. Electrocardiographic findings include ST-T-wave changes, first-degree and more severe forms of heart block, atrioventricular dissociation, and other arrhythmias. Myocarditis may present abruptly with congestive heart failure and circulatory collapse or insidiously with progressive dyspnea and weakness. Damage to the nervous system may be manifest as local paralysis of the soft palate and posterior pharynx, cranial neuropathy, or peripheral motor disorders involving proximal muscle groups in the extremities and extending distally. Mortality rates, ranging from 3 to 12%, are highest in the very young, the very old, and those who are incompletely immunized.

Cutaneous diphtheria may be manifest as chronic nonhealing ulcers covered by a gray membrane, or it may appear similar to chronic dermatitis such as eczema or psoriasis. Systemic manifestations of toxin production are rare.

Corynebacterium jeikeium and Corynebacterium Group D2

Both Corynebacterium jeikeium (formerly Corynebacterium group JK) and corynebacteria of group D2 are resistant to many antimicrobial agents (penicillins, cephalosporins, aminoglycosides) and are responsible for an increasing number of serious infections among hospitalized and immunocompromised persons.

Corynebacterium jeikeium, first recognized in 1976, is a minor component of the normal skin flora, especially of the groins, axillae, and rectum (43–45). Males are colonized more frequently than females, suggesting that growth of the organism may be promoted by free fatty acids, which are present in greater quantities on the skin of men. Broad-spectrum antimicrobial therapy of hospitalized persons with malignancies or other serious diseases also favors colonization (46).

Most infections with Corynebacterium jeikeium are hospital acquired and affect severely immunocompromised patients. Risk factors include prolonged hospitalization, prolonged neutropenia, treatment with multiple antimicrobial agents, and disruption of the integument. Bacteremia, often associated with skin or soft tissue infection, is most common in those with hematologic malignancies. Other reported infections include endocarditis, pneumonia, peritonitis, shunt infections, and wound infections (47–50).

Corynebacterium group D2, a urea-splitting organism, most commonly causes cystitis, bacteriuria, and pyelonephritis, primarily in elders who have a history of urologic abnormalities, instrumentation, and treatment with broad-spectrum antimicrobial agents, but it has caused bacteremia and pneumonia in hospitalized patients (51–54). The organisms frequently colonize the skin and mucous membranes, especially the groin and rectum of females (55). Infection with Corynebacterium group D2 causes alkaline urine, promoting the formation of ammonium-magnesium-phosphate (struvite) stones in the bladder.

Corynebacterium ulcerans

Corynebacterium ulcerans was first isolated in 1926 from the throat of persons who had a diphtheria-like illness (56). Infection is most common during the summer in persons living in rural areas and those exposed to horses and cattle, which asymptomatically harbor the organism. C. ulcerans has been recovered from milk and milk containers, and some infected persons report ingesting raw milk; person-to-person transmission of the organism does not occur (57). Infection with C. ulcerans has been recognized in several countries, but most reports have come from England. Clinical manifestations are due to the production of diphtheria toxin, dermonecrotic toxin, or both.

Most isolates of Corynebacterium ulcerans have been from throats of asymptomatic persons, but the organism may cause exudative pharyngitis, a diphtheria-like disease with pseudomembrane formation and cardiac and neurologic manifestations, skin ulcer, and possibly pneumonia (58,59).

Corynebacterium minutissimum

In 1961, Corynebacterium minutissimum was recognized as the agent of erythrasma, a superficial skin infection characterized by pruritic, scaling, reddish brown macular patches in intertriginous areas (60). The infection is diagnosed by observing coral red fluorescence of involved skin examined under Wood's lamp and finding pleomorphic gram-positive bacilli in smears of skin scrapings stained with Gram stain. Rare cases of breast abscess, endocarditis, and fatal septicemia caused by C. minutissimum in persons without erythrasma have been reported (61–63).

Corynebacterium pseudotuberculosis

Corynebacterium pseudotuberculosis, a common animal pathogen, has caused suppurative granulomatous lymphadenitis in humans who had a history of contact with animals, handling animal hides, or consuming raw milk (57,64,65). Nearly all strains of the organism produce a dermonecrotic toxin; and although some isolates produce diphtheria toxin, no cases of diphtheria attributed to infection with C. pseudotuberculosis have been reported.

Other Corynebacterium Species

Corynebacterium pseudodiphtheriticum, a commensal of the human nasopharynx, is a rare cause of endocarditis and necrotizing tracheitis (34,57,66). Rare cases of endocarditis, bacteremia, pneumonia, and surgical wound infections due to Corynebacterium xerosis, a commensal of the conjunctival sac, nasopharynx, and skin, have been reported (34,57). Corynebacterium bovis, a common commensal of the bovine udder, is a rare cause of infections of the central nervous system, infections of prosthetic valves, chronic otitis media and mastoiditis, and chronic leg ulcers in humans (34,57). The source of human infection with C. bovis is unknown; humans are not colonized with the organism, and infected persons often do not report exposure to animals.

Laboratory Diagnosis

Specimens necessary for diagnosis of infection with the species of Corynebacterium are listed in Table 29–4 (67).

Table 29–4. Infections Produced by Corynebacteria and Specimens for Diagnosis

Infection	Species	Specimen
Diphtheria	C. diphtheriae, ulcerans	
Respiratory		Nasopharyngeal and throat swab*
Cutaneous		Swab of ulcer base
Pharyngitis	C. ulcerans	Throat swab
Cutaneous ulcers, wounds	C. ulcerans, xerosis, bovis, jeikeium	Aspirate or swab of exudate, tissue biopsy
Sepsis	C. jeikeium, pseudodiphtheriticum, xerosis, bovis	Blood
Pneumonia	C. jeikeium, xerosis	Sputum, transtracheal aspirate, bronchoalveolar lavage fluid, pleural fluid (if present), blood, lung tissue
Erythrasma	C. minutissimum	Skin scrapings
Lymphadenitis	C. pseudotuberculosis	Lymph node aspirate, biopsy

* Both specimens should be collected for optimal detection of C. diphtheriae.

Collection, transport, and processing of these specimens are discussed in Part III. Identification of the most important human pathogens is reviewed here; features of other species are described elsewhere (34,68).

Corynebacterium diphtheriae. Colonies of C. diphtheriae are black or gunmetal gray on cystine-tellurite agar and gray-black, surrounded by dark brown halos, on modified Tinsdale medium. Cultural typing (biotyping) of C. diphtheriae—gravis, intermedius, and mitis—initially reflected the severity of disease produced by each type during major epidemics in Europe during the early 1900s, but now is used principally as an epidemiologic tool, because the correlation between type and disease severity no longer is clear. The lipophilic intermedius strains require blood, serum, or Tween 80 for growth and produce flat, creamy, transparent, nonhemolytic colonies on blood agar. Colonies of gravis and mitis strains are larger, convex, and surrounded by a zone of weak β-hemolysis.

The cellular structure of the three cultural types grown on Loeffler slants and stained with Loeffler methylene blue is distinct: bacilli of the mitis strain—long, pleomorphic, rigid rods in cuneiform arrangements—have intensely staining metachromatic granules; bacilli of type intermedius strain vary in size and often have swollen ends containing large terminal granules; cells of the gravis type are uniformly staining, short, often coccoid or pyriform bacilli.

Biochemical tests for identification of the species of Corynebacterium are described in references 34 and 68. All isolates of Corynebacterium diphtheriae must be tested for toxin production, which most often is done in a reference laboratory in vitro by the modified Elek immunodiffusion test or in vivo by the guinea pig lethality test (68). In the Elek test a filter paper strip impregnated with diphtheria antitoxin is placed just below the surface of a special agar plate immediately before the agar hardens. Test isolates of C. diphtheriae and known toxigenic and nontoxigenic strains are streaked on the agar surface in straight lines perpendicular to the paper strip; the plate is incubated 24 to 72 hours at 37° C and examined for precipitin lines at a 45-degree angle to the streaks (Fig. 29-3), indicating that the organism produced toxin which reacted with the homologous antitoxin.

Corynebacterium jeikeium. Corynebacterium jeikeium forms white, smooth, pinpoint colonies with a metallic sheen on blood agar. A smear stained with the Gram stain shows small, beaded gram-positive bacilli in a cuneiform pattern or coccal forms resembling streptococci (Chapter 28). These organisms are catalase positive, ferment glucose and galactose in serum-supplemented peptone broth, and give negative reactions for oxidase, urease, nitrate reduction, and motility. Moreover, their antibiogram often is a useful identifying characteristic: isolates frequently are resistant to penicillins, cephalosporins, and aminoglycosides but consistently are susceptible to vancomycin. Certain commercially available kit systems accurately identify C. jeikeium and corynebacteria of group D2, but they are less reliable for other species of Corynebacterium (34,69).

Corynebacterium Group D2. On blood agar, colonies of Corynebacterium group D2 are pinpoint, white, opaque, smooth, and nonhemolytic after 48 hours. A smear stained with the Gram stain shows pleomorphic gram-positive bacilli, typical of diphtheroids, and coccobacilli. The organisms are nonmotile, catalase- and urease positive, and oxidase- and indole negative. They do not ferment glucose, lactose, sucrose, maltose, mannitol, D-xylose, or starch, or reduce nitrates to nitrites.

Treatment and Prevention

Corynebacterium diphtheriae. Persons with diphtheria should be hospitalized in strict isolation and treated with antitoxin to neutralize unbound toxin and with erythromycin to halt production of toxin and eliminate respiratory tract colonization. Antitoxin is available only as horse serum, so serum sickness is a potential complication of treatment. The manifestations of diphtheria can be prevented by immunization with formalin-inactivated toxin. Beginning at 6 to 8 weeks of age, infants should be given three intramuscular injections of diphtheria-pertussis-tetanus (DPT) vaccine at 4- to 8-week intervals and a fourth dose 6 to 12 months after the third. A DPT booster should be given at the time of entry into school, after which diphtheria-tetanus boosters are given every 10 years.

Other Corynebacterium Species. Treatment of infections with other species of Corynebacterium is based on the antibiogram of the specific organism. Many species are susceptible to penicillin, but Corynebacterium jeikeium and Corynebacterium of group D2 usually are resistant to most antimicrobial agents except vancomycin. Infected foreign devices often must be removed.

Arcanobacterium

Arcanobacterium haemolyticum (formerly Corynebacterium haemolyticum) first was isolated in the South Pacific during World War II from throats of American soldiers who had nasopharyngeal and skin infections, and has been associated with chronic skin ulcers, cellulitis, brain abscesses, septicemia, and osteomyelitis (70–74). Humans are the most likely reservoir of infection: the organism is found in the pharynx and on the skin of healthy persons and only rarely is isolated from animals. Infection probably is transmitted by aerosol droplets. In studies of pharyngitis, A. haemolyticum is recovered from 2% or fewer throat cultures, predominantly from persons 10 to 30 years of age, of whom approximately a third have a history of recurrent tonsillitis (75,76). Affected persons have pharyngeal erythema with or without a patchy white tonsillar exudate; 40% have low-grade fever; and almost half have bilateral, tender anterior cervical or submandibular lymphadenopathy. An erythematous, macular, blanching rash, frequently associated with fine (1-mm) papules, often appears 1 to 4 days after the onset of pharyngitis. The rash generally involves the distal extremities first, spreads centrally over 2 to 3 days, sparing the face, palms, and soles, and then desquamates during resolution.

Colonies of Arcanobacterium haemolyticum on sheep blood agar are very small (0.1 mm and 0.5 mm after 24 and 48 hours, respectively) and surrounded by a narrow zone of complete hemolysis that may not be apparent after only 24 hours. On rabbit blood agar and on human blood agar colonies are larger and surrounded by a wide zone of β-hemolysis. The microscopic appearance of cells from Loeffler medium resembles that of Corynebacterium diphtheriae. Biochemical tests for identification of Arcanobacterium haemolyticum are described elsewhere (34,68,74).

Rothia

The genus Rothia, created in 1967, contains one species, Rothia dentocariosa, a constituent of the normal human oral flora that has been recovered from gingival crevices of persons with periodontal disease and has caused abscesses and endocarditis (77). In smears stained with the Gram stain cells are coccoid, becoming branched after incubation in broth for several days. Rothia grows well on nutrient agar, producing smooth colonies that become rough or globose with age. The organism is catalase- and Voges-Proskauer positive and lactose negative

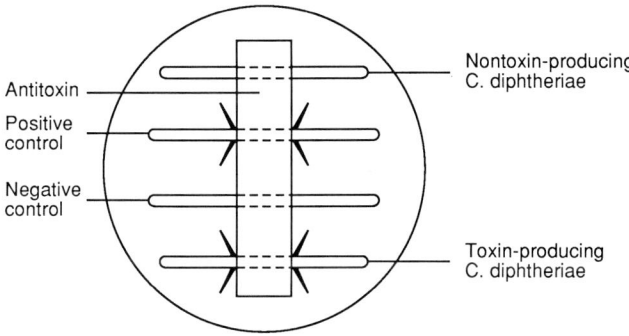

Fig. 29–3. Diagram of the Elek in vitro toxigenicity test for Corynebacterium diphtheriae.

and is susceptible to penicillin, erythromycin, the cephalosporins, and the aminoglycosides (78).

NOCARDIOFORMS AND AEROBIC ACTINOMYCETES

Included in this section are the aerobic gram-positive bacteria that in smears stained with the Gram stain usually appear as branching filaments, occasionally fragmenting into rod-shaped and short coccoid forms. Members of Nocardia are characteristic of this group of organisms, hence the name "nocardioform," a term used only to describe their cellular appearance. These gram-positive bacilli usually grow more slowly than most of the aerobic and facultative bacilli discussed previously, and they grow well on media commonly used to recover fungi. The nocardiae are reviewed in detail; Actinomadura, Streptomyces, Nocardiopsis, Dermatophilus, Oerskovia, and Rhodococcus are discussed briefly.

Nocardia

Nocardia was first described in 1888 by Edmund Nocard, who isolated a slowly growing gram-positive bacillus exhibiting filamentous growth and true branching (initially called Streptothrix farcinica) from cattle on the island of Guadeloupe that had bovine farcy, a granulomatous disease with multiple abscesses, draining sinuses, pulmonary involvement, emaciation, and eventually death (79). In 1891, Eppinger described the first human case in a person with pulmonary disease and brain abscesses (80). The responsible organism was renamed Cladothrix asteroides by Eppinger, and in 1896 the name was changed to Nocardia asteroides (81).

Epidemiology

Nocardia is found in soil and organic material worldwide and causes disease in many animals and in fish. Nocardiosis most commonly is acquired via inhalation of the organism; however, cutaneous and ocular infections caused by primary inoculation may follow trauma and contact with contaminated soil, and the organism may enter via the gastrointestinal tract when contaminated material comes in contact with an area of mucosal ulceration. Infection with Nocardia, reported in persons aged 1 month to 87 years (average, 45 years), affects males two to three times as often as females, possibly owing to hormonal effects on bacterial growth or virulence (82,83). Of the Nocardia recognized as human pathogens, Nocardia asteroides is responsible for 80 to 90% of human infections, Nocardia brasiliensis for 5 to 6%, most often in tropical and subtropical parts of the world, and Nocardia caviae (also called Nocardia otitidiscaviarum) for about 3%. Nocardia transvalensis is an extremely rare human pathogen (84). In the United States, an estimated 500 to 1000 cases of nocardiosis occur annually, and recipients of organ transplants account for about 13% (83).

Pathogenesis and Pathology

In the lungs, Nocardia organisms are phagocytosed by alveolar macrophages and grow within cells; this elicits a mixed inflammatory response (neutrophils, lymphocytes, and macrophages), eventually resulting in abscess or, occasionally, granuloma formation. In animals infected with the organism in the laboratory, virulent strains inhibit phagosome-lysosome fusion, reduce intracellular levels of lysosomal acid phosphatase, and produce superoxide dismutase and catalase, which may mediate resistance to killing by neutrophils (85,86). In vitro, studies of the host defenses against Nocardia have indicated that neutrophils, activated macrophages, and cytotoxic T cells are involved (85,87–90). Although neutrophils do not kill virulent Nocardia they inhibit their growth, possibly suppressing the infection until macrophages are fully activated. In animal models of infection with Nocardia, T cells and activated macrophages promote clearance of the organism and prevent its dissemination from the lungs, and resistance to infection may be transferred with spleen cells and splenic T lymphocytes derived from immune mice (87,90). If the organism is not contained within the lung, spread to other tissues occurs by advancing growth, producing empyema, chest wall involvement, and draining sinuses, or by hematogenous dissemination, resulting in abscess formation, especially in the brain, subcutaneous tissues, and kidneys.

The primary host factor associated with increased risk of nocardiosis is cellular immune dysfunction, although immunoglobulin deficiencies and leukocyte defects also predispose to disease (91–93). Recipients of organ transplants; persons with leukemia, lymphoma, pancytopenia, abnormal leukocyte function, dysgammaglobulinemias, chronic granulomatous disease of childhood, and Cushing's syndrome; and persons receiving steroid therapy are among those at greatest risk of infection (83). Chronic illnesses associated with nocardiosis include chronic obstructive pulmonary disease (present in as many as 12% of cases), pulmonary alveolar proteinosis, tuberculosis, diseases associated with steroid use (systemic lupus erythematosus, mixed connective tissue disease, rheumatoid arthritis, and inflammatory bowel disease), diabetes, and malignancy (83). Recently, nocardiosis has been reported in persons with the acquired immunodeficiency syndrome (AIDS) (94). Many persons infected with Nocardia, however, have no recognized cellular or humoral immune defect (82,95).

Clinical Manifestations

Pulmonary disease is the most frequent manifestation of nocardiosis, occurring in about 75% of cases (82). Symptoms include fever, anorexia, weight loss, productive or nonproductive cough, dyspnea, and pleuritic chest pain. Manifestations of skin and subcutaneous disease vary: pyoderma, cellulitis, single or multiple abscesses, lymphocutaneous disease resembling sporotrichosis (see Chapter 45), or nodules may develop. In Central and South America, primary infections of the skin with Nocardia brasiliensis may produce actinomycetoma, a localized, indurated granulomatous mass with sinus tracts that drain pus and "sulfur" granules, typically on the lower extremities. Disseminated disease, almost always due to Nocardia asteroides, originates in the lung in 60 to 80% of cases and most commonly is manifested as one or more abscesses involving the central nervous system and causing gradual or sudden onset of headache, lethargy, seizures, peripheral paresthesias, nuchal rigidity, confusion, aphasia, tremor, and paresis (in order of decreasing frequency) (82,83). The skin is the second most common site of dissemination, followed by kidney, liver, and lymph nodes (82,83).

Other Nocardioforms

Species of Actinomadura, Streptomyces and, less commonly, Nocardiopsis and Dermatophilus may cause actinomycetomas (described earlier) involving the skin, mucous membranes, and subcutaneous tissue (96). Oerskovia turbata and Oerskovia xanthineolytica, soil saprophytes, have been recovered from cardiac valve vegetations, blood, cerebrospinal fluid, wounds, and in an individual receiving peritoneal dialysis, peritoneal fluid (97–102). Rhodococcus equi, formerly Corynebacterium equi, is an animal pathogen widely distributed in soil and a rare cause of necrotizing pneumonia in humans who have diminished T-cell immunity, such as those receiving corticosteroid therapy and those who have AIDS (103–107). Infection usually follows exposure to animals and most likely is acquired via the respiratory route.

Laboratory Diagnosis

Specimens for diagnosis of infections with the branching, filamentous gram-positive bacilli vary according to the clinical presentation. For pulmonary disease, sputum, bronchoalveolar lavage fluid, material obtained by transthoracic aspiration of a nodule or abscess visualized in a roentgenograph of the chest, or lung tissue may be submitted. For extrapulmonary disease, exudate, pus, granules, biopsy or autopsy tissue, and scrapings from ulcers should be collected; swabs are not recommended. Cerebrospinal fluid and blood specimens also may be obtained. Specimen collection, transport, and processing are discussed in Part III. Organism identification is reviewed here.

Nocardia Species. In smears of sputum and purulent material stained with the Gram stain Nocardia appear as long, thin (0.5 to 1.2 μm diameter), beaded, branching gram-positive bacilli (Plate IIIE). The most distinguishing quality of the nocardiae is their partial acid-fastness (Plate IF): cells stain positively with a modified acid fast (Ziehl-Neelsen or Kinyon) stain (see Appendix, Procedure 7), differentiating them from Actinomyces (Chapter 30), which often have a similar Gram stain appearance (Plate IIIF). Partial acid-fastness, which may be difficult to demonstrate, can be enhanced by growing the organism to be tested and fresh subcultures of known positive (Nocardia asteroides) and negative (Actinomadura madurae) controls for about 4 days on Middlebrook 7H11 agar or in litmus milk broth.

Nocardia grows aerobically on many media: sheep blood, chocolate, and modified Thayer-Martin agar; Sabouraud dextrose agar without chloramphenicol (the antimicrobial agent inhibits Nocardia); and Lowenstein-Jensen or Middlebrook media, typically used for recovery of mycobacteria (see Chapter 40). Incubation in the presence of 10% carbon dixoide enhances the growth of Nocardia, and incubating at least one primary isolation medium at 45° C may increase the recovery of Nocardia asteroides. Nocardia generally survive the decontamination procedures used for recovery of mycobacteria (see Chapter 57); however, one study has shown that decontamination with benzalkonium chloride trisodium phosphate may be toxic to the organisms (108).

Nocardia may grow in 48 hours, but colonies typically appear in 5 to 20 days as waxy, bumpy, or velvety, rugose forms, usually with yellow to orange pigment (Plate IVA). Observing partially acid-fast branching filaments distinguishes Nocardia from the mycobacteria. Nocardia are differentiated from Streptomyces by testing for resistance to the action of lysozyme (Nocardia are resistant, Streptomyces susceptible), described in reference 35. Species of Nocardia are identified according to the characteristics shown in Table 29–5.

Other Nocardioforms. Species of Actinomadura form waxy, cerebriform, tough, membranous colonies that vary in color (white, yellow, pink, or red). Colonies of Streptomyces are dry to chalky, heaped or folded, gray-white to yellow, and have a musty-basement odor. Cells of Nocardiopsis have a unique appearance: zigzag chains of spores within a sheathlike structure. Dermatophilus congolensis forms rough colonies, initially whitish gray and becoming orange to yellow on heart infusion agar and β-hemolytic on horse blood agar, but it does not grow on Sabouraud dextrose agar. Its branching filaments, 0.5 to 1.5 μm in diameter, divide longitudinally and transversely, forming packets of 8 coccoid or cuboid cells (or spores) that become motile (14).

Species of Oerskovia produce yellow-pigmented colonies. These organisms have many characteristics similar to those of Corynebacterium, but esculin hydrolysis and motility tests, positive with Oerskovia and negative with most corynebacteria, may differentiate the two. Rhodococcus equi grows well on ordinary media, producing large, mucoid, pale salmon-pink colonies and may be partially acid fast when stained with the modified Kinyon stain, similar to the Nocardia.

Treatment

Sulfonamides are the antimicrobial agents of choice for infections with Nocardia, although trimethoprim-sulfamethoxazole also may be used. Minocycline is an acceptable alternative, and amikacin and imipenem may be effective. Actinomycetomas require therapy with two antimicrobial agents: streptomycin plus dapsone or trimethoprim-sulfamethoxazole. Optimal treatment for the

Table 29–5. Differentiation of Nocardia

Nocardia Species	Hydrolysis of:			
	Casein	Hypoxanthine	Tyrosine	Xanthine
N. asteroides	−	−	−	−
N. brasiliensis	+	+	+	−
N. caviae	−	+	±	+

Abbreviations: +, ≥90% of strains are positive; −, ≥90% of strains are negative; ±, results vary.

remaining nocardioforms is unknown because few infections in humans have been reported.

REFERENCES

1. Ezzel JW: Anthrax—Pasteur to the present. Clin Microbiol Newslett, *10*:113, 1988.
2. Centers for Disease Control: Human cutaneous anthrax—North Carolina, 1987. MMWR, *37*:413, 1988.
3. Curtis JR, Wing AJ, and Coleman JC: Bacillus cereus bacteremia—a complication of intermittent hemodialysis. Lancet, *i*:136, 1976.
4. Ihde DC, and Armstrong D: Clinical spectrum of infection due to Bacillus species. Am J Med, *55*:839, 1973.
5. Tuazon CU, Hill R, Sheagren JN: Microbiologic study of street heroin and injection paraphernalia. J Infect Dis, *129*:327, 1974.
6. William RP: Bacillus anthracis and other aerobic spore-forming bacilli. *In* Medical Microbiology and Infectious Diseases. Edited by A Braude. Philadelphia, WB Saunders, 1981.
7. Cotton DJ, et al: Clinical features and therapeutic interventions in 17 cases of Bacillus bacteremia in an immunocompromised patient population. J Clin Microbiol, *25*:672, 1987.
8. Farrar WE: Serious infections due to "non-pathogenic" organisms of the genus Bacillus: Review of their status as pathogens. Am J Med, *34*:134, 1963.
9. Davey RT, Jr, and Tauber WB: Posttraumatic endophthalmitis: The emerging role of Bacillus cereus infection. Rev Infect Dis, *9*:110, 1987.
10. Bekemeyer WB, and Zimmerman GA: Life-threatening complications associated with Bacillus cereus pneumonia. Am Rev Respir Dis, *131*:466, 1985.
11. Sliman R, Rehm S, and Shlaes DM: Serious infections caused by Bacillus species. Medicine, *66*:218, 1987.
12. Terranova W, and Blake PA: Bacillus cereus food poisoning. N Engl J Med, *298*:143, 1978.
13. Turnbull PCB, and Kramer JM: Bacillus. *In* Manual of Clinical Microbiology. 5th ed. Edited by A Balows, et al. Washington, DC, American Society for Microbiology, 1991.
14. Koneman EW, et al (eds): The aerobic gram-positive bacilli. *In* Color Atlas and Textbook of Diagnostic Microbiology. 3rd ed. Philadelphia, JB Lippincott, 1988.
15. Bejsen-Moller J: Human listeriosis, diagnostic, epidemiological, and clinical studies. Acta Pathol Microbiol Scand, *229*(suppl):1, 1972.
16. Fleming DW, et al: Pasteurized milk as a vehicle of infection in an outbreak of listeriosis. N Engl J Med, *312*:404, 1985.
17. Linnan MJ, et al: Epidemic listeriosis associated with Mexican-style cheese. N Engl J Med, *319*:823, 1988.
18. Schlech WF, et al: Epidemic listeriosis: Evidence for transmission by food. N Engl J Med, *308*:203, 1983.
19. Bula C, et al: Epidemic foodborne listeriosis in Wesern Switzerland: I. Description of the 58 adult cases. *In* Abstracts of the 28th Interscience Conference on Antimicrobial Agents and Chemotherapy. Washington, DC, American Society for Microbiology, 1988.
20. Gellin BG, and Broome CV: Listeriosis. JAMA, *261*:1313, 1989.
21. Gray ML, and Killinger AH: Listeria monocytogenes and listeric infections. Bacteriol Rev, *30*:309, 1966.
22. Bassan R: Bacterial endocarditis produced by Listeria monocytogenes: Case presentation and review of the literature. Am J Clin Pathol, *63*:522, 1975.
23. Snead JW, et al: Listeria monocytogenes and ophthalmitis. Am J Ophthalmol, *84*:337, 1977.
24. Breckenridge RL, et al: Listeria monocytogenes septic arthritis. Am J Clin Pathol, *73*:140, 1980.
25. Houang ET, Williams CJ, and Wrigley PFM: Acute Listeria monocytogenes osteomyelitis. Infection, *4*:113, 1976.
26. Al-Dajani O, and Khatib R: Cryptogenic liver abscess due to Listeria monocytogenes. J Infect Dis, *147*:961, 1983.
27. Gordon S, and Singer C: Listeria monocytogenes cholecystitis. J Infect Dis, *154*:918, 1986.
28. Case 35-1974, Case records of Massachusetts General Hospital: Weekly clinicopathological exercises. N Engl J Med, *291*:516, 1974.
29. Ananthraman A, Israel RN, and Magnussen CR: Pleural-pulmonary aspects of Listeria monocytogenes infection. Respiration, *44*:153, 1983.
30. Owen CR, et al: A case of primary cutaneous listeriosis. N Engl J Med, *262*:1026, 1960.
31. McClain JB: Erysipelothrix rhusiopathiae. *In* Principles and Practice of Infectious Diseases. 3rd ed. Edited by GL Mandell, RG Douglas, Jr, and JE Bennett. New York, Churchill Livingstone, 1990.
32. Sussman JI, et al: Clinical manifestations and therapy of Lactobacillus endocarditis: Report of a case and review of the literature. Rev Infect Dis, *8*:771, 1986.
33. Baron EJ, and Finegold SM (eds): Aerobic, non-spore-forming gram-positive bacilli. *In* Bailey and Scott's Diagnostic Microbiology. 8th ed. St. Louis, CV Mosby, 1990.
34. Coyle MB, and Lipsky BA: Coryneform bacteria in infectious diseases: Clinical and laboratory aspects. Clin Microbiol Rev, *3*:227, 1990.
35. Pitcher DG: Rapid identification of cell wall components as a guide to the classification of aerobic coryneform bacteria from human skin. J Med Microbiol, *10*:439, 1977.
36. Loeffler F: Untersuchungen Über die Bedeutung der Mikroorganismen für die Entstehung der Diphtherie. Mitt Kaiserlichen Gesundheitsamt, *2*:421, 1884.
37. Heath CW, and Zusman J: An outbreak of diphtheria among skid-row men. N Engl J Med, *267*:809, 1962.
38. Pedersen AHB, et al: Diphtheria on skid road, Seattle, Washington, 1972–75. Public Health Rep, *92*:336, 1977.
39. Koopman JS, and Campbell J: The role of cutaneous diphtheria infections in a diphtheria epidemic. J Infect Dis, *131*:239, 1975.
40. Belsey MA, et al: Corynebacterium diphtheriae skin infections in Alabama and Louisiana. N Engl J Med, *280*:135, 1969.
41. Centers for Disease Control: Annual summary, 1984. MMWR, *33*:23, 1986.
42. Pappenheimer AM: The diphtheria bacillus and its toxin: A model system. J Hyg (Camb), *93*:397, 1984.
43. Telander B, Lerner R, Palmblad J, and Ringertz O: Corynebacterium group JK in a hematological ward: Infections, colonization and environmental contamination. Scand J Infect Dis, *20*:55, 1988.
44. Wichmann S, Wirsing von Koening CH, Becker-Boost E, and Finger H: Group JK corynebacteria in skin flora of healthy persons and patients. Eur J Clin Microbiol, *4*:502, 1985.
45. Larson E, et al: Skin colonization with antibiotic-resistant (JK group) and antibiotic-sensitive lipophilic diphtheroids in hospitalized and normal adults. J Infect Dis, *153*:701, 1986.
46. Gill VJ, et al: Antibiotic-resistant group JK bacteria in hospitals. J Clin Microbiol, *13*:472, 1981.
47. Van Bosterhaut B, et al: Corynebacterium jeikeium (group

47. (cont.) JK diphtheroids) endocarditis. A report of five cases. Diagn Microbiol Infect Dis, *12*:265, 1989.
48. Waters BL: Pathology of culture-proven JK corynebacterium pneumonia. Am J Clin Pathol, *91*:616, 1989.
49. Dan M, Somer J, Knobel B, and Gutman R: Cutaneous manifestations of infection with Corynebacterium group JK. Rev Infect Dis, *10*:1204, 1988.
50. Pierard D, et al: Group JK corynebacterium peritonitis in a patient undergoing continuous ambulatory peritoneal dialysis. J Clin Microbiol, *18*:1011, 1983.
51. Soriano F: Corynebacterium group D2 as a cause of alkaline-encrusted cystitis: Report of four cases and characterization of the organisms. J Clin Microbiol, *21*:788, 1985.
52. Aguado JM, Ponte C, and Soriano F: Bacteriuria with a multiply resistant species of Corynebacterium (Corynebacterium group D2): An unnoticed cause of urinary tract infection. J Infect Dis, *156*:144, 1987.
53. Marshall RJ, Routh KR, and MacGowan AP: Corynebacterium CDC group D-2 bacteraemia. J Clin Pathol, *40*:813, 1987.
54. Marty N, et al: Corynebacterium group D2 etude clinique, identification biochimique et sensibilite aux antibiotiques. Path Biol., *36*:460, 1988.
55. Soriano F, et al: Skin colonization by Corynebacterium group D2 and JK in hospitalized patients. J Clin Microbiol, *26*:1878, 1988.
56. Gilbert R, and Stewart FC: Corynebacterium ulcerans: A pathogenic microorganism resembling C. diphtheriae. J Lab Clin Med, *12*:756, 1926.
57. Lipsky BA, Goldberger AC, Tompkins LS, and Plorde JJ: Infections caused by nondiphtheria corynebacteria. Rev Infect Dis, *4*:1220, 1982.
58. Siegel SM, and Haile CA. Corynebacterium ulcerans pneumonia. South Med J, *78*:1267, 1985.
59. Brown AE: Other corynebacterium. *In* Principles and Practice of Infectious Diseases. 3rd ed. Edited by GL Mandell, RG Douglas, Jr, and JE Bennett. New York, Churchill Livingstone, 1990.
60. Sarkany I, Taplin D, and Blank H: The etiology and treatment of erythrasma. J Invest Dermatol, *37*:283, 1961.
61. Berger SA, et al: Recurrent breast abscesses caused by Corynebacterium minutissimum. J Clin Microbiol, *20*:1219, 1984.
62. Guarderas J, Karnad A, Alvarez S, and Berk SL: Corynebacterium minutissimum bacteremia in a patient with chronic myeloid leukemia in blast crisis. Diagn Microbiol Infect Dis, *5*:327, 1986.
63. Herschorn BJ, and Brucker A: Embolic retinopathy due to Corynebacterium minutissimum endocarditis. Br J Ophthalmol, *69*:29, 1985.
64. House RW, Schousboe M, Allen JP, and Grant CC: Corynebacterium ovis (pseudotuberculosis) lymphadenitis in a sheep farmer: A new occupational disease in New Zealand. N Z Med J, *99*:659, 1986.
65. Richards M, and Hurse A: Corynebacterium pseudotuberculosis abscesses in a young butcher. Aust N Z Med, *15*:85, 1985.
66. Colt HG, Morris JF, Marston BJ, and Sewell DL: Necrotizing tracheitis caused by Corynebacterium pseudodiphtheriticum: Unique case and review. Rev Infect Dis, *13*:73, 1991.
67. Lyman ED, and Youngstrom JA: Diphtheria cases and contacts: Is it necessary to take cultures from both nose and throat? Nebr State Med J, *41*:361, 1956.
68. Krech T, and Hollis DG: Corynebacterium and related organisms. *In* Manual of Clinical Microbiology. 5th ed. Edited by A Balows, et al. Washington, DC, American Society for Microbiology, 1991.
69. Tillotson G, Arora M, Robbins M, and Holton J: Identification of Corynebacterium jeikeium and Corynebacterium CDC group D2 with the API 20 strep system. Eur J Microbiol Infect Dis, *7*:675, 1988.
70. MacLean PD, Liebow AA, and Rosenberg AA: A hemolytic corynebacterium resembling Corynbacterium ovis and Corynebacterium pyogenes in man. J Infect Dis, *79*:69, 1946.
71. Altman G, and Bogokovsky B: Brain abscess due to Corynebacterium haemolyticum. Lancet, *i*:378, 1973.
72. Ceilley RI: Foot ulceration and vertebral osteomyelitis with Corynebacterium haemolyticum. Arch Dermatol, *113*:646, 1977.
73. Ben Jaacob D, et al: Septicemia due to Corynebacterium haemolyticum. Isr J Med Sci, *20*:431, 1984.
74. Clarridge JE: The recognition and significance of Arcanobacterium haemolyticum. Clin Microbiol Newslett, *11*:41, 1989.
75. Banck G, and Nyman M: Tonsillitis and rash associated with Corynebacterium haemolyticum. J Infect Dis, *154*:1037, 1986.
76. Miller RA, Brancato F, and Holmes KK: Corynebacterium hemolyticum as a cause of pharyngitis and scarlatiniform rash in young adults. Ann Intern Med, *105*:867, 1986.
77. Schafer EJ, Wing EJ, and Norden CW: Infectious endocarditis caused by Rothia dentocariosa. Ann Intern Med, *91*:747, 1979.
78. Barksdale L: Identifying Rothia dentocariosa. Ann Intern Med, *91*:786, 1979.
79. Nocard E: Note sur la maladie de boeufs de la Guadeloupe: Connue sous le nom de facin. Ann Inst Pasteur, *2*:293, 1988.
80. Eppinger H: Über eine neue pathogene Cladothrix and einedurch sie hervorgerufene Pseudotuberculosis (Cladothrishica). Beitr Pathol Anat Allg Pathol, *9*:287, 1891.
81. Blanchard R: Parasites végétaux a l'exclusion des bactéries. *In* Traité de Pathologie Générale. Vol. 2. Edited by C Bouchard. Paris, 1895.
82. Palmer DL, Harvey RL, and Wheeler JK: Diagnostic and therapeutic considerations in Nocardia asteroides infection. Medicine, *53*:391, 1974.
83. Wilson JP, Turner AP, Kirchner KA, and Chapman SW: Nocardial infections in renal transplant recipients. Medicine, *68*:38, 1989.
84. Badhdadlian H, et al: Nocardia transvalensis pneumonia in a child. Pediatr Infect Dis J, *8*:470, 1989.
85. Beaman BL, Black CM, Doughty F, and Beaumant L: Role of superoxide dismutase and catalase as determinants of pathogenicity of Nocardia asteroides: Importance in resistance to microbicidal activities of human polymorphonuclear neutrophils. Infect Immun, *47*:135, 1985.
86. Black CM, Beaman BL, Donovan RM, and Goldstein E: Effect of virulent and less virulent strains of Nocardia asteroides on acid-phosphatase activity in alveolar and peritoneal macrophages maintained in vitro. J Infect Dis, *148*:117, 1983.
87. Beaman BL, et al: Lung response of congenitally athymic (nude), heterozygous, and Swiss Webster mice to aerogenic and intranasal infection by Nocardia asteroides. Infect Immun, *22*:867, 1978.
88. Filice GA: Inhibition of Nocardia asteroides by neutrophils. J Infect Dis, *151*:47, 1985.
89. Filice GA, Beaman BL, and Krick JA: Effects of human neutrophils and monocytes on Nocardia asteroides: Failure of

killing despite occurrence of the oxidative metabolic burst. J Infect Dis, *142*:432, 1980.
90. Deem RI, Beaman BL, and Gershwin ME: Adoptive transfer of immunity to Nocardia asteroides in nude mice. Infect Immun, *38*:914, 1982.
91. Young LS, Armstrong D, Blevins A, and Lieberman P: Nocardia asteroides infection complicating neoplastic disease. Am J Med, *50*:356, 1971.
92. Murray JF, Finegold SM, Froman S, and Will DW: The changing spectrum of nocardiosis, a review and presentation of nine cases. Am Rev Respir Dis, *83*:315, 1961.
93. Bryak JS, Ottesen EA, and Dinarello CA: Nocardiosis in a child with chronic granulomatous disease. J Pediatr, *83*:98, 1973.
94. Rodriguez JL, Barrio JL, and Pitchenik AE: Pulmonary nocardiosis in the acquired immunodeficiency syndrome, diagnosis with bronchoalveolar lavage and treatment with nonsulfur containing drugs. Chest, *90*:912, 1986.
95. Curry WA: Human nocardiosis, a clinical review with selected case reports. Arch Intern Med, *140*:818, 1980.
96. Emmons CW, et al: Medical Mycology. 3rd ed. Philadelphia. Lea & Febiger, 1977.
97. Rihs JD, McNeil MM, Brown JM, and Yu VL: Oerskovia xanthineolytica implicated in peritonitis associated with peritoneal dialysis: Case report and review of Oerskovia infections in humans. J Clin Microbiol, *28*:1934, 1990.
98. Cruickshank JG, Gawler AH, and Shaldon C: Oerskovia species: rare opportunistic pathogens. J Med Microbiol, *12*:513, 1979.
99. Guss WJ, and Ament ME: Oerskovia infection caused by contaminated home parenteral nutrition solution. Arch Intern Med, *149*:1457, 1989.
100. Kailath EJ, Goldstein E, and Wagner FH: Case report: Meningitis caused by Oerskovia xanthineolytica. Am J Med Sci, *295*:216, 1988.
101. LeProwse CR, McNeil MM, and McCarthy JM: Catheter-related bacteremia caused by Oerskovia turbata. J Clin Microbiol, *27*:571, 1989.
102. Reller LB, Maddoux GL, Eckman MR, and Pappas G: Bacterial endocarditis caused by Oerskovia turbata. Ann Intern Med, *83*:664, 1975.
103. Bishopric GA, et al: Pulmonary pseudotumour due to Corynebacterium equi in a patient with the acquired immunodeficiency syndrome. Thorax, *43*:486, 1988.
104. Fierer J, et al: Nonpulmonary Rhodococcus equi infections in patients with acquired immunodeficiency syndrome (AIDS). J Clin Pathol, *40*:556, 1987.
105. MacGregor JH, Samuelson WH, Sane DC, and Goodwin JD: Opportunistic lung infection caused by Rhodococcus (Corynebacterium) equi. Radiology, *160*:83, 1986.
106. Sane DC, and Durack DT: Infection with Rhodococcus equi in AIDS. N Engl J Med, *314*:56, 1986.
107. Harvey RL, and Sunstrum JC: Rhodococcus equi infection in patients with and without human immunodeficiency virus infection. Rev Infect Dis, *13*:139, 1991.
108. Murray PR, Geeren RL, and Niles AC: Effect of decontamination procedures on recovery of Nocardia species. J Clin Microbiol, *25*:2010, 1987.

Chapter 30

ANAEROBIC GRAM-POSITIVE BACTERIA

The anaerobic gram-positive bacteria of medical importance are discussed in this chapter: the spore-forming bacilli, Clostridium; the non–spore-forming bacilli, Actinomyces, Bifidobacterium, Eubacterium, Lactobacillus, and Propionibacterium; and the cocci, Peptostreptococcus and Peptococcus.

SPORE-FORMING ANAEROBIC BACILLI (CLOSTRIDIUM)

Species of Clostridium are spore-forming obligate anaerobes that usually stain gram-positive. Individual species, however, vary in their relationships to oxygen (for example, Clostridium haemolyticum and Clostridium novyi are strict obligate anaerobes, whereas Clostridium histolyticum and Clostridium tertium are aerotolerant) and some, such as Clostridium ramosum, typically stain gram-negative. Clostridia are ubiquitous in the environment, in soil, sewage, marine sediments, decaying animal and plant products, and the intestinal tract of many animals and humans, and they can easily contaminate wounds and foods. Of the more than 80 species of Clostridium, fewer than 20 are encountered in specimens pertaining to illness or infections in humans (1). In this chapter, Clostridium botulinum, Clostridium tetani, Clostridium perfringens, and Clostridium difficile are reviewed; Clostridium sordellii, Clostridium novyi, Clostridium histolyticum, Clostridium septicum, Clostridium bifermentans, Clostridium sporogenes, Clostridium tertium, Clostridium ramosum, Clostridium butyricum, and Clostridium baratii are discussed briefly.

Clostridium botulinum

Clostridium botulinum is responsible for almost all cases of botulism, of which three forms are recognized (foodborne, wound, and infant botulism), although in some cases of botulism in adults no source of the organism or its toxin is identified. Seven distinct types of botulinal toxin, designated A through G, are known, and types A, B, and E are responsible for most cases of human disease. Clostridium botulinum is divided into four groups based on culture characteristics (described later): Group I includes all strains of C. botulinum type A, almost all type B strains isolated in the United States, and about half of type F strains recovered from the environment in the United States. These organisms produce very heat-resistant spores and, therefore, are responsible for most of the botulism associated with home-canned foods. Group II includes all type E strains described, most type B strains that cause botulism in Europe, and about half the type F strains. These organisms grow optimally at 30° C, which may reduce their ability to cause wound botulism or colonize the intestine, and they produce spores that are less resistant to heat than those of Group I. Organisms of Group III produce types C and D toxins and are associated almost exclusively with botulism in avian and animal species. Organisms in Group IV, for which the name Clostridium argentinense has been proposed, produce type G toxin or are nontoxigenic (2).

Epidemiology

Clostridium botulinum commonly is found in samples of soil and aquatic sediments. Types A and B predominate in the soils of the continental United States, and type E predominates in the soils of Alaska, northern Europe, and Japan and in aquatic sediments (3). Type F strains have been recovered from marine sediments from the Pacific Coast and from crabs in Chesapeake Bay, and type G organisms have been found in a few soil samples in Argentina and in Switzerland (1,4–6).

Foodborne botulism is uncommon in the United States; typically, fewer than 50 cases are reported each year (7,8). From 1957 to 1975, 170 outbreaks were reported; and of the 125 for which information was available 110 (88%) were related to home-canned or home-processed foods (predominantly canned items but also frozen potpies [mishandled at home], commercially packaged fish, and potato salad) and only one occurred in a restaurant (9). Between 1976 and 1984 in about 125 outbreaks involving more than 300 persons more than 20 deaths were reported from 36 states, the incidence rates being highest in Alaska, Washington, Oregon, and California (9). Toxin types A, B, and E were identified in 60%, 30%, and 10% of cases, respectively. The implicated vehicles were vegetables in 70% of cases, usually home canned, and meat or fish in 30%. Of the outbreaks caused by E toxin, 90% occurred in Alaska, and all were associated with home-processed fish or meat from marine mammals. Commercially canned foods, implicated in 3% of outbreaks, accounted for 2% of cases. Foods served in restaurants were responsible for 4% of outbreaks and 42% of all cases. Of the four large restaurant-associated outbreaks, type B toxin was identified in one associated with home-canned food (involving 60 persons in Michigan in 1977, the largest outbreak ever recorded in the United States). The other three, due to type A toxin, were associated with foods such as sauteed onions and potato salad made from leftover baked potatoes that were cooked, allowed to stand at room temperature or in slightly warmed ovens at least overnight, and then eaten without reheating (9).

In Portugal between 1970 and 1984, 13 outbreaks affecting 50 persons were reported; 30 persons were hospitalized but none died (10). All outbreaks were associated with home-prepared foods, predominantly smoked ham, though bacon, sausage, and mussels were implicated in one case each. In all cases in which bacteriologic studies were performed type B toxin was identified.

Wound botulism first was described in 1943 (11). In the United States between 1976 and 1984 16 cases, of which two were fatal, were reported to the Centers for Disease Control (CDC) from California, Washington, Texas, Maryland, Pennsylvania, and New York (9). Type A toxin or organisms were identified in 11 cases, type B in four, and both in one. Disease was associated with compound fractures or crush injuries to an extremity in 11 cases and with lesions induced by intravenous drug use in 2 cases.

Infant botulism, affecting infants younger than 1 year, first was recognized in 1976 and has become the most common form of botulism confirmed in the United States; 50 to 100 cases are reported annually (1,7,12,13). Foods implicated in infant botulism include honey and corn syrup, but in many cases no source is identified (1,14). Rarely, a similar form of botulism occurs in adults who have predisposing factors such as a surgical procedure involving the gastrointestinal tract, gastric achlorhydria, and antimicrobial therapy (15,16).

Pathogenesis

The clinical manifestations of all forms of botulism are caused by the action of botulinal neurotoxin, a heat-labile toxin inactivated by heating at 100° C for 10 minutes. The toxin binds to receptors (possibly a ganglioside) on peripheral nerve endings, a portion of the molecule is internalized, and by an unknown process prevents the release of acetylcholine from the nerve ending (1). The muscle response to a nerve impulse thus is blocked because no neurotransmitter is released to excite the muscle (1). With foodborne botulism, preformed toxin is ingested; with wound botulism, toxin is produced by Clostridium botulinum growing in a wound; and with infant botulism (and rare cases of botulism in adults), toxin is produced by toxigenic strains of C. botulinum colonizing the intestinal tract. Healthy persons ingest spores of C. botulinum without deleterious effects; therefore, infants probably become colonized because they have not established a stable normal intestinal flora that inhibits the germination of ingested spores and outgrowth of the organism. Similarly, adults who have conditions that predispose to alteration of the intestinal flora (discussed earlier) are at increased risk of disease.

Clinical Manifestations

Symptoms of foodborne botulism typically begin after an incubation period of 18 to 36 hours (range, a few hours to 8 days). Fever is absent early but may develop later if the illness is complicated by pneumonia or other infection. Most persons are responsive and oriented but some are anxious, agitated, or somnolent. The neurologic manifestations are those of a descending symmetric motor paralysis that first affects muscles supplied by the cranial nerves without causing sensory disturbance or paresthesia. Common symptoms and signs include diplopia, dysarthria, dysphagia, dilated and fixed pupils, depressed deep tendon reflexes, dry mucous membranes and dizziness or vertigo. Occasionally urine retention or incontinence develops, and a third of affected persons have abdominal pain, cramps, and fullness, with diarrhea or constipation. Respiratory failure or aspiration pneumonia may occur later in the illness.

Symptoms of wound botulism appear after an incubation period of 4 to 14 days and are similar to those of foodborne botulism with the following exceptions: fever may be present, gastrointestinal symptoms generally are absent, unilateral sensory changes may be associated with the trauma or infection, and the wound usually drains purulent material.

The spectrum of illness in infant botulism varies from subclinical infection to fulminant, fatal disease. Most cases begin gradually with constipation, followed by lethargy, listlessness, decreased appetite, diminished suck and gag reflexes, and a weak, feeble cry. The infant may drool, owing to dysphagia, and loss of head control, ptosis, and other cranial nerve palsies may develop. Undiagnosed botulism has been implicated as one possible cause of the sudden infant death syndrome, but this theory is controversial because data from several studies have not confirmed the association (1,17–20).

Clostridium tetani

Clostridium tetani, a ubiquitous organism worldwide in soil, in animal and human feces, and in house dust, is the agent of tetanus, a disease recognized since ancient times (21). In 1884 tetanus was transmitted from a human with the disease to a rabbit by injecting material from the person's infected wound (22). In 1890 tetanus was produced in animals infected in the laboratory with bacteria-free filtrates of C. tetani cultures, demonstrating that the disease is toxin mediated. That same year animals were immunized with modified tetanus toxin, and neutralizing antitoxin antibodies were detected in their sera. Commercial antitoxin for passive immunization, produced in horses and cows, was used widely during World War I, and active immunization with tetanus toxoid was suggested in the late 1920s.

In dry earth, spores of Clostridium tetani survive for many years but die slowly when exposed to air and sunlight. Spores are very resistant to antiseptics and fairly resistant to heat. Most spores are killed after 1 hour in water at 100° C but because some are unusually resistant, sterility is ensured only after boiling for 4 hours or autoclaving at 121° C for 10 minutes.

Epidemiology

Despite the availability of an effective vaccine, tetanus remains an important health problem worldwide. Most cases are attributed to contamination of a wound (typically punctures and lacerations of the hands and feet, although any type of wound may precede the illness), contamination of a newborn's umbilical stump, or contamination of the puerperal uterus after inexpert attempts to remove a retained placenta. Skin infections may predispose to tetanus, and in India tetanus due to chronic otitis is common (23). Iatrogenic tetanus may follow intramuscular injections, especially with necrotizing materials such as quinine, or use of nonsterile surgical instruments and dressings during procedures such as abortion, ear piercing, and ritual scarification. In about 10% of cases the portal of entry of the organism is unknown.

The prevalence of tetanus, inversely related to socioeconomic conditions, is greatest in underdeveloped countries. In areas where the per capita income is less than $100 annually an estimated 10% of newborn infants die from tetanus, making it the second most common cause of neonatal death, after prematurity (24). But because neonatal tetanus often occurs after delivery at home, many cases are not reported, so the true frequency of the disease probably is much greater than estimated.

The reported incidence of tetanus in the United States declined steadily between 1947 and 1976, and continued to fall thereafter at a slower rate. The decline is attributed to the widespread use of tetanus toxoid and improved wound management (25). Most cases of tetanus occur in rural areas of the southeastern and south central states, possibly reflecting more frequent outdoor work and contact with soil (which may explain the peak prevalence in summer and spring), poorer medical care, and lower levels of immunization. In urban areas the majority of cases involve intravenous drug users (26).

In the United States in 1987 and 1988 101 cases of tetanus (48 in 1987 and 53 in 1988) from 35 states were reported to the Centers for Disease Control, for an average annual incidence rate of 0.02 per 100,000 population, compared with 0.39 per 100,000 in 1947, when national reporting began (25). Five states in the Rocky Mountain region reported no cases, a pattern that was constant during the 1980s (27,28). The incidence of tetanus increased with age (Fig. 30–1), and no cases were reported in neonates. Thirty-one of the 46 persons whose immunization status was known were not immunized. The overall case-fatality rate was 21%.

Pathogenesis

The clinical manifestations of tetanus result from the action of tetanospasmin, a powerful (estimated lethal dose, 130 μg) selective neurotoxin that acts on motor end plates in skeletal muscle, in the spinal cord, in the brain, and in the sympathetic nervous system, inhibiting the release of acetylcholine from nerve terminals in muscle, thus impairing neuromuscular transmission (1,24). In the spinal cord the toxin causes dysfunction of polysynaptic reflexes with subsequent unopposed muscle contraction. Seizures may be due to fixation of the toxin by cerebral gangliosides. The toxin may spread from the site of infection to the central nervous system by adsorption at myoneural junctions and migration through the perineural tissue spaces of nerve trunks or by passage from tissue spaces to the lymphatics and the blood; however, the exact mechanism is unknown (25).

Clinical Manifestations

The signs and symptoms of tetanus may become apparent 24 hours to several months after an injury, but the usual incubation period is 3 to 21 days. Early signs of disease include tension or cramps in the muscles around a wound, increased reflexes in the injured extremity, mild pains in the facial muscles, stiffness of the muscles of the neck and jaw, slight difficulty in swallowing, and anxious facies. Four forms of tetanus are recognized. *Local tetanus*, an uncommon, relatively benign form of the disease, is characterized by stiffness and rigidity of muscles around the site of injury. *Cephalic tetanus*, the rarest form, characterized by facial or oculomotor palsy and dysphagia (manifestations of dysfunction of cranial nerves III, IV, IX, X and XII), develops 1 to 2 days after an infection of

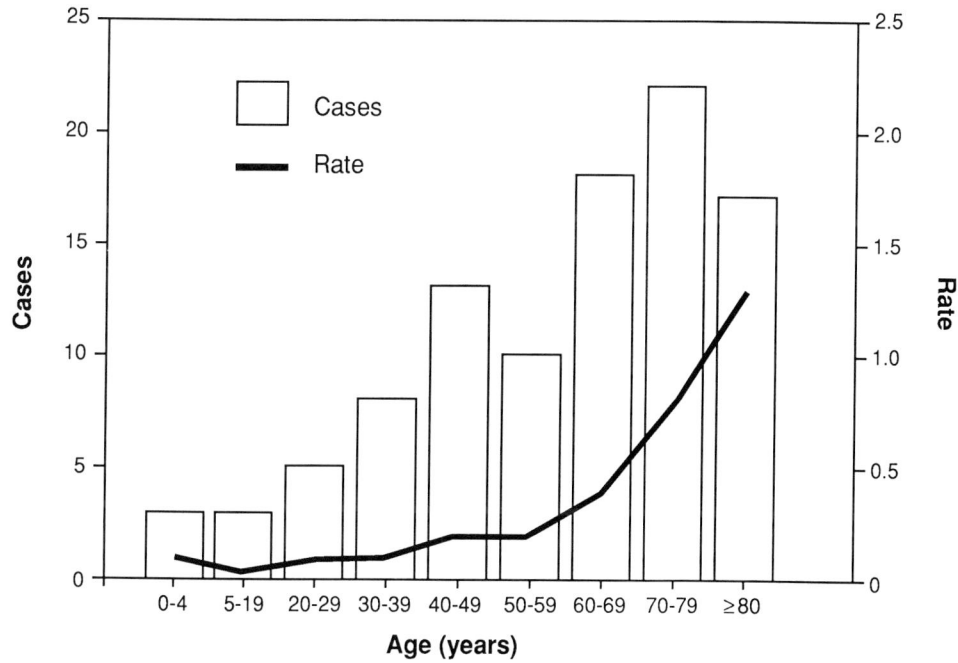

Fig. 30–1. Age distribution of reported cases of tetanus and the average annual age-specific incidence per million population in the United States, 1987 and 1988. (From Centers for Disease Control: Tetanus—United States, 1987 and 1988. MMWR, 39:37, 1990.)

the head or face. *Generalized tetanus*, the most common form, may be mild, characterized by muscle stiffness and rigidity; moderate, with recurrent muscle spasms occurring spontaneously or in response to various stimuli (cold air, noise, light, touch); or severe, characterized by sudden contractions of muscle groups causing opisthotonos, flexion and adduction of the arms, extension of the legs and feet, and clenching of the fist on the chest. Spasms of the larynx, diaphragm, and intercostal muscles may cause acute respiratory failure, and autonomic nervous system involvement may produce tachycardia, labile hypertension, sweating, cardiac arrhythmias and, terminally, hypotension, hyperpyrexia, and pulmonary edema. Pneumonia is the most common cause of death. The risk of death is inversely related to the incubation period: periods under 7 days are associated with the greatest mortality rate. *Otogenous tetanus*, a less severe form of generalized or local tetanus, follows chronic otitis media.

Neonatal tetanus most commonly occurs after infection of the umbilical cord, usually is generalized, and typically has a short incubation period, with symptoms peaking 6 to 7 days after birth. The infant suddenly is unable to suck, the body becomes stiff, and generalized spasms occur. Laryngeal spasms result in inability to swallow, and spasms of the respiratory muscles may cause apnea. Aspiration pneumonia and gastroenteritis are common complications. Most deaths occur after 4 to 14 days.

Clostridium perfringens

Clostridium perfringens, the most prevalent pathogenic bacterium and the species of Clostridium most commonly isolated from humans, is found in soil samples and intestinal contents of animals and humans (1). The organism is associated with several diseases, including myonecrosis (gas gangrene), food poisoning, enterotoxin-associated diarrhea, and enteritis necroticans.

Epidemiology

Factors that predispose to clostridial myonecrosis are extensive laceration or devitalization of muscles (especially large muscle groups of the lower extremities and buttocks), impairment of the main blood supply to a limb or muscle group, contamination by foreign bodies, and failure to provide prompt surgical management. A surgical procedure of the gallbladder or bowel or the upper female genital tract may precede clostridial myonecrosis of the abdominal wall or uterus, respectively.

Clostridium perfringens is the third most common cause of foodborne disease in the United States, after Salmonella (Chapter 34) and Staphylococcus aureus (Chapter 28). Disease often occurs in outbreaks and is associated with food such as meat, poultry, or gravy that was previously cooked, allowed to cool slowly or to remain unrefrigerated (conditions optimal for bacterial multiplication) and then reheated (8). Between 1970 and 1980 about 570 outbreaks of foodborne illness due to C. perfringens were confirmed in England, and about 25 outbreaks were reported yearly in the United States; but because the illness is mild, many cases are not reported (1).

Enterotoxin-associated diarrhea predominantly affects elderly persons who have received antimicrobial therapy (29,30). Enteritis necroticans, a disease endemic in New Guinea but reported only sporadically in Western countries, occurs almost exclusively in the setting of massive pork feasting (8).

Pathogenesis

Alpha toxin, believed the major factor responsible for the tissue damage in myonecrosis, is a phospholipase produced in large amounts by type A strains of Clostridium perfringens. The toxin hydrolyzes phosphatidylcholine and sphingomyelin, increases vascular permeability, and affects myocardial function, causing hypotension and bradycardia with subsequent shock, a common and frequently fatal manifestation of gas gangrene (1). Enterotoxin, produced predominantly by type A strains of C. perfringens but also by type C and D strains, is responsible for the diarrhea associated with ingesting food heavily contaminated with the organism and with antimicrobial therapy. The enterotoxin apparently binds directly to receptors on the surface of intestinal epithelial cells (principally in the ileum in animal models of the disease) and is inserted into the cell membrane without being internalized into the cell, causing a change of ion fluxes that affects cellular metabolism (1). As intracellular calcium levels increase, membrane permeability is altered, allowing the loss of cellular fluid, ions, and moderate-sized molecules (31,32).

Beta toxin, produced by type B and C strains of Clostridium perfringens, is responsible for the lesions of enteritis necroticans, which in animal models of the disease develop only when a protease inhibitor is introduced into the gut. These findings in animals support the hypothesis that enteritis necroticans occurs in persons whose gastrointestinal protease activity is low (owing to a normally low-protein diet). Disease develops when the level of protease activity is further reduced by protease inhibitors, which are present in sweet potatoes (consumed in large quantities at the New Guinea feast), and pork contaminated with C. perfringens is ingested (8).

Clinical Manifestations

Clostridial myonecrosis is a rapidly advancing, sometimes rapidly fatal, infection that begins suddenly with pain in the area of a wound. The pain increases in severity but remains localized to the wound and spreads as the infection progresses. Local swelling, edema, and a hemorrhagic exudate appear, accompanied by tachycardia. The skin is tense, cold, and white, often with areas of blue or bronze discoloration. Bullae filled with dark red or purplish fluid appear; and small amounts of gas develop. Later the affected person becomes hypotensive, weak, incoherent, and disoriented. The involved muscle is pale and edematous early, becoming pasty with red and purple mottling, and finally diffusely gangrenous, dark greenish purple or black, friable, and occasionally liquefied. Jaundice, associated with clostridial bacteremia and intravascular hemolysis, develops occasionally.

Symptoms of clostridial food poisoning—abdominal pain, nausea, and watery diarrhea without fever—begin 8 to 24 hours after eating contaminated food and resolve spontaneously in 24 hours. Enterotoxin-associated diarrhea following antimicrobial therapy in hospitalized patients occasionally is bloody and lasts about 7 days. Abdominal pain occurs in about half the cases, but vomiting is uncommon. Enteritis necroticans often is a fulminant illness with anorexia, abdominal pain, bloody diarrhea and vomiting, progressing to peritonitis and shock.

Clostridium difficile

Clostridium difficile is the major cause of nosocomial diarrhea and the primary pathogen responsible for pseudomembranous colitis, a disease characterized by pseudomembranes or microabscesses in the colon. Pseudomembranous colitis was first recognized in 1893 by Finney, who described a "diphtheritic membrane" in the small bowel of a young woman who developed severe, eventually fatal, diarrhea after a surgical procedure (33). It was uncommon in the preantibiotic era but became more frequent as antimicrobial agents were introduced (34). Clindamycin initially was the predominant agent implicated, but it soon was recognized that treatment with other antimicrobials could produce the disease (35). Staphylococcus aureus was recovered from the stool of persons with pseudomembranous colitis in the 1960s and, therefore, initially was believed to be the agent of the disease (36). Subsequently this was disproven, and the role of S. aureus in these early cases now is questioned.

Hall and O'Toole isolated Clostridium difficile from the stools of healthy newborn infants in 1935 and showed that it was toxigenic; but because C. difficile was not known to be a pathogen, its toxin was not studied in detail until the late 1970s, when the organism was associated with pseudomembranous colitis (37). Cytotoxic activity, neutralized by antiserum against toxin produced by Clostridium sordellii, was demonstrated in stools from persons with pseudomembranous colitis; however, C. sordellii almost never was isolated from persons who had the disease. Clostridium difficile then was identified in large numbers in persons with pseudomembranous colitis; and its cytotoxin, neutralized by Clostridium sordellii antiserum, was shown to be almost identical to that produced by C. sordellii (35).

Epidemiology

Carriage rates of Clostridium difficile and its toxins are high (50% or more) among neonates but disease is rare (35). Colonization, with or without toxin production, may be maintained for several months, but when the adult flora becomes established at age 6 to 12 months, colonization rates fall, and only about 3% of normal healthy adults are colonized with the organism (35).

Clostridium difficile almost always is acquired in the hospital via direct or indirect exposure to human or inanimate reservoirs. Persons with diarrhea caused by C. difficile excrete the organism in their feces, readily contaminating clothing and room fixtures. Once in the environment, C. difficile produces spores that persist for months. Hospitalized patients may be directly exposed to an environment contaminated with spores, or spores may be spread on the hands of hospital personnel.

After a person is exposed to Clostridium difficile various factors predispose to diarrhea. A strong association exists between C. difficile colonization and older age, more severe underlying disease, and increased length of stay in the hospital, although the latter may reflect increased opportunity to acquire the organism owing to longer exposure to a potentially contaminated environment and more frequent contacts with hospital personnel. In a recent prospective study of hospitalized patients significant independent predictors of asymptomatic carriage of C. difficile were the use of antacids, which may facilitate passage of the organism through the normally inhibitory acid pH of the stomach and into the colon; and the use of stool softeners, perhaps by altering the osmotic balance in the lumen of the colon (38). Risk factors significantly associated with diarrhea due to C. difficile were the use of penicillins or cephalosporins, gastrointestinal stimulants, stool softeners, and enemas, all of which alter the normal gastrointestinal flora, an important barrier against colonization with or overgrowth of C. difficile. Although the penicillins and cephalosporins are implicated most frequently, any antimicrobial agent may trigger C. difficile–associated disease. Disease rarely occurs without antibiotic exposure, and cases have been reported following therapy with antineoplastic agents that have antibacterial activity (35).

Pathogenesis

Exposure to the organism and alteration of the normal microflora of the gastrointestinal tract by one or more of the mechanisms discussed earlier are essential for the development of Clostridium difficile–associated disease. Pseudomembranous colitis is a toxin-mediated illness in which microbial invasion of the mucosa is not known to occur. C. difficile produces two toxins. Toxin A, weakly cytopathic, is predominantly responsible for the enterotoxic activity of the organism. In a hamster model of disease, injection of toxin A elicits an infiltration of neutrophils into the ileum and the release of inflammatory mediators, causing fluid secretion, altered membrane permeability, and hemorrhagic necrosis; and in vitro toxin A is a powerful chemotactic agent for human neutrophils (35). Toxin B, a potent cytotoxin, appears to play a minor role in human disease. In the hamster model of pseudomembranous colitis, animals must be vaccinated against both toxin A and B to be completely protected, suggesting that toxin B also is important in the disease in hamsters and that a similar situation might occur in humans (35,39,40). A motility-altering factor that causes altered motor activity in the intestine has been described in filtrates of C. difficile cultures, but its role in disease is unknown.

Clinical Manifestations

Persons with pseudomembranous colitis have diarrhea, which may be watery or bloody and may be accompanied by abdominal cramps, leukocytosis, and fever. Severe complications include toxic megacolon, marked electrolyte imbalance, colonic perforation, or hypoalbuminemia with anasarca. Clostridium difficile is estimated to cause about 25% of cases of antibiotic-associated diarrhea, though the exact role of the organism in the latter disease is not clear (35). In addition to its involvement in gastrointestinal diseases, C. difficile is a rare cause of abscesses, wound infections, osteomyelitis, pleuritis, peritonitis, septicemia, and urogenital tract infections (41–43).

Other Clostridia

Clostridium sordellii which produces a β-toxin, may cause gas gangrene–like infections and fatal infections associated with episiotomy incisions, endometritis, and deep lacerations (44–47). Clostridium novyi causes more than one third of cases of gas gangrene, a disease caused by the production of α toxin, which alters capillary permeability, causing massive edema (1). Clostridium histolyticum, which has been isolated from gangrenous and nongangrenous war wounds, produces a lethal toxin and a mixture of collagenases and other proteolytic enzymes that convert tissue proteins to amino acids and peptides (1).

Clostridium septicum may infect wounds, producing gas gangrene, and is the one species of Clostridium that may cause spontaneous myonecrosis. The latter occurs predominantly in persons with a colonic (especially cecal) or hematologic malignancy which, in over a third of cases, is occult when the myonecrosis develops (48). Different factors have been suggested to explain the association of C. septicum with malignancy, but certain aspects are ill-understood. For example, persons with injured colonic mucosa, whether from primary colon cancer or enterocolitis (in those with leukemia), have a suitable port of entry for the organism, but why C. septicum is not associated with other disease states in which the bowel mucosa is compromised (such as ulcerative colitis or Crohn's disease) is unknown. The anaerobic and acidic environment in a necrotic tumor provides conditions favorable for the germination of clostridial spores; however, why C. septicum, and not other species of Clostridium, is so closely associated with malignancy remains unclear. The pathogenicity of C. septicum is related to the production of α toxin and the enzymes hyaluronidase, fibrinolysin, and deoxyribonuclease, which may enhance its invasiveness.

Clostridium bifermentans, Clostridium sporogenes, and Clostridium tertium uncommonly cause gas gangrene, and C. tertium is a cause of bacteremia in neutropenic persons (49). Clostridium ramosum, the second most frequently isolated species of Clostridium, is particularly common in intra-abdominal infections but has been found in severe infections in almost all body sites.

Clostridium butyricum, which often is found in the stool of normal infants, has been associated with neonatal necrotizing enterocolitis, a disease possibly caused by high concentrations of butyric acid, a major end product of C. butyricum metabolism (1,50). Moreover, a few cases of type E infant botulism due to neurotoxigenic C. butyricum have been reported (51,52). Clostridium baratii, which has been recovered from feces of normal infants and adults and from soil samples, generally has low virulence because it does not produce any lethal toxins, but a neurotoxigenic strain has been implicated as the cause of type F infant botulism (53,54).

Laboratory Diagnosis

Specimens for diagnosis of infections caused by clostridia are listed in Table 30–1. Specimen collection, transport, and processing are discussed in Part III. General guidelines for the identification of anaerobes and features characteristic of the clostridia are discussed here.

General Guidelines for Identification of Anaerobes

The first step in identification of an isolate suspected to be an anaerobe is the aerotolerance test to determine the relationship of that isolate to oxygen. This is done for two reasons: a colony recovered on a medium incubated anaerobically may be an obligate or a facultative anaerobe, and the tolerance of anaerobes to oxygen is useful for identification. To perform the aerotolerance test, each colony type is subcultured to three blood agar plates; one each is incubated anaerobically, in an atmosphere of 5 to 10% carbon dioxide, and in ambient air. Anaerobic bacte-

Table 30–1. Diseases Caused by Clostridium and Specimens for Diagnosis

Disease	Species of Clostridium		Specimens
	Common	Uncommon	
Botulism			
Foodborne	C. botulinum		Serum (15–20 ml), gastric contents, stool (25–50 g), vomitus; food samples; at autopsy, serum, gastric and intestinal contents
Wound	C. botulinum		Serum; exudate, tissue or swab of wound
Infant	C. botulinum	C. butyricum, -baratii	Feces, serum, return from sterile water enema; food and environmental samples; at autopsy, intestinal contents
Tetanus*	C. tetani		Exudate, tissue from wound
Gas gangrene	C. perfringens, -novyi, -septicum	C. sordellii, -histolyticum, -bifermentans	Exudate, tissue from wound; blood
Food poisoning*	C. perfringens		Food, stool
Diarrhea	C. difficile, -perfringens		Stool†

* Diagnosis most commonly is based on clinical presentation.
† A rectal swab may be submitted to detect colonization with C. difficile but is not acceptable for toxin detection.

ria grow only on the plate incubated anaerobically, although aerotolerant anaerobes also show slight growth on plates incubated in carbon dioxide and ambient air. Evaluating resistance to a 5-μg metronidazole disk also may help determine an organism's atmospheric requirements, especially those of facultative bacteria that require a reduced-oxygen environment for initial or good growth. The test is performed as described for disk diffusion in Chapter 24 except that the agar plate is incubated anaerobically. Most obligate anaerobes are susceptible (defined as any zone of inhibition) to metronidazole, whereas facultative anaerobes are resistant (no zone of inhibition).

Colony appearance and the Gram reaction often are useful identifying characteristics. One problem associated with the Gram stain, however, is the tendency of gram-positive organisms (especially anaerobes) to decolorize, resulting in misclassification as gram-negative bacteria. Two rapid techniques that may distinguish gram-positive from gram-negative bacteria are the potassium hydroxide (KOH) solubility test (see Appendix, Procedure 18) and the vancomycin disk susceptibility test (55). In the KOH test, exposure of gram-negative bacteria to dilute alkaline solutions disrupts their cell walls, releasing unfragmented threads of DNA and forming a viscous suspension. The KOH reaction is a useful complement to the Gram stain but may yield false-negative results; therefore, routine use of the vancomycin disk susceptibility test should be considered. To perform the latter, a 5-μg vancomycin disk (commercially available) is placed on the surface of a blood agar plate inoculated with a lawn of the test isolate, and the plate is incubated at 35° to 37° C anaerobically for 24 to 48 hours. Gram-negative organisms are resistant to vancomycin and gram-positive organisms are susceptible (defined as any zone of inhibition).

The cellular structure and the presence or absence of spores also are key features used to identify anaerobic bacteria. Typically, anaerobes are more pleomorphic than aerobic and facultative bacteria. In a smear stained with the Gram stain, endospores usually appear as round or oval unstained portions of the cell (Plate IVB). Finding spores in a Gram-stained smear of an isolate shown by the aerotolerance test to be an anaerobe identifies the bacterium as a Clostridium. However, some species of Clostridium (Clostridium tertium, Clostridium histolyticum) are aerotolerant and could be confused with species of Bacillus (see Chapter 29). Isolates of these two genera may be distinguished by their catalase reaction and colony appearance: species of Clostridium are catalase negative and produce larger colonies and more spores when grown in an anaerobic than in an aerobic environment; species of Bacillus are catalase positive and form larger colonies when grown in ambient air.

Clostridium perfringens and Clostridium ramosum generally do not produce spores when grown in the laboratory and, therefore, could be confused with a non–spore-forming anaerobic gram-positive bacillus (discussed later). These two species, however, usually are recognized by their characteristic cellular or colony structure (described below), and if necessary, spores may be induced by performing the ethanol spore test. Isolated colonies of the organism to be tested are inoculated into chopped meat or thioglycolate broth and incubated 48 hours at 35° to 37° C and then at room temperature for 24 hours. One milliliter of the broth culture is mixed with an equal volume of 95% ethanol and allowed to stand for 30 to 45 minutes. The ethanol-broth mixture and the original broth culture are subcultured to a sheep blood agar plate and incubated anaerobically at 35° to 37° C for 48 hours. Growth on both plates indicates that the organism forms spores; growth only from the original broth culture indicates that spores are not produced; if no growth occurs on either plate the test is inconclusive and should be repeated.

Once an isolate is recognized as an anaerobe and classified as gram-positive or gram-negative and as a spore-former or non–spore-former, various methods may be used for identification. The reference method includes determining reactions in a series of conventional carbohydrate broths and biochemicals and using gas-liquid chromatography to identify volatile and nonvolatile acidic metabolic products. The conventional carbohydrate and biochemical media rarely are used in the clinical microbiology laboratory today and, therefore, are not discussed here, but excellent reviews are provided elsewhere (56–60). Gas-liquid chromatography is not mandatory to presumptively classify or to identify most anaerobes encountered in the clinical microbiology laboratory, but it may be useful in identifying some species of Clostridium and some of the anaerobic non–spore-forming gram-positive bacilli. Therefore, a basic understanding of the technique is important; details of test performance are provided elsewhere (56–60). Peptone-yeast extract–glucose broth is inoculated with isolated colonies from an anaerobic blood agar plate and incubated anaerobically for 48 hours or until adequate growth is obtained. Short-chain volatile fatty acids—acetic, propionic, isobutyric, butyric, isovaleric, valeric, isocaproic, and caproic—are extracted in ether, in which they are soluble. Nonvolatile acids—pyruvic, lactic, and succinic—are methylated (in methanol) and then extracted in chloroform. Volatile and nonvolatile acids produced by an organism are identified by injecting the extracts into a gas chromatograph and comparing elution times of known standards chromatographed on the same day.

In most clinical microbiology laboratories isolates of anaerobic bacteria are identified by using one of the commercially available kit systems. Systems based on biochemical test and carbohydrate fermentation reactions of actively growing organisms provide results after anaerobic incubation for 24 to 48 hours; however, these systems often require supplemental tests (such as gas-liquid chromatography) to correctly identify nonsaccharolytic or weakly saccharolytic organisms (59–61). Rapid enzyme test systems, inoculated with a heavy suspension of fresh growth and incubated aerobically for 4 hours, accurately identify most clinically encountered anaerobes, including those that are nonsaccharolytic or weakly reactive, but occasionally additional tests are required (59–64).

Useful identifying characteristics of the commonly encountered species of Clostridium are shown in Table 30–2, and features of Clostridium botulinum, Clostridium tetani, Clostridium perfringens, and Clostridium difficile are discussed in more detail. The anaerobic non–spore-forming gram-positive bacilli and the anaerobic gram-positive cocci are reviewed later, and the gram-negative anaerobes are discussed in Chapter 38.

Identifying Features

Clostridium botulinum. Botulism is so rare that diagnostic investigations of potential cases are performed best in a specialized reference laboratory (such as the CDC). But because the organism may be encountered in the clinical laboratory, particularly in a wound specimen when the diagnosis of botulism is not being considered, features of the four culturally distinct groups of C. botulinum (described earlier) are reviewed briefly. Organisms in group I are strongly proteolytic, and they liquefy gelatin, ferment glucose and maltose, produce lipase on egg yolk agar, and hydrolyze esculin. Organisms in group II are saccharolytic but nonproteolytic. They liquefy gelatin, ferment many sugars, and produce lipase on egg yolk agar, but they do not hydrolyze esculin. Organisms in group III are lipase positive and liquefy gelatin. Organisms in group IV hydrolyze gelatin but, in contrast to other strains of C. botulinum, are lipase negative and asaccharolytic (hence the proposal that they be called Clostridium argentinense). The metabolic end products for each group are listed in Table 30–2.

The mouse bioassay (described in reference 65) is the method of choice for detection of botulinal neurotoxins in investigative specimens (food, stool, vomitus, serum). Experimental methods for detecting toxin in vitro include immunodiffusion, reversed passive hemagglutination, radioimmunoassay, and enzyme-linked immunosorbent assay (ELISA) (65). Smears of stool stained with fluorescent antibodies that detect organisms of group I toxin types A, B, and F (currently not commercially available) may provide a presumptive diagnosis of infant botulism. The antibodies may react with nontoxigenic strains, however, and do not differentiate the toxin types; therefore, confirmation of toxigenicity and toxin typing should be done by the mouse bioassay.

Clostridium tetani. Tetanus usually is diagnosed on the basis of characteristic clinical manifestations (described earlier). The diagnosis may be confirmed bacteriologically by isolating the organism from the infected wound, but C. tetani is recovered only from about one-third of wounds cultured (25). It is a strict anaerobe and grows best at 37° C, at 25° C or 42° C there is little or no growth. Bacilli are slender, 2 to 18 μm long and 0.5 to 1.5 μm wide; often possess round, terminal endospores, producing a "drumstick" appearance (Plate IVB); and in cultures older than 24 hours are easily decolorized, appearing gram negative. Vegetative forms are motile via numerous flagella. Colonies on blood agar, which may not be apparent for 48 hours, are 4 to 6 mm in diameter, flat, translucent, gray with a matte surface and irregular, rhizoid margins, and surrounded by a narrow zone of complete hemolysis. Occasionally growth may appear as a film rather than as discrete colonies because of swarming due to vigorous motility. Most biochemical tests are negative (no sugars are fermented; milk is not digested; neither lecithinase nor lipase is produced; nitrate is not reduced), except for hydrogen sulfide production, indole, and gelatin liquefication (which may require up to 1 week for completion). The gas-liquid chromatography profile is shown in Table 30–2.

Clostridium perfringens. Smears of exudate from cases of myonecrosis caused by C. perfringens stained with the Gram stain typically show large gram-positive bacilli (1 to 19 μm long by 0.5 to 2.5 μm wide) with square ends and no spores and few intact polymorphonuclear leukocytes, which generally have been distorted by clostridial toxins. C. perfringens grows optimally at 45° C (range, 20° to 50° C) and generally does not produce spores when grown on laboratory media. On blood agar colonies typically are surrounded by a double zone of β hemolysis—an inner clear zone and an outer hazy zone. On egg yolk agar, colonies are surrounded by a wide circular opaque zone owing to the production of lecithinase. The organisms are nonmotile, reduce nitrate; ferment glucose, lactose (responsible for "stormy fermentation" in milk), maltose, and sucrose; and liquefy gelatin.

One of the following criteria are required to confirm foodborne disease caused by Clostridium perfringens: greater than 10^5 colonies per gram of suspected food, a median spore count greater than 10^6 per gram of feces from a group of affected persons, or recovery of C. perfringens of a common serotype from stools from groups of affected persons and from suspected food. Enterotoxin-associated diarrhea is diagnosed by detecting enterotoxin in feces of affected persons; a test is commercially available but data on its sensitivity, specificity, and accuracy are not available (1). Moreover, C. perfringens in large quantities (more than 10^7 cfu per gram) generally is present in the stool of these persons.

Clostridium difficile. Colonization with C. difficile is recognized by recovery of the organism from feces or a rectal swab specimen. Cycloserine-cefoxitin-fructose-egg yolk agar, a commercially available selective and differential medium, is used most frequently, but other media such as cycloserine-mannitol agar or cycloserine-mannitol-blood agar may be used (66). To isolate C. difficile from feces, dilutions of the stool sample (1:200, 1:400) are cultured to inhibit overgrowth of the organism by the many other bacteria present. After 48 hours colonies of C. difficile on cycloserine-cefoxitin-fructose-egg yolk agar are yellow, about 4 mm in diameter, have rhizoid margins and crystalline internal structures, show yellow-green fluorescence under long-wave ultraviolet light, and emit an odor like that of a horse barn. C. difficile is motile, liquefies gelatin, ferments fructose, glucose, mannitol, mannose, and usually xylose, and is negative for lecithinase and lipase. Of its metabolic products (Table 30–2), isocaproic acid and p-cresol are produced uncommonly by other organisms and, therefore, have been suggested as markers for C. difficile (especially p-cresol), but their detection lacks the specificity required for definitive identification (35).

The diagnosis of Clostridium difficile–associated disease is based on toxin detection, for which the reference method is cell culture, an assay that principally measures the cytotoxic activity of toxin B in filtrates of stool speci-

Table 30-2. Identifying Characteristics of the Commonly Encountered Clostridia

Clostrium Species	Spores	Aerobic Growth	Lecithin	Lipase	Gelatin Hydrolysis	Indole	Principal Metabolic Products	Comments
C. botulinum								
Group I	OS	−	−	+	+	−	A, P, IB, B, IV, (v), (ic)	
Group II	OS	−	−	+	+	−	A, B	
Group III	OS	−	+	+	+	−	A, P, B	
Group IV	OS	−	−	−	+	−	A, IB, B, IV, PA	Proposed name: C. argentinense
C. tetani	RT	−	−	−	+	v	A, p, B	May swarm on blood agar
C. perfringens	OS	−	+	−	+	−	A, (p), B	Spores seldom observed; produces double zone of hemolysis on blood agar; nonmotile
C. difficile	OS	−	−	−	v	−	A, p, IB, B, IV, V, IC	
C. sordellii	OS	−	+	−	+	+	A, f, (p), (ib), (b), (iv), (ic)	Urease positive
C. novyi A	OS	−	+	+	+	−	A, P, B, (v)	Extremely sensitive to O_2; β-hemolytic on blood agar
C. novyi B	OS	−	+	−	+	−	A, P, B, (v)	
C. histolyticum	OS	v	−	−	+	−	A	Asaccharolytic
C. septicum	OS	−	−	−	+	−	A, B	May swarm on blood agar
C. bifermentans	OS	−	+	−	+	+	A, (p), (ib), (b), (iv), (v), (ic)	Urease negative
C. sporogenes	OS	−	−	+	+	−	A, (p), (ib), B, IV, (ic)	
C. tertium	OT	+	−	−	−	−	A, B	
C. ramosum	R/OT	−	−	−	−	−	A	Spores seldom observed; frequently stains gram-negative
C. butyricum	OS	−	−	−	−	−	A, (p), B	
C. baratii	R/OS/T	−	+	−	−	−	A, B, L, (p), (s)	

Key: +, positive reaction; −, negative reaction; v, variable reaction; /, either/or; O, oval; R, round; S, subterminal; T, terminal. Fermentation products: A, acetic, B, butyric; F, formic; IB, isobutyric; IC, isocaproic; IV, isovaleric; P, propionic; V, valeric; L, lactic; PA, phenylacetic; S, succinic. ( ), May or may not be present; capital letters indicate major peaks; lower case letters indicate minor peaks.

mens. Toxin detection by cell culture has several drawbacks. The assay is not standardized, so comparing data from different studies is difficult. The technique is labor intensive; and unless commercially available multiwell culture plates seeded with indicator cells are used, laboratory personnel performing the test must be familiar with cell culture. The turnaround time is 24 to 48 hours, and the sensitivity of the assay is less than 100% (67). Because of these problems, alternative methods for toxin detection have been developed.

A commercially available latex aggutination test, initially marketed for the detection of Clostridium difficile toxin A in stool specimens, is technically simple to perform and provides results in 30 minutes or less. The test, however, detects glutamate dehydrogenase, not toxin A, and gives positive reactions with nontoxigenic isolates of C. difficile, with strains of C. botulinum and C. sporogenes, and with other anaerobes (Peptostreptococcus anaerobius and Bacteroides asaccharolyticus) (35,68,69). In addition to the potential for false-positive reactions, false-negative results also may be a problem. The sensitivity of the latex test compared with the cell culture assay has been as low as 75 to 80%; though other data suggest that the test results correlate with C. difficile–associated diarrhea (70,71).

In preliminary evaluations of a commercially available ELISA that detects cytotoxin A in stool specimens the sensitivity of the test ranged from 85 to 97% and the specificity from 98 to 99% (72,73). Advantages of this test are its technical simplicity, the elimination of the filtration step required in the cell culture assay, a turnaround time less than 2.5 hours, and minimal hands-on time. Nucleic acid hybridization and gene amplification via the polymerase chain reaction currently are being evaluated in research laboratories. The results are promising, and the techniques may be used in the clinical microbiology laboratory in the future (74,75).

Treatment and Prevention

Clostridium botulinum. All persons known or suspected to have ingested food contaminated with botulism toxin should be hospitalized; if exposure occurred within several hours, vomiting should be induced and gastric lavage performed. Treatment of symptomatic botulism includes supportive care—monitoring respiratory function, mechanical ventilatory assistance when necessary, nasogastric or parenteral nutritional support—and administration of antitoxin (a trivalent type A, B, and E product of equine origin currently is available in the United States). In the case of wound botulism, the wound should be débrided and antitoxin plus penicillin given.

Foodborne botulism can be prevented by adequately heating the food (100° C for 10 minutes), which inactivates the toxin, and foods that must be held for long periods should be refrigerated rather than kept at room temperature. To prevent infant botulism infants under 1 year of age should not be fed honey. Laboratory personnel working with Clostridium botulinum and its toxin should be immunized with pentavalent toxoids (ABCDE).

Clostridium tetani. The objectives of therapy for tetanus are to provide supportive care until the toxin fixed to neural tissue has been metabolized, to neutralize circulating toxin, and to remove the source of the toxin. Patients should be admitted to an intensive care unit and, if necessary, supported by tracheostomy, curarization, and artificial respiration. Decreased external stimuli and sedation diminish reflex spasms. Tetanus immune globulin is given to neutralize tetanus toxin. Wound débridement and drainage are performed, and patients are given penicillin.

Tetanus is completely preventable with proper immunization. For infants and children less than 7 years of age, tetanus toxoid is administered in an adsorbed vaccine in combination with diphtheria toxoid and pertussis vaccine (DPT). In this age group the principal immunization series consists of four doses of DPT vaccine, beginning at age 6 to 8 weeks: the first three doses are given 4 to 8 weeks apart and the fourth 1 year after the third. A booster is recommended at 4 to 6 years of age and additional boosters with tetanus and reduced-dose diphtheria toxoids (Td) every 10 years thereafter. For anyone older than 7 years immunization with Td is recommended because the frequency of reactions to full doses of diphtheria toxoid increases with age. A series of three doses of Td is recommended: the second dose is given 4 to 8 weeks after the first, and the third 6 to 12 months after the second; boosters are given every 10 years.

Neonatal tetanus can be prevented by improving obstetric and neonatal care. Antibodies to tetanus toxoid cross the placenta, and a newborn can be protected by administering a single booster of Td to a previously immunized woman or two injections at least 1 month apart to an unimmunized woman, preferably during the first 6 months of pregnancy. Tetanus prophylaxis for persons with wounds includes appropriate wound care (cleansing, drainage, débridement), penicillin therapy, and immunoprophylaxis with Td and tetanus immune globulin, according to the individual's vaccination history and the type of wound (see reference 76 for guidelines).

Clostridium perfringens. The most important component of therapy for clostridial gas gangrene is extensive surgical débridement of all involved tissues. Currently, the antimicrobial agent of choice for cases caused by C. perfringens is penicillin, although occasional isolates are resistant. The use of hyperbaric oxygen is controversial (76).

Food poisoning caused by Clostridium perfringens is a self-limited illness that requires only supportive care. Enterotoxin-associated diarrhea caused by C. perfringens has been treated successfully with metronidazole. Treatment of enteritis necroticans includes fluid and electrolyte support, administration of penicillin or chloramphenicol, and surgical intervention for persistent toxicity, intestinal obstruction, suspected perforation, and severe recurrent bleeding.

Clostridium difficile. Frequently, C. difficile–associated diarrhea and some cases of pseudomembranous colitis resolve when the offending antimicrobial agent is discontinued. Most often, however, pseudomembranous colitis is treated with oral vancomycin, oral metronidazole, or less commonly, oral bacitracin (35). Because C. difficile–associated disease is hospital acquired and may be transmitted from patient to patient by hospital personnel, enforcing appropriate handwashing technique may prevent spread of the organism.

Other Clostridia. Surgical débridement and drainage are essential in the treatment of clostridial myonecrosis and abscesses. In general, penicillin is the antimicrobial agent of choice for infections caused by Clostridium; however, isolates of some species, especially Clostridium ramosum and Clostridium tertium, are resistant to penicillin. Clindamycin is active against most commonly encountered anaerobes, but isolates of Clostridium ramosum and Clostridium tertium frequently are resistant. Metronidazole, chloramphenicol, and imipenem are active against almost all species of Clostridium.

NON–SPORE-FORMING GRAM-POSITIVE ANAEROBIC BACILLI

Non–spore-forming gram-positive anaerobic bacilli are members of the genera Actinomyces, Bifidobacterium, Eubacterium, Lactobacillus, and Propionibacterium. The genus Arachnia has been eliminated, and Arachnia propionicus now belongs in the genus Propionibacterium (Propionibacterium propionicus). Most members of these genera are obligate anaerobes, but some are aerotolerant or microaerophilic and grow in an atmosphere of increased carbon dioxide. These organisms are part of the normal flora of the upper respiratory tract, oral cavity, gastrointestinal tract, vagina, and, in the case of Propionibacterium, the skin. They usually are isolated from clinical specimens with many other organisms, and many are considered nonpathogenic.

Actinomyces

Species of Actinomyces that cause actinomycosis in humans—Actinomyces israelii (the most common and most important organism), Actinomyces naeslundii, Actinomyces odotolyticus, Actinomyces viscosus, and Actinomyces meyeri—are normal flora in the mouth and the female genital tract. These organisms generally have low virulence and act as endogenous opportunists. They typically cause invasive disease, usually associated with other bacteria, when the intact mucosal barriers are disrupted by infection, trauma, or surgical injury.

Epidemiology

Actinomycosis occurs at all ages. In a series of almost 200 persons, two thirds were between ages 30 and 60 years (range, 10 to 90 years), and infection was more common in males (male-female ratio, 4:1) (77). In children, both sexes are affected equally (78). Typically, antecedent disease or trauma predisposes to infection, but often no such event is identified (77). Cervicofacial actinomycosis follows dental infections and manipulations, surgical injury, or trauma to the oral mucosa. Thoracic actinomycosis is most common in persons with periodontal disease who aspirate oral secretions. Abdominal infections frequently originate in the appendix, but they also may follow perforation of a colonic diverticulum or duodenal ulcer, a gunshot wound, or cholecystectomy. Pelvic actinomycosis is associated with intrauterine contraceptive devices (79–83).

Pathogenesis and Pathology

As previously mentioned, the actinomycetes are opportunistic pathogens that typically cause disease only when a break in the normal mucosa occurs, and almost always they are found with other bacteria. Mechanisms of host resistance and immunity to these organisms are unknown.

Typical lesions are single or multiple indurated masses with fibrous walls, central necrosis, and sinus tracts that extend to the surface of the skin or mucous membranes or into organs and drain pus that contains "sulfur granules"—hard, gritty, yellow, dull white, or light brown masses averaging 2 mm in diameter. Histologically, lesions show granulation tissue with foamy macrophages; and the granules, composed of aggregates of gram-positive branching filaments, appear as round or oval, basophilic or amphophilic masses (Fig. 30–2) with eosinophilic clubs on the surface.

Clinical Manifestations

Cervicofacial actinomycosis usually evolves as a slowly growing, painless, fluctuant swelling at the lower border of the mandible that develops draining cutaneous fistulous tracts, or as a painful, widespread infection in the submandibular or paramandibular area, but these presentations can overlap. Many affected persons have poor oral hygiene, dental decay, periodontal disease, and gingivitis. Primary infection of the bone is rare, but the infection may spread into bone from adjacent soft tissues. Thoracic actinomycosis involves the lungs, pleura, mediastinum, or chest wall and occasionally extends to involve the ribs, sternum, shoulder girdle, or vertebrae. Clinically, the infection is characterized by empyema or a chest wall fistula draining purulent material with granules.

Abdominal involvement, which accounts for about 25 to 50% of cases of actinomycosis, most frequently involves the ileocecal region and, therefore, may be mistaken for Crohn's disease, carcinoma, tuberculosis, amebiasis, or chronic appendicitis (84,85). It may be localized or spread by contiguity to involve the subcutaneous tissues of the abdominal wall or the pelvic or perirectal tissues. In general, sinus tracts are uncommon but they may form when the infection spreads to the pelvic or perirectal tissues. Pelvic actinomycosis associated with an intrauterine contraceptive device is a localized infection that may present as simple vaginal discharge, or it may mimic pelvic inflammatory disease with tubo-ovarian abscess or a malignancy (80).

Actinomycosis may involve the central nervous system by direct extension from a cervicofacial focus; via hematogenous seeding from a primary site of infection in the lungs, mouth, abdomen, or pelvis; or, rarely, as a primary infection. The most common manifestation is a single brain abscess, although multiple abscesses may develop. Meningitis, meningoencephalitis, actinomycomas mimicking a tumor, subdural empyema, and epidural abscess are less common. Actinomycosis of the muscles of an extremity usually results from local spread of a thoracic or abdominal infection or from hematogenous dissemination, but rarely the infection is primary, in which case trauma is a common preceding event (86).

Other Non–Spore-Forming Gram-Positive Anaerobic Bacilli

Species of Bifidobacterium, normal flora in the gastrointestinal tract and the oral cavity, are rare human pathogens, but Bifidobacterium dentium (formerly Bifidobacterium eriksonnei) is an uncommon cause of thoracic actinomycosis. Species of Eubacterium (Eubacterium lentum is isolated most often), which are normal flora in the gastrointestinal tract and oral cavity, have been recovered with other bacteria from abscesses, wounds, blood, and dental and pulmonary infections and rarely have caused endocarditis and actinomycosis (87). Species of Lactobacillus (briefly reviewed in Chapter 29), are normal flora in the vagina, colon, and to a lesser extent, the oral cavity. They are uncommon human pathogens but have caused pleuropulmonary disease (generally as part of a mixed bacterial infection) and chorioamnionitis. Species of Propionibacterium, the most common of the non–spore-forming, anaerobic gram-positive bacilli encountered in clinical specimens, are normal flora on the skin and in the gastrointestinal, upper respiratory, and urogenital tract. These organisms, especially Propionibacterium acnes but also Propionibacterium granulosum and Propionibacterium avidium, often are contaminants of blood cultures and other sterile body fluids; but they have caused endocarditis, infections of prosthetic devices (artificial joints and ventricular shunts), osteomyelitis, and meningitis (88–90). Moreover, Propionibacterium acnes is associated with acne and with uveitis, endophthalmitis, or both following surgical removal of cataracts; and Propionibacterium propionicus may cause actinomycosis. Propionibacterium acnes produces hyaluronidase, chondroitin sulfatase, neuraminidase, and a lipase that causes release of

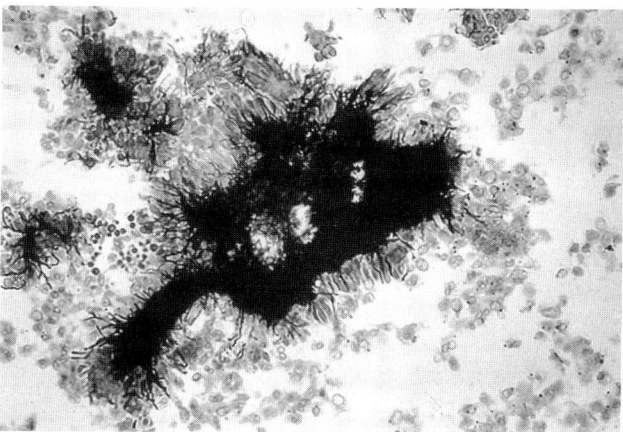

Fig. 30–2. Section of spleen showing a sulfur granule of Actinomyces israelii (Gomori's methenamine silver/hematoxylin and eosin, ×128).

long-chain fatty acids in the skin, potentially contributing to the formation of acne pustules.

Laboratory Diagnosis

Specimens for diagnosis of infections with the non–spore-forming gram-positive bacilli depend on the clinical manifestations. To diagnose actinomycosis, aspirated pus, granules, or a biopsy specimen of involved tissue is preferred. Sputum or bronchoalveolar lavage fluid may be submitted for diagnosis of thoracic actinomycosis; however, detection of the organism (sulfur granules) in smears of respiratory specimens stained with the Gram or Papanicolaou stain does not necessarily correlate with disease because the Actinomyces are normal flora in the oral cavity. Pelvic actinomycosis is diagnosed by direct microscopic detection of the organism in smears of endocervical secretions stained with the Papanicolaou stain or in smears of aspirated purulent material stained with the Gram stain or by recovering the organism from endocervical swab specimens or purulent material.

Specimen collection, transport, and processing are discussed in Part III. The non–spore-forming gram-positive anaerobic bacilli are identified by following the general guidelines for identification of anaerobes discussed earlier. Tests that presumptively differentiate these organisms are shown in Table 30–3; the individual genera are discussed in more detail below.

Identifying Features

***Actinomyces* species.** In smears stained with the Gram stain, cells of most Actinomyces are branching and beaded (Plate IIIF), but occasionally cocci and forms resembling corynebacteria (see Chapter 29) are seen, and cells of Actinomyces meyeri typically are small and nonbranching. Sulfur granules stained with the Gram stain show a tangled mass of long filaments.

The colony appearance of two species of Actinomyces is characteristic: colonies of Actinomyces israelii usually are white, heaped, rough, and lobate, resembling a molar tooth, but occasionally they are smooth or breadcrumb-like, and those of Actinomyces odontolyticus generally become red on sheep blood agar after several days and may be surrounded by a zone of β hemolysis. Colonies of other species of Actinomyces are smooth, flat to convex, gray-white, and translucent with entire margins. Because the Actinomyces grow slowly, agar plates should be incubated at least 7 days, and, if Actinomyces israelii is strongly suspected, 14 days. In broth some species of Actinomyces produce tight aggregates (balls). Most species of Actinomyces are microaerophilic, but many grow better anaerobically, and Actinomyces meyeri is an obligate anaerobe.

***Bifidobacterium* species.** In smears stained with the Gram stain, cells of Bifidobacterium are wider than those of Actinomyces and vary in shape: many have clubbed or bifurcated ends, but branching forms and forms resembling corynebacteria may be observed. Bifidobacterium dentium forms white, convex, shiny colonies with irregular edges on blood agar and shows diffuse growth in broth. Some isolates grow aerobically in the presence of carbon dioxide.

***Eubacterium* species.** In smears stained with the Gram stain, cells of Eubacterium vary in appearance: pleomorphic rods, coccobacilli in pairs or short chains, and straight uniform or curved rods may be seen. Cells of Eubacterium nodatum may appear as beaded, filamentous, branching rods, mimicking the Actinomyces. Colonies of Eubacterium are raised to convex and transparent to translucent, without distinct characteristics; however, colonies of Eubacterium nodatum may resemble those of Actinomyces israelii (described earlier).

***Lactobacillus* species.** In smears stained with the Gram stain, cells of Lactobacillus usually are straight and uniform with rounded ends (Plate IIIC), occasionally forming chains, but may be short and coccobacillary, resembling cells of Streptococcus (see Chapters 28 and 29). These microaerophilic organisms usually form larger colonies when grown anaerobically. On sheep blood agar incubated in an atmosphere of increased carbon dioxide, colonies are small and occasionally cause greening of the agar.

***Propionibacterium* species.** Cells of Propionibacterium resemble those of corynebacteria: irregular, pleomorphic, and often club-shaped, with one rounded and one tapered end, and occasionally short branching and beaded forms are seen. On blood agar colonies are small and white to gray-white, but may become yellow with age, and sometimes surrounded by a zone of complete hemolysis. Many species are aerotolerant but grow better anaerobically. An anaerobic gram-positive bacillus with

Table 30–3. Characteristics for Presumptive Differentiation of Anaerobic, Non–spore-forming, Gram-positive Bacilli

Genus	Cellular Structure*	Relation to Oxygen	Catalase	Nitrate Reduction	Metabolic Products
Actinomyces	Branching filaments; diphtheroidal	F, M, OA	− (+ for A. viscosus)	V	A, L, S
Bifidobacterium	Thin rods, bifid or bulbous ends	OA, rarely M	−	−	A, L, (A > L)
Eubacterium	Thin to plump, short rods; may be coccoidal or diphtheroidal	OA	−	V	V
Lactobacillus	Short rods in chains or singly	M	−	−+	A, L (L > A)
Propionibacterium	Diphtheroidal	F, OA	+−	V	A, P

* For organisms grown in thioglycolate broth.
Key: +, positive reaction for ≥90% of strains tested; −, negative reaction for ≥90% of strains tested; superscripts, reaction with rare strains; V, variable reaction; F, facultative anaerobe, M, microaerophilic; OA, obligate anaerobe; A, acetic acid; L, lactic acid; P, propionic acid; S, succinic acid

the cellular structure described above that reduces nitrate and is indole positive is Propionibacterium acnes, although a few isolates give negative results for these tests.

Treatment

Penicillin is the antimicrobial agent of choice for infections caused by anaerobic non–spore-forming gram-positive bacilli. For persons allergic to penicillin, tetracycline is recommended; and chloramphenicol, cefoxitin, and clindamycin show excellent activity in vitro against Actinomyces israelii and Propionibacterium acnes. Metronidazole shows poor activity against all of these organisms.

ANAEROBIC GRAM-POSITIVE COCCI

The anaerobic gram-positive cocci encountered in the clinical microbiology laboratory are the species of Peptostreptococcus (Peptostreptococcus magnus, Peptostreptococcus asaccharolyticus, Peptostreptococcus prevotii, Peptostreptococcus anaerobius, and Peptostreptococcus micros), Peptococcus niger, microaerophilic species of Streptococcus, and Staphylococcus saccharolyticus (formerly Peptococcus saccharolyticus). Major changes in the taxonomy of gram-positive cocci were made in the early 1980s (90). Based on DNA guanine-plus-cytosine content, all of the former species of Peptococcus, except Peptococcus niger, were reclassified in the genera Peptostreptococcus or Staphylococcus, and a new species, Peptostreptococcus tetradius, was proposed to replace those organisms previously designated "Gaffkya anaerobia." Moreover, gram-positive cocci that grow optimally under anaerobic conditions but will grow in an atmosphere of 5 to 10% carbon dioxide and produce large quantities of lactic acid during carbohydrate fermentation were members of the genera Peptostreptococcus or Peptococcus but were reclassified in the genus Streptococcus. Other genera of anaerobic gram-positive cocci—Ruminococcus, Coprococcus, Gemella, and Sarcinia—rarely if ever are recovered from clinical specimens and are not discussed here.

Epidemiology and Pathogenesis

The anaerobic, gram-positive cocci are normal flora in the oral cavity, upper respiratory tract, large intestine, and the female genital tract and may be found on the skin. As a group, these organisms are the second most commonly encountered anaerobes in the clinical microbiology laboratory, after the Bacteroides (see Chapter 38); the most frequent clinical isolates are Peptostreptococcus magnus, P. anaerobius, P. micros, P. prevotii, and the microaerophilic streptococci. Infections with these organisms are endogenous. Little is known of their relative pathogenic potential and virulence factors, but lipopolysaccharides, hyaluronidase, collagenase, and capsules have been described.

Clinical Manifestations

The anaerobic gram-positive cocci typically are involved in polymicrobial infections such as pleuropulmonary infections; intra-abdominal abscesses; infections of the female genital tract (endometritis, pyometra, pelvic abscess, abscess of Bartholin's gland, puerperal sepsis, infections following a surgical procedure, and pelvic inflammatory disease), skin and soft tissue infections, including necrotizing fasciitis, necrotizing synergistic gangrene, and infections of foot ulcers and decubiti of diabetics; osteomyelitis and septic arthritis; and bacteremia and endocarditis (8,91).

Laboratory Diagnosis

Specimens for diagnosis vary depending on the clinical manifestations, but in general aspirated pus or a biopsy specimen of involved tissue is optimal, although a swab sample transported in an anaerobic collection system may be submitted if exudate cannot be obtained. To diagnose bacteremia and endocarditis, blood should be collected; joint fluid should be submitted to diagnose septic arthritis; and a bone biopsy specimen is necessary to diagnose osteomyelitis.

In a smear stained with the Gram stain the cells of the anaerobic gram-positive cocci vary in appearance: many resemble Staphylococcus (see Chapter 28); cells of Peptostreptococcus anaerobius are large coccobacilli, often in chains; cells of Peptostreptococcus tetradius typically form tetrads. Cells of Peptostreptococcus magnus are greater than 0.7 μm in diameter and occur singly or in masses; cells of Peptostreptococcus micros typically are smaller and often form short chains, although the size difference between it and Peptostreptococcus magnus is not a reliable identifying feature. Colonies of the anaerobic gram-positive cocci are small (less than 0.5 mm to 2 mm in diameter), convex, gray to white, and translucent to opaque, occasionally appearing stippled or pock marked, with an entire edge, and usually appear on blood agar after 48 hours. Colonies of Peptostreptococcus anaerobius are larger and more opaque and have a sweet, fetid odor; and those of Peptococcus niger are black pigmented. Peptostreptococcus anaerobius is the only anaerobic gram-positive coccus that is sensitive to sodium polyanethol sulfonate (SPS disk) by disk diffusion, which therefore is a useful identifying feature.

Treatment

Penicillin is the antimicrobial agent of choice for treating infections involving Peptostreptococcus. Clindamycin, chloramphenicol, and imipenem also are active against these organisms, although occasional strains are resistant to clindamycin. The activity of metronidazole against Peptostreptococcus is unpredictable; up to 10% of isolates are very resistant.

REFERENCES

1. Hatheway CL: Toxigenic clostridia. Clin Microbiol Rev, 3: 66, 1990.
2. Suen JC, Hatheway CL, Steigerwalt AG, and Brenner DJ: Clostridium argentinense sp. nov.: A genetically homogeneous group composed of all strains of Clostridium botulinum toxin type G and some nontoxigenic strains previously identified as Clostridium subterminale or Clostridium hastiforme. Int J Syst Bacteriol, 38:375, 1988.

3. Smith LDS: The occurrence of Clostridium botulinum and Clostridium tetani in the soil of the United States. Health Lab Sci, 15:74, 1978.
4. Williams-Walls NJ: Clostridium botulinum type F: Isolation from crabs. Science, 162:375, 1968.
5. Eklund MW, and Poysky FT: Clostridium botulinum type F from marine sediments. Science, 149:306, 1965.
6. Gimenez DF, and Ciccarelli AS: Another type of Clostridium botulinum. Zentralbl Bakteriol Parasitenkd Infektionskr, Abt. 1 Orig. Reihe A, 215:215, 1970.
7. Centers for Disease Control: Summary of notifiable diseases, United States, 1989. MMWR, 38(54):1, 1989.
8. Finegold SM, George WL, and Mulligan ME: Anaerobic infections. Part II. Disease a Month, 31(11):1, 1985.
9. MacDonald KL, Cohen ML, and Blake PA: The changing epidemiology of adult botulism in the United States. Am J Epidemiol, 124:794, 1986.
10. Lecour H, Ramos HH, Almeida B, and Barbosa R: Food-borne botulism—a review of 13 outbreaks. Arch Intern Med, 148:578, 1988.
11. Davis JB, Mattman LH, and Wiley M: Clostridium botulinum in a fatal wound infection. JAMA, 146:646, 1951.
12. Pickett J, Berg B, Chaplin E, and Brunstetter MA: Syndrome of botulism in infancy: Clinical and electrophysiologic study. N Engl J Med, 295:770, 1976.
13. Midura TF, and Arnon SS: Infant botulism: Identification of Clostridium botulinum and its toxin in faeces. Lancet, ii:934, 1976.
14. Arnon SS, et al: Honey and other environmental risk factors for infant botulism. J Pediatr, 94:331, 1979.
15. Chia JK, et al: Botulism in an adult associated with food-borne intestinal infection with Clostridium botulinum. N Engl J Med, 315:239, 1986.
16. Bartlett JC: Infant botulism in adults. N Engl J Med, 315:254, 1986.
17. Arnon SS, et al: Intestinal infection and toxin production by Clostridium botulinum as one cause of sudden infant death syndrome. Lancet, i:1273, 1978.
18. Sonnabend OA, et al: Continuous microbiological study of 70 sudden and unexpected infant deaths: Toxigenic intestinal Clostridium botulinum infection in 9 cases of sudden infant death syndrome. Lancet, ii:237, 1985.
19. Gurwith MJ, Langston C, and Citron DM: 1981. Toxin-producing bacteria in infants. Am J Dis Child, 135:1104, 1981.
20. Heinzel G, Lenk V, and Schneider V: Ergebnesse bakteriologischer Untersuchungen zum plotzlichen unerwarteten Sauglingstod, unter besonderer Berucksichtigung des Sauglingsbotulismus. Beitr Gerichtl Med, 43:378, 1985.
21. Adams EB, Lawrence DR, and Smith JWG: Tetanus. Oxford, Blackwell Scientific Publications, 1969.
22. Kobel T and Marti MC: Decouverete du bacille de tetanos (1884). Rev Med Suisse Romande, 105:547, 1985.
23. Schofield F: Selective primary health care: Strategies for control of disease in the developing world. XXII. Tetanus: a preventable problem. Rev Infect Dis, 8:144, 1986.
24. Stoll BJ: Tetanus. Ped Clin North Am, 26:415, 1979.
25. Centers for Disease Control: Tetanus—United States, 1987 and 1988. MMWR, 39:37, 1990.
26. Furste W: Tetanus statistics. JAMA, 228:28, 1974.
27. Centers for Disease Control: Tetanus—United States, 1982–1984. MMWR, 34:602, 1985.
28. Centers for Disease Control: Tetanus—United States, 1985–1986. MMWR, 36:477, 1987.
29. Larson HE, and Borriello SP: Infectious diarrhea due to Clostridium perfringens. J Infect Dis, 157:390, 1988.
30. Borriello SP, et al: Enterotoxigenic Clostridium perfringens: A possible cause of antibiotic-associated diarrha. Lancet, i:305, 1984.
31. McClane BA, Wnek AP, Hulkower KI, and Hanna PC: Divalent cation involvement in the action of Clostridium perfringens type A enterotoxin. J Biol Chem, 263:2423, 1988.
32. McClane BA, Hanna PC, and Wnek AP: Clostridium perfringens enterotoxin. Microb Pathogen, 4:317, 1988.
33. Finney JM: Gastro-enterostomy for cicatrizing ulcer of the pylorus. Johns Hopkins Hosp Bull, 11:53, 1893.
34. Goulston SJ, and McGovern VJ: 1965. Pseudomembranous colitis. Gut, 6:207, 1965.
35. Lyverly DM, Krivan HC, and Wilkins TC: Clostridium difficile: Its disease and toxins. Clin Microbiol Rev, 1:1, 1988.
36. Hummel RP, Altemeir WA, and Hill EO: Iatrogenic staphylococcal enterocolitis. Ann Surg, 160:551, 1964.
37. Hall IC, and O'Toole E: Intestinal flora in newborn infants. Am J Dis Child, 49:390, 1935.
38. McFarland LV, Surawicz CM, and Stamm WE: Risk factors for Clostridium difficile carriage and C. difficile–associated diarrhea in a cohort of hospitalized patients. J Infect Dis, 162:678, 1990.
39. Fernie DS, Thomson RO, Batty I, and Walker PD: Active and passive immunization to protect against antibiotic associated caecitis in hamsters. Dev Biol Stand, 53:325, 1983.
40. Libby JM, Jortner BS, and Wilkins TD: Effects of the two toxins of Clostridium difficile in antibiotic-associated cecitis in hamsters. Infect Immun, 36:822, 1982.
41. Hafiz S, Morton RS, McEntegart MG, and Waitkins SA: Clostridium difficile in the urogenital tract of males and females. Lancet, i:420, 1975.
42. Levett PN: Clostridium difficile in habitats other than the human gastrointestinal tract. J Infect, 12:253, 1986.
43. Saginur R, et al: Splenic abscess due to Clostridium difficile. J Infect Dis, 147:1105, 1983.
44. McGregor JA, Soper DE, Lovell G, and Todd JK: Maternal deaths associated with Clostridium sordellii infection. Am J Obstet Gynecol, 161:987, 1989.
45. Soper DD: Clostridial myonecrosis arising from an episiotomy. Obstet Gynecol, 68:265, 1986.
46. Hogan SF, and Ireland K: Fatal acute spontaneous endometritis resulting from Clostridium sordellii. Am J Clin Pathol, 91:104, 1989.
47. Browdie DA, et al: Clostridium sordellii infection. J Trauma, 15:515, 1975.
48. Kornbluth AA, Danzig JB, and Bernstein LH: Clostridium septicum infection and associated malignancy: Report of 2 cases and review of the literature. Medicine, 68:30, 1989.
49. Thaler M, Gill V, and Pizzo PA: Emergence of Clostridium tertium as a pathogen in neutropenic patients. Am J Med, 81:596, 1986.
50. Howard FM, et al: Outbreak of necrotizing enterocolitis caused by C. butyricum. Lancet, ii:1099, 1977.
51. Aureli P, et al: Two cases of type E infant botulism caused by neurotoxigenic Clostridium butyricum in Italy. J Infect Dis, 154:201, 1986.
52. McCroskey LM, et al: Characterization of an organism that produces type E botulinal toxin but which resembles Clostridium butyricum from the feces of an infant with type E botulism. J Clin Microbiol, 23:201, 1986.
53. Hall JD, McCroskey LM, Pincomb BJ, and Hatheway CL: Isolation of an organism resembling Clostridium barati which produces type F botulinal toxin from an infant with botulism. J Clin Microbiol, 21:654, 1985.
54. Hoffman, RE, Pincomb BJ, and Skeels MR: Type F infant botulism. Am J Dis Child, 136:270, 1982.
55. Bourgault A, and Lamothe F: Evaluation of the KOH test and

the antibiotic disk test in routine clinical anaerobic bacteriology. J Clin Microbiol, 26:2144, 1988.
56. Holdeman LV, Cato EP, and Moore WEC: Anaerobe Laboratory Manual. 4th ed. Blacksburg, VA, Virginia Polytechnic Institute and State University Anaerobe Laboratory, 1977.
57. Dowell VR Jr, and Hawkins TM: Laboratory methods in anaerobic bacteriology. In CDC Laboratory Manual publication number (CDC) 78-8272. Atlanta, GA, U.S. Department of Health, Education and Welfare, 1977.
58. Sutter VL, et al: Wadsworth Anaerobic Bacteriology Manual. 4th ed. Belmont, CA, Star Publishing, 1985.
59. Allen SD, Siders JA, and Marler LM: Isolation and examination of anaerobic bacteria. In Manual of Clinical Microbiology. 4th ed. Edited by EH Lennette, A Balows, WJ Hausler, Jr., and HJ Shadomy. Washington, DC, American Society for Microbiology, 1985.
60. Koneman EW, et al (eds): The anaerobic bacteria. In Color Atlas and Textbook of Clinical Microbiology. 3rd ed. Philadelphia, JB Lippincott, 1988.
61. Appelbaum PC: Advances in rapid preliminary and definitive identification of anaerobes. Clin Microbiol Newslett, 11:89, 1989.
62. Quentin C, Desailly-Chanson M-A, and Bebear C: Evaluation of AN-Ident. J Clin Microbiol, 29:231, 1991.
63. Celig DM, and Schreckenberger PC: Clinical evaluation of the Rapid-ANA II panel for identification of anaerobic bacteria. J Clin Microbiol, 29:457, 1991.
64. Marler LM, et al: Evaluation of the new Rapid ANA-II system for the identification of clinical anaerobic isolates. J Clin Microbiol, 29:874, 1991.
65. Hatheway CL: Botulism. In Laboratory Diagnosis of Infectious Diseases—Principles and Practice. Edited by A Balows, WJ Hausler, Jr, M Ohaski, and A Turano. New York, Springer-Verlag, 1988.
66. Iwen PC, Booth SJ, and Woods GL: Comparison of media for screening of diarrheic stools for the recovery of Clostridium difficile. J Clin Microbiol, 27:2105, 1989.
67. Gerding DN: Disease associated with Clostridium difficile infection. Ann Intern Med, 110:255, 1989.
68. Borriello SP, et al: Analysis of latex agglutination test for Clostridium difficile toxin A (D-1) and differentiation between C. difficile toxins A and B and latex reactive protein. J Clin Pathol, 40:573, 1987.
69. Lyerly DM, Barroso LA, and Wilkins TD: Identification of the latex reactive protein of Clostridium difficile as glutamate dehydrogenase. J Clin Microbiol, 29:2639, 1991.
70. Woods GL, and Iwen PC: Comparison of a dot immunobinding assay, latex agglutination, and cytotoxin assay for laboratory diagnosis of Clostridium difficile–associated diarrhea. J Clin Microbiol, 28:855, 1990.
71. Kelly MT, et al: Commercial latex agglutination test for detection of Clostridium difficile–associated diarrhea. J Clin Microbiol, 25:1244, 1987.
72. Gilligan P, et al: Evaluation of the PREMIER Clostridium difficile toxin A enzyme immunoassay. In Program and Abstracts of the 30th Interscience Conference on Antimicrobial Agents and Chemotherapy. Washington, DC, American Society for Microbiology, 1990.
73. DeGirolami PC, et al: Multicenter evaluation of a new enzyme immunoassay for detection of Clostridium difficile enterotoxin A. J Clin Microbiol 30:1085, 1992.
74. Wren BW, Clayton CL, Castledine NB, and Tabaqchali S: Identification of toxigenic Clostridium difficile strains by using a toxin A gene-specific probe. J Clin Microbiol, 28:1808, 1990.
75. Kato N, et al: Detection of toxigenic Clostridium difficile by the polymerase chain reaction. In Program and Abstracts of the Interscience Conference on Antimicrobial Agents and Chemotherapy. Washington, DC, American Society for Microbiology, 1990.
76. Cate TR: Clostridium tetani (tetanus). In Principles and Practice of Infectious Diseases. 3rd ed. Edited by GL Mandell, RG Douglas, Jr, and JE Bennett. New York, Churchill Livingstone, 1990.
77. Brown JR: Human actinomycosis. A study of 181 subjects. Hum Pathol, 4:319, 1973.
78. Drake DP, and Holt RJ: Childhood actinomycosis. Report of 3 recent cases. Arch Dis Child, 51:979, 1976.
79. Schiffer MA, et al: Actinomycosis infections associated with intrauterine contraceptive devices. Obstet Gynecol, 45:67, 1975.
80. Spagnuolo RJ, and Fransiolli M: Intrauterine device-associated actinomycosis simulating pelvic malignancy. Am J Gastroenterol, 75:144, 1981.
81. Persson E, et al: Actinomyces israelii in the genital tract of women with and without intrauterine contraceptive devices. Acta Obstet Gynecol Scand, 62:563, 1983.
82. Gupta PK: Intrauterine contraceptive devices. Vaginal cytology, pathological changes and clinical implications. Acta Cytol, 26:571, 1982.
83. Persson E: Genital actinomycosis and Actinomyces israelii in the female genital tract. Adv Contracept, 3:115, 1987.
84. Weese WC, and Smith JM: A study of 57 cases of actinomycosis over a 36-year period. Arch Intern Med, 135:1562, 1975.
85. Eastridge CE, et al: Actinomycosis. South Med J, 65:839, 1972.
86. Reiner SL, et al: Primary actinomycosis of an extremity: A case report and review. Rev Infect Dis, 9:581, 1987.
87. Hill GB, Ayers OM, and Kohan AP: Characteristics and sites of infection of Eubacterium nodatum, Eubacterium timidum, Eubacterium brachy and other asaccharoytic eubacteria. J Clin Microbiol, 25:1540, 1987.
88. Beeler BA, Crowder JG, Smith JW, and White A: Propionibacterium acnes: Pathogen in central nervous system shunt infection. Am J Med, 61:935, 1976.
89. Felner JM, and Dowell VR Jr: Anaerobic bacterial endocarditis. N Engl J Med, 283:1188, 1970.
90. Ezaki T, et al: Transfer of Peptococcus indolicus, Peptococcus asaccharolyticus, Peptococcus prevotii, and Peptococcus magnus to the genus Peptostreptococcus and proposal of Peptostreptococcus tetradius sp. nov. Int J Syst Bacteriol, 33:683, 1983.
91. Finegold SM, George WL, and Mulligan ME: Anaerobic infections. Part I. Disease a Month, 31(10):1, 1985.

Chapter 31

NEISSERIA AND BRANHAMELLA

The species of Neisseria are gram-negative cocci classified in the family Neisseriaceae. Other genera currently in the family are Kingella, Moraxella, and Acinetobacter (discussed in Chapter 32, because they often appear as coccobacilli rather than cocci, and they are identified by using systems typically used for identification of the group of organisms called glucose "nonfermenters"). A proposal has been made, however, to exclude the latter two genera from the family (1). Moraxella (Branhamella) catarrhalis initially was classified in the genus Neisseria (Neisseria catarrhalis), subsequently was placed in a separate genus (Branhamella), and currently is a subgenus of Moraxella (2). However, the name Branhamella catarrhalis continues to be used by most clinical pathologists, microbiologists, and infectious disease clinicians and is used in this chapter.

NEISSERIA

Species of Neisseria are true cocci and in smears stained with the Gram stain appear as gram-negative cocci in pairs (diplococci), with adjacent sides of the cells flattened (Plate IC), except for Neisseria elongata, which is rod shaped. These organisms grow best on enriched media incubated at 35° to 37° C in a humid atmosphere of 2 to 8% carbon dioxide, but the commensal species of Neisseria—Neisseria lactamica, Neisseria sicca, Neisseria subflava, Neisseria mucosa, Neisseria flavescens, Neisseria cinerea, Neisseria polysaccbareae, and Neisseria elongata—also grow at room temperature and on nutrient agar. Neisseria gonorrhoeae is fastidious and requires the added nutrients of chocolate agar or special enrichments for growth, although occasional isolates are recovered on sheep blood agar. Other species of Neisseria, including Neisseria meningitidis, grow well on blood agar. The primary human pathogens, Neisseria gonorrhoeae and Neisseria meningitidis—are reviewed in detail; the commensal species rarely cause human disease and, therefore, are discussed briefly.

Neisseria gonorrhoeae

Neisseria gonorrhoeae is the agent of gonorrhea (from Greek *gonos* and *rhoia*, seed and flow). The bacterium was described in purulent urethral and conjunctival exudates by Neisser in 1879, was first cultivated by Leistikow and Loeffler in 1882, and in 1885 was proven by Bumm to be responsible for the disease (3).

Structure

Within the outer membrane of Neisseria gonorrhoeae are several proteins. Protein I, the principal protein, acts as a porin, providing channels through which aqueous solutes can pass. It shows stable interstrain antigenic variation and forms the basis of the system most commonly used to serotype isolates of Neisseria gonorrhoeae. Protein II, the designation for several related outer membrane proteins, is present in variable amounts or may be absent. It is present in most isolates from mucosal surfaces, which form opaque colonies, but absent from isolates from normally sterile sites, which form transparent colonies. Protein III is found in all N. gonorrhoeae in close association with protein I and the lipo-oligosaccharide. The latter is composed of lipid A and a core oligosaccharide that lacks the O-antigenic side chains that are present in most other gram-negative bacteria. Other outer membrane proteins are linked with iron utilization and transport, and traversing the membrane are proteins termed pili.

Epidemiology

The prevalence of gonorrhea is known only for the few countries that have a reporting system that permits a reasonable estimate of the disease, a figure that is often lower than the actual prevalence owing to incomplete reporting. In the United States the number of reported cases of gonorrhea rose from about 250,000 in the early 1960s to over 1 million in 1978 and then slowly declined to about 780,000 in 1987 (4–6). In contrast, the incidence of gonorrhea in Sweden peaked around 1970 and then declined to a much lower level: about 30 cases per 100,000 population were reported in 1987 (3). The prevalence of gonorrhea in developing countries is unknown, but most likely it is higher than in the United States.

In the United States sexually active men and women aged 20 to 24 years have the highest attack rates of gonorrhea, but 15- to 19-year old women are at the greatest risk of developing disease. More cases of gonorrhea are reported in men; partially this reflects the greater proportion of undiagnosed cases in women than in men. The prevalence of gonorrhea is 8 to 10 times greater among persons of nonwhite races than among whites. Lower socioeconomic status, less education, urban residence, and being unmarried also are associated with increased risk of gonorrhea (7). Moreover, the prevalence of gonorrhea fluctuates seasonally, with the peak between July and September and the trough between January and April.

The predominant mechanism of spread of Neisseria gonorrhoeae is via sexual intercourse with an infected partner. The risk of transmission from an infected woman is about 20% per episode of vaginal intercourse and 60 to 80% after four or more exposures (8,9). The risk of spread from males to females probably is about 50% per exposure and at least 90% after several exposures (10). The efficiencies of transmission during other modes of sexual contact are unknown, but spread via rectal intercourse apparently is efficient, and transmission from oropharynx to urethra and vice versa is uncommon (11,12). N. gonorrhoeae also may be transmitted from an infected mother to her infant during delivery.

Penicillinase-producing strains of Neisseria gonorrhoeae (PPNG), which carry a plasmid (designated Pc^r) that specifies production of a β-lactamase (see Chapter 24), were first documented in 1975 to 1976 almost simultaneously in the United States, western Europe, the Philippines, and western Africa, but probably were responsible for some penicillin treatment failures in parts of Asia, the Western Pacific, and Africa during the preceding several years (13,14). The prevalence of infections due to PPNG in the United States increased slowly between 1976 and 1981, with foci in Los Angeles, Miami, and New York City, and then increased over five-fold from 1981 to 1986, prompting the recommendation that penicillins not be used as single-dose, primary therapy for gonorrhea (15,16). In 1989 PPNG accounted for 7.4% of isolates (range, 1.2 to 31.7%; median, 5.0%) from 21 sexually transmitted disease clinics participating in the Gonococcal Isolate Surveillance Project implemented by the Centers for Disease Control; and between 1988 and 1989 statistically significant increases in the percentage of PPNG occurred in Atlanta, Birmingham, Boston, Long Beach, Philadelphia, San Antonio, and San Diego (5).

Tetracycline-resistant strains of Neisseria gonorrhoeae, which carry a 25.2-megadalton conjugative plasmid into which the *tet*M transposon has been inserted, were first described in the United States in 1985 (17). Currently, infections with these strains appear to be most common in the eastern United States; but sexually transmitted disease clinics in St. Louis and Denver reported substantial increases in the percentage of tetracycline-resistant N. gonorrhoeae, suggesting that further spread from eastern to western cities is likely (5).

Chromosomally mediated resistance to penicillin in strains of Neisseria gonorrhoeae, which results from mutations that reduce the permeability of the organism's outer membrane or alter penicillin-binding protein 2 to reduce the affinity for penicillin, is relatively common in the Far East but was rare in the United States until the early 1980s (18). In 1983 an outbreak of gonorrhea caused by such a strain occurred in North Carolina, and since then similar strains of N. gonorrhoeae have been reported from 23 states (19,20).

Pathogenesis

Several surface components of Neisseria gonorrhoeae contribute to its pathogenicity. Pili allow the bacterium to attach to human mucosal surfaces and to resist killing by neutrophils (21–23). Protein I may trigger invasion by facilitating endocytosis of the organism, and certain protein I serovars are associated with resistance to the bactericidal effect of nonimmune human serum and, consequently, with increased ability to cause bacteremia (21,24–27). Protein II may enhance attachment to buccal epithelial cells and neutrophils; and in vitro it increases the association between bacterial cells, an event that in vivo may reduce the need for an individual bacterium to adhere to an epithelial surface (26). Loss of protein II has been associated with resistance to killing by neutrophils (27). Protein III appears to stimulate blocking antibodies, reducing the serum bactericidal activity against N. gonorrhoeae (28).

The lipo-oligosaccharide of the outer membrane has endotoxic activity, is lethal for animals inoculated in the laboratory, and mediates loss of cilia and death of adjacent uninfected cells in the fallopian tube explant model of infection with Neisseria gonorrhoeae (21,29). Antigenically variable components of the oligosaccharide are associated with resistance to serum bactericidal activity, and possibly with the severity of the disease (30,31). Immunoglobulin (Ig) A$_1$ proteases presumably protect the organism from secretory IgA at mucosal surfaces, but this is unproven. The peptidoglycan layer of the cell wall, located beneath the outer membrane, is toxic to ciliated cells lining the fallopian tube (32).

Neisseria gonorrhoeae predominantly infects noncornified epithelium. Bacteria attach to the mucosal surface, a process mediated by pili and protein II, and within 24 to 48 hours penetrate between and through the epithelial cells to the submucosal tissues, causing sloughing of the epithelium and eliciting infiltration of neutrophils, which eventually form submucosal microabscesses. If treatment is not initiated, neutrophils gradually are replaced by macrophages and lymphocytes, and after several weeks organisms cannot be identified microscopically or recovered by culture.

Clinical Manifestations

Urogenital gonorrhea is manifest after a 2- to 5-day incubation period as purulent urethral discharge and dysuria in males, and in women who have symptoms as vaginal discharge, dysuria, urinary frequency, labial pain or swelling, abnormal uterine bleeding, lower abdominal pain, or a combination of these. Pelvic examination may show a purulent exudate in the cervical os. Ten to 20% of women with acute urogenital gonorrhea develop acute pelvic inflammatory disease (PID) via upward spread of Neisseria gonorrhoeae from the cervix. In the United States during the 1980s N. gonorrhoeae was associated with about 20 to 40% of cases of acute PID in urban areas; however, the proportion of cases associated with gonorrhea varies in different geographic regions (33). Symptoms typically begin a few days after the onset of menses; bilateral lower abdominal pain usually is present, and about two thirds of patients are febrile. Acute perihepatitis (called Fitz-Hugh-Curtis syndrome) occurs primarily by spread of N. gonorrhoeae or Chlamydia trachomatis (Chapter 25) from the fallopian tube through the peritoneal cavity to the liver capsule, and uncommonly results from lymphangitic or hematogenous spread. Symptoms include abdominal pain and right-side upper quadrant tenderness. Ascending infection with N. gonorrhoeae during pregnancy may cause septic abortion before the twelfth week of gestation and chorioamnionitis after the sixteenth week. Possible complications of the latter are premature rupture of membranes and premature labor (34–36).

Anorectal gonorrhea occurs in about 40% of women with uncomplicated disease and in about 40% of infected homosexual men. It may be asymptomatic or cause acute proctitis with anal pruritus, anal discharge, bleeding, anorectal pain, tenesmus, and constipation (3). Pharyngeal infection with Neisseria gonorrhoeae develops in 10 to 20% of heterosexual women, 10 to 20% of homosexual men, and 3 to 7% of heterosexual men with gonorrhea. Affected persons usually are asymptomatic but may have pharyngitis and cervical lymphadenitis (3,12).

Disseminated disease, which occurs in 0.5 to 3% of persons infected with Neisseria gonorrhoeae, is characterized by fever, skin lesions, and joint involvement. Skin lesions, usually fewer than 20 tender papules or petechiae that evolve into hemorrhagic or necrotic pustules, are located peripherally on the extremities. Asymmetric arthralgias, tenosynovitis, or arthritis most frequently involves the knees, and less often the elbows, ankles, wrists, and small joints of the hands and the feet. Uncommon manifestations include hepatitis, myocarditis, and osteomyelitis; acute endocarditis and meningitis are extremely rare (3,36). Properties of N. gonorrhoeae associated with disseminated disease are resistance to the bactericidal action of nonimmune human serum, AHU$^-$ auxotype (described later), specific IA serovars, and marked susceptibility to penicillin, features typical of isolates that cause asymptomatic infection in men (37,38). Host risk factors associated with dissemination include the homozygous deficiency of complement components C5, C6, C7, or C8 (see Chapter 2) (accounting for about 5% of such infections), female sex, menstruation, and possibly pharyngeal infection and pregnancy (3,36,39).

Conjunctivitis caused by Neisseria gonorrhoeae in the newborn (called ophthalmia neonatorum) generally becomes apparent within a week (typically, 2 to 3 days) after delivery. This once was the most common cause of blindness in the United States, and it remains a problem in developing countries (40). Uncommon manifestations of infection in the newborn are septicemia and arthritis. In prepubertal girls, purulent vaginitis is the predominant manifestation of gonorrhea.

Neisseria meningitidis

Clinical descriptions of meningococcal meningitis date back to the sixteenth century, but epidemic cerebrospinal meningitis (called "malignant purpuric fever") was first reported in 1805 in Geneva (41). The agent, Neisseria meningitidis, was isolated from cerebrospinal fluid by Weichselbaum in Vienna in 1887 (42). Healthy persons were recognized as carriers of the organism in 1896, and in 1909 different serotypes of N. meningitidis were identified (43,44). National and worldwide epidemics of meningococcal meningitis occurred from 1928 to 1930 and in 1941 (45–47). Sulfonamides, introduced in 1937, improved the outcome of the infection significantly and, when used as prophylaxis, eradicated the carrier state and prevented epidemics, especially in crowded army barracks (48,49). Strains of N. meningitidis resistant to sulfonamides emerged in the early 1940s, become a clinically significant problem during meningococcal epidemics in 1963, and subsequently spread worldwide (50–52).

Structure

Neisseria meningitidis possesses a polysaccharide capsule that forms the basis of the serogroup typing system. Currently 13 serogroups are recognized: A,B,C,D,X,Y,Z, W135, 29E, and the newly described serogroups H,I,K,L (53,54). Groups A,B,C,Y, and W135 account for most isolates in the United States (55–57).

The outer membrane of Neisseria meningitidis is similar in structure to that of other gram-negative bacteria. It contains the lipo-oligosaccharide and several outer membrane proteins, both of which are useful for serotyping. Moreover, cells of N. meningitidis possess pili (described earlier for Neisseria gonorrhoeae).

Epidemiology

Epidemic meningitis occurs on all continents, but the classic endemic area is the meningitis belt in central Africa (Fig. 31–1) (58). Meningococcal disease is infrequent in the United States; approximately 3000 cases are reported annually. Disease caused by Neisseria meningitidis in industrialized countries during nonepidemic conditions is most common in children under school age, but in the meningitis belt in Africa the prevalence peaks in young school-aged children. During epidemics the age distribution often shifts toward older groups (58). The overall prevalence of disease is slightly higher among males, owing at least in part to the high incidence among the military recruits.

Neisseria meningitidis is recovered most commonly from the throat or nasopharynx of asymptomatic persons who chronically, intermittently, or transiently carry the organisms, usually for only a few months but potentially as long as 2 years (59). Because the organism survives poorly in the environment and infects only humans,

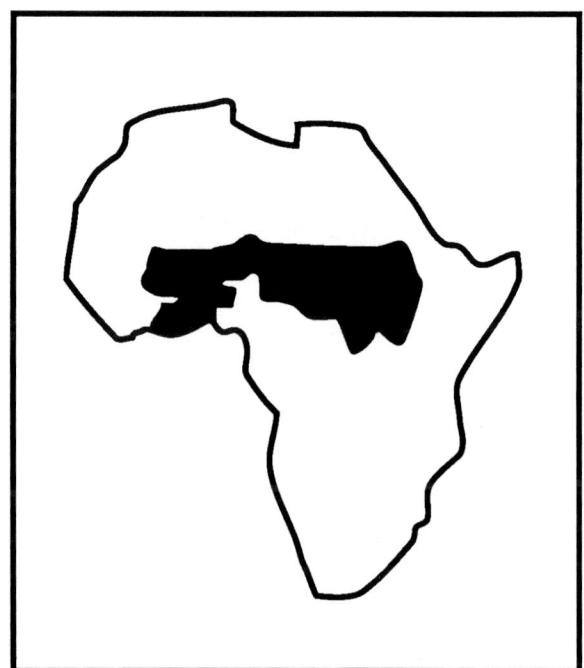

Fig. 31–1. Location of the area endemic for epidemic meningitis, termed the "meningitis belt," in central Africa. (From Peltola, H: Meningococcal disease: Still with us. Rev. Infect. Dis., 5:71, 1983.)

human carriers are the major reservoir of infection. Transmission of N. meningitidis from carrier to carrier probably occurs by direct contact with respiratory tract secretions or by airborne droplets contaminated with the organism, but this has not been proven. In one study conducted under nonepidemic conditions, N. meningitidis was found in 11% of children under 15 years of age, in 3% of persons over age 65 years, and in 30% of 15- and 16-year old boys entering naval school (60). Of the isolates of N. meningitidis 51% were groupable, and group B accounted for the majority (63%). In another study of carriage rates in families during a nonepidemic period, 18% of those evaluated were carriers at least once; the median duration of carriage was almost 10 months but exceeded 16 months in 38%; and adult men had the highest rate of carriage (19 to 33%) (61). Of the isolates of N. meningitidis, 88% were groupable, and group B was the most common.

Pathogenesis

Both bacterial and host factors are involved in the pathogenesis of disease caused by Neisseria meningitidis. Bacterial pili probably facilitate attachment to human cells. Production of IgA_1 protease, an enzyme that separates the Fc fragment of IgA from the Fab portion of the molecule (see Chapter 2), may protect the organism from secretory IgA at mucosal surfaces, but this is speculative. The disseminated intravascular coagulation and shock that may develop during disease presumably is related to or initiated by endotoxin in the bacterial cell wall, but this has not been proven.

The high level of natural immunity to meningococcal disease in neonates, the high level of susceptibility among infants beginning at about 6 months of age when the level of serum immunoglobulins is lowest, and the return to a lower level of susceptibility in older children and adults suggest that humoral antibodies are important in protecting against disease. The percentage of persons that have serum bactericidal activity against Neisseria meningitidis, which apparently is mediated by antibodies to the capsular polysaccharide and cell wall antigens, varies inversely with the frequency of meningococcal meningitis during the first 12 years of life (62,63). At birth about 50% of infants have bactericidal antibodies, due to maternal transfer. Antibody titers decline after birth, reach a nadir between 6 and 24 months of age, and then steadily increase until 12 years of age. In early adulthood, the prevalence of bactericidal antibodies varies with the serogroup, ranging from 67% for group A to 86% for group B. During an epidemic, bactericidal antibodies protect against homologous serogroups.

The meningococcal carrier state is an immunizing process, and within 2 weeks of colonization antibodies to Neisseria meningitidis can be detected (62,63). Nontypable strains of N. meningitidis, frequently found in colonized children, contain antigens that cross-react with those of encapsulated strains; and during colonization, bactericidal antibodies are produced against colonizing strains and against specific serogroups. Serologic cross-reactions also occur between the meningococcal group A polysaccharide and antigens of Bacillus pumilis, and the group B capsular polysaccharide is immunologically and chemically identical to the K1 antigen of Escherichia coli (see Chapter 34). This immunologic similarity and identity may be important in the development of natural immunity of N. meningitidis, and ultimately in protection against virulent strains.

Specific factors that determine whether or not infection with Neisseria meningitidis will result in disease are unknown. An estimated one in every 1000 to 5000 infections with N. meningitidis culminates in disease (64). Persons with deficiencies in the terminal complement proteins are at increased risk of disease (see Chapter 2); and overcrowding, poor general health, poor living conditions, acute respiratory tract disease, the absence of serum bactericidal activity, or a combination of these factors may be predisposing factors (58,59). Persons who have high levels of IgA antibodies to the meningococcal capsular polysaccharide may be at increased risk, possibly because the IgA antibodies block serum bactericidal activity (65).

Clinical Manifestations

The clinical manifestations of meningococcal disease range from transient fever and bacteremia to fulminant disease resulting in death within a few hours of the onset of clinical symptoms. Four clinical situations are described: bacteremia without sepsis, overwhelming meningococcal sepsis without meningitis (called the Waterhouse-Friderichsen syndrome), meningitis with or without meningococcemia, and meningoencephalitis. Possible complications of meningococcemia include arthritis, pericarditis, and osteomyelitis.

A common harbinger of meningococcal disease is a petechial rash, characterized by discrete 1- to 2-mm diameter lesions, typically on the trunk and lower portions of the body, that may coalesce, forming large ecchymoses. The petechiae correlate with the degree of thrombocytopenia and are a clinical indicator of disseminated intravascular coagulation (DIC). Occasionally, a non-pruritic, transient, maculopapular rash develops, similar to that associated with rubella (see Chapter 17), or a vesicular rash that desquamates during recovery. In persons with meningitis, evidence of meningeal irritation (headache, stiff neck, vomiting) is common except in the very young and the very old, but focal neurologic signs and seizures are unusual (59). Shock frequently dominates and is an ominous prognostic sign, especially when accompanied by DIC.

Other manifestations of infection with Neisseria meningitidis include persistent bacteremia with low-grade fever, rash, and arthritis; pneumonia, especially in older persons with pre-existing pulmonary disease; conjunctivitis, urethritis, cervicitis, and proctitis (66–72).

Other Species of Neisseria

Neisseria lactamica, which is frequently isolated from the nasopharynx of infants and children, is a rare cause of meningitis and sepsis, and it has been recovered from the urogenital tract (73–77). Neisseria sicca, Neisseria subflava, Neisseria flavescens, Neisseria cinerea, Neisseria mucosa, Neisseria elongata (which now includes bacteria that formerly were designated Centers for Disease Control [CDC] group M-6), and Neisseria polysaccharea colonize the human nasopharynx (78). All have low virulence but rarely cause disease—meningitis, endocarditis, osteomyelitis, bacteremia, pericarditis, ocular infections, proctitis, and visceral botryomycosis (79–94).

BRANHAMELLA CATARRHALIS

Branhamella catarrhalis is a common saprophyte of the human upper respiratory tract, and occasionally of the female genital tract. It produces a capsule, and extending from its outer membrane are pili that serve as adhesins. In its outer membrane are eight major proteins, phospholipids, and a lipo-oligosaccharide. The latter is composed of lipid A, which has endotoxic activity (see Chapter 2), and a polysaccharide that lacks the O antigen present in enteric bacteria, thus increasing the permeability of the outer membrane and enhancing the organism's susceptibility to erythromycin and rifampin (2). The most common diseases associated with B. catarrhalis are laryngitis, tracheitis, pneumonia (especially in those with underlying chronic lung disease), acute bronchitis, exacerbations of bronchitis, otitis media, and maxillary sinusitis (2,95–99). Moreover, B. catarrhalis is an uncommon cause of meningitis, sepsis, endocarditis, bacteremia, keratitis, urogenital infections, ophthalmia neonatorum, arthritis, and pericarditis (2,100–108).

Laboratory Diagnosis

Specimens for diagnosis of infections caused by the species of Neisseria and Branhamella catarrhalis depend on the clinical manifestations (Table 31–1). Specimen collection, transport and processing are discussed in Part III, but in general, specimens for recovery of Neisseria gonorrhoeae or Neisseria meningitidis should be transported to the laboratory as rapidly as possible and processed immediately. Organisms collected on swabs remain viable up to 12 hours in tube transport systems containing holding medium (commercially available), provided they are not exposed to temperature extremes. Alternatively, swab specimens collected for recovery of Neisseria gonorrhoeae may be inoculated immediately to a transport system using growth medium in a chamber that provides the appropriate carbon dioxide atmosphere (commercially available) and incubated up to 24 hours before transport (109,110). Specimens for recovery of N. gonorrhoeae and Neisseria meningitidis must never be refrigerated.

In this section, the microscopic features and colony characteristics of the species of Neisseria and Branhamella catarrhalis are reviewed, and methods of identification and susceptibility testing are discussed.

Microscopic Features and Colony Characteristics

Neisseria gonorrhoeae. The Gram stain is recommended for direct examination of smears prepared from urethral discharge of males with urethritis. The presence of gram-negative kidney bean–shaped diplococci found extracellularly and intracellularly within neutrophils (Plate IC) and few, if any, other bacteria is presumptive evidence of gonorrhea. Smears of cervical discharge stained with the Gram stain may show intracellular gram-negative diplococci; but because similar-looking organisms are part of the normal flora of the female genital tract, accurate interpretation of the smear is difficult. The sensitivity of the Gram stain for diagnosing gonococcal cervicitis is only 50 to 70%, so culture must be performed to diagnose urogenital infections in females and to diagnose extragenital gonococcal disease (111).

To isolate Neisseria gonorrhoeae from a nonsterile site (cervix, urethra, rectum, pharynx), a selective medium that prevents overgrowth by other more rapidly growing micro-organisms must be inoculated. Media that may be used and their composition are listed in Table 31–2 (109,112). Vancomycin-susceptible strains of N. gonorrhoeae, which may not grow on selective media containing that antimicrobial agent, have been reported in certain geographic locales, and in those areas inoculation of both selective and nonselective (chocolate agar) media is recommended (113,114).

After 24 hours, colonies of Neisseria gonorrhoeae are 0.5 to 1 mm in diameter, gray to white, opaque, raised, and glistening. On translucent agar, different colony types may be distinguished. Fresh clinical isolates initially form colony types P^+ and P^{++} (formerly called T1 and T2), composed of piliated bacterial cells. With repeated subcultures, larger and flatter P^- (formerly called T3 and T4) colonies, comprised of nonpiliated cells, predominate.

Neisseria meningitidis. Meningococcal meningitis may be diagnosed presumptively when gram-negative diplococci, which may vary in size and staining intensity, are seen within neutrophils and extracellularly in a smear of cerebrospinal fluid stained with the Gram stain. Isolates that cause meningitis usually have a capsule, so cells may be surrounded by a distinct pink halo, and they may appear gram-positive because the capsule increases their resistance to decolorization. In persons with meningococcal pneumonia, smears of respiratory tract specimens (sputum, tracheal aspirates, or bronchoalveolar lavage fluids) stained with the Gram stain may show many neutrophils and a predominance of gram-negative diplococci, often within neutrophils, though, this is not specific because infections with Branhamella catarrhalis are associated with similar findings (Plate IVC).

On agar media, colonies of Neisseria meningitidis are nonpigmented or gray to white, round, convex, smooth, and generally larger than those of Neisseria gonorrhoeae, measuring 1 mm or more in diameter after overnight incubation. Colonies of serogroups A and C may appear mucoid. On blood agar the medium beneath and adjacent to the colonies often exhibits greenish discoloration. Young cultures have a butyrous consistency; but with continued incubation, the organisms "autolyse" and the colonies become sticky and rubbery.

Other Neisseria species and Branhamella catarrhalis. The microscopic features of these organisms are identical to features discussed earlier for Neisseria gonorrhoeae. Their colony morphology is described in Table 31–3. This often is the only feature that differentiates isolates of Neisseria subflava (biovar perflava), which form smooth and easily emulsified colonies, from those of Neisseria sicca, which form nonpigmented colonies that adhere to the agar surface and with prolonged incubation become wrinkled.

Table 31–1. Diseases Caused by Species of Neisseria and Branhamella Catarrhalis and Specimens Required for Diagnosis

Disease	Organisms		Specimens*
	Common	Uncommon	
Urogenital infection	N. gonorrhoeae	N. meningitidis B. catarrhalis	Female: *endocervix*; rectum, urethra, pharynx, Bartholin's duct Male: urethra (plus rectum and pharynx if homosexual)
Proctitis	N. gonorrhoeae	N. cinerea N. meningitidis	Rectum
Ophthalmia neonatorum	N. gonorrhoeae	N. cinerea B. catarrhalis	Conjunctiva
Pelvic inflammatory disease	N. gonorrhoeae		Endocervix†
Arthritis-dermatitis	N. gonorrhoeae		Blood, joint fluid, skin lesions‡
Septicemia	N. meningitidis	N. gonorrhoeae N. lactamica N. subflava N. flavescens	Blood
Meningitis	N. meningitidis	N. gonorrhoeae N. lactamica N. sicca N. subflava	*Cerebrospinal fluid*, blood
Pneumonia	B. catarrhalis	N. meningitidis	Sputum, tracheal or transtracheal aspirate, bronchoalveolar lavage fluid, blood
Otitis media, sinusitis	B. catarrhalis		Tympanocentesis fluid, aspirate of sinus
Endocarditis		N. gonorrhoeae N. meningitidis N. subflava N. sicca N. mucosa	Blood, valve tissue

* Swab specimens are collected from mucosal sites; specimen in italics is preferred.
† The presence of N. gonorrhoeae in the cervix does not prove that it is responsible for salpingitis or exclude coinfection with other organisms; moreover, given that cervical cultures are insensitive for diagnosis of pelvic infections, failure to isolate N. gonorrhoeae does not exclude its involvement in the ascending infection.
‡ Blood usually is positive during the polyarthritis-dermatitis stage; synovial fluid usually is positive during the septic arthritis stage; organisms may be demonstrated by immunochemical methods in skin biopsy specimens, but cultures usually are negative.

Organism Identification

An isolate from a urogenital specimen (urethra, cervix) showing the appropriate colony appearance (described earlier) on a selective medium (see Table 31–2) presumptively may be called Neisseria gonorrhoeae based on results of the following tests: Gram stain, oxidase (see Chapter 34), and catalase (see Appendix, Procedure 9). Gram-stained smears prepared from colonies of Neisseria gonorrhoeae should show typical gram-negative diplococci, but organisms occasionally occur in tetrads, especially cells from young cultures; and cells from older cultures may be swollen and show variable intensity of the safranin counterstain. Species of Moraxella have a similar appearance but can be differentiated from N. gonorrhoeae by the penicillin disk test (see Chapter 32). All species of Neisseria are oxidase positive, and all except Neisseria elongata are catalase positive. Because species of Neisseria other than Neisseria gonorrhoeae may be recovered from urogenital sites, confirmatory testing is strongly recommended and is required for all isolates from extragenital

Table 31–2. Selective Media Used to Recover N. Gonorrhoeae from Nonsterile Sites

Medium	Composition	Comments
Thayer-Martin (TM)	Supplemented chocolate agar (TM medium) with vancomycin, colistin, nystatin	
Modified Thayer-Martin (MTM)	Thayer-Martin plus trimethoprim	Inhibits swarming Proteus
Martin-Lewis	Similar to MTM with increased concentration of vancomycin and anisomycin instead of nystatin	
New York City agar (NYC)	Proteose peptone-cornstarch agar with lysed horse erythrocytes, citrated horse plasma, yeast dialysate, dextrose, vancomycin, colistin, trimethoprim, amphothericin B	Supports growth of genital mycoplasmas (see Chapter 27); translucent
Modified NYC agar	NYC without lysed horse erythrocytes	Provides good growth of N. gonorrhoeae, less expensive than NYC
GC Lect	Not available from manufacturer	Similar to MTM for isolating N. gonorrhoeae but superior for suppressing normal flora

Table 31–3. Characteristics of Neisseria Species and B. Catarrhalis

Species	Colony Morphology	Growth on: MTM, ML, or NYC Medium	Growth on: Chocolate or Blood Agar at 22° C	Growth on: Nutrient Agar at 35° C	Acid Production from: Glucose	Maltose	Lactose	Sucrose	Fructose	Reduction of: NO_3	NO_2	Polysaccharide Synthesis	DNase
N. gonorrhoeae	Gray to white, smooth, five colony types on subculture from primary	+	0	0	+	0	0	0	0	0	0	0	0
N. meningitidis	Nonpigmented or gray to white, some yellowish, smooth, transparent, encapsulated strains mucoid	+	0	0	+	+	0	0	0	0	V	0	0
N. lactamica	Nonpigmented or yellowish, smooth, transparent	+	V	+	+	+	+	0	0	0	+	0	0
N. sicca	Nonpigmented, wrinkled, coarse and dry, adherent	0	V	+	+	+	0	+	+	0	+	+	0
N. subflava	Greenish, yellow, smooth, adherent	0	V	V	+	+	0	V	V	0	+	V	0
N. mucosa	Sometimes yellowish, mucoid appearance due to capsule	0	+	+	+	+	0	+	+	+	+	+	0
N. flavescens	Yellow, opaque, smooth	0	+	+	0	0	0	0	0	0	+	+	0
N. cinerea	Grayish-white, slightly granular	V	V	+	0	0	0	0	0	0	+	0	0
N. elongata*	Grayish-white, slight yellow tinge, flat, glistening, dry, claylike consistency	0	+	+	0	0	0	0	0	0	+	0	0
N. polysaccharea	Nonpigmented, translucent	+	V	+	+	+	0	V	0	0	0	+	0
B. catarrhalis	Nonpigmented or gray, opaque, smooth	0	+	+	0	0	0	0	0	+	+	0	+

* Rod-shaped organism; weakly positive or negative catalase test, whereas other species of Neisseria and B. catarrhalis are catalase positive.
Key: MTM, modified Thayer Martin; ML, Martin Lewis; NYC, New York City; +, typically positive but negative strains are encountered occasionally; 0, most strains negative; V, variable characteristic.
(Modified from Morello JA, Janda WM, and Bohnhoff M: Neisseria and Branhamella. In Manual of Clinical Microbiology. 4th ed. Edited by EH Lennette, A Balows, WJ Hausler, Jr, HJ Shadomy. Washington, DC, American Society for Microbiology, 1985.)

sites. Moreover, confirmatory testing, preferably by more than one method, must be done for all Neisseria isolated from children because sexual abuse may be suspected.

Confirmation of Neisseria gonorrhoeae and identification of the other Neisseria species and Branhamella catarrhalis are based on growth and biochemical characteristics. The standard method of identification is detection of acid production from carbohydrates in a cystine-tryptic acid (CTA) base medium and other conventional biochemical tests (see Table 31–3) (115). However, given the drawbacks of the conventional methods (discussed later), more rapid techniques (summarized in Table 31–4) to identify isolates have been developed and are used in most clinical laboratories. In addition, tests for direct detection of Neisseria gonorrhoeae and Neisseria meningitidis in clinical specimens are available. Typing isolates of Neisseria gonorrhoeae and Neisseria meningitidis is done principally for epidemiologic studies.

Conventional Biochemical Tests. With the standard method of identification, acid production from glucose, maltose, lactose, sucrose, and fructose in a CTA-based medium and a carbohydrate-free control are tested, although the o-nitrophenyl-β-D-glactopyranoside (ONPG) test (see Chapter 34) may be substituted for lactose. Tubes of semisolid agar containing 1% filter-sterilized carbohydrate are inoculated with the test isolate, incubated at 35° to 37° C in ambient air, and examined at 24-hour intervals until reactions are interpretable or for 72 hours. Expected results for the species of Neisseria and Branhamella catarrhalis are shown in Table 31–3. Occasionally, however, an isolate of Neisseria meningitidis yields aberrant carbohydrate reactions: glucose-negative, maltose-negative, or asaccharolytic (116,117). If N. meningitidis is strongly suspected in these cases the identification often can be confirmed by slide agglutination, using pooled polyvalent grouping antisera or sera specific for individual serogroups (109). One drop of a dense suspension of the organism prepared in phosphate-buffered saline from an 18-hour subculture on blood agar is mixed with one drop of antiserum on a glass slide and rotated for 2 to 4 minutes. Agglutination indicates a positive result.

In addition to conventional carbohydrate degradation tests, reduction of nitrates and nitrites, polysaccharide synthesis (described later), and deoxyribonuclease (DNAse) production should be evaluated. The latter is especially useful for identification of Branhamella catarrhalis, which is DNase positive, whereas the Neisseria species are negative. Moreover, most clinical isolates of B. catarrhalis produce β-lactamase and are positive for tributyrin (a rapid test is commercially available), features that distinguish it from respiratory isolates of Neisseria species, most of which do not produce β-lactamase and are tributyrin negative.

Drawbacks to conventional carbohydrates are the requirement for a heavy inoculum, the need to work with pure cultures, the need to use reagent-grade carbohydrates, long turnaround time (results may not be available for 96 hours), and failure of some fastidious strains of

Table 31-4. Methods for Identification of Neisseria Species and Branhamella catarrhalis

Method	Turnaround Time (hr)*	Comments
CTA sugars and conventional biochemicals	≤120	Fastidious N. gonorrhoeae may not grow
Commercial carbohydrate degradation	48	Acid reactions of some N. gonorrhoeae may be hard to interpret; some N. cinerea may give a positive glucose reaction; some N. flava, N. subflava, and N. polysaccharea may be misidentified as N. meningitidis; do not identify many commensal species
Chromogenic enzyme substrates	48	Recommended only for oxidase-positive, gram-negative diplococci recovered on a selective medium; useful for identifying maltose-negative N. meningitidis; color changes may be hard to interpret
Combined enzyme and modified conventional tests	48	Can be used to identify Neisseria species isolated on nonselective media; some systems also identify Haemophilus (see Chapter 36)
Immunologic tests Coagglutination and immunofluorescent antibodies for N. gonorrhoeae	24	Recommended for oxidase-positive, gram-negative diplococci recovered on selective media
Direct-detection tests ELISA for N. gonorrhoeae	4	Used only for urethral and endocervical swabs; recommended for high-risk groups
DNA probe for N. gonorrhoeae	3	Used for urethral and endocervical swabs and urine from males
Particle agglutination for N. meningitidis	1	Sensitivity about equal to Gram stain for CSF

* From the time specimen is received in laboratory.

Neisseria gonorrhoeae to grow. For these reasons, one of the alternative methods of identification described in this section is used in most clinical laboratories.

Commercial Carbohydrate Degradation Kits. Several commercially available systems detect acid production from carbohydrates (glucose, maltose, lactose, and sucrose), usually in 1 to 4 hours; but because the inoculum for these tests must be prepared from a pure culture of the isolate, identification usually is available 24 hours after isolation (73,109). In general, results of these tests are comparable to those of the CTA carbohydrates, though problems have been encountered with the rapid carbohydrate degradation tests, and when used alone they will not identify many of the commensal species of Neisseria.

Acid reactions of some strains of Neisseria gonorrhoeae (and to a lesser extent Neisseria meningitidis) may be difficult to interpret with some of these kits, and strains of Neisseria gonorrhoeae that are weak producers of acid from glucose may appear to be glucose negative (73,118,119). Some strains of Neisseria cinerea, which does not produce acid from glucose, can give positive glucose reactions in certain systems, possibly by rapidly overoxidizing glucose to carbon dioxide (120,121). To accurately interpret results of commercial carbohydrate degradation kits adequate controls must be included. Moreover, if the glucose reaction is equivocal, additional tests such as colistin susceptibility by disk diffusion (see Chapter 24) using a 10-μg disk should be performed to differentiate Neisseria gonorrhoeae (resistant, growing up to the edge of the disk) from Neisseria cinerea (susceptible, showing a zone of 10 mm or more).

An isolate of Neisseria meningitidis may yield aberrant carbohydrate reactions, as discussed earlier for conventional carbohydrate testing. Moreover, with the commercial rapid carbohydrate test systems isolates of Neisseria flava, Neisseria subflava, and Neisseria polysaccharea may be identified as Neisseria meningitidis. Isolates of Neisseria flava and Neisseria subflava should be distinguished by colony morphology (see Table 31-3). Moreover, they are susceptible to colistin (Neisseria meningitidis is resistant), and they typically are not isolated on gonococcal selective media, whereas Neisseria meningitidis is. Isolates of Neisseria polysaccharea are differentiated from Neisseria meningitidis by their ability to produce polysaccharide from sucrose (73,109). Brain-heart infusion agar containing 5% sucrose is inoculated with the test organism; and after incubation at 35° C for 48 hours a 1:4 dilution of fresh Lugol iodine is added to the plate. A blue color forms around the colonies when polysaccharides are present, indicating a positive result.

Chromogenic Enzyme Substrate Tests. Enzyme substrate tests for rapid identification (1 to 4 hours) of Neisseria gonorrhoeae, Neisseria meningitidis, Neisseria lactamica, and Branhamella catarrhalis use biochemical reagents that, when hydrolyzed by bacterial enzymes, produce a colored end product visualized with or without the addition of a detection reagent (73,109). Isolates of oxidase-positive, gram-negative diplococci *recovered on a selective medium* (see Table 31-2) are inoculated into tubes or onto filter paper disks containing chromogenic substrates that detect production of β-D-galactosidase (positive only for Neisseria lactamica), γ-glutamyl-aminopeptidase (positive only for Neisseria meningitidis), or hydroxyprolylaminopeptidase (positive for Neisseria lactamica and Neisseria gonorrhoeae). An isolate that lacks all of these enzymes presumptively is called Branhamella catarrhalis, and this can be confirmed by a positive test for DNAse or tributyrin (discussed earlier).

The enzyme substrate tests are valuable for differentiating maltose-negative strains of Neisseria meningitidis from Neisseria gonorrhoeae, but problems with these tests exist (122,123). For example, with the test using filter paper disks, the substrate for γ-glutamylaminopeptidase changes from red to purple, a change that may be subtle and if misinterpreted could cause isolates of Neisseria meningitidis and other species of Neisseria to be incorrectly identified as Neisseria gonorrhoeae. Moreover, strains of Neisseria cinerea, Neisseria perflava, and Kingella denitrificans (see Chapter 32) that grow on gonococcal-selective media could be misidentified as Neisseria gonorrhoeae if not confirmed with other procedures (73).

Commercially available products that combine enzyme substrate tests with modified conventional tests provide accurate identification of species of Neisseria (including those isolated on nonselective media) and species of Haemophilus (see Chapter 36) (115,124).

Immunologic Tests. Commercially available immunologic tests used specifically for culture confirmation of Neisseria gonorrhoeae are coagglutination and fluorescent antibody tests. With these tests colonies from the primary isolation plate may be evaluated without subculturing to obtain a pure culture; therefore, an isolate may be identified 24 hours earlier than is possible with the rapid carbohydrate or enzyme-substrate tests, which require inoculation with a suspension prepared from a pure culture. However, each technique is associated with potential problems. With coagglutination, reactions may be difficult to interpret, and false-positive results may occur when the organism suspension is too heavy or when the suspension is prepared in saline that has a pH less than 7.2 (115). False-positive and false-negative reactions, depending on the reagents, have been associated with the fluorescent antibody test. Polyclonal antibodies cross-reacted with other species of Neisseria and did not detect all strains of N. gonorrhoeae; therefore, they are no longer used (125–127). Fluorescent tests using monoclonal antibodies are highly specific and sensitive for N. gonorrhoeae, but false-positive results with other species of Neisseria and with Kingella denitrificans and nonspecific Fc binding to other bacteria, including some Staphylococcus aureus, have been reported (73,128,129). Therefore, using the latter reagents to test only gram-negative oxidase-positive organisms recovered on gonococcal-selective media is suggested. One monoclonal antibody reagent failed to detect isolates of Neisseria gonorrhoeae belonging to the serovar IA-4 (129).

Direct Detection Tests. An enzyme-linked immunosorbent assay (ELISA) for detection of Neisseria gonorrhoeae directly in urethral and endocervical swab specimens is commercially available. For urethral swab specimens from men its sensitivity and specificity are about equal to those of a smear stained with the Gram stain. The ELISA, however, is less sensitive than cervical culture for women and has yielded false-positive reactions with other species of Neisseria; therefore, the test should be used only to detect N. gonorrhoeae in specimens from persons in high-risk groups, and results should be considered presumptive (73,130).

Recently, a chemiluminescent nucleic acid probe for detection of Neisseria gonorrhoeae became commercially available. When used for culture confirmation, the probe appears to be highly specific and sensitive for testing colonies from 24-hour cultures but less sensitive for testing older cultures (131). Evaluations of the reliability of the probe for detecting N. gonorrhoeae directly in clinical swab specimens currently are limited, but in one study of symptomatic and asymptomatic women the sensitivity and specificity of the DNA probe test were equivalent to those of endocervical culture (132).

Neisseria meningitidis–induced meningitis may be diagnosed by using particle agglutination for detection of capsular polysaccharide antigens in clinical specimens. Cerebrospinal fluid is preferred, but urine and serum also may be tested (discussed in more detail in Chapter 24). Currently, latex and coagglutination reagents that detect N. meningitidis serogroups A, B, C, Y, and W135 are commercially available. Given the immunologic and chemical similarity between N. meningitidis group B and Escherichia coli K1, the two organisms cannot be distinguished by particle agglutination. Antigen detection tests always should be used to supplement Gram stain and culture. Positive results provide a rapid presumptive diagnosis, allowing early administration of appropriate antimicrobial therapy; however, false-positive results with the latex agglutination test for Neisseria meningitidis groups A and Y have been attributed to contamination of the specimen with povidone-iodine, and negative results do not exclude the diagnosis of meningococcal meningitis (133).

Typing of Isolates. Characterization of strains of Neisseria gonorrhoeae by auxotyping and serotyping is used predominantly to study the pathogenesis and epidemiology of diseases caused by the organism. Auxotyping, which separates strains of N. gonorrhoeae according to their requirements for one or more metabolites, has been used extensively but is too complex to perform routinely in the clinical microbiology laboratory. Organisms are inoculated onto a variety of synthetic media from which individual specific substances (primarily amino acids and nitrogenous bases) have been omitted; and an isolate that does not grow on a medium requires the omitted substance for growth. Of the more than 30 identified auxotypes, the one referred to most frequently is AHU^-, which requires arginine, hypoxanthine, and uracil for growth, a type usually sensitive to penicillin, resistant to the bactericidal activity of nonimmune human serum, and more likely than other auxotypes to cause asymptomatic urethritis in males and disseminated disease in females. The most widely used serotyping system is based on the antigenic variation of protein I. It separates isolates of N. gonorrhoeae into two groups, IA and IB, which in turn are divided into serovars based on coagglutination reactions using monoclonal antibodies that react with variable epitopes of protein IA or IB.

Serologic classification of isolates of Neisseria meningitidis based on capsular polysaccharides is useful for epidemiologic studies. Agglutination is the most reliable and routinely used technique. Grouping antisera is commercially available, but if N. meningitidis is recovered only rarely it may be most cost effective to send isolates to a reference laboratory for typing. Almost all isolates of N. meningitidis that cause systemic infections are groupable by this technique, whereas isolates recovered from the nasopharynx of carriers may be ungroupable.

Susceptibility Testing

All isolates of Neisseria gonorrhoeae should be tested for their ability to produce β-lactamase, a plasmid-mediated enzyme responsible for resistance to penicillin. Testing growth from the primary isolation plate by the chromogenic cephalosporin method (see Chapter 24) is preferred. Additional susceptibility testing must be performed to detect chromosomally mediated resistance to penicillin and resistance to other antimicrobial agents. Disk diffusion susceptibility testing of isolates of N. gonorrhoeae against penicillin (10-U disk), tetracycline (30-μg disk), spectinomycin (100-μg disk), and ceftriaxone (30-μg disk) using GC agar with a "XV-like" supplement lacking cysteine, which may inactivate some of the newer β-lactam compounds, is recommended (134). Plates are incubated at 35° C in 3 to 7% carbon dioxide for 20 to 24 hours, after which the diameters of the zones of inhibition are measured and interpreted as follows:

Penicillin: susceptible, ≥47mm; resistant, ≤26mm
Tetracycline: susceptible, ≥38mm; resistant, ≤30mm
Spectinomycin: susceptible, ≥18mm; resistant, ≤14mm
Ceftriaxone: susceptible, ≥35mm; no resistance category

Antimicrobial susceptibility testing of isolates of Neisseria meningitidis usually is not necessary because most are very susceptible to penicillin. However, penicillin-resistant strains have been reported, so, isolates of N. meningitidis from patients who do not respond well to penicillin therapy warrant susceptibility testing by disk diffusion or agar dilution and a β-lactamase test (135–137).

Isolates of Branhamella catarrhalis should be tested for β-lactamase production by the nitrocefin-based chromogenic cephalosporin assay (see Chapter 24). Additional susceptibility testing should not be performed routinely because B. catarrhalis appears to be uniformly resistant to vancomycin, clindamycin, and trimethoprim alone and uniformly susceptible to most other antimicrobial agents (138). However, if the activity of a specific antimicrobial agent against an isolate of B. catarrhalis must be evaluated, disk diffusion or dilution tests should be performed according to guidelines provided by the National Committee for Clinical Laboratory Standards (139,140).

Treatment

Neisseria gonorrhoeae. Owing to the increasing prevalence of penicillinase-producing N. gonorrhoeae, penicillin no longer is the recommended initial treatment for uncomplicated gonorrhea in adults. Ceftriaxone is the agent of choice unless active surveillance shows that PPNG and isolates with chromosomally mediated resistance account for fewer than 1% and 5%, respectively, of isolates of N. gonorrhoeae in the community (141). Ceftriaxone is effective therapy for infection at all anatomic sites, is safe and effective for pregnant women, and appears to abort incubating syphilis, but it is costly and must be given intramuscularly (142). Alternatively, spectinomycin may be used for genital and rectal gonorrhea, but it is ineffective for pharyngeal infection and does not inhibit Treponema pallidum. Both ceftriaxone and spectinomycin must be followed by 7 to 10 days' treatment with doxycycline, tetracycline, or erythromycin. Recommended treatment regimens for pelvic inflammatory disease include doxycycline plus cefoxitin followed by doxycycline or clindamycin plus gentamicin with continued clindamycin for hospitalized patients and ceftriaxone followed by doxycycline for outpatients. Disseminated gonorrhea is treated with 7 to 10 days' ceftriaxone or, if the isolate is fully susceptible to penicillin or tetracycline, one of the latter drugs may be used. Partners of persons with gonorrhea should be treated regardless of whether they have clinical disease.

Other Species of Neisseria and Branhamella catarrhalis. Infections caused by Neisseria meningitidis are treated with penicillin or, if the organism is resistant to penicillin, with chloramphenicol. Commensal species of Neisseria usually are susceptible to penicillin and ampicillin; but β-lactamase production by these organisms has rarely been reported (91). Isolates of Branhamella catarrhalis usually are susceptible to erythromycin, tetracycline, and trimethoprim-sulfamethoxazole, but most are resistant to penicillin, ampicillin, and amoxicillin owing to production of β-lactamase (2).

Prevention and Control

Neisseria gonorrhoeae. Properly used, condoms protect against the transmission or acquisition of gonorrhea; diaphragms and topical spermicides containing nonoxynol-9 probably are effective, but less so than condoms (143). Research to develop a vaccine is ongoing, but to date vaccines containing purified pili or recombinent protein I have not provided complete protection (3,27).

Neisseria meningitidis. Currently, chemoprophylaxis with rifampin is recommended for household contacts of persons who have meningococcal disease, because the attack rate in this group is 500 to 800 times greater than in the general population (144). Similar high-risk situations in which chemoprophylaxis is indicated are closed populations such as college dormitories, long term care hospitals, nursery schools, and military barracks. Immunoprophylaxis with a quadrivalent polysaccharide vaccine against serotypes A, C, Y, and W135, which appears to provide protection for at least 2 years in persons over 2 years of age, is recommended for military personnel, for persons living in epidemic areas of developing countries and for those with a nonfunctional or absent spleen (145).

REFERENCES

1. Rossau R, et al: Ribosomal ribonucleic acid cistron similarities and deoxyribonucleic acid homologies of Neisseria, Kingella, Eikenella, Simonsiella, Alysiella, and Centers for Disease Control groups EF-4 and M-5 in the emended family Neisseriaceae. Int J Syst Bacteriol *39*:185, 1989.
2. Catlin BW: Branhamella catarrhalis: An organism gaining respect as a pathogen. Clin Microbiol Rev, *3*:293, 1990.
3. Handsfield HH: Neisseria gonorrhoeae. *In* Principles and Practice of Infectious Diseases. 3rd ed. Edited by GL Mandell, RG Douglas, Jr, and JE Bennett. New York, Churchill Livingstone, 1990.
4. Centers for Disease Control: Summary of notifiable diseases, United States 1987. MMWR, *36*:1, 1987.
5. Centers for Disease Control: Plasmid-mediated antimicrobial resistance in Neisseria gonorrhoeae—U.S., 1988 and 1989. MMWR, *39*:284, 1990.
6. Centers for Disease Control: Summary of notifiable diseases, United States, 1989. MMWR, *38*(54):22, 1989.

7. Rice RJ, et al: Gonorrhea in the United States 1975–1984: Is the giant only sleeping? Sex Transm Dis, *14*:83, 1987.
8. Hooper RR, et al: Cohort study of venereal disease: I. The risk of gonorrhea transmission from infected women to men. Am J Epidemiol, *108*:136, 1978.
9. Holmes KK, Johnson DW, and Trostle JH: An estimate of the risk of men acquiring gonorrhea by sexual contact with infected females. Am J Epidemiol, *91*:170, 1970.
10. Thin RNT, Williams IA, and Nicol CS: Direct and delayed methods of immunofluorescent diagnosis of gonorrhea in women. Br J Vener Dis, *47*:27, 1971.
11. Tice RW, and Rodriguez VL: Pharyngeal gonorrhea. JAMA, *246*:2717, 1981.
12. Wiesner PJ, et al: Clinical spectrum of pharyngeal gonococcal infection. N Engl J Med, *288*:181, 1973.
13. Elwell LP, et al: Plasmid-mediated β-lactamase production in Neisseria gonorrhoeae. Antimicrob Agents Chemother, *11*:528, 1977.
14. Perine PL, et al: Epidemiology and treatment of penicillinase-producing Neisseria gonorrhoeae. Sex Transm Dis, *6*(suppl):152, 1979.
15. Whittington WL, and Knapp JS: Trends in antimicrobial resistance in Neisseria gonorrhoeae in the United States. Sex Transm Dis, *15*:202, 1988.
16. Centers for Disease Control: Policy guidelines for the detection, management, and control of antibiotic-resistant strains of Neisseria gonorrhoeae. MMWR, *36*(5S):1, 1987.
17. Centers for Disease Control: Tetracycline-resistant Neisseria gonorrhoeae—Georgia, Pennsylvania, New Hampshire. MMWR, *34*:563, 1985.
18. Brown S, et al: Antimicrobial resistance of Neisseria gonorrhoeae in Bangkok: Is single-drug treatment passe? Lancet, *ii*:1366, 1982.
19. Faruki H, Kohmescher RN, McKinney WP, and Sparling PF: A community-based outbreak of infection with penicillin-resistant Neisseria gonorrhoeae not producing penicillinase (chromosomally mediated resistance). N Engl J Med, *313*:607, 1985.
20. Rice RJ, et al: Chromosomally mediated resistance in Neisseria gonorrhoeae in the United States: Results of surveillance and reporting, 1983–84. J Infect Dis, *153*:340, 1986.
21. McGee ZA, Johnson AP, and Taylor-Robinson D: Pathogenic mechanisms of Neisseria gonorrhoeae: Observations on damage to human fallopian tubes in organ culture by gonococci of colony type 1 or type 4. J Infect Dis, *143*:413, 1981.
22. Ofek I, Beachy EH, and Bisno AL: Resistance of Neisseria gonorrhoeae to phagocytosis: Relationship to colonial morphology and surface pili. J Infect Dis, *129*:310, 1974.
23. Dilworth JA, Hendley JO, and Mandell GL: Attachment and ingestion of gonococci by neutrophils. Infect Immun, *11*:512, 1975.
24. Heckels JE: Molecular studies on the pathogenesis of gonorrhea. J Med Microbiol, *18*:293, 1984.
25. Blake MS, and Gotschlich EC: Gonococcal membrane proteins: Speculation on their role in pathogenesis. Prog Allergy, *33*:298, 1983.
26. Britigan BE, Cohen MS, and Sparling PF: Gonococcal infections: A model of molecular pathogenesis. N Engl J Med, *312*:1683, 1985.
27. Virji M, and Heckels JE: The effect of protein II and pili on the interaction of Neisseria gonorrhoeae with human polymorphonuclear leucocytes. J Gen Microbiol, *132*:503, 1986.
28. Rice PA, et al: Immunoglobulin G antibodies directed against protein III block killing of serum-resistant Neisseria gonorrhoeae by immune serum. J Exp Med, *164*:1735, 1986.
29. Gregg CR, et al: Toxic activity of purified lipopolysaccharide of Neisseria gonorrhoeae for human fallopian tube mucosa. J Infect Dis, *143*:432, 1981.
30. Rice PA, and Kasper DL: Characterization of serum resistance of Neisseria gonorrhoeae that disseminate: Roles of blocking antibody and outer membrane proteins. J Clin Invest, *70*:157, 1982.
31. Apicella MA, et al: Bactericidal antibody response of normal human serum to the lipo-oligosaccharide of Neisseria gonorrhoeae. J Infect Dis, *153*:520, 1986.
32. Rosenthal RS, et al: Resistance of O-acetylated gonococcal peptidoglycan to human peptidoglycan–degrading enzymes. Infect Immun, *40*:903, 1983.
33. Sweet RL: Pelvic inflammatory disease and infertility in women. Infect Dis Clin North Am, *1*:199, 1987.
34. Edwards LE, et al: Gonorrhea in pregnancy. Am J Obstet Gynecol, *132*:637, 1978.
35. Handsfield HH, Hodson WA, and Holmes KK: Neonatal gonococcal infections: I. Orogastric contamination with Neisseria gonorrhoeae. JAMA, *225*:697, 1973.
36. Hook EH, and Holmes KK: Gonococcal infections. Ann Intern Med, *102*:229, 1985.
37. Bohnhoff M, Morello JA, and Lerner SA: Auxotypes, penicillin susceptibility and serogroups of Neisseria gonorrhoeae from disseminated and uncomplicated infections. J Infect Dis, *154*:225, 1986.
38. Knapp JS, and Holmes KK: Disseminated gonococcal infection caused by Neisseria gonorrhoeae with unique nutritional requirements. J Infect Dis, *132*:204, 1975.
39. Petersen BH, et al: Neisseria meningitidis and Neisseria gonorrhoeae bacteremia associated with C6, C7, or C8 deficiency. Ann Intern Med, *90*:917, 1979.
40. Laga M, et al: Single-dose therapy of gonococcal ophthalmia neonatorum with ceftriaxone. N Engl J Med, *315*:1382, 1986.
41. Vieusseaux M: Memoire sur le maladie qui a regne a Geneve au printemps de 1805. J Med Chir Pharmacol, *11*:163, 1805.
42. Weichselbaum A: Üeber die Aetiologie der akuten Meningitis cerebrospinalis. Fortschr Med, *5*:573, 1887.
43. Kiefer F: Zur differential Diagnose des Erregers der epidemischen Cerebrospinalmeningitis und der Gonorrhoe. Berl Klin Wochenschr, *33*:628, 1896.
44. Dopter C: Etude de quelques germes isoles du rhino-pharynx, voisans du meningocoque (parameningocoques). C R Soc Biol (Paris), *67*:74, 1909.
45. Norton JF, and Gordon JE: Meningococcal meningitis in Detroit in 1928–1929. I. Epidemiology. J Prev Med, *4*:207, 1930.
46. French MR: Epidemiological study of 383 cases of meningococcus meningitis in the city of Milwaukee, 1927–1928 and 1929. Am J Public Health, *21*:130, 1931.
47. Pizzi M: A severe epidemic of meningococcus meningitis in Chile, 1941 and 1942. Am J Public Health, *34*:231, 1944.
48. Schwentker FF, Gelman S, and Long PH: The treatment of meningococcic meningitis with sulfonamide. Preliminary report. JAMA, *108*:1407, 1937.
49. Kuhns DM, et al: The prophylactic value of sulfadiazine in the control of meningococcic meningitis. JAMA, *123*:335, 1943.
50. Schoenback EB and Phair JJ: The sensitivity of meningococci to sulfadiazine. Am J Hyg, *47*:177, 1948.
51. Gauld JR, et al: Epidemiology of meningococcal meningitis at Fort Ord. Am J Epidemiol, *82*:56, 1965.
52. Bristow MW, Van Peenen PFD, and Volk R: Epidemic meningitis in naval recruits. Am J Public Health, *55*:1039, 1965.
53. Ding S, Ye R, and Zhang H. Three new serogroups of Neisseria meningitidis. J Biol Stand, *9*:305, 1981.

54. Ashton FE, et al: A new serogroup (L) of Neisseria meningitidis. J Clin Microbiol, 17:722, 1983.
55. Brandstetter RD, Blaikr RJ, and Roberts RB: Neisseria meningitidis serogroup W-135 disease in adults. JAMA, 246: 2060, 1981.
56. DeVoe IW: The meningococcus and mechanisms of pathogenicity. Microbiol Rev, 46:162, 1982.
57. Galaid EI, et al: Meningococcal disease in New York City, 1973–1978. Recognition of groups Y and W135 as frequent pathogens. JAMA, 224:2167, 1980.
58. Peltola H: Meningococcal disease: Still with us. Rev Infect Dis, 5:71, 1983.
59. Apicella MA: Neisseria meningitidis. In Principles and Practice of Infectious Diseases. 3rd ed. Edited by GL Mandell, RG Douglas, Jr, and JE Bennett. New York, Churchill Livingstone, 1990.
60. Fraser PK, et al: The meningococcal carrier rate. Lancet, i:1235, 1973.
61. Greenfield S, Sheede PR, and Feldman HA: Meningococcal carriage in a population of "normal" families. J Infect Dis, 123:67, 1971.
62. Goldschneider I, Gotschlich EC, and Artenstein MS: Human immunity to the meningococcus. I. The role of humoral antibody. J Exp Med, 129:1307, 1969.
63. Goldschneider I, Gotschlich EC, and Artenstein MS: Human immunity to the meningococcus. II. Development of natural immunity. J Exp Med, 129:1327, 1969.
64. Hedrich AW: Recent trends in meningococcal disease. Public Health Rep, 67:411, 1952.
65. Kayhty H, Jousimies-Somer H, Peltola H, and Makela PH: Antibody response to capsular polysaccharides of groups A and C Neisseria meningitidis and Haemophilus influenzae type b during bacteremic disease. J Infect Dis, 143:32, 1981.
66. Saslaw S: Chronic meningococcemia: Report of a case. N Engl J Med, 266:605, 1962.
67. Rompalo AM, et al: The acute arthritis dermatitis syndrome. The changing importance of Neisseria gonorrhoeae and Neisseria meningitidis. Arch Intern Med, 147:281, 1987.
68. Putsch RW, Hamilton JD, and Wolinsky E: Neisseria meningitidis, a respiratory pathogen. J Infect Dis, 121:48, 1970.
69. Irwin RS, Woelk WK, and Coudon WL: Primary meningococcal pneumonia. Ann Intern Med, 82:493, 1975.
70. Miller M, et al: Neisseria meningitidis urethritis: A case report. Arch Intern Med, 242:1656, 1979.
71. Faur YC, Weisburd MH, and Wilson ME: Isolation of Neisseria meningitidis from the genitourinary tract and anal canal. J Clin Microbiol, 2:178, 1975.
72. Barquet N, et al: Primary meningococcal conjunctivitis: Report of 21 patients and review. Rev Infect Dis, 12:838, 1990.
73. Knapp JS: Historical perspectives and identification of Neisseria and related species. Clin Microbiol Rev, 1:415, 1988.
74. Gold R, et al: Carriage of Neisseria meningitidis and Neisseria lactamica in infants and children. J Infect Dis, 137: 112, 1978.
75. Hansman D: Meningitis caused by Neisseria lactamica. N Engl J Med, 299:491, 1978.
76. Wilson DH, and Overman DL: Septicemia due to Neisseria lactamica. J Clin Microbiol, 4:214, 1976.
77. Jephcott AE, and Morton RS: Isolation of Neisseria lactamica from a genital site. Lancet, ii:739, 1972.
78. Grant PE, et al: Neisseria elongata subsp. nitroreducens subsp. nov., formerly CDC Group M-6, a gram-negative bacterium associated with endocarditis. J Clin Microbiol, 28:2591, 1990.
79. Gay RM, and Sevier RE: Neisseria sicca endocarditis: Report of a case and review of the literature. J Clin Microbiol, 8: 729, 1978.
80. Doern GV, et al: Neisseria sicca osteomyelitis. J Clin Microbiol, 16:595, 1982.
81. Gilrane T, et al: Neisseria sicca pneumonia. Report of two cases and review of the literature. Am J Med, 78:1038, 1985.
82. Demmler GJ, Couch RS, and Taber LH: Neisseria subflava bacteremia and meningitis in a child: Report of a case and review of the literature. Pediatr Infect Dis, 4:286, 1985.
83. Scott RM: Bacterial endocarditis due to Neisseria flava. J Pediatr, 78:673, 1971.
84. Clark H, and Patton RD: Postcardiotomy endocarditis due to Neisseria perflava on a prosthetic aortic valve. Ann Intern Med, 68:386, 1968.
85. Pollack S, Mogtader A, and Lange M: Neisseria subflava endocarditis. Case report and review of the literature. Am J Med, 76:752, 1984.
86. Stricker RB, et al: Neisseria subflava endophthalmitis. Am J Ophthalmol, 94:423, 1982.
87. Fainstain V, Musher DM, and Young EJ: Purulent pericarditis due to Neisseria mucosa. Chest, 74:476, 1978.
88. Carter KD, Morgan CM, and Otto MH: Neisseria mucosa endophthalmitis. Am J Ophthalmol, 104:663, 1987.
89. Washburn RG, et al: Visceral botryomycosis caused by Neisseria mucosa in a patient with chronic granulomatous disease. J Infect Dis, 151:563, 1985.
90. Wertlake PT, and Williams TW: Septicaemia caused by Neisseria flavescens. J Clin Pathol, 21:437, 1968.
91. Sinave CP, and Ratzan KR: Infective endocarditis caused by Neisseria flavescens. Am J Med, 82:163, 1987.
92. Southern PM, and Kutscher AE: Bacteremia due to Neisseria cinerea: Report of two cases. Diagn Microbiol Infect Dis, 7:143, 1987.
93. Dossett JH, Appelbaum PC, Knapp JS, and Totten TA: Proctitis associated with Neisseria cinerea misidentified as Neisseria gonorrhoeae in a child. J Clin Microbiol, 21:575, 1985.
94. Bourbeau P, Holla V, and Piemontese S: Ophthalmia neonatorum caused by Neisseria cinerea. J Clin Microbiol, 28: 1640, 1990.
95. Hager H, et al: Branhamella catarrhalis respiratory infections. Rev Infect Dis, 9:1140, 1987.
96. Schalen L, et al: High isolation rate of Branhamella catarrhalis from the nasopharynx in adults with acute laryngitis. Scand J Infect Dis, 12:277, 1980.
97. Ernst TN, and Philp M: Bacterial tracheitis caused by Branhamella catarrhalis. Pediatr Infect Dis J, 6:574, 1987.
98. VanHare GF, et al: Acute otitis media caused by Branhamella catarrhalis: Biology and therapy. Rev Infect Dis, 9:16, 1987.
99. Brorson J-E, Axelsson A, and Holm SE: Studies on Branhamella catarrhalis (Neisseria catarrhalis) with special reference to maxillary sinusitis. Scand J Infect Dis, 8:151, 1976.
100. Cocchi P, and Ulivelli A: Meningitis caused by Neisseria catarrhalis. Acta Paediatr Scand, 57:451, 1968.
101. Baron J, and Shapiro ED: Unsuspected bacteremia caused by Branhamella catarrhalis. Pediatr Infect Dis, 4:100, 1985.
102. Spark RP, Dahlberg DW, and LaBelle JW: Pseudogonococcal ophthalmia neonatorum. Am J Clin Pathol, 72:471, 1979.
103. Ahmad F, et al: Urinary tract infection caused by Branhamella catarrhalis. J Infect, 10:176, 1985.
104. Doern GV, and Gantz NM: Isolation of Branhamella (Neisseria) catarrhalis from men with urethritis. Sex Transm Dis, 9:202, 1982.
105. Jacobson SH, and Björklind A: Symptomatic bacteriuria caused by Branhamella catarrhalis. J Infect, 18:192, 1989.

106. Izraeli S, et al: Branhamella catarrhalis as a cause of suppurative arthritis. Pediatr Infect Dis J, 8:256, 1989.
107. Kostiala AAI, and Honkanen T: Branhamella catarrhalis as a cause of acute purulent pericarditis. J Infect, 19:291, 1989.
108. Turner HR, Taylor MR, and Lockwood WR: Branhamella catarrhalis endocarditis in a patient receiving hemodialysis. South Med J, 78:1021, 1985.
109. Koneman EW, et al (eds): Color Atlas and Textbook of Diagnostic Microbiology. 3rd ed. Philadelphia, JB Lippincott, 1988.
110. Deveaux DL, et al: Comparison of the Gono Pak System™ with the candle extinction jar for recovery of Neisseria gonorrhoeae. J Clin Microbiol, 25:571, 1987.
111. Lossick JG, Smeltzer MP, and Curran JW: The value of the cervical Gram stain in the diagnosis of gonorrhea in women in a sexually transmitted disease clinic. Sex Transm Dis, 9:124, 1982.
112. Reichart CA, Rupkey LM, Brady WE, Hook EW III: Comparison of GC-Lect and modified Thayer-Martin media for isolation of Neisseria gonorrhoeae. J Clin Microbiol, 27:808, 1989.
113. Mirret S, Reller LB, and Knapp JS: Neisseria gonorrhoeae strains inhibited by vancomycin in selective media and correlation with auxotype. J Clin Microbiol, 14:94, 1981.
114. Windall JJ, et al: Inhibitory effects of vancomycin on Neisseria gonorrhoeae in Thayer-Martin medium. J Infect Dis, 142:775, 1980.
115. Morello JA, Janda WM, and Bohnhoff M: Neisseria and Branhamella. In Manual of Clinical Microbiology. 4th ed. Edited by EH Lennette, A Balows, WJ Hausler, Jr, and HJ Shadomy. Washington, DC, American Society for Microbiology, 1985.
116. Granato PA, et al: Meningitis caused by maltose-negative variant of Neisseria meningitidis. J Clin Microbiol, 11:270, 1980.
117. Watanakunakorn C, and Thomson RB, Jr: Septicemia due to a maltose-positive, glucose-negative strain of group C Neisseria meningitidis. J Clin Microbiol, 18:436, 1983.
118. Welch DW, and Cartwright G: Fluorescent monoclonal antibody compared with carbohydrate utilization for rapid identification of Neisseria gonorrhoeae. J Clin Microbiol, 26:293, 1988.
119. Morello JA, Lerner SA, and Bohnhoff M: Characteristics of atypical Neisseria gonorrhoeae from disseminated and localized infections. Infect Immun, 13:1510, 1976.
120. Knapp JS, Totten PA, Mulks MH, and Minshew BH: Characterization of Neisseria cinerea, a nonpathogenic species isolated on Martin-Lewis medium selective for pathogenic Neisseria spp. J Clin Microbiol, 19:63, 1984.
121. Boyce JM, Taylor MR, Mitchell EB, Jr, and Knapp JS: Nosocomial pneumonia caused by a glucose-metabolizing strain of Neisseria cinerea. J Clin Microbiol, 21:1, 1985.
122. Morello JA, Janda WH, and Doern GV: Neisseria and Branhamella. In Manual of Clinical Microbiology. 5th ed. Edited by A Balows et al. Washington, DC, American Society for Microbiology, 1991.
123. Saez-Nieto JA, Fenoll A, Vazquez J, and Casal J: Prevalence of maltose-negative Neisseria meningitidis variants during an epidemic period in Spain. J Clin Microbiol, 15:78, 1982.
124. Janda WM, Malloy PJ, and Schreckenberger PC: Clinical evaluation of the Vitek Neisseria-Haemophilus identification card. J Clin Microbiol, 25:37, 1987.
125. Pollock HM: Evaluation of rapid identification of Neisseria gonorrhoeae in a routine clinical laboratory. J Clin Microbiol, 4:19, 1976.
126. Thin RNT: Immunofluorescent method for the diagnosis of gonorrhoeae in women. Br J Vener Dis, 46:27, 1970.
127. Hare MJ: Comparative assessment of microbiological methods for the diagnosis of gonorrhoeae in women. Br J Vener Dis, 50:437, 1974.
128. Dillon JR, Carballo M, and Pauze M: Evaluation of eight methods for identification of pathogenic Neisseria species: Neisseria-Kwik, RIM-N, Gonobio-Test, Minitek, Gonochek II, GonoGen, Phadebact monoclonal GC OMNI test, and Syva Microtrak Test. J Clin Microbiol, 26:493, 1988.
129. Minshew BH, Beardsley JL, and Knapp JS: Evaluation of GonoGen coagglutination test for serodiagnosis of Neisseria gonorrhoeae: Identification of problem isolates by auxotyping, serotyping, and with a fluorescent antibody reagent. Diagn Microbiol Infect Dis, 3:41, 1985.
130. Schachter J, et al: Enzyme immunoassay for diagnosis of gonorrhea. J Clin Microbiol, 19:57, 1984.
131. Lewis JS, Kranig-Brown D, and Trainor DA: DNA probe confirmatory test for Neisseria gonorrhoeae. J Clin Microbiol, 28:2349, 1990.
132. Panke ES, et al: Comparison of Gen-Probe DNA probe test and culture for the detection of Neisseria gonorrhoeae in endocervical specimens. J Clin Microbiol, 29:883, 1991.
133. D'amato RF, Hochstein L, and Fay EA: False-positive latex agglutination test for Neisseria meningitidis groups A and Y caused by povidone-iodine antiseptic contamination of cerebrospinal fluid. J Clin Microbiol, 28:2134, 1990.
134. Jones RN, et al: Standardization of disk diffusion and agar dilution susceptibility tests for Neisseria gonorrhoeae: Interpretive criteria and quality control guidelines for ceftriaxone, penicillin, spectinomycin, and tetracycline. J Clin Microbiol, 27:2758, 1989.
135. Dillon JR, Pauze M, and Yeung KH: Spread of penicillinase-producing and transfer plasmids from the gonococcus to Neisseria meningitidis. Lancet, i:779, 1983.
136. Sprott MS, Kearns AM, and Field JM: Penicillin-insensitive Neisseria meningitidis. Lancet, 1:1167, 1988.
137. Campos J, et al: Detection of relatively penicillin G–resistant Neisseria meningitidis by disk susceptibility testing. Antimicrob Agents Chemother, 31:1478, 1987.
138. Doern GV, and Jones RN: Antimicrobial susceptibility tests: fastidious and unusual bacteria. In Manual of Clinical Microbiology. 5th ed. Edited by A Balows, et al. Washington DC, American Society for Microbiology, 1991.
139. National Committee for Clinical Laboratory Standards: Performance Standards for Antimicrobial Disk Susceptibility Tests. Approved Standard M2-A4. Villanova, PA, National Committee for Clinical Laboratory Standards, 1990.
140. National Committee for Clinical Laboratory Standards: Dilution Procedures for Susceptibility Testing of Aerobic Bacteria. Approved Standard M7-A2. Villanova, PA, National Committee for Clinical Laboratory Standards, 1990.
141. Centers for Disease Control: Antibiotic-resistant strains of Neisseria gonorrhoeae: Policy guidelines for detection, management, and control. MMWR, 36(Suppl):1S, 1987.
142. Hook EW III, Roddy RE, and Handsfield HH: Ceftriaxone therapy for incubating and early syphilis. J Infect Dis, 158:881, 1988.
143. Stone KM, Grimes DA, and Magder LS: Personal protection against sexually transmitted diseases. Am J Obstet Gynecol, 155:180, 1986.
144. The Meningococcal Disease Surveillance Group: Analysis of endemic meningococcal disease by serogroup and evaluation of chemoprophylaxis. J Infect Dis, 134:2011, 1976.
145. Centers for Disease Control: Availability of meningococcal vaccine in single-dose vials for travelers and high-risk persons. MMWR, 39:763, 1990.

Chapter 32

AEROBIC, NONFERMENTATIVE GRAM-NEGATIVE BACILLI AND COCCOBACILLI

The aerobic nonfermentative gram-negative bacilli and coccobacilli are a group of non–spore-forming bacteria that degrade carbohydrates via metabolic pathways other than fermentation or do not utilize carbohydrates as a source of energy. In general, these organisms do not have special growth requirements and are easily cultured on media used routinely to isolate bacteria in the clinical microbiology laboratory, features that distinguish them from the "fastidious" gram-negative bacteria discussed in Chapter 33, which usually require special media for isolation. The nomenclature and taxonomic classification of the nonfastidious non–glucose-fermenting gram-negative bacilli and coccobacilli have undergone many changes over the years; Table 32–1 shows the most recent classification of the clinically significant members (1). The genera reviewed in this chapter are Pseudomonas (including Xanthomonas maltophilia), Acinetobacter, and Flavobacterium; Alcaligenes, Moraxella, Kingella, Weeksella, Agrobacterium, Sphingobacterium, and Bordetella bronchiseptica (the nonfastidious member of the genus) are discussed briefly.

Pseudomonas aeruginosa is the nonfermenter most commonly isolated in the clinical microbiology laboratory, accounting for about 75% of all nonfermenters encountered; Acinetobacter baumannii, the second most frequently recovered nonfermenter, accounts for 10 to 20% (2). Xanthomonas maltophilia and species of Pseudomonas other than Pseudomonas aeruginosa, predominantly Pseudomonas cepacia, account for about 5% of the nonfermenters isolated, and species of Flavobacterium and Moraxella each account for 1 to 2%.

PSEUDOMONAS

Members of the genus Pseudomonas are straight or slightly curved, strictly aerobic gram-negative bacilli; most are motile by means of one or more polar flagella (although Pseudomonas mallei is nonmotile); most utilize glucose and other carbohydrates oxidatively (although certain asaccharolytic species are nonoxidizers); and they are cytochrome oxidase positive, although Xanthomonas maltophilia (formerly Pseudomonas maltophilia) is oxidase negative. These organisms are found in soil and water and colonize plants, animals, and occasionally humans. On the basis of RNA/DNA homology studies, the species of Pseudomonas are divided into five RNA homology groups, which include several smaller DNA homology groups (see Table 32–1). The key characteristics of the major groups are listed in Table 32–2. In this section, the species of Pseudomonas of medical importance—Pseudomonas aeruginosa, Pseudomonas cepacia, Pseudomonas mallei, and Pseudomonas pseudomallei—are discussed; Xanthomonas maltophilia also is included because, until recently, it was a member of the genus Pseudomonas.

Pseudomonas aeruginosa

Epidemiology

Pseudomonas aeruginosa is ubiquitous in the environment; it is recovered from soil, water, plants, and animals and has a predilection for moist habitats. The organism has survived in water at about 37° C for 300 days and, in one study was cultured from distilled water (3,4). Moisture is critical to the development of reservoirs of P. aeruginosa, which in the hospital have included respiratory support equipment, cleaning solutions, medicines, disinfectants, sinks, mops, food mixers, and vegetables and outside the hospital swimming pools, whirlpools, hot tubs, and contact lens solutions (5).

Pseudomonas aeruginosa may be part of the normal human microbial flora, especially at moist sites such as the perineum, axillae, and ears, but the frequency of colonization in healthy persons outside of or upon entry to hospitals is low: 0 to 2% on the skin, 0 to 3% on the nasal mucosa, 0 to 7% in the throat, and 3 to 24% in the stool (6). Hospitalization increases the rate of carriage, especially on the skin of patients with serious burns, in the lower respiratory tract of patients supported by mechanical ventilation, in the gastrointestinal tract of patients receiving chemotherapy for malignancies, and at almost any site in persons who take antimicrobial drugs. The risk of disease is considerably greater among colonized patients, especially certain groups of them (Table 32–3), whose common factor is an interruption of the natural barriers that protect against invasion by bacteria (discussed in Chapter 2). Other risk factors include neutropenia; cancer, possibly owing to the selective pressures of extensive antibiotic use in cancer hospitals; hypogammaglobulinemia, complement deficiency, and iatrogenic immunosuppressed states.

Although colonization by Pseudomonas aeruginosa often antedates disease, the original source of the organism and the mechanism of transmission frequently are not known. Uncooked vegetables, hospital sinks, and flowers in patients' rooms are potential reservoirs of the organism and may be the sources of some infections. Nosocomial outbreaks have been traced to respiratory equipment, endoscopes, transvenous pacemakers, antiseptics, orthopedic plaster, operating room suction apparatus, contaminated nursery formula, and physiotherapy pools (5). Transmission of the organism from patient to patient via the hands of hospital personnel or by fomites is possible but rarely proven.

Table 32–1. Nonfastidious, Glucose-nonfermenting Gram-negative Bacilli Encountered in Clinical Bacteriology

Name	Comments	Name	Comments
Family: Alcaligenaceae		Unidentified fluorescent	
Genus: Alcaligenes		Species:	
Species:		Pseudomonas sp.	
A. piechaudii		Stutzeri group	
A. xylosoxidans subsp. xylosoxidans	Previously Achromobacter xylosoxidans	Species:	
		P. stutzeri	
A. xylosoxidans subsp. denitrificans	Previously Alcaligenes denitrificans	CDC group Vb-3	
		P. mendocina	
A. faecalis	Previously Alcaligenes odorans	Alcaligenes group	
"A. faecalis types I, II"		Species:	
Genus: Bordetella		P. alcaligenes	
Species:		Pseudomonas sp. group 1	
B. avium			
B. bronchiseptica		P. pseudoalcaligenes	
Bordetella-like species		RNA Group II	
Family: Cytophagaceae		Pseudomallei group	
Genus: Flavobacterium		Species:	
Species:		P. mallei	
F. breve		P. pseudomallei	
F. gleum	Previously CDC group IIb	P. cepacia	
F. indologenes		P. gladioli	
F. meningosepticum		P. pickettii	
F. odoratum		RNA Group IV	
Flavobacterium sp. group IIe	Previously CDC group IIe	Diminuta group	
		Species:	
Flavobacterium sp. group IIh	Previously CDC group IIh	P. diminuta	
		P. vesicularis	
Flavobacterium sp. group IIi	Previously CDC group IIi	Genus: Shewanella	
		Species:	
Genus: Sphingobacterium		S. putrefaciens	
Species:		Genus: Xanthomonas	
S. multivorum	Previously Flavobacterium multivorum, CDC group IIk-2	RNA Group V	
		Species:	
S. spiritivorum	Previously Flavobacterium spiritivorum, Sphingobacterium versatilis	X. maltophilia	Previously Pseudomonas maltophilia
		Unknown nucleic acid homology	
S. mizutaii	Previously Flavobacterium mizutae	Species:	
		P. paucimobilis	
S. thalpophilum		P. pertucinogena	
S. yabuuchiae		Pseudomonas-like group 2	
Genus: Weeksella			
Species:		Family: Rhizobiaceae	
W. virosa	Previously Flavobacterium genitale, CDC group IIf	Genus: Agrobacterium	
		Species:	
W. zoohelcum	Previously CDC group IIj	Agrobacterium tumefaciens	Previously Agrobacterium radiobacter
Family: Methylococcaceae			
Genus: Methylobacterium		Taxonomic position uncertain	
Species:		Genus: Acinetobacter	
Methylobacterium spp.		Species:	
Family: Pseudomonadaceae		Acinetobacter spp.	Includes Acinetobacter baumannii and Acinetobacter lwoffi; previously Mima polymorpha
Genus: Chryseomonas			
Species:			
C. luteola			
Genus: Comamonas		Genus: Moraxella	
RNA Group III		Species:	
Species:		M. lacunata	
C. acidovorans	Previously Pseudomonas acidovorans	M. nonliquefaciens	
		M. atlantae	
C. terrigena		M. phenylpyruvica	
C. testosteroni	Previously Pseudomonas testosteroni	M. osloensis	
		Genus: Ochrobacterium	
Pseudomonas delafieldii		Species:	
Genus: Flavimonas		Ochrobacterium anthropi	
Species:			
Flavimonas oryzihabitans		Genus: Oligella	
Genus: Pseudomonas		Species:	
RNA Group I		O. urethralis	Previously Moraxella urethralis
Fluorescent group		O. ureolytica	Previously CDC group IVe
Species:		Genus: Psychrobacter	
P. aeruginosa		Species:	
P. fluorescens		P. immobilis	
P. chlororaphis		CDC group IVc-2	
P. putida		CDC group EO-2	

Table 32–2. Key Characteristics of the Major Groups of Pseudomonas

Group	Characteristics
Flourescent	Produce water-soluble pyoverdin pigments that fluoresce under short wavelength (254-nm) ultraviolet light
Stutzeri	Grow anaerobically in media containing nitrate, producing nitrogen gas; are motile via polar monotrichous flagellae; grow with ammonia as sole source of nitrogen and acetate as sole source of carbon for energy
Alcaligenes	Motile via peritrichous flagellae; do not utilize glucose in OF glucose medium; oxidase positive; do not produce pigments
Pseudomallei	Utilize carbohydrates, amino acids, amines polyalcohols, and aromatic compounds as sole sources of carbon and energy; resistant to polymyxin antibiotics
Acidovorans	Motile via polar tuft (up to 6) of flagellae with distinctive morphology; do not produce acid from glucose in OF medium
Diminuta	Motile via single, tightly coiled, monotrichous flagellum; produce acids from primary alcohols but otherwise show minimal biochemical reactivity

In the United States, Pseudomonas aeruginosa is the fourth most frequently isolated nosocomial pathogen, responsible for 10% of all hospital-acquired infections, the leading cause of nosocomial pneumonia (accounting for 17% of all pneumonias), the third most common cause of urinary tract infections, and the fourth most common cause of surgical wound infections and of primary gram-negative bacteremias (7,8).

Pathogenesis

Both host and bacterial factors are involved in the pathogenesis of disease caused by Pseudomonas aeruginosa, an opportunistic pathogen that generally becomes invasive only after the normal host defenses are altered. Cellular and extracellular bacterial factors responsible for adherence to mucosal and epithelial surfaces, evasion of host immune defenses, invasiveness, and toxigenicity are listed

Table 32–3. Conditions That Predispose to Infection with Pseudomonas Aeruginosa

Condition	Most Prevalent Infections
Diabetes mellitus	Malignant otitis externa
Intravenous drug use	Endocarditis, osteomyelitis
Leukemia	Septicemia, typhlitis, perirectal abscess
Malignancy	Pneumonia, septicemia
Burns	Cellulitis, septicemia
Cystic fibrosis	Pneumonia
Surgical procedure involving central nervous system	Meningitis
Tracheostomy	Pneumonia
Neonatal period	Diarrhea
Corneal ulcer	Panophthalmitis
Vascular catheterization	Suppurative thrombophlebitis
Urinary catheterization	Urinary tract infection

(Modified from Bodey GP, Bolivar R, Fainstein V, and Jadeja L: Infections caused by Pseudomonas aeruginosa. Rev Infect Dis, 5:279, 1983.)

in Table 32–4 (5,9–14). Bacterial adherence is aided by the loss of fibronectin in the host. Fibronectin, a protein that normally coats epithelial cells and protects against bacterial attachment, is present in much lower levels during illness in general, and in persons with cystic fibrosis and other chronic lung diseases it apparently is degraded by the high levels of protease in respiratory tract secretions (15). Bacterial proteases that cleave immunoglobulins and inactivate complement probably provide mechanisms by which blood isolates of P. aeruginosa resist the direct bactericidal activity of serum, because the production of antibodies to bacterial cell components and toxins, especially to exotoxin A, correlates with survival (16).

Clinical Manifestations

Infections caused by Pseudomonas aeruginosa affect several organ systems (3,5). A large variety of dermatologic manifestations are possible. The green-nail syndrome, a paronychial infection of persons whose hands are frequently immersed in water, results from the diffusion of pigments produced by the organism into the nail plate. Pyoderma, a purulent skin infection characterized by a bluish green exudate (that when caused by P. aeruginosa has a distinctive grape odor) typically affects persons with eczema, tinea pedis, and bedsores. Cellulitis presents as an area of erythema with a violaceous center and may extend to involve the subcutaneous tissues or muscle. Ecthyma gangrenosum, a unique skin lesion almost always caused by P. aeruginosa (Staphylococcus aureus, Aeromonas hydrophila, Serratia marcescens, Xanthomonas mal-

Table 32–4. Virulence Factors of Pseudomonas Aeruginosa

Factor	Biological Effects
Cellular	
Surface pili	Adherence to epithelial cells
Polysaccharide capsule	Enhance adherence to epithelial cells; protects from host immune defenses (phagocytic cells, antibodies, complement)
Lipid A moiety of endotoxin	Activates clotting, fibrinolytic, kinin, and complement systems; stimulates production of prostaglandins and leukotrienes; promotes release of β-endorphins; induces production and release of tumor necrosis factor, a mediator of endotoxic shock
Extracellular	
Proteases (elastase, alkaline protease)	Destroy basement membrane—associated laminin, disrupt respiratory cilia, cleave human type III and IV collagen, solubilize human lung elastin; alter host defenses via inactivating complement factors and cleaving IgG
Cytotoxin	? Inhibits neutrophil function
Hemolysins (glycolipid and phospholipase C)	Break down lipids and lecithin; degrade lung surfactant (phospholipase C)
Exotoxin A	Inhibits mammalian protein synthesis, causing cell damage
Exoenzyme S	Toxic to mice; cytopathic in vitro for tissue culture cells; target in humans is unknown

tophilia, Aspergillus, and the zygomycetes occasionally have been implicated), begins as a localized area of erythema and edema, usually in the axilla, groin, or perianal region, and rapidly progresses to a bluish bulla that ruptures, producing the typical blue to black area of central necrosis surrounded by an erythematous halo. Histologically, lesions show vasculitis with bacilli in the media and adventitia of the vessel; thrombosis is absent, and often the neutrophil response is minimal. Skin lesions associated with pseudomonas septicemia include clusters of painful vesicles, pink maculopapular plaques or nodules involving the trunk, and painful subcutaneous nodules (17–20). Pseudomonas aeruginosa also is a common cause of burn wounds during the second to third week after thermal injury.

Pseudomonas aeruginosa may cause minor and serious infections in the head and neck. It is a rare cause of blepharoconjunctivitis, an infection that usually accompanies septicemia in immunosuppressed persons who have a malignancy, and orbital cellulitis, a disease principally associated with ethmoid sinusitis in children, but it is the most common gram-negative bacillus infecting corneal ulcers, producing an infection that rapidly progresses to panophthalmitis if not treated appropriately (3). P. aeruginosa causes about 70% of cases of otitis externa, predominantly in swimmers in hot climates, and is the most frequent cause of chronic otitis media (3). The most serious ear infection due to P. aeruginosa is malignant otitis externa, principally a disease of elderly diabetes patients. The infection, characterized by constant pain, edema, and tenderness of the soft tissues of the ear, and purulent drainage, may spread anteriorly, causing necrosis of the facial nerve, or posteriorly, producing osteomyelitis of the base of the skull (21–24).

In the central nervous system, Pseudomonas aeruginosa is responsible for about 5% of cases of bacterial meningitis in neonates and about 10% of cases in persons with cancer (3,25). Recurrent or chronic meningitis caused by P. aeruginosa usually is associated with an alteration of cranial anatomy due to trauma, a surgical procedure, or malignant disease; indwelling catheters, shunts, or reservoirs; prosthetic materials; active or undrained parameningeal infections; and cerebrospinal fluid leaks.

Infections of the cardiovascular system caused by Pseudomonas aeruginosa include endocarditis, predominantly in intravenous drug users, and bacteremia, which most often occurs at the extremes of age (26,30). Signs and symptoms of bacteremia depend on the primary site of infection but generally include fever, tachycardia, and tachypnea, often accompanied by disorientation, hypotension, jaundice, renal failure, and occasionally respiratory failure. Mortality rates, ranging from about 35% to about 75%, exceed those associated with bacteremias caused by all other gram-negative bacilli (3).

In the gastrointestinal tract, Pseudomonas aeruginosa has been responsible for epidemics of diarrhea in newborns, during which the organism was introduced via contaminated equipment (31). "Shanghai fever," a syndrome resembling typhoid fever (see Chapter 34), is a Pseudomonas-induced enteritis characterized by prostration, headache, fever, skin rash, and diarrhea or constipation (32,33). The most important gastrointestinal infection caused by P. aeruginosa (and other gram-negative bacilli) is typhlitis, a necrotizing colitis that frequently is localized to the cecum, most often occurs in children with acute leukemia, and clinically is manifested by the abrupt onset of fever, abdominal distention, and pain. P. aeruginosa also may cause perirectal abscesses, primarily in neutropenic persons with acute leukemia or another malignancy (35).

Lower respiratory tract infections with Pseudomonas aeruginosa predominantly affect persons whose local respiratory or systemic host defense mechanisms are compromised. Primary pneumonia develops in persons with chronic lung disease, congestive heart failure, or both who become colonized with P. aeruginosa in the upper respiratory tract and then aspirate oral secretions; alternatively, organisms may be introduced directly via contaminated respiratory inhalation equipment. This fulminant, often fatal infection is characterized by diffuse bronchopneumonia with microabscess formation and focal hemorrhage. Bacteremic pneumonia caused by P. aeruginosa, which occurs principally in neutropenic persons after cancer chemotherapy, is a fulminant disease, typically fatal 3 to 4 days after the first signs or symptoms of pulmonary or extrapulmonary infection. Bacteria are introduced by the respiratory route, produce disease in the lungs, and invade the blood, occasionally spreading to other viscera. Two types of pulmonary lesions are seen. Poorly defined hemorrhagic nodules, sometimes with an area of central necrosis, characterized histologically by alveolar hemorrhage and necrosis without inflammation, develop around small and medium-sized pulmonary arteries, often just beneath the pleura. Firm, yellow-tan, necrotic, 2- to 15-mm diameter umbilicated nodules with a narrow rim of hemorrhage microscopically show abscesses, coagulative necrosis, and necrotic small arteries and veins with bacteria in their walls (Plate IVD).

Colonization of the lower respiratory tract with mucoid strains of Pseudomonas aeruginosa in association with cystic fibrosis appears to be a function of age: most patients over age 18 years are so affected, but few children younger than 5 years. This colonization is associated with acute exacerbations and chronic progression of the disease, manifest clinically by chronic productive cough and low-grade fever, and it appears to correlate with the pathologic changes in the bronchial airways. Airway obstruction, beginning as bronchiolitis with mucus plugging, is followed by infections, which produce more mucus plugging and lead to chronic suppuration and, eventually, bronchiectasis, atelectasis, and fibrosis.

Urinary tract infections caused by Pseudomonas aeruginosa usually are acquired during hospitalization after manipulation of the genitourinary tract, insertion of a catheter, or antimicrobial therapy. P. aeruginosa infections of bone and joints result from hematogenous spread, most often in intravenous drug users or in association with infections of the urinary tract or pelvis; or from extension of contiguous foci, usually related to penetrating trauma, a surgical procedure, or adjacent soft tissue infections. Children, elders, chronically debilitated persons, and those with underlying diseases or other predisposing factors are affected most frequently.

Pseudomonas cepacia

Epidemiology

Pseudomonas cepacia is ubiquitous in the environment, associated with soil, water, and plants, and like Pseudomonas aeruginosa, it has a predilection for moist environments and can proliferate in tap- and distilled water. Outbreaks of pulmonary colonization and infection with Pseudomonas cepacia have been associated with contaminated topical anesthetics and solutions used in bronchoscopy, aerosolized antibiotics, and contaminated nebulizers (36–39). Data from several centers indicate that in persons with cystic fibrosis rates of colonization of the respiratory tract with P. cepacia have increased (40). Although the exact mechanism of initial colonization in cystic fibrosis patients is unknown exposure to the organism probably occurs in the community, and colonization may be favored by the selective pressure of the prolonged antibiotic therapy required to suppress their pulmonary tract infections. Moreover, evidence suggests that many persons with cystic fibrosis acquire P. cepacia either in the hospital or from colonized siblings (41,42).

Pathogenesis

Pseudomonas cepacia is virtually nonpathogenic in normal, healthy persons but can cause serious disease in those whose host defenses are impaired. However, the exact mechanism by which P. cepacia produces disease in humans is unknown. In animal models of infection this pathogen is much less virulent than Pseudomonas aeruginosa (41). In vitro, 50 to 80% of strains of P. cepacia have protease (or gelatinase) activity, which may allow the organism to enter the blood; most strains produce lipase; but neither exotoxin A nor exotoxin S–like activity has been detected (41). Some strains synthesize phenazine pigments similar to those produced by P. aeruginosa, which may inhibit lymphocyte proliferation (43).

Clinical Manifestations

In persons whose host defenses are altered or who have indwelling catheters or other medical devices, Pseudomonas cepacia has caused endocarditis (especially in intravenous drug users), bacteremia, postoperative and burn wound infections, peritonitis, osteomyelitis and septic arthritis, and lung abscesses and pneumonia (36,41,44–49). Data from one study indicates that persons with cystic fibrosis who are infected with P. cepacia have significantly poorer overall pulmonary function than those infected with Pseudomonas aeruginosa alone, often are hospitalized longer, and die sooner (40).

Pseudomonas mallei

Epidemiology

Pseudomonas mallei is the pathogen of glanders, a disease that principally affects horses, mules, and donkeys, and occasionally goats, sheep, cats, and dogs. Infection with P. mallei in horses may produce a systemic illness with prominent pulmonary involvement (glanders) or subcutaneous ulcerative lesions that spread along the lymphatics (farcy). In animals, the infection may be transmitted via inhalation, ingestion, or breaks in the skin, but the exact mechanism is unknown. Human disease occurs predominantly in persons who have close contact with horses, mules, or donkeys, probably via inoculation through broken skin or the nasal mucosa with contaminated discharges. Several infections have been reported in laboratory personnel; presumably these were acquired via inhalation of infectious aerosols (50).

Thanks to improved sanitation, the prevalence of glanders has decreased in most countries. No naturally acquired infections have been reported in the United States since 1938, but sporadic cases still occur in Asia, Africa, and other parts of the Americas. Almost 60% of affected persons are between 20 and 40 years of age, and nearly all are males (51).

Clinical Manifestations

Human disease may be categorized as acute localized suppurative, acute septicemic, acute pulmonary, or chronic suppurative infection, although groups overlap. Acute localized suppurative infection, acquired via inoculation of a break in the skin or mucous membranes, presents after an incubation period of 1 to 5 days as a nodule with associated acute lymphangitis. The septicemic form, acquired via inhalation, manifests after an incubation period of 10 to 14 days as fever, rigors, myalgias, fatigue, headache, and pleuritic chest pain, and usually it is fatal within 7 to 10 days. Acute pulmonary disease is characterized by lobar or bronchopneumonia with abscess formation. Persons with the chronic suppurative form develop multiple subcutaneous and intramuscular abscesses, most often on the arms and legs, accompanied by involvement of the lymphatics in about half the cases, the skin in about a third, and viscera in no more than a quarter.

Pseudomonas pseudomallei

Epidemiology

Pseudomonas pseudomallei is the agent of melioidosis, a glanders-like infectious disease of humans and animals first described in 1912 (52). The organism is an environmental saprophyte found in soil, stagnant streams, ponds, rice paddies, and market produce in endemic areas of Southeast Asia, especially Vietnam, Cambodia, Laos, Thailand, Malaysia, and Burma. Indigenously acquired human disease also has been reported from China, Hong Kong, India, Borneo, the Philippines, Guam, Indonesia, Ceylon, New Guinea, and North Queensland; and cases in animals or humans have been reported from Madagascar, Kenya, central West Africa, Iran, and Turkey (51). Human disease is rare in the Western hemisphere but has been reported from Mexico, Panama, Ecuador, Haiti, Brazil, Peru, Guyana, Hawaii, Georgia, and possibly Oklahoma (53–56).

Pseudomonas pseudomallei has caused epizootics among sheep, goats, swine, horses, and seals, and it occasionally infects cows, rodents, and cats; but animals apparently are not a reservoir for human disease. Humans probably become infected by soil contamination of skin abrasions; or possibly by ingestion or inhalation; one case of human-to-human transmission was reported (57). Disease can recur months or years after apparent cure or develop after several years of latency, an event often related to intercurrent illness, injury, or stress (51).

Clinically evident human melioidosis is rare; however, serologic surveys indicate that mild or inapparent infection is not uncommon. For example, 6 to 20% of the indigenous population of Vietnam, Thailand, Malaysia, and Northern Australia, 2% of Europeans living in Vietnam, 1 to 2% of healthy or nonwounded United States Army troop personnel returning to the United States after spending 6 to 12 months in Vietnam, and approximately 225,000 of the 2.5 million United States citizens at risk while serving in Vietnam are seropositive (58–62).

Clinical Manifestations

Illness may be manifested after an as yet undefined incubation period, as an acute, subacute, or chronic process; and subclinical infections may remain latent for years before disease becomes apparent. Infection by inoculation of a break in the skin generally results in a nodule accompanied by acute lymphangitis, regional lymphadenopathy, fever, and malaise. This may progress to an acute septicemic illness, often accompanied by arthritis, meningitis, and cutaneous pustules on the head, trunk, and extremities. Despite appropriate therapy, the mortality rate for septicemic melioidosis is 50% or more.

The most common form of melioidosis is acute pulmonary disease, which varies from mild bronchitis with pharyngitis to overwhelming necrotizing pneumonia with consolidation and cavitation (63). In the chronic suppurative form of disease, abscesses develop in the skin, brain, lung, myocardium, liver, spleen, bones, joints, lymph nodes, or eyes.

Xanthomonas maltophilia

Epidemiology

Xanthomonas maltophilia has been recovered from many environmental, animal, and human sources, including water, soil, sewage, hospital disinfectant solutions, raw milk, frozen fish, and rabbit and human feces (64). The organism is primarily a nosocomial pathogen, predominantly infecting patients treated with antimicrobial agents; community-acquired infections are rare. In recent years the number of isolates of X. maltophilia—and the number of clinically significant infections with the organism—have increased, a trend probably related to the increasing number of debilitated patients and the selective pressure of broad-spectrum antimicrobial agents (64,65).

Pathogenesis

Little is known about the pathogenic and virulence factors of Xanthomonas maltophilia. Like Pseudomonas aeruginosa, Xanthomonas maltophilia is an opportunistic pathogen; but unlike Pseudomonas aeruginosa, most strains of Xanthomas maltophilia do not produce extracellular proteases and hemolysins that promote tissue invasion and necrosis. However, production of proteases and elastase has been demonstrated by one strain of X. maltophilia associated with bacteremia and ecthyma gangrenosum (66).

Clinical Manifestations

Xanthomonas maltophilia has been recovered from many clinical specimens, including blood, respiratory tract secretions, urine, wounds, skin lesions, cerebrospinal fluid, pericardial fluid, and pus; but in many cases these isolates are part of a mixed culture and very likely are not clinically significant. The frequency of recovery of X. maltophilia from respiratory tract secretions of persons with cystic fibrosis appears to be increasing, but its role in disease progression is unclear (67,68). Infections specifically attributed to X. maltophilia include endocarditis involving prosthetic valves and native valves of intravenous drug users, meningitis, primary bacteremia, ecthyma gangrenosum, traumatic and postoperative wound infections, mastoiditis, epididymitis, cellulitis, abscesses, intravascular line–associated bacteremia, and purulent conjunctivitis (64,69). Major hospital epidemics of infections caused by X. maltophilia have been traced to contaminated calibration devices and transducers used in arterial and central venous monitoring lines, and to contaminated hospital disinfectants (70,71).

ACINETOBACTER

Acinetobacter probably was first isolated and described in 1908 as Diplococcus mucosus, and since then has undergone several changes in taxonomic classification (72). Based on biochemical and genetic data Acinetobacter is classified in the family Neisseriaceae (Chapter 31). Isolates most frequently encountered in the laboratory are Acinetobacter baumannii (formerly Acinetobacter calcoaceticus var anitratus) and Acinetobacter lwoffi (formerly Acinetobacter calcoaceticus var lwoffi), which are differentiated based on acid production from dextrose: Acinetobacter baumannii is dextrose positive; Acinetobacter lwoffi, negative.

Epidemiology

Species of Acinetobacter are free living, found in almost all soil and water samples, and have been isolated from pasteurized milk, frozen foods, chilled poultry, foundry and hospital air, vaporized mist, tap water faucets, peritoneal dialysate baths, bedside urinals, washcloths, angiography catheters, ventilators, plasma protein fractions, and sink basins (72). These organisms colonize the skin of as many as 25% of healthy ambulatory adults and transiently colonize the pharynx of about 7%. They are the most common gram-negative bacteria persistently carried on the skin of hospital personnel, and in one study they colonized about 45% of in-patient tracheostomy sites (73–76). Acinetobacter lwoffi has a predilection for the genitourinary tract, and Acinetobacter baumannii is recovered more frequently from all other sites (77). In the 1984 report of the National Nosocomial Infection Study, Acinetobacer was identified as a pathogen in 0.6% of all hospital-acquired infections in the United States reported to the Centers for Disease Control (78). The incidence of infections caused by Acinetobacter peaks in the summer, and about 40% occur in children younger than 10 years (78,79).

Pathogenesis

Acinetobacter is an opportunistic pathogen: it causes disease only after normal host defenses are disrupted. No virulence factors except the cell wall lipopolysaccharide have been identified. The capsule may inhibit phagocytosis and assist in adherence to epithelial and mucosal surfaces, but this has not been evaluated. Moreover, its production of bacteriocins—factors that inhibit the growth of other bacteria—may afford a selective advantage.

Clinical Manifestations

Acinetobacter baumannii has caused suppurative infections of almost every organ system, predominantly in persons with altered host defenses, but occasionally in otherwise healthy ones. Specific infections include cystitis and pyelonephritis, principally in persons who have an indwelling bladder catheter or nephrolithiasis, meningitis and intracranial abscesses (generally associated with recent neurosurgical procedures), community-acquired or nosocomial pulmonary infections (in healthy children or adults with altered host defenses or underlying pulmonary disease), cellulitis associated with intravascular catheters, wound infections, bacteremia, ocular infections, endocarditis, osteomyelitis, septic arthritis, or pancreatic or liver abscesses (72).

FLAVOBACTERIUM

Epidemiology and Pathogenesis

Species of Flavobacterium are widely distributed in nature—in fresh and marine waters, soil and ocean sediments, and foods such as raw meats and poultry, vegetables, and dairy products—and they have been recovered from hospital environments including nebulizers, incubators, water baths, drinking fountains, sink faucets, distilled water lines, saline solutions, and hemodialysis systems (80). Although not part of the normal human flora these organisms may colonize wounds and the upper respiratory, gastrointestinal, or urogenital tract. Species of Flavobacterium produce proteases and gelatinase, which may enhance their virulence.

Clinical Manifestations

Flavobacterium meningosepticum is a cause of meningitis, primarily in neonates but also in adults who have an underlying disease that predisposes them to infection. Although neonatal meningitis due to F. meningosepticum is very uncommon, its recognition is important because epidemics may occur in nurseries and the mortality rate may be as high as 55% (2). F. meningosepticum also may cause septicemia, endocarditis, and pneumonia, predominantly in debilitated or immunosuppressed hospital patients, and cases of meningitis and septicemia have been attributed to Flavobacterium glenum (formerly CDC group IIb) (80).

OTHER NONFERMENTERS

Species of Alcaligenes are opportunistic pathogens which cause disease principally in immunocompromised hosts. Because these organisms have a predilection for moist environments and are resistant to many disinfectants and antimicrobial agents they frequently colonize aqueous fluids in the hospital environment such as those in nebulizers and respirators, and lavage fluids. In particular, Alcaligenes xylosoxidans (formerly Achromobacter xylosoxidans) has been associated with colonization and disease linked to dialysis fluids, nonbacteriostatic saline, contaminated mouthwash solutions, incubator condensates, and certain disinfectants (quaternary ammonium compounds and alcohol solutions) (81). Infections caused by Alcaligenes xylosoxidans include bacteremia, meningitis, peritonitis, wound infections, pneumonia, infections of the ear, eye, and urinary or biliary tract, and nosocomial infections involving aortic grafts and prosthetic heart valves. Alcaligenes faecalis is most often recovered from blood, sputum, or urine.

Species of Moraxella reside in the upper respiratory tract and on the skin of humans and animals; Oligella urethralis (formerly Moraxella urethralis) is part of the normal flora of the human genitourinary tract. These organisms generally are considered nonpathogens, contaminants, or organisms with low pathogenic potential, but they may cause serious disease in humans, including pericarditis, lung abscesses, osteomyelitis, ocular infections, pyoderma, urogenital tract disease, sinusitis, endocarditis, meningitis, and septicemia (82). The three species of Kingella—Kingella kingae, Kingella indologenes, Kingella denitrificans—are normal flora in the human oropharynx. Of the three, Kingella kingae is the most common human pathogen, causing septic arthritis, bacteremia, and skin lesions, particularly in children; Kingella indologenes is a rare cause of ocular infections, and the pathogenicity of Kingella denitrificans is unknown (2,82).

Weeksella zoohelcum (formerly CDC group IIj) has been recovered from human wounds, especially dog bites (83). Agrobacterium tumefaciens (formerly Agrobacterium radiobacter) has been isolated from sputum, blood, and wounds (2). Sphingobacterium multivorum (formerly Flavobacterium multivorum) is a rare human pathogen but has caused peritonitis in a person with alcoholic liver disease and septicemia in a patient undergoing hemodialysis (80). Bordetella bronchiseptica, predominantly an animal pathogen, rarely causes symptomatic infections of the upper or lower respiratory tract of humans, principally animal caretakers, and one case of fatal septicemia and bronchopneumonia, in a malnourished alcoholic, has been reported (2,84).

Laboratory Diagnosis

Specimens required to diagnose infections caused by the aerobic, nonfastidious, non–glucose-fermenting gram-negative bacilli and coccobacilli are shown in Table 32–5. Specimen collection, transport, and processing are discussed in Part III. Identifying features of the organisms reviewed earlier in this chapter are described below.

General Characteristics

Features of an isolate of a gram-negative bacillus suggestive of a nonfermenter are a positive cytochrome oxidase

Table 32–5. Diseases Caused by the Aerobic, Nonfermenting Gram-negative Bacilli and Specimens for Diagnosis

Disease or Lesion	Organisms	Specimens
Cutaneous lesions, abscesses	P. aeruginosa X. maltophilia P. mallei P. pseudomallei Acinetobacter	Aspirate (or swab) of pus or fluid, tissue biopsy
Burn wounds	P. aeruginosa	Aspirate (or swab) of pus or fluid, tissue biopsy
Eye infections		
Corneal ulcers	P. aeruginosa	Corneal scrapings
Conjunctivitis	Moraxella	Conjunctival scrapings (or swab)
Ear infections		
Otitis externa	P. aeruginosa	Not necessary*
Malignant otitis externa	P. aeruginosa	Scrapings of external auditory canal; soft tissue or bone
Meningitis	P. aeruginosa F. meningosepticum Acinetobacter Alcaligenes X. maltophilia	Cerebrospinal fluid
Bacteremia/septicemia	P. aeruginosa Acinetobacter X. maltophilia P. mallei P. pseudomallei Moraxella Alcaligenes Flavobacterium	Blood
Endocarditis	P. aeruginosa X. maltophilia	Blood, valve tissue, prosthetic valve
Gastrointestinal infections		
Enteritis	P. aeruginosa	Feces, biopsy of involved mucosa
Rectal abscess	P. aeruginosa	Aspirate (or swab) of pus or fluid
Pneumonia	P. aeruginosa P. cepacia P. mallei P. pseudomallei Acinetobacter Alcaligenes	Sputum or tracheal aspirate, transtracheal aspirate, bronchoalveolar aspirate fluid, blood, pleural fluid (if present), lung tissue
Urinary tract infections	P. aeruginosa Acinetobacter Oligella	Urine
Osteomyelitis/arthritis	P. aeruginosa	Bone tissue/joint fluid

* Diagnosis usually is made by physical examination alone.

reaction, lack of evidence for glucose fermentation (see Chapter 34), and for some organisms, failure to grow on MacConkey agar. The nonfermenters produce much weaker acids than the mixed acids derived from fermentative bacteria; and in media containing large amounts of peptones and other protein sources nonfermenters utilize peptones preferentially, producing alkaline end products that overshadow pH indicator changes that might result from acid production. Therefore, a low-peptone medium called oxidative-fermentative (OF) medium, designed by Hugh and Leifson to accommodate the metabolic properties of the nonfermentative bacilli, should be used in the laboratory to determine the ability of these organisms to utilize carbohydrates as follows (Fig. 32–1): Two tubes of each carbohydrate medium are inoculated by picking material from isolated colonies and stabbing each medium about 5 mm deep at least four times. The medium in one of the two tubes is overlayed with sterile melted petrolatum or vaspar (melted paraffin combined with an equal volume of petroleum jelly) about 1 mm deep. Sterile mineral oil is not recommended as an overlay because some lots are acidic and, so, may cause false-positive results. Tubes are incubated up to 4 days at 35° C in ambient air and examined daily for acid production, indicated by a change in the color of the medium from green to yellow. Fermentative organisms produce acid in both the overlaid and open tubes; oxidative organisms produce acid only in the open tube, and asaccharolytic organisms that do not utilize carbohydrates produce no color change in either tube.

The aerobic, glucose-nonfermentative bacilli and coccobacilli are identified by a series of biochemical reactions, performed using oxidative-fermentative media and other conventional tube media (see Chapter 34), commercially available kit systems, or a combination of both (85). Key characteristics of the nonfermenters discussed in this chapter are described in the following section; a more complete list of their expected biochemical reactions and those of infrequently encountered nonfermenters may be found elsewhere (2,83,86–88).

Organism Identification

Pseudomonas aeruginosa. P. aeruginosa grows on most media used routinely in the clinical laboratory and produces a characteristic grapelike odor. On 5% sheep blood agar colonies are flat, 1 to 2 mm in diameter after 24 hours' incubation, often have a rough- or ground-glass appearance, and are surrounded by a zone of complete hemolysis (Plate IVE). Some isolates, especially those from persons with cystic fibrosis, have thick capsules (Plate IVF) and produce very mucoid colonies. Most strains of P. aeruginosa produce pyocyanin, a water-soluble green phenazine pigment that imparts a green color to uncolored culture media such as Mueller-Hinton agar. Because this pigment is not synthesized by any other nonfermenter, its presence identifies an isolate as P. aeruginosa. Some isolates of P. aeruginosa produce other pigments—pyoverdins (yellow), pyorubin (red), and pyomelanin (brown)—that may mask the pyocyanin. P. aeruginosa and other species of Pseudomonas isolated from humans (Pseudomonas fluorescens and Pseudomonas putida) often produce water-soluble fluorescent pigments, visualized by observing fluorescence of growth on certain commercially available media (King's medium B, Sellers' medium, Pseudomonas F agar, Flo agar, GNF agar, Mueller-Hinton agar) under short-wave ultraviolet light; a standard Wood's lamp, emitting light at 365 nm, may be used, but the fluorescence of pseudomonads is best observed with 254 nm light.

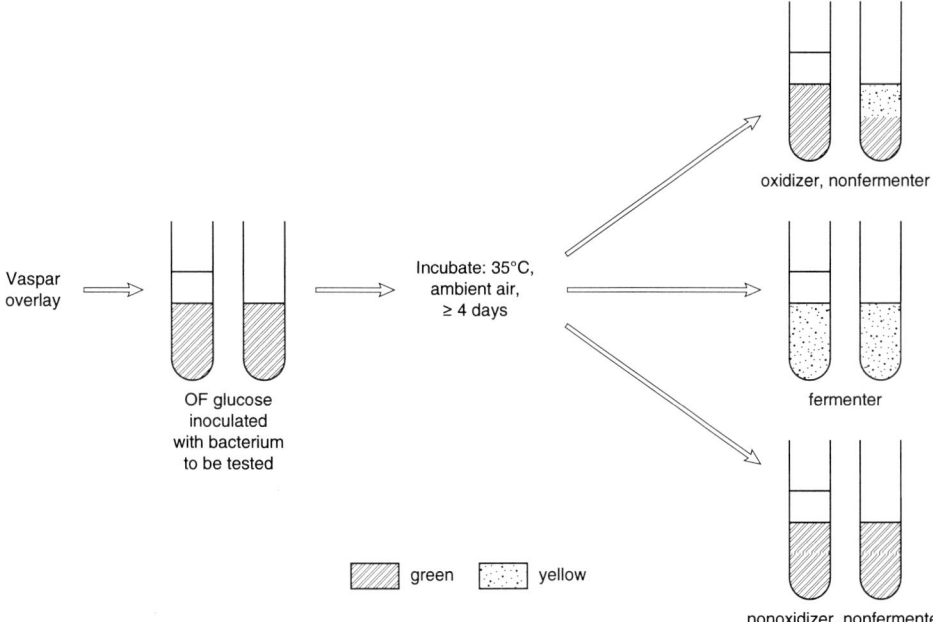

Fig. 32–1. Reactions of a glucose oxidizer, a glucose fermenter, and an organism that neither ferments nor oxidizes glucose in OF medium.

All isolates of Pseudomonas aeruginosa grow at 42° C, are oxidase positive, motile via a polar monotrichous flagellum, able to oxidize glucose but not maltose in oxidative-fermentative medium, able to dihydrolyze arginine, and unable to decarboxylate lysine or ornithine. Practically, isolates on sheep blood agar that exhibit the characteristic colony morphology (previously described), have the typical grapelike odor, grow at 42° C, and are oxidase positive presumptively may be called P. aeruginosa.

Pseudomonas cepacia. Recovery of P. cepacia from respiratory tract specimens may require a selective medium (several are available commercially). On sheep blood agar colonies are convex, opaque, glistening, and butyrous. Some strains produce a sweet odor similar to that associated with Pseudomonas aeruginosa, and some produce a sulfur-yellow or green, water-soluble, chloroform-soluble, nonfluorescent phenazine pigment. Optimal growth occurs at 30° C, and some strains grow poorly at 35° C. Pseudomonas cepacia is motile via a tuft of three to eight polar flagella; oxidizes glucose, lactose, maltose, and mannitol; and is resistant to polymyxin B.

Pseudomonas mallei. P. mallei, the only nonmotile species of Pseudomonas, grows slowly, forming white to cream-colored colonies. It does not produce nitrogen gas, hydrolyze gelatin, or grow at 42° C.

Pseudomonas pseudomallei. P. pseudomallei grows slowly on sheep blood agar, forming mucoid and smooth to rough and wrinkled colonies that are bright orange to cream in color. Growth is characterized by an odor of putrefaction followed by an aromatic, pungent smell. Organisms are motile via a polar tuft of three or more flagella, grow at 42° C, hydrolyze gelatin, dihydrolyze arginine, and oxidize glucose, lactose, and maltose.

Xanthomonas maltophilia. On sheep blood agar, colonies of X. maltophilia are rough, develop a lavender-green color, may cause slight greenish discoloration of the agar, and have an ammonia-like odor. The organism is motile via a polar tuft of three or more flagella, is oxidase negative, oxidizes maltose and glucose, and yields positive reactions for lysine decarboxylase, esculin, DNase, and gelatin.

Acinetobacter species. Cells of Acinetobacter appear as gram-negative cocci or coccobacilli in smears of primary specimens stained with the Gram stain but often appear more rodlike in smears prepared from broth or agar cultures. These organisms grow well on MacConkey agar, on which colonies occasionally have a bluish tint. On sheep blood agar, colonies are convex, gray to white, 2 to 3 mm in diameter after 48 hours, and may be surrounded by a zone of complete hemolysis. Acinetobacter is oxidase negative, immotile, and lysine decarboxylase negative. Acinetobacter baumanii oxidizes glucose and 10% lactose, whereas Acinetobacter lwoffi is biochemically inactive.

Flavobacterium meningosepticum. On sheep blood agar after incubation for 24 to 48 hours F. meningosepticum forms 0.5- to 1.5-mm diameter colonies with a yellow pigment that often is augmented by incubation at room temperature for an additional 24 hours. Most strains grow slowly on MacConkey agar. The organism is nonmotile, gives positive reactions for oxidase, DNase, and indole (when tested with the Ehrlich reagent described in Chapter 34), is resistant to polymyxin, and produces acid oxidatively from glucose, fructose, maltose, and mannitol.

Alcaligenes species. On sheep blood agar colonies of Alcaligenes are small (0.5 to 1.5 mm in diameter), translucent, smooth, and colorless after 24 hours. Some isolates of Alcaligenes faecalis cause green discoloration of the surrounding medium and have a sweet, fruity odor described as resembling strawberries or pared apples. All species grow well on MacConkey agar, use citrate as the sole carbon source, are oxidase positive, and motile via peritrichous flagella. A. faecalis is nonsaccharolytic; Alcaligenes xylosoxidans oxidizes xylose and glucose.

Moraxella and Oligella species. On sheep blood agar colonies of Moraxella and Oligella are smaller than 0.5 mm diameter after 24 hours, and on MacConkey agar growth is poor. In smears stained with the Gram stain, bacterial cells appear as cocci or small bacilli in pairs, occasionally resembling Neisseria (see Chapter 31). To distinguish the two genera, a smear of growth from the outer zone of inhibition around a penicillin susceptibility disk is stained with the Gram stain and examined: species of Moraxella are elongate and pleomorphic cells, whereas cells of Neisseria retain their coccal form. Moraxella and Oligella are oxidase positive, catalase positive, asaccharolytic, and immotile, and most isolates are sensitive to low concentrations of penicillin.

Kingella species. On sheep blood agar, colonies of Kingella kingae typically are small, surrounded by a zone of complete hemolysis, but occasionally colonies pit the agar, assuming a "fried egg" appearance with a thin spreading haze of growth around the central colony. Growth appears to be enhanced by increased carbon dioxide and initially may not become apparent for several days. In smears stained with the Gram stain, cells appear as short, plump bacilli with squared ends, occasionally forming chains. All species are oxidase positive and immotile, most are catalase negative, and about a third of isolates grow on MacConkey agar. These organisms do not grow well in triple sugar iron agar, and supplementation of oxidative-fermentative carbohydrate media with 5% horse serum may be necessary to allow sufficient growth. Because a unique feature of Kingella denitrificans is its ability to grow on Thayer-Martin medium it may be confused with Neisseria gonorrhoeae (see Chapter 31): both are oxidase positive and produce acid from glucose. The nitrate reduction test should distinguish the two organisms: Kingella denitrificans reduces nitrate and Neisseria gonorrhoeae does not.

Treatment

Antimicrobial agents selected to treat infections caused by the nonfermenters are based on results of susceptibility testing. Invasive infections with Pseudomonas aeruginosa generally are treated with two agents: an aminoglycoside plus an extended-spectrum penicillin (mezlocillin or piperacillin), an antipseudomonal cephalosporin such as ceftazidime, or aztreonam, ciprofloxacin, or imipenem. Therapy with the latter four agents has been associated with the emergence of resistant strains of P. aeruginosa.

Antimicrobial therapy for infections with Pseudomonas cepacia is a challenge because this organism is resistant to many agents, including the aminoglycosides, ticarcillin (an antipseudomonal penicillin), and trimethoprim-sulfamethoxazole. Potentially effective antimicrobials include ceftazidime, imipenem, aztreonam, and ciprofloxacin.

Sulfadiazine is effective treatment for infections with Pseudomonas mallei. Recommended therapy for infections caused by Pseudomonas pseudomallei includes trimethoprim-sulfamethoxazole (imipenem may be considered for strains resistant to trimethoprim-sulfamethoxazole) plus a third-generation cephalosporin such as ceftazidime for septicemic infections, and single-agent therapy with tetracycline, chloramphenicol, sulfisoxazole, or trimethoprim-sulfamethoxazole for less serious forms of disease.

Like Pseudomonas cepacia, Xanthomonas maltophilia is resistant to multiple antimicrobial agents, including aminoglycosides and β-lactams (penicillins, cephalosporins, imipenem). Trimethoprim-sulfamethoxazole is recommended as initial empiric therapy. Alternative or additional agents such as chloramphenicol, doxycycline, ceftazidime, or ciprofloxacin might be considered, based on the results of susceptibility testing.

Species of Acinetobacter are resistant to many antimicrobials, but Acinetobacter lwoffi usually is more sensitive than Acinetobacter baumannii. Almost all isolates are resistant to penicillin, ampicillin, and the first-generation cephalosporins; susceptibility to second- and third-generation cephalosporins and trimethoprim-sulfamethoxazole varies. Aminoglycosides, imipenem, and ciprofloxacin usually are effective, and the synergistic combination of an aminoglycoside and ticarcillin or piperacillin may be useful for serious infections.

Species of Flavobacterium usually are susceptible to trimethoprim-sulfamethoxazole, rifampin, third-generation cephalosporins, and clindamycin but resistant to aminoglycosides, penicillins, and chloramphenicol. Alcaligenes is uniformly resistant to the penicillins, and most species are resistant to the aminoglycosides. The third-generation cephalosporins, trimethoprim-sulfamethoxazole, and the quinolones show the most activity in vitro against these organisms. Species of Moraxella are susceptible in vitro to penicillin, ampicillin, chloramphenicol, and the aminoglycosides. Penicillin is the antimicrobial agent of choice for treating infections caused by Kingella kingae, and gentamicin and chloramphenicol have been used successfully to treat septic arthritis.

Prevention

Most of the bacteria discussed in this chapter are opportunistic pathogens, except Pseudomonas mallei and Pseudomonas pseudomallei. Because the infections they cause are acquired from the hospital environment, preventing infections requires an appreciation of the hospital sources of these organisms and what environments are likely to be colonized. Proper attention to hand-washing techniques may minimize patient-to-patient spread of these organisms via hospital personnel. Sterility of aqueous fluids used to irrigate wounds should be ensured. In procedures involving the implantation of artificial materials, sodium hypochlorite or povidone-iodine disinfectant should be used rather than alcohol or quaternary ammonium compounds, in which organisms such as Alcaligenes xylosoxidans and Pseudomonas cepacia can grow.

Prevention of human infections with Pseudomonas mallei requires avoiding contact with diseased horses; infected humans should be placed in isolation. To prevent infection due to Pseudomonas pseudomallei, vigorous cleansing of abrasions and lacerations sustained in endemic areas (discussed earlier) is recommended (89).

REFERENCES

1. Gilardi GL: Update on taxonomy of nonfastidious, glucose-nonfermenting gram-negative bacill. Clin Microbiol Newslett, *12*:73, 1990.

2. Koneman EW, et al: The nonfermentative gram-negative bacilli. *In* Color Atlas and Textbook of Diagnostic Microbiology. 3rd ed. Philadelphia, JB Lippincott, 1988.
3. Bodey GP, Bolivar R, Fainstein V, and Jadeja L: Infections caused by Pseudomonas aeruginosa. Rev Infect Dis, 5:279, 1983.
4. Favero MS, Carson LA, Bond WW, and Petersen NJ: Pseudomonas aeruginosa: Growth in distilled water from hospitals. Science, 173:836, 1971.
5. Pollack M: Pseudomonas aeruginosa. *In* Principles and Practice of Infectious Diseases. 3rd ed. Edited by GL Mandell, RG Douglas, Jr, and JE Bennett. New York, Churchill Livingstone, 1990.
6. Morrison AJ and Wenzel RP: Epidemiology of infections due to Pseudomonas aeruginosa. Rev Infect Dis, 6(suppl):627, 1984.
7. Centers for Disease Control: Nosocomial infection surveillance, 1980–1982. *In* CDC Surveillance Summaries, 32(No. 4SS):15S, 1983.
8. Craven DE, Steger KA, and Barber TW: Preventing nosocomial pneumonia: state of the art and perspectives for the 1990s. Am J Med, 91(S3B):44S, 1991.
9. Ramphal R, McNiece MT, and Polack FM: Adherence of Pseudomonas aeruginosa to the injured cornea: A step in the pathogenesis of corneal infections. Ann Ophthalmol, 13:421, 1981.
10. Baltimore RS, and Mitchell M: Immunologic investigations of mucoid strains of Pseudomonas aeruginosa: Comparison of susceptibility to opsonic antibody in mucoid and nonmucoid strains. J Infect Dis, 141:238, 1980.
11. Hingley ST, et al: Disruption of respiratory cilia by proteases including those of Pseudomonas aeruginosa. Infect Immun, 54:379, 1986.
12. Heck LW, et al: Specific cleavage of human type III and IV collagens by Pseudomonas aeruginosa elastase. Infect Immun, 51:115, 1986.
13. Bishop MB, et al: The effect of Pseudomonas aeruginosa cytotoxin and toxin A on human polymorphonuclear leukocytes. J Med Microbiol, 24:315, 1987.
14. Pollack M: The virulence of Pseudomonas aeruginosa. Rev Infect Dis, 6(suppl):617, 1984.
15. Woods DE, et al: Role of salivary protease activity in adherence of gram-negative bacilli to mammalian buccal epithelial cells in vivo. J Clin Invest, 68:1435, 1981.
16. Pollack M, and Young LS: Protective activity of antibodies to exotoxin A and lipopolysaccharide at the onset of Pseudomonas aeruginosa septicemia in man. J Clin Invest, 63:276, 1979.
17. Schlossberg D: Multiple erythematous nodules as a manifestation of Pseudomonas aeruginosa septicemia. Arch Dermatol, 116:446, 1980.
18. Bagel J, and Grossman ME: Subcutaneous nodules in Pseudomonas sepsis. Am J Med, 80:528, 1986.
19. Fleming MG, Milburn PB, and Prose NS: Pseudomonas septicemia with nodules and bullae. Pediatr Dermatol, 4:18, 1987.
20. Hall JH, et al: Pseudomonas aeruginosa in dermatology. Arch Dermatol, 97:312, 1968.
21. Chandler JR: Malignant external otitis. Laryngoscope, 78:1257, 1968.
22. Zaky DA, et al: Malignant external otitis: A severe form of otitis in diabetic patients. Am J Med, 61:298, 1976.
23. Doroghazi RM, et al: Invasive external otitis. Report of 21 cases and review of the literature. Am J Med, 71:603, 1981.
24. Rubin J, and Yu VL: Malignant external otitis: insights into pathogenesis, clinical manifestations, diagnosis, and therapy. Am J Med, 85:391, 1988.
25. Chernik NL, Armstrong D, and Posner JB: Central nervous system infections in patients with cancer. Medicine, 52:563, 1973.
26. Cohen PS, Maguire JH, and Weinstein L: Infective endocarditis caused by gram-negative bacteria: A review of the literature, 1945–1977. Prog Cardiovasc Dis, 22:205, 1980.
27. Wieland M, et al: Left-sided endocarditis due to Pseudomonas aeruginosa. A report of 10 cases and review of the literature. Medicine, 65:180, 1986.
28. Levine DP, Crane LR, and Zervos MJ: Bacteremia in narcotic addicts at the Detroit Medical Center. II. Infectious endocarditis: A prospective comparative study. Rev Infect Dis, 8:374, 1986.
29. Kreger BE, et al: Gram-negative bacteremia III. Reassessment of etiology, epidemiology and ecology in 612 patients. Am J Med, 68:332, 1980.
30. Whimbey EA, et al: Bacteremia and fungemia in patients with neoplastic disease. Am J Med, 82:723, 1987.
31. Florman AL, and Schifrin N: Observations on a small outbreak of infantile diarrhea associated with Pseudomonas aeruginosa. J Pediatr, 36:758, 1950.
32. Dold H: On pyocyaneus sepsis and intestinal infections in Shanghai due to Bacillus pyocyaneus. Chin Med J, 32:435, 1918.
33. Chakravarti DN, and Tyagi NN: Pyrexia simulating that of enteric fever caused by Pseudomonas pyocyaneus in children. Indian Med Gaz, 72:367, 1937.
34. Sherman NJ, and Woolley MM: The ileocecal syndrome in acute childhood leukemia. Arch Surg, 107:39, 1973.
35. Schimpff SC, Wiernik PH, and Block JB: Rectal abscesses in cancer patients. Lancet, ii:844, 1972.
36. Poe RH, Marcus HR, and Emerson GL: Lung abscesses due to Pseudomonas cepacia. Am Rev Respir Dis, 115:861, 1977.
37. Martone WH, et al: Pseudomonas cepacia: Implications and control of epidemic nosocomial colonization. Rev Infect Dis, 3:708, 1981.
38. Nolan G, et al: Antibiotic prophylaxis in cystic fibrosis: Inhaled cephaloridine as an adjunct to oral cloxacillin. J Pediatr, 101:626, 1982.
39. Gelbart SM, Reinhardt GF, and Greenlee HB: Pseudomonas cepacia strains isolated from water reservoirs of unheated nebulizers. J Clin Microbiol, 3:62, 1976.
40. Isles A, et al: Pseudomonas cepacia infection in cystic fibrosis: An emerging problem. J Pediatr, 104:206, 1984.
41. Goldman DA and Klinger JD: Pseudomonas cepacia: Biology, mechanisms of virulence, epidemiology. J Pediatr, 108;806, 1986.
42. Thomassen MJ, et al: Pseudomonas cepacia colonization among patients with cystic fibrosis. Am Rev Respir Dis, 131:791, 1985.
43. Sorensen RU, et al: In vitro inhibition of lymphocyte proliferation by Pseudomonas aeruginosa phenazine pigments. Infect Immun, 41:321, 1983.
44. Noriega ER, et al: Subacute and acute endocarditis due to Pseudomonas cepacia in heroin addicts. Am J Med, 59:29, 1975.
45. Brauner A, et al: Pseudomonas cepacia septicemia in patients with burns: Report of two cases. Scand J Infect Dis, 17:63, 1985.
46. Berkelman RL, et al: Pseudomonas cepacia peritonitis associated with contamination of automatic peritoneal dialysis machines. Ann Intern Med, 96:456, 1982.
47. Smith MA, Trowers NRH, and Klein RS: Cervical osteomyelitis caused by Pseudomonas cepacia in an intravenous-drug abuser. J Clin Microbiol, 21:445, 1985.
48. Darby CP: Treating Pseudomonas cepacia meningitis with

trimethoprim-sulfamethoxazole. Am J Dis Child, *130*:1365, 1976.
49. Weinstein AJ, Moellering RC Jr, Hopkins CC, and Goldblatt A: Pseudomonas cepacia pneumonia. Am J Med Sci, *265*: 491, 1973.
50. Howe C, and Miller WR: Human glanders: Report of six cases. Ann Intern Med, *26*:93, 1947.
51. Sanford JP: Peudomonas species including melioidosis and glanders. *In* Principles and Practice of Infectious Diseases. 3rd ed. Edited by GL Mandell, RG Douglas, Jr, and JE Bennett. New York, Churchill Livingstone, 1990.
52. Whitmore A, and Krishnaswami CS: An account of the discovery of a hitherto undescribed infective disease occurring among the population of Rangoon. Indian Med Gaz, *47*:262, 1912.
53. Barnes PF, Appleman MD, and Cosgrove MM: A case of melioidosis originating in North America. Am Rev Respir Dis, *134*:170, 1986.
54. Osteraas GR, et al: Neonatal melioidosis. Am J Dis Child, *122*:446, 1971.
55. Nussbaum JJ, Hull DS, and Carter MJ: Pseudomonas pseudomallei in an anophthalmic orbit. Arch Ophthalmol, *98*: 1224, 1980.
56. McCormick JB, et al: Wound infections by an indigenous Pseudomonas pseudomallei–like organism isolated from the soil: Case report and epidemiologic study. J Infect Dis, *135*: 103, 1977.
57. McCormick JB, et al: Human-to-human transmission of Pseudomonas pseudomallei. Ann Intern Med, *83*:512, 1975.
58. Strauss JM, et al: Melioidosis in Malaysia. III. Antibodies to Pseudomonas pseudomallei in the human population. Am J Trop Med Hyg, *18*:703, 1969.
59. Ashdown JR, and Guard RW: The prevalence of human melioidosis in northern Queensland. Am J Trop Med Hyg, *33*: 474, 1984.
60. Brygoo ER: Contribution a l'etude des agglutinine naturelles pour le bacille de Whitmore. Bull Soc Pathol Exot Filiales, *46*:347, 1953.
61. Sanford JP, and Moore WL, Jr: Recrudescent melioidosis: A Southeast Asian legacy. Am Rev Respir Dis, *104*:452, 1971.
62. Clayton AJ, Lisella RS, and Martin DG: Melioidosis: A serological survey in military personnel. Milit Med, *138*:24, 1973.
63. Everett ED, and Nelson R: Pulmonary melioidosis: Observations in thirty-nine cases. Am Rev Respir Dis, *112*:331, 1975.
64. Marshall WF, Keating MR, Anhalt JP, and Steckelberg JM: Xanthomonas maltophilia: An emerging nosocomial pathogen. Mayo Clin Proc, *64*:1097, 1989.
65. Elting LS, and Bodey GP: Septicemia due to Xanthomonas species and nonaeruginosa Pseudomonas species: Increasing incidence of catheter-related infections. Medicine, *69*: 296, 1990.
66. Bottone EJ, et al: Pseudomonas maltophilia exoenzyme activity as correlate in pathogenesis of ecthyma gangrenosum. J Clin Microbiol, *24*:995, 1986.
67. Klinger JD, and Thomassen MJ: Occurrence and antimicrobial susceptibility of gram-negative nonfermentative bacilli in cystic fibrosis patients. Diagn Microbiol Infect Dis, *3*:149, 1985.
68. Bauernfeind A, et al: Qualitative and quantitative microbiological analysis of sputa of 102 patients with cystic fibrosis. Infection, *15*:270, 1987.
69. Muder RR, et al: Infections caused by Pseudomonas maltophilia—expanding clinical spectrum. Arch Intern Med, *147*:1672, 1987.
70. Fisher MC, et al: Pseudomonas maltophilia bacteremia in children undergoing open heart surgery. JAMA, *246*:1571, 1981.
71. Wishart MW, and Riley TV: Infection with Pseudomonas maltophilia hospital outbreak due to contaminated disinfectant. Med J Aust, *2*:710, 1976.
72. Allen DM, and Hartman BJ: Acinetobacter species. *In* Principles and Practice of Infectious Diseases. 3rd ed. Edited by GL Mandell, RG Douglas, Jr, and JE Bennett. New York, Churchill Livingstone, 1990.
73. Al-Khoja MS, and Darrell JH: The skin as the source of Acinetobacter and Moraxella species occuring in blood cultures. J Clin Pathol, *32*:497, 1979.
74. Rosenthal S, and Tager IB: Prevalence of gram-negative rods in the normal pharyngeal flora. Ann Intern Med, *83*:355, 1975.
75. Larson EL: Persistent carriage of gram-negative bacteria on hands. Am J Infect Control, *9*:112, 1986.
76. Rosenthal SL: Sources of Pseudomonas and Acinetobacter species found in human culture materials. Am J Clin Pathol, *62*:807, 1974.
77. Hoffmann S, Mabeck CE, and Vejlsgaard R: Bacteriuria caused by Acinetobacter calcoaceticus biovars in a normal population and in general practice. J Clin Microbiol, *16*:443, 1982.
78. Centers for Disease Control: Nosocomial Infection Surveillance Summary. MMWR, *35*:17, 1987.
79. Reynolds RC, and Cluff LE: Infection of man with Mimeae. Ann Intern Med, *58*:759, 1963.
80. Gilardi GL: Flavobacterium. Clin Microbiol Newslett, *8*:143, 1986.
81. Schoch PE, and Cunha BA: Nosocomial Achromobacter xylosoxidans infections. Infect Control Hosp Epidemiol, *9*:84, 1988.
82. Graham DR, et al: Infections caused by Moraxella, Moraxella urethralis, Moraxella-like groups M-5 and M-6, and Kingella kingae in the United States, 1953–1980. Rev Infect Dis, *12*: 423, 1990.
83. Baron EJ, and Finegold SM: Nonfermentative gram-negative bacilli and coccobacilli. In Bailey and Scott's Diagnostic Microbiology. 8th ed. St. Louis, CV Mosby, 1990.
84. Ghosh JK, and Tranter J: Bordetella bronchiseptica infections in man: Review and case report. J Clin Pathol, *32*:546, 1979.
85. Appelbaum PC, and Leathers DJ: Evaluation of the rapid NFT system for identification of gram-negative, nonfermenting rods. J Clin Microbiol, *20*:730, 1984.
86. Gilardi GL: Identification of glucose-nonfermenting gram-negative bacilli. Clin Microbiol Newslett, *6*:115, 1984.
87. Gilardi GL: Pseudomonas and related genera. *In* Manual of Clinical Microbiology. 5th ed. Edited by A Balows, et al. Washington, DC, American Society for Microbiology, 1991.
88. Pickett MJ, Hollis DG, and Bouttone EJ: Miscellaneous gram-negative bacteria *In* Manual of Clinical Microbiology. 5th ed. Edited by A Balows, et al. Washington, DC, American Society for Microbiology, 1991.
89. Dance DAB: Melioidosis: The tip of the iceberg? Clin Microbiol Rev, *4*:52, 1991.

Chapter 33

FASTIDIOUS AEROBIC GRAM-NEGATIVE BACILLI AND COCCOBACILLI

The aerobic, gram-negative bacteria discussed in this chapter—Francisella tularensis, the species of Brucella, Bordetella pertussis and Bordetella parapertussis, and the species of Legionella—have specific growth requirements and, for cultivation in vitro, require special media or prolonged incubation, or both.

FRANCISELLA TULARENSIS

The disease now known as tularemia probably was described first in 1837 by a Japanese physician; however, little attention was given to the illness until Ohara, in 1925, described three Japanese who developed a febrile illness after skinning, cooking, and eating a dead hare, which he postulated was the source of the illness (1). To prove his theory, Ohara rubbed the hearts removed from dead hares on the hand of a human volunteer (his wife), who in four days developed fever and chills followed by axillary lymphadenopathy on the affected side. The lymph nodes, excised and cultured, yielded a new bacterium, called the Ohara-Haga's coccus (1).

In 1911, a new organism responsible for a plague-like illness in ground squirrels was identified by McCoy and named Bacterium tularense after Tulare County, in California, where the infected squirrels were found (2). The first bacteriologically confirmed human case of infection with B. tularense—conjunctivitis and lymphadenopathy in a meat cutter—was described 3 years later (3). The role of ticks in the transmission of tularemia was recognized in 1924, and a few years later the discovery of transovarial transmission of the organism in ticks established the tick as a reservoir of infection (4,5). Edward Francis confirmed that the disease reported by Ohara (previously discussed) was tularemia, and in 1928 he described the clinical manifestations and epidemiology of the disease, based on his experience with more than 800 cases (6). In his honor, the genus name of the organism was changed to Francisella in 1959 (7).

Francisella tularensis is a small, immotile, encapsulated, gram-negative coccobacillus that requires cysteine or cystine (or sulfhydryl compounds) for growth in vitro. All isolates of F. tularensis are serologically identical but they may be divided into two categories. Type A (Nearctica), recovered from many rodents and blood-sucking arthropods, is highly virulent in humans and rabbits, uses glycerol, and is citrulline ureidase positive. Type B (Palaearctica), more commonly isolated from water and from aquatic animals, is less virulent in humans and rabbits, does not utilize glycerol, and is citrulline ureidase negative.

Epidemiology

Francisella tularensis, found throughout the northern hemisphere except in the United Kingdom, between 30° and 70° north latitude, has been isolated from about 100 species of wild mammals, several species of domestic animals, birds, some amphibians and fish, many invertebrates, mud, and water from streams and wells. The most important reservoir hosts in the United States are ticks, rabbits, and hares. Tularemia is most often transmitted to humans during the bite of a tick (although the organism probably is transmitted in the feces, because F. tularensis has not been found in the salivary glands) or via contact with tissues or body fluids of an infected mammal (usually a rabbit) and less commonly by inhaling infectious aerosols, by ingesting contaminated water or inadequately cooked meat from an infected animal, or by animal bites (cat, coyote, squirrel) (6,8–11).

In the United States the incidence of human tularemia peaked in 1939 at about 20 per million population and then steadily declined to about one case per million population in the late 1960s; fewer than 200 cases have been reported annually since 1967 (12,13). Tularemia occurs in all states except Hawaii, but in the past several years almost half the cases have been reported from Arkansas, Tennessee, Texas, Oklahoma, and Missouri (14). The seasonal distribution of cases depends on the mechanism of transmission: tick-borne cases predominate in spring and summer and rabbit-associated ones in winter. Since 1950 the number of rabbit-associated cases has declined, and currently about 60% of cases occur between May and September. All races and all ages are susceptible to infection, but attack rates are highest among adults, and men account for 65 to 75% of all cases.

Pathogenesis and Pathology

In humans, 10 virulent organisms injected subcutaneously and 10 to 50 given by aerosol produce disease, but about 10^8 organisms must be ingested to cause infection (14). Francisella tularensis most frequently enters the body through small breaks in the skin or mucous membranes but probably does not penetrate intact skin. Bacteria then enter the blood and localize in the cells of the monocyte/macrophage system, where they survive inside cells for long periods. Early lesions are characterized by foci of necrosis and an infiltrate of many polymorphonuclear leukocytes and few macrophages, but later macrophages and T lymphocytes predominate and caseating granulomas, with or without multinucleate giant cells, may develop. The bacterial capsule is antiphagocytic, and neutrophils are incapable of phagocytosing and killing F. tularensis without opsonizing antibodies. Because these antibodies are not produced until later in the infection, neutrophils probably play a minor role in the host defense against this organism. In contrast, macrophages and lymphocytes are essential.

Clinical Manifestations

Typically, tularemia begins abruptly with fever, chills, malaise, fatigue, and one of several clinical syndromes. The ulceroglandular form (75 to 85% of cases) is characterized by painful regional lymphadenopathy and a cutaneous ulcer. In more than 90% of rabbit-associated cases the skin lesion involves the finger or hands, and in tick-borne disease it is on the lower extremities or perianal area in 50% of cases, on the trunk in 30%, and the head in 5 to 10%. Persons who have contact with many infected animals can have multiple ulcers (12). Axillary or epitrochlear nodes are affected in 80 to 90% of persons with rabbit-associated disease, and the inguinal or femoral nodes in 60 to 70% of those with tick-borne tularemia. Glandular tularemia, characterized by fever and tender lymphadenopathy without a skin ulcer, accounts for 5 to 10% of cases. The typhoidal form—fever, prostration, and weight loss without lymphadenopathy—accounts for 5 to 15% of cases. Oculoglandular tularemia, which accounts for 1 to 2% of cases, is characterized by unilateral, painful, purulent conjunctivitis with preauricular or cervical lymphadenopathy. Oropharyngeal tularemia, an acute exudative or membranous pharyngotonsillitis with cervical lymphadenopathy, accounts for the remainder.

Pneumonia, characterized by nonproductive cough and patchy, ill-defined infiltrates in one or more lobes on chest roentgenogram, occurs in 30 to 80% of persons with typhoidal tularemia and some 10 to 15% of those with ulceroglandular disease. As many as 20% of persons develop a macular, maculopapular, pustular, or blotchy rash several days after the onset of illness. Occasionally, hepatomegaly and abnormal liver function tests develop; transient renal failure and rhabdomyolysis are uncommon; pericarditis, peritonitis, meningitis, and osteomyelitis are rare (14).

Laboratory Diagnosis

Tularemia usually is diagnosed serologically, but the organism may be recovered in the laboratory. If culture is attempted, what specimens are required for diagnosis depends on the clinical presentation. For draining lymph nodes and pustular skin lesions, suppurative material is aspirated with a needle and syringe or a small pipette, and if biopsy is performed the tissue is cultured. For oculoglandular tularemia conjunctival scrapings are collected with a swab. During the systemic phase of all forms of tularemia, Francisella tularensis may be recovered from blood (collected without anticoagulant), sputum, or gastric and throat washings; the latter three should be collected early in the morning before the patient eats, drinks, or brushes the teeth. When typhoidal or pulmonary tularemia is suspected, culture of bronchial secretions and pleural fluid (if present) in addition to blood, sputum, and gastric and throat washings should be considered. After collection, specimens should be processed immediately; however, if a delay is unavoidable specimens (except blood) should be refrigerated to prevent overgrowth by normal flora. Laboratory personnel should wear gloves, gown, and mask when handling specimens or cultures suspected to contain F. tularensis.

Because Francisella tularensis requires cysteine or cystine for growth, specimens must be inoculated to special media. Glucose cystine agar or cystinc hcart agar containing 5% sheep or rabbit blood, chocolate or blood agar enriched with supplements containing cysteine or cystine, GC base medium with hemoglobin, and charcoal yeast extract agar supplemented with α-ketoglutarate (used for recovery of Legionella, discussed later) will support its growth. F. tularensis rarely grows on Thayer-Martin agar after prolonged incubation but does not grow on MacConkey agar. Incubation in an atmosphere of increased carbon dioxide is not required but is not harmful. Although pinpoint colonies may be visible in 24 hours, typical colonies—transparent to gray, smooth, convex, mucoid, pearly, 1 to 2 mm in diameter—usually form in 48 to 72 hours. Slight greening of the agar often occurs immediately beneath the colony. A smear of the colony stained with the Gram stain shows small, gram-negative bacilli with bipolar staining, a feature more apparent in preparations stained with Giemsa stain.

Francisella tularensis is weakly catalase positive, oxidase negative, and produces acid but not gas from glucose, maltose, mannose, and fructose. Biochemical testing, however, requires supplemented media, and because working with the organism in the laboratory is dangerous it is recommended that suspicious cultures be sent to a reference laboratory such as the Centers for Disease Control (CDC) for confirmation with a slide agglutination or direct fluorescent antibody test.

A serologic diagnosis of tularemia is based on a fourfold rise in agglutination titers between acute- and convalescent-phase serum samples. A single convalescent-phase titer of 1:160 or greater indicates past or current infection. Agglutination titers, usually negative in the first week of illness, are positive after 2 weeks in 50 to 70% of infected persons, peak in 4 to 8 weeks, and may remain elevated at diagnostic titers for several years after the acute infection. Because serum from persons with tularemia or brucellosis (discussed later) may show cross-reactions, a control with Brucella antigen should be included when serologic tests are done to diagnose tularemia; if agglutination occurs with both organisms to the same or a similar titer, agglutinin absorption tests should be performed.

Treatment and Prevention

Streptomycin is the antimicrobial agent of choice for all forms of tularemia; gentamicin may be an acceptable alternative (12,14). The mortality rate, 5 to 15% before antibiotics became available, has decreased to 1 to 3% in recent years (12).

To reduce the risk of acquiring tularemia, gloves should be worn while skinning or eviscerating rabbits and other wild animals, and tick-infested areas should be avoided if possible or tick repellents used. Ticks should be removed promptly without squeezing the body, because excretions may be infectious. A live attenuated tularemia vaccine, recommended for laboratory personnel exposed to Francisella tularensis and for persons whose vocation requires repeated contact with wild animals or arthropod vectors in tularemia-enzootic areas, does not provide complete protection against infection but reduces the severity of the illness (12).

BRUCELLA

The organism now known as Brucella melitensis first was recovered from the spleens of British Army personnel who died of an illness called Malta fever in 1887 by Sir David Bruce, who named the agent Micrococcus melitensis. The same organism was isolated from goats on Malta in 1905, and soon thereafter Brucella was recognized as a cause of infectious abortion in cattle and was identified in domesticated livestock in many countries.

Six species of Brucella currently are recognized: Brucella abortus (a pathogen of cattle), Brucella melitensis (goats), Brucella suis (pigs), Brucella canis (dogs), Brucella ovis (sheep), and Brucella neotomae (recovered from rats); the first four also cause disease in humans. The cell walls of Brucella abortus, Brucella suis, and Brucella melitensis contain two major surface antigens, A and M, and endotoxin, which has a chemical structure and biologic activity different from those of the endotoxins produced by many enteric bacilli.

Epidemiology

Brucellosis is predominantly a zoonotic disease, causing contagious abortion or other reproductive problems in domesticated animals (see above). Humans acquire the infection by direct contact of infected tissues or body fluids with conjunctivae or broken skin, by ingestion of contaminated meat or dairy products, and by inhalation of infectious aerosols. The disease occurs worldwide, affecting about 500,000 people annually. In the United States implementation in 1945 of the Federal-State Cooperative Brucellosis Eradication Program (requiring that cattle be tested for brucellosis and slaughtered if infected), immunization of cattle with live, attenuated Brucella abortus vaccine, and mandatory pasteurization of dairy products have much reduced the prevalence of brucellosis in humans. Over 6000 cases were reported in 1945, and 200 or fewer cases annually since 1980.

In recent years more than half the reported cases of brucellosis in the United States occurred in Texas, California, Virginia, and Florida, and from 1980 to 1986 Texas and California reported almost 40% of all cases (15). Between 1960 and 1974 swine were the most common source of human brucellosis, and from 1975 to 1978 cattle (16–18). Ingestion of unpasteurized dairy products accounted for about 10% of cases reported annually between 1965 and 1978, and accidental inoculation of veterinarians or livestock raisers with the Brucella abortus vaccine and exposure to the organism in the laboratory each accounted for 1 to 2% of all cases. During the past decade many cases of brucellosis reported from Texas and California were associated with ingestion of unpasteurized goats' milk cheese (contaminated with Brucella melitensis) from Mexico (19).

Brucellosis acquired by direct contact with animals is predominantly a disease of men aged 20 to 60 years who have certain occupations—abattoir employees, especially those working in areas where carcasses are skinned, sawn into pieces, and washed, livestock producers, and veterinarians. In contrast, about half of those who acquire disease by ingesting unpasteurized goats' milk cheese are younger than 20 years and 50 to 60% are female.

Pathogenesis

Brucellae are facultative intracellular pathogens that enter the body via breaks in the skin or mucous membranes or via inhalation. Brucella abortus and Brucella melitensis may be opsonized by normal human serum, promoting their phagocytosis by polymorphonuclear leukocytes. Polymorphonuclear leukocytes can kill Brucella abortus but not Brucella melitensis, and normal human serum has good bactericidal activity against Brucella abortus but not against Brucella melitensis, factors that probably account for the greater virulence of the latter. Organisms not killed by polymorphonuclear leukocytes travel to regional lymph nodes, then enter the circulation, and localize in organs of the monocyte/macrophage system, where they are ingested by macrophages. Some organisms survive and multiply inside cells; but when macrophages are activated, intracellular organisms are killed, releasing endotoxin from their cell walls.

In animals infected in the laboratory lymphokines produced by sensitized T lymphocytes about 7 to 10 days after infection activate macrophages, which become more efficient at killing intracellular bacteria. About the same time granulomas form in the liver and spleen, and delayed-type hypersensitivity develops to Brucella antigens (20).

Clinical Manifestations

The clinical manifestations of brucellosis depend on the overall health of the person and the species involved: disease caused by Brucella melitensis usually is most severe, followed by Brucella suis infection; disease due to Brucella abortus or Brucella canis generally is the least severe. Infection may be subclinical, diagnosed during serologic surveys of high-risk groups or during the investigation of an outbreak such as might occur in a meat-packing plant. Disease, manifest 1 week to several months after exposure (average, 2 to 3 weeks), usually begins gradually but may begin abruptly, with sweats, chills, fever, and weakness, often accompanied by malaise, headache, and anorexia. Weight loss, myalgias, arthralgias, and back pain develop in 25 to 50% of cases, splenomegaly in 20 to 30%, and lymphadenopathy in 10 to 20% (15). Disease recurs, owing to relapse or reinfection, in about 5% of cases (21). Complications of acute brucellosis, reported in as many as 30% of cases, are most likely to develop when infection is present longer than 2 months before antimicrobial therapy is begun, and they may affect almost any organ system (Table 33–1) (15,21–30).

Table 33–1. Complications of Acute Brucellosis

Organ System	Manifestations	Comments (references)
Musculoskeletal	Sacroilitis, arthritis, spondylitis, osteomyelitis, tenosynovitis, bursitis, paraspinal abscess	Most common with B. melitensis (22,23)
Neurologic	Meningoencephalitis, myelitis, paresis, paresthesias, depression, psychosis	(24,25)
Genitourinary	Epididymo-orchitis; rarely interstitial nephritis, pyelonephritis, prostatitis, cystitis	(15,26)
Cardiovascular	Endocarditis, usually involving aortic valve	Occurs in <2% of cases, but is the most common cause of death (27,28)
Gastrointestinal	Granulomatous hepatitis; rarely hepatic abscess, cholecystitis	Granulomas may be noncaseating or caseating (29)
Monocyte/macrophage; hematologic	Splenic abscess; anemia, leukopenia, thrombocytopenia, pancytopenia	Most common with B. melitensis (15)
Pulmonary	Hilar adenopathy, perihilar infiltrates, nodular lesions, lung abscess, pleural effusion	(15)
Cutaneous	Erythema nodosum; papular, eczematous, rubeoliform, and scarlatiniform rashes; soft tissue abscess	(30)
Ocular	Corneal ulcers, keratitis, iridocyclitis, uveitis	(21)

Laboratory Diagnosis

To diagnose brucellosis multiple blood cultures and acute- and convalescent-phase serum samples always should be collected, and culture of bone marrow should be considered. Involved tissues (such as liver in a person with elevated liver function test values) and abscess material should be cultured; and occasionally Brucella is recovered from cerebrospinal fluid, pleural or peritoneal fluid, joint fluid, or urine. Specimens should be processed as soon as possible in a biologic safety cabinet, and they should be refrigerated if transport to a reference laboratory for culture is necessary.

Species of Brucella grow on sheep blood– and chocolate agar and some isolates grow on MacConkey agar; however, Brucella agar or some type of infusion base agar supplemented with 5% heated horse or rabbit serum provides optimal recovery. Agar plates should be incubated at 35° C in a humidified atmosphere containing 5 to 10% carbon dioxide. Biphasic blood culture bottles (Castaneda type with an agar slant and broth) are recommended. Brucellae grow in commercially available broth blood culture systems; but frequently evidence of bacterial growth is lacking and blind subculture to Brucella broth or an agar medium is necessary for detection. Agar plates are held 3 weeks and blood cultures 4 weeks before being discarded as negative.

Brucellae grow slowly, forming pinpoint, translucent, convex, smooth, nonhemolytic colonies with a glistening surface after 3 to 7 days. Smears of a colony stained with the Gram stain (performed by counterstaining with safranin for at least 2 minutes) show gram-negative coccobacilli without bipolar staining. The organisms are immotile, catalase positive, and oxidase positive; most hydrolyze urea rapidly, but they do not ferment lactose or glucose. Isolates that exhibit these reactions should be tested for agglutination in anti–smooth Brucella serum (available commercially), which will detect Brucella abortus, Brucella suis, and Brucella melitensis, but not Brucella canis. Characteristics used to differentiate the species of Brucella that infect humans are shown in Table 33–2; but because Brucella is isolated infrequently in most clinical laboratories, suspected isolates should be sent to a reference laboratory for confirmation.

Treatment and Prevention

Currently, doxycycline plus rifampin is the treatment recommended by the World Health Organization. Rifampin is used to treat pregnant women, and trimethoprim-sulfamethoxazole has been used in children. Rifampin plus a third-generation cephalosporin has been recommended to treat central nervous system involvement (15).

One of the most effective means of preventing human brucellosis is controlling brucellosis in livestock, for example by routine vaccination of cattle with Brucella abortus strain 19 vaccine in conjunction with serologic testing of cattle and slaughter of infected animals. Effective vaccines against Brucella melitensis and Brucella suis have been developed but currently are not used widely in some areas where brucellosis in goats is enzootic. Pasteurization of dairy products also is important in preventing human brucellosis. Vaccines have been used for per-

Table 33–2. Differentiation of Species of Brucella That Infect Humans

| Characteristic | Species | | | |
	B. melitensis	B. abortus	B. suis	B. canis
CO_2 required for growth	−	+/−	−	−
H_2S produced*	+	+	−	−
Time to urease positive (hr)	2	2	1/4	1/4
Growth on dye medium containing:				
Basic fuschin 1:100,000	+	+	−	−
Thionin 1:100,000	+	−	+	+

* Detected by suspending a lead acetate paper strip over the inoculated surface of a tryptose agar slant and incubating for 4 days.
Key: +, >90% of isolates positive; −, >90% of isolates negative; +/−, variable result.

sons at high risk of contracting brucellosis in Russia, China, and France, but currently no vaccine is available for human use in the United States (31,32).

BORDETELLA

Three species of Bordetella—Bordetella pertussis, Bordetella parapertussis, and Bordetella bronchiseptica—cause disease in humans, although the latter is predominantly an animal pathogen. Bordetella bronchiseptica is discussed briefly in Chapter 32 because it does not require special media or prolonged incubation for recovery and it is identified by methods typically used to identify the nonfermenters. Bordetella pertussis, the most important human pathogen, is discussed in detail. The cultural characteristics of Bordetella parapertussis, a rare cause of pertussis, are reviewed briefly.

Bordetella pertussis

Bordetella pertussis causes an acute and chronic respiratory illness termed whooping cough, or pertussis, primarily in infants and young children, a disease recognized since the 1500s but first described in 1640 (33). The organism, a fastidious, nonmotile, aerobic gram-negative coccobacillus, was recovered from a person who had pertussis by Bordet and Gengou in 1906 (34). A whole-cell vaccine, introduced in the 1940s, was responsible for a decline in the prevalence of the disease; however, pertussis remains a major health problem in developing countries, and a recent decrease in the vaccination rate has been associated with increased prevalence of the disease in the United States (Fig. 33–1), the United Kingdom, and Sweden (35–37).

Epidemiology

Bordetella pertussis, a pathogen only for humans, is found worldwide, causing an estimated 51 million cases of pertussis and 600,000 deaths annually (38). In most populations pertussis is endemic, and epidemics, cycling at 3- to 4-year intervals, are superimposed on the background level of disease. Infected humans, especially adults with atypical undiagnosed pertussis, are the only reservoir of infection, which is transmitted principally via aerosol droplets produced during coughing (39). The attack rate is over 90% in unimmunized persons (40).

Before pertussis vaccine was introduced disease occurred almost exclusively among children 1 to 5 years of age; maternally acquired antibodies apparently provided passive protection in the first year of life. With the introduction of the whole-cell vaccine the prevalence of pertussis decreased, the peak age shifted to infants and children under one year of age, and up to 10 to 15% of cases involved persons over age 15 years (Fig. 33–2). Vaccine immunity usually lasts less than 12 years; therefore, fully immunized children are well-protected, but adults have little or no immunity for passive transfer to infants, who are at the greatest risk for morbidity and mortality but are unprotected.

Pathogenesis

Bordetella pertussis produces toxins and enzymes that may play a role in the pathogenesis of disease. Pertussis toxin (also called pertussigen, lymphocytosis-promoting factor, histamine-sensitizing factor, and islet-activating factor), the most extensively studied factor, induces leukocytosis, lymphocytosis, histamine sensitization, lethality, mitogenicity, adjuvant effects, and insulin secretion in vivo (41). Structurally, pertussis toxin resembles cholera toxin (see Chapter 35), possessing an A subunit responsible for toxicity by virtue of its adenosine diphosphate ribosylating activity, and a 5- to 7-component B subunit, responsible for cell binding and entry and for stimulating lymphocyte mitosis (42,43). Antibodies specific for pertussis toxin protect animals infected with B. pertussis in the

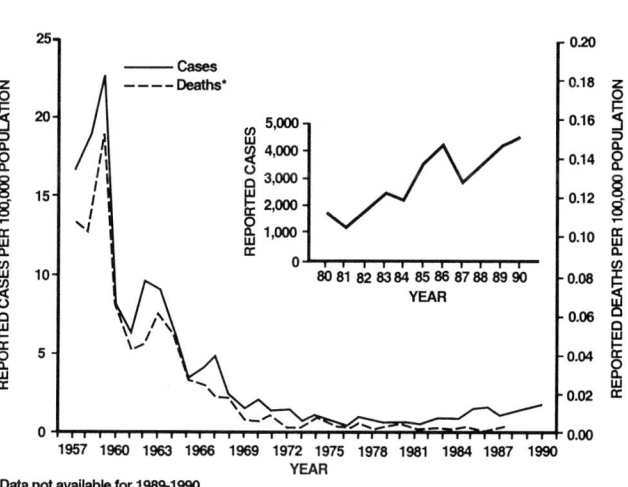

Fig. 33–1. Incidence of reported cases of pertussis in the United States, 1957–1990. (From Centers for Disease Control: Summary of notifiable diseases, United States, 1990. MMWR, 39:1, 1990.)

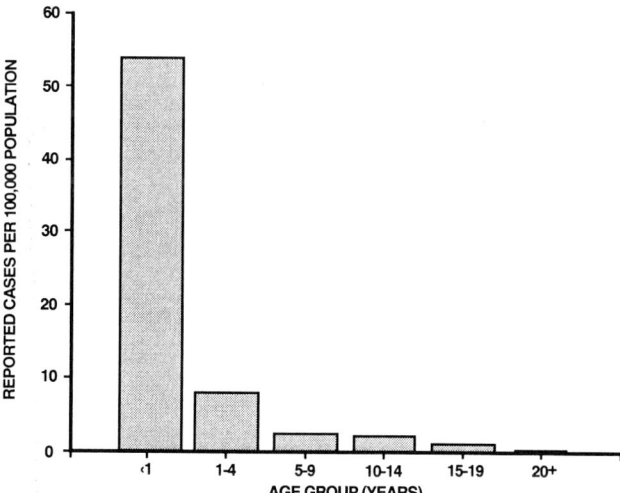

Fig. 33–2. Reported cases of pertussis by age group in the United States, 1990. (From Centers for Disease Control: Summary of notifiable diseases, United States, 1990. MMWR, 39:1, 1990.)

laboratory against disease, and in humans antitoxin antibody titers correlate with immunity to infection with B. pertussis (44,45).

Tracheal cytotoxin, a small glycopeptide, causes ciliostasis and specifically damages ciliated cells in hamster tracheal ring cultures by inhibiting DNA synthesis, suggesting its potential role in secondary bacterial infections in pertussis by impairing normal pulmonary mucociliary clearance mechanisms (46). Bacterial adenylate cyclase is hypothesized to enter polymorphonuclear leukocytes and macrophages, become activated by the eucaryotic regulatory protein calmodulin, and induce high levels of cyclic adenosine monophosphate (cAMP), which subsequently impairs bactericidal functions, possibly allowing the bacteria to survive and multiply. Heat-labile dermonecrotic toxin, an intracellular protein not actively secreted by Bordetella pertussis, produces inflammation and necrotic skin lesions in mice after subcutaneous injection in small doses and is lethal in large doses; however, its exact role in human disease is unknown.

Cell wall and surface components of Bordetella pertussis also may be involved in the pathogenesis of disease. The cell wall lipopolysaccharide has the same biologic activity as endotoxin from other gram-negative bacteria—pyrogenicity, toxicity, and induction of cytokine production (41,46). The filamentous hemagglutinin, a surface filament-like protein that agglutinates red blood cells, and surface fimbriae may initiate attachment and adherence of B. pertussis to ciliated epithelial cells of the upper respiratory tract (41).

Clinical Manifestations

Pertussis is divided into catarrhal, paroxysmal, and convalescent stages. After an incubation period of 6 to 20 days the catarrhal stage begins with symptoms of the common cold—rhinorrhea, conjunctivitis, coryza, low-grade fever, mild cough—that may last several weeks. Increasing episodes of severe, violent coughing mark the beginning of the paroxysmal stage, characterized by 15 to 25 paroxysmal coughing episodes during a 24-hour period. During the coughing attacks the rapid inspiration of air into the lungs past the swollen glottis produces the classic "whoop"; but because this does not occur in all cases, the term pertussis, rather than whooping cough, is preferred. The paroxysmal stage may last 1 to 4 weeks and is followed by the convalescent stage, during which coughing paroxysms may occur sporadically for up to 6 months after infection. Potential complications of the paroxysmal stage include vomiting with subsequent weight loss, dehydration, and malnutrition; hemorrhagic events, hernia, pneumothorax, seizures, encephalopathy, secondary bacterial infections, and death (38). The mortality rate is highest for children under 12 months of age, and secondary bacterial infections are the major cause of death.

Pertussis may be atypical in infants, partially immunized children, and adults (47,48). Infants may present with apneic spells and later develop a paroxysmal cough without the classic whoop. Partially immunized children may have a short catarrhal phase (or none), and the whoop often is absent. Adults may have only common cold–like symptoms. In persons infected with human immunodeficiency virus, Bordetella pertussis may cause prolonged paroxysmal cough and dyspnea (49).

Laboratory Diagnosis

Bordetella pertussis. Collection of two pernasal nasopharyngeal swabs (one for culture and one to prepare a smear for direct staining with fluorescent antibodies) is recommended for diagnosis of pertussis. A calcium alginate or dacron swab on a fine, flexible wire is inserted via the nostril to the nasopharynx and held for up to a minute; cotton swabs contain fatty acids that may inhibit the growth of B. pertussis and should not be used (50). Throat swabs specimens, aspirates of nasopharyngeal secretions, bronchial washings, and transtracheal aspirates also may be used for culture. If specimen transport is necessary, Regan-Lowe or Jones-Kendrick transport medium and storage at 4° C are recommended (41).

Culture is the most sensitive method for detection of Bordetella pertussis; however, its sensitivity is adversely affected by a prolonged interval between disease onset and specimen collection (B. pertussis is most likely to be recovered during the catarrhal stage), by antimicrobial therapy, and by prolonged interval between specimen collection and planting. Regan-Lowe or charcoal horse blood agar is recommended for isolation of B. pertussis (41). Adding antibiotics such as methicillin or cephalexin inhibits overgrowth by normal nasopharyngeal flora, but because some strains of B. pertussis may be inhibited by penicillins or cephalexin, both selective and nonselective media should be used (51). Plates should be incubated at 35° to 37° C in a humidified atmosphere; increased carbon dioxide is not necessary. Small, smooth, convex, mucoid colonies with a pearly luster, resembling drops of mercury, and often surrounded by a narrow zone of complete hemolysis (when grown on blood-containing agar), appear in 3 to 7 days. A smear of a colony stained with the Gram stain (counterstained with safranin for 2 minutes) shows faint gram-negative coccobacilli arranged singly and in pairs. Isolates suspected to be B. pertussis are confirmed by staining a smear with specific fluorescent-labeled antibodies (discussed later). B. pertussis does not grown on MacConkey agar or on sheep blood agar on primary isolation. It is immotile, catalase- and oxidase positive, and urease- and nitrate negative.

The direct fluorescent antibody test, utilizing polyclonal fluorescein-labeled antibodies to Bordetella pertussis, for detection of the bacteria directly in smears prepared from nasopharyngeal specimens or for confirmation of isolates showing typical colony and cellular morphology, is positive when short rods with a rim of bright green fluorescence are seen (41). Results are available within a few hours of receiving the specimen, but the test has limited sensitivity, owing to the large number of organisms necessary for microscopic visualization, and it is associated with a large percentage of false-positive results, ranging from about 7 to 40%, a problem due to variability among technologists in interpreting results, poor-quality smears, and nonspecific reagents (41). Recently developed diagnostic tests that may be valuable in the future include an enzyme-linked immunosorbent assay (ELISA) for detection of specific immunoglobulin (Ig) A in nasopharyngeal secretions, tests that detect B. pertussis toxin or its adenylate cyclase enzyme, and nucleic acid hybridization (41,52–54).

Bordetella parapertussis. B. parapertussis may be cultured from the same specimens submitted for isolation of Bordetella pertussis. The organism grows more rapidly (1 or 2 days) than B. pertussis on Regan-Lowe agar, forming grayer and less domed colonies. On primary isolation, Bordetella parapertussis grows on sheep blood agar, producing opaque, smooth colonies surrounded by a zone of β-hemolysis; and it forms a brown, soluble pigment when grown on tyrosine agar. B. parapertussis is immotile, oxidase negative, and urease- and citrate positive.

Treatment and Prevention

The estolate ester of erythromycin, the antimicrobial agent of choice, reduces the severity and duration of pertussis even when therapy is not begun until the paroxysmal phase of the disease.

Currently, the vaccine recommended by the World Health Organization and used throughout most of the world is a killed, whole-cell vaccine combined with diphtheria and tetanus toxoids and aluminum-containing adjuvants (DPT vaccine). The standard immunization schedule includes three primary doses given at 2-month intervals beginning at 6 to 8 weeks of age and booster doses given 6 to 12 months after the third dose and at 4 to 6 years of age. This vaccine is believed to be over 80% effective in preventing pertussis, but the duration of protection is limited, and the attack rate is about 95% 12 years or more postimmunization (40). A major limitation of the vaccine is its potential to cause adverse reactions. Compared with the diphtheria-tetanus toxoid vaccine, DPT is associated with more local and systemic reactions, including pain, swelling, fever, anorexia, fretfulness, and vomiting (55). Encephalopathy and permanent neurologic sequelae have been associated temporally with DPT administration, but few of these cases actually are caused by the vaccine (56). Despite the potential adverse effects of the whole-cell vaccine, its benefits outweigh the risks, and it continues to be recommended (57).

Because of the reactions associated with the whole-cell vaccine, an acellular vaccine containing inactivated pertussis toxin, filamentous hemagglutinin, agglutinogens, and reduced levels of endotoxin was developed and has been used since 1981 in Japan in children 24 months and older, with apparent efficacy (58). In Sweden pertussis toxoid, alone or combined with filamentous hemagglutinin, administered to children beginning at 6 months of age, provided partial protection against infection and good protection against severe disease (59).

LEGIONELLA

In the summer of 1976, during the bicentennial celebration of the Declaration of Independence in Philadelphia, an outbreak of an acute respiratory tract illness that clinically resembled influenza involved over 180 members of the Pennsylvania American Legion, of whom almost 30 died. The epidemiologic and microbiologic investigation of this outbreak continued for 6 months until Joseph McDade discovered the agent, first named the Legionnaires' disease bacterium and now known as Legionella pneumophila (60). Diagnostic tests then were developed; and using these techniques to retrospectively study unsolved epidemics, investigators were able to attribute outbreaks of acute respiratory disease from as far back as the late 1950s to the Legionnaires' disease bacterium (61–63). Moreover, this agent was shown to be responsible for an epidemic of a mild acute respiratory disease, Pontiac fever, that afflicted employees and visitors in a health department in Pontiac, Michigan. The latter outbreak provided the best documentation that L. pneumophila can produce epidemic illness by aerosol dissemination and demonstrated that the bacterium causes two distinct clinical syndromes. (1) Legionnaires' disease is a potentially fatal, severe respiratory illness associated with pneumonia and has an attack rate of less than 5% for exposed persons. (2) Pontiac fever is a mild, self-limited respiratory tract disease without pneumonia that is associated with an attack rate of 95% for persons exposed (64).

During the investigation of an outbreak of respiratory disease among immunocompromised patients in Pittsburgh, Pennsylvania in 1979, a bacterium distinct from Legionella pneumophilia, initially designated the "Pittsburgh pneumonia agent" and now known as Legionella micdadei, was identified (65,66). Further study of these "new agents" revealed that the earliest recorded isolate of a species of Legionella was a strain of L. micdadei recovered by Hugh Tatlock during an outbreak of Fort Bragg fever in 1943 (65). Moreover, in the late 1940s F. Marilyn Bozeman had isolated two organisms subsequently recognized as the first recorded isolates of Legionella pneumophila and Legionella bozemanii (60,67).

During an international symposium held in 1978 at the CDC a nomenclature for the Legionnaires' disease bacterium based on DNA homology was proposed: a new family, Legionellaceae, containing one genus, Legionella, named for the Philadelphia victims, and, at that time, one species, Legionella pneumophila, named for the predilection of the organism for the lungs (68). Since that time, the serologic diversity of L. pneumophila has been recognized, and many new species of Legionella have been described. Currently, 30 species have been named, several of which have more than one serotype (including L. pneumophila, which has 14), and 13 of the 30 have been recovered from clinical specimens (Table 33–3) (66,69–87).

Species of Legionella are aerobic, non–spore-forming, unencapsulated gram-negative bacteria, 2 to 20 μm long by 0.3 to 0.9 μm wide. However, bacterial cells may appear coccobacillary, measuring 1 to 2 μm in diameter, in clinical specimens (including tissue) and elongated and filamentous when cultured in vitro. Cells stain faintly with the Gram stain, particularly when basic fuchsin rather than safranin is the counterstain, but are more easily visualized when stained with the Gimenez stain. In formalin-fixed, paraffin-embedded tissue, organisms are seen by staining with the Dieterle or Warthin-Starry silver stain; and Legionella micdadei stains acid fast, a feature unique

Table 33-3. Currently Recognized Species of Legionella

Source	Species of Legionella
Clinical specimens	L. pneumophila, -micdadei, -bozemanii, -dumoffii, -longbeachae, -jordanis, -gormanii, -feeleii, -hackeliae, -maceachernii, -birminghamensis, -cincinnatiensis, -oakridgensis, -wadsworthii, -tucsonensis
Environment	L. anisa,* -cherrii,* -rubrilucens,* -sainthelensi,* -brunensis, -erythra, -israelensis, -jamestowniensis, -moravica, -parisiensis, -santicrucis, -spiritensis, -steigerwaltii, -fairfieldensis, -adelaidensis

* These organisms have been implicated as potential human pathogens by serologic studies only[70].

among the Legionella. These organisms are nutritionally fastidious; for primary isolation in vitro, L-cysteine is essential, and ketoacids and ferric ions together stimulate growth. In nature Legionella pneumophila survives in temperatures ranging from 0° to 63° C, at a pH of 5.0 to 8.5, and it can survive years in water samples at 2° to 8° C.

Epidemiology

The apparent natural habitats for Legionella pneumophila are bodies of water such as rivers, lakes, and streams, where the organism typically is present in small numbers. L. pneumophila also has been recovered from river banks and mud, but not from dry soil. In the environment, it is believed to exist in symbiosis with other micro-organisms, such as freshwater amoebae and ciliated protozoa, rather than as a free-living aquatic bacterium (88–90). Because it is tolerant of chlorination, it can survive the usual water-treatment process and colonize various manmade habitats, such as cooling towers and water distribution systems, that provide an appropriate temperature, sediment accumulation, and commensal microflora (91–94). L. pneumophila prefers higher temperatures, and in storage tanks it is most likely to be found in the bottom of the tank, on the surface of sediment. The sediment apparently stimulates the growth of commensal bacteria, which in turn stimulate the growth of L. pneumophila (91).

The source of human infection with Legionella pneumophila has been shown by epidemiologic studies to be contaminated water-distribution systems such as evaporative condensers, cooling towers, and potable water-distribution systems in hospitals (60,94–100). Community-acquired Legionnaires' disease has been linked to contaminated residential and industrial water supplies (101,102). The exact mechanism of transmission of L. pneumophila is uncertain, but airborne spread by aerosolization is the favored hypothesis. Aerosols created by air conditioning systems, shower heads, and nebulizers have been implicated (103–107). Moreover, aspiration of contaminated water or contaminated oropharyngeal secretions has been suggested as a potential mechanism of transmission (108,109).

Most species of Legionella other than Legionella pneumophila inhabit natural bodies of water; however, Legionella wadsworthii, Legionella hackeliae, Legionella birminghamensis, and Legionella cincinnatiensis have not been isolated from the environment. Moreover, Legionella micdadei, Legionella bozemanii, Legionella dumoffii, and Legionella feeleii have been recovered from water-distribution systems (80,110–112). Outbreaks of nosocomial pneumonia caused by Legionella dumoffii and by Legionella bozemanii have been linked to contaminated respiratory therapy equipment and room humidifiers and to contamination of the hospital water-distribution system, respectively (80,111). The mechanism of transmission of the species of Legionella other than Legionella pneumophila is unknown, but aspiration of contaminated water or oropharyngeal secretions is possible.

The prevalence of infection with Legionella depends on the extent to which water sources are contaminated with the organisms, the susceptibility of individuals exposed to that water, and the intensity of the exposure. Legionella pneumophila, especially serogroup 1, is responsible for about 85% of human lung infections, Legionella micdadei for about 6% and Legionella bozemanii, Legionella dumoffii, and Legionella longbeachae for most of the remainder (69). Pontiac fever has been caused by Legionella pneumophila and by Legionella feeleii (60,81).

Epidemics of Legionnaires' disease have occurred on three continents (113). In prospective studies of community-acquired pneumonias, the prevalence of sporadic Legionnaires' disease has ranged from 1 to 15% and the prevalence of nosocomial disease from 1 to 40% (94). Risk factors for Legionnaires' disease or for fatal infection include cigarette smoking, advanced age, chronic lung disease, and immunosuppression, especially associated with organ transplantation; in some studies, excessive alcohol intake has been a risk factor; and surgery is a major predisposing factor for nosocomial infection (60,94,114). Legionnaires' disease primarily affects adults, but it has been reported in immunosuppressed children.

Pathogenesis and Pathology

Once Legionella organisms reach the upper respiratory tract they probably are cleared by the mucociliary process, a theory supported by the fact that conditions associated with impaired mucociliary clearance—cigarette smoking, chronic pulmonary disease, alcoholism—are consistent factors that predispose to Legionnaires' disease. After bacteria reach the alveoli, the outcome of the infection depends on the virulence of the bacteria and the immune response of the host. The first line of host defense, and the most critical component, is the alveolar macrophage, which readily ingests the bacteria, although phagocytosis is enhanced by specific opsonizing antibodies (60,94). Inside the macrophage virulent Legionella pneumophila, enclosed in a specialized phagosome, inhibit phagolysosomal fusion and acidification of the phagosome, thus escaping the microbicidal mechanisms of the macrophage. The bacteria multiply within cells until the cell ruptures, releasing additional bacteria to be phagocytosed by newly recruited macrophages.

The second phase of defense begins with an influx of polymorphonuclear leukocytes into the lungs. Monocytes then are recruited from the blood and transform into macrophages, resulting in an infiltrate of nearly equal numbers of neutrophils and mononuclear cells. Legionella organisms fix to their surfaces the complement component C3, which acts as a ligand available for binding to the C3 receptor on the monocyte, facilitating phagocytosis of the organism, a process enhanced by specific opsonizing antibodies (115,116). The exact role of neutrophils in defense against Legionella is unclear.

Cell-mediated immunity apparently is the primary host defense against Legionella, as it is for other intracellular pathogens. Legionnaires' disease is more common and more severe in persons with depressed cell-mediated immunity and those with hairy cell leukemia, a malignancy characterized by monocyte deficiency and dysfunction (117). Specific cell-mediated immunity develops during the first 2 weeks of infection (94,118–120). Mononuclear cells respond to Legionella pneumophila antigens by proliferating and generating the monocyte-activating cytokines interferon α and interleukin 1 (121,122). Activated macrophages inhibit intracellular multiplication, but killing of the organisms is not enhanced (123). However, mononuclear cells infected with L. pneumophila are killed by natural killer–like cells activated by interleukin 2 (124). Humoral immunity appears to play only a secondary role in host defense, promoting modest killing of L. pneumophila by phagocytes (116,123).

Strains of Legionella pneumophila differ in virulence; however virulence factors of the organism have not been elucidated completely. L. pneumophila produces a protease that may damage tissue (125). Recently, a gene designated *mip* that encodes a surface protein (molecular weight, 24,000) was shown to be necessary for full virulence of the organism (126).

The lungs of persons with Legionnaires' disease typically show multifocal bronchopneumonia, occasionally with abscess formation, but Legionella pneumophila may produce lobar pneumonia resembling disease caused by Streptococcus pneumoniae (see Chapter 28) (127). Histologic examination of involved tissue shows a mixed inflammatory infiltrate composed of polymorphonuclear leukocytes and macrophages, usually with one cell type predominating, in the alveoli, respiratory bronchioles, and terminal bronchioles, sparing the proximal bronchioles. Lysis of the inflammatory exudate is characteristic, but not pathognomonic, of infection with Legionella pneumophila and may suggest the correct diagnosis. Diffuse alveolar damage with hyaline membranes occurs occasionally, and infrequently the airspaces are filled with proteinaceous material but few cells.

Clinical Manifestations

Infection with Legionella is manifest in two different forms, Pontiac fever and Legionnaires' disease. Why these different forms occur is not known, but the inoculum, mode of transmission, and host factors may be important. Pontiac fever, an acute, self-limited, flulike illness without pneumonia, begins after an incubation period of 24 to 48 hours with malaise, myalgia, fever, chills, and headache, occasionally accompanied by nonproductive cough, dizziness, and nausea. Symptoms generally resolve within a week.

Symptoms of Legionnaires' disease range from mild cough with low-grade fever to coma with multilobar pneumonia and multisystem failure. Typically, the illness begins after an incubation period of 2 to 10 days with nonspecific symptoms of fever, malaise, myalgia, anorexia, and headache, followed in 1 to 2 days by cough that is productive of nonpurulent, occasionally bloody or watery sputum, chest pain, and sometimes shaking chills. Diarrhea occurs in 25 to 50% of cases and nausea, vomiting, and abdominal pain in 10 to 20%. Neurologic symptoms range from headache and lethargy to encephalopathy, but a change in mental status is the most common (128). The mortality rate is low in immunocompetent persons treated with appropriate antimicrobial therapy, but it approaches 50% in nosocomial infections, especially if therapy is delayed (94).

Laboratory Diagnosis

Specimens that may be submitted for diagnosis of infections caused by Legionella include sputum, other types of respiratory secretions (transtracheal aspirate, bronchial washings, bronchoalveolar lavage fluid, pleural fluid), lung and transbronchial biopsy tissue (fresh tissue, imprints of fresh tissue, frozen sections, and formalin-fixed paraffin-embedded tissue), blood, serum, and urine. Sputum specimens are preferable to specimens collected by bronchoscopy, because the latter are diluted by saline and may contain small amounts of inhibitory local anesthetic. Screening sputum specimens to determine their adequacy is not necessary. In persons with Legionnaires' disease organisms generally can be detected in respiratory secretions, even for several days after antimicrobial therapy is instituted; therefore, the initial specimen from an infected individual often demonstrates the organism. However, if the disease is strongly suspected, additional samples should be collected. All specimens should be transported to the laboratory without transport medium, buffers, or saline, which may inhibit the growth of Legionella, within 60 minutes of collection or stored in the refrigerator if a longer delay is anticipated. Specimen processing is discussed in Chapter 57.

The reference method for diagnosis of infections caused by Legionella is culture, which has a sensitivity of 50 to 90% and a specificity of 100% (60). On buffered charcoal yeast extract (BCYE) agar containing α-ketoglutaric acid (the recommended nonselective medium for isolating Legionella), glistening, convex, circular colonies with a multifaceted surface, often described as resembling cut glass, usually appear after incubation for 2 to 5 days at 35° C in a humid atmosphere, in ambient air, or in a candle jar. Growth of Legionella gormanii only is stimulated by carbon dioxide, and concentrations of carbon dioxide over 5% may inhibit some Legionella; therefore, incubation in air is preferred. Colonies of Legionella bozemanii, Legionella dumoffii, and Legionella gormanii fluoresce blue-white under long-wave (366 nm) ultraviolet light. Isolates that have colony and cellular structures and growth characteristics typical of Legionella and are weakly catalase positive should be subcultured to sheep blood– and BCYE agar. If growth occurs only on BCYE agar, further characterization by staining a smear with commercially available fluorescein-conjugated antibodies or by nucleic acid hybridization (discussed later) should be performed. Isolates not identified by one of these methods should be sent to a reference laboratory for definitive characterization.

Because the sensitivity of culture for detection of Legionella is less than 100% and because growth usually is not apparent for several days, performing culture and either the direct fluorescent antibody test or nucleic acid hybridization on specimens from persons suspected to have Legionnaires' disease is recommended (129–131). The direct immunofluorescence assay (DFA) using commercially available polyvalent antisera or monoclonal antibodies has a sensitivity of 20 to 70% and a specificity of 90 to 95%, depending on the experience of the microbiologist interpreting the test and the quality of the microscope (130–132). Some isolates of Staphylococcus aureus, Streptococcus pneumoniae, and other species of Streptococcus may fluoresce owing to natural antibodies in the conjugate or to the nonspecific reaction of IgG with components in the cell walls of the bacteria; however, the coccal forms of these organisms generally are easily distinguished from the coccobacillary to rod-shaped Legionella (132). Some species of Pseudomonas, Xanthomonas maltophilia, a few strains of Bacteroides fragilis, and some strains of Bordetella pertussis cross-react with the polyclonal reagents, potentially causing false-positive test results (133–136). The interpretation of the DFA is based on the source of the specimen and the number of positive organisms observed in the smear, using the 25 × objective (Table 33–4) (132).

A genus-specific nucleic acid probe that detects Legionella ribosomal ribonucleic acid is commercially available. Results may be available within a few hours of receiving the specimen; and its sensitivity appears to be comparable to that of the direct immunofluorescence assay, although false-positive results have been reported (137). An advantage of the probe is that all species and serotypes of Legionella are detected, whereas the number of species and serotypes identified by available antisera is limited. The probe cannot replace culture but may be used as an alternative to DFA, depending on the cost-effectiveness of the two methods (138).

Table 33–4. Guidelines for Interpretation of the Legionella DFA

Specimen	Bacteria* (No)	Interpretation
Smear of lung tissue	≥25	Positive
	<25	Report number seen
	0	Negative
Sputum and other respiratory secretions	≥5	Positive
	<5	Negative

* Strongly fluorescing bacteria with a consistent cellular morphology.
(Data from Koneman EW, et al (eds): Legionella. In Color Atlas and Textbook of Diagnostic Microbiology. 3rd ed. Philadelphia, JB Lippincott, 1988.)

A soluble antigen of Legionella pneumophila serogroup 1 may be detected in urine during the illness and for months thereafter by radioimmunoassay, ELISA, and latex agglutination (139–141). The sensitivity of these tests for diagnosing infection with L. pneumophila serogroup 1 ranges from 75 to 90%, and the specificity is 100%. The primary drawback of antigen detection for diagnosis is that only infections with L. pneumophila serogroup 1 are recognized; however, this organism causes about 70% of cases of Legionnaires' disease (142).

Infections by Legionella may be diagnosed by detecting specific antibodies in serum, using indirect immunofluorescence or ELISA. The sensitivity of the indirect immunofluorescence assay is 75 to 80% and the specificity about 96%; cross-reactions have occurred in persons with infections caused by other organisms—Mycoplasma pneumoniae, Coxiella burnetii, Francisella tularensis, Bacteroides fragilis, and Pseudomonas aeruginosa (94,132). The major drawback of serologic testing is that acute- and convalescent-phase serum samples collected 4 to 8 weeks apart must be tested, which significantly delays diagnosis. A fourfold or greater rise in antibody titer, to 1:128 or higher, indicates recent infection with Legionella (142). A single titer of 1:256 or greater may suggest recent infection during an outbreak but does not indicate recent infection with Legionella in a person who has sporadic pneumonia, because titers of this level may persist in healthy persons who have no current clinical evidence of legionellosis (132).

Treatment and Prevention

Currently, erythromycin is the treatment of choice for legionellosis. Alternatively, tetracyclines (especially doxycycline), trimethoprim-sulfamethoxazole, imipenem, and ciprofloxacin have been used successfully (94,143). Symptoms generally improve in 3 to 5 days.

Nosocomial Legionnaires' disease linked to water-distribution systems can be prevented by eradicating Legionella from the water system. Disinfection modalities include hyperchlorination, thermal eradication, instantaneous steam heating, ozonation, ultraviolet light, and metal ionization; an excellent discussion of the costs, advantages, and disadvantages associated with each is provided in reference 144.

REFERENCES

1. Ohara S: Studies on Yato-Byo (Ohara's disease, tularemia in Japan), report I. Jpn J Exp Med, 24:69, 1954.
2. McCoy GW: Plague-like disease of rodents. Public Health Bull, 43:53, 1911.
3. Wherry WB, and Lamb BH: Infection of man with Bacterium tularense. J Infect Dis, 15:331, 1914.
4. Parker RR, Spencer RR, and Francis E: Tularemia XI: Tularemia infection in ticks of the species Dermacentor andersoni, stiles in the Bitterroot Valley, Montana. Public Health Rep, 39:1057, 1924.
5. Parker RR, and Spencer RR: Hereditary transmission of tularemia infection by the wood tick, Dermacentor andersoni, Stiles. Public Health Rep, 41:1403, 1926.
6. Francis E: A summary of the present knowledge of tularemia. Medicine (Baltimore), 7:411, 1928.

7. Rockwood SW: Tularemia: What's in a name? Am Soc Microbiol News, *48*:63, 1983.
8. Warring WB, and Ruffin JS, Jr: A tick-borne epidemic of tularemia. N Engl J Med, *234*:137, 1946.
9. Klock LE, Olsen PF, and Fukushima T: Tularemia epidemic associated with the deerfly. JAMA, *226*:149, 1973.
10. Syrjala H, et al: Airborne transmission of tularemia in farmers. Scand J Infect Dis, *17*:371, 1985.
11. Teutsch SM, et al: Pneumonic tularemia on Martha's Vineyard. N Engl J Med, *301*:826, 1979.
12. Evans ME, Gregory DW, Schaffner W, and McGee ZA: Tularemia: A 30-year experience with 88 cases. Medicine, *64*:251, 1985.
13. Centers for Disease Control: Summary of notifiable diseases, United States, 1989. MMWR, *38*(54):1, 1989.
14. Boyce JM: Francisella tularensis (tularemia). *In* Principles and Practice of Infectious Diseases. 3rd ed. Edited by GL Mandell, RG Douglas, Jr, and JE Bennett. New York, Churchill Livingstone, 1990.
15. Mikolich DJ, and Boyce JM: Brucella species. *In* Principles and Practice of Infectious Diseases. 3rd ed. Edited by GL Mandell, RG Douglas, Jr, and JE Bennett. New York, Churchill Livingstone, 1990.
16. Fox MD, and Kaufmann AF: Brucellosis in the United States, 1964–1974. J Infect Dis, *136*:312, 1977.
17. Centers for Disease Control: Brucellosis Surveillance. Annual Summary, 1975. Atlanta, Centers for Disease Control, 1976.
18. Centers for Disease Control: Brucellosis Surveillance. Annual Survey, 1978. Atlanta, Centers for Disease Control, 1979.
19. Thapar MK, and Young EJ: Urban outbreak of goat cheese brucellosis. Pediatr Infect Dis, *5*:640, 1986.
20. Meyer ME: Brucellosis. *In* Immunological Diseases. Edited by M Samter. Boston, Little, Brown, 1978.
21. Buchanan TM, Faber LC, and Feldman RA: Brucellosis in the United States, 1960–1972. An abattoir-associated disease. Part I. Clinical features and therapy. Medicine, *53*:403, 1974.
22. Lulu AR, Araj GF, and Khateeb MI: Human brucellosis in Kuwait: A prospective study of 400 cases. Q J Med, *249*:39, 1988.
23. Mousa ARM, et al: Osteoarticular complications of brucellosis: A study of 169 cases. Rev Infect Dis, *9*:531, 1987.
24. Mousa ARM, et al: Brucella meningitis: Presentation, diagnosis and treatment—a prospective study of ten cases. Q J Med, *223*:873, 1986.
25. Bouza E, et al: Brucellar meningitis. Rev Infect Dis, *9*:810, 1987.
26. Ibrahim AIA, Awad R, and Shetty SD: Genitourinary complications of brucellosis. Br J Urol, *61*:294, 1988.
27. Al-Kasab S, et al: Brucella infective edocarditis. Successful combined medical and surgical therapy. Thorac Cardiovasc Surg, *95*:862, 1988.
28. Perry TM, and Belter LF: Brucellosis and heart disease II. Fatal brucellosis. A review of the literature and report of new cases. Am J Pathol, *36*:673, 1960.
29. Cervantes F, et al: Liver disease in brucellosis. A clinical and pathological study of 40 cases. Postgrad Med J, *58*:346, 1982.
30. Berger TG, Guill MA, and Goette DK: Cutaneous lesions in brucellosis. Arch Dermatol, *117*:40, 1981.
31. Joint FAO/WHO Expert Committee on Brucellosis. Geneva, World Health Organization, 1986.
32. Plommet M, Serre A, and Fensterbank R: Vaccines, vaccination in brucellosis. Ann Inst Pasteur Microbiol, *138*:117, 1987.
33. Major RH: A History of Medicine. Vol. 1. Springfield, IL, Charles C Thomas, 1954.
34. Bordet J, and Gengou O: Le microbe de la coqueluche. Ann Inst Pasteur, *20*:731, 1906.
35. Centers for Disease Control: Summary of notifiable diseases, United States, 1990. MMWR, *39*(53):1, 1990.
36. Cherry JD: The epidemiology of pertussis and pertussis immunization in the United Kingdom and the United States. A comparative study. Curr Prob Pediatr, *14*:1, 1984.
37. Romanus V, Jonsell R, and Bergquist SO: Pertussis in Sweden after the cessation of general immunization in 1979. Pediatr Infect Dis J, *6*:364, 1987.
38. Hewlett EL: Bordetella species. *In* Principles and Practice of Infectious Diseases. 3rd ed. Edited by GL Mandell, RG Douglas, Jr, and JE Bennett. New York, Churchill Livingstone, 1990.
39. Biellik RJ, et al: Risk factors for community- and household-acquired pertussis during a largescale outbreak in central Wisconsin. J Infect Dis, *157*:1134, 1988.
40. Lambert HJ: Epidemiology of a small pertussis outbreak in Kent County, Michigan. Public Health Rep, *80*:365, 1965.
41. Friedman RL: Pertussis: The disease and new diagnostic methods. Clin Microbiol Rev, *1*:365, 1988.
42. Tamura M, et al: A role of the B-oligomer moiety of islet-activating protein, pertussis toxin, in development of the biological effects on intact cells. J Biol Chem, *258*:6756, 1983.
43. Tamura M, et al: Subunit structure of islet-activating factor, pertussis toxin, in conformity with the A-B model. Biochemistry, *21*:5516, 1982.
44. Sato H, and Sato Y: Bordetella pertussis infection in mice: Correlation of specific antibodies against two antigens, pertussis toxin, and filamentous hemagglutinin with mouse protectivity in an intracerebral or aerosol challenge system. Infect Immun, *46*:415, 1984.
45. Granstrom M, Granstrom G, Gillenius P, and Askelof P: Neutralizing antibodies to pertussis toxin in whooping cough. J Infect Dis, *151*:646, 1985.
46. Weiss AA, and Hewlett EL: Virulence factors of Bordetella pertussis. Annu Rev Microbiol, *40*:661, 1986.
47. Centers for Disease Control: Pertussis—United States, 1982 and 1983. MMWR, *33*:573, 1984.
48. Linnemann CC, Jr, and Nasenbeny J: Pertussis in the adult. Annu Rev Med, *38*:177, 1977.
49. Doebbeling BN, Feilmeier NL, and Herwaldt LA: Pertussis in an adult man infected with the human immunodeficiency virus. J Infect Dis, *161*:1296, 1990.
50. Gilchrist MJR: Bordetella. *In* Manual of Clinical Microbiology. 5th ed. Edited by A Balows, et al. Washington, DC, American Society for Microbiology, 1991.
51. Stauffer LR, Brown DR, and Sandstrom RE: Cephalexin-supplemented Jones-Kendrick charcoal agar for selective isolation of Bordetella pertussis: Comparison with previously described media. J Clin Microbiol, *17*:60, 1983.
52. Goodman YE, Wort AJ, and Jackson FL: Enzyme-linked immunosorbent assay for detection of pertussis immunoglobulin A in nasopharyngeal secretions as an indicator of recent infection. J Clin Microbiol, *132*:286, 1981.
53. Confer DL, and Eaton JW: Bordetella adenylate cyclase: Host toxicity and diagnostic utility. Dev Biol Stand, *61*:3, 1985.
54. Friedman RS, Paulaitis S, and McMillan JW: Development of a rapid diagnostic test for pertussis: direct detection of pertussis toxin in respiratory secretions. J Clin Microbiol, *27*:2466, 1989.
55. Cody CL, et al: Nature and rates of adverse reactions associ-

ated with DTP and DT immunizations in infants and children. Pediatrics, 68:650, 1981.
56. Cherry JD, et al: Report of the task force on pertussis and pertussis immunization—1988. Pediatrics, 81(suppl):939, 1988.
57. Hinman AR, and Koplan JP: Pertussis and pertussis vaccine: Reanalysis of benefits, risks and costs. JAMA, 251:3109, 1984.
58. Isomura S: Efficacy and safety of acellular pertussis vaccine to Aichi Prefecture, Japan. Pediatr Infect Dis, 7:258, 1988.
59. Ad Hoc Group for the Study of Pertussis Vaccines: Placebo-controlled trial of two acellular pertussis vaccines in Sweden—protective efficacy and adverse effects. Lancet, i: 955, 1988.
60. Winn WC, Jr: Legionnaires' disease: Historical perspective. Clin Microbiol Rev, 1:60, 1988.
61. Osterholm M, et al: A 1957 outbreak of Legionnaires' disease associated with a meat-packing plant. Am J Epidemiol, 117:60, 1983.
62. Terranova W, Cohen ML, and Fraser DW: 1974 outbreak of Legionnaires' disease diagnosed in 1977. Clinical and epidemiological features. Lancet, ii:122, 1978.
63. Thacker SB, et al: An outbreak in 1965 of severe respiratory illness caused by Legionnaires' disease bacterium. J Infect Dis, 138:512, 1978.
64. Glick TH, et al: Pontiac fever. An epidemic of unknown etiology in a health department. I. Clinical and epidemiologic aspects. Am J Epidemiol, 107:149, 1978.
65. Hebert GA, et al: The rickettsia-like organisms TATLOCK (1943) and HEBA (1959): Bacteria phenotypically similar to but genetically distinct from Legionella pneumophila and the WIGA bacterium. Ann Intern Med, 92:45, 1980.
66. Pasculle AW, et al: Pittsburgh pneumonia agent: Direct isolation from human lung tissue. J Infect Dis, 141:727, 1980.
67. McDade JE, Brenner DJ, and Bozeman FN: Legionnaires' disease bacterium isolated in 1947. Ann Intern Med, 90: 659, 1979.
68. Brenner DJ, Steigerwalt AG, and McDade JE: Classification of the Legionnaires' disease bacterium: Legionella pneumophila, genus novum, species nova, of the family Legionellaceae, familia nova. Ann Intern Med, 90:656, 1979.
69. Fang GD, Yu VL, and Vickers RM: Disease due to the Legionellaceae (other than Legionella pneumophila): Historical microbiological, clinical and epidemiological review. Medicine, 68:116, 1989.
70. Fang GD, and Tu VL: Other Legionella species. In Principles and Practice of Infectious Diseases. 3rd ed. Edited by GL Mandell, RG Douglas, Jr, and JE Bennett. New York, Churchill Livingstone, 1990.
71. Thacker WL, et al: Second serogroup of Legionella feeleii strains isolated from humans. J Clin Microbiol, 22:1, 1985.
72. Wilkinson HW, et al: Fatal Legionella maceachernii pneumonia. J Clin Microbiol, 22:1055, 1985.
73. Edelstein PH, et al: Legionella wadsworthii species nova: A cause of human pneumonia. Ann Intern Med, 97:809, 1982.
74. Tang PW, Toma S, and MacMillan LG: Legionella oakridgenis: Laboratory diagnosis of a human infection. J Clin Microbiol, 21:462, 1985.
75. Mehta P, Patel JD, and Milder JE: Legionella micdadei (Pittsburgh pneumonia agent): Two infections with unusual clinical features. JAMA, 249:1620, 1983.
76. Fang GD, Yu VL, and Vickers RM: Infections caused by the Pittsburgh pneumonia agent. Semin Respir Infect, 2:262, 1987.
77. Wilkinson HW, et al. Second serogroup of Legionella hackeliae isolated from a patient with pneumonia. J Clin Microbiol, 22:488, 1985.
78. Griffith ME, et al: First isolation of Legionella gormanii from human disease. J Clin Microbiol, 26:380, 1988.
79. Baron EJ, and Finegold SM (eds): Unclassified or unusual but easily cultivated etiologic agents of infectious disease. In Bailey and Scott's Diagnostic Microbiology. 8th ed. St. Louis, CV Mosby, 1990.
80. Parry MF, et al: Waterborne Legionella bozemanii and nosocomial pneumonia in immunosuppressed patients. Ann Intern Med, 103:205, 1985.
81. Herwaldt LA, et al: A new Legionella species, Legionella feeleii species novo, causes Pontiac fever in an automobile plant. Ann Intern Med, 100:333, 1984.
82. Wilkinson HW, et al: Legionella birminghamensis sp. nov. isolated from cardiac transplant recipient. J Clin Microbiol, 25:2120, 1987.
83. Thacker WL, et al: Legionella cincinnatiensis sp. nov. isolated from a patient with pneumonia. J Clin Microbiol, 26: 418, 1988.
84. Brenner DJ, Steigerwalt A, and Gorman GW: Legionella bozemanii, sp. nov. and Legionella dumoffii sp. nov.: Classification of two additional species of Legionella associated with human pneumonia. Curr Microbiol, 4:111, 1980.
85. McKinney RM, et al: Legionella longbeachae species novo, another etiologic agent of human pneumonia. Ann Intern Med, 94:739, 1981.
86. Thacker WL, et al: Legionella jordanis isolated from a patient with fatal pneumonia. J Clin Microbiol, 28:1400, 1988.
87. Benson RF, et al: Legionella adelaidensis, a new species isolated from cooling tower water. J Clin Microbiol, 29: 1004, 1991.
88. Rowbotham TJ: Isolation of L. pneumophila from clinical specimens via amoebae, and the interaction of those and other isolates with amoebae. J Clin Pathol, 36:978, 1983.
89. Holden EP, et al: Intracellular growth of L. pneumophila within Acanthamoeba casteanni neff. Infect Immun, 45:18, 1984.
90. Fields BS, et al: Proliferation of Legionella pneumophila as an intracellular parasite of the ciliated protozoan, Tetrahymena pyriformis. Appl Environ Microbiol, 47:467, 1984.
91. Stout JE, Yu VL, and Best M: Ecology of Legionella pneumophila within water distribution systems. Appl Environ Microbiol, 49:221, 1985.
92. Lee TC, Stout JE, and Yu VL: Factors predisposing to L. pneumophila colonization in residential water systems. Arch Environ Health, 43:59, 1988.
93. Groothuis DG, Veenendaal HR, and Dijkstra HL: Influence of temperature on the number of Legionella pneumophila in hot water systems. J Appl Bacteriol, 59:529, 1985.
94. Yu VL: Legionella pneumophila (Legionnaires' disease). In Principles and Practice of Infectious Diseases. 3rd ed. Edited by GL Mandell, RG Douglas, Jr, and JE Bennett. New York, Churchill Livingstone, 1990.
95. Mangione EJ, et al: An outbreak of Pontiac fever related to whirlpool use, Michigan, 1982. JAMA, 77:535, 1985.
96. Friedman S, et al: Pontiac fever outbreak associated with a cooling tower. Am J Public Health, 77:568, 1987.
97. Girod JC, et al: Pneumonic and nonpneumonic forms of legionellosis. The result of a common-source exposure to Legionella pneumophila. Arch Intern Med, 142:545, 1982.
98. Fraser DW: Potable water as a source for legionellosis. Environ Health Perspect, 62:337, 1985.
99. Dondero TJ, et al: An outbreak of Legionnaires' disease associated with a contaminated air-conditioning cooling tower. N Engl J Med, 302:365, 1980.
100. Arnow PM, et al: Nosocomial Legionnaires' disease caused

100. by aerosolized tap water from respiratory devices. J Infect Dis, *146*:460, 1982.
101. Stout J, Yu VL, and Muraca P: Legionnaires' disease acquired from the water supply within the homes of two patients. JAMA, *257*:1215, 1987.
102. Centers for Disease Control: Legionnaires' disease outbreak associated with a grocery store mist machine—Louisiana, 1989. MMWR, *39*:108, 1990.
103. Bollin GE, et al: Aerosols containing Legionella pneumophila generated by shower heads and hot water faucets. Appl Environ Microbiol, *50*:1128, 1985.
104. Woo AH, Yu VL, and Goetz A: Potential in-hospital mode of transmission for Legionella pneumophila: Demonstration experiments for dissemination by showers, humidifiers, and rinsing of ventilation bag apparatus. Am J Med, *80*:567, 1986.
105. Dennis P, et al: Legionella pneumphila in aerosols from shower baths. J Hyg, *93*:349, 1984.
106. Zuravleff JJ, et al: Legionella pneumophila contamination of a hospital humidifier: Demonstration of aerosol transmission and subsequent subclinical infection in exposed guinea pigs. Am Rev Respir Dis, *138*:657, 1983.
107. Mastro TD, et al: Nosocomial Legionnaires' disease and use of medication nebulizers. J Infect Dis, *163*:667, 1991.
108. Yu VL, Stout J, and Zuravleff JJ: Aspiration of contaminated water may be a mode of transmission for Legionella pneumophila [abstract]. *In* Program and Abstracts of 21st Interscience Conference on Antimicrobial Agents and Chemotherapy. Chicago, American Society for Microbiology, 1981.
109. Marrie T, et al: Nasogastric tubes flushed with contaminated potable water are a risk factor for nosocomial Legionella pneumophila [abstract]. *In* Program and Abstracts of the 28th Interscience Conference on Antimicrobial Agents and Chemotherapy. Los Angeles, American Society for Microbiology, 1988.
110. Best M, et al: Legionellaceae in the hospital water supply—epidemiological link with disease and evaluation of a method of control of nosocomial Legionnaires' disease and Pittsburgh pneumonia. Lancet, *ii*:307, 1983.
111. Joly JR, et al: Legionnaires' disease caused by Legionella dumoffii in distilled water. Can Med Assoc J, *135*:1274, 1986.
112. Palutke WA, et al: Legionella feeleii–associated pneumonia in humans. Am J Clin Pathol, *86*:348, 1986.
113. Bartlett CLR, Macrae AD, and Macfarlane JT: Legionella infections. London, Edward Arnold, 1986.
114. Dowling JN, et al: Infections caused by Legionella micdadei and Legionella pneumophila among renal transplant recipients. J Infect Dis, *149*:703, 1984.
115. Payne NR, and Horwitz MA: Phagocytosis of Legionella pneumophila is mediated by human monocyte complement receptors. J Exp Med, *166*:1377, 1987.
116. Horwitz MA, and Silverstein SC: Interaction of the Legionnaires' disease bacterium (Legionella pneumophila) with human phagocytes. I. L. pneumophila resists killing by polymorphonuclear leukocytes, antibody, and complement. J Exp Med, *153*:386, 1981.
117. Cordonnier C, Farcet JP, and Desforges L: Legionnaires' disease and hairy-cell leukemia. Arch Intern Med, *144*: 2373, 1984.
118. Friedman H, et al: Cellular immunity to L. pneumophila in guinea pigs assessed by direct and indirect migration inhibition; reaction in vitro. Infect Immun, *41*:1132, 1983.
119. Wong KH, et al: Detection of hypersensitivity to L. pneumophila in guinea pigs by skin test. Curr Top Microbiol Immunol, *4*:105, 1980.
120. Horwitz MA: Cell-mediated immunity in Legionnaires' disease. J Clin Invest, *71*:1686, 1983.
121. Bhardwaj N, Nash T, and Horwitz MA: Interferon-γ–activated human monocytes inhibit the intracellular multiplication of L. pneumophila. J Immunol, *137*:2662, 1986.
122. Klein TW, et al: Induction of interleukin 1 by Legionella pneumophila antigens in mouse and human mononuclear leukocyte cultures. Zentralbl Bakteriol Mikrobiol Hyg [A], *265*:462, 1987.
123. Nash TW, Libby D, and Horwitz MA: Interaction between the Legionnaires' disease bacterium (L. pneumophila) and human alveolar macrophages: Influence of antibody, lymphokines, and hydrocortisone. J Clin Invest, *74*:771, 1984.
124. Blanchard DK, et al: Cytolytic activity of human peripheral blood leukocytes against Legionella pneumophila–infected monocytes: Characterization of the effector. J Immunol, *139*:551, 1987.
125. Baskerville A, Conlan JW, Ashworth LA, and Dowsett AB: Pulmonary damage caused by a protease from Legionella pneumophila. Br J Exp Pathol, *67*:527, 1986.
126. Cianciotto NP, Eisenstein BI, Mody CH, and Engleberg NC: A mutation in the *mip* gene results in an attenuation of Legionella pneumophila virulence. J Infect Dis, *162*:121, 1990.
127. Winn WC, Jr, and Myerowitz RL: The pathology of the Legionella pneumonias. Hum Pathol, *12*:401, 1981.
128. Johnson JD, Raff M, and VanArsdall J: Neurologic manifestations of Legionnaires' disease. Medicine, *63*:303, 1984.
129. Rodgers FG, and Pasculle AW: Legionella. *In* Manual of Clinical Microbiology. 5th ed. Edited by A Balows, et al. Washington, DC, American Society for Microbiology, 1991.
130. Edelstein PH, Meyer RD, and Finegold SM: Laboratory diagnosis of Legionnaires' disease. Am Rev Respir Dis, *121*:317, 1980.
131. Winn WC, Jr, and Pasculle AW: Laboratory diagnosis of infections caused by Legionella species. Clin Lab Med, *2*: 343, 1982.
132. Koneman EW, et al: Legionella. *In* Color Atlas and Textbook of Diagnostic Microbiology. 3rd ed. Edited by EW Koneman, et al. Philadelphia, JB Lippincott, 1988.
133. Orrison LH, Bibb WF, Cherry WB, and Thacker L: Determination of antigenic relationships among legionellae and nonlegionellae by direct flurescent-antibody and immunodiffusion tests. J Clin Microbiol, *17*:332, 1983.
134. Edelstein PH, and Edelstein MA: Evaluation of the Merifluor-Legionella immunofluorescent reagent for identifying and detecting 21 Legionella species. J Clin Microbiol, *27*: 2455, 1989.
135. Benson RE, Lanier-Thacker W. Plikaytis BB, and Wilkinson HW. Cross-reactions in Legionella antisera and Bordetella pertussis strains. J Clin Microbiol, *25*:594, 1987.
136. Laboratory Center for Disease Control: Cross-reactivity noted between a strain of Bordetella pertussis and Legionella antisera. Can Dis Weekly Rep, *13*:196, 1987.
137. Laussucq S, et al: False-positive DNA probe for Legionella species associated with a cluster of respiratory illnesses. J Clin Microbiol, *26*:1442, 1988.
138. Doebbeling BN, et al: Prospective evaluation of the Gen-Probe assay for detection of Legionellae in respiratory specimens. Eur J Clin Microbiol Infect Dis, 7:748, 1988.
139. Kohler RB: Antigen detection for the rapid diagnosis of Mycoplasma and Legionella pneumonia. Diagn Microbiol Infect Dis, *4*(suppl 3):47, 1986.
140. Kohler RB, Winn WC, and Wheat LJ: Onset and duration of urinary antigen excretion in Legionnaires' disease. J Clin Microbiol, *20*:605, 1984.

141. Kohler RB: Legionella antigenuria: Testing and interpretation. Clin Microbiol Newslett, *12*:185, 1990.
142. Wilkinson HW, et al: Reactivity of serum from patients with suspected legionellosis against 29 antigens of Legionellaceae and Legionella-like organisms by indirect immunofluorescence assay. J Infect Dis, *147*:23, 1983.
143. Miller AC: Erythromycin in Legionnaires' disease: A reappraisal. J Antimicrob Chemother, 7:217, 1981.
144. Muraca PW, Yu VL, and Goetz A: Disinfection of water distribution systems for Legionella: A review of application procedures and methodologies. Infect Control Hosp Epidemiol, *11*:79, 1990.

Chapter 34

ENTEROBACTERIACEAE

Members of the family Enterobacteriaceae are facultative gram-negative bacilli that ferment glucose and share several characteristics that differentiate them from other glucose-fermenting facultative gram-negative bacilli, most of which belong to the families Vibrionaceae and Pasteurellaceae (Chapters 35 and 36). The Enterobacteriaceae are oxidase negative, reduce nitrates to nitrites (except some Enterobacter, Erwinia, Klebsiella, and Yersinia); do not require sodium chloride for growth nor does it enhance their growth; and (except Tatumella) are motile by peritrichous flagella or are immotile. The negative oxidase or lack of sodium chloride requirement, or both, distinguish Enterobacteriaceae from Vibrionaceae; and negative oxidase or no requirement for organic nitrogen sources, or both, separate them from Pasteurellaceae.

The Enterobacericeae are found on plants, in the soil, and as a component of the normal flora in the intestines of animals and humans. These organisms uncommonly are normal flora of other sites of healthy persons, but they frequently colonize the oral cavity, and occasionally the skin of hospital patients. Members of the Enterobacteriaceae are the organisms most frequently isolated from clinical specimens, accounting for up to 80% of clinically significant isolates of gram-negative bacilli, up to 50% of cases of septicemia, 60 to 70% of cases of bacterial gastroenteritis, and more than 70% of urinary tract infections (1).

More than 20 genera and more than 100 species are classified in the family Enterobacteriaceae, and additional species are confirmed constantly (2). Members of the Enterobacteriaceae that have been isolated from clinical specimens are listed in Table 34–1 (3). This chapter focuses on the genera most commonly encountered in the clinical microbiology laboratory.

ESCHERICHIA

Escherichia is the type genus for the Enterobacteriaceae, and Escherichia coli is the type species for the genus. In this section, the epidemiology, pathogenesis, and clinical manifestations of the most common diseases caused by E. coli are reviewed. Other species of Escherichia—Escherichia hermannii, Escherichia vulneris, and Escherichia fergusonii—are uncommon in the clinical laboratory and are not discussed further. Genetically, the genera Shigella and Escherichia are related, but because much confusion would result from renaming the Shigella, that genus name has been retained.

Escherichia coli first was described by Theodore Escherich in 1885 as a commensal organism present in feces; however, its pathogenic potential gradually became recognized, and today it is known to cause many diseases. Isolates of E. coli may be serotyped on the basis of lipopolysaccharide O, flagellar H, and polysaccharide (capsular) K antigens. Currently, 171 O and 56 H serotypes are recognized, constituting the O:H system commonly used to study the epidemiology and pathogenesis of disease due to E. coli (Table 34–2).

Intestinal Infections. Four major categories of diarrheagenic Escherichia coli are recognized: *enterotoxigenic*, most frequently responsible for travelers' diarrhea and a major cause of infant diarrhea in developing countries; *enteroinvasive*, a cause of dysentery; *enteropathogenic*, an important cause of infant diarrhea; and *enterohemorrhagic*, a cause of hemorrhagic colitis and hemolytic uremic syndrome (4). Enteroadherent or enteroaggregative E. coli is a less well-defined, possibly heterogeneous, fifth category identified by the pattern of adherence of the organisms to HEp-2 cells in cell culture (5,6).

Enterotoxigenic Escherichia coli (ETEC) were recognized as an important cause of diarrhea in developing countries in the late 1960s and early 1970s (4,7). These organisms are the most common agents of travelers' diarrhea but are encountered infrequently in the United States and other developed countries (8,9). The pathogenicity of the ETEC is due to two factors. First, three fimbrial colonization factors (CFA/I, CFA/II, and CFA/IV) allow the bacteria to colonize the proximal small intestine. Second, after infection is established organisms produce heat-labile enterotoxin (LT) or heat-stable enterotoxin (ST), or both (4). Stable toxin is a small molecule that causes elevation of cyclic guanine monophosphate within the mucosal cells of the small intestine with subsequent altered ion transport and markedly increased fluid excretion. Labile toxin, a large molecule almost identical to the cholera toxin of Vibrio cholerae (Chapter 35), has two components: B binds to a galactoglycoprotein on the mucosal surface of the epithelial cells of the small intestine, allowing entry of the A molecule, which catalyzes the adenosine diphosphate ribosylation of the guanyl nucleotide–dependent component of adenylate cyclase. The subsequent elevated levels of cyclic adenosine monophosphate (cAMP) alter electrolyte transport, causing excessive fluid excretion by mucosal cells.

Enteroinvasive strains of Escherichia coli (EIEC), first described in 1971, have several features similar to Shigella (discussed later) (10–12). Both invade and proliferate within epithelial cells, predominantly in the colonic mucosa, eventually causing cell death. For both, the property of invasiveness depends on the presence of large (about 140-Md) plasmids that code for the production of several outer membrane proteins. The proteins of EIEC and Shigella are antigenically closely related (if not identical), and cross-reactions among their O antigens occur. Moreover, both organisms are nonmotile and unable to fer-

Table 34–1. Members of the Enterobacteriaceae Isolated from Humans

Genus	Species	Comments
Budvicia	B. aquatica	Isolated from feces
Cedecea	C. davisae	Isolated from respiratory tract, wounds
	C. lapagei	
	C. neteri	
Citrobacter	C. freundii	Normal flora in GIT; nosocomial pathogens isolated from wounds, urine, blood, CSF
	C. diversus	
	C. amalonaticus	
Edwardsiella	E. tarda	Associated with diarrhea, wound infections, sepsis
	E. hoshinae	
	E. ictaluri	
Enterobacter	E. cloacae	Normal flora in GIT; nosocomial pathogens associated with sepsis wound infections, pneumonia, UTI, meningitis (E. sakazakii), contaminated pharmaceutical solutions
	E. aerogenes	
	E. agglomerans	
	E. sakazakii	
	E. gergoviae	
	E. amnigenus	
	E. taylorae	
Escherichia	E. coli	Normal flora in GIT; E. coli associated with diarrhea, UTI, meningitis, sepsis; E. vulneris isolated from wounds; E. hermannii isolated from wounds, blood, CSF
	E. fergusonii	
	E. hermannii	
	E. vulneris	
Ewingella	E. americanus	Isolated from respiratory tract, blood
Hafnia	H. alvei	Nosocomial pathogen isolated from respiratory tract
Klebsiella	K. pneumoniae	Normal flora in GIT; nosocomial pathogens isolated from respiratory tract, wounds, blood, urine
	K. oxytoca	
	K. ozaenae	
	K. rhinoscleromatis	
	K. planticola	
Kluyvera	K. ascorbata	Probably normal GIT flora; isolated from respiratory tract, blood, urine
	K. cryocrescens	
Koserella	K. trabulsii	Isolated from feces, wounds, respiratory tract, joint fluid
Leclercia	L. adecarboxylata	Isolated from respiratory tract, blood, urine, wounds
Leminorella	L. grimontii	Isolated from human feces, not known to be pathogenic for humans
	L. richardii	
Moellerella	L. wisconsensis	Isolated from stool; not known to be pathogenic for humans
Morganella	M. morganii	Normal flora of GIT; isolated from urine, blood
Proteus	P. mirabilis	Normal flora of GIT; isolated from urine, wounds, blood
	P. vulgaris	
	P. penneri	
Providencia	P. alcalifaciens	Normal flora in GIT; isolated from urine, wounds, blood. P. rustigianii not known to be pathogenic for humans
	P. rettgeri	
	P. rustigianii	
	P. stuartii	
Rhanella	R. aquatilis	Only one human isolate reported; not known to be pathogenic for humans
Salmonella	S. (enterica) >2000 serovars	Cause of gastroenteritis and enteric fever
Serratia	S. marcescens	S. marcescens is the only known pathogen and is associated with nosocomial infections of respiratory and urinary tracts, sepsis, meningitis
	S. ficaria	
	S. liquefaciens	
	S. odorifera	
	S. plymuthica	
	S. rubidaea	
Shigella	S. boydii	Cause of gastroenteritis and bacterial dysentery
	S. dysenteriae	
	S. flexneri	
	S. sonnei	
Tatumella	T. ptyseos	Isolated from respiratory tract, urine, blood
Yersinia	Y. aldovae	Y. pestis causes plague; Y. enterocolitica and Y. pseudotuberculosis cause gastroenteritis and other infections (isolated from stool, blood, urine, wounds)
	Y. enterocolitica	
	Y. pseudotuberculosis	
	Y. frederiksenii	
	Y. intermedia	
	Y. kristensenii	
	Y. pestis	

Key: GIT, gastrointestinal tract; CSF, cerebrospinal fluid, UTI, urinary tract infection.
(Modified from Baron EJ and Finegold SM (eds): Enterobacteriaceae. *In* Bailey and Scott's Diagnostic Microbiology. 8th ed. St. Louis, CV Mosby, 1990.)

Table 34–2. Serogroups of Escherichia coli Associated with Intestinal and Extraintestinal Infections

Infection	Serogroups
Intestinal	
ETEC	06, 08, 011, 015, 020, 025, 027, 063, 078, 080, 085, 0114, 0115, 0126, 0128ac, 0139, 0148, 0153, 0159, 0166, 0167
EPEC	018, 026, 044, 055, 086, 0111ab, 0112, 0114, 0119, 0125ac, 0127, 0128ab, 0142, 0158
EIEC	028ac, 029, 0112ac, 0115, 0124, 0135, 0136, 0143, 0144, 0152, 0164, 0167
EHEC	026, 0111, 0157
Urinary tract	01, 02, 04, 06, 07, 08, 09, 011, 018, 022, 025, 062, 075
Bacteremia	01, 02, 04, 06, 07, 08, 09, 011, 018, 022, 025, 075
Meningitis	01, 06, 07, 016, 018, 083

Key: ETEC, enterotoxigenic E. coli; EPEC, enteropathogenic E. coli; EIEC, enteroinvasive E. coli; EHEC, enterohemorrhagic E. coli.
(Data from Farmer JJ III, and Kelly MT: Enterobacteriaceae. In Manual of Clinical Microbiology, 5th ed. Edited by A Balows, et al. Washington DC, American Society for Microbiology, 1991; and Riley LW: Infectious diseases associated with Escherichia coli. In Laboratory Diagnosis of Infectious Diseases—Principles and Practice. Edited by Balows, WJ Hawsler, Jr, M Ohashi, and A Turano. New York, Springer Verlag, 1988.)

ment lactose. Infection with EIEC causes fever, severe abdominal cramps, and watery diarrhea, consisting of scanty stools containing blood, mucus, and polymorphonuclear leukocytes. The illness probably is less common than disease caused by ETEC, but the true prevalence of EIEC in the United States is unknown because no assay to detect these strains is available that is suitable for use in the clinical laboratory.

Enteropathogenic strains of Escherichia coli (EPEC), which were epidemiologically associated with infant diarrhea in the 1950s, are among the most common causes of bacterial diarrhea in infants in South America (13,14). These organisms cause a distinct lesion in the human intestines, recognized by electron microscopy: the bacteria, which adhere closely to, and often become partially enveloped by, the enterocyte membrane, destroy the microvilli without invading the cell (4). Almost all important EPEC serotypes (Table 34–2) possess a plasmid that encodes a 94-kd protein, termed EPEC adherence factor (EAF), giving these strains the property of adhesiveness to HEp-2 cells (15). The few strains of EAF-negative EPEC that cause diarrhea and produce typical lesions in enterocytes are considered a separate class (class II) within the EPEC (16). Illness produced by EPEC—fever, vomiting, and diarrhea containing mucus but no gross blood—is more severe than many other diarrheal infections in infants and may persist 2 weeks or longer.

Enterohemorrhagic Escherichia coli (EHEC) 0157:H7 was recognized as a new enteric pathogen in 1982, during the investigation of a multistate outbreak of hemorrhagic colitis (bloody diarrhea, without fecal leukocytes, in afebrile persons) and later implicated as a cause of the hemolytic uremic syndrome, a microangiopathic hemolytic anemia associated with renal failure (17–19). Since its recognition, EHEC has become an enteric pathogen of public health importance in the United States and Canada, causing outbreaks of hemorrhagic colitis, hemolytic uremic syndrome, and diarrhea in nursing homes, day care centers, schools, and the community (4,17–21). The EHEC (0157:H7 and, less commonly, 026:H11) elaborate phage-encoded cytotoxins active on HeLa cells and Vero cells in vitro (4,19). Almost all produce a toxin called Shiga-like toxin 1 or Verotoxin 1, apparently identical to the Shiga toxin produced by Shigella dysenteriae type 1, and many also elaborate a cytotoxin termed Shiga-like toxin 2 or Verotoxin 2. Another virulence factor of the EHEC is a 60-Md plasmid that encodes the production of a fimbria that appears to mediate attachment to epithelial cells in cell culture (4).

Isolates of Escherichia coli may show any of three distinct patterns of adherence in the HEp-2 cell assay: localized (typical of EPEC, described earlier), diffuse, and aggregative, of which the latter two are newly recognized categories associated with diarrhea (22). In particular, the enteroaggregative E. coli (originally called enteroadherent-aggregative E. coli) may induce persistent diarrhea in infants in developing countries (5,6). These strains do not produce cytotoxins, invade epithelial cells, or possess EPEC adherence factor plasmids.

All groups of diarrheagenic Escherichia coli may be transmitted by ingesting contaminated food; and ETEC, EIEC, and EPEC strains also may be spread by contaminated water. Contaminated milk or dairy products have been the source of outbreaks of diarrhea caused by EPEC, EIEC, ETEC, and EHEC (23,24). In institutional settings, person-to-person transmission is an important mode of spread of infection and any diarrhea-producing E. coli may be involved.

In tropical climates the prevalence of diarrhea due to ETEC and EPEC peaks in the rainy season. In Canada, diarrhea caused by EHEC occurs most frequently during the summer. Although Escherichia coli reside in the intestines of humans, other mammals, and birds, the reservoirs of most pathogenic E. coli are unknown. Strains of ETEC that cause diarrhea in animals are not pathogenic in humans, and strains that cause diarrhea in humans rarely are recovered from farm animals. However, E. coli 0157:H7 has been isolated from cattle, and this finding, plus the frequent association between ingestion of undercooked beef and hemorrhagic colitis, suggest that cattle may be a reservoir of EHEC (23).

Urinary Tract Infections. Uropathogenic Escherichia coli (see Table 34–2) account for more than 90% of community-acquired and more than 30% of hospital-acquired infections of the urinary tract in the United States (25). In most cases, infection is initiated by E. coli from the host's fecal flora. These bacteria spread to the urethra and into the bladder, where they multiply, a process most likely facilitated by fimbrial and nonfimbrial adhesins of the organism (24). Host factors associated with decreased urinary clearance, such as obstruction to flow or vesicoureteral reflux, predispose to urinary tract infections, and for nosocomial infections, instrumentation of the urinary tract is an important risk factor. Moreover, the frequency of acquiring infections of the urinary tract depends on sex and age. From birth to age 3 months urinary tract infections, predominantly caused by E. coli, are more common in males, but after infancy females are affected more frequently (25).

Infections of the urinary tract include asymptomatic bacteriuria, cystitis, and acute pyelonephritis. These infections typically produce dysuria, urgency, frequency, and lower abdominal pain; and fever, rigors, nausea, vomiting, and lower back or flank pain also are present with pyelonephritis. Potential complications of acute urinary tract infections are chronic pyelonephritis (which may progress to renal failure or hypertension), sepsis, and in men prostatitis or epididymitis.

Bacteremia. Escherichia coli was an unusual cause of bacteremia in the United States and Europe until the 1950s, when it replaced the gram-positive bacteria as the organism most frequently responsible for bacteremia in neonates and adults (24). In the 1986 report of the National Nosocomial Infections Surveillance System (incorporating data from 51 hospitals in the United States), E. coli was the third most common agent of bacteremia, after coagulase-negative staphylococci and Staphylococcus aureus (26).

In neonates, about 20% of bacteremias caused by Escherichia coli follow infection or manipulation of the urinary tract, but usually no primary source of infection is apparent (24). Risk factors include premature delivery, premature rupture of membranes, maternal infection in the peripartum period, traumatic delivery, hypoxia, and low birth weight. The latter is related to an immature immune response (see Chapter 2) and decreased levels of the iron-binding proteins lactoferrin and transferrin, which may protect against bacteremia because iron promotes the growth of E. coli in serum. In adults who have E. coli bacteremia, the principal source of infection is the genitourinary tract in 40 to 60% of cases, the gastrointestinal tract in 25 to 30%, and it is inapparent in about 25% (27). The risk of bacteremia in adults is higher for those who have an underlying disease and is increased by urologic instrumentation or a surgical procedure.

Most Escherichia coli serogroups associated with bacteremia also are associated with urinary tract infections (see Table 34–2). Certain O polysaccharide antigens may promote survival of the bacteria in the blood by rendering them resistant to the bactericidal properties of serum (28). Bacterial endotoxin (see Chapter 2) is responsible for many clinical features of bacteremia.

Bacteremia caused by E. coli cannot be distinguished clinically from that produced by other bacteria. In neonates, anorexia, thermal instability, respiratory distress, apnea, vomiting, diarrhea, jaundice, hepatomegaly, and lethargy are common. Adults may present with fever, rigors, changes in mental status, hypotension, oliguria or anuria, respiratory distress, or a combination of these findings.

Meningitis. Escherichia coli is one of the most common agents of meningitis among neonates but is a rare cause in adults, in whom the infection almost always is a complication of head trauma or an intracranial surgical procedure. The incidence of neonatal disease is less than 1 per 1000 live births per year, and in most studies is higher in male infants (29–31).

Neonatal meningitis caused by Escherichia coli almost always is a complication of bacteremia. It develops in 10 to 40% of neonates who are bacteremic with E. coli of certain serotypes (see Table 34–2), the majority of which possess the polysaccharide capsule antigen K1. The K1 antigen is chemically and immunologically related to the capsular polysaccharide of Neisseria meningitidis type B (see Chapter 31), but its pathogenic relationship to meningitis is unknown. Of the risk factors associated with bacteremia due to Escherichia coli in neonates (discussed earlier), low birth weight is the most important predisposing factor to meningitis.

The clinical manifestations of meningitis caused by Escherichia coli—fever, lethargy, vomiting, diarrhea, respiratory distress, jaundice, changes in consciousness, hyperactivity, and occasionally seizures—are not diagnostic. The mortality rate varies from 12% in neonates with no known risk factors to more than 35% in those whose gestational age is less than 35 weeks, birth weight under 2500 g, or who have congenital defects. Of the survivors, 20 to 50% suffer neurologic sequelae (24).

SHIGELLA

Shigellae first were recognized in the stools of persons with dysentery (described later) by Shiga in 1898 (32). Two years later, Flexner identified a similar but serologically different organism (33).

Species of Shigella genetically belong in the genus Escherichia, but to avoid confusion the genus Shigella has remained separate. The 39 serotypes of Shigella are grouped into four species based on serologic similarity and biochemical reactions: Shigella dysenteriae (serogroup A, the prototype of the genus), Shigella flexneri (serogroup B), Shigella boydii (serogroup C), and Shigella sonnei (serogroup D). All shigellae are capable of causing bacillary dysentery, but the severity of the illness, the mortality rate, and the epidemiology vary for each species.

Epidemiology

Shigellosis occurs worldwide and is most prevalent where poverty, crowding, poor personal hygiene, inadequate water supply, and malnutrition are common. Endemic shigellosis is predominantly a disease of children between ages 6 months and 10 years. Recently, however, the prevalence of shigellosis in the United States has increased significantly in women over 20 years of age (34). The incidence of shigellosis is about 750 to 2000 cases per 1000 children per year in developing countries and about 5 to 15 per 1000 population in the United States, but the latter figures are based on bacteriologically confirmed cases reported to the Centers for Disease Control (CDC) and, therefore, probably are an underestimate (35,36). Shigellosis may be a serious problem among adults in custodial institutions and in homosexual males, and outbreaks have been associated with the consumption of raw oysters (37,38).

Major shifts in the predominant species of Shigella that cause disease in the world have occurred over the past 80 years. Shigella dysenteriae, originally associated with epidemic dysentery, predominated until World War I, when it was replaced by Shigella flexneri. Shigella sonnei replaced Shigella flexneri after World War II in developed, but not in developing, countries. By the late 1950s, Shigella dysenteriae had become a minor component of endemic shigellosis, but over the past 20 years it has been responsible for major epidemics in Latin America, Central Africa, Asia, and India (39). Currently, in the United States, Shigella sonnei accounts for 60 to 70% of isolates of Shigella and Shigella flexneri for most of the remainder; Shigella boydii and Shigella dysenteriae comprise about 2% of isolates, and most infections caused by S. dysenteriae are acquired during foreign travel (35,38,40). In developing countries S. dysenteriae and Shigella boydii are isolated most frequently, followed by Shigella flexneri and Shigella sonnei.

Humans are the only important source of Shigella, and carriers, who shed organisms in their feces, are the reservoir. The carrier state usually lasts 1 to 4 weeks but may be prolonged. From the carriers, organisms are spread from person to person by fingers, food, water, feces, and flies, a process facilitated by the ability of a very small inoculum (as few as 200 to 300 viable cells) to induce infection. Outbreaks occur in closed populations such as families, institutions for the mentally handicapped, Indian reservations, day-care centers, prisons, and cruise ships (38,41). Rates of secondary transmission are high, especially in children younger than 1 year.

Pathogenesis

The colitis that characterizes dysentery caused by Shigella is a consequence of the organism's ability to invade epithelial cells, to escape from the phagocytic vesicle into the cytoplasm, to multiply within cells, and to invade adjacent cells (42). Growth of the organism causes death of the intestinal epithelial cells and subsequent mucosal ulceration and inflammation. The genes required for invasion, intracellular multiplication, and cell-to-cell spread are on the bacterial chromosome and plasmids, and all are necessary for full virulence. All virulent shigellae have large (120- to 140-Mda) plasmids that code for shared outer membrane proteins. Distinct loci of importance include *ipa* (invasion plasmid antigen), which specifies outer membrane proteins presumably involved in epithelial cell recognition; *inv* (invasion), which may regulate insertion of *ipa* gene products into the outer membrane; *vir*F, which regulates surface charge; and *vir*G, which allows the bacterium to escape from the phagosome into the cytoplasm and spread from cell to cell.

A potential factor in the pathogenesis of dysentery produced by shigellae is the cytotoxin, of which Shiga toxin is the prototype, that causes fluid secretion in animal intestinal loop models in the laboratory (43). The A subunit of the toxin, an enzyme with glycosidase activity, cleaves the 28S ribosomal RNA of the 60S ribosomal subunit of eukaryotic cells, causing irreversible inhibition of protein synthesis and cell death. Linked to the A subunit are five B subunit monomers that mediate binding of the toxin to the cell receptor, globotriaosylceramide, which is found in rabbit jejunal villus, but not crypt cells (35). Binding of toxin by the villus cell inhibits protein synthesis in that cell, the consequence being impaired sodium absorption. Decreased sodium and water absorption cause a net fluid accumulation in the intestinal lumen.

Clinical Manifestations

The spectrum of shigellosis varies from asymptomatic infection to severe bacillary dysentery with high fever, chills, seizures, abdominal cramps, tenesmus, and frequent bloody stools. Typically, after an incubation period of 1 to 3 days, fever and malaise develop, followed by watery diarrhea (usually 10 to 25 stools per day) that may progress within hours to a few days to bloody diarrhea or dysentery. The classic stool consists of a small amount of blood and mucus, but stools may be partially formed and mixed with blood and mucus. Abdominal cramps may be severe, and tenesmus due to proctitis may cause rectal prolapse. Mucosal ulcerations predominate in the rectum and distal colon. Previously healthy adults may recover spontaneously in 2 to 7 days, but in young or old or malnourished persons the disease lasts longer, and the mortality rate due to dehydration and electrolyte imbalance is higher. Severe infections with S. dysenteriae type 1, and occasionally with S. flexneri, may be complicated by life-threatening local problems such as toxic megacolon with perforation and protein-losing enteropathy. Systemic complications of shigellosis include the hemolytic-uremic syndrome, seizures, bacteremia, meningitis, and osteomyelitis (44–46).

SALMONELLA

The taxonomy of the genus Salmonella is complicated by the different nomenclatures used over the years. In the early 1930s Kauffman and White categorized Salmonella according to their antigen composition, a scheme by which over 1800 serotypes were identified (47). Two antigens—O, the somatic, heat-stable cell wall polysaccharide, and H, the diphasic, heat-labile flagellar proteins—are found in almost all serotypes, and some salmonellae possess heat-labile surface polysaccharides (such as the Vi antigen of Salmonella typhi) that prevent O agglutination. The major division of the salmonellae is into groups (designated by capital letters and numbers), and within each group, members share a common somatic antigen. Almost all serotypes isolated from all sources in the United States belong to group A, B, C_1, C_2, D, E_1, E_2, E_3, E_4, F, G, or H, and most human isolates are members of groups A through E_4.

In 1963, Ewing proposed a classification system based on the biochemical reactions given by large numbers of isolates of each genus and species within the Enterobacteriaceae. Using this scheme the genera Salmonella, Arizona, and Citrobacter were placed in the tribe Salmonellae, and three biochemically distinct species of Salmonella were recognized: Salmonella typhi, -choleraesuis, and -enteritidis (48). The first two were serologically homogeneous, whereas S. enteritidis contained numerous serotypes.

Based on recent DNA hybridization studies the two genera, Salmonella and Arizona, now are classified as a single genus, Salmonella, which contains one species of seven distinct subgroups (49):

Genus: Salmonella
Species: choleraesuis

Subspecies:	Subgroup
choleraesuis	1
salamae	2
arizonae	3a
diarizonae	3b
houtenae	4
bongori	5
indica	6

Almost all strains of Salmonella isolated in the clinical laboratory and implicated in human and animal disease belong to subgroup 1.

In 1983 the proposal was made that the Salmonella serotype name (as designated in the Kauffman and White classification) be used in reporting and that designations of Salmonella in scientific communications artificially treat the serotypes as species (49). This practical approach to nomenclature is advocated by the CDC, is accepted in much of the world, and is used in this text.

Epidemiology

Salmonella typhi, the agent of typhoid fever, is uniquely adapted to humans, and human carriers are the only known reservoir. Organisms are excreted from convalescent carriers for a short time but are shed for over 1 year in the feces of "chronic" carriers (principally older women who had a diseased biliary tract, where the bacteria reside in gallstones or scars). S. typhi is transmitted by ingesting contaminated food or water. Water-borne typhoid fever is a problem where sanitation fails in modern water-distribution systems (50). Food usually becomes contaminated with S. typhi by a food handler who is an asymptomatic carrier of the organism or by sewage.

In the United States, the incidence of typhoid fever decreased from about 1 per 100,000 in 1955 to about 0.2 per 100,000 in 1989, owing to control of carriers, chlorination of water, and proper sewage disposal (36). In developing countries that lack adequate control measures typhoid fever, especially waterborne disease, remains a major public health problem, with an annual incidence of 300 to 500 cases per 100,000 population in some areas. Persons who travel to these countries account for about 70% of all cases of typhoid fever in the United States (51).

Species of Salmonella other than Salmonella typhi are principally pathogens of animals, and animals are the principal sources of human infections, although person-to-person transmission may occur. The nontyphoidal salmonellae have been recovered from most animal species, including poultry (chickens, turkeys, and ducks), cows, pigs, turtles, cats, dogs, mice, guinea pigs, hamsters, birds, sheep, seals, donkeys, lizards, and snakes (52). Some Salmonella serotypes are highly host adapted: Salmonella paratyphi A, Salmonella schottmuelleri (paratyphi B), Salmonella hirschfeldii (paratyphi C), and Salmonella sendai principally infect humans, and chickens and other birds are the major reservoirs of Salmonella gallinarum-pullorum.

Poultry and poultry products (chiefly eggs) are the most important sources of human infection, accounting for about 50% of the common-vehicle epidemics (53). Salmonella in the feces of infected hens may contaminate the surface of shell eggs or penetrate into the egg's interior through hairline cracks, and in hens with ovarian infection organisms may gain access to the yolk. In an attempt to decrease the prevalence of salmonellosis in the United States associated with bulk egg products and eggs with cracked shells, the Egg Products Inspection Act, requiring pasteurization of all bulk egg products and federally supervised inspection of shell eggs for cracks, was passed in 1970. The frequency of outbreaks associated with eggs subsequently decreased, but eggs or foods containing raw or undercooked eggs (homemade eggnog, grilled egg-dipped bread, caesar salad, pasta made with eggs, hollandaise sauce) remain sources of outbreaks (54,55). From 1985 to 1988 state health departments reported 140 outbreaks of salmonellosis; contaminated food was implicated in 89 (64%), and 65 (73%) of these were associated with grade A shell eggs (55).

Meats, particularly beef and pork, account for about 13% of outbreaks of salmonellosis and dairy products, including raw and powdered milk, for about 4% (56). Pasteurized 2% milk was responsible for a massive outbreak that affected 150,000 to 200,000 persons in Illinois in 1985 (57). Pets, especially turtles, are implicated in about 3% of outbreaks. As a result of the Food and Drug Administration's ban on interstate shipment of pet turtles in 1975 the frequency of salmonellosis acquired from turtles declined but it was not eliminated (58). Fruits and vegetables are infrequent sources of infection with Salmonella but in 1990 and 1991 were the vehicles responsible for three large outbreaks of salmonellosis: two nationwide outbreaks associated with contaminated cantaloupes and one multistate outbreak associated with contaminated tomatoes (59).

Although most cases of nontyphoidal salmonellosis are acquired via ingestion of contaminated food, other mechanisms of spread occur infrequently. In 1981 an outbreak due to contact with marijuana, apparently contaminated with animal manure, was reported (60). Transmission by inadequately sterilized fiberoptic instruments has occurred among persons undergoing gastrointestinal endoscopy, and outbreaks have been related to pharmacologic or diagnostic preparations (61,62). Food handlers rarely are identified as sources of outbreaks (63).

In the United States most outbreaks of salmonellosis occur in homes; and if one family member is infected, about a third of household or family contacts are as well (63,64). Ranking second to homes are institutions. Acute-care hospitals, pediatric wards, and neonatal nurseries account for about two thirds of reported institutional outbreaks, and nursing homes, psychiatric hospitals, and institutions for the mentally handicapped for the remainder (65). Other sources of outbreaks are banquets, restaurants, food stores, and schools. Contaminated food or water is responsible for about 85% of all outbreaks, and most of the remainder are spread by cross-infection.

The number of Salmonella isolates from humans reported to the CDC has increased progressively since the late 1970s, probably as a result of better reporting, processing foods in bulk and distributing the products over wide geographic areas, an increasing number of persons whose resistance to infection is impaired, and the widespread use of antimicrobial agents, which enhance susceptibility to enteric infection. The rates of reported Salmonella isolates in the United States are highest for infants 1 to 6 months of age, decrease during early childhood, remain constant through the adult years, and increase slightly in elders (66). Infections caused by Salmonella occur with greatest frequency between July and November in the United States, and worldwide peak during warm weather.

Pathogenesis

The development of disease after ingestion of Salmonella depends on the inoculum size, the virulence of the organisms, and host factors. In general about 10^6 to 10^9 organisms must be ingested to produce symptomatic infection; however, if the organisms are unusually virulent or if the person's resistance is impaired, a smaller inoculum may cause disease.

Local factors in the stomach and upper small intestine (see Chapter 2) influence the outcome of the infection. Factors that neutralize the acid pH of the stomach or decrease the time the organism is exposed to the acid diminish the local bactericidal activity, increasing the likelihood that the ingested organisms will reach the small intestine. Therefore, the risk of severe enterocolitis caused by salmonellae is increased in persons who have achlorhydria, who have undergone gastrectomy, gastroenterostomy, or vagotomy, or who receive oral buffering compounds. Antibiotic administration alters the normal flora of the small intestine, which reduces the size of the inoculum required to produce disease, prolongs the convalescent carrier state, and increases the risk of infection with antibiotic-resistant strains of Salmonella (67,68).

Age is an important determinant in the development of disease. Newborns and infants younger than 1 year are especially susceptible to enterocolitis caused by salmonellae, possibly reflecting an immature immune system, decreased antibacterial action of the normal intestinal flora, high frequency of fecal-oral contamination, or a combination of these factors. Increased resistance with age sometimes is related to immunity acquired from previous exposure to the organism.

Persons with impaired cellular and humoral immune mechanisms as a result of malnutrition, malignancy, infection with human immunodeficiency virus, or therapy with corticosteroids or immunosuppressants are at increased risk of salmonellosis (69,70), as are those who have malaria, bartonellosis, or a sickle hemoglobinopathy. The marked susceptibility of persons with sickle hemoglobinopathies to bacteremia and osteomyelitis caused by salmonellae may be due to a defect in the alternate complement pathway (71).

The various serotypes of Salmonella produce different clinical syndromes. Salmonella anatum generally produces asymptomatic infection or mild diarrhea; Salmonella typhi usually penetrates the intestinal mucosa, causing enteric fever; and Salmonella choleraesuis penetrates the intestinal mucosa, producing bacteremia, often associated with localized infection but without the manifestations of enteric fever.

Diarrhea produced by salmonellae probably results from infection with mucosal invasion, and possibly from elaboration of an enterotoxin that acts on upper intestinal transport; however, the mechanisms involved have not been unequivocally defined. In infections induced in the laboratory mucosal invasion alone does not account for the intestinal fluid, but mucosal invasion may trigger local inflammatory cells to produce mediators that stimulate electrolyte secretion and smooth muscle contraction (72).

The pathogenesis of enteric fever has been studied more extensively. Although the site at which Salmonella typhi penetrate the intestinal mucosa is unknown, the bacteria apparently attach to specific receptors on the microvilli and invade through Peyer's patches. They then are transported to intestinal lymphoid follicles, where they multiply in mononuclear cells, causing hyperplasia of lymphoid follicles (Fig. 34–1) and a monocytic infiltrate (73). Organisms reach the mesenteric lymph nodes, enter the thoracic duct and then the blood, and eventually are removed by the monocyte/macrophage cells in the liver, spleen, and bone marrow; although some organisms reach the gallbladder, multiply, and secondarily seed the intestine via the bile (62). The prolonged fever and toxic symptoms of enteric fever have been attributed to endotoxin in the bacterial cell wall and to mediators released from mononuclear cells (see Chapter 2), but neither hypothesis has been proven (74,75). The surface Vi antigen on most S. typhi organisms and some other serotypes of Salmonella may inhibit phagocytosis and serum bactericidal activity, and it appears to correlate with invasiveness and the ability to produce disease (73).

Localization of salmonellae in bone, meninges, heart, lungs, kidneys, spleen, and other organs or tissues, a condi-

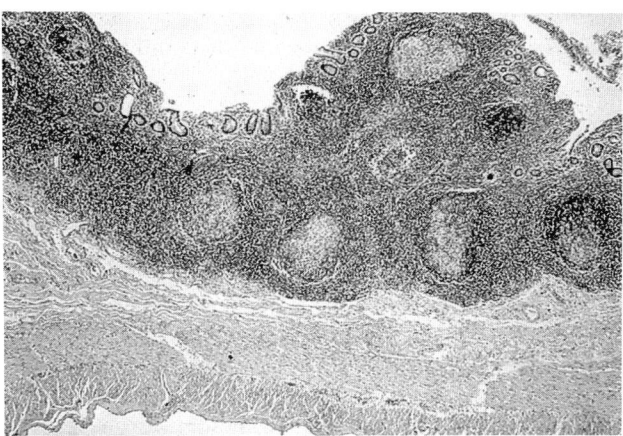

Fig. 34–1. Micrograph of section of ileum from a patient with typhoid fever shows prominent hyperplasia of lymphoid follicles (hematoxylin and eosin, ×10).

tion favored by pre-existing necrosis or scarring, elicits a neutrophilic response and abscess formation. Gallbladder disease, especially gallstones, favors persistence of Salmonella in the biliary tract, predisposing to the chronic carrier state; and infection with Schistosoma haematobium (see Chapter 52) is associated with increased frequency of carriage of Salmonella in the urinary tract.

Clinical Manifestations

Acute enterocolitis is the most common clinical manifestation of infection with Salmonella. The illness begins 6 to 48 hours after ingestion of contaminated food or water, with nausea, vomiting, myalgia, headache, fever, abdominal cramps, and diarrhea. Leukocytes, and occasionally red blood cells, are present in feces, but gross blood is rare. In most cases fever resolves in less than 2 days and the diarrhea in less than 1 week, but stool cultures often are positive though the patient is without symptoms during the second or third week after the onset of illness. The disease is more severe in children, in elders, and in persons with conditions associated with impaired resistance (described earlier).

Enteric fever, produced by Salmonella typhi and occasionally Salmonella paratyphi A, Salmonella schottmuelleri, and Salmonella hirschfeldii, begins insidiously after an incubation period of 10 to 14 days (range, 7 to 21 days) with fever, malaise, anorexia, headache, and myalgias. Constipation or diarrhea may occur and may be accompanied by respiratory tract symptoms such as cough and sore throat. Confusion, dizziness, seizures, or acute psychotic behavior occasionally is prominent. Rose spots, transient 2- to 4-mm erythematous maculopapular lesions that blanch on pressure, appear in less than 50% of cases, typically in crops of 10 on the upper abdomen. Hepatomegaly develops in 25 to 50% of cases, and splenomegaly in 40 to 60%. The lymphoid tissue in the ileocecal area of the intestinal tract undergoes sequential changes: hyperplasia occurs during the first week of symptoms and may regress after 7 to 10 days or progress to necrosis and sloughing of the mucosa, forming ulcers that parallel the long axis of the ileum and usually heal completely with little scarring. Major hemorrhage occurs in the second or third week of illness in 1 to 2% of cases, and perforation, most frequently of the terminal ileum, complicates 1% of cases or fewer during the same period. Disease relapses in 8 to 12% of persons not treated with antimicrobial therapy, and perhaps in a larger percentage of persons treated with antibiotics, especially chloramphenicol.

Bacteremia may be caused by any serotype of Salmonella. In the United States Salmonella typhimurium is implicated most commonly, because the frequency of infection with this serotype is so great, although only a small fraction of S. typhimurium isolates are from the blood. Salmonella choleraesuis, which appears to be especially virulent, is isolated more frequently from blood than from stool. Salmonella bacteremia is common in persons with the acquired immunodeficiency syndrome (AIDS) and may be the initial manifestation of the disease (69). Recently, bacteremia due to Salmonella arizonae in persons with AIDS has been associated with ingesting rattlesnake meat (70).

Localized infections with Salmonella include meningitis, a rare complication, almost exclusively of infants; pneumonia, empyema, or lung abscess, usually in elders or persons who have underlying disease; endocarditis and pericarditis; arteritis; osteomyelitis, associated primarily with sickle hemoglobinopathies, systemic lupus erythematosus, hematopoietic malignancies, immunosuppressive therapy, a surgical procedure or trauma, and hepatic cirrhosis; septic arthritis; and abscesses of the spleen, liver, or soft tissues. The chronic carrier state (defined earlier) develops in 1 to 3% of persons with typhoid and in far fewer than 1% of persons with nontyphoidal salmonellosis.

YERSINIA

Infections caused by the pathogenic species of Yersinia—Yersinia enterocolitica, -pseudotuberculosis, and -pestis—are zoonoses that predominantly affect rodents, pigs, and birds; humans are accidental hosts. In humans, Yersinia enterocolitica and sometimes Yersinia pseudotuberculosis causes fever, diarrhea, and abdominal pain, mimicking acute appendicitis; Yersinia pestis is the agent of plague.

Yersinia enterocolitica and Yersinia pseudotuberculosis
Epidemiology

First described as a human pathogen in the late 1930s, Yersinia enterocolitica has been recovered from humans in many countries of the world, but it is found most frequently in cooler climates, a distribution that may reflect differences in reservoirs or culinary practices, or more intensive surveillance in these areas (76,77). The true incidence and prevalence of infection with Y. enterocolitica are unknown; however, the rate of recovery of the organism from stool of persons who have diarrhea ranges from zero to almost 3% (78–81). In Europe, infections often cluster during the fall and winter, but outbreaks involving three or more cases have not been clustered seasonally (79,82–86). Y. enterocolitica serotype 0:3, which has an important reservoir in pigs, is the predominant serotype in Scandinavia, Japan, Canada, and parts of Europe; and in Belgium, the country reporting the highest incidence of yersiniosis, infections with Y. enterocolitica 0:3 have been linked to ingesting raw pork (84,87–90). In the United States, limited data from outbreaks and from the CDC indicate that, before 1980, Y. enterocolitica 0:8 was the predominant serotype and Y. enterocolitica 0:3 was relatively uncommon; however, in the past decade Y. enterocolitica 0:3 has become the predominant serotype among isolates submitted to the CDC from all areas of the United States (91).

Yersinia enterocolitica has been recovered from many animals and insects, including birds, frogs, fish, flies, fleas, snails, crabs, oysters, and various mammals; from animal products such as raw milk, whipped cream, ice cream, beef, lamb, pork, and poultry; and from inanimate reservoirs including lakes, streams, well water, soil, and vegetables (86). Swine are a recognized reservoir for pathogenic Y. enterocolitica in Europe, Japan, and recently the United

States (91). The serotypes of Y. enterocolitica isolated from environmental sources often are different from those that cause human infections, suggesting that environmental reservoirs may be unrelated to human disease.

Transmission of Yersinia enterocolitica occurs principally by ingestion of contaminated foods (especially pork and milk) and water, and infection may be spread from dogs, cats, and swine to humans, possibly via the fecal-oral or oral-oral route (86). Spread of infection via transfusion of blood products has been documented; and reports of nosocomial infection suggest that direct person-to-person transmission may occur, but this has not been proven (83,85,86,92).

Human infection with Yersinia pseudotuberculosis is rare. The organism is distributed worldwide, with reservoirs in rodents, deer, farm animals, and birds, and is presumed to be transmitted to humans by ingestion of contaminated food or water. Most cases of human infection have been reported from Europe, primarily in boys 5 to 15 years of age during the winter.

Pathogenesis

Bacterial and host factors are involved in the pathogenesis of disease caused by Yersinia enterocolitica. Differences in virulence exist among strains of Y. enterocolitica. Pathogenic strains isolated from persons with disease contain 40- to 48-Mda plasmids that are responsible for virulence in animals infected in the laboratory (86). The expression of plasmid-encoded proteins of the outer membrane of Y. enterocolitica is associated with resistance to complement-mediated opsonization, to neutrophil phagocytosis, and to the bactericidal activity of human serum (86). The invasiveness of Y. enterocolitica is a chromosomally mediated property. In animals infected in the laboratory by intragastric inoculation bacteria invade the ileal mucosa, multiply in Peyer's patches, and drain into mesenteric lymph nodes, whence they may disseminate (93).

The virulence of Yersinia enterocolitica is enhanced by iron loading, so iron overload and deferoxamine therapy increase the risk of systemic infection with the organism (86). Persons who have undergone stomach resection also are at increased risk of bacteremia with Y. enterocolitica, suggesting that gastric acidity may be an important host defense against the organism (94).

Clinical Manifestations

The clinical manifestations of infection with Yersinia enterocolitica depend at least in part on the age and physical state of the host. Enterocolitis, characterized by diarrhea, low-grade fever, and abdominal pain, typically in young children, is the most common presentation. Leukocytes and red blood cells may be present in the stool, and in as many as 25% of cases stools are grossly bloody. The illness usually is self-limited but may be complicated by appendicitis, diffuse ulceration of the small and large intestine, intestinal perforation, peritonitis, ileocolonic intussusception, toxic megacolon, cholangitis, and mesenteric vein thrombosis with gangrene of the small bowel (78,86,95). The pseudoappendicular syndrome, mimicking appendicitis with fever, abdominal pain, right-side lower quadrant tenderness, and leukocytosis, occurs principally in older children and young adults (86,96,97). Laparotomy in such patients reveals mesenteric lymphadenitis and terminal ileitis, and Y. enterocolitica can be cultured from involved tissue.

Postinfection manifestations of disease caused by Yersinia enterocolitica—arthritis and erythema nodosum—occur mainly in adults. Polyarticular arthritis, which most frequently involves the weight-bearing joints of the lower extremities, typically begins 1 to 2 weeks after the onset of gastrointestinal symptoms and persists 1 to 4 months. Cultures of synovial fluid are sterile, but microbial antigens may be detected (98). Reiter's syndrome (arthritis, urethritis, and conjunctivitis) also has been reported, and it and polyarticular arthritis are most likely to develop in persons with the HLA-B27 histocompatibility antigen (99,100). Lesions of erythema nodosum appear on the legs and trunk 2 to 20 days after the onset of fever and abdominal pain, principally in women, and generally resolve spontaneously within a month.

Bacteremia with Yersinia enterocolitica usually occurs in persons who have a predisposing underlying condition: immunosuppression, diabetes mellitus, alcoholism, malnutrition, and iron overload such as that that occurs with cirrhosis, hemochromatosis, acute iron poisoning, transfusion-dependent blood dyscrasias, and deferoxamine therapy (86). The fatality rate is 34 to 50%; however, blood donors who have Y. enterocolitica bacteremia at the time of donation have been asymptomatic, suggesting that it can cause unrecognized transient bacteremia. Spread of organisms to extraintestinal sites during bacteremia may result in a spectrum of complications: hepatic, renal, and splenic abscesses; endocarditis; mycotic aneurysm; meningitis; peritonitis; osteomyelitis; and pulmonary, ocular, and skin infections (86). Focal extraintestinal infections that may occur in the absence of detectable bacteremia include pharyngitis, osteomyelitis, lymphadenitis, pyomyositis, cellulitis, wound infections, conjunctivitis, urinary tract infections, renal abscesses, pneumonia, and lung abscess (86).

The most common manifestation of infection with Yersinia pseudotuberculosis is mesenteric adenitis (described earlier). Erythema nodosum and polyarthritis have been described, and fewer than 30 cases of septicemia, half in persons with cirrhosis, hemochromatosis, or diabetes mellitus, have been reported (101).

Yersinia pestis

The first documented pandemic of plague began about 540 AD in Egypt or Ethiopia and spread far over the next 60 years, killing approximately 100 million persons. The second pandemic, called the Black Death, started in the fourteenth century in central Asia and was spread via rats and infectious droplets from persons with pneumonic disease throughout Europe (where nearly a fourth of the entire population died), the Near East, India, and China. The current pandemic began in China in the 1860s, spread to Hong Kong in the 1890s, and subsequently was spread by rats transported on ships to California, South America, Africa, and Asia. The pathogen, Yersinia pestis (formerly called Pasteurella pestis), was isolated by Alexander Yersin in Hong Kong in 1894.

Epidemiology

Currently over 90% of cases of plague in the world occur in Southeast Asia, especially South Vietnam, Burma, Nepal, and Indonesia, and another major focus is in Brazil. The first human case of plague in the United States occurred in 1900 in San Francisco. Permanent foci of plague in the United States extend from the West Coast east to Kansas, Oklahoma, and Texas and to approximal areas of Canada and Mexico and involve almost 60 wild rodent species and their fleas.

Plague is perpetuated by three cycles. *Sylvatic plague* (also called wild plague), the only form prevalent in the United States, is transmitted among commensal rodents and from rodents to humans by the bite of a flea or by contaminated mouth parts of a flea, the most efficient vector being Xenopsylla cheopis, the Oriental rat flea. *Urban rat plague* (also called domestic plague) is the principal cause of massive epidemics of plague in recent history, especially in seaports. The epidemic is preceded by an epizootic among rodents (particularly black rats); and when approximately 10% of rats are infected, infected fleas move from rodents to humans living nearby. *Pneumonic plague,* the clinical form of disease that has greatest potential for rapid dissemination, and the only directly contagious form, is transmitted via infected aerosol droplets exhaled from a person with pulmonary involvement.

In the United States an average of one or two cases of plague were reported annually before 1965; but since the 1965 outbreak of seven cases in a Navajo reservation in New Mexico, the number of cases has increased, averaging nearly 20 per year (102). Most cases of human plague occur between May and October in New Mexico, Arizona, California, Colorado, and Oregon. Of the nearly 300 persons who contracted plague between 1956 and 1987, 30% were American Indians, primarily Navajos; 20% Caucasian-Hispanics; and 50% Caucasians. Slightly more than half were males, and about 55% were younger than 20 years. Risk factors for disease include living in an area with a high concentration of vector fleas and rodents that are susceptible to plague (particularly prairie dogs and squirrels) and lifestyle—sheep herding, hunting prairie dogs and rabbits, and living in rude dwellings that may attract rodents. Although the primary mechanism of transmission of plague to humans is the bite of a flea or contact with the mouth parts of an infected flea, cases have been acquired by close contact with animals infected with Yersinia pestis, for example while preparing a prairie dog for food or by caring for a cat ill with pneumonic plague (103,104).

Pathogenesis

When a flea infected with Yersinia pestis attempts to ingest a blood meal from a human, numerous bacteria are regurgitated into the person's skin. These organisms migrate by cutaneous lymphatics to regional lymph nodes, and because flea-borne bacilli possess only a small amount of the envelope (F-1) antigen, they are phagocytosed by polymorphonuclear leukocytes and monocytes. Virulence factors of Y. pestis are associated with resistance to intracellular killing by phagocytic cells and with invasiveness. V and W antigens, which always are produced together early in the infection, are associated with the ability of the organism to proliferate rapidly and cause overwhelming septicemia. Moreover, these antigens apparently allow small numbers of bacilli to establish infection in animals. Calcium dependence, a plasmid-mediated major virulence factor, is associated in vitro with a nutritional requirement for calcium at room temperature. When deprived of calcium, bacterial cells undergo metabolic shutdown, accompanied by the expression of V and W antigens and several major outer membrane proteins. Mutants that lack these outer membrane proteins are avirulent, but the specific role of the proteins is unknown. The envelope (F-1) antigen, which is produced at 37° C (not at the ambient temperature in the flea) in regional lymph nodes and during the incubation period when bacteria are replicating in mononuclear cells, is antiphagocytic. Endotoxin may be responsible for shock.

Clinical Manifestations

Bubonic plague, the only form of disease that occurs in humans after infection from a wild focus, begins abruptly after an incubation period of 2 to 8 days with high fever, chills, malaise, confusion, nausea, pain in the limbs and back, and a painful swelling (a bubo) 1 to 10 cm in diameter, in one anatomic region of lymph nodes, usually a groin, axilla, or neck. Almost all affected persons have intermittent low-grade bacteremia. Septicemic plague is characterized by a high level of bacteremia early in the disease, often before a local bubo evolves, frequently accompanied by disseminated intravascular coagulation.

Pneumonic plague most often is secondary to hematogenous spread of bacteria from a bubo, but occasionally it is primary, following exposure to a person with plague who has a cough. This highly contagious form of disease, characterized by cough, chest pain, and often hemoptysis in a person who has fever and lymphadenopathy, is associated with a high mortality rate. Rare manifestations of plague are meningitis and pharyngitis.

OTHER ENTEROBACTERIACEAE

Klebsiella species

Four species of Klebsiella—Klebsiella pneumoniae, -oxytoca, -ozaenae, and -rhinoscleromatis—are human pathogens. Klebsiella pneumoniae and Klebsiella oxytoca, the species most commonly encountered, colonize the human gastrointestinal tract and are a major cause of nosocomial and opportunistic infections. A notable characteristic of these organisms is their prominent polysaccharide capsule, of which more than 70 serotypes have been identified. Factors associated with virulence are the capsule, which prevents phagocytosis and retards leukocyte migration into infected areas, and endotoxin.

An important but uncommon primary infection caused by Klebsiella pneumoniae is community-acquired lobar pneumonia, which affects persons with an underlying condition that impairs respiratory tract host defenses, such as alcoholism, diabetes mellitus, or chronic obstructive pulmonary disease. This destructive infection commonly results in abscess formation, cavitation, empyema, and pleural adhesions. The more frequent pulmonary disease caused by K. pneumoniae, however, is hospital-acquired bronchopneumonia or bronchitis.

Most isolates of Klebsiella pneumoniae are associated with infections of the urinary tract. In one study, K. pneumoniae and Klebsiella oxytoca were responsible for 9% of urinary tract infections and 14% of primary bacteremias in hospital patients, and they have been implicated in 8% of nosocomial bacterial infections, most often involving the urinary, respiratory, or biliary tract or surgical wound sites (105,106). Factors that predispose to nosocomial infection include urinary catheters, endotracheal tubes, and intravascular catheters.

Klebsiella ozaenae and Klebsiella rhinoscleromatis are encountered infrequently in the United States but have been associated with upper respiratory tract infections in other parts of the world. Klebsiella ozaenae has been implicated, but not proven, as a cause of chronic atrophic rhinitis. Rhinoscleroma, a common infection in areas of eastern Europe, central Africa, Latin America, and southern Asia, is a chronic granulomatous disease caused by Klebsiella rhinoscleromatis that involves the mucosa of the upper respiratory system and may involve bone, causing airway obstruction (107,108).

Enterobacter species

Of the eight species of Enterobacter isolated from clinical specimens, Enterobacter cloacae and Enterobacter aerogenes are responsible for most human infections. Enterobacter organisms are widely distributed in the environment, found in soil, water, and sewage, and are part of the normal flora of the human gastrointestinal tract. These opportunistic pathogens rarely cause primary disease, but they frequently colonize hospitalized patients, especially those receiving antimicrobial agents, and they may be spread horizontally in the hospital on the hands of hospital personnel who do not practice proper hand-washing technique. In 1984 species of Enterobacter accounted for about 6% of all nosocomial infections in United States hospitals participating in the National Nosocomial Infections Surveillance System, and more than 6% of all nosocomial bacteremias (109). In addition to bacteremia, these organisms may cause infections of burns, wounds, and the respiratory and urinary tracts. Enterobacter sakazakii has been associated with meningitis and cerebral abscesses in neonates; and Enterobacter cloacae and Enterobacter agglomerans have caused major outbreaks of infections associated with contaminated pharmaceutical products (110,111).

Serratia marcescens

Serratia marcescens, the most important species of Serratia isolated from humans, is a saprophyte found in soil, water, and sewage and on plants. The organism first was described by Bizio in 1819, and since the 1960s it has been recognized as an opportunistic pathogen, primarily of hospitalized patients and intravenous drug users (112). The organism is most likely to colonize the respiratory or urinary tract of hospitalized adults and gastrointestinal tract of neonates. Spread of the organism on the hands of hospital personnel is the most important factor in nosocomial transmission.

Serratia marcescens is responsible for about 4% of nosocomial bacteremias and pneumonias and 2% of infections of the urinary tract, surgical wounds, and skin; and it may cause meningitis and conjunctivitis in newborns (105,112). Factors that predispose to infection include urinary catheters, respiratory support equipment, intravenous catheters, arterial monitoring devices, and a history of a neurosurgical procedure. S. marcescens also has been associated with contaminated intravenous solutions (113). Among intravenous drug users S. marcescens is an important cause of endocarditis and osteomyelitis; and in persons receiving intra-articular injections for diagnostic or therapeutic purposes it has caused septic arthritis, which in one outbreak was linked to contaminated benzalkonium chloride antiseptic used to soak cotton balls (113–117).

Proteus and Providencia species

The species of Proteus that swarm—Proteus mirabilis and Proteus vulgaris—are primary pathogens in the urinary tract and are the second most common of the Enterobacteriaceae (after Escherichia coli) encountered in the clinical microbiology laboratory (105). One characteristic of Proteus that contributes to its uropathogenicity is the production of urease, an enzyme that splits urea to ammonium hydroxide, raising the pH of the urine to a level that favors the formation of struvite stones, which obstruct urine flow and act as a nidus for persistance of infection. Additional microbial virulence factors are surface fimbriae, which are important for colonization of the uroepithelium; flagella, which promote spread of infection in the urinary tract; and possibly hemolysins (118,119).

Proteus mirabilis, the more frequently encountered of the species, causes up to 10% of all urinary tract infections and in debilitated persons may cause wound infections, pneumonia, and septicemia. The reservoir of nosocomial infections due to Proteus, many of which are caused by Proteus vulgaris, is the gastrointestinal tract of persons who later become infected. In residents of nursing homes who have chronic indwelling catheters, Providencia stuartii, which typically is resistant to multiple antimicrobial agents, is a common cause of bacteriuria (120).

Citrobacter species

All three species of Citrobacter—Citrobacter diversus, -freundii, and -amalonaticus—have been associated with human disease, almost exclusively nosocomial infections involving the urinary or respiratory tract of debilitated patients. These organisms also may cause endocarditis and hospital-acquired bacteremia, and in neonates, Citrobacter diversus is an important cause of meningitis and brain abscesses (105). Isolates of C. diversus recovered from persons with meningitis possess an outer membrane protein not found in nonpathogenic bacteria and in an animal model of infection appear to be more virulent than isolates not associated with meningitis (121).

Laboratory Diagnosis

Specimens for diagnosis of infections with the Enterobacteriaceae are listed in Table 34–3. Specimen collection, transport, and processing are discussed in Part III. Clinical samples suspected to contain Yersinia pestis may be hazardous; therefore, such specimens or cultures should be sent to a laboratory that has appropriate facilities for handling the organism. Because members of the Enterobacteriaceae as a group are the organisms most frequently encountered in the clinical laboratory, understanding the methods used for identification is important. Therefore, the key tests for identification are reviewed and features of the organisms discussed in this chapter are described.

Tests for Identification

Cells of the Enterobacteriaceae are short, fat, gram-negative bacilli (Plate VA). Most produce large (2 to 3 mm diameter after 24 hours), dull gray, dry or mucoid colonies on sheep blood agar and grow well on MacConkey agar. Preliminary test results that identify a gram-negative bacillus with this colony appearance as a member of the Enterobacteriaceae are negative oxidase, glucose fermentation, and nitrate reduction.

An isolate known to be a member of the Enterobacteriaceae is identified by the presence or absence of various enzymes that direct bacterial metabolism. Enzymes are detected in vitro by inoculating culture media that contain substrates upon which the enzymes react and an indicator that detects substrate utilization or specific metabolic end products. Currently, this is done in most laboratories by using a commercially available identification system (discussed in detail in reference 122), which provides results in 4 to 24 hours. Understanding the biochemical reactions, however, allows a more accurate assessment of the reliability of the different systems, more timely recognition of problems (or errors) that may develop once a system is in use, and selection of appropriate additional tests to perform if the system does not provide an identification. Therefore, some of the classic biochemical tests used to identify the Enterobacteriaceae are reviewed. Additional biochemical reactions are shown in Table 34–4. Biochemical profiles of the less commonly encountered Enterobacteriaceae are found elsewhere (1,122,123).

Oxidase Test. The oxidase test detects cytochrome oxidase, an iron-containing porphyrin enzyme that participates in the electron transport mechanism and in the nitrate metabolic pathways of some bacteria. The test may be performed by dropping the oxidase reagent (1% tetramethyl-*p*-phenylenediamine dihydrochloride, prepared in house or available commercially) on suspect colonies on an agar plate, but it is interpreted most easily when a portion of a colony from a blood agar plate is transferred by platinum wire or wooden stick to a piece of filter paper moistened with several drops of oxidase reagent. Color change to blue or purple within 10 seconds constitutes a positive reaction. Because colonies growing on plates containing dyes such as MacConkey agar may obscure the results they should not be used. Moreover, inoculating loops or wires of stainless steel or nichrome should be avoided because trace amounts of iron oxide on the flamed surface may yield false-positive reactions.

Glucose Fermentation. The ability of an organism to utilize glucose anaerobically, forming acidic end products (fermentation) is tested by inoculating portions of a colony to a Kligler's iron agar (KIA) or triple sugar iron agar (TSIA) medium. Both media are nutritionally enriched and support growth of all but the most fastidious aerobic and facultative bacteria. Other characteristics detected by

Table 34–3. Diseases Caused by the Enterobacteriaceae and Specimens Required for Diagnosis

Disease	Organisms Involved*		Specimens†
	Common	Uncommon	
Diarrhea	E. coli Salmonella spp. Shigella spp.	Yersinia spp.	*Stool*, rectal swab, ?serum (Yersinia)
Enteric fever	S. typhi		Bone marrow (1st month), blood (1st 2 weeks), stool (week 3)
Plague	Y. pestis		Blood, aspirate of bubo, sputum
Septicemia, bacteremia	E. coli S. typhi Klebsiella Enterobacter	Salmonella spp. Shigella Serratia Proteus Providencia Y. pestis	Blood
Meningitis	E. coli E. sakazakii C. diversus	Salmonella typhi Salmonella spp. Serratia	CSF
Urinary tract infection	E. coli Proteus Klebsiella Providencia Enterobacter	Serratia	Urine
Wound infection	E. coli Klebsiella Enterobacter Proteus	Serratia	*Aspirated pus, biopsy tissue,* swab
Lung infection	Klebsiella Enterobacter E. coli Serratia	Salmonella typhi Salmonella spp. Proteus Y. pestis Yersinia spp.	Sputum, BAL, lung tissue, transtracheal aspirate, blood, pleural fluid (if present)
Osteomyelitis, arthritis	Salmonella spp. Yersinia spp.	Serratia	Bone biopsy, joint fluid
Mesenteric adenitis	Yersinia spp.		Mesenteric lymph node

* Salmonella spp, species of Salmonella other than S. typhi; Yersinia spp, Y. enterocolitica, Y. pseudotuberculosis
† Specimens in *italics* are preferred.
Key: CSF, cerebrospinal fluid; BAL, bronchoalveolar lavage fluid.

Table 34–4. Biochemical Reactions of the Enterobacteriaceae That Are the Most Important in Human Infections or Are Frequently Isolated from Clinical Specimens*

Species	Indole Production	Methyl Red	Voges-Proskauer	Citrate (Simmons')	Hydrogen Sulfide (TSI)	Urea Hydrolysis	Phenylalanine Deaminase	Lysine Decarboxylase	Arginine Dihydrolase	Ornithine Decarboxylase	Motility (36°C)	Gelatin Hydrolysis (22°C)	D-Glucose, Gas	Lactose Fermentation	Sucrose Fermentation	D-Mannitol Fermentation	Dulcitol Fermentation	Adonitol Fermentation	D-Sorbitol Fermentation	L-Arabinose Fermentation	Raffinose Fermentation	L-Rhamnose Fermentation	D-Xylose Fermentation	Melibiose Fermentation	DNase, 25°C	ONPG†
Escherichia coli	98	99	0	1	1	1	0	90	17	65	95	0	95	95	50	98	60	5	94	99	50	80	95	75	0	95
Shigella serogroups A, B, and C	50	100	0	0	0	0	0	0	5	1	0	0	2	0	0	93	2	0	30	60	50	5	2	50	0	2
Shigella sonnei	0	100	0	0	0	0	0	0	2	98	0	0	2	1	1	99	0	0	2	95	3	75	2	25	0	90
Salmonella, most serotypes	1	100	0	95	95	1	0	98	70	97	95	0	96	1	1	100	96	0	95	99	2	95	97	95	2	2
Salmonella typhi	0	100	0	0	97	0	0	98	3	0	97	0	0	1	0	100	0	0	99	2	0	0	82	100	0	0
Salmonella paratyphi A	0	100	0	0	10	0	0	0	15	95	95	0	99	0	0	100	0	0	95	100	0	100	0	95	0	0
Citrobacter freundii	5	100	0	95	80	70	0	0	65	20	95	0	95	50	30	99	55	0	98	100	30	99	99	50	0	95
Citrobacter diversus	99	100	0	99	0	75	0	0	65	99	95	0	98	35	45	100	50	98	99	100	0	100	100	0	0	96
Klebsiella pneumoniae	0	10	98	98	0	95	0	98	0	0	0	0	97	98	99	99	30	90	99	99	99	99	99	99	0	99
Klebsiella oxytoca	99	20	95	95	0	90	1	99	0	0	0	0	97	100	100	99	55	99	99	98	100	100	100	99	0	100
Enterobacter aerogenes	0	5	98	95	0	2	0	98	0	98	97	0	100	95	100	100	5	98	100	100	99	99	100	99	0	100
Enterobacter cloacae	0	5	100	100	0	65	0	0	97	96	95	0	100	93	97	100	15	25	95	100	97	92	99	90	0	99
Hafnia alvei	0	40	85	10	0	4	0	100	6	98	85	0	98	5	10	99	0	0	0	95	2	97	98	0	0	90
Serratia marcescens	1	20	98	98	0	15	0	99	0	99	97	90	55	2	99	99	0	40	99	0	2	0	7	0	98	95
Proteus mirabilis	2	97	50	65	98	98	98	0	0	99	95	90	96	2	15	0	0	0	0	0	1	1	98	0	50	0
Proteus vulgaris	98	95	0	15	95	95	99	0	0	0	95	91	85	2	97	0	0	0	0	0	1	5	95	0	80	1
Providencia rettgeri	99	93	0	95	0	98	98	0	0	0	94	0	10	5	15	100	0	100	1	1	5	70	10	5	0	5
Providencia stuartii	98	100	0	93	0	30	95	0	0	0	85	0	2	50	10	0	0	5	1	1	7	0	7	0	10	10
Providencia alcalifaciens	99	99	0	98	0	0	98	0	0	1	96	0	85	0	15	2	0	98	1	1	1	0	1	0	0	1
Morganella morgani	98	97	0	0	5	98	95	0	0	98	95	0	90	1	0	0	0	0	0	0	0	0	0	0	0	5
Yersinia enterocolitica	50	97	2	0	0	75	0	0	0	95	2	0	5	5	95	98	0	0	99	98	5	1	70	1	5	95
Yersinia pestis	0	80	0	0	0	5	0	0	0	0	0	0	0	0	0	97	0	0	50	100	0	1	90	20	0	50
Yersinia pseudotuberculosis	0	100	0	0	0	95	0	0	0	0	95	0	0	0	0	100	0	0	0	50	15	70	100	70	0	70

* Numbers represent the percentage of positive reactions after 2 days of incubation at 36°C. Most positive reactions occur within 24 hr.
† ONPG, o-Nitrophenyl-β-D-galactopyranoside.
Reported with permission from Farmer JJ III, et al: Biochemical identification of new species and biogroups of Enterobacteriaceae isolated from clinical specimens. J Clin Microbiol 21:46, 1985.)

these media include the production of gas from the fermentation of sugars (indicated by the formation of bubbles or cracks in the agar), the fermentation of lactose in KIA or lactose and sucrose in TSIA, and the production of hydrogen sulfide gas, using sodium thiosulfate as the sulfur source (Plate VB). The latter is visualized by the formation of a black precipitate containing iron when hydrogen sulfide gas reacts with ferrous sulfate.

To inoculate these tubes the tops of isolated colonies are touched with an inoculating needle, which is stabbed down the center of the agar into the lower, relatively anaerobic portion (called the butt or deep) of the tube, extending within 3 to 5 mm of the bottom, without touching the walls. When the inoculating needle is removed from the butt, the surface of the slant is streaked with a back-and-forth motion. Inoculated tubes are loosely capped and incubated 18 to 24 hours in ambient air at 35°C. The reactions that occur with different bacteria are illustrated in Figure 34–2 and Plate VB and are discussed in more detail below.

The concentration of lactose in TSIA and KIA is ten times greater than that of glucose (and in TSIA, the ratio of sucrose to glucose also is 10:1). Organisms that ferment glucose metabolize that sugar first, both aerobically on the slant and anaerobically in the butt, because glucose-utilizing enzymes are present constitutively and the bacteria gain the most energy from using the simplest sugar. Once all of the available glucose is reduced, the product, pyruvate, is further metabolized on the slant via the aerobic Krebs cycle, producing acidic end products. The acid in the medium causes the phenol red pH indicator to become yellow; therefore, after about 6 hours the slant and butt of a TSIA or a KIA tube inoculated with a glucose-fermenting organism will be yellow.

Organisms that utilize glucose but do not ferment lactose or sucrose produce energy by metabolizing proteins and amino acids, an aerobic process that occurs primarily on the surface of the slant. Because the by-products of peptone breakdown, such as ammonia, are alkaline, the phenol red indicator reverts to its original red color; and after incubation for 18 to 24 hours (when the tubes are examined) the TSIA or KIA slant will be red and the butt yellow, a reaction called alkaline over acid (K/A). However, organisms that ferment lactose (or sucrose) do so after the glucose is depleted. This continued production of acidic end products causes the slant and butt of the TSIA or KIA tube to remain yellow after 18 to 24 hours, a reaction called acid over acid (A/A).

Inoculation of a glucose nonfermenter (Chapter 32) causes the butt to remain red or become alkaline (evidenced by a slightly deeper red color), indicating that the organism is not a member of the Enterobacteriaceae. Glucose nonfermenters may utilize peptones on the slant, producing alkaline products. Such reactions are termed alkaline over alkaline (K/K).

Nitrate Reduction. All Enterobacteriaceae isolated from humans except certain biotypes of Enterobacter agglomerans reduce nitrate to nitrite. Nitrate reduction, however, requires up to 24 hours and, therefore, generally is used to confirm the correct classification of an unknown

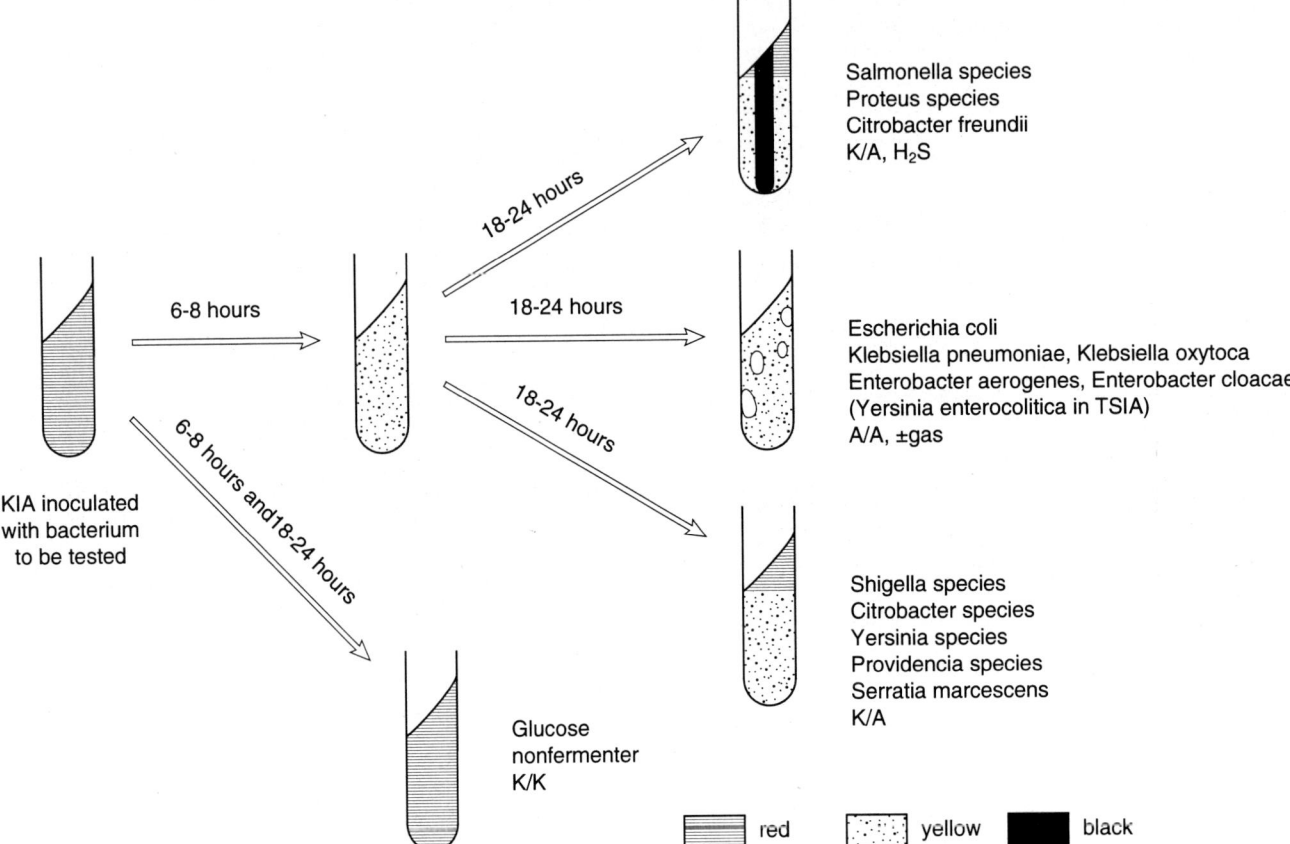

Fig. 34–2. Reactions produced in Kligler's iron agar (KIA) by common gram-negative bacilli. Key: K/A, alkaline slant and acid butt; TSIA, triple sugar iron agar; A/A, acid slant and butt; K/K, alkaline slant and butt.

isolate or to help identify a bacterial species rather than as a screening test. To perform the nitrate reduction test, nitrate broth or a nitrate agar slant (available commercially) is inoculated and incubated at 35° C in ambient air for 24 hours. Three drops of reagent A (sulfanilic acid) and then three drops of reagent B (N,N-dimethyl-1-naphthylamine) are added; a red color develops if nitrites are present, indicating nitrate reduction. The absence of a red color indicates that nitrates were not reduced or that the reaction continued, yielding nitrogen gas from nitrites. To distinguish the two, a pinch of zinc dust (available commercially) is added; a red color develops if nitrates are present.

Methyl Red and Voges-Proskauer Tests. Organisms that ferment glucose produce abundant acidic end products such as formate and acetate from pyruvic acid, or they metabolize pyruvic acid to the more neutral products acetoin and butanediol (Fig. 34–3). The methyl red (MR) and Voges-Proskauer (VP) tests determine which metabolic pathway is used. For both tests the same substrate broth (MR/VP broth, commercially available) is inoculated below the surface of the medium with the organism then incubated 48 hours in ambient air at 35° C. The broth is divided into two equal aliquots, one each for the MR and VP tests. To perform the VP test 0.6 ml (6 drops) of VP reagent A (α-naphthol) and then 0.2 ml (2 drops) of VP reagent B (40% potassium hydroxide) are added.

The solution is mixed and allowed to sit up to 15 minutes. The formation of a pink to red color, indicating the presence of acetoin, is a positive reaction; negative reactions are colorless or yellow. To perform the MR test 0.5 ml (5 drops) of the methyl red reagent is added; no change in the red color is a positive result; a change to yellow,

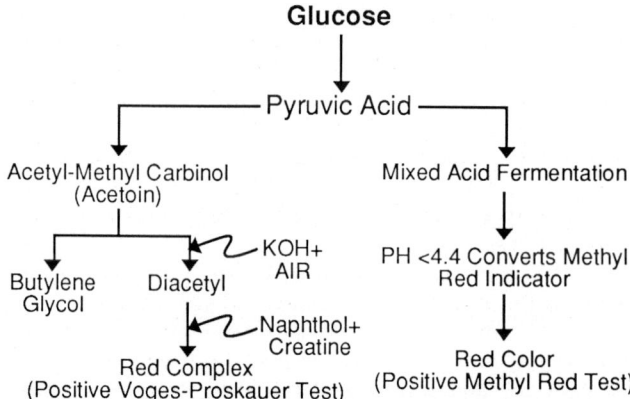

Fig. 34–3. Mixed acid (methyl red) and butylene glycol (Voges-Proskauer) pathways of glucose fermentation. (From Koneman EW, et al. (eds.): The Enterobacteriaceae. In Color Atlas and Textbook of Diagnostic Microbiology. 3rd ed. Philadelphia, JB Lippincot, 1988.)

indicating pH above 6.0, is a negative result; and an orange color indicates that the test must be repeated after a longer initial incubation period. In general, members of the genera Klebsiella, Enterobacter, and Serratia are VP positive and MR negative (at 35° to 37°C), and the remaining Enterobacteriaceae are VP negative, MR positive.

o-Nitrophenyl β-D-galactopyranoside Test. To detect fermentation of lactose, a disaccharide composed of glucose and galactose joined by a β-galactoside bond, on media such as MacConkey, TSIA or KIA, an organism must produce two enzymes: β-galactoside permease, responsible for actively transporting lactose across the bacterial cell wall, and β-galactosidase, the enzyme required to hydrolyze the β-galactoside bond between glucose and galactose moieties. An organism that lacks the permease enzyme but possesses β-galactosidase ferments lactose only after the sugar diffuses across the cell membrane. This process generally takes several days; therefore, in the clinical laboratory an organism with these features usually appears unable to ferment lactose. The *o*-nitrophenyl β D-galactopyranoside (ONPG) test allows rapid detection of β-galactosidase. The ONPG compound, which is structurally similar to lactose except that the glucose is replaced by an *o*-phenyl group, permeates the bacterial cell wall more readily than lactose, and if the enzyme is present is hydrolyzed by β-galactosidase into galactose and *o*-nitrophenol. The latter is a chromophore that produces a pale yellow color when it is released into the medium. To perform the test an ONPG disk (commercially available) is reconstituted in a small volume of water, heavily inoculated with the test organism, incubated overnight at 35° to 37°C, and examined for the color change.

Indole. Bacteria that possess the enzyme tryptophanase cleave tryptophan, producing indole, pyruvic acid, and ammonia. To detect indole production, a medium containing tryptophan (such as tryptophan broth, sulfide-indole-motility agar, or motility-indole-ornithine agar; all commercially available) is inoculated with the organism and incubated at 35°C in ambient air for 24 hours, after which an aldehyde indicator is added. The reaction of the aldehyde with indole forms a pink ring at the interface between the medium and the reagent. One of two aldehyde indicators may be used: Kovac's reagent, *p*-dimethylaminobenzaldehyde in amyl alcohol, or Ehrlich's reagent, *p*-dimethylaminobenzaldehyde in ethyl alcohol. When the latter is used, xylene must be added first to extract the indole. Ehrlich's reagent, a more sensitive indicator, is preferred for testing organisms that produce minimal amounts of indole, such as nonfermentative gram-negative bacilli and anaerobes (Chapters 32 and 38).

Alternatively, indole production by bacteria growing in pure culture on a nonselective medium such as sheep blood or chocolate agar may be evaluated by a spot test. A portion of the colony to be tested is transferred to a strip of filter paper saturated with a *p*-dimethylaminocinnamaldehyde solution (commercially available). A positive reaction is indicated by immediate development of a blue color.

Citrate Utilization. To determine whether an organism can utilize sodium citrate as the sole source of carbon for metabolism and growth the surface of a Simmons' citrate agar slant (commercially available), a medium containing buffers, salts, cations, and a bromthymol blue pH indicator, is slightly inoculated. The tube is loosely capped and incubated at 35°C in ambient air for 24 hours. Growth of the organism on the slant and a color change from green to blue is a positive test (Plate VC). Rarely, a citrate-positive organism utilizes the substrate without producing enough alkaline end products to change the pH indicator; therefore, good growth on the slant without a blue color may be positive but the test should be repeated with a minimal inoculum.

Urease Production. The ability of an organism to hydrolyze urea to ammonia and carbon dioxide may be determined by inoculating one of two media. Stuart's broth (commercially available), a heavily buffered medium (pH 6.8) in which relatively large amounts of ammonia must be generated to elevate the pH above 8.0, is virtually selective for species of Proteus. Christensen's urea agar (commercially available), a less buffered medium containing peptones and glucose that supports growth of many bacteria that cannot grow in Stuart's broth, is used most frequently in the laboratory. Either medium should be heavily inoculated, incubated at 35° to 37°C in a water bath or ambient air incubator, and examined at 15, 30, and 60 minutes and at 4 and 24 hours. A change from a yellow or salmon color to pink or red is a positive result (Plate VD). Rapid urease tests, in which substrates are impregnated into filter paper disks or tablets, also are commercially available.

Decarboxylation and Dihydrolation of Amino Acids. Definitive tests for lysine and ornithine decarboxylases and arginine dihydrolase are performed in broth media developed by Moeller (called Moeller's decarboxylase medium), containing glucose, bromcresol purple, a nitrogen source, cresol red indicator, the enzyme activator pyridoxal, and the amino acid to be tested. For each test a tube containing the amino acid to be evaluated and a control tube containing only the basal medium must be inoculated to determine if the organism forms alkaline end products in the absence of the amino acid. Media are inoculated with a small amount of growth from isolated colonies by emulsifying the inoculum below the broth surface and then are overlayed with sterile mineral oil or vaspar (melted paraffin combined with an equal volume of petroleum jelly) to a depth of 1 cm, to prevent the introduction of oxygen. Tubes are incubated up to 14 days at 35°C in ambient air, although reactions may be interpreted earlier (usually at 4 days). Breakdown of the amino acid (a positive result) forms alkaline amino end products, causing a shift in the pH indicators and a purple color. A yellow color indicates that only glucose was utilized, forming acid. The control tube should remain its original pale purple color or, if the test organism ferments glucose, turn yellow.

Lysine iron agar (LIA), which contains glucose, lysine, ferric ammonium citrate, sodium thiosulfate, and bromcresol purple pH indicator, detects lysine decarboxylation and deamination and hydrogen sulfide formation and often is used to differentiate species of Salmonella from members of the normal bowel flora (such as species of Proteus) that produce hydrogen sulfide (see Chapter 59).

The LIA tube is inoculated and incubated as described earlier for KIA, except that the butt is stabbed several times. The presence of a black precipitate indicates hydrogen sulfide production; however, LIA is less sensitive than KIA or TSIA for detecting hydrogen sulfide. Lysine decarboxylation occurs anaerobically in the butt, producing alkaline end products and a purple color. Bacteria that do not decarboxylate lysine but ferment glucose yield acid by-products, causing the butt to turn yellow. Lysine deamination, characteristic of Proteus, Providencia, and Morganella, is indicated by a change in the color of the slant from purple to red (called R/A). Reactions produced by different organisms are illustrated in Figure 34–4.

Phenylalanine (or Tryptophan) Deaminase Production. Deamination of phenylalanine to phenylpyruvic acid differentiates Proteus, Morganella, and Providencia, which produce this reaction, from almost all other gram-negative bacilli. The only other human isolates that may yield a positive result are Enterobacter agglomerans (up to 20% of isolates) and Enterobacter sakazakii (up to 50% of isolates). To perform the test an agar slant containing phenylalanine, salts, yeast extract, and buffers (commercially available) is inoculated with the test organism and incubated overnight in ambient air at 35° C; 0.5 ml (5 drops) of ferric chloride is added, and the immediate development of a green color indicates a positive result. Rather than phenylalanine, many of the commercially available identification systems use tryptophan, which is deaminated to indole pyruvic acid. The method is identical to that described for phenylalanine, except an orange-brown end product indicates a positive result.

Hydrogen Sulfide Production. To detect the release of sulfur from sulfur-containing amino acids in the form of hydrogen sulfide, a source of sulfur and a hydrogen sulfide detector must be present in the medium. Sulfur sources include the sulfur-containing amino acids cysteine and methionine and the inorganic compound sodium thiosulfate, which often is added as a supplemental sulfur source. Ferrous sulfate, ferric citrate, ferric ammonium sulfate, ferric ammonium citrate, peptonized iron, or lead acetate may act as the hydrogen sulfide detector. Sulfide released from the sulfur source couples with hydrogen ions, forming hydrogen sulfide. The latter reacts with iron, bismuth, or lead, producing insoluble heavy metal sulfides that appear as a black precipitate (Plate VB). Media vary in their ability to detect hydrogen sulfide. Lead acetate, the most sensitive indicator, should be used to test bacteria that produce small amounts of hydrogen sulfide. Incorporating lead acetate in media, however, may inhibit bacterial growth, so a filter paper strip impregnated with lead acetate is draped under the cap of a tube of KIA. Sulfide-indole-motility medium is more sensitive than KIA, possibly because it is semisolid, lacks carbohydrates (which suppress hydrogen sulfide formation), and uses peptonized iron as the indicator. Kligler's iron agar is more sensitive than TSIA, probably because the sucrose in TSIA suppresses the enzymes responsible for hydrogen sulfide production.

Motility. The fastest, most direct method of detecting motility is to place a drop of broth culture medium incubated at room temperature for 2 to 4 hours onto a microscope slide and view it under oil immersion. Purposeful and directed movement of one or many bacteria, rather than the flowing movement of all bacteria in a field, indicates motility. Motility also may be detected by inoculating a semisolid medium (commercially available): the center of the agar butt is stabbed vertically to a depth of about 2 cm with a straight wire carrying the inoculum and incubated overnight at the temperature preferred by the organism. Motility is indicated by a haze of growth extending from the stab line into the agar. Incorporating a colored growth indicator such as tetrazolium salts is not recommended because it may inhibit certain bacteria.

Features of Commonly Encountered Enterobacteriaceae

Escherichia coli. Colonies of E. coli on sheep blood agar are gray, 2 to 3 mm in diameter, and often surrounded by a zone of complete hemolysis. On MacConkey agar, colonies are pink, owing to lactose fermentation, and the surrounding agar often contains a dark pink precipitate (Plate VE). Reactions of E. coli in KIA are acid slant and acid butt (A/A) with gas formation. Additional biochemi-

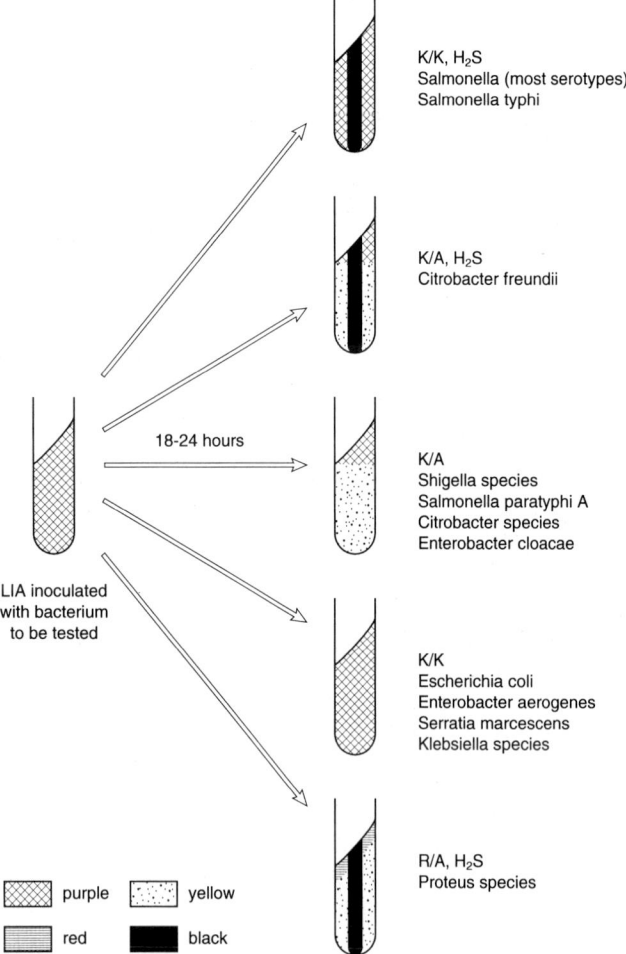

Fig. 34–4. Reactions produced in lysine iron agar (LIA) by common Enterobacteriaceae.

cal reactions typical of E. coli are positive indole, methyl red, and lysine and ornithine decarboxylase; and negative Voges-Proskauer, citrate, and urease. In the clinical laboratory, isolates recovered in pure culture (as from urine specimens) presumptively are called E. coli based on the appearance of colonies of MacConkey agar and a positive spot indole test (described earlier).

The identification of strains of Escherichia coli that cause diarrhea requires additional testing. Infection with ETEC is diagnosed by detecting heat-labile or heat-stable toxin, or both. Traditionally, E. coli culture supernatants have been tested in the Chinese hamster ovary or Y1 adrenal cell culture assay (for LT) and in the suckling mouse assay (for ST), procedures that are time consuming, costly, and unsuitable for large-scale epidemiologic studies (24). Recently, genes that code for LT and ST have been characterized, and specific fragments have been cloned and used to identify ETEC; however, currently these probes are not commercially available and testing must be performed in a specialized reference laboratory (4,24). In addition, an enzyme-linked immunosorbent assay for detecting LT has been developed but is not yet commercially available (24). Conventional techniques for detecting EIEC are the Sereney test (or guinea pig conjunctivitis test) and the HEp-2 or HeLa cell invasion assay (4,24). Radiolabeled and biotinylated probes cloned from the large plasmid associated with invasiveness also detect EIEC, but these tests are not available commercially (4). Enteropathogenic E. coli are identified by their pattern of adherence in the HEp-2 or HeLa cell adhesion assay or by using a radiolabeled DNA probe cleaved from the entero-adhesiveness factor (4). Enteroaggregative E. coli are detected by their pattern of adherence in the HEp-2 cell assay, and a DNA probe prepared from the 60-megadalton plasmid necessary for expression of this phenotype may prove valuable for diagnosis (124).

To detect EHEC, stool samples must be inoculated onto sorbitol-MacConkey agar plates (MacConkey agar containing sorbitol in place of lactose). Strains of EHEC do not ferment sorbitol, and almost all other strains of Escherichia coli do. Clear colonies (indicating that sorbitol was not fermented) identified biochemically as E. coli (described earlier) are serotyped by a slide-agglutination test using E. coli 0157 antiserum (commercially available), and the H7 flagellar antigen is detected by an immobilization test in semisolid motility agar containing H7 antiserum (commercially available) (125). Direct staining of colonies from sorbitol-MacConkey agar with fluorescein-labeled, polyclonal antibodies to E. coli 0157:H7 appears to be a reliable method of identification, but data are limited (126). Detecting toxin production in the Vero cell culture assay also is important because strains of E. coli other than 0157:H7, in particular 026:H11, may cause hemorrhagic colitis (4,19). A DNA probe prepared from a segment of the 60-Mda plasmid that encodes a fimbrial antigen and promotes attachment to epithelial cells reliably identifies EHEC, but currently it is not available commercially (127).

Shigella species. Species of Shigella do not ferment lactose, thus forming colorless colonies on MacConkey agar and green colonies on Hektoen enteric agar. Reactions in KIA are alkaline slant and acid butt (K/A) with neither hydrogen sulfide nor gas formation, except for certain gas-producing biogroups of Shigella flexneri. Species of Shigella are nonmotile, and typically they are biochemically inert: negative for methyl red, Voges-Proskauer, citrate, urease, and lysine decarboxylase, and variable for indole (about half of serogroups A, B, and C are positive). Additional biochemical reactions are shown in Table 34–4.

Isolates of Shigella should be examined for agglutination in polyvalent antisera (commercially available) for each of the four species by testing a suspension of bacteria prepared from a KIA slant. Agglutination within 30 seconds is a positive reaction. If a suspension of bacteria with biochemical reactions characteristic of Shigella fails to agglutinate, the suspension should be boiled for 30 minutes, cooled, and retested, because many Shigella, particularly isolates of groups A and C, possess heat-labile envelope or capsular antigens that inhibit agglutination of unheated bacteria in O antisera. All isolates of Shigella should be reported to the State Department of Health.

Salmonella species. Species of Salmonella produce hydrogen sulfide but do not ferment lactose; therefore, colonies are clear on MacConkey agar and are green with a black center on Hektoen enteric agar. Reactions in KIA are alkaline slant and acid butt (K/A) with production of hydrogen sulfide and gas. Most serotypes of Salmonella are motile; positive for methyl red, citrate, and lysine decarboxylase; and negative for indole, urease, and malonate. Additional biochemical reactions are listed in Table 34–4.

Isolates of Salmonella should be serotyped on the basis of heat-stable O antigens of the cell wall, found in many other genera; heat-labile H antigens of the flagella, specific to the salmonellae; and the Vi surface polysaccharide antigen, present in Salmonella typhi and in some species of Citrobacter. The O and Vi antigens are easily detected in the clinical microbiology laboratory by slide agglutination using saline suspensions of live organisms; H antigen detection via tube agglutination is not performed routinely. Organisms that possess the Vi antigen may not agglutinate in homologous O antisera but may be rendered agglutinable by boiling a saline suspension of the organism for 30 minutes. The Salmonella are assigned to groups based on the predominant O antigen, and most clinical laboratories test antisera (commercially available) that will detect the groups to which most human isolates belong: polyvalent O antiserum, O antisera for serogroups A, B, C_1, C_2, D, and E (a mixed antiserum that agglutinates all members of E_1, E_2, E_3, and E_4), and a Vi antiserum. All isolates of Salmonella must be reported to the State Department of Health.

Yersinia species. Colonies of Yersinia are clear on MacConkey agar, indicating failure to ferment lactose, but most Yersinia enterocolitica and many Yersinia pseudotuberculosis give a positive result with ONPG (described earlier). The reactions in KIA are alkaline slant and acid butt (K/A) without gas or hydrogen sulfide production. In TSIA, Yersinia enterocolitica produces an acid slant and acid butt (A/A) because it ferments sucrose; whereas Yersinia pestis and Yersinia pseudotuberculosis do not ferment sucrose and produce an alkaline slant and acid butt. All species of Yersinia are motile and Voges-Proskauer positive at 25° C but nonmotile and Voges-Proskauer negative at 35° to 37° C, a key identifying feature. Almost all Y. pseudotuberculosis and about 75% of Yersinia enterocolitica are urease positive. Because handling Yersinia pestis is hazardous, suspect cultures may be mailed to the CDC for identification. Serologic tests have been used to detect antibodies to Yersinia enterocolitica and Yersinia pestis, but these are not commercially available. A fluorescent antibody stain to detect Y. pestis in tissue is available only in specialized reference laboratories.

Klebsiella species. On blood agar, the Klebsiella form large, gray-white mucoid colonies, and on MacConkey agar colonies are mucoid and dark pink owing to lactose fermentation (Plate VF). Reactions in KIA are acid slant and acid butt (A/A) with gas formation. All species of Klebsiella are nonmotile and characteristically give negative reactions for arginine dihydrolase, ornithine decarboxylase, methyl red, and hydrogen sulfide and positive reactions for Voges-Proskauer, citrate, and urease. Moreover, uniform resistance to ampicillin and carbenicillin are useful identifying features. Klebsiella pneumoniae does not produce indole, whereas Klebsiella oxytoca does. Other biochemical tests useful for identifying these two species are shown in Table 34–4; references 1, 122, and 123 describe tests useful for identifying other species.

Enterobacter species. In general, on blood agar colonies of Enterobacter appear similar to those of Klebsiella but usually are less mucoid, and colonies of Enterobacter agglomerans and Enterobacter sakazakii are yellow. Most isolates of Enterobacter cloacae and Enterobacter aerogenes ferment lactose, but for the other species the lactose reaction is variable. Therefore, reactions in KIA may be acid slant and acid butt (A/A) with gas production or alkaline slant and acid butt (K/A) with gas formation. Most species of Enterobacter are motile; give positive reactions for ornithine decarboxylase, Voges-Proskauer, and citrate; ferment arabinose, raffinose, and rhamnose; and are negative for DNase, hydrogen sulfide, and indole. Moreover, these organisms are resistant to ampicillin and cephalothin. Additional biochemical reactions to identify Enterobacter cloacae and Enterobacter aerogenes are shown in Table 34–4, and reactions helpful for identifying other species are found in references 1, 122, and 123.

Serratia species. Colonies of Serratia marcescens are 1 to 2 mm in diameter, gray-white, and smooth on blood agar after incubation for 24 hours at 35° C and may become red pigmented if incubated an additional 24 to 48 hours at room temperature. Most isolates of S. marcescens do not ferment lactose, so colonies on MacConkey agar are colorless. Reactions in KIA are alkaline slant and acid butt (K/A), with or without gas production. Most species of Serratia are resistant to colistin, motile, and give negative reactions for arginine dihydrolase, hydrogen sulfide, and urease, and positive reactions for citrate and Voges-Proskauer. Unique among the Enterobacteriaceae, these organisms produce the enzymes DNase, gelatinase, and lipase. Additional tests to identify S. marcescens are shown in Table 34–4; the biochemical profiles of other Serratia species are found elsewhere (1,122,123).

Proteus and Providencia species. Proteus mirabilis and Proteus vulgaris are unique in their ability to swarm on blood agar (Plate VIA). These organisms produce hydrogen sulfide but do not ferment lactose, so colonies are colorless on MacConkey agar and green with a black center on Hektoen agar (identical to those of Salmonella). Reactions in KIA are alkaline slant and acid butt (K/A), with blackening in the butt or throughout the tube. Typically, Proteus are motile, positive for methyl red, phenylalanine (and tryptophan) and lysine deaminase, and urease; negative for lysine decarboxylase; and resistant to colistin and nitrofurantoin. Proteus mirabilis is indole negative and ornithine decarboxylase positive; Proteus vulgaris is indole positive and ornithine negative. Species of Providencia give negative reactions for lactose and hydrogen sulfide; therefore colonies are colorless on MacConkey agar, and reactions in KIA are alkaline slant and acid butt (K/A), with or without gas formation. Providencia typically are positive for motility, citrate, phenylalanine deaminase, and indole and negative for arginine dihydrolase and lysine and ornithine decarboxylase. For additional biochemical reactions to identify to Proteus and Providencia the reader is referred to Table 34–4 and references 1, 122, and 123.

Citrobacter species. Species of Citrobacter are motile, positive for citrate, and produce gas from glucose. They are negative for lysine decarboxylase and Voges-Proskauer and yield variable reactions for lactose. About 80% of Citrobacter freundii are hydrogen sulfide positive. Additional biochemical reactions to identify the species of Citrobacter are found in Table 34–4 and references 1, 122, and 123.

Treatment and Prevention

Escherichia coli. The mainstay of therapy for most cases of diarrhea caused by E. coli is fluid and electrolyte replacement. Antimicrobial therapy (e.g., ampicillin, trimethoprim-sulfamethoxazole, or norfloxacin) generally is indicated only for enteroinvasive disease. Vaccines based on the major virulence determinants of diarrheagenic E. coli have been developed and currently are being evaluated. In one study, oral administration of a live, nontoxigenic fimbriated strain of E. coli induced a secretory immunoglobulin A response in the intestines and was protective against diarrhea, but further evaluations of this type of vaccine should be conducted because recent data indicate that strains of ETEC that lack colonization factors can produce diarrhea (128,129).

Antimicrobial agents are essential in the treatment of extraintestinal infections with Escherichia coli. Urinary tract infections generally respond to ampicillin, amoxicillin, or trimethoprim-sulfamethoxazole, and for community-acquired lower urinary tract infections susceptibility testing may not be necessary, except in cases of clinical failure. Susceptibility testing always should be performed on isolates of E. coli from other body sites, and therapy should be based on the antibiogram. Many isolates are susceptible to ampicillin and the cephalosporins, and almost all are susceptible to the aminoglycosides. Meningitis caused by E. coli is treated with ampicillin plus an aminoglycoside, but in the presence of renal failure a third-generation cephalosporin that achieves optimal levels in the cerebrospinal fluid (such as cefotaxime or ceftriaxone) may be substituted for the aminoglycoside.

***Shigella* species.** Treatment of shigellosis includes supportive care, maintaining fluid and electrolyte balance, and administration of an antimicrobial. Ampicillin, trimethoprim-sulfamethoxazole, or norfloxacin usually is effective, but some organisms are resistant and therapy should be based on the results of susceptibility testing.

Good hand-washing practices and maintaining safe water supplies and effective sewage systems are important for disease prevention. Two types of oral vaccine are being evaluated: attenuated strains of Salmonella and an Escherichia coli K12 strain, each carrying the 140-Mda plasmid necessary for invasion, to which the genes that encode the Shigella somatic antigens have been conjugally transferred (130).

***Salmonella* species.** Antimicrobial therapy is not indicated for most persons with enterocolitis or for transient intestinal carriers but is necessary for persons with enteric fever, bacteremia, or localized infections caused by Salmonella. Effective therapy includes chloramphenicol, ampicillin (which may terminate the chronic carrier state and is the agent of choice for intravascular infections), trimethoprim-sulfamethoxazole, certain third-generation cephalosporins, and possibly ciprofloxacin (131). Antimicrobial therapy has been complicated by the emergence of strains of Salmonella that are resistant to multiple antimicrobial agents, a phenomenon caused by the widespread use of antimicrobials in humans and animals. Supportive therapy for enterocolitis and enteric fever includes fluid and electrolyte balance and maintenance of nutrition. If the chronic carrier state is not eradicated with ampicillin (or amoxicillin), cholecystectomy should be considered.

Control of salmonellosis transmitted by animals requires controlling infection in the animal reservoirs, reducing contamination of foodstuffs prepared from animals, and enforcing standards for processing and preparing food in commercial and private kitchens. Control of disease acquired by person-to-person spread depends on good personal hygiene habits (especially hand washing), maintaining a supply of uncontaminated water, proper sewage disposal, and identifying, treating, and following chronic carriers.

Typhoid vaccine, a saline suspension of acetone- or heat- or phenol-killed Salmonella typhi, has an efficacy rate of 51 to 67%, but the degree of resistance to infection it confers can be overcome by increasing the inoculum (73,132). A live attenuated oral vaccine prepared from the Ty 21a strain of S. typhi, which had an efficacy rate about 67% in one field trial, appears to be as effective as the conventional parenteral whole cell vaccine but is associated with fewer side effects (132–134). Using the capsular polysaccharide Vi antigen of S. typhi as a parenteral typhoid vaccine also is being evaluated (135). Immunization against serotypes of Salmonella other than S. typhi is not effective in humans.

***Yersinia* species.** Antimicrobial therapy usually is not indicated for uncomplicated enterocolitis or the pseudoappendicular syndrome caused by Yersinia enterocolitica or Yersinia pseudotuberculosis, but it is necessary for systemic infections, focal extraintestinal infections, and enterocolitis in compromised hosts. Doxycycline or trimethoprim-sulfamethoxazole is recommended for complicated gastrointestinal and focal extraintestinal infections, and the combination of doxycycline and an aminoglycoside is appropriate therapy for bacteremia. The quinolones may prove to be the agents of choice, but this requires documentation by further investigation.

To prevent infection with Yersinia enterocolitica reservoirs must be eliminated and the frequency of ingesting contaminated food, especially raw pork and beverages, reduced. Environmental sources and common vehicles of transmission should be located during outbreaks. Enteric precautions are recommended for hospitalized persons who have Y. enterocolitica–induced diarrhea.

The estimated mortality rate for untreated plague is over 50%, so after appropriate cultures are obtained prompt institution of effective antimicrobial therapy is essential. Streptomycin is the agent of choice; tetracycline and chloramphenicol are acceptable alternatives. Maintaining fluid and electrolyte balance also is important. Persons with cough or other signs of pneumonia must be placed in strict isolation for a minimum of 48 hours after antimicrobial therapy is instituted, or until sputum culture is negative. Contacts of a person who has plague pneumonia should be given prophylactic tetracycline or sulfadiazine.

A formalin-killed vaccine is available for travelers to endemic or hyperendemic areas, for persons who must live and work in close contact with rodents, and for laboratory personnel who must handle live cultures of Yersinia pestis. Urban plague has been controlled successfully in many cities in the world by quarantine, rat control, and insecticides; however, sylvatic plague is difficult to control owing to the wide-ranging and diverse wild rodent reservoirs.

Other Enterobacteriaceae. Resistance to multiple antimicrobials is common among isolates of Enterobacter, Serratia, Proteus vulgaris, Providencia, and Citrobacter, and therapy for infections they cause is based on the antibiogram. For serious infections, treatment often consists of an aminoglycoside plus an extended-spectrum penicillin such as mezlocillin or a third-generation cephalosporin such as cefotaxime or ceftriaxone; and for very resistant organisms, imipenem or ciprofloxacin should be considered. Because the predominant mode of transmission of these organisms in the hospital is the hands of personnel, proper hand washing should prevent spread. Catheter-associated urinary tract infections may be avoided by maintaining a closed draining system, limiting irrigations, and removing the catheter as soon as possible. To limit spread of Serratia marcescens, patients whose urinary or respiratory tract is colonized or infected should be separated from uncolonized patients.

REFERENCES

1. Farmer JJ III, and Kelly MT: Enterobacteriaceae. *In* Manual of Clinical Microbiology. 5th ed. Edited by A Balows, et

al. Washington, DC, American Society for Microbiology, 1991.
2. Miller JM, and Farmer JJ III: Recent additions to the Enterobacteriaceae. Clin Microbiol Newslett, 9:173, 1987.
3. Baron EJ, and Finegold SM (eds): Enterobacteriaceae. In Bailey and Scott's Diagnostic Microbiology. 8th ed. St. Louis, CV Mosby, 1990.
4. Levine MM: Escherichia coli that cause diarrhea: Enterotoxigenic, enteropathogenic, enteroinvasive, enterohemorrhagic, and enteroadherent. J Infect Dis, 155:377, 1987.
5. Bhan MK, et al: Escherichia coli associated with persistent diarrhea in a cohort of rural children in India. J Infect Dis, 159:1061, 1989.
6. Vial PA, et al: Characterization of enteroadherent-aggregative Escherichia coli, a putative agent of diarrheal disease. J Infect Dis, 158:70, 1988.
7. Sack RB: Enterotoxigenic Escherichia coli: Identification and characterization. J Infect Dis, 142:279, 1980.
8. Merson MH, et al: Traveler's diarrhea in Mexico. A prospective study of physicians and family members attending a congress. N Engl J Med, 294:1299, 1976.
9. Rosenberg ML, et al: Epidemic diarrhea at Crater Lake from enterotoxigenic Escherichia coli. A large waterborne outbreak. Ann Intern Med, 86:714, 1977.
10. DuPont HL, et al: Pathogenesis of Escherichia coli diarrhea. N Engl J Med, 285:1, 1971.
11. Harris JR, Wachsmuth IK, Davis BR, and Cohen ML: High–molecular weight plasmid correlates with Escherichia coli enteroinvasiveness. Infect Immun, 37:1295, 1982.
12. Hale TL, et al: Characterization of virulence plasmids and plasmid-associated outer membrane proteins in Shigella flexneri, Shigella sonnei, and Escherichia coli. Infect Immun, 40:340, 1983.
13. Robins-Browne RM: Traditional enteropathogenic Escherichia coli of infantile diarrhea. Rev Infect Dis, 9:28, 1987.
14. Gomes TAT, Blake PA, and Trabulsi LR: Prevalence of Escherichia coli strains with localized, diffuse, and aggregative adherence to HeLa cells in infants with diarrhea and matched controls. J Clin Microbiol, 27:266, 1989.
15. Levine MM, et al: The diarrheal response of humans to some classic serotypes of enteropathogenic Escherichia coli is dependent on a plasmid encoding and enteroadhesiveness factor. J Infect Dis, 152:550, 1985.
16. Nataro JP, et al: Detection of an adherence factor of enteropathogenic Escherichia coli with a DNA probe. J Infect Dis, 152:560, 1985.
17. Riley LW, et al: Hemorrhagic colitis associated with a rare Escherichia coli serotype. N Engl J Med, 308:681, 1982.
18. Spika JS, et al: Hemolytic uremic syndrome and diarrhea associated with Escherichia coli 0157:H7 in a day care center. J Pediatr, 109:287, 1986.
19. Karmali MA: Infection by verotoxin-producing Escherichia coli. Clin Microbiol Rev, 2:15, 1989.
20. Pai CH, Gordon R, Sims HV, and Bryan LE: Sporadic cases of hemorrhagic colitis associated with Escherichia coli 0157:H7. Clinical, epidemiologic, and bacteriologic features. Ann Intern Med, 101:738, 1984.
21. Stewart PJ, Desormeaux W, and Chene J: Hemorrhagic colitis in a home for the aged: Ontario. Can Dis Weekly Rep, 9:29, 1983.
22. Nataro JP, et al: Patterns of adherence of diarrheagenic Escherichia coli to HEp-2 cells. Pediatr Infect Dis J, 6:829, 1987.
23. Martin ML, et al: Isolation of Escherichia coli 0157:H7 from dairy cattle associated with two cases of hemolytic-uremic syndrome. Lancet, ii:1043, 1986.
24. Riley LW: Infectious diseases associated with Escherichia coli. In Laboratory Diagnosis of Infectious Diseases—Principles and Practice. Edited by A Balows, WJ Hausler, Jr, M Ohashi, and A Turano. New York, Springer-Verlag, 1988.
25. Rubin RH: Infections of the urinary tract. Inf Dis Sci Am, 7:1, 1987.
26. Centers for Disease Control: Surveillance summaries 1986. MMWR, 35:17SS, 1986.
27. Weinstein MP, Murphy JR, Reller LB, and Lichtenstein KA: The clinical significance of positive blood cultures: A comprehensive analysis of 500 episodes of bacteremia and fungemia in adults. II. Clinical observations with special reference to factors influencing prognosis. Rev Infect Dis, 5:54, 1983.
28. McCabe WR, et al: Escherichia coli in bacteremia: K and O antigens and serum sensitivity of strains from adults and neonates. J Infect Dis, 138:33, 1978.
29. Mulder CJJ, van Alphen L, and Zanen HC: Neonatal meningitis caused by Escherichia coli in the Netherlands. J Infect, 9:177, 1984.
30. Speer CP, Hauptmann D, Stubbe P, and Gahr M: Neonatal septicemia and meningitis in Göttingen, West Germany. Ped Infect Dis, 4:36, 1985.
31. McCracken GH Jr, et al: Moxalactam therapy for neonatal meningitis due to gram-negative bacilli. JAMA, 252:1427, 1984.
32. Shiga K: Observations on the epidemiology of dysentery in Japan. Philippine J Sci, 1:485, 1906.
33. Flexner S: On the etiology of tropical dysentery. Philadelphia Med J, 6:417, 1990.
34. Lee LA, Shapiro CN, Hargrett-Bean N, and Tauxe RV: Hyperendemic shigellosis in the United States: A review of surveillance data for 1967–1988. J Infect Dis, 164:894, 1991.
35. Keusch GT, and Bennish ML: Shigellosis: Recent progress, persisting problems, and research issues. Pediatr Infect Dis J, 8:713, 1989.
36. Centers for Disease Control: Summary of notifiable diseases, United States, 1989. MMWR, 38(54):1, 1989.
37. Reeve G, et al: An outbreak of shigellosis associated with the consumption of raw oysters. N Engl J Med, 321:224, 1989.
38. Kao NL, Stein DS, and Koneman EW: Shigellosis: Not exclusively a pediatric problem. Clin Microbiol Newslett, 10:172, 1988.
39. Keusch GR, and Bennish ML: Shigellosis. In Bacterial diseases of humans. 2nd ed. Edited by AS Evans and P Brachman. New York: Plenum, 1989.
40. Centers for Disease Control: Shigellosis—United States, 1984. MMWR, 34:600, 1985.
41. Levine MM, et al: Shigellosis in custodial institutions. J Pediatr, 84:803, 1974.
42. Hale TL, Oaks V, and Formal SB: Identification and antigenic characterization of virulence-associated, plasmid-coded proteins of Shigella spp. and enteroinvasive Escherichia coli. Infect Immun, 50:620, 1985.
43. Keusch GT, et al: Pathogenesis of shigella diarrhea. II. Enterotoxin-induced acute enteritis in the rabbit ileum. J Infect Dis, 126:92, 1972.
44. Koster F, et al: Haemolytic-uremic syndrome after shigellosis. N Engl J Med, 298:927, 1978.
45. Jackson HP, and Kilgore DG, Jr: Purulent meningitis caused by Shigella flexneri. SC Med Assoc J, 67:347, 1971.
46. Morduchowicz G, et al: Shigella bacteremia in adults—a report of five cases and review of the literature. Arch Intern Med, 147:2034, 1987.
47. Silliker JH, and Gabis DA: Salmonellosis. In Laboratory Di-

agnosis of Infectious Diseases—Principles and Practice. Edited by A Balows, WJ Hausler, Jr, M Ohashi, and A Turano. New York, Springer-Verlag, 1988.
48. Ewing WH: An outline of nomenclature of the family Enterobacteriaceae. Int Bull Bacteriol Nomencl Taxon, 13: 95, 1963.
49. Farmer JJ III, McWhorter AC, Brenner DJ, and Morris GK: The Salmonella-Arizona group of Enterobacteriaceae: Nomenclature, classification, and reporting. Clin Microbiol Newslett, 6:63, 1984.
50. Feldman RE, et al: Epidemiology of Salmonella typhi infections in a migrant labor camp in Dade County, Florida. J Infect Dis, 130:334, 1974.
51. Ryan CA, Hargrett-Bean NT, and Blake PA: Salmonella typhi infections in the United States, 1975–1984: Increasing role of foreign travel. Rev Infect Dis, 11:2, 1989.
52. Bennett IL, Jr, and Hook EW: Infectious diseases (some aspects of salmonellosis). Annu Rev Med, 10:1, 1959.
53. Aserkoff B, Schroeder SA, and Brechman PS: Salmonellosis in the United States—a five-year review. Am J Epidemiol, 92:13, 1970.
54. Centers for Disease Control: Update: Salmonella enteritidis infections and grade A shell eggs. MMWR, 37:490, 1988.
55. Centers for Disease Control: Update: Salmonella enteritidis infections and grade A shell eggs—United States, 1989. MMWR, 38:877, 1990.
56. Tacket CO, et al: An outbreak of multiple drug–resistant Salmonella enteritis from raw milk. JAMA, 253:2058, 1985.
57. Ryan CA, et al: Massive outbreak of antimicrobial-resistant salmonellosis traced to pasteurized milk. JAMA, 258:3269, 1987.
58. Cohen ML, et al: Turtle-associated salmonellosis in the United States. JAMA, 243:1247, 1980.
59. Centers for Disease Control: Multistate outbreak of Salmonella poona infections—United States and Canada, 1991. MMWR, 40:549, 1991.
60. Taylor DN, et al: Salmonellosis associated with marijuana. N Engl J Med, 306:1249, 1982.
61. Dean AG: Transmission of Salmonella typhi by fiberoptic endoscopy. Lancet, ii:134, 1977.
62. Hook EW: Salmonella species (including typhoid fever). In Principles and Practice of Infectious Diseases. 3rd ed. Edited by GL Mandell, RG Douglas, Jr, and JE Bennett. New York, Churchill Livingstone, 1990.
63. Pether JVS, and Scott RJD: Salmonella carriers; are they dangerous? A study to identify finger contamination with Salmonellae by convalescent carriers. J Infect, 5:81, 1982.
64. Rosenstein BJ: Salmonellosis in infants and children: Epidemiologic and therapeutic considerations. J Pediatr, 70:1, 1967.
65. Baine WB, et al: Institutional salmonellosis. J Infect Dis, 128:357, 1973.
66. Centers for Disease Control: Salmonella isolates from humans in the United States, 1984–1986. MMWR, 37(SS-2): 25, 1988.
67. Riley LW, et al: Importance of host factors in human salmonellosis caused by multiresistant strains of Salmonella. J Infect Dis, 149:878, 1984.
68. Holmberg SD, Osterholm MT, Senger KA, and Cohen ML: Drug-resistant Salmonella from animals fed antimicrobials. N Engl J Med, 311:617, 1984.
69. Sperber SJ, and Schleupner CJ: Salmonellosis during infection with human immunodeficiency virus. Rev Infect Dis, 9:925, 1987.
70. Noskin GA, and Clarke JT: Salmonella arizonae bacteremia as the presenting manifestation of human immunodeficiency virus infection following rattlesnake meat ingestion. Rev Infect Dis, 12:514, 1990.
71. Hand WL, and King NL: Serum opsonization of Salmonella in sickle cell anemia. Am J Med, 64:388, 1978.
72. Musch MW, et al: Stimulation of colonic secretion by lipoxygenase metabolites of arachidonic acid. Science, 217: 1255, 1982.
73. Hornick RB, et al: Typhoid fever: Pathogenesis and immunologic control. N Engl J Med, 283:686, 1970.
74. Edelman R and Levine MM: Summary of an international workshop on typhoid fever. Rev Infect Dis, 8:329, 1986.
75. Hornick RB and Greisman S: On the pathogenesis of typhoid fever. Arch Intern Med, 138:357, 1978.
76. Schleifstein JI, and Coleman MB: An unidentified microorganism resembling B. lignieri and Past. pseudotuberculosis, and pathogenic for man. NY State J Med, 39:1749, 1939.
77. Mollaret HH, Bercovier H, and Alonso JM: Summary of the data received at the WHO Reference Center for Yersinia enterocolitica. Contrib Microbiol Immunol, 5:174, 1979.
78. Marks MI, et al: Yersinia enterocolitica gastroenteritis: A prospective study of clinical, bacteriologic, and epidemiologic features. J Pediatr, 96:26, 1980.
79. Hoogkamp-Korstanje JA, de Koning J, and Samson J: Incidence of human infection with Yersinia enterocolitica serotypes 0:3, 0:8, and 0:9 and the use of indirect immunofluorescence in diagnosis. J Infect Dis, 153:138, 1986.
80. Dajani AS, and Mauer MJ: Is Yersinia enterocolitica gastroenteritis a Canadian disease? J Pediatr, 97:165, 1980.
81. Mingrone MG, Fantasia M, Figura N, and Guglielmetti P: Characteristics of Yersinia enterocolitica isolated from children with diarrhea in Italy. J Clin Microbiol, 25:1301, 1987.
82. Black RE, et al: Epidemic Yersinia enterocolitica infection due to contaminated chocolate milk. N Engl J Med, 298: 76, 1978.
83. Toivanen P, Toivanen A, Olkkonen L, and Anantaa S: Hospital outbreak of Yersinia enterocolitica infection. Lancet, i: 801, 1973.
84. Tauxe RV, et al: Yersinia enterocolitica infections and pork: The missing link. Lancet, i:1129, 1987.
85. Ratnam S, et al: A nosocomial outbreak of diarrheal disease due to Yersinia enterocolitica serotype 0:5, biotype 1. J Infect Dis, 145:242, 1982.
86. Cover TL, and Aber RC: Yersinia enterocolitica. N Engl J Med, 321:16, 1989.
87. Miroshi Z: Epidemiologic aspects of yersiniosis in Japan. In Yersinia enterocolitica. Edited by EJ Buttone. Boca Raton, Florida, CRC Press, 1981.
88. Van Noyen R, Vandepitte J, Wauters G, and Selderslaghs R: Yersinia enterocolitica: Its isolation by cold enrichment from patients and healthy subjects. J Clin Pathol, 34:1052, 1981.
89. de Groote G, Vandepitte J, and Wauters G: Surveillance of human Yersinia enterocolitica infections in Belgium: 1963–1978. J Infect, 4:189, 1982.
90. Christensen SG: The Yersinia enterocolitica situation in Denmark. Contrib Microbiol Immunol, 9:93, 1987.
91. Lee LA, et al: Yersinia enterocolitica 0:3 infections in infants and children, associated with the household preparation of chitterlings. N Engl J Med, 322:984, 1990.
92. Jacobs J, et al: Yersinia enterocolitica in donor blood: A case report and review. J Clin Microbiol, 27:1119, 1989.
93. Carter PB: Pathogenicity of Yersinia enterocolitica for mice. Infect Immun, 11:164, 1975.
94. Foberg U, et al: Yersinia enterocolitica septicemia: Clinical and microbiological aspects. Scand J Infect Dis, 18:269, 1986.

95. Gutman LT, et al: An inter-familial outbreak of Yersinia enterocolitica enteritis. N Engl J Med, 288:1372, 1973.
96. Jepsen OB, et al: Yersinia enterocolitica infection in patients with acute surgical abdominal disease: A prospective study. Scand J Infect Dis, 8:189, 1976.
97. Nilehn B, and Sjostrom B: Studies on Yersinia enterocolitica: occurrence in various groups of acute abdominal disease. Acta Pathol Microbiol Scand, 71:612, 1967.
98. Granfors K, et al: Yersinia antigens in synovial fluid cells from patients with reactive arthritis. N Engl J Med, 320:216, 1989.
99. Aho K, et al: HLA-27 in reactive arthritis: A study of yersinia arthritis and Reiter's disease. Arthritis Rheum, 17:521, 1974.
100. Laitinen O, Leirisalo, M, and Skylv G: Relation between HLA-B27 and clinical features in patients with yersinia arthritis. Arthritis Rheum, 20:1121, 1977.
101. Butler T: Yersinia species (including plague). In Principles and Practice of Infectious Diseases. 3rd ed. Edited by GL Mandell, RG Douglas, Jr, and JE Bennett. New York, Churchill Livingstone, 1990.
102. Barnes AM, Quan TJ, Beard ML, and Maupin GO: Plague in American Indians, 1956–1987. MMWR, 37(SS-3):11, 1988.
103. Weniger BG, et al: Human bubonic plague transmitted by a domestic cat scratch. JAMA, 251:927, 1984.
104. Werner SB, et al: Primary plague pneumonia contracted from a domestic cat scratch. JAMA, 251:929, 1984.
105. Einstein BI: Enterobacteriaceae. In Principles and Practice of Infectious Diseases. 3rd ed. Edited by GL Mandell, RG Douglas, Jr, and JE Bennett. New York, Churchill Livingstone, 1990.
106. de la Torre MG, et al: Klebsiella bacteremia: An analysis of 100 cases. Rev Infect Dis, 7:143, 1985.
107. Reyes E: Rhinoscleroma. Observations based on a study of two hundred cases. Arch Dermatol Syph, 54:531, 1946.
108. Muzyka MM and Gubina KM: Problems of the epidemiology of scleroma. J Hyg Epidemiol Microbiol Immunol, 15:233, 1971.
109. Centers for Disease Control: Nosocomial infection surveillance, 1984. MMWR, 33(Suppl 3SS):17, 1984.
110. Willis J and Robinson JE: Enterobacter sakazakii meningitis in neonates. Pediatr Infect Dis J, 7:196, 1988.
111. Gaston MA: Enterobacter: An emerging nosocomial pathogen. J Hosp Infect, 11:197, 1988.
112. Yannelli B, Schoch PE, and Cunha BA: Serratia marcescens. Clin Microbiol Newslett, 9:157, 1987.
113. Maki DG, and Martin WT: Nationwide epidemic septicemia caused by contaminated infusion products. IV. Growth of microbial pathogens in fluids for intravenous infusion. J Infect Dis, 131:267, 1975.
114. Mills J, and Drew E: Serratia marcescens endocarditis: A regional illness associated with intravenous drug abuse. Ann Intern Med, 84:29, 1976.
115. Ashby ME: Serratia osteomyelitis in heroin users. J Bone Joint Surg, 158A:132, 1976.
116. Dorwar BB, Abrutyn E, and Schumacher HR: Serratia arthritis. JAMA, 225:1642, 1973.
117. Nakashima AK, et al: Epidemic septic arthritis caused by Serratia marcescens and associated with a benzalkonium chloride antiseptic. J Clin Microbiol, 25:1014, 1987.
118. Mosher DM, et al: Role of urease in pyelonephritis resulting from urinary tract infection with Proteus. J Infect Dis, 131:177, 1975.
119. Wray SK, et al: Identification and characterization of a uropathogenic isolate of Proteus mirabilis. Infect Immun, 54:43, 1986.
120. Warren JW: Providencia stuartii: A common cause of antibiotic-resistant bacteriuria in patients with long-term indwelling catheters. Rev Infect Dis, 8:61, 1986.
121. Kline MW, Mason EO, Jr, and Kaplan SL: Characterization of Citrobacter diversus strains causing neonatal meningitis. J Infect Dis, 157:101, 1988.
122. Koneman EW, et al (eds): The Enterobacteriaceae. In Color Atlas and Textbook of Diagnostic Microbiology. 3rd ed. Philadelphia, JB Lippincott, 1988.
123. Farmer JJ III, et al: Biochemical identification of new species and biogroup of Enterobacteriaceae from clinical specimens. J Clin Microbiol, 21:46, 1985.
124. Baudry B, et al: A sensitive and specific DNA probe to identify enteroaggregative Escherichia coli, a recently discovered diarrheal pathogen. J Infect Dis, 161:1249, 1990.
125. Marshall WF, et al: Results of a 6-month survey of stool cultures for Escherichia coli 0157:H7. Mayo Clin Proc, 65:787, 1990.
126. Tison DL: Culture confirmation of Escherichia coli serotype 0157:H7 by direct immunofluorescence. J Clin Microbiol, 28:612, 1990.
127. Levine MM, et al: A DNA probe to identify enterohemorrhagic Escherichia coli of 0157:H7 and other serotypes that cause hemorrhagic colitis and hemolytic uremic syndrome. J Infect Dis, 156:175, 1987.
128. Svennerholm AM, et al: Mucosal immunity in the gastrointestinal tract in relation to ETEC vaccine development. In Progress in Vaccinology. Edited by GP Tarwar. New York, Springer-Verlag, 1989.
129. Lopez-Vidal Y, et al: Enterotoxins and adhesions of enterotoxigenic Escherichia coli: Are they risk factors for acute diarrhea in the community? J Infect Dis, 162:442, 1990.
130. Formal SB, Hale TL, and Kapfer C: Shigella vaccines. Rev Infect Dis, 11(S3):S547, 1989.
131. Ramirez CA, et al: Open, prospective study of the clinical efficacy of ciprofloxacin. Antimicrob Agents Chemother, 28:128, 1985.
132. Levine MM, et al: Chilean Typhoid Committee. Large-scale field trial of Ty21a live oral typhoid vaccine in enteric-coated capsule formulation. Lancet, i:1049, 1987.
133. Wahdan MH, Serie C, and Cerisier Y: A controlled field trial of live Salmonella typhi strain TY 21a oral vaccine against typhoid: Three-year results. J Infect Dis, 145:292, 1982.
134. Woodward TE, and Woodward WE: A new oral vaccine against typhoid fever. J Infect Dis, 145:289, 1982.
135. Acharya IL, et al: Prevention of typhoid fever in Nepal with the Vi capsular polysaccharide of Salmonella typhi. N Engl J Med, 317:1101, 1987.

Chapter 35

VIBRIONACEAE

The Vibrionaceae, a family of facultative, oxidase-positive, glucose-fermenting, curved, gram-negative bacilli, includes Vibrio, Aeromonas, Plesiomonas, and Photobacterium. Differentiating features of the first three genera, which infect humans, are shown in Table 35–1; members of the latter genus do not infect humans and are not discussed further here.

VIBRIO

Vibrios are among the organisms most commonly found in ocean and estuary waters. Ten species cause human infections. Vibrio cholerae, the agent of cholera and the most important human pathogen, is discussed in detail; the remaining species are reviewed briefly.

Vibrio cholerae

Epidemics of the disease now called cholera were described on the Indian subcontinent in the late fifteenth century. The first pandemic begin in the Ganges River delta in 1816 and 1817, after which six additional pandemics occurred at approximately 10- to 15-year intervals through the late 1800s. The most recent pandemic, in 1961, was caused by the El Tor variant of Vibrio cholerae.

Vibrio cholerae is a curved or comma-shaped bacterium that measures 1 to 5 μm by 0.5 μm. It is vigorously motile by a monotrichous flagellum and grows well at 30° to 40° C (optimum, 37° C) on media used routinely in the laboratory and between pH 6 and 9.6, although the ideal pH range for growth is 7.6 to 9.0. Vibrio cholerae does not require sodium chloride for growth, unlike other species of Vibrio, but it cannot grow in 8% sodium chloride. When excreted from the body into water, V. cholerae survives only 4 to 7 days, and not that long in the presence of competing bacteria. The organism does not withstand drying or mildly acidic conditions and survives better in brackish than fresh water.

Two serovars of Vibrio cholerae are recognized: the 01 group of V. cholerae, named "cholera vibrios," agglutinate in vibrio group 0:1 antiserum; the non-0:1 group of V. cholerae, also called noncholera vibrios or nonagglutinable vibrios, do not. The 01 group of V. cholerae is divided into three serotypes (subtypes) based on somatic (O) antigens designated A through C: Ogawa (A,B), Inaba (A,C), and Hikojima (A,B,C); and two biovars (biotypes) according to biologic characteristics (Table 35–2): classical and El Tor, the latter named after the place where it was first isolated (1). The El Tor variant, first recognized in 1905, was responsible for the 1961 cholera pandemic and for the current cholera epidemic in South America, which began in Peru in January, 1991 (2–4). Since the 1960s the El Tor variant has replaced the classical biotype as the predominant variant in several parts of the world, a phenomenon due, at least in part, to prolonged carriage of the El Tor variant after infection and its ability to survive longer in the environment.

Epidemiology

The 01 group of Vibrio cholerae is endemic in India, especially in the area of the Ganges River delta (the heartland of cholera), in underdeveloped areas in Asia, the Middle East, and Africa, and in parts of Europe; they rarely cause disease in the United States (4,5). The non-01 group of V. cholerae inhabit surface waters worldwide and have been recovered from sewage, untreated well water, a home storage tank for treated water, and raw seafood.

During epidemics, contact with water that is contaminated with stool of persons with cholera and that is used for washing, swimming, cooking, or drinking is the principal mechanism by which disease is spread. Persons with mild illness or in convalescence are an important source of infection; no animal reservoirs or vectors are known. Outbreaks of disease in the Philippines, Thailand, and Italy and sporadic cases of cholera in the United States have been linked to the ingestion of Vibrio cholerae–contaminated shellfish (4,6). Where the organism resides between epidemics is not known, but limited evidence suggests that the surface of chitinous plankton and water plants are potential reservoirs (7,8). Although long-term carriers of 01 V. cholerae have not been described, it is possible that they are simply indetectable by methods used to date.

Persons at greatest risk of disease during an outbreak are household contacts of persons who have cholera. In cholera-endemic areas attack rates are ten times greater for children between age 1 and 5 years than for adults; infants under 1 year of age generally are not affected. In areas where cholera has been introduced only recently attack rates are similar in all age groups. Persons who have undergone gastrectomy and those who are hypochlorhydric are at increased risk of disease.

Pathogenesis

Group 01 Vibrio cholerae, an acid-sensitive organism swallowed with water or food, must survive the acid environment of the stomach and reach the small intestine, where it must overcome the propulsive gut motility and locate an environment suitable for proliferation. Bacterial factors that promote colonization of the small intestine are the combined effect of very active motility, production of mucinase and proteases, and chemotaxis directed toward the gut mucosa. Once the organism penetrates the mucus layer and colonizes the lining epithelium the epithelial cells secrete an alkaline, bile-rich solution, providing ideal growth conditions for the vibrios. Disease results from the production of an enterotoxin—cholera

Table 35-1. Characteristics of the Genera of Vibrionaceae

Characteristic	Genus		
	Vibrio	Aeromonas	Plesiomonas
DNA guanine-plus-cytosine content (mol%)	38–51	57–63	51
NaCl required for or stimulates growth	+	–	–
Sensitive to vibriostatic compound 0129*	+	–	+
Ferments D-mannitol	+	±	–
Ferments inositol	–	+	–
Sheathed polar flagella	+	–	–

* 2,4-diamino-6,7-diisopropylpteridine (150 μg)

Table 35-2. Properties That Distinguish Biovars of Vibrio Cholerae

Property	Classical	El Tor
Voges-Proskauer	–	+
Polymyxin B (50 U)	S	R
Hemolysis of sheep blood	–	+
Agglutination of chicken RBC	–	+
Bacteriophage IV	S	R

Key: +, positive reaction; –, negative reaction; S, susceptible; R, resistant; RBC, red blood cells

toxin, composed of 5 binding B subunits arranged in a circular form, the active A_1 subunit, and a bridging piece A_2 that links A_1 to the B subunits (9,10). The B subunit binds to a specific receptor, monosialosyl ganglioside (GM_1 ganglioside), allowing entry of the A molecule. The latter catalyzes the adenosine ribosylation of the guanyl nucleotide–dependent component of adenylate cyclase, resulting in elevated levels of cyclic adenine monophosphate (cAMP) and subsequent altered electrolyte transport and excessive fluid excretion by the crypt cells.

Natural infection with Vibrio cholerae induces systemic and local immune responses. Of the circulating antibodies detected, including those against the toxin (mainly the B subunit) and the H (flagellar) and O (somatic) antigens, the vibriocidal antibodies, which are directed against O antigens, correlate with resistance to infection but probably are not the predominant mediator of protection (11,12). Antibodies produced locally that act at the surface of the intestine most likely play the major role in defense against clinical illness and infection.

The mechanisms by which the non-01 Vibrio cholerae cause disease are ill-understood. The organism may produce a cholera-like toxin, which appears to be associated with the severity of diarrheal disease, enterotoxins, and at least two distinct cytotoxins/hemolysins; however, not all strains produce all toxins, and how the enterotoxins and cytotoxins/hemolysins affect pathogenicity is unknown (13,14). Host susceptibility appears to play an important role in the development of severe disease, because an underlying predisposing condition is present in almost all persons who develop septicemia (15).

Clinical Manifestations

Typically, cholera begins after an incubation period of a few hours to 5 days (average, 2 to 3 days) with a sense of fullness in the abdomen, rapidly followed by colorless, rice water diarrhea and vomiting. Fluid loss may amount to 10 L per day, resulting in severe dehydration, hypokalemia, acidosis, and circulatory collapse. The illness lasts for a few hours to several days, depending on the adequacy of treatment. In addition to the typical syndrome, infection with the 01 Vibrio cholerae may be asymptomatic or cause only mild diarrhea.

The non-01 Vibrio cholerae have been associated with a spectrum of gastrointestinal illnesses ranging from mild watery diarrhea to enteritis with bloody diarrhea and fever. Moreover, in contrast to the 01 V. cholerae, which rarely cause extraintestinal infection, the non-01 V. cholerae have been associated with systemic disease such as septicemia and meningitis, especially in immunocompromised persons (15).

Other Vibrio Species

The epidemiology and clinical manifestations of the pathogenic species of Vibrio other than Vibrio cholerae are summarized in Table 35–3. The pathogenesis of infections caused by several of these organisms has not been evaluated in detail or is unknown. Vibrio parahaemolyticus and Vibrio vulnificus, the most important of the species, are discussed in more detail.

Vibrio parahaemolyticus

Vibrio parahaemolyticus, a halophilic (salt-requiring) vibrio, is the major cause of acute diarrheal disease in Japan, is responsible for as much as 20% of acute diarrheal illnesses in underdeveloped countries, and has caused outbreaks of food poisoning along the Atlantic and Gulf coasts and on Caribbean cruise ships (16–18). Infection is acquired by ingesting inadequately cooked contaminated seafood that is allowed to remain several hours at ambient temperatures, raw seafood (rare), or food contaminated with seawater. Attack rates approach 50% in exposed populations; but the rarity of secondary spread suggests that a large infective dose is necessary to cause disease (19). Vibrio parahaemolyticus produces an enterotoxin and causes mucosal inflammation in the small intestine, virulence factors believed to be responsible for the clinical illness. Generally, the disease is self-limited, characterized by explosive watery diarrhea and cramping abdominal pain, typically within 24 hours of ingesting the contaminated seafood, but death has occurred in very young children and elderly persons who have an underlying disease.

Vibrio vulnificus

Vibrio vulnificus is part of the normal bacterial flora of estuaries along the Gulf Coast of the United States and the Atlantic and Pacific coasts and is concentrated in "filter feeders" such as oysters (20). This organism, unique among vibrios because of the frequency with which it causes severe, invasive disease, has been associated with

Table 35-3. *Characteristics of Vibrios Other Than Vibrio Cholerae*

Species	Epidemiology	Clinical Manifestations
V. parahaemolyticus*	Distributed worldwide in fresh- and seawater; endemic in Japan; infection acquired by ingesting contaminated raw seafood	Acute gastroenteritis; wound infections and septicemia
V. vulnificus	Distributed in coastal waters and estuaries; infection acquired by ingesting contaminated raw oysters or by exposing broken skin to infected marine animals or contaminated water	Cellulitis, necrotizing vasculitis; septicemia
V. alginolyticus	Distributed in marine waters; infection acquired by exposing broken skin to seawater or infected animals	Infections of soft tissue and wounds; otitis and otitis externa
V. mimicus*	Distributed in coastal waters; infection acquired by ingesting undercooked seafood (especially oysters)	Diarrhea; swimmers' ear
V. hollisae†	Distributed in marine environment in Gulf Coast and Chesapeake Bay states; organism acquired by ingesting contaminated raw seafood	?Diarrhea, gastroenteritis
V. fluvialis*	Distributed worldwide; endemic in Bangladesh and the United States (Gulf Coast, New York, and Pacific Northwest estuaries); infection acquired by ingestion of or contact with contaminated water	Cholera-like gastroenteritis
V. furnisii†	Endemic in marine waters and estuaries in the Orient; infection acquired by ingestion of or contact with contaminated water	?Diarrhea, gastroenteritis
V. damsela‡	Distributed in marine waters; infection acquired by contact of broken skin with infected marine animals or contaminated seawater	Wounds
V. metschnikovii*	Distributed worldwide in fresh and brackish marine waters, rivers, sewage; may contaminate seafood; infection acquired by ingesting contaminated water or seafood	?Septicemia, urinary tract infections, wounds, peritonitis

* Disease probably caused by an enterotoxin.
† These organisms have been recovered from clinical specimens, but their pathogenic role in human disease has not been documented.
‡ Placement of V. damsela in the genus Listonella has been proposed (49).

two clinical syndromes (21,22). Primary septicemia, acquired by ingestion of contaminated shellfish, is a rapidly progressive illness characterized by bullous skin lesions. It generally occurs in persons with a chronic underlying condition such as hemochromatosis, cirrhosis, hematopoietic or other disorders associated with immunosuppression, renal failure, and diabetes, and is fatal in over 50% of cases. Wound infections, associated with exposure of wounds to seawater, may be mild and self-limited or may rapidly progress to severe cellulitis and myositis, mimicking gas gangrene.

The severity of infections caused by Vibrio vulnificus depends on bacterial and host factors. Potential bacterial virulence factors are its capsule, which in vitro confers resistance to the bactericidal activity of human serum and to phagocytosis, and several enzymes, including a cytotoxin-hemolysin, an elastolytic protease, collagenase, and various phospholipases, that may contribute to the invasiveness of the organism (23–27). Encapsulated isolates of V. vulnificus are extremely sensitive to iron, which may at least partially explain the greater risk of severe disease in persons with hemochromatosis and other states of iron overload. The association between cirrhosis (especially alcoholic cirrhosis) and illness is unclear, but it may be related to increased levels of available iron, problems with opsonization, neutrophil and macrophage dysfunction, and leakage of the organism across the gut wall or impaired clearance from the enterohepatic circulation. Immunocompromised persons are at increased risk of developing sepsis and severe wound infections.

Laboratory Diagnosis

What specimens are required for diagnosis of infections caused by vibrios depends on the clinical presentation. Collection, transport, and processing of specimens are discussed in Part III. To diagnose cholera and other gastrointestinal illnesses, liquid stool, a rectal swab specimen, or vomitus should be collected as early in the illness as possible. Wound infections are diagnosed by culturing exudate or tissue biopsy specimens, although a swab of the exudate is acceptable; blood cultures are required to diagnose septicemia. Specimens other than blood should be transported in closed containers to preserve moisture (vibrios are very sensitive to drying) and planted onto culture media as rapidly as possible. Specimens that cannot be processed immediately should be transported in Cary-Blair transport medium; buffered glycerol saline transport medium should be avoided.

Organism Identification

Species of Vibrio typically form smooth, convex, creamy colonies that on sheep blood agar often are surrounded by a zone of complete hemolysis. Growth on MacConkey agar is variable. On thiosulfate citrate–bile salts–sucrose agar (TCBS, the most commonly used selective agar, see Chapters 54 and 59), colonies of sucrose-fermenting vibrios (Vibrio cholerae, Vibrio vulnificus, Vibrio alginolyticus, Vibrio fluvialis, Vibrio furnisii, and Vibrio metschnikovii) are yellow; colonies of the vibrios that do not ferment sucrose appear olive green. In a smear prepared from a colony on TCBS agar and stained with Gram stain, straight or curved gram-negative bacilli are seen; curved cells are best observed during the early, stationary phase of growth in broth culture. If stool and rectal swab specimens from a person with severe watery diarrhea grow many sucrose-positive colonies on TCBS agar, yellow colonies should be subcultured to blood agar, and when good growth is apparent, tested with polyvalent antisera to Vibrio cholerae serogroup 01. An isolate showing agglutination presumptively may be called V. cholerae, but the identification must be confirmed by biochemical testing.

The media and tests designed to identify isolates of Enterobacteriacea (see Chapter 34), including the commercially manufactured biotyping systems, are used to identify the species of Vibrio. However, for identification of the halophilic vibrios (species other than Vibrio cholerae and Vibrio mimicus), sodium chloride (1 to 3%) may have to be added to media and prepackaged commercial systems to obtain proper reactions, although systems that utilize a saline-suspended inoculum may support the growth of some of the clinically important species of Vibrio without added salt.

All species of Vibrio ferment glucose, but only Vibrio furnisii produces gas from glucose. All species except Vibrio metschnikovii are oxidase positive and reduce nitrate to nitrite in the presence of 1% sodium chloride. Vibrio vulnificus and half the isolates of Vibrio metschnikovii ferment lactose; the remaining species do not. Only Vibrio cholerae and Vibrio mimicus grow in nutrient broth containing 0% sodium chloride. Additional biochemical characteristics are discussed elsewhere (28).

Treatment and Prevention

Vibrio cholerae. Treatment of cholera requires prompt fluid and electrolyte replacement and antimicrobial therapy, which shortens the duration of diarrhea, reducing fluid loss. The tetracyclines are the agents of choice, and chloramphenicol, trimethoprim-sulfamethoxazole, and furazolidone are effective alternatives; however, owing to the emergence of resistant strains, susceptibility testing (disk diffusion, see Chapter 24) should be performed.

Cholera could be prevented if opportunities for water or food to become contaminated with Vibrio cholerae did not exist; however, in developing countries implementing methods usually advocated to control contamination is almost impossible. Transmission of V. cholerae via food can be eliminated by thorough cooking (core temperature, 70° C) and by preventing contamination of cooked foods by contact with raw foods or with infected food handlers, and transmission via water can be eliminated by boiling (3). Several approaches to developing a safe, effective, oral vaccine against V. cholerae are being pursued (29). The currently available vaccine protects about 50% of vaccinated persons for 3 to 6 months and is not recommended for travelers to an endemic area (4).

Other Vibrio species. Gastroenteritis caused by Vibrio parahaemolyticus typically is self-limited and does not require therapy. The illness can be prevented by preparing seafood at temperatures high enough to kill the organisms and refrigerating cooked seafood that is not to be eaten immediately.

Infections caused by Vibrio vulnificus require prompt antimicrobial therapy. Most isolates are susceptible to gentamicin, tetracycline, and chloramphenicol, but susceptibility testing (by disk diffusion using Mueller-Hinton agar without added salt) should be performed. To prevent infection, persons in high-risk groups (described earlier) should avoid raw shellfish and limit seawater exposure. Efforts to increase reporting and tracing of oysters associated with cases are under way, and restricting oyster harvest during "high-risk" summer months has been suggested (20).

AEROMONAS

In the genus Aeromonas are 10 validated or proposed species: Aeromonas hydrophila, Aeromonas sobria, Aeromonas caviae, Aeromonas salmonicida, Aeromonas media, Aeromonas veronii (biogroups sobria and veronii), Aeromonas schubertii, Aeromonas eucrenophila, Aeromonas jandaei, and a newly recognized ampicillin-susceptible species, Aeromonas trota (30–35). All species except Aeromonas salmonicida and Aeromonas eucrenophila have been isolated from clinical specimens. Currently, Aeromonas is classified in the Vibrionaceae family. Molecular genetic evidence indicates that the evolutionary history of the species of Aeromonas is sufficiently different from that of the Vibrionaceae to warrant its removal from that family, and the creation of a new family—Aeromonadaceae—to accommodate the species of Aeromonas has been proposed (36).

Aeromonas hydrophila first was isolated from eggs in 1937 and soon thereafter was recognized as a pathogen of fish and reptiles (37). Species of Aeromonas have been known opportunistic pathogens in immunocompromised persons since 1968 and were first implicated in cases of severe gastroenteritis in 1981 (38,39). Since then, these organisms have been associated with several cases of gastroenteritis; however, their role in gastrointestinal disease is controversial, at least in part because the mechanism of the diarrhea is unclear (40–42).

Epidemiology and Pathogenesis

In nature, species of Aeromonas are ubiquitous inhabitants of fresh- and seawater, where they commonly infect cold-blooded aquatic animals. These organisms also reside in sink traps and drain pipes and have been recovered from tap water faucets and distilled water supplies. Injury with direct exposure to contaminated water is a common event preceding wound infections, cellulitis, osteomyelitis, and myonecrosis caused by Aeromonas. Risk factors for acquiring Aeromonas-related gastroenteritis include drinking untreated water, current gastrointestinal or liver disease, decreased gastric acidity, and recent antimicrobial therapy.

Aeromonas veronii (formerly Aeromonas sobria) and Aeromonas hydrophila demonstrate invasiveness in cell culture and produce a cholera-like extractable toxin (Asao toxin) that causes watery diarrhea plus several other extracellular enzymes, including protease, amylase, lipase, and nuclease. However, the involvement of the toxin in gastroenteritis is controversial, and the role of the enzymes in the pathogenesis of disease caused by Aeromonas is unknown (42). Adherence has been proposed as a virulence factor, but this has not been proven.

Clinical Manifestations

Four clinical syndromes resulting from infection with Aeromonas have been described (39). (1) Cellulitis and wound infections follow exposure to contaminated water, soil, and food, principally during warm seasons. Serious wound infections also follow medicinal leech therapy (40). (2) Diarrhea, the most commonly associated clinical manifestation, usually occurs during the summer and may present as a mild to severe illness of short duration or a more chronic illness, especially in persons over 12 years of age (39,41–44). (3) Septicemia, occasionally accompanied by necrotizing myositis and skin lesions, most commonly occurs in persons with hepatobiliary disease and those who are immunocompromised (45). (4) Less frequently encountered infections include intra-abdominal abscesses, infections of the hepatobiliary tract, spontaneous bacterial peritonitis, meningitis, endocarditis, osteomyelitis, pneumonia, urinary tract infections, otitis media, and surgical wound infections.

Laboratory Diagnosis

Specimens required for diagnosis of infections caused by Aeromonas depend on the clinical syndrome and include pus or a swab of the exudate to diagnose cutaneous and soft tissue infections, stool or a rectal swab to diagnose diarrhea, and blood to diagnose septicemia. Specimen collection, transport, and processing are reviewed in Part III; organism identification is discussed here.

Organism Identification

Species of Aeromonas grow well on media used routinely in the clinical laboratory, including sheep blood agar and MacConkey agar, but growth of some isolates is inhibited on selective media commonly used to isolate Salmonella, Shigella, and Campylobacter (see Chapters 54 and 59). Using a selective sheep blood agar containing ampicillin or modified CIN (cefsulodin-irgasan-novobiocin agar containing 4 µg/ml cefsulodin) and incubating at 25° to 30° C may enhance recovery of Aeromonas from stool (46). On blood agar many isolates of Aeromonas produce colonies surrounded by a large zone of complete hemolysis, although some isolates (some Aeromonas caviae and some Aeromonas trota) are not hemolytic. Most isolates do not ferment lactose and therefore produce clear colonies on MacConkey agar, but occasional isolates are lactose positive.

Species of Aeromonas are identified using media and tests designed to identify the Enterobacteriaceae, including commercially available systems (see Chapter 34). They are oxidase positive, which distinguishes them from the Enterobacteriaceae; resistant to the vibriostatic agent 0/129, which differentiates them from the Vibrio and from Plesiomonas shigelloides (discussed later); and utilize glucose fermentatively and are indole positive, which distinguishes them from species of Pseudomonas. Additional biochemical test reactions are described elsewhere (46–48).

Treatment

Diarrhea caused by Aeromonas typically is self-limited and is not treated. Invasive disease, however, requires antimicrobial therapy. Susceptibility testing should be performed, but most isolates are resistant to the penicillins and first- and second-generation cephalosporins, and are susceptible to aminoglycosides, trimethoprim-sulfamethoxazole, the quinolones, and the third-generation cephalosporins.

PLESIOMONAS

Plesiomonas shigelloides, the only species in the genus, first was isolated in 1947 and named C27. At that time the organism was believed to belong to the Enterobacteriaceae, but later it was renamed and placed in the family Vibrionaceae. Reassignment to the tribe Proteaceae in the Enterobacteriaceae has been proposed (49–51).

Epidemiology and Pathogenesis

Plesiomonas shigelloides is ubiquitous in soil and in surface water, predominantly fresh water or estuaries in temperate and tropical climates, but during warm months it also may be isolated from seawater. The organism commonly infects or colonizes cold-blooded and warm-blooded animals, including frogs, snakes, turtles, lizards, cows, pigs, poultry, dogs, and cats, and in tropical and subtropical climates may colonize fish and shellfish, all of which may be sources of human infection. Humans also become infected by ingesting contaminated water or unwashed food such as oysters, shrimp, or chicken (52). P. shigelloides rarely is recovered from human feces, except in Thailand, where the carrier rate is as high as 6.2% among hospital patients (53).

Several potential virulence factors of P. shigelloides have been identified (52). Cytotoxins and enterotoxins may act in the gastrointestinal tract, causing fluid accumulation. Endotoxin, toxic to mice and rabbits in vitro, may activate complement in vivo. Adhesins may facilitate adherence to the mucosa of the gastrointestinal tract, and elastase may degrade connective tissue. The organism's invasiveness, demonstrated in vitro by invasion of HeLa cells, may allow invasion of the mucosal lining of the gastrointestinal tract.

Clinical Manifestations

Plesiomonas shigelloides probably causes gastroenteritis, and, infrequently, extraintestinal disease. Isolated cases of Plesiomonas-induced gastroenteritis have been reported in children and adults, although the prevalence usually is greater among adults; and several food-borne outbreaks have been described, most in Japan (52,54). Because the exact enteropathogenic mechanism has not been determined and disease has not been induced in volunteers, the relationship between P. shigelloides and diarrhea is not firmly established. Gastrointestinal disease varies from mild, self-limited illness to mucoid, bloody diarrhea and polymorphonuclear leukocytes in smears of feces. In the United States the infection is significantly associated with consuming raw seafood and with foreign travel, especially to Mexico (55).

Extraintestinal infections caused by Plesiomonas shigelloides are rare but severe, especially in immunosuppressed persons. Meningitis, the most frequent extraintestinal infection, principally affects neonates and is associated with a high fatality rate (80%) (52,56). Sepsis, cellulitis, arthritis, endophthalmitis, osteomyelitis, cholecystitis, and pancreatic abscesses also have been reported (39,57,58). Although the port of entry of the organism in these cases usually is not known, P. shigelloides may disseminate hematogenously from the gastrointestinal tract or organisms in the environment may be introduced during trauma and then enter the blood (59).

Laboratory Diagnosis

Plesiomonas shigelloides is usually recovered from stool or a rectal swab specimen. Specimens required to diagnose extraintestinal disease depend on the clinical presentation. Collection, transport, and processing of specimens are discussed in Part III; organism identification is reviewed here.

Organism Identification

Plesiomonas shigelloides grows well on sheep blood agar and most enteric agars, including MacConkey and Hektoen agars, at 30° to 35° C, although growth is optimal at 30° C. After incubation for 24 hours, colonies are gray and not hemolytic, averaging 1.5 mm in diameter, on sheep blood agar and clear (lactose-negative) on MacConkey agar. Plesiomonas shigelloides is identified by using biochemical tests and commercial systems designed to identify the Enterobacteriaceae (see Chapter 34). The organism ferments glucose and gives positive reactions for oxidase, indole, arginine dihydrolase, and lysine and ornithine decarboxylase. A more complete biochemical profile is provided in reference 46.

Treatment

Plesiomonas shigelloides usually is susceptible to chloramphenicol, tetracycline, trimethoprim-sulfamethoxazole, the aminoglycosides, the quinolones, imipenem, and the third-generation cephalosporins, but it is becoming more resistant to the penicillins. Oral therapy with tetracycline, trimethoprim-sulfamethoxazole, or the quinolones is recommended for gastroenteritis; parenteral therapy based on results of susceptibility testing is necessary for extraintestinal infections.

REFERENCES

1. Gotschlich F: Vibrios Choleriques isoles au campement de Tor. Retour du pelerinage de l'annee, 1905. Report addresse au President du Conseil quarante naine d'Egypt. Alexandria. Quoted in Bull Inst Louis Pasteur, 3:726, 1905.
2. Centers for Disease Control: Cholera—Peru 1991. MMWR, 40:108, 1991.
3. Centers for Disease Control: Update: Cholera outbreak—Peru, Ecuador, and Colombia. MMWR, 40:225, 1991.
4. Centers for Disease Control: Cholera—New Jersey and Florida MMWR, 40:287, 1991.
5. Centers for Disease Control: Cholera—worldwide, 1989. MMWR, 39:365, 1990.
6. de Lorenzo F, et al: Epidemic of cholera El Tor in Naples 1973. Lancet, i:669, 1974.
7. Huq A, et al: Ecological relationships between V. cholerae and planktonic crustacean copepods. Appl Environ Microbiol, 45:275, 1983.
8. Blake PA, et al: Cholera—a possible endemic focus in the United States. N Engl J Med, 302:305, 1980.
9. Finkelstein RA: Cholera enterotoxin (choleragen): An historical perspective. In Topics in Infectious Disease: Cholera. Edited by D Barua and WB Greenough III. New York, Plenum Press, 1990.
10. Gill DM, and Woolkalis M: Toxins which activate adenylate cyclase. In Microbial Toxins and Diarrhoeal Disease. Edited by D Evered and J Whelan. Ciba Foundation Symposium 112. London, Pittman, 1985.
11. Sack RB, et al: Vibriocidal and agglutinating antibody patterns in cholera patients. J Infect Dis, 116:630, 1966.
12. Mosley WH: The role of immunity in cholera. A review of epidemiological and serological studies. Tex Rep Biol Med, 27(suppl. 1):227, 1969.
13. Spira WM, Fedorka-Cray PJ, and Pettebone P: Colonization of the rabbit small intestine by clinical and environmental isolates of non-01 Vibrio cholerae and Vibrio mimicus. Infect Immun, 41:1175, 1983.
14. Ichinose Y, et al: Enterotoxicity of El Tor–like hemolysin of non-01 Vibrio cholerae. Infect Immun, 55:1090, 1987.
15. Safrin S, et al: Non-0:1 Vibrio cholerae bacteremia: case report and review. Rev Infect Dis, 10:1012, 1988.
16. Zen-Yoji H, et al: Epidemiology, enteropathogenicity, and classification of Vibrio parahemolyticus. J Infect Dis, 115:436, 1965.
17. Barker WH, et al: Vibrio parahemolyticus gastroenteritis outbreak in Covington, Louisiana, in August 1972. Am J Epidemiol., 100:316, 1974.
18. Centers for Disease Control: Gastroenteritis caused by Vibrio parahaemolyticus aboard a cruise ship. MMWR, 27:67, 1978.
19. Dadisman TA, et al: Vibrio parahemolyticus gastroenteritis in Maryland. I. Clinical and epidemiological aspects. Am J Epidemiol, 96:414, 1973.
20. Morris JE, Jr: Vibrio vulnificus—a new monster of the deep? Ann Intern Med, 109:261, 1988.
21. Morris JG, Jr, and Black RE: Cholera and other vibrioses in the United States. N Engl J Med, 312:343, 1985.
22. Tacket CO, Brenner F, and Blake PA: Clinical features and an epidemiological study of Vibrio vulnificus infections. J Infect Dis, 149:558, 1984.
23. Yoshida S, Ogawa M, and Mizuguchi Y: Relation of capsular materials and colony opacity to virulence of Vibrio vulnificus. Infect Immun, 47:446, 1985.
24. Grzay LD, and Kreger AS: Purification and characterization of an extracellular cytolysin produced by Vibrio vulnificus. Infect Immun, 48:62, 1985.
25. Kothary MH, and Kreger AS: Purification and characterization of an elastolytic protease of Vibrio vulnificus. J Gen Microbiol, 133:(pt 7):1783, 1985.
26. Smith GC, and Merkel JR: Collagenolytic activity of Vibrio vulnificus: Potential contribution to its invasiveness. Infect Immun, 35:1155, 1982.
27. Testa J, Danile LW, and Kreger AS: Extracellular phospholipase A2 and lysophospholipase produced by Vibrio vulnificus. Infect Immun, 45:458, 1984.
28. Kelly MT, Hickman-Brenner FW, and Farmer JJ III: Vibrio. In Manual of Clinical Microbiology. 5th ed. Edited by A Balows, et al. Washington, DC, American Society for Microbiology, 1991.
29. Kaper JB: Vibrio cholerae vaccines. Rev Infect Dis, 11(S3):S568, 1989.
30. Kuijper EJ, et al: Phenotypic characterization and DNA relatedness in human fecal isolates of Aeromonas spp. J Clin Microbiol, 27:132, 1989.
31. Hickman-Brenner FW, et al: Aeromonas schubertii, a new

mannitol-negative species found in human clinical specimens. J Clin Microbiol, 26:1561, 1988.
32. Carnahan A, Fanning GR, and Joseph SW: Aeromonas jandaei (formerly genospecies DNA group 9 A. sobria), a new sucrose-negative species isolated from clinical specimens. J Clin Microbiol, 29:560, 1991.
33. Joseph SW, et al: Aeromonas jandaei and Aeromonas veronii dual infection of a human wound following aquatic exposure. J Clin Microbiol, 29:565, 1991.
34. Carnahan AM, et al: Aeromonas trota sp. nov., an ampicillin-susceptible species isolated from clinical specimens. J Clin Microbiol, 29:1206, 1991.
35. Altwegg M, et al: Biochemical identification of Aeromonas geno-species isolated from humans. J Clin Microbiol, 28:258, 1990.
36. Colwell RR, MacDonell MT, and de Ley J: Proposal to recognize the family Aeromonadaceae fam. nov. Int J System Bacteriol, 36:473, 1986.
37. Miles AA, and Halnan ET: A new species of micro-organism (Proteus melanovogenes) causing black rot in eggs. J Hyg (Camb), 37:79, 1937.
38. VonGraevenitz A, and Mersh A: The genus Aeromonas in human bacteriology: Report of 30 cases and review of the literature. N Engl J Med, 278:587, 1968.
39. McGowan JE, Jr, and del Rio C: Other gram-negative bacilli. In Principles and Practice of Infectious Diseases. 3rd ed. Edited by GL Mandell, RG Douglas, Jr, and JE Bennett. New York, Churchill Livingstone, 1990.
40. Abrutyn E: Hospital-associated infection from leeches. Ann Intern Med, 109:356, 1988.
41. Holmberg SD, et al: Aeromonas intestinal infections in the United States. Ann Intern Med, 105:683, 1986.
42. Agger WA, McCormick JD, and Gurwith MJ: Clinical and microbiological features of Aeromonas hydrophila–associated diarrhea. J Clin Microbiol, 21:909, 1985.
43. Holmberg SD, and Farmer JJ III: Aeromonas hydrophila and Plesiomonas shigelloides as causes of intestinal infections. Rev Infect Dis, 6:633, 1984.
44. Kuijper EJ, Zanen HC, and Peeters MF: Aeromonas associated diarrhea in the Netherlands. Ann Intern Med, 106:640, 1987.
45. Ketover BP, Young LS, and Armstrong D: Septicemia due to Aeromonas hydrophila: Clinical and immunological aspects. J Infect Dis, 127:284, 1973.
46. VonGraevenitz A and Altwegg M: Aeromonas and Pleiomonas. In Manual of Clinical Microbiology. 5th ed. Edited by A Balows, et al. Washington DC, American Society for Microbiology, 1991.
47. Carnahan AM: Update on Aeromonas identification. Clin Microbiol Newslett, 13:169, 1991.
48. Janda JM: Recent advances in the study of the taxonomy, pathogenicity, and infectious syndromes associated with the genus Aeromonas. Clin Microbiol Rev, 4:397, 1991.
49. MacDonell MT, and Colwell RR: Phylogeny of the Vibrionaceae, and recommendation for two new genera, Listonella and Shewanella. System Appl Microbiol, 6:171, 1985.
50. Basu S, Tharanathan RN, Kontrohr T, and Mayer H: Chemical structure of the lipid A component of Plesiomonas shigelloides and its taxonomical significance. FEMS Microbiol Lett, 28:7, 1985.
51. McDonell MT, et al: Ribosomal RNA phylogenies for the vibrio-enteric group of eubacteria. Microbiol Sciences, 3:172, 1986.
52. Brenden RA, Miller MA, and Janda JM: Clinical disease spectrum and pathogenic factors associated with Plesiomonas shigelloides infections in humans. Rev Infect Dis, 10:303, 1988.
53. Pitarangsi C, et al: Enteropathogenicity of Aeromonas hydrophila and Plesiomonas shigelloides: Prevalence among individuals with and without diarrhea in Thailand. Infect Immun, 35:666, 1982.
54. Tsukamoto T, Kinoshita Y, Shimada T, and Sakazaki R: Two epidemics of diarrhoeal disease possibly caused by Plesiomonas shigelloides. J Hyg (Camb), 80:275, 1978.
55. Holmberg SD, et al: Plesiomonas enteric infections in the United States. Ann Intern Med, 105:690, 1986.
56. Pathak A, Custer JR, and Levy R: Neonatal septicemia and meningitis due to Plesiomonas shigelloides. Pediatrics, 71:389, 1983.
57. Gordon DL, Philpot CR, and McGuire C: Plesiomonas shigelloides septic arthritis complicating rheumatoid arthritis. Aust NZ J Med, 13:275, 1983.
58. Nolte FS, et al: Proctitis and fatal septicemia caused by Plesiomonas shigelloides in a bisexual man. J Clin Microbiol, 26:388, 1988.
59. Ellner PD, and McCarthy LR: Aeromonas shigelloides bacteremia: A case report. Am J Clin Pathol, 59:216, 1973.

Chapter 36

HAEMOPHILUS AND OTHER FACULTATIVE GRAM-NEGATIVE BACILLI

Organisms discussed in this chapter are facultative gram-negative bacilli not of the families Enterobacteriaceae or Vibrionaceae, including species of Haemophilus, Pasteurella, Actinobacillus, and Capnocytophaga; Cardiobacterium hominis, Chromobacterium violaceum, Eikenella corrodens, and bacteria given the Centers for Disease Control (CDC) group designation EF-4, HB-5, and DF-3. Many of these bacteria are part of the normal flora of humans, and some are normal flora of animals. Species of Haemophilus are encountered most frequently in the clinical laboratory and are discussed in detail; the remaining organisms are reviewed briefly.

HAEMOPHILUS

Members of the genus Haemophilus are nonmotile, gram-negative coccobacilli to filamentous rods that require growth factors present in blood, thus the genus name (from Greek *haima, philein*, "blood-loving"). Some species of Haemophilus require X factor, a group of heat-stable tetrapyrrole compounds provided by iron-compounds such as hemin and hematin that are used in the cytochrome electron transport system and to synthesize catalases and peroxidases. These species cannot synthesize protoporphyrin from δ-aminolevulinic acid, a biochemical reaction used for identification (described later) (1). Certain species of Haemophilus require V factor, a heat-labile coenzyme supplied by nicotinamide adenine dinucleotide (NAD, coenzyme I) or nicotinamide adenine dinucleotide phosphate (NADP, coenzyme II) and synthesized in large amounts by micro-organisms such as Staphylococcus aureus and yeasts. A few species require both X and V factors, and one species, Haemophilus aphrophilus, requires neither.

Both X and V factors are present in erythrocytes, including sheep red blood cells used to prepare the blood agar plates used routinely in clinical microbiology laboratories. However, blood from sheep and certain other animals often contains enzymes that slowly hydrolyze and inactivate V factor, so species of Haemophilus that require V factor do not grow on sheep blood agar in which erythrocytes are intact unless organisms that provide V factor, such as Staphylococcus aureus, also are present. In the latter case, pinpoint colonies of Haemophilus surround colonies of S. aureus, a phenomenon called satelliting. Species of Haemophilus grow on media containing lysed sheep red blood cells, such as chocolate agar, the medium most often used to recover Haemophilus from clinical specimens; on media prepared with unlysed 5% horse or rabbit blood, on which some species are β hemolytic; and on media containing Fildes supplement, a peptic digest of sheep blood rich in X and V factors.

Classification

Currently, Haemophilus is classified in the family Pasteurellaceae, which also includes Pasteurella and Actinobacillus; but because the genetic analyses of many organisms in these genera is incomplete the present classification is considered tentative and may be redefined when more data are available. Of the eight species of Haemophilus found in humans, Haemophilus influenzae and Haemophilus ducreyi are the most important pathogens and are discussed in detail; characteristics of the remaining species are reviewed briefly.

Haemophilus influenzae

Robert Koch first detected Haemophilus-like organisms in the early 1880s, in conjunctival exudates of persons with Egyptian eye disease (2). The essential characteristics of this organism were described a few years later by Weeks, who reported outbreaks of acute conjunctivitis in the United States (3). Subsequently, similar epidemics were reported from Europe and South America (4,5). Richard Pfeiffer isolated Haemophilus influenzae from sputum and lung tissue of persons who died during the 1892 influenza pandemic and proposed that the organism was the pathogen of influenza, a claim disproven when human influenza virus was discovered in 1933. Six antigenically distinct capsular types of H. influenzae, designated a through f, were described by Pittman in 1931 (6).

The agent of acute conjunctivitis has had many names, including the Koch-Weeks bacillus (after the persons who first described the organism), Bacillus aegyptius, Haemophilus conjunctivitidis, and Haemophilus aegyptius (7). Recently, DNA hybridization studies demonstrated that phylogenetically Haemophilus influenzae and Haemophilus aegyptius are one species, but to account for their clinical differences (discussed later) the name Haemophilus influenzae biogroup aegyptius is used for the organisms previously named Haemophilus aegyptius (8,9).

Epidemiology

Haemophilus influenzae, indigenous to humans, is normal flora in the pharynx and may colonize the mucosa of the conjunctivae and genital tract. Because as many as 80% of persons of all ages are carriers of one or more strains of H. influenzae for days to months, isolating the organism from the upper respiratory tract is normal. Most persons are colonized with unencapsulated strains, but in 3 to 5% of cases the colonizing organism is encapsulated, most commonly serotype b, the one responsible for most serious, invasive infections in young children (10). H. influenzae is transmitted from person to person by airborne droplets or by direct contact with infected secretions. Epidemiologic features associated with the different infections caused by H. influenzae are discussed under Clinical Manifestations.

Pathogenesis

Bacterial and host factors are involved in the pathogenesis of the disease that follows infection with Haemophilus influenzae. Microbial factors responsible for colonization are not defined clearly, but they may be related to surface fimbriae that facilitate attachment to human buccal epithelial cells in vitro (11). Several potential virulence factors have been identified. H. influenzae produces immunoglobulin (Ig) A_1 proteases, which have unknown biologic significance, and two factors that inhibit the ciliary activity of human epithelial cells in vitro—a lipopolysaccharide and a currently unidentified factor of low molecular weight, most likely a heat-stable glycoprotein (12,13). The most important virulence factor in the pathogenesis of invasive disease is the type b capsule, composed of repeating units of ribosyl-ribitol phosphate (PRP) and the only one of the six capsular types that contains a pentose (ribose) rather a hexose as its subunit carbohydrate component. Why organisms of H. influenzae serotype b are especially virulent and able to cause rapidly progressive, potentially life-threatening disease is not completely understood, but the capsule probably allows the organism to resist phagocytosis and intracellular killing by neutrophils (14–16).

The humoral immune response is the predominant host factor that affects the outcome of infection with Haemophilus influenzae. Serum antibodies specific for the PRP unit of the type b capsule, which activate complement-mediated bactericidal and opsonic activity in vitro, are the major mediators of protection against invasive disease (17–19). Antibodies to the cell wall lipopolysaccharide and outer membrane proteins demonstrate protective potential in laboratory-induced infections and probably are involved in protection against natural infection (20). However, the mechanisms that determine the age-related, natural acquisition of antibodies to PRP, which are detected in most persons by age 3 to 4 years (see Chapter 2), are incompletely understood. Exposure to commensal bacteria or foods that possess epitopes that cross-react with the PRP unit may provide the antigenic stimulus for production of specific antibodies, a theory supported by the fact that human volunteers fed Escherichia coli K100, a normal commensal of the gastrointestinal tract with a capsular polysaccharide immunologically similar to PRP, respond with increased levels of specific bactericidal and opsonizing antibodies to Haemophilus influenzae (21).

Other important components in the host defense against disease caused by Haemophilus influenzae are the complement system and phagocytic cells (see Chapter 2). Congenital deficiencies of certain complement components are associated with increased risk of pyogenic infections with H. influenzae type b (22). Because the monocyte/macrophage system is principally responsible for clearing H. influenzae from the blood, persons who lack a spleen or have decreased splenic function (as in sickle cell disease) are more susceptible to H. influenzae–induced sepsis and meningitis (23,24).

The role of local mucosal immunity in host defense against infection with Haemophilus influenzae is controversial. Secretory antibodies may block attachment of the organism to the respiratory mucosa, but this has not been proven (25). Conversely, data from one study suggest that high titers of local or serum IgA may block the activity of other antibodies, increasing susceptibility to infection (26).

Susceptibility to infection may also have a genetic basis. For example, absence of the G2m(n) phenotype, a heavy-chain marker for antibodies of the IgG_2 subclass, appears to correlate with a low antibody responder phenotype (27). The prevalence of the G2m(n) phenotype is low in blacks and Hispanics, and these racial groups have higher rates of disease than whites. Moreover, serum concentrations of IgG_2 are predictive of antibody responses to immunization with polysaccharide antigens.

Clinical Manifestations

The clinical manifestations of disease caused by Haemophilus influenzae are discussed according to the type of infecting isolate: type b, encapsulated isolates of other serotypes, H. influenzae biogroup aegyptius, and unencapsulated (or nontypable) isolates.

Type b. At least 20,000 cases of invasive disease caused by Haemophilus influenzae type b occur annually in the United States, predominantly in young children, resulting in about 1000 deaths (28). In the United States and many other countries, H. influenzae type b is the most common cause of meningitis; the attack rate peaks before 1 year of age (29). H. influenzae type b is the most common cause of bacterial meningitis in children between the ages of 1 month and 2 years but an infrequent cause in neonates and persons older than 6 years. Between ages of 2 and 6 years meningitis due to H. influenzae and to Neisseria meningitidis (Chapter 31) are about equally frequent. Meningitis caused by Haemophilus influenzae type b occurs more often in the winter, in males, in families of low socioeconomic status, and in certain ethnic groups (American Indians, Eskimos, Aleuts, blacks, and Hispanics) (20,30). Outbreaks have occurred in day care centers and in other closed populations, indicating that disease is contagious (31,32). Adults with meningitis caused by H. influenzae type b usually have an underlying predisposing condition—rhinorrhea secondary to head trauma, a recent neurosurgical procedure, chronic sinusitis or otitis, diabetes, chronic alcoholism, or an immunodeficiency such as hypogammaglobulinemia (33).

Clinical signs of meningitis—fever and altered central nervous system function with or without nuchal rigidity—frequently follow symptoms of an upper respiratory tract infection or otitis media. Seizures or coma may develop as the infection progresses. With appropriate therapy the overall mortality rate is less than 5%, but permanent sequelae—hearing loss, language delay or, less commonly, mental retardation, cerebral palsy, and continuing seizures—affect as many as 50% of survivors (34,35).

The second most common manifestation of disease caused by Haemophilus influenzae type b is epiglottitis, a potentially lethal condition rarely caused by other bacteria (see Chapter 57). The illness, which typically affects children 2 to 6 years of age but also some adults, begins abruptly with sore throat, fever, and dyspnea, progressing rapidly to dysphagia, pooling of oral secretions, and drooling of saliva (20,36). Deterioration within a few hours is common and results in death from airway obstruction if adequate therapy is not begun. Physical examination, which should be performed only in a setting where an airway can be placed, reveals a red, swollen epiglottis, resembling a cherry obstructing the pharynx at the base of the tongue.

Haemophilus influenzae type b is the second most common cause, after Streptococcus pneumoniae, of bacteremia with no evidence of a local infection in children 6 to 36 months of age, especially those who have sickle cell disease or no spleen (37). It is the most common cause of septic arthritis, usually involving a single, large, weight-bearing joint, in children under age 2 years, but the infection may occur in adults, most of whom have a predisposing condition such as alcoholism, trauma, rheumatoid arthritis, systemic lupus erythematosus, diabetes mellitus, asplenia, multiple myeloma, lymphoma, or hypogammaglobulinemia (38). Haemophilus influenzae type b also may cause cellulitis, typically on the cheek or in the periorbital region of young children, and it is an uncommon cause of pneumonia (in children) and endocarditis.

Other Capsular Types. Rarely, Haemophilus influenzae organisms possessing capsular serotypes other than b cause systemic disease. Examples include neonatal sepsis caused by type c; pneumonia and bacteremia in adults associated with types a and d; and pneumonia, epiglottitis, nosocomial bacteremia, infection of a prosthetic vascular graft, and meningitis in adults, most of whom had a predisposing condition, due to type f (39–43).

Biotype aegyptius. Haemophilus influenzae biotype aegyptius causes seasonal epidemics of highly contagious conjunctivitis, also called pinkeye, predominantly in hot climates, and recently has been associated with Brazilian purpuric fever, a potentially fatal septicemia resembling meningococcemia (Chapter 31) (44,45). To date, Brazilian purpuric fever has been recognized only in São Paulo State in Brazil and in one Brazilian city outside São Paulo; whether the disease occurs in other, less developed areas of Brazil where cases might not be diagnosed is unknown. Moreover, a possible case was reported in Australia (46). Outbreaks of Brazilian purpuric fever are most common at the onset of warmer weather and are less likely to occur during the Brazilian winter. The median age of affected children has been 30 to 36 months; no cases have occurred in persons over 10 years of age. About 90% of children have a history of conjunctivitis, which often has resolved 10 to 60 days (mean, 7 to 16 days) before the onset of Brazilian purpuric fever, an illness that ranges from mild fever alone to fever with toxic, systemic symptoms and a rash without petechiae. The overall fatality rate is about 70%.

Unencapsulated Strains. Unencapsulated (or non-typable) strains of Haemophilus influenzae are important pathogens of adults and children. These organisms cause chronic bronchitis and pneumonia, especially in elders, alcoholics, persons who have lung disease, and those infected with human immunodeficiency virus, and they are a frequent cause of acute otitis media in children (47,48). During the postpartum period they may cause bacteremia in women and meningitis and septicemia in neonates. In adults, unencapsulated strains rarely cause meningitis, epiglottitis, pericarditis, cellulitis, septic arthritis, osteomyelitis, endocarditis, or bacteremia without a recognized source of infection (47).

Haemophilus ducreyi

The agent of chancroid (also called soft chancre), now known as Haemophilus ducreyi, first was described in 1889 by Ducrey, who inoculated the skin of the forearm of three persons with purulent material from their own genital ulcers (49). Each subsequently developed an ulcer, and in exudate and tissue from the lesion, short, compact, bacilli (1.5 by 0.5 μm) with rounded ends were found, singly (in secretions) and in chains (in tissue), both within and outside neutrophils. Ducrey, however, was unable to culture the organism in vitro. His observations were confirmed in 1892, and H. ducreyi first was isolated in culture in the late 1890s (50).

Epidemiology

Chancroid occurs worldwide and typically is associated with low socioeconomic status and poor hygiene. This sexually transmitted disease is prevalent in developing countries of Asia and Africa but uncommon in developed countries. In the United States the reported number of cases of chancroid peaked at about 9500 in 1947 and then declined until 1978, when the downward trend reversed. In 1987 about 5000 cases were reported, more than six times the number reported in 1984 (49). From 1981 to 1986 more than 90% of cases were reported from New York, Texas, California, Florida, and Georgia. Since 1981, nine large outbreaks, which principally affected black and Hispanic heterosexual males, were reported from six states—California, Florida, New York, Massachusetts, Texas, and Pennsylvania (51). Prostitutes, most of whom had genital ulcers, were important in transmitting the infection in outbreaks outside Florida, and in Florida disease was most common among very sexually active black males who had no known contact with prostitutes. The role of asymptomatic carriers in the epidemiology of chancroid is controversial.

Pathogenesis and Pathology

The classic test of virulence for Haemophilus ducreyi is the rabbit intradermal test: virulent strains produce a necrotic lesion with eschar formation, and avirulent strains produce no cutaneous lesion (52,53). Virulent strains are resistant to the bactericidal action of 50% normal rabbit serum and 50% pooled normal human serum and to phagocytosis and killing by human neutrophils, whereas avirulent strains are sensitive to the bactericidal activity of serum, which is mediated at least in part by the classical complement pathway, and they are readily ingested and killed by human neutrophils (54). The cell wall lipopolysaccharide of H. ducreyi, which is chemically different for virulent and avirulent strains, appears to be an important determinant of the susceptibility of the organism to human serum (55,56).

The histologic findings in sections of a chancroid ulcer are nonspecific mucosal ulceration with interstitial edema and an infiltrate of neutrophils and mononuclear cells. Involved regional lymph nodes show microabscesses, which often coalesce.

Clinical Manifestations

After an incubation period of 1 day to several weeks (median, 5 to 7 days), the lesion of chancroid begins as a tender papule with surrounding erythema. The papule becomes pustular and then ruptures, forming a painful, nonindurated, sharply circumscribed ulcer with ragged, undermined edges and a granular base, often covered with a necrotic exudate. In males lesions usually are single and most often involve the distal prepuce, the mucosal surface of the prepuce on the frenulum, or the coronal sulcus. In females lesions may be multiple, and most occur at the entrance to the vagina on the fourchette, labia, vestibule, and clitoris (49). In about half the cases, the ulcer is accompanied by unilateral painful, tender, enlarged inguinal lymph nodes, which may become fluctuant and spontaneously rupture, forming an inguinal ulcer. Extragenital chancroid, involving the mouth, fingers, or breasts, is rare.

Other Species of Haemophilus

Species of Haemophilus other than Haemophilus influenzae and Haemophilus ducreyi are normal flora in the mouth, pharynx, and occasionally the genital tract. From sites of colonization these organisms may cause local or systemic disease, but because their pathogenic potential is much lower than that of Haemophilus influenzae, disease is uncommon. Haemophilus parainfluenzae is the most frequent pathogen, followed by Haemophilus aphrophilus and Haemophilus paraphrophilus. Haemophilus segnis, which has been isolated in pure and mixed cultures from a few patients with acute appendicitis, Haemophilus haemolyticus, and Haemophilus parahaemolyticus are rare human pathogens and are not discussed further here (57).

Haemophilus parainfluenzae, Haemophilus aphrophilus, and Haemophilus paraphrophilus are recovered from persons with endocarditis more frequently than Haemophilus influenzae, and together they account for about 5% of all cases of infective endocarditis (58). Factors that predispose to endocarditis caused by these organisms are dental disease, dental procedures, oral trauma, sinusitis, pneumonia, and intravenous drug use. The disease typically resembles endocarditis caused by viridans streptococci (Chapter 28)—subacute onset in a young to middle-aged adult who has underlying valvular heart disease or a prosthetic valve—but a distinguishing feature is the formation of large vegetations and, consequently, a high frequency of clinically significant arterial emboliza-

tion: in 50 to 60% of cases, compared with about 25% of all cases of subacute endocarditis (58). In addition to endocarditis, Haemophilus parainfluenzae, Haemophilus aphrophilus, and Haemophilus paraphrophilus may cause epiglottitis, otitis, conjunctivitis, septic arthritis, osteomyelitis, pneumonia, empyema, bacteremia, meningitis, brain abscess, and infections of the genitourinary tract (58).

Laboratory Diagnosis

Specimens for diagnosis of infections caused by the species of Haemophilus are listed in Table 36–1. Specimen collection, transport, and processing are discussed in Part III, but in general, specimens should not be refrigerated and swab specimens should be kept moist, because these organisms are sensitive to cold and to desiccation. In this section, organism identification and susceptibility testing are reviewed.

Table 36–1. Diseases Caused by Species of Haemophilus and Specimens Required for Diagnosis

Disease	Haemophilus Species*	Specimens
Meningitis	H. influenzae type b	CSF, blood
Epiglottitis	H. influenzae type b	Blood, laryngeal secretions, throat swab
Bronchitis	H. influenzae (nontypable)	Sputum, TTA, bronchial washings
Pneumonia	H. influenzae (nontypable); H. influenzae type b	Sputum, TTA, bronchial washings, BAL, lung tissue
Acute sinusitis	H. influenzae (nontypable)	Sinus aspirate or tissue biopsy
Conjunctivitis	H. influenzae biogroup aegyptius	Conjunctival scraping or swab specimen
Otitis media	H. influenzae (nontypable)	Tympanocentesis fluid†
Endocarditis	H. parainfluenzae, -aphrophilus, -paraphrophilus	Blood, valve tissue
Genital tract infection, postpartum bacteremia, neonatal sepsis with meningitis	H. influenzae (nontypable)	Urethral and endocervical swab specimens; blood, CSF, fetal tissue
Brazilian purpuric fever	H. influenzae biogroup aegyptius	Blood
Chancroid	H. ducreyi	Swab of genital ulcer; aspirate of involved lymph node
Cellulitis	H. influenzae type b	Blood, aspirate from margin of the involved area
Septic arthritis	H. influenzae type b	Joint fluid
Bacteremia	H. influenzae type b	Blood

* Includes species most commonly involved.
† Acute otitis media usually is diagnosed on the basis of clinical presentation, without collecting tympanocentesis fluid for microbiologic studies.
Key: CSF, cerebrospinal fluid; TTA, transtracheal aspirate, BAL, bronchoalveolar lavage fluid.

Organism Identification

Haemophilus influenzae. In a smear of a specimen such as the sediment of centrifuged cerebrospinal fluid (CSF), a blood culture broth, or sputum stained with the Gram stain, cells of H. influenzae appear as small pale-staining gram-negative coccobacilli (Plate VI B), or occasionally as slender filaments of variable staining intensity. After incubation at 35° C in 5 to 10% carbon dioxide for 18 to 24 hours (or 2 to 4 days for H. influenzae biogroup aegyptius), colonies on chocolate agar are gray, semiopaque, smooth, flat, and convex with an entire edge. Clinical isolates that have colony and cellular structures suggestive of Haemophilus usually are named presumptively based on catalase and oxidase reactions, growth requirements for X and V factors, and perhaps their hemolytic reaction on horse blood agar (Table 36–2).

Growth requirements are determined in several ways. One method involves placing filter-paper disks or strips impregnated with X factor, V factor, and both X and V factors 1 to 2 cm apart onto a lawn of the test isolate inoculated on a medium deficient in growth factors, such as trypticase soy agar (which in one study was superior to brain-heart infusion agar), nutrient agar, or Mueller-Hinton agar (59). Suspending colonies from the primary culture in broth deficient in X and V factors before transferring them to the agar plate is recommended to prevent carry-over of growth factors from the chocolate agar or other blood-containing media and consequent false-positive results. The plate is incubated 18 to 24 hours at 35° C in 5 to 7% carbon dioxide, and the patterns of growth around the strips or disks are observed. The test is easy to perform and interpretation usually is clear cut, though inconsistent results in X factor determinations can cause Haemophilus influenzae to be misidentified as Haemophilus parainfluenza and vice versa in 20 to 30% of cases (43).

Requirements for X and V factors also may be evaluated by testing for satelliting around colonies of Staphylococcus aureus. To perform this test, one medium deficient in both X and V factors (such as trypticase soy agar) and one blood agar medium containing only X factor (such as chocolatized blood agar held at 60° C for 1 hour after the first 80° C heat treatment, which lyses the erythrocytes to inactivate V factor) are inoculated with a lawn of the test isolate and then streaked with a strain of S. aureus that produces V factor. Plates are incubated 18 to 24 hours at 35° C in 5 to 7% carbon dioxide and examined for tiny, moist colonies adjacent to the steak of S. aureus. Growth around the streak on both media indicates a V factor requirement only, because X factor is not present in trypticase soy agar, and growth around the streak on the chocolatized agar indicates a requirement for both X factor (in the agar) and V factor (provided by the S. aureus).

The δ-aminolevulinic acid (ALA)–porphyrin test is a rapid, accurate method of determining the X-factor requirement. When supplied with δ-ALA, species of Haemophilus that do not require X factor (see Table 36–2) excrete porphobilinogen and porphyrins, which are intermediates in the heme biosynthetic pathway; whereas species that require X factor for growth lack enzymes involved in the synthesis of heme and, so, do not excrete these compounds. To perform the test, substrate prepared in house (43,60) or a commercially available ALA-impregnated filter paper disk or growth medium containing the ALA reagent is inoculated with the test organism. The substrate (if heavily inoculated) and the disk are incubated at 35° C for 4 hours and the agar plate is incubated overnight, after which each is exposed to ultraviolet light (Wood's light, 360 nm). Brick-red fluorescence indicates that the isolate does not require X factor.

Alternate approaches to identification include an agar system (quad-plate, composed of horse blood agar, an X factor–enriched medium, V factor–enriched medium, and medium containing both X and V factors) and rapid enzymatic biochemical systems, both commercially available (59,61,62). Moreover, conventional biochemical tests may be done to confirm the identification based on growth requirements and hemolysis on horse blood agar (see Table 36–2). Sugar fermentation tests are performed in 1% solutions of the carbohydrate in phenol red broth base supplemented with X and V factors (10 mg each per liter) after autoclaving or by using commercial disks containing substrate; reactions are interpreted after 24 hours' incubation (60).

Isolates identified as Haemophilus influenzae may be

Table 36–2. Identification of Species of Haemophilus Isolated from Humans

Species	Hemolysis*	Catalase	Oxidase	Porphyrin Test	Factor Requirements	Production of Acid from:				
						Glucose	Fructose	Sucrose	Lactose	Mannose
H. influenzae	−	+	+	−	X, V	+	−	−	−	−
H. parainfluenzae	−	±	+	+	V	+	+	+	−	+
H. haemolyticus	+	+	+	−	X, V	+	w	−	−	−
H. parahaemolyticus	+	±	+	+	V	+	+	+	−	−
H. aphrophilus	−	−	−	w	None	+	+	+	+	+
H. paraphrophilus	−	−	+	+	V	+	+	+	+	+
H. segnis	−	±	−	+	V	w	w	w	−	−
H. ducreyi	−	+	+	−	X	−	−	−	−	−

* Hemolysis on horse blood agar
Key: +, 90% or more of strains are positive; −, 10% or less of strains are positive; w, weakly positive reactions; ±, reaction is variable
(Modified from Koneman EW, et al (eds): Haemophilus. In Color Atlas and Textbook of Diagnostic Microbiology. 3rd ed. Philadelphia, JB Lippincott, 1988.)

further evaluated by serotyping, biotyping, or subtyping for epidemiologic purposes. Serotyping is performed by slide agglutination or by coagglutination using commercially available reagents. The biotype (designated I through VI), which is related to the source of isolation, is based on indole production, urease activity, and ornithine decarboxylase activity (see references 43 and 60 for test methods and expected reactions). Biotyping, however, is a less sensitive epidemiologic tool than subtyping isolates by their outer membrane proteins or lipopolysaccharides and, therefore, is rarely performed in the clinical microbiology laboratory.

Systemic infections with Haemophilus influenzae type b may be diagnosed rapidly by detecting type b PRP antigen directly in CSF, serum (or blood culture broth showing small gram-negative bacilli suggestive of H. influenzae), or urine by using a commercially available latex agglutination test (Chapter 24). Latex agglutination must not replace culture, however, because the organism must be recovered to perform susceptibility testing.

Haemophilus ducreyi. The value of direct examination of smears of exudate stained with the Gram stain for diagnosis of chancroid is controversial. Sensitivity of 62 to 92% and specificity of 51 to 99% have been reported (49). The "school of fish" arrangement—extracellular or intracellular bacilli grouped in long, parallel columns between cells or shreds of mucus—and long chains of bacilli have been considered typical of H. ducreyi; however, these findings are more characteristic of smears prepared from colonies on an agar plate and are infrequently seen in smears prepared from clinical material (49). Monoclonal antibodies specific for H. ducreyi have been developed and in the future may be useful for diagnosis, allowing direct detection of the organism in smears of clinical specimens (63,64).

In endemic areas the positive predictive value of a diagnosis of chancroid based on clinical presentation among males with genital ulcers is about 84%, but in nonendemic areas where the prevalence of chancroid is low the positive predictive value is much lower, and accurate diagnosis requires isolation of the organism (65). The culture medium recommended for recovery of Haemophilus ducreyi from clinical specimens is GC agar base containing 1 to 2% hemoglobin, 5% fetal bovine serum, and vancomycin (3 μg/ml) (49). Colonies, pinpoint-sized after 24 hours' incubation at 33° to 35° C in 5 to 7% carbon dioxide and 1 to 2 mm in diameter after 48 to 72 hours, are tan, yellow, or grayish yellow, transparent to opaque, nonmucoid, raised, compact, and granular, and often can be pushed intact across the surface of solid medium with an inoculating loop. Identifying characteristics are shown in Table 36–2. Tests are performed as described earlier for Haemophilus influenzae.

Other Species of Haemophilus. Cells of Haemophilus parainfluenzae, Haemophilus aphrophilus, and Haemophilus paraphrophilus in smears prepared from clinical specimens or colonies and stained with the Gram stain resemble those of Haemophilus influenzae. Colonies of Haemophilus parainfluenzae are up to 3 mm in diameter after 24 hours and are flat, gray, semiopaque, and smooth or rough and wrinkled. Haemophilus aphrophilus and Haemophilus paraphrophilus form rough, raised colonies 1 to 2 mm in diameter and are identified as shown in Table 36–2. Haemophilus parainfluenza may be subdivided into four biotypes (I through IV) based on indole production, urease activity, and ornithine decarboxylase activity (43,60).

Susceptibility Testing

The prevalence of ampicillin resistance, usually due to plasmid-mediated production of β-lactamase, among isolates of Haemophilus influenzae and other species of Haemophilus (especially Haemophilus parainfluenzae) is increasing, so all isolates of Haemophilus should be tested for β-lactamase production, preferably by the chromogenic cephalosporin disk test (Chapter 24). Some β-lactamase–negative strains of Haemophilus influenzae are resistant to ampicillin by virtue of altered penicillin-binding proteins and decreased permeability of the outer membrane to the antimicrobial agent, chromosomally mediated traits not detected by β-lactamase tests. Therefore, susceptibility testing (discussed later) of isolates of H. influenzae from sterile body sites (CSF, blood, joint fluid) is recommended. A small proportion of isolates of H. influenzae are resistant to chloramphenicol (an agent effective in treating meningitis). This resistance almost always is due to production of the enzyme chloramphenicol acetyltransferase, which alters active sites on the chloramphenicol molecule, but it may also result from the loss of a major outer membrane protein that serves as a porin, allowing chloramphenicol to enter the bacterial cell (66). A disk test for detection of chloramphenicol acetyltransferase is commercially available, but because it does not detect all chloramphenicol-resistant strains and its sensitivity has been questioned, broth dilution or disk diffusion susceptibility testing is recommended (67).

To perform susceptibility testing of isolates of Haemophilus influenzae, the routine methods described in Chapter 24 must be modified. For disk diffusion, Haemophilus Test Medium (commercially available) is inoculated with a suspension of the test organism prepared in Mueller-Hinton broth directly from overnight growth on chocolate agar and adjusted to equal the turbidity of a 0.5 McFarland standard (68). Susceptibility to ampicillin, chloramphenicol, cefotaxime, and ceftriaxone (at a minimum) should be tested; zone diameters are interpreted according to the guidelines recommended by the National Committee for Clinical Laboratory Standards (NCCLS). Haemophilus Test Medium also should be used to determine the minimum inhibitory concentration (MIC) by broth dilution (69). A suspension of the test isolate is prepared from overnight growth on chocolate agar and adjusted to equal the turbidity of a 0.5 McFarland standard. The final inoculum should be 5×10^5 cfu/ml in each well or tube. Because higher concentrations of inoculum often cause inappropriately high MICs with certain cephalosporin antimicrobials, performing colony counts on inoculum suspensions at regular intervals (once a month) is recommended. The MIC interpretive standards recommended by the NCCLS are published in reference 69.

Treatment and Prevention

Haemophilus influenzae. Without appropriate antimicrobial therapy, meningitis and epiglottitis caused by H. influenzae can rapidly be fatal. Empiric therapy with chloramphenicol and ampicillin, discontinuing the chloramphenicol if the isolate is susceptible to ampicillin, is effective in most places where the prevalence of chloramphenicol resistance is low, such as the United States. However, owing to the increasing prevalence of resistance to chloramphenicol in some parts of the world and the agent's potential bone marrow toxicity, a third-generation cephalosporin such as cefotaxime or ceftriaxone often is given initially, and ampicillin is substituted if the isolate turns out to be susceptible. For less severe infections caused by H. influenzae, such as sinusitis, otitis, and bronchitis, ampicillin or amoxicillin usually is effective; alternatives include erythromycin-sulfisoxazole, cefaclor, trimethoprim-sulfamethoxazole, and amoxicillin-clavulanate.

A vaccine consisting of purified Haemophilus influenzae type b polysaccharide (PRP) was licensed for use in North America in 1985 and was recommended as a routine immunization for susceptible children 2 years or older based on the estimated 90% efficiacy demonstrated in a vaccine trial in Finland (17). Data from subsequent studies of the efficacy of the vaccine in North America, however, indicated that it was less effective than was initially predicted (70). Conjugate vaccines, therefore, were developed to enhance the immunogenicity of PRP by covalent linkage or complexing of the oligosaccharides to protein, and in 1987 a conjugate vaccine (PRP-D) was licensed in the United States and recommended for routine use in infants aged 18 months or older. Early data indicated that PRP-D protects infants against invasive type b disease; however, recent evaluations of this vaccine in Apache children and Alaska Native infants demonstrated limited efficacy in these populations, primarily owing to the failure of these persons to develop an antibody response to the type b polysaccharide (18,71,72). In 1990, the Food and Drug Administration approved two additional Haemophilus b conjugate vaccines for use in a two-dose or three-dose (depending on the vaccine) primary immunization schedule for infants, beginning at 2 months of age, with a booster dose at 1 year (73). The H. influenzae type b routine vaccination schedule currently recommended by the Immunization Practices Advisory Committee is shown in Table 36–3.

Haemophilus ducreyi. Effective treatment for persons with chancroid and their contacts includes oral erythromycin, a single intramuscular injection of ceftriaxone, or amoxicillin-clavulanic acid. Trimethoprim-sulfamethoxazole is effective in areas where trimethoprim resistance is not prevalent. A properly used condom should help prevent the disease.

OTHER FACULTATIVE GRAM-NEGATIVE BACILLI

Pasteurella species

Species of Pasteurella, which are classified in the family Pasteurellaceae, include Pasteurella multocida (which has three subspecies, Pasteurella multocida, -septica, and -gallicida), Pasteurella dagmatis, Pasteurella gallinarum, Pasteurella canis, Pasteurella stomatis, Pasteurella anatis, Pasteurella langaa, Pasteurella avium, Pasteurella volantium, and several unnamed species. The previously described species, Pasteurella aerogenes, Pasteurella haemolytica, Pasteurella ureae, and Pasteurella pneumotropica, were shown by DNA homology studies to be significantly different from other species of Pasteurella and more closely related to the genus Actinobacillus (74). Pasteurella multocida is the most common human pathogen; the remaining species rarely infect humans (infected wounds, osteomyelitis, endocarditis, pneumonia, and septicemia) and are not discussed further here (74).

Epidemiology and Pathogenesis

Pasteurella multocida, which is part of the normal flora of the respiratory and gastrointestinal tract of many domestic and wild animals and birds, causes disease in animals and humans. Most human infections are acquired by a dog- or cat bite or scratch, however, infections of the respiratory tract may be acquired via inhalation of the organism, and some infections occur in the absence of known exposure to animals or animal tissues. The virulence of P. multocida is related to its polysaccharide capsule, which allows the organism to resist phagocytosis, and virulence may be enhanced by the organism's ability to utilize free iron.

Clinical Manifestations

Infections caused by Pasteurella multocida are divided into three groups (75). Local infections of wounds inflicted by animal bites or scratches (cats account for 60 to 80% of cases and dogs for most others) are most common. Such infections are characterized by the rapid appearance of erythema, warmth, tenderness, and purulent drainage and occasionally are complicated by abscess formation, tenosynovitis, septic arthritis (especially in persons with

Table 36–3. Detailed Vaccination Schedule for Haemophilus b Conjugate Vaccines

Vaccine	Age at First Dose (mo)	Primary Series (No. Doses/Interval [mo])	Age at Booster Dose*
HbOC	2–6	3/2	15 mo
	7–11	2/2	15 mo
	12–14	1	15 mo
	15–59	1	—
PRP-OMP	2–6	2/2	12 mo
	7–11	2/2	15 mo
	12–14	1	15 mo
	15–59	1	—
PRP-D	15–59	1	—

* At least 2 months after previous dose
Key: HbOC, Haemophilus b conjugate vaccine; PRP-OMP, Haemophilus b conjugate vaccine (meningococcal protein conjugate); PRP-D, Haemophilus b conjugate vaccine (diphtheria toxoid conjugate).
(From Centers for Disease Control: Haemophilus b conjugate vaccines for prevention of Haemophilus influenzae type b disease among infants and children two months of age and older. MMWR, 40(RR-1):1, 1991.)

previously damaged joints), and osteomyelitis. Respiratory tract infections, including sinusitis, bronchitis, pneumonia, and empyema, typically occur in association with underlying pulmonary disease and a history of animal exposure. However, recovery of P. multocida from a respiratory tract specimen such as sputum does not always indicate that the organism is causing disease, as it may be a commensal in persons who have underlying pulmonary disease. Systemic infections include bacteremia, meningitis, brain abscess, spontaneous bacterial peritonitis, and intra-abdominal abscess. In most of these cases P. multocida is an opportunistic pathogen, with a predilection for causing bacteremia in persons with liver dysfunction and meningitis in very young or elderly persons.

Laboratory Diagnosis

Pasteurella multocida most frequently is detected in drainage, aspirated pus, or a swab specimen collected from a bite wound. Respiratory specimens—sputum, transtracheal aspirates, bronchial washings, bronchoalveolar lavage fluid, lung tissue, pleural fluid—are the next most common sources of P. multocida. The organism also may be recovered from blood, CSF, joint fluid, peritoneal fluid, bone biopsy specimens, and pus aspirated from an abscess.

In smears stained with the Gram stain Pasteurella multocida appears as a small, gram-negative rod, often with bipolar staining. The organism grows well on sheep blood agar but does not grow on MacConkey agar. Colonies are small (1 to 2 mm diameter), smooth, moist to mucoid, nonhemolytic, often cause green or brown discoloration of the surrounding agar, and have a musty odor. Pasteurella multocida gives positive reactions for oxidase (but occasionally this requires several subcultures), catalase, indole, nitrate reduction, glucose and sucrose fermentation, and ornithine decarboxylation. It is nonmotile, urease negative, and negative for hydrogen sulfide production in Kligler's iron (KIA) and triple sugar iron (TSIA) agars, but a positive hydrogen sulfide reaction often is observed on lead acetate paper draped over a KIA or a TSIA slant. Characteristics helpful for differentiating other species of Pasteurella are described elsewhere (62,76).

Treatment

Penicillin is the antimicrobial agent of choice for all infections caused by Pasteurella multocida. For the rare penicillin-resistant isolates, tetracycline and chloramphenicol are effective, and cephalothin may be used for infections of bite wounds. Aminoglycosides, erythromycin, and clindamycin are not recommended.

Actinobacillus species

Species of Actinobacillus include Actinobacillus actinomycetemcomitans, Actinobacillus lignieresii, Actinobacillus equuli, and Actinobacillus suis. The proposal to reassign Actinobacillus actinomycetemcomitans to the genus Haemophilus has been made but has not been well-received (77). Actinobacillus actinomycetemcomitans is the species that most often causes disease in humans; the rest predominantly infect domesticated animals and are not discussed further here (76).

Epidemiology and Pathogenesis

Actinobacillus actinomycetemcomitans, named for its frequent association with Actinomyces israelii (Chapter 30), is part of the normal flora of the human oral cavity. Material from its capsule inhibits DNA and collagen synthesis, features that suggest that the capsule may be involved in the tissue destruction associated with periodontal disease (78). The organism also produces a leukotoxin that kills neutrophils and may contribute to its pathogenicity, and a bacteriocin that is inhibitory to other bacteria in the mouth (79).

Clinical Manifestations

Infections caused by Actinobacillus actinomycetemcomitans are endogenous in origin. A. actinomycetemcomitans is recovered from persons with periodontal disease, especially juvenile periodontitis, a severe and destructive localized infection of adolescents (80). It often is isolated with Actinomyces israelii from submucous or subcutaneous suppurative lesions, but its role in these mixed infections is difficult to determine. The organism also may cause endocarditis (especially on damaged or prosthetic valves), wound infections and rarely meningitis, osteomyelitis, infections of the urinary tract, and pericarditis (81).

Laboratory Diagnosis

Actinobacillus actinomycetemcomitans most often is recovered from aspirated pus or a swab specimen collected from a periodontal lesion or from purulent material obtained from subcutaneous or soft tissue lesions (actinomycosis). It also may be recovered from blood, and rarely from CSF, urine, or pericardial fluid. Direct immunofluorescence has been used to detect A. actinomycetemcomitans in smears prepared from dental plaque, but reagents are not commercially available and culture generally is required for identification (82).

The organism grows on chocolate or sheep blood agar in 3 to 7 days, especially when plates are incubated in an atmosphere of increased carbon dioxide, but it does not grow on MacConkey agar. On blood agar colonies are small, translucent with an opaque center, smooth with a slightly wrinkled surface, and frequently adhere to the agar surface. With further incubation they develop a characteristic four- to six-pointed star shape, a feature best seen on a clear medium such as brain-heart infusion agar. In broth media the organism forms granules that adhere to the walls of the bottle or tube, but the broth remains clear. A smear of a colony or granule from broth stained with the Gram stain demonstrates small gram-negative coccoid to coccobacillary organisms that often appear more bacillary in smears prepared from older cultures. Biochemical characteristics useful for identifying Actinobacillus actinomycetemcomitans are no growth on MacConkey agar, positive catalase reaction, negative urease, indole, and motility tests, and fermentation of glucose but not lactose or sucrose. A more complete biochemical profile can be found in references 62 and 76.

Treatment

Most isolates of Actinobacillus actinomycetemcomitans are susceptible in vitro to newer cephalosporins, rifampin, trimethoprim-sulfamethoxazole, aminoglycosides, ciprofloxacin, tetracycline, and chloramphenicol, but susceptibility testing should be performed because results vary (81). A. actinomycetemcometans usually appears susceptible or relatively resistant to penicillin in vitro, but results do not always correlate with patient outcome (83,84). Endocarditis generally is treated with penicillin plus an aminoglycoside.

Capnocytophaga species

Species of Capnocytophaga (previously known as Bacteroides ochraceus and DF-1 ["dysgonic fermenter"]) are fastidious gram-negative gliding bacteria that grow optimally in an atmosphere of increased carbon dioxide. Until recently, three species—Capnocytophaga ochracea, Capnocytophaga sputigena, and Capnocytophaga gingivalis—and one unnamed group were recognized. In 1989, the organism designated DF-2 was renamed Capnocytophaga canimorsus and Capnocytophaga cynodegmi was described (85).

Epidemiology, Pathogenesis, and Clinical Manifestations

Capnocytophaga ochracea, Capnocytophaga sputigena, and Capnocytophaga gingivalis are part of the normal flora of the oral cavity and commonly are isolated from the gingival sulcus of persons who may or may not have periodontal disease and from periodontal lesions in persons with juvenile periodontitis. These organisms may cause systemic disease, including bacteremia and endocarditis, in immunocompromised hosts (particularly granulocytopenic persons who have oral ulcers) and rarely in immunocompetent persons, and they have been recovered from sputum, cerebrospinal fluid, pleural fluid, amniotic fluid, the female genital tract, and the eye (81,86–88).

The exact reservoir of Capnocytophaga canimorsus is unknown, but because most infected persons have a history of exposure to oral secretions of a dog and about half the cases follow a dog bite, the infections probably are zoonotic (89,90). In one survey the organism was found in the gingival crevices of about 20% of dogs and cats examined (91). Some infections with C. canimorsus are not associated with a history of close animal contact (92). Persons without a spleen, alcoholics, and those receiving corticosteroids are at increased risk of severe disease, characterized by shock and disseminated intravascular coagulation. If the spleen is intact, the illness generally is milder. Isolated cases of meningitis, endocarditis, pneumonia, cellulitis, corneal perforation, and septic arthritis caused by C. canimorsus have been reported (81).

Laboratory Diagnosis

Capnocytophaga ochraceae, Capnocytophaga sputigena, and Capnocytophaga gingivalis most commonly are recovered from purulent material or swab specimens obtained from mucosal ulcers or periodontal lesions and from blood of immunocompromised persons, although they may be isolated from other sites (described earlier). These organisms grow on sheep blood agar, chocolate agar, and Thayer-Martin medium incubated anaerobically or in an atmosphere of increased carbon dioxide; they do not grow in ambient air or on MacConkey agar. Colonies, which usually do not become apparent for 48 to 72 hours, are shiny, opaque, nonhemolytic and either dry and adherent to the agar surface or mucoid and nonadherent. Occasionally, the gliding motility of these organisms is observed as outgrowths from the colony or as a haze on the agar surface, a feature that is influenced by the composition of the agar medium and is best appreciated on media containing 3% agar (62). On blood agar colonies may appear gray to white, but when they are scraped onto a cotton or Dacron swab a yellow pigment becomes apparent. In smears prepared from a colony and stained with the Gram stain, cells are long, thin, gram-negative bacilli with tapered ends.

The most useful identifying characteristics of these three species of Capnocytophaga are the requirement of carbon dioxide for growth, slow growth, cellular structure, negative catalase, oxidase, and indole reactions, and fermentation of glucose and sucrose. Patterns of carbohydrate fermentation and nitrate reduction differentiate the species: Capnocytophaga ochraceae ferments lactose, is nitrate negative, and most isolates ferment galactose; Capnocytophaga sputigena does not ferment galactose, most isolates are nitrate positive, and lactose fermentation is variable; Capnocytophaga gingivalis gives negative reactions in all three tests. Moreover, these species are identified by many commercially available anaerobic identification systems (see Chapter 30).

Capnocytophaga canimorsus typically is recovered from blood. Smears prepared from growth in a broth culture and stained with the Gram stain reveal long, uniform, frequently curved, gram-negative bacilli, filaments with tapered ends, and occasional sickle- and cigar-shaped cells. Subcultures from broth media should be incubated in an atmosphere of increased carbon dioxide, although growth occurs, but less vigorously, under anaerobic conditions. The organism grows on chocolate agar, but growth is better on heart-infusion agar with 5% rabbit blood. Pinpoint colonies appear on chocolate agar after incubation for about 4 days, and on heart-infusion agar with 5% rabbit blood colonies are larger (2 to 3 mm diameter), convex, smooth, and circular. The organism is nonmotile; it does not grow on MacConkey agar or reduce nitrates to nitrites. It gives positive reactions for oxidase, catalase, and o-nitrophenyl-β-D-galactopyranoside and negative reactions for indole and urease; and it ferments glucose, lactose, and maltose, though addition of 3% rabbit serum may be necessary for growth in carbohydrate broth.

Treatment

Capnocytophaga ochraceae, Capnocytophaga sputigena, and Capnocytophaga gingivalis are susceptible in vitro to clindamycin, penicillin, ampicillin, imipenem, erythromycin, tetracycline, chloramphenicol, ciprofloxacin, third-generation cephalosporins, and metronidazole but are resistant to trimethoprim and aminoglycosides. Isolates of Capnocytophaga canimorsus are susceptible to penicillin, cephalothin, chloramphenicol, clindamycin, imipenem, and carbenicillin but resistant to aminoglycosides.

Cardiobacterium hominis

Cardiobacterium hominis, first named in 1964, is part of the normal flora of the nose, mouth, and throat, occasionally is found on other mucous membranes, and may be present in the gastrointestinal tract. Virtually the only disease caused by C. hominis is endocarditis. The infection involves previously diseased heart valves or prosthetic valves and is characterized by large vegetations that commonly embolize (81). Many affected persons have had severe periodontitis and prior dental procedures without prophylaxis. The illness characteristically begins insidiously, with minor and vague symptoms that progress slowly over several months, and often the diagnosis is delayed because recovering the organism is difficult.

Laboratory Diagnosis

Almost all clinical isolates of Cardiobacterium hominis are from blood, and the organism can be recovered in most commercial blood culture media. Smears prepared from broth cultures and stained with the Gram stain show pleomorphic, gram-negative bacilli with bulbous ends and occasional slender filaments and teardrop forms arranged in pairs, short chains, and loose rosettes. The cells may retain the crystal violet stain at the swollen ends, giving a metachromatic appearance. C. hominis grows well on sheep blood and chocolate agar but does not grow on MacConkey agar. Growth is enhanced by incubation in an atmosphere of increased humidity and elevated (3 to 5%) carbon dioxide. After incubation for 48 hours at 35° to 37° C, colonies are pinpoint to 1 mm in diameter, smooth, round, glistening, and opaque, and they may cause slight greening of the surrounding agar. Observation of colonies grown on trypticase soy agar without blood under a stereomicroscope reveals a central intertwining network of bacilli, some of which appear to stream from the periphery of the colony, in contrast to the central stellate imprint of colonies of Actinobacillus actinomycetemcomitans described earlier.

Cardiobacterium hominis appears to be correctly identified by commercially available systems. It is oxidase-positive, weakly indole positive after incubation for 48 hours and extraction with xylene (a key characteristic), and negative for catalase, urease, and nitrate reduction. Determination of carbohydrate utilization often requires the addition of 10% horse serum to allow sufficient growth.

Treatment

Penicillin appears to be the agent of choice for Cardiobacterium hominis–induced infections. In vitro susceptibility testing is difficult because the organism grows slowly and has specific growth requirements. When it is performed, C. hominis usually is susceptible to penicillin, ampicillin, cephalothin, chloramphenicol, tetracycline, and the aminoglycosides.

Chromobacterium violaceum

Epidemiology and Pathogenesis

Chromobacterium violaceum is found in soil and water, principally in tropical areas. In the United States most human infections occur in the southeastern states, especially Florida. Infection in humans, usually acquired via soil or water contamination of a wound or, less commonly, by ingestion of contaminated water, is characterized by bacteremia; a primary focus may or may not be obvious. Persons with an underlying neutrophil dysfunction, such as chronic granulomatous disease, appear to be at increased risk of infection with C. violaceum; however, infection occurs in persons who have no known immune disorder (81). Virulence factors of C. violaceum are not well-studied, but the organism produces extracellular proteases that could promote invasiveness.

Clinical Manifestations

Persons infected with Chromobacterium violaceum typically develop high fever, and, as a result of hematogenous spread of the organism, secondary foci of infection such as osteomyelitis; abscesses in the lung, liver, or abdomen; and skin manifestations, including pustular dermatitis, cellulitis, or ulceration, are common. In the United States, the overall mortality rate approaches 60% despite appropriate therapy (93).

Laboratory Diagnosis

Specimens useful for diagnosis of infections with Chromobacterium violaceum are blood and pus aspirated from an abscess or skin lesion, although a swab specimen collected from an abscess or skin lesion is acceptable. Smears prepared from a broth culture that shows growth or directly from purulent material and stained with the Gram stain show short to medium-length, occasionally slightly curved, gram-negative bacilli that frequently give a bipolar staining reaction. The organism grows on sheep blood, chocolate, and MacConkey agars incubated at 30° to 35° C, although growth is optimal at 25° C. Colonies, which may smell of ammonium cyanide, are 0.5 to 1.5 mm in diameter, convex, smooth, and have a violet pigment (hence the species name), but occasional strains produce nonpigmented colonies. C. violaceum is motile, ferments glucose (usually without producing gas), and gives positive reactions for nitrate reduction, catalase, and oxidase. The latter is best demonstrated by subculturing violet colonies anaerobically, which inhibits pigment production. Urease and citrate reactions are variable, and some nonpigmented isolates are weakly indole positive. Reference 76 provides a more complete biochemical profile.

Treatment

Isolates of Chromobacterium violaceum usually are susceptible in vitro to chloramphenicol, tetracycline, trimethoprim-sulfamethoxazole, gentamicin, and erythromycin; variably susceptible to the penicillins and other aminoglycosides; and resistant to most cephalosporins (81). In one series those who survived were treated with gentamicin, with or without chloramphenicol (94).

Eikenella corrodens

Epidemiology and Pathogenesis

Eikenella corrodens (formerly known as HB-1) is part of the normal flora of the mouth and upper respiratory tract of humans and may inhabit the gastrointestinal tract. The most significant factor that predisposes to infection with this organism is trauma to a mucous membrane surface, which allows the bacteria to gain access to surrounding tissue and potentially to enter the blood and establish secondary foci of infection elsewhere in the body.

Clinical Manifestations

Typically, Eikenella corrodens is recovered with other organisms as a component of a mixed bacterial infection, frequently involving the head and neck or the abdominal region, although the organism may be the only pathogen of infections such as septicemia (especially following tooth extraction and in immunocompromised hosts and drug users), endocarditis, meningitis, subdural empyema, septic arthritis, pneumonia, postsurgical infections, and soft tissue abscesses (81). Moreover, E. corrodens is associated with dental infections, causing periapical abscesses and necrosis of root canals, and with infections of human bite wounds, which may extend to the underlying bone, resulting in osteomyelitis (95).

Laboratory Diagnosis

Eikenella corrodens may be recovered from purulent material aspirated from abscesses or wounds, blood, sputum, CSF, and joint fluid. When incubated aerobically, it requires hemin for growth and grows slowly on sheep blood or chocolate agar but does not grow on MacConkey agar. Growth is enhanced by incubation in an atmosphere of 3 to 10% carbon dioxide. Colonies generally are pinpoint sized after 24 hours and measure 0.5 to 1.0 mm at 48 hours. On blood agar, E. corrodens forms slightly yellow, dry, flat, radially spreading colonies with an irregular periphery that cause green discoloration of the agar and have an odor similar to that of bleach. About half the isolates cause pitting of the agar surface. In broth media, growth usually is poor, appearing as a faint granular band about 1 cm below the surface after 3 to 4 days' incubation at 35° C. Smears prepared from broth cultures or colonies on agar plates and stained with the Gram stain show slender gram-negative bacilli or coccobacilli with parallel sides and rounded ends.

Eikenella corrodens is nonmotile, oxidase positive, lysine- and ornithine decarboxylase positive, and catalase negative, although rare isolates may be weakly catalase positive. Most isolates reduce nitrates to nitrites. The organism lacks oxidative and fermentative capabilities and gives negative reactions for indole, urease, and hydrogen sulfide production.

Treatment

The recommended method of susceptibility testing of isolates of Eikenella corrodens is agar dilution using Mueller-Hinton agar supplemented with Fildes extract and incubating at 35° to 37° C for 48 hours, although broth dilution using Mueller-Hinton broth supplemented with Fildes extract or lysed horse blood also is acceptable (95). Most isolates are susceptible to tetracycline, ampicillin, penicillin, and second- and third-generation cephalosporins and are resistant to clindamycin and the aminoglycosides.

Centers for Disease Control Group EF-4

Gram-negative bacilli belonging to the CDC group EF-4 are "eugonic fermenters" (organisms that grow well by carbohydrate fermentation) not yet known by genus and species and currently defined by the CDC system of letters and numbers (EF-4, the fourth group of eugonic fermenters described). Most human infections caused by these organisms are wounds due to dog or cat bites; bacteremia not associated with an animal bite is rare (96).

In smears stained with the Gram stain cells of group EF-4 appear as gram-negative coccobacilli, often in short chains. These organisms grow well on sheep blood agar, forming small, nonhemolytic or slightly α-hemolytic, yellow-pigmented colonies with a popcorn odor, but they grow poorly if at all on MacConkey agar. Bacilli of group EF-4 are oxidase- and catalase positive, ferment glucose, reduce nitrates to nitrites, and are urease- and indole negative. Additional biochemical reactions are described elsewhere (76). Isolates tested have been susceptible to β-lactam agents, chloramphenicol, tetracycline, and some aminoglycosides; however, the clinical relevance of in vitro susceptibility test results is unknown (96).

Centers for Disease Control Group HB-5

The designation group HB-5 describes fermentative gram-negative coccoid to rod-shaped bacteria of medium length with uniform biochemical characteristics. Most clinical isolates of the HB-5 group referred to the CDC have been recovered from the genitourinary tract; other sources include blood, finger lesions, rectal abscess, perianal furuncle, appendectomy wound infection, and leg abscess.

Bacilli of group HB-5 require increased carbon dioxide for primary isolation. After 24 hours colonies on blood agar are smooth, convex, occasionally mottled, 0.5 to 1.0 mm in diameter, and may cause slight green discoloration of the surrounding agar. About a third of isolates grow poorly on MacConkey agar after 48 hours, and about half grow after 7 days. The organisms are catalase negative, oxidase negative or weakly oxidase positive, weakly indole positive, and reduce nitrate to nitrite. They ferment glucose, fructose, and mannose, producing small amounts of gas, and are negative for urease and lysine and ornithine decarboxylation. Additional biochemical reactions are listed in reference 76.

Centers for Disease Control Group DF-3

Gram-negative coccobacilli that belong to the CDC group DF-3 are dysgonic fermenters, so named to reflect their fastidious nature and poor growth. The organism has been associated with soft tissue infections, bacteremia, and diarrhea, although a causal relationship with the latter has not been established (97–99).

DF-3 organisms grow on sheep blood and chocolate agar but not on MacConkey agar or other media used for isolation of pathogens from stool specimens (see Chapter 59). Therefore, to recover DF-3 from feces, the specimen must be inoculated onto a selective medium such as sheep blood agar containing cefoperazone, vancomycin, and amphotericin B (commercially available). Colonies of DF-3 are pinpoint sized after incubation for 24 hours at 35° C in an atmosphere of 5% carbon dioxide, and after 48 to 72 hours they are gray or white, 2 to 3 mm in diameter, and have a sweet, fruity odor. Key biochemical characteristics are negative reactions for catalase, oxidase, indole, and nitrate reduction; positive reaction for esculin hydrolysis; and fermentation of glucose, lactose, maltose, xylose, and sucrose, but not mannitol.

Most infections with DF-3 have responded clinically to clindamycin or tetracycline. Clinical failures, however, have been associated with isolates that, in vitro, were resistant or intermediate in susceptibility to these antimicrobial agents (99).

REFERENCES

1. Kilian M: A rapid method for the differentiation of Haemophilus strains: The porphyrin test. Acta Pathol Microbiol Immunol Scand [B], 82:935, 1974.
2. Koch R: Report on the activities of the German Cholera Commission in Egypt and East India. Wien Med Worchenschr, 33:1548, 1883.
3. Weeks JE: The bacillus of acute conjunctival catarrh, or "pink eye." Arch Ophthalmol, 15:441, 1886.
4. Weeks JE: The status of our knowledge of the aetiological factors in acute conjunctivitis. NY Eye Infirmary Rep, Jan: 24, 1895.
5. Monteiro Salles FJ: Bacterioscopia das secrecoes conjunctivais. Rev Med Cirurg Sao Paulo, 1:105, 1941.
6. Pittman M: Variation and type specificity in the bacterial species Haemophilus influenzae. J Exp Med, 53:471, 1931.
7. Holt JG (ed): Bergey's manual of systematic bacteriology. Baltimore, Williams & Wilkins, 1984.
8. Brenner DJ, et al: Biochemical, genetic, and epidemiologic characterization of Haemophilus influenzae biogroup aegyptius (Haemophilus aegyptius) strains associated with Brazilian purpuric fever. J Clin Microbiol, 26:1524, 1988.
9. Casin I, Grimont F, and Grimont PAD: Deoxyribonucleic acid relatedness between Haemophilus aegyptius and Haemophilus influenzae. Ann Inst Pasteur Microbiol, 137B: 155, 1986.
10. Moxon ER: The carrier state: Haemophilus influenzae. J Antimicrob Chemother, 18[suppl A]:17, 1986.
11. van Alphen L, van den Berghe N, and van den Broek LG: Interaction of Haemophilus influenzae with human erythrocytes and oropharyngeal epithelial cells is mediated by common fimbrial epitope. Infect Immun, 56:1800, 1988.
12. Mulks MH, Kornfeld SJ, and Plaut AG: Specific proteolysis of human IgA by Streptococcus pneumoniae and Haemophilus influenzae. J Infect Dis, 141:450, 1980.
13. Wilson R, and Moxon ER: Molecular mechanisms of Haemophilus influenzae pathogenicity in the respiratory tract. In Bacterial Infections of Respiratory and Gastrointestinal Mucosae. Edited by W Donachie, E Griffiths, and J Stephen: Washington, DC, IRL Press, 1988.
14. Robbins JB, et al: Haemophilus influenzae type b: Disease and immunity in humans. Ann Intern Med, 78:259, 1973.
15. Anderson P, Johnston R, and Smith DH: Human serum activities against Haemophilus influenzae type b. J Clin Invest, 51: 31, 1972.
16. Kilian M: Haemophilus. In Infectious Diseases and Medical Microbiology. 2nd ed. Edited by AI Braude. Philadelphia, WB Saunders, 1986.
17. Peltola H, et al: Prevention of Haemophilus influenzae type b bacteremic infections with the capsular polysaccharide vaccine. N Engl J Med, 310:1561, 1984.
18. Eskola J, et al: Efficacy of Haemophilus influenzae type b polysaccharide–diphtheria toxoid conjugate vaccine in infancy. N Engl J Med, 317:717, 1987.
19. Kayhty M, Peltola H, Karanko V, and Makela PH: The protective level of serum antibodies to the capsular polysaccharide of Haemophilus influenzae type b. J Infect Dis, 147:1100, 1983.
20. Moxon ER: Haemophilus influenzae. In Principles and Practice of Infectious Diseases. 3rd ed. Edited by GL Mandell, RG Douglas, Jr, and JE Bennett. New York, Churchill Livingstone, 1990.
21. Schneerson R, and Robbins JB: Induction of serum Haemophilus influenzae type b capsular antibodies in adult volunteers fed cross-reacting Escherichia coli 075.K100:H5. N Engl J Med, 29:1093, 1975.
22. Moxon ER, and Winkelstein JA: Interaction of Haemophilus influenzae with complement. In Bacteria, Complement and the Phagocytic Cell. Edited by FC Cabello and C Pruzzo. Berlin, Springer-Verlag, 1988.
23. Barrett-Connor E: Bacterial infection and sickle-cell anemia: An analysis of 250 infections in 166 patients and review of literature. Medicine, 50:97, 1971.
24. Weitzman SA, et al.: Impaired humoral immunity in treated Hodgkin's disease. N Engl J Med, 297:245, 1977.
25. Pichichero ME and Insel RA: Relationship between naturally occurring human mucosal and serum antibody to the capsular polysaccharide of Haemophilus influenzae type b. J Infect Dis, 146:243, 1983.
26. Kayhty H, et al: Antibody response to capsular polysaccharides of groups A and C Neisseria meningitidis and Haemophilus influenzae type b during bacteremic disease. J Infect Dis, 143:32, 1981.
27. Ambrosino DM, et al: Correlation between G2m(n) immunoglobulin allotype and human antibody response and susceptibility to polysaccharide encapsulated bacteria. J Clin Invest, 75:1935, 1985.
28. Ward J, and Cochi S: Haemophilus influenzae vaccines. In Vaccines. Edited by SA Plotkin and EA Mortimer, Jr. Philadelphia, WB Saunders, 1988.
29. Schlech WF, et al: Bacterial meningitis in the United States, 1978 through 1981: The National Bacterial Meningitis Surveillance Study. JAMA, 253:1749, 1985.
30. Ward JI, et al: Haemophilus influenzae disease in Alaskan Eskimos: Characteristics of a population with an unusual incidence of invasive disease. Lancet, i:1281, 1981.
31. Glode MP, et al: Haemophilus influenzae type b meningitis: A contagious disease of children. Br Med J, 280:899, 1980.
32. Marks MI, and Dorchester WL: Secondary rates of Hae-

mophilus influenzae type b disease among day care contacts. J Pediatr, 111:305, 1987.
33. Spagnuolo PJ, et al: Haemophilus influenzae meningitis: The spectrum of disease in adults. Medicine (Baltimore), 61:74, 1982.
34. Sell SH, et al: Long-term sequelae of Haemophilus influenzae meningitis. Pediatrics, 49:206, 1972.
35. Ferry PC, et al: Sequelae of Haemophilus influenzae meningitis: preliminary report of a long-term follow-up study. In Haemophilus influenzae, Epidemiology, Immunology and Prevention of Disease. Edited by SH Sell and PF Wright. New York, Elsevier, 1982.
36. MayoSmith MF, Hirsch PJ, Wodzinski SF, and Schiffman FJ: Acute epiglottitis in adults. An eight-year experience in the state of Rhode Island. N Engl J Med, 314:1133, 1986.
37. Marshall R, Teele DW, and Klein JD: Unsuspected bacteremia due to Haemophilus influenzae: Outcome in children not initially admitted to hospital. J Pediatr, 95:690, 1979.
38. Borenstein DG, and Simon GI: Haemophilus influenzae septic arthritis in adults. A report of four cases and a review of the literature. Medicine, 65:191, 1986.
39. Slater LN, Guarnaccia J, Makintubee S, and Istre GR: Bacteremic disease due to Haemophilus influenzae capsular type f in adults: Report of five cases and review. Rev Infect Dis, 12:628, 1990.
40. Barton LL, DeLa Cruz R, and Walentik C: Neonatal Haemophilus influenzae type c sepsis. Am J Dis Child, 136:463, 1972.
41. Buck LL, and Douglas GW: Meningitis due to Haemophilus influenzae type e. J Clin Microbiol, 4:381, 1976.
42. Denis FA, et al: Meningitis caused by Haemophilus influenzae type c. J Pediatr, 91:1064, 1979.
43. Koneman EW, et al (eds): Haemophilus. In Color Atlas and Textbook of Diagnostic Microbiology. 3rd ed. Philadelphia, JB Lippincott Co., 1988.
44. Harrison LH, et al: Epidemiology and clinical spectrum of Brazilian purpuric fever. J Clin Microbiol, 27:599, 1989.
45. Swaminathan B, et al: Microbiology of Brazilian purpuric fever and diagnostic tests. J Clin Microbiol, 27:605, 1989.
46. McIntyre P, Wheaton G, and Erlich J: Brasilian purpuric fever in central Australia. Lancet, ii:112, 1987.
47. Murphy TF, and Apicella MA: Nontypable Haemophilus influenzae: A review of clinical aspects, surface antigens, and the human immune response to infection. Rev Infect Dis, 9:1, 1987.
48. Schlamm HT, and Yancovitz SR: Haemophilus influenzae pneumonia in young adults with AIDS, ARC, or risk for AIDS. Am J Med, 86:11, 1989.
49. Morse SA: Chancroid and Haemophilus ducreyi. Clin Microbiol Rev, 2:137, 1989.
50. Sullivan M: Chancroid. Am J Syph Gonorrhea Vener Dis, 24:482, 1940.
51. Schmid GP, Sanders LL, Jr, Blount JH, and Alexander ER: Chancroid in the United States. Reestablishment of an old disease. JAMA, 258:3265, 1987.
52. Dienst RB: Virulence and antigenicity of Haemophilus ducreyi. Am J Syph Gonorrhea Vener Dis, 32:289, 1948.
53. Feiner RR, and Mortara F: Infectivity of Haemophilus ducreyi for the rabbit and the development of skin hypersensitivity. Am J Syph Gonorrhea Vener Dis, 29:71, 1945.
54. Odumeru JA, Wiseman GM, and Ronald AR: Virulence factors of Haemophilus ducreyi. Infect Immun, 43:607, 1984.
55. Odumeru JA, Wiseman GM, and Ronald AR: Role of lipopolysaccharide and complement in susceptibility of Haemophilus ducreyi to human serum. Infect Immun, 50:495, 1985.
56. Odumeru JA, Wiseman GM, and Ronald AR: Relationship between lipopolysaccharide composition and virulence of Haemophilus ducreyi. J Med Microbiol, 23:155, 1987.
57. Welch WD, Southern PM, and Schneider NR: Five cases of Haemophilus segnis appendicitis. J Clin Microbiol, 24:851, 1986.
58. Hand WL: Haemophilus species. In Principles and Practice of Infectious Diseases. 3rd ed. Edited by GL Mandell, RG Douglas, Jr, and JE Bennett. New York, Churchill Livingstone, 1990.
59. Doern GJ, and Chapin KC: Laboratory identification of Haemophilus influenzae: Effects of basal media on the results of the satellitism test and evaluation of the Rapid NH system. J Clin Microbiol, 20:599, 1984.
60. Kilian M: Haemophilus. In Manual of Clinical Microbiology. 5th ed. Edited by A Balows, et al. Washington, DC, American Society for Microbiology, 1991.
61. Durfee KK, et al: Comparison of methods for identification of Haemophilus influenzae. Lab Med, 17:275, 1986.
62. Baron EJ, and Finegold SM: Gram-negative facultatively anaerobic bacilli and coccobacilli. In Bailey and Scott's Diagnostic Microbiology. 8th ed. St. Louis, CV Mosby, 1990.
63. Borchardt KA, and Hoke AW: Simplified laboratory technique for diagnosis of chancroid. Arch Dermatol, 102:188, 1970.
64. Choudhary BP, Kumari S, Bhati R, and Agarwal DS: Bacteriological study of chancroid. Indian J Med Res, 76:379, 1982.
65. Fast MV, et al: The clinical diagnosis of genital ulcer disease in men in the tropics. Sex Transm Dis, 11:72, 1984.
66. Burns JL, et al: A permeability barrier as a mechanism of chloramphenicol resistance in Haemophilus influenzae. Antimicrob Agents Chemother, 27:46, 1986.
67. Doern GV, Daum GS, and Tubert TA: In vitro chloramphenicol susceptibility testing of Haemophilus influenzae: Disk diffusion procedures and assays for chloramphenicol acetyltransferase. J Clin Microbiol, 25:1453, 1987.
68. National Committee for Clinical Laboratory Standards: Performance standards for antimicrobial disk susceptibility tests. Tentative Standard NCCLS Publication M2-T4. 4th ed. Villanova, PA, NCCLS, 1988.
69. National Committee for Clinical Laboratory Standards: Dilution procedures for susceptibility testing of aerobic bacteria. Approved Standard NCCLS Publication M2-T4. 2nd ed. Villanova, PA, NCCLS, 1990.
70. Gilsdorf JR: Haemophilus influenzae type b vaccine efficacy in the United States. Pediatr Infect Dis J, 7:147, 1988.
71. Eskola J, et al: A randomized, prospective field trial of a conjugate vaccine in the protection of infants and young children against invasive Haemophilus influenzae type b disease. N Engl J Med, 323:1381, 1990.
72. Ward J, et al: Limited efficacy of a Haemophilus influenzae type b conjugate vaccine in Alaska native infants. N Engl J Med, 323:1393, 1990.
73. Centers for Disease Control: Haemophilus b conjugate vaccines for prevention of Haemophilus influenzae type b disease among infants and children two months of age and older. MMWR, 40(RR-1):1, 1991.
74. Mutters R, et al: Reclassification of the genus Pasteurella Trevisan 1887 on the basis of deoxyribonucleic acid homology, with proposals for the new species Pasteurella dagmatis, Pasteurella canis, Pasteurella stomatis, Pasteurella anatis, and Pasteurella langaa. Int J Syst Bacteriol, 35:309, 1985.
75. Weber DJ, Wolfson JS, Swartz MN, and Hooper DC: Pasteurella multocida infections: Report of 34 cases and review of the literature. Medicine, 63:133, 1984.
76. Pickett MJ, Hollis DG, and Bottone EJ: Miscellaneous gram-

negative bacteria. *In* Manual of Clinical Microbiology. 5th ed. Edited by A Balows, et al. Washington DC, American Society for Microbiology, 1991.

77. Potts TV, Zambon JJ, and Genco RJ: Reassignment of Actinobacillus actinomycetemcomitans to the genus Haemophilus as Haemophilus actinomycetemcomitans comb. nov. Int J Syst Bacteriol, *35*:337, 1985.
78. Kamin S, et al: Inhibition of fibroblast proliferation and collagen synthesis by capsular material from Actinobacillus actinomycetemcomitans. J Med Microbiol, *22*:245, 1986.
79. Hammond BF, Lillard SE, and Stevens RH: A bacteriocin of Actinobacillus actinomycetemcomitans. Infect Immun, *55*: 686, 1987.
80. Asikainen S, et al: Certain bacterial species and morphotypes in localized juvenile peridontitis and in matched controls. J Periodontol, *58*:224, 1987.
81. McGowan JE, and Del Rio C: Other gram-negative bacilli. *In* Principles and Practice of Infectious Diseases. 3rd ed. Edited by GL Mandell, RG Douglas, Jr, and JE Bennett. New York, Churchill Livingstone, 1990.
82. Bonta Y, et al: Rapid identification of periodontal pathogens in subgingival plaque; comparison of indirect immunofluorescence microscopy with bacterial culture for detection of Actinobacillus actinomycetemcomitans. J Dent Res, *64*:793, 1985.
83. Horowitz EA, et al: Pericarditis caused by Actinobacillus actinomycetemcomitans. J Infect Dis, *155*:152, 1987.
84. Pierce CS, et al: Endocarditis due to Actinobacillus actinomycetemcomitans serotype c and patient immune response. J Infect Dis, *149*:479, 1984.
85. Brenner DJ, Hollis DG, Fanning GR, and Weaver RE: Capnocytophaga canimorsus sp. nov. (formerly CDC Group DF-2), a cause of septicemia following dog bite, and C. cynodegmi sp. nov., a cause of localized wound infection following dog bite. J Clin Microbiol, *27*:231, 1989.
86. Warren JS, and Allen SD: Clinical, pathogenic and laboratory features of Capnocytophaga infections. Am J Clin Pathol, *86*: 513, 1986.
87. Parenti DM, and Syndman DE: Capnocytophaga species: Infections in nonimmunocompromised and immunocompromised hosts. J Infect Dis, *151*:140, 1985.
88. Matlow A, and Vellend H: Capnocytophaga: A pathogen in immunocompetent hosts. J Infect Dis, *152*:233, 1985.
89. Hicklin H, Verghese A, and Alvarez S: Dysgonic fermenter 2 septicemia. Rev Infect Dis, *9*:884, 1987.
90. Elliot DL, et al: Pet-associated illness. N Engl J Med, *313*:985, 1985.
91. Westwell AJ, Spencer MB, and Kerr KG: DF-2 bacteremia following cat bites. Am J Med, *83*:1170, 1987.
92. Butler T, et al: Unidentified gram-negative rod infection: A new disease of man. Ann Intern Med, *86*:1, 1977.
93. Baron EJ, and Finegold SM: Unclassified or unusual but easily cultivated etiologic agents of infectious diseases. *In* Bailey and Scott's Diagnostic Microbiology. 8th ed. St. Louis, CV Mosby, 1990.
94. Macher AM, Casale TM, and Fauci AS: Chronic granulomatous disease of childhood and Chromobacterium violaceum infections in the southeastern United States. Ann Intern Med, *97*:51, 1982.
95. Koneman EW, et al (eds.): Miscellaneous and fastidious gram-negative bacilli. *In* Color Atlas and Textbook of Diagnostic Microbiology. 3rd ed. Philadelphia, JB Lippincott, 1988.
96. Dul MJ, Shalaes DM, and Lerner PI: EF-4 bacteremia in a patient with hepatic carcinoid. J Clin Microbiol, *18*:1260, 1983.
97. Aronson N, and Zbick CJ: Dysgonic fermenter 3 bacteremia in a neutropenic patient with acute lymphocytic leukemia. J Clin Microbiol, *26*:2213, 1988.
98. Bangsborg JM, Frederiksen V, and Bruun B: Dysgonic fermenter 3–associated abscess in a diabetic patient. J Infection, *20*:237, 1990.
99. Blum RN, et al: Clinical illness associated with isolation of dysgonic fermenter 3 from stool samples. J Clin Microbiol, *30*:398, 1992.

Chapter 37

CAMPYLOBACTER AND HELICOBACTER

The species of Campylobacter and Helicobacter pylori are small (0.5 to 8 μm long by 0.2 to 0.5 μm wide), motile non–spore-forming, curved (comma-shaped) or S-shaped, gram-negative bacilli that in general grow optimally in an atmosphere containing 5 to 10% oxygen and, therefore, are considered microaerophilic. Until recently, H. pylori was classified in the genus Campylobacter because of its spiral shape, microaerophilic nature, and guanine-plus-cytosine ratio (36 to 37 mol%). However, owing to significant morphologic differences between "Campylobacter" pylori (cells that have smooth surfaces, rounded ends, and one to six polar flagella covered with a membrane sheath) and other species of Campylobacter (cells that have ruffled surfaces, pointed ends, depressions in the end, and one unsheathed polar flagellum or one flagellum at each end) and differences in the fatty acid composition of the cell, whole-cell protein profiles examined by polyacrylamide gel electrophoresis, and ribosomal RNA sequences, "C. pylori" was placed in a separate genus, Helicobacter (1–4).

CAMPYLOBACTER

Campylobacter (from Greek *kampylos, bactērion* curved rod) organisms were isolated originally from aborted sheep fetuses in 1909 and named Vibrio fetus. However, because these bacteria do not ferment carbohydrates and their guanine-plus-cytosine DNA content differs from that of true vibrios (Campylobacter, 28 to 38 mol%; Vibrio, 38 to 51 mol%), a new genus, Campylobacter, was created. Of the 13 species of Campylobacter recognized currently, Campylobacter jejuni and Campylobacter fetus subspecies fetus are the most important pathogens and are discussed in detail. The remaining species, which uncommonly cause human disease or are not known to be human pathogens, are reviewed briefly in Tables 37–1 and 37–2 (5–12).

Campylobacter jejuni

Campylobacter jejuni (formerly Campylobacter fetus subspecies jejuni) first was recognized as a human pathogen in 1972, when it was isolated from children with enteritis (13). The relationship between this organism and enteritis was confirmed in 1977, and since then Campylobacter jejuni has become the most common cause of diarrhea in the United States and in England (14,15).

Epidemiology

Campylobacter jejuni is worldwide a common commensal of the gastrointestinal tract of wild or domesticated cattle, sheep, swine, goats, dogs, cats, and many varieties of fowl, especially turkeys and chickens. In animals, primary infections with C. jejuni occur early in life, and although infection may cause morbidity and mortality, in most animals a lifelong carrier state with specific immunity develops. This animal reservoir probably is the major source of most human infections. Meat from infected animals often is contaminated with intestinal contents during slaughter, and excreta from infected animals may contaminate soil or water.

Most human infections with Campylobacter jejuni are acquired by consuming contaminated food, especially undercooked poultry, or water. Several outbreaks of enteritis caused by C. jejuni have been linked to unpasteurized milk or to defects in municipal water systems (15–20). Household pets have been implicated as potential vectors, and fecal-oral, person-to-person transmission has been reported (15,19). Perinatal transmission and parenteral transmission (via blood transfusion) are rare (21,22).

In developed countries infections caused by Campylobacter jejuni occur year round, but peak in summer and early fall; in tropical countries the seasonal variation is influenced by rainfall. In the United States and England, C. jejuni organisms are isolated more frequently than Salmonella or Shigella from stool specimens of persons with diarrhea and rarely are recovered from healthy persons (15,23). Enteritis caused by C. jejuni affects all ages and both sexes equally, but the peak prevalence is in children younger than 1 year and in persons 15 to 29 years of age (14). In developing countries C. jejuni is isolated more often from healthy persons, especially during the first 5 years of life. These early infections often are symptomatic, whereas infections that occur later typically are not recognized, principally owing to age- or exposure-related immunity (25).

Pathogenesis and Pathology

Two important factors that determine whether infection with Campylobacter jejuni results in disease are the dose of organisms that reaches the small intestine and the specific immunity of the host. C. jejuni is susceptible to hydrochloric acid; and in human volunteers who ingest fewer than 10^4 organisms rarely induces disease (15,26). Persons infected with C. jejuni develop specific immunoglobulin (Ig) G, IgM, and IgA in serum, and IgA in intestinal secretions (27,28). Volunteers infected with C. jejuni and rechallenged with homologous organisms again develop infection but do not become ill, which suggests that humoral immunity is protective (27).

Campylobacter jejuni organisms multiply in bile and may adhere to epithelial cells, factors that aid colonization of the bile-rich upper small intestine early in infection. The organism produces a cytotoxin and an enterotoxin,

Table 37–1. Epidemiology and Clinical Manifestations of Infections Caused by Campylobacter

Species	Natural Habitat	Human Disease (Reference)
C. jejuni	GIT of wild and domesticated animals and fowl	Gastroenteritis (14–20)
C. fetus subsp. fetus	GIT and GUT of sheep and cattle	Bacteremia (38)
C. fetus subsp. venerealis	GUT of cattle	? Rarely recovered from stool of homosexual men and from women with vaginosis (15)
C. hyointestinalis	GIT of swine	? Proctitis, ? diarrhea (5,8,9)
C. coli	As for C. jejuni	Gastroenteritis (40)
C. lari	Seagulls	Diarrhea, bacteremia (10)
C. cinaedi and fennelliae*	ND	Proctitis, proctocolitis, enteritis in homosexual men (11)
C. cryaerophila	GUT and GIT of swine and cattle	? Diarrhea (6)
C. concisus	Normal flora in human oral cavity	? Peridontal disease (12)
C. sputorum subsp. sputorum	Normal flora in human oral cavity	? Diarrhea (40) ? Skin infection (15,40)
C. sputorum subsp. bubulis	GUT of cattle	—
C. sputorum subsp. fecalis	GUT of cattle	—
C. mucosalis	Swine	—
C. nitrofigilis	Roots of plants in salt marshes	—

* C. cinaedi and C. fennelliae are more closely related to Helicobacter pylori than to other species of Campylobacter and in the future may be transferred to the genus Helicobacter.
Key: GIT, gastrointestinal tract; GUT, genitourinary tract; ?, association with the disease has not been proven; ND, not determined; —, no known association with disease in humans.

but their significance in vivo is unknown (28,29). Lipopolysaccharides present in the outer membranes possess typical endotoxic activities. Because the clinical signs of enteritis caused by C. jejuni (described later) are characteristic of infection with an invasive organism, the invasiveness of C. jejuni is believed to be an important virulence factor; and in vitro monoclonal antibodies directed against an unidentified surface antigen inhibit invasiveness, a fact that supports this theory (30).

Ulcers produced by Campylobacter jejuni may be found in the jejunum, ileum, and colon. Microscopic examination of involved tissue shows nonspecific colitis with a mixed inflammatory infiltrate (neutrophils, mononuclear cells, and eosinophils) in the lamina propria, loss of goblet cells, crypt abscesses, and focal mucosal ulceration.

Clinical Manifestations

After an incubation period of 2 to 4 days (range, 1 to 7 days), acute enteritis begins after a brief prodrome of fever, headache, myalgia, and malaise followed by cramping abdominal pain and diarrhea, varying from loose stools to massive watery stools or grossly bloody stools. The illness is self-limiting, and symptoms gradually improve over several days but last longer than 1 week in 10 to 20% of persons who seek medical attention and may relapse in 5 to 10% of untreated patients (15). Infrequently, acute enteritis is accompanied by bacteremia, an event most likely to occur in very young, elderly, or immunocompromised persons (31). Potential complications of enteritis caused by Campylobacter jejuni include cholecystitis, pancreatitis, cystitis, reactive arthritis in persons with HLA-B27 histocompatibility antigens, hepatitis, interstitial nephritis, the hemolytic-uremic syndrome, and, rarely, the Guillain-Barré syndrome (32–36). C. jejuni also may cause septic abortion.

Campylobacter fetus subspecies fetus

In 1909, an organism named Vibrio fetus ovis (shortened to Vibrio fetus in 1919) was identified as an agent of

Table 37–2. Differential Characteristics of Species of Campylobacter Isolated from Clinical Specimens

Species	Growth 25°C	Growth 42°C	Hippurate Hydrolysis	Catalase	H₂S In TSI	Indoxyl Acetate Hydrolysis	Nitrate to Nitrite	Susceptibility Cephalothin	Susceptibility Nalidixic Acid
C. cinaedi*	−	±	−	+	−	−	+	S	S
C. coli	−	+	−	+	±	+	+	R	S
C. concisus	−	+	−	−	+	ND	+	R	R
C. cryaerophila	+	−	−	+	−	+	+	R	S
C. fennelliae*	−	−	−	+	−	+	−	S	S
C. fetus subsp. fetus†	+	∓	−	+	−	−	+	S	R
C. hyointestinalis	±	+	−	+	+	−	+	S	R
C. jejuni‡	−	+	+	+	−	+	+	R	S
C. lari	−	+	−	+	−	−	+	R	R
C. sputorum	−	+	−	∓	+	−	+	S	R
C. upsaliensis	−	+	−	−/weak +	−	+	+	S	S

* C. cinaedi and C. fennelliae are more closely related to Helicobacter pylori than to other species of Campylobacter and may be transferred to the genus Helicobacter in the future.
† Cephalothin-resistant isolates of C. fetus subsp. fetus have been reported.
‡ Hippurate-negative isolates and nalidixic acid–resistant isolates of C. jejuni have been reported.
Key: +, most isolates positive; −, most isolates negative; ±, variable results; S, susceptible; R, resistant; TSI, triple sugar iron agar; ND, not determined.

epizootic abortion in domesticated animals (37). Since the 1950s this organism, now called Campylobacter fetus subspecies fetus, has been recognized as an uncommon cause of septicemia and other infections, principally in persons who have an underlying disease (38). C. fetus subsp fetus has a predilection for the cardiovascular system, involving the vascular endothelium, particularly in the presence of pre-existing vascular damage (39).

Epidemiology

The major habitat of Campylobacter fetus subsp fetus is the intestines of sheep and cattle, and recovery of the organism from healthy sheep and cattle is not uncommon. C. fetus subsp fetus also may be found in the genital tract of sheep and cattle, their placentas, the gastric contents of their aborted fetuses, and less frequently in other animals and birds (40). Animals probably acquire infection by ingesting food or water contaminated with bacteria from feces, aborted fetuses, or vaginal discharge of an aborting animal. Organisms in the intestine enter the circulation and, because they have high affinity for placental tissue, invade the uterus and multiply in the fetus. An infected fetus usually is aborted, but those born live die within a few days.

Human infections caused by Campylobacter fetus subsp fetus occur worldwide. Clusters of cases have been reported in South Africa, Nepal, France, Germany, and the United States (41). About 75% of affected persons are over age 45 years, and a similar proportion have a chronic underlying illness such as alcoholism, hepatic or renal failure, cirrhosis, diabetes mellitus, tuberculosis, chronic lymphocytic leukemia, systemic lupus erythematosus, or agammaglobulinemia (38). In children, both sexes are affected equally; but, for reasons unknown, among adults the infection predominates in males. The mechanisms of transmission of C. fetus subsp fetus are not understood completely. Direct contact with an infected animal is possible, but fewer than a third of infected persons have a history of environmental or occupational exposure (41). Contaminated food or water may be a vehicle for infection, or infection may originate from an endogenous source (42). The organism may be a normal commensal in the oral cavity, and dental disease or manipulation might predispose to bacteremia (41). Alternatively, C. fetus subsp fetus might colonize the intestinal tract, becoming invasive in the setting of decreased host immunity or resistance.

Pathogenesis

The surface (S) protein of Campylobacter fetus subsp fetus appears to be a major virulence factor. Functioning as a capsule, the S protein disrupts binding of the C3b component of complement to the organism, which might explain its resistance to serum bactericidal activity and phagocytosis. The mechanism responsible for the organism's vascular tropism is unknown, but two theories have been proposed. The organism may produce a local procoagulant that promotes thrombus formation, or it may bind to the endothelium via a surface receptor that has affinity for endothelial cells and induce local injury, promoting thrombus formation (43).

Clinical Manifestations

Most often, infection with Campylobacter fetus subsp fetus is manifest as bacteremia marked by fever, chills, night sweats, malaise, and weight loss. In more than half the cases the bacteremia is secondary to a localized infection such as septic arthritis, pelvic inflammatory disease, meningitis, endocarditis, pneumonia, thrombophlebitis, or mycotic aneurysm. In the remainder, bacteremia is a cryptogenic, isolated event that responds readily to antimicrobial agents; or it is a chronic, relapsing illness that persists up to several months (38). The mortality rate ranges from 17 to 43% and is higher in persons who have secondary bacteremia and localized infections than in those with cryptogenic bacteremia. Infection with C. fetus subsp fetus also may cause a diarrheal illness clinically similar to that caused by Campylobacter jejuni (15).

Laboratory Diagnosis

The optimal specimen for diagnosis of enteritis caused by Campylobacter jejuni or other Campylobacter species is stool, but a rectal swab specimen is an acceptable alternative. Infection caused by Campylobacter fetus subsp fetus most often is diagnosed by recovering the organism from blood. Specimen collection, transport, and processing are reviewed in Part III. Characteristics of Campylobacter jejuni and Campylobacter fetus subsp fetus are discussed below; features of other Campylobacter species that are suspected or known human pathogens are shown in Table 37-2.

Campylobacter jejuni. Enteritis caused by C. jejuni is diagnosed most frequently by recovering the organism from stool or a rectal swab specimen. The presence of the organism in diarrheal stool specimens, however, may be suggested by observing characteristic darting motility in a fresh (≤ 2 hours) sample examined by phase-contrast or darkfield microscopy or by finding comma- or S-shaped gram-negative bacilli in a smear stained with the Gram stain.

After incubation for 48 hours on Campy-blood agar, a selective medium commonly used to recover the organism from stool samples, typical colonies of Campylobacter jejuni are gray to pink and mucoid, occasionally showing a tailing effect of growth along the streak line, but they may appear flat, dry, and irregular in shape. Hemolysis is not observed on blood agar. A smear prepared from young colonies and stained with the Gram stain shows gram-negative, curved, S-shaped, gull-winged, or long spiral forms (Plate VI C), but a smear prepared from an older culture, especially one exposed to ambient air, often shows coccoid forms (44). In a wet-mount preparation of a suspected colony examined by phase-contrast or darkfield microscopy, organisms demonstrate a characteristic darting motility. Organisms that are recovered on a selective medium at 42° C, show the typical cellular structure and that give positive results for catalase and oxidase presumptively are called Campylobacter. C. jejuni is hippurate positive (see Appendix, Procedure 14), hydrolyzes indoxyl acetate, and is susceptible to nalidixic acid and resistant to cephalothin (45). Antimicrobial susceptibility is determined by inoculating a 5% sheep blood or Mueller-Hinton agar plate with a suspension of the organism showing turbidity equal to that of a 0.5 McFarland standard, as for agar disk diffusion (see Chapter 24). A 30-μg disk of each of the two agents is placed on the agar surface, and plates are incubated at 37° C in a microaerophilic atmosphere. Additional identifying characteristics are shown in Table 37–2. A nucleic acid probe that detects the thermophilic campylobacters (C. jejuni, Campylobacter coli, Campylobacter lari) but does not distinguish each species is commercially available (46).

Campylobacter fetus subsp fetus. C. fetus subsp fetus, and other species of Campylobacter, grow in most blood culture broth media, although growth may not be detected for up to 2 weeks, and they are detected by commercially available carbon dioxide monitoring instruments (see Chapter 58). Because visible turbidity often is absent, performing blind subcultures (to 5% sheep blood or chocolate agar incubated in a microaerophilic atmosphere) or Gram stain may be necessary to detect the organism.

On blood agar after incubation for 48 to 72 hours, colonies of Campylobacter fetus subsp fetus are 0.5 to 1.0 mm in diameter, smooth, slightly convex, translucent, and nonhemolytic. Like other campylobacters, C. fetus subsp fetus is oxidase- and catalase positive. Other helpful identifying features are shown in Table 37–2.

Treatment

Treatment of enteritis caused by species of Campylobacter includes fluid and electrolyte replacement; and for persons with high fever, bloody diarrhea, more than eight stools per day, or symptoms that persist longer than a week, antimicrobial therapy is recommended. Erythromycin is the agent of choice; ciprofloxacin, norfloxacin, tetracycline, and clindamycin are effective alternatives. Isolates of Campylobacter cinaedi and Campylobacter coli may be resistant to erythromycin and tetracycline (47). Systemic infections with Campylobacter fetus subsp fetus require parenteral therapy; gentamicin is the agent of choice for bacteremia and other nonenteric infections except meningitis, for which chloramphenicol is recommended (30).

HELICOBACTER

Spiral bacteria were described in gastric tissue of humans since the early 1900s, but because no correlation between their presence and a specific pathologic condition was demonstrated in early investigations, interest waned until the late 1970s. During the early 1980s, Warren and Marshall examined antral biopsy specimens from many persons who had gastric symptoms, and they demonstrated a strong relationship between these spiral bacteria and gastritis and peptic ulcers, especially duodenal ulcers. Soon thereafter they recovered the pathogen (which initially was named Campylobacter pyloridis, though subsequently the designation was amended to Campylobacter pylori and recently changed to Helicobacter pylori) by culturing clinical specimens in microaerophilic conditions, an approach adopted because the organisms in biopsy tissue appeared similar to campylobacters (1,48–50).

Epidemiology

Helicobacter pylori occurs worldwide, but currently the reservoir of infection and its mechanism of transmission are unknown. An animal reservoir is unlikely because the organism has not been reported in animals other than nonhuman primates (51). H. pylori has not been isolated from periodontal pockets of persons with gastritis, but highly sensitive methods of detection, such as DNA probes, have not been used (1). The prevalence of gastritis associated with H. pylori increases with age, suggesting that the organism is acquired as people grow older, though the prevalence also may depend on ethnic or geographic differences (52). Person-to-person transmission has been suggested but not proven (1).

Pathogenesis

Factors involved in the establishment of Helicobacter pylori in the stomach and the production of inflammation are ill-defined. Production by the organism of large amounts of urease could create an alkaline microenvironment, providing protection from gastric acid until it establishes itself under the layer of mucus. The bacteria apparently attach to the surface of epithelial cells, possibly by surface hemagglutinin or by attachment pedestals similar to those of the enteropathogenic Escherichia coli (see Chapter 34). Microvilli on the epithelial cells appear to become depleted, and the bacteria aggregate at intercellular junctions, which subsequently are disrupted. This mild tissue damage may elicit a leukocyte response, producing gastritis. Approximately half of H. pylori isolates elaborate a cytotoxin that has nonlethal effects on various mammalian cells; however, its role in the pathogenesis of disease is questionable (53).

Evidence associating Helicobacter pylori with peptic ulcer disease is only circumstantial; however, various theories of how the organism might be involved have been proposed. Wyatt and coworkers showed that almost 90% of persons with duodenitis had both H. pylori and gastric metaplasia in the duodenum, that metaplasia occurred only in persons whose gastric pH was less than 2.5, and that in the duodenum bacteria were found only in areas of gastric metaplasia (54). Based on these findings they suggested that gastric metaplasia could develop in the duodenum of persons with high gastric acid output and become colonized with H. pylori originating from the antrum, colonization that could elicit an inflammatory response that eventually would cause ulcer formation. Alternatively, H. pylori could alter the gastric environment by rapid urea hydrolysis at intercellular junctions, preventing normal passage of hydrogen ions and causing back-diffusion with subsequent hypochlorhydria and tissue damage; or the organism could disrupt the protective mucus barrier via its proteolytic activity that degrades mucin, allowing acid to damage underlying epithelial cells (55,56).

Clinical Manifestations

A very significant relationship exists between Helicobacter pylori and chronic and chronic active type B gastritis (gastritis that principally involves the antrum but occasionally extends into the body of the stomach and affects the mucus-secreting cells). Evidence confirming this association includes these findings: Ingestion of H. pylori by human volunteers results in chronic gastritis. Inoculation of animals with H. pylori in the laboratory produces chronic gastritis, simulating human infection. Gastritis resolves with antimicrobial therapy that clears the infection. Moreover, titers of specific antibodies decrease with therapy, contemporaneously with resolution of the inflammation.

Gastritis associated with Helicobacter pylori, manifested by epigastric pain, nausea, and vomiting, most commonly occurs in adults, increasing in prevalence with age, but has been reported in children (1). H. pylori also has been implicated as a cause of nonulcer dyspepsia (a condition marked by symptoms of peptic ulcer—epigastric pain, bloating, nausea, vomiting—but no ulcer) and duodenal ulcers; however, these associations have not been confirmed (1).

Laboratory Diagnosis

Methods that may be used to diagnose infection with Helicobacter pylori include histologic examination of biopsy tissue, culture, direct Gram stain, serologic tests, and the urea breath test. Gastric biopsy specimens, typically taken from involved areas of the antrum, are required for histologic diagnosis. Specimens generally show glandular atrophy, epithelial degeneration and metaplasia, an infiltrate of neutrophils in the epithelium; neutrophils, lymphocytes, and plasma cells in the lamina propria, and spiral organisms in the layer of mucus on the epithelium (Fig. 37–1). Organisms may be visualized with the hematoxylin and eosin, Warthin-Starry, Dieterle, tissue Gram, or Giemsa stain, but the latter appears to provide the best combination of simplicity and accuracy (57). The sensitivity of histologic examination is better than 90%, but an invasive procedure is necessary to obtain the specimen and only a small area of the stomach can be evaluated.

Helicobacter pylori may be cultured from gastric biopsy specimens or brushings of the gastric epithelium. Specimens should be transported to the laboratory immediately for processing (see Chapter 59), but if delay is unavoidable, storage at 4° C in isotonic saline or 20% glucose solution is acceptable (58). Several types of media support the growth of H. pylori: 5 to 10% horse blood agar, 5 to 10% sheep blood agar, chocolate agar, Skirrow medium, and Thayer-Martin agar (1,58). Incorporating antibiotics into the medium to suppress contaminating bacteria is useful; however, cephalothin should be omitted because H. pylori usually are susceptible to this agent. Small, clear, weakly β-hemolytic colonies generally become apparent after incubation for 2 to 5 days at 35° to 37° C in a microaerophilic atmosphere, but occasionally incubation for a week is necessary. Isolates that have catalase, oxidase, and urease activity, that do not hydrolyze hippurate or indoxyl acetate, and that are susceptible to cephalothin but resistant to nalidixic acid by disk diffusion presumptively are called H. pylori. Culture is sensitive, but prolonged incubation is required and an invasive procedure is required to collect the specimen. Rapid urease tests, performed by inoculating biopsy specimens directly into urease broth or onto a gel pellet containing urea and incubating up to 24 hours, have been suggested as a sensitive and specific alternative to culture (59–61). A positive result provides presumptive evidence that H. pylori is present.

Examination of a direct Gram-stained biopsy tissue specimen has a sensitivity of 65 to 85% if a single antral specimen is evaluated, and of 92 to 100% if tissue from

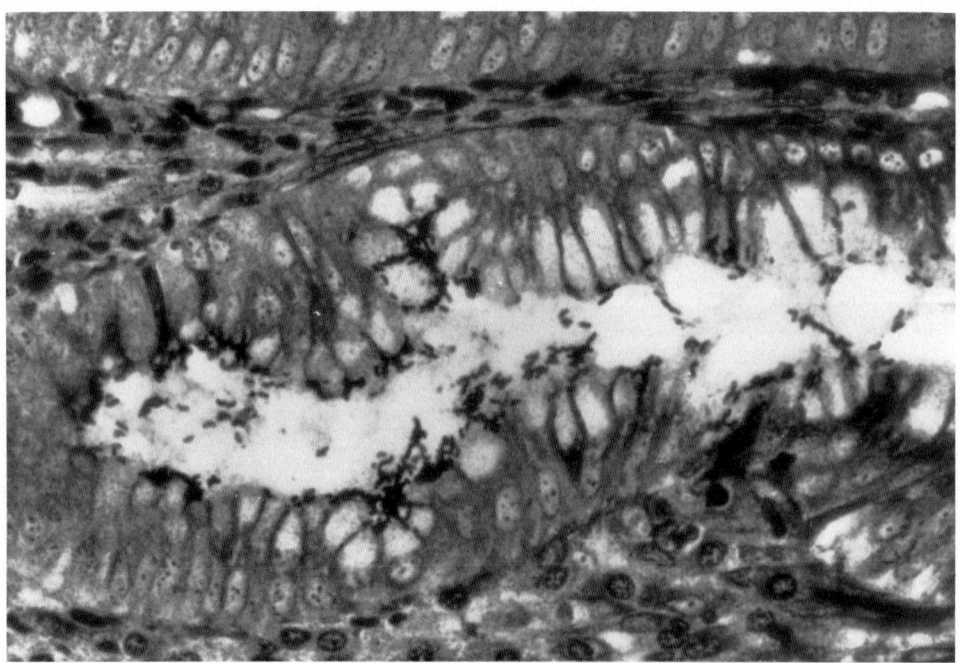

Fig. 37–1. Micrograph of gastric biopsy specimen showing curved bacteria in the mucus layer on the epithelium (Giemsa, ×600). (Courtesy of Miles McFarland, MD, Medical College of Pennsylvania, Philadelphia, PA).

the antrum and fundus are examined (62,63). Data from one study suggest that the rinse-imprint technique (rinse the biopsy in dextrose phosphate broth, blot it onto sterile gauze or filter paper, and press it onto the surface of a sterile glass slide) is preferred to examining smears prepared from ground tissue (63).

Serum IgG and IgA specific for Helicobacter pylori are detected in persons infected with the organism but rarely are detected in persons with normal gastric mucosa. The sensitivity of serologic assays has ranged from 81 to 100%, depending on the antigen preparation (1). Advantages of serologic tests are that an invasive procedure is not required and that the potential for sampling error (a problem with biopsy) does not exist. Enzyme-linked immunosorbent assays that detect specific IgG, IgA, and IgM currently are commercially available; however, few comprehensive evaluations of these products have been done.

To perform the urea breath test, the patient ingests urea labeled with carbon-13 or -14 and, after a time, the level of labeled urea is determined in a breath sample by mass spectrometry (^{13}C) or with a scintillation counter (^{14}C) (64,65). This test is sensitive, rapid, and not invasive but requires special, expensive equipment.

Treatment

Whether all persons infected with Helicobacter pylori require treatment—and with which agents—currently are unknown. In vitro, H. pylori is resistant to sulfonamides and susceptible to erythromycin, rifampin, amoxicillin, tetracycline, metronidazole, and bismuth salts. Treatment with furazolidone or metronidazole (but not erythromycin) results in clearance of the organisms and improvement in the histologic findings in gastric biopsy specimens; but after therapy is terminated the organisms usually recur and gastric tissue assumes its pretreatment appearance (66). Although results with combination therapy generally are better, disease still may recur (67).

REFERENCES

1. Buck GE: Campylobacter pylori and gastroduodenal disease. Clin Microbiol Rev, *3*:1, 1990.
2. Goodwin CS, McCulloch RK, Armstrong JA, and Wee SH: Unusual cellular fatty acids and distinctive ultrastructure in a new spiral bacterium (Campylobacter pyloridis) from the human gastric mucosa. J Med Microbiol, *19*:257, 1985.
3. Jones DM, et al: Antibody to the gastric campylobacter-like organism ("Campylobacter pyloridis")—clinical correlations and distribution in the normal population. J Med Microbiol, *22*:57, 1986.
4. Paster BJ, and Dewhirst FE: Phylogeny of campylobacters, wolinellas, Bacteroides gracilis, and Bacteroides ureolyticus by 16S ribosomal ribonucleic acid sequencing. Int J Syst Bacteriol, *38*:56, 1988.
5. Edmonds P, et al: Campylobacter hyointestinalis associated with human gastrointestinal disease in the United States. J Clin Microbiol, *25*:685, 1987.
6. Tee W, Baird R, Dyall-Smith M, and Dwyer B: Campylobacter cryaerophila isolated from a human. J Clin Microbiol, *26*:2469, 1988.
7. Patton CM, et al: Human disease associated with "Campylobacter upsaliensis" (catalase-negative or weakly positive Campylobacter species) in the United States. J Clin Microbiol, *27*:66, 1989.
8. Minet J, Grosbois B, and Megraud F: Campylobacter hyointestinalis: An opportunistic enteropathogen? J Clin Microbiol, *26*:2659, 1988.
9. Fennell CL, et al: Characterization of Campylobacter-like organisms isolated from homosexual men. J Infect Dis, *149*:58, 1986.
10. Tauxe RV, et al: Illness associated with Campylobacter laridis, a newly recognized Campylobacter species. J Clin Microbiol, *21*:222, 1985.
11. Totten PA, et al: Campylobacter cinaedi (sp. nov.) and Campylobacter fennelliae (sp. nov.): Two new Campylobacter species associated with enteric disease in homosexual men. J Infect Dis, *151*:131, 1985.
12. Badger SJ, and Tanner ACR: Serological studies of Bacteroides fragilis, Campylobacter concisus, Wolinella recta, and Eikenella corrodens, all from humans with periodontal disease. Int J System Bacteriol, *31*:446, 1981.
13. Butzler JP, Dekeyser P, Detrain M, and DeHaen F: Related vibrios in stools. J Pediatr, *82*:493, 1973.
14. Skirrow MB: Campylobacter enteritis: A "new" disease. Br Med J, *2*:9, 1977.
15. Blaser MJ: Campylobacter species. *In* Principles and Practice of Infectious Diseases. 3rd ed. Edited by GL Mandell, RG Douglas, Jr, and JE Bennett. New York, Churchill Livingstone, 1990.
16. Blaser MJ, Taylor DN, and Feldman RA: Epidemiology of Campylobacter jejuni infections. Epidemiol Rev, *5*:157, 1983.
17. Taylor DN, et al: Campylobacter enteritis associated with drinking untreated water in back-country areas of the Rocky Mountains. Ann Intern Med, *99*:38, 1983.
18. Mentzing L-O: Waterborne outbreaks of Campylobacter enteritis in central Sweden. Lancet, *ii*:352, 1981.
19. Deming MS, et al: Campylobacter enteritis at a university: Transmission from eating chicken and from cats. Am J Epidemiol, *126*:526, 1987.
20. Vogt RL, et al: Serotyping and serology studies of campylobacteriosis associated with consumption of raw milk. J Clin Microbiol, *20*:998, 1984.
21. Vesikari T, Huttunen L, and Maki R: Perinatal Campylobacter fetus ss jejuni enteritis. Acta Paediatr Scand, *70*:261, 1981.
22. Pepersack F, et al: Campylobacter jejuni posttransfusional septicaemia. Lancet, *ii*:911, 1979.
23. Blaser MJ, et al: Campylobacter enteritis in the United States. A multicenter study. Ann Intern Med, *98*:360, 1983.
24. Centers for Disease Contol: Campylobacter isolates in the United States, 1982–1986. MMWR, *37*(SS-2):1, 1988.
25. Glass RI, et al: Epidemiologic and clinical features of endemic Campylobacter jejuni infection in Bangladesh. J Infect Dis, *148*:292, 1983.
26. Blaser MJ, et al: Survival of Campylobacter fetus subsp. jejuni in biological milieus. J Clin Microbiol, *11*:309, 1980.
27. Black RE, et al: Experimental Campylobacter jejuni infection in humans. J Infect Dis, *157*:472, 1988.
28. Walker RI, et al: Pathophysiology of Campylobacter enteritis. Microbiol Rev, *50*:81, 1986.
29. Johnson WM, and Lior H: Cytotoxic and cytotonic factors produced by Campylobacter jejuni, Campylobacter coli, and Campylobacter laridis. J Clin Microbiol, *24*:275, 1986.
30. Konkel ME, Babakhani F, and Jones LA: Invasion-related antigens of Campylobacter jejuni. J Infect Dis, *162*:888, 1990.
31. Dhawan VK, et al: Campylobacter jejuni septicemia—epidemiology, clinical features, and outcome. West J Med, *144*:324, 1986.

32. Gallagher P, et al: Acute pancreatitis associated with Campylobacter infection. Br J Surg, 68:383, 1981.
33. Feder HM, Rasoulpour M, and Rodriquez AJ: Campylobacter urinary tract infection. Value of the urine Gram stain. JAMA, 256:2389, 1986.
34. Kosunen TU, et al: Reactive arthritis after Campylobacter jejuni enteritis in patients with HLA-B27. Lancet, i:1312, 1980.
35. Kaldor J, and Speed BR: Guillain-Barré syndrome and Campylobacter jejuni: A serological study. Br Med J, 288:1867, 1984.
36. Mertens A, and DeSmet M: Campylobacter cholecystitis. Lancet, i:1092, 1979.
37. McFaydean F, and Stockman S: Report of the Departmental Committee Appointed by the Board of Agriculture and Fisheries to Inquire into Epizootic Abortion. Vol. 3. London, His Majesty's Stationery Office, 1909.
38. Morrison VA, Lloyd BK, Chia JKS, and Tuazon CU: Cardiovascular and bacteremic manifestations of Campylobacter fetus infection: Case report and review. Rev Infect Dis, 12:387, 1990.
39. Geffen DB, Gill VJ, and Chabner BA: Campylobacter thrombophlebitis [letter]. Ann Intern Med, 99:126, 1983.
40. Penner JL: The genus Campylobacter: A decade of progress. Clin Microbiol Rev, 1:157, 1988.
41. Rettig PJ: Campylobacter infections in human beings. J Pediatr, 94:855, 1979.
42. Guerrant RL, Lahita RG, Winn WC, and Roberts RB: Campylobacteriosis in man: Pathogenic mechanisms and review of 91 bloodstream infections. Am J Med, 65:584, 1978.
43. Carbone KM, Heinrich MC, and Quinn TC: Thrombophlebitis and cellulitis due to Campylobacter fetus ssp. fetus: Report of four cases and a review of the literature. Medicine, 64:244, 1985.
44. Karmali MA, et al: Evaluation of a blood-free, charcoal-based, selective medium for the isolation of Campylobacter organisms from feces. J Clin Microbiol, 23:456, 1986.
45. Popovic-Uroic T, Patton CM, Nicholson MA, and Kiehlbauch JA: Evaluation of the indoxyl acetate hydrolysis test for rapid differentiation of Campylobacter, Helicobacter, and Wolinella species. J Clin Microbiol, 28:2335, 1990.
46. Popovic-Uroic, et al: Evaluation of an oligonucleotide probe for identification of Campylobacter species. Lab Med, 22:533, 1991.
47. Taylor DN, et al: Erythromycin-resistant Campylobacter infections in Thailand. Antimicrob Agents Chemother, 31:438, 1987.
48. Marshall BJ, et al: Original isolation of Campylobacter pyloridis from human gastric mucosa. Microbiol Lett, 25:83, 1984.
49. Marshall BJ, and Warren JR: Unidentified curved bacilli in the stomach of patients with gastritis and peptic ulceration. Lancet, i:1311, 1984.
50. Marshall BJ, and Goodwin CS: Revised nomenclature of Campylobacter pyloridis. Int J Syst Bacteriol, 37:68, 1987.
51. Baskerville A, and Newell DG: Naturally occurring chronic gastritis and C. pylori infection in the rhesus monkey: A potential model for gastritis in man. Gut, 29:465, 1988.
52. Rauws EAJ, et al: Campylobacter pyloridis–associated chronic active antral gastritis. Gastroenterology, 94:33, 1988.
53. Leunk RD, et al: Cytotoxic activity in broth-culture filtrates of Campylobacter pylori. J Med Microbiol, 26:93, 1988.
54. Wyatt JI, Rathbone BJ, Dixon MF, and Heatley RV: Campylobacter pyloridis and acid induced gastric metaplasia in the pathogenesis of duodenitis. J Clin Pathol, 40:841, 1987.
55. Hazell SL, and Lee A: Campylobacter pyloridis, urease, hydrogen ion back-diffusion, and gastric ulcers. Lancet, ii:15, 1986.
56. Slomiany BL, et al: Campylobacter pyloridis degrades mucin and undermines gastric mucosal integrity. Biochem Biophys Res Commun, 14:307, 1987.
57. Madan E, et al: Evaluation of staining methods for identifying Campylobacter pylori. Am J Clin Pathol, 90:450, 1988.
58. Edmonds P, Kassman N, Judd RL, and Rudert CS: Clinical and microbiologic features of Campylobacter pylori–associated gastric ulcers in humans. Clin Microbiol Newslett, 10:97, 1988.
59. Czinn SJ, and Carr H: Rapid diagnosis of Campylobacter pyloridis–associated gastritis. J Pediatr, 110:569, 1987.
60. Borromeo M, Lambert JR, and Pinkard KJ: Evaluation of "CLO-test" to detect Campylobacter pyloridis in gastric mucosa. J Clin Pathol, 40:462, 1987.
61. Marshall BJ, et al: Rapid urease test in the management of Campylobacter pyloridis–associated gastritis. Am J Gastroenterol, 82:200, 1987.
62. Montgomery EA, Martin DF, and Peura DA: Rapid diagnosis of Campylobacter pylori by Gram's stain. Am J Clin Pathol, 90:606, 1988.
63. Parsonnet J, et al: Simple microbiologic detection of Campylobacter pylori. J Clin Microbiol, 26:948, 1988.
64. Marshall BJ, et al: Carbon-14 urea breath test for the diagnosis of Campylobacter pylori–associated gastritis. J Nucl Med, 29:11, 1988.
65. Graham DY, et al: Campylobacter pylori detected noninvasively by the ^{13}C-urea breath test. Lancet, i:1174, 1987.
66. McNulty CAM, et al: Campylobacter pyloridis and associated gastritis: Investigator-blind, placebo-controlled trial of bismuth salicylate and erythromycin ethylsuccinate. Br Med J, 293:645, 1986.
67. Blaser MJ: Helicobacter pylori and the pathogenesis of gastroduodenal inflammation. J Infect Dis, 161:626, 1990.

Chapter 38

ANAEROBIC GRAM-NEGATIVE BACTERIA

The anaerobic gram-negative bacteria include the genera of bacilli—Anaerorhabdus, Anaerovibrio, Bacteroides, Bilophila, Butyrivibrio, Centipeda, Desulfomonas, Fusobacterium, Leptotrichia, Mitsukella, Mobiluncus, Porphyromonas, Prevotella, Selenomonas, Succinimonas, Succinivibrio, and Wolinella—and the genera of cocci—Acidaminococcus, Megasphaera, and Veillonella. These organisms are part of the normal flora of the mouth and the upper respiratory, gastrointestinal, and genital tract of humans and animals. Members of the genera Bacteroides (predominantly Bacteroides fragilis and Bacteroides thetaiotaomicron) Porphyromonas, Prevotella, and Fusobacterium account for almost all gram-negative anaerobes encountered in the clinical laboratory. The remaining organisms are uncommon pathogens or are not known to cause disease and are not discussed further here (1–3).

The taxonomy of the anaerobic gram-negative bacilli recently was revised. It was proposed that only members of the Bacteroides fragilis group be retained in the genus Bacteroides, because they share biochemical and physiologic characteristics that are distinct from other species that formerly were included in the genus (4). The genus Porphyromonas was created for the pigmenting, asaccharolytic species of Bacteroides, and the genus Prevotella was proposed for the saccharolytic or partially saccharolytic species (Table 38–1) (5,6). Moreover, data from ribosomal RNA sequencing studies suggest that Bacteroides gracilis and Bacteroides ureolyticus are not "true" Bacteroides species (7).

Diseases caused by the medically important anaerobic gram-negative bacilli are similar, so, their epidemiology and pathogenesis, and the clinical manifestations of the infections they cause are discussed as a group.

Epidemiology

Infections with the anaerobic gram-negative bacilli are endogenous (sites where these organisms are normal flora are listed in Table 38–1), and often polymicrobial. Host factors that predispose to infection include disruption of normal cutaneous or mucosal barriers, tissue injury via accidental trauma or a surgical procedure, impaired blood supply, tissue necrosis, obstruction of a hollow viscus, the presence of a foreign body, and malignancies, especially carcinoma of the lung, colon, and uterus.

Pathogenesis

Potential virulence factors have been identified for some of the anaerobic gram-negative bacilli. Species of Bacteroides and Fusobacterium adhere to host cells as the first step in invasion (8). Capsules, produced by Bacteroides fragilis and probably by Prevotella melaninogenica, Prevotella intermedius, and Prevotella oralis, inhibit macrophage migration, are antiphagocytic, and promote abscess formation. Superoxide dismutase, produced by Bacteroides fragilis, may counteract the toxic effect of superoxide radicals produced by neutrophils (see Chapter 2), thus facilitating bacterial survival until a reduced environment favorable for anaerobes is generated (9). Other enzymes produced by B. fragilis include neuraminidase, hyaluronidase, and fibrinolysin, all of which may promote tissue digestion or dissolution. Porphyromonas gingivalis binds and degrades human fibrinogen and produces collagenase; the latter may play a role in periodontal disease (10,11). Release of phospholipase A by Prevotella melaninogenica, Prevotella intermedia, and Fusobacterium necrophorum may disrupt the integrity of epithelial cell membranes, resulting in cell death (12). Cells of Bacteroides fragilis contain an endotoxin that differs structurally from endotoxin of other gram-negative bacteria and has weaker biologic activity, whereas the endotoxin of Prevotella bivia and species of Fusobacterium has potent biologic activity. Fusobacteria produce a leukocidin that is cytopathic for various mammalian cells and a lysophospholipase, which may allow the organism to spread through tissues.

The host immune response to infection with the anaerobic gram-negative bacilli has been evaluated most extensively for the Bacteroides fragilis group. In vitro, the alternate complement pathway (Chapter 2) is essential for effective opsonization of B. fragilis and Bacteroides thetaiotaomicron; and in animals infected in the laboratory with Bacteroides fragilis, T lymphocytes are required for protection against the development of intra-abdominal abscesses (13,14).

Clinical Manifestations

The anaerobic gram-negative bacilli are found in a variety of infections (see Table 38–1) whose hallmark is abscess formation. Anaerobes, especially Bacteroides fragilis and Bacteroides thetaiotaomicron, play a major role in intra-abdominal (peritoneal or visceral) abscesses such as appendicitis with perforation and abscess formation, diverticulitis with perforation and abscess formation or generalized peritonitis, and liver abscess.

Brain abscesses almost always are associated with a predisposing condition: an adjacent infection such as sinusitis, otitis, or mastoiditis; trauma or a surgical procedure; hematogenous seeding from a pulmonary infection; or congenital heart disease with right-to-left shunting. Typically, the clinical presentation is subacute or chronic, with headache and altered mental status in about 70% of cases, fever, nausea, and vomiting in about 50%, and seizures in about 30% (15).

Infections of the head and neck that commonly involve

Table 38–1. Anaerobic Gram-Negative Bacilli Encountered in Clinical Specimens and Associated Diseases

Organism	Normal Habitat	Associated Diseases
Bacteroides fragilis group, -fragilis, -thetaiotaomicron, -vulgatus, -distasonis, -uniformis, -caccae, -ovatus, -merdae, -stercoris	Large intestine	Intra-abdominal and pelvic abscesses, bacteremia, infected decubitus ulcers; arthritis, osteomyelitis and infections of the central nervous system are less common
Bacteroides ureolyticus, -gracilis	Oral cavity, gastrointestinal and genitourinary tract	Infections of the lower respiratory and female genital tract, head and neck, bone, and soft tissues
Porphyromonas asaccharolytica, -endodontalis, -gingivalis	Oral cavity, especially dental structures	Gingivitis, periodontitis, infections of the head and neck, aspiration pneumonia
Prevotella melaninogenica, -intermedia, -loescheii, -denticola, -bivia, -disiens, -oralis, -buccalis, -veroralis, -corporis, -oulora	Oropharynx and upper respiratory, gastrointestinal and genitourinary tract	Infections of the head and neck, female genital tract, (especially P. bivia and -disiens), and bite wounds; pleuropulmonary infections; osteomyelitis (less common)
Fusobacterium nucleatum, -necrophorum	Oral cavity and gastrointestinal, lower respiratory, and genital tract	Gingivitis, periodontitis, infections of the head and neck, aspiration pneumonia, bite wounds; pleuropulmonary infections; osteomyelitis and infections of the female genital tract (less common)

anaerobes are chronic otitis media, chronic mastoiditis, chronic sinusitis, peritonsillar abscesses, Vincent's angina (pseudomembrane formation on one or both tonsils associated with ulceration and purulent drainage), odontogenic infections (periapical abscess, periodontitis and abscess, gingivitis, stomatitis), and all infections of the deep neck space. Pharyngotonsillitis caused by Fusobacterium necrophorum, an especially virulent organism, often is associated with local complications (peritonsillar abscess, periapical abscess, and septic thrombophlebitis of the jugular vein) or bacteremia and subsequent distant infections (empyema, arthritis, or abscesses in the liver or lungs).

Pleuropulmonary infections such as aspiration pneumonia, necrotizing pneumonia, lung abscess, and empyema commonly involve anaerobes, especially pigmenting species of Prevotella and Fusobacterium nucleatum. These infections follow aspiration of the oropharyngeal secretions, and thus have a predilection for dependent segments of lung (especially the superior segments of the lower lobes and the posterior segments of the upper lobes). Typically, lesions are based on a pleural surface and have a pyramidal shape, with the apex toward the hilum. Conditions that predispose to infection include abuse of alcohol or other drugs, seizure disorders, general anesthesia, cerebrovascular accidents, esophageal disease, nasogastric tube feeding, periodontal disease, and gingivitis. Symptoms of fever, malaise, dry cough, and pleuritic pain usually begin abruptly, but occasionally the onset is more insidious, with weeks to months of malaise, low-grade fever, cough, and weight loss.

Pelvic infections caused by anaerobic gram-negative bacilli, particularly Bacteroides fragilis, are pelvic inflammatory disease with tubo-ovarian abscess and infections that occur post partum. Bacteremias with these organisms, most frequently B. fragilis and other species in the B. fragilis group, almost always are associated with a localized source of infection, predominantly in the abdomen, but decubitus ulcers or the female genital tract may be the primary focus (16). The mortality rate approaches 50% when the portal of entry is an intra-abdominal infection and ranges from 0 to about 15% when associated with other primary sources of infection (15).

Infections of the skin and soft tissues produced by the anaerobic gram-negative bacilli include infected foot ulcers of persons with diabetes mellitus, infected decubitus ulcers, human and animal bite wounds, and wounds associated with surgical procedures in the abdomen. Gram-negative anaerobic bacteria may cause osteomyelitis (most commonly Bacteroides fragilis, followed by Prevotella melaninogenica), septic monarticular arthritis (especially Fusobacterium necrophorum and Bacteroides fragilis), and endocarditis (primarily members of the Bacteroides fragilis group and less commonly species of Fusobacterium). The latter often occurs in the presence of an underlying source of bacteremia (such as an intra-abdominal abscess caused by species of Bacteroides), and is characterized by large vegetations and septic emboli involving large vessels.

Laboratory Diagnosis

Specimens required for diagnosis of infections caused by the anaerobic gram-negative bacilli vary with the site involved (Table 38–2). Specimen collection, transport, and processing are discussed in Part III, but in general, whenever an infection with an anaerobe is suspected, specimens must be collected in a way that avoids contamination by normal flora and must be transported in a way that prevents exposure of anaerobes to the deleterious effects of oxygen. Ideally, specimens for anaerobic culture should be collected with a needle and syringe. Purulent material is aspirated into the syringe, all air is expelled from the syringe, the needle is removed, and the syringe is capped and transported immediately to the laboratory, where it should be processed as rapidly as possible. Swabs should be discouraged, but if a swab is necessary, it must be transported in an appropriate anaerobic transport device (several are commercially available).

The general approach to identification of anaerobes in the clinical laboratory is discussed in Chapter 30. In addi-

Table 38–2. Specimens Recommended for Optimal Recovery of Anaerobic Gram-Negative Bacilli

Infection	Specimen
Abscess	Aspirate of purulent material using needle and syringe
Pulmonary	Percutaneous transtracheal aspirate or material collected by direct lung puncture
Pleural	Thoracentesis fluid
Female genital	Aspirate of purulent material via culdocentesis (after decontaminating vagina); double catheter and bronchial brush or sterile swab for specimens from uterine cavity (except for diagnosing postpartum endometritis)
Sinus tract or draining wound	Tissue from deep in the wound or aspirate from deep in the wound using syringe and catheter
Bacteremia	Blood
Endocarditis	Blood, vegetation

tion, most medically important gram-negative bacilli can be placed into groups based on susceptibility to special-potency antibiotic disks: kanamycin (1000 μg), vancomycin (5 μg), and colistin (10 μg). For all three disks, a zone diameter less than 10 mm is considered resistant. Specific features of the anaerobic gram-negative bacilli are presented here (see references 17–19 for more detail).

Bacteroides fragilis group. In smears prepared directly from clinical material and stained with the Gram stain, cells of the members of the B. fragilis group are pale, pleomorphic gram-negative bacilli that have rounded ends, vacuoles, and often stain irregularly (Plate VID). On blood agar, colonies of the B. fragilis group are 1 to 4 mm in diameter, smooth, gray to white, translucent to semiopaque, and not hemolytic. Colonies of Bacteroides thetaiotaomicron often are whiter than those of Bacteroides fragilis, and colonies of Bacteroides ovatus frequently are mucoid. Key features of the B. fragilis group are growth in 20% bile and resistance to kanamycin, vancomycin, and colistin (using disks as described earlier).

Other Bacteroides species. Cells of Bacteroides ureolyticus and Bacteroides gracilis are thin, gram-negative rods with rounded ends. On blood agar, colonies are small and translucent or transparent. They are smooth and convex, pitting, or spreading (although more than one colony type may grow in a single culture), and may cause greening of the agar. These organisms do not grow in 20% bile, are susceptible to kanamycin and colistin but resistant to vancomycin, and require supplementation of broth media with formate and fumarate for growth. Bacteroides ureolyticus is urease positive; Bacteroides gracilis is urease negative.

Porphyromonas species. Cells of Porphyromonas are pale-staining coccobacilli or pleomorphic bacilli, and in smears prepared from young cultures cells may appear gram-positive to gram-variable. Colonies are mucoid and dark brown to black on blood agar, especially laked rabbit blood agar, which allows the earliest and most reliable pigment production. Some colonies fluoresce brick red, yellow-green, or coral under long-wave (365-nm) ultraviolet light, a feature that may not be detected after pigment is produced. These organisms are inhibited by 20% bile, usually are susceptible to vancomycin and resistant to kanamycin and colistin, and are indole positive and asaccharolytic.

Prevotella species. Cells of Prevotella resemble those of Porphyromonas. The colony appearance varies: Prevotella intermedia produces dark brown to black, dry colonies; Prevotella melaninogenica, Prevotella loescheii, and Prevotella denticola produce light tan or buff, smooth colonies; colonies of the remaining species are not pigmented. Pigment production, most reliably detected when the organisms are grown on laked rabbit blood agar, may not become apparent for 2 weeks or more, especially for Prevotella melaninogenica. Before pigment is produced colonies of some isolates fluoresce under ultraviolet light, similar to that described earlier for colonies of Porphyromonas. Growth of these organisms is inhibited by 20% bile. The species of Prevotella are resistant to kanamycin and vancomycin and vary in susceptibility to colistin.

Fusobacterium species. Cells of Fusobacterium nucleatum are long, slender, spindle-shaped, gram-negative filaments that have tapered ends (Plate VIE). They often occur in pairs or an end-to-end arrangement and occasionally have spherical swellings. On blood agar colonies are 1 to 2 mm in diameter, slightly convex, α-hemolytic, and have a characteristic flecked internal structure. Cell of Fusobacterium necrophorum are pleomorphic, frequently curved, irregularly stained forms with spherical swellings. Colonies are umbonate and nonhemolytic on blood agar but often cause greening of the surrounding agar after exposure to air. Species of Fusobacterium are inhibited by 20% bile, are resistant to vancomycin and susceptible to kanamycin and colistin, produce a large amount of the metabolic end product butyric acid, and are indole positive. F. necrophorum is the only lipase-positive species of Fusobacterium.

Treatment

One of the most important aspects of treatment of infections caused by the anaerobic gram-negative bacilli is drainage of any abscess that may be present. In addition, antimicrobial therapy must be given. Members of the Bacteroides fragilis group are resistant to the penicillins (mediated by production of cephalosporinases that also hydrolyze penicillins), and resistance to cefoxitin and clindamycin is increasing (approaching 20% in some places), especially among isolates of Bacteroides thetaiotaomicron and Bacteroides distasonis (20). Metronidazole and chloramphenicol are active against essentially all isolates of the Bacteroides fragilis group, and only rare isolates are resistant to imipenem. Bacteroides gracilis and Bacteroides ureolyticus also are resistant to the penicillins, and 25 to 35% of isolates of Bacteroides gracilis are resistant to clindamycin, cefoxitin, and piperacillin, and a very small percentage appear resistant to imipenem and metronidazole (1).

Because many isolates of Porphyromonas and Prevotella produce β-lactamase, penicillin G no longer is the agent of choice for treatment of aspiration pneumonia, an infection in which these organisms typically are found.

Species of Porphyromonas and Prevotella are susceptible to metronidazole, chloramphenicol, and imipenem, and most to clindamycin. In general, the species of Fusobacterium are more susceptible to antimicrobial agents than are the species of Bacteroides, but some isolates of Fusobacterium nucleatum produce β-lactamase. Most fusobacteria are susceptible to cefoxitin, clindamycin, chloramphenicol, imipenem, and metronidazole.

REFERENCES

1. Baquero F, et al: Capnophilic and anaerobic bacteremia in neutropenic patients: An oral source. Rev Infect Dis, 12(Suppl 2):S157, 1990.
2. Johnson CC, and Finegold SM: Uncommonly encountered, motile, gram-negative bacilli associated with infection. Rev Infect Dis, 9:1150, 1987
3. Sutter VL, Citron DM, Edelstein MAC, and Finegold SM: Wadsworth Anaerobic Bacteriology Manual. 4th ed. Belmont, CA, Star Publishing, 1985.
4. Shah HN, and Collins MD: Proposal to restrict the genus Bacteroides (Castellani and Chalmers) to Bacteroides fragilis and closely related species. Int J Syst Bacteriol, 39:85, 1989.
5. Shah HN, and Collins MD: Proposal for reclassification of Bacteroides asaccharolyticus, Bacteroides gingivalis, and Bacteroides endodontalis in a new genus, Porphyromonas. Int J Syst Bacteriol, 38:128, 1988.
6. Shah HN, and Collins MD: Prevotella, a new genus to include Bacteroides melaninogenicus and related species formerly classified in the genus Bacteroides. Int J Syst Bacteriol, 40:205, 1990.
7. Paster BJ, and Dewhirst FE: Phylogeny of campylobacters, wolinellas, Bacteroides gracilis, and Bacteroides ureolyticus by 16S ribosomal ribonucleic acid sequencing. Int J Syst Bacteriol, 38:56, 1988.
8. Styrt B, and Gorbach SL: Recent developments in the understanding of the pathogenesis and treatment of anaerobic infections. N Engl J Med, 321:240, 1989.
9. Tally FP, et al: Superoxide dismutase in anaerobic bacteria of clinical significance. Infect Immun, 16:20, 1977.
10. Lantz MS, et al: Interactions of Bacteroides gingivalis with fibrinogen. Infect Immun, 54:654, 1986.
11. McKee AS, et al: Effect of hemin on the physiology and virulence of Bacteroides gingivalis W50. Infect Immun, 52:349, 1986.
12. Bulkacz J, et al: Phospholipase A activity of extracellular products from Bacteroides melaninogenicus on epithelium tissue cultures. J Periodont Res, 20:146, 1985.
13. Bjornson AB, et al: Opsonization of Bacteroides by the alternative complement pathway reconstructed from isolated plasma proteins. J Exp Med, 164:777, 1987.
14. Onderdonk AB, et al: Evidence for T cell–dependent immunity to Bacteroides fragilis in an intraabdominal abscess model. J Clin Invest, 69:9, 1982.
15. Finegold SM, George WL, and Mulligan ME: Anaerobic infections, Part 1. Disease a Month, 31(10):1, 1985.
16. Brook I: Anaerobic bacterial bacteremia: 12-year experience in two military hospitals. J Infect Dis, 160:1071, 1989.
17. Koneman EW, et al (eds): Color Atlas and Textbook of Diagnostic Microbiology. 3rd ed. Philadelphia, JB Lippincott, 1988.
18. Edelstein MAC: Anaerobic gram-negative bacilli. In Bailey & Scott's Diagnostic Microbiology. 8th ed. Edited by EJ Baron and SM Finegold. St. Louis, CV Mosby, 1990.
19. Jousimies-Somer HR, and Finegold SM: Anaerobic gram-negative bacilli and cocci. In Manual of Clinical Microbiology. 5th ed. Edited by A Balows, et al. Washington, DC, American Society for Microbiology, 1991.
20. Appleman MD, Heseltine PNR, and Cherubin CE: Epidemiology, antimicrobial susceptibility, pathogenicity, and significance of Bacteroides fragilis group organisms isolated at Los Angeles County—University of Southern California Medical Center. Rev Infect Dis, 13:12, 1991.

Chapter 39

SPIROCHETES

The spirochetes of human importance are the pathogenic species of Treponema and Borrelia, Leptospira interrogans, the anaerobic spirochetes, and Spirillum minor. These helical organisms, 0.1 to 0.5 μm wide and 5 to 30 μm long, have a multilayered outer envelope; a protoplasmic cylinder composed of a peptidoglycan layer, a cytoplasmic membrane, and the enclosed cytoplasmic contents; and periplasmic fibrils or axial filaments. The latter flagellum-like organelles are attached near the ends of the organism by insertion disks located in the cell wall between the outer envelope and the protoplasmic cylinder and they extend along the body of the spirochete toward the opposite poles, permitting winding, corkscrew motility. Spirochetes are gram negative, but because they stain poorly if at all with the Gram or Giemsa stain, silver stains (Plate VIF) or direct visualization using darkfield or phase optics are necessary to demonstrate the organisms in clinical specimens.

TREPONEMA

The pathogenic Treponema species are microaerophilic, antigenically similar organisms, 6 to 15 μm long and 0.1 to 0.2 μm wide, with pointed ends and three periplasmic fibrils attached at each end, whereas the nonpathogenic Treponema are anaerobic, wider (0.15 to 0.25 μm), and have blunt ends and one to eight fibrils per cell. The pathogenic treponemes, Treponema pallidum and its subspecies and Treponema carateum, are discussed here; the anaerobic treponemes are reviewed briefly later.

Treponema pallidum

Treponema pallidum has 4 to 14 spirals. These organisms are readily inactivated by heat, cold, desiccation, most disinfectants, and osmotic changes; and they do not grow on artificial media or in tissue culture but can be maintained in vitro for 1 to 6 days using maintenance (Nelson) medium containing rabbit serum, reducing agents, vitamins, cofactors, amino acids, and salts (1). Based on DNA homology studies, T. pallidum is divided into three subspecies—Treponema pallidum-pallidum, -pertenue, and -endemicum—the agents of veneral syphilis, yaws, and nonvenereal endemic syphilis, respectively.

Treponema pallidum subspecies pallidum

Venereal syphilis was recognized as a unique entity in Europe when Columbus' crew returned to Spain in 1493, after his second voyage. As initially described, syphilis was a much more severe illness than it is currently: death resulted in about 25% of cases during the early stages of infection (2). The organism responsible for the disease was first recognized in 1905, when Metchnikoff and Roux infected monkeys with extracts of infected tissues from persons with syphilis, and Schaudinn and Hoffman identified a nearly transparent spiral-shaped organism which they named Spirocheta pallida (3). In 1906, Landsteiner introduced darkfield microscopy as a means to visualize this organism.

Epidemiology

Humans are the only natural hosts for Treponema pallidum subsp. pallidum. Infected persons are most infectious early in the disease, particularly when a chancre, mucous patch, or condyloma lata (described below) are present. They become less infectious with time and are unable to spread the disease by sexual contact 4 years after acquiring it. In addition to sexual contact, syphilis may be spread by kissing or by touching an active lesion; by transfusing fresh blood or blood products (the organism cannot survive more than 24 to 48 hours under conditions of blood bank storage) collected from an individual with the disease, a rare occurrence where blood from donors who have a reactive nontreponemal blood test (described later) is not used; and by accidental direct inoculation during a needlestick or when handling infected clinical material (4,5). Congenital syphilis may be acquired during passage through an infected birth canal but most frequently is transmitted in utero. The latter may occur in any untreated mother but is most likely during the early stages of infection. Fetal infection is rare before the fourth month of gestation, and treating the mother during the first 4 months of pregnancy generally ensures that the fetus will not be infected.

In the United States the number of cases of primary and secondary syphilis peaked during World War II, reached the nadir in the mid-1950s, rose in 1960, and remained relatively stable until 1986; since then, the prevalence has continued to rise (6). A disproportionate number of cases occurred in homosexual men until the 1980s, when the prevalence among this cohort began to decline because they adapted safer sex practices in an attempt to prevent the spread of the acquired immunodeficiency syndrome (AIDS). Concurrently, the number of cases rose among heterosexual women, an increase linked to the use of crack cocaine and the practice of trading sex with multiple partners for these drugs, and it was paralleled by a similar rise in the number of cases of congenital syphilis (Fig. 39–1) (7).

Pathogenesis and Pathology

Treponema pallidum subsp pallidum penetrates intact mucous membranes or gains access to the tissues through abraded skin, multiplies locally, dividing about every 30 hours, enters the lymphatics and blood, and disseminates

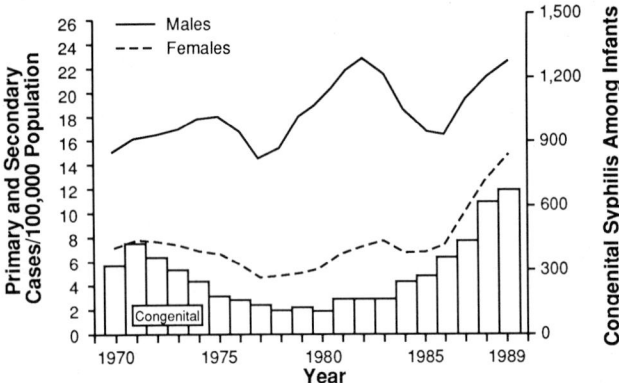

Fig. 39–1. Cases of primary and secondary syphilis among males and females and of congenital syphilis (patient younger than 1 year), United States, 1970–1989. (From Centers for Disease Control: Summary of notifiable diseases, United States. MMWR, 38:40, 1990.)

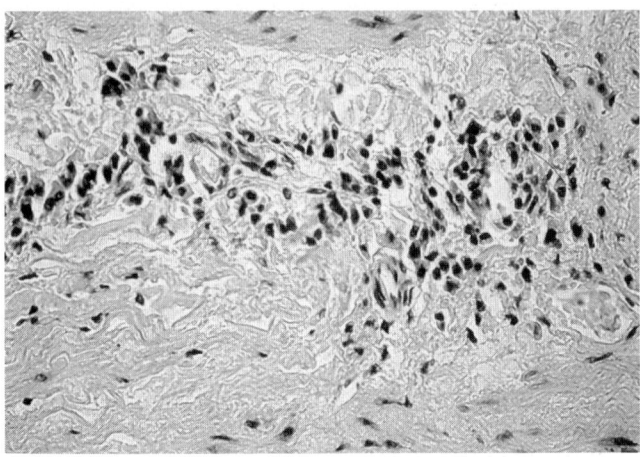

Fig. 39–2. Micrograph of tissue involved with syphilitic aortitis, characterized by obliterative endarteritis (hematoxylin and eosin, ×100).

throughout the body, including the central nervous system (CNS). The necessary infectious dose varies, but in rabbits inoculated in the laboratory as few as four spirochetes can establish an infection. Clinical lesions appear when a critical concentration of organisms (about 10^7 per gram of tissue) is reached; therefore, the incubation period is directly proportional to the size of the inoculum. The spirochetemia may persist weeks or months; therefore, new lesions may develop long after the initial contact with the organism.

Four clinical stages of syphilis are recognized. The *primary stage* consists of the primary lesion, the chancre, which develops at the site of inoculation. The *secondary or disseminated stage*, characterized by parenchymal, constitutional, and mucocutaneous manifestations, occurs 2 to 12 weeks (mean, 6 weeks) after contact, when the greatest number of organisms are present in the body, particularly in the blood. During this phase, the immune response of the host becomes active and immune complexes may form. The *latent period* follows the secondary stage and is divided into the early latent stage, during which relapses of secondary syphilis may occur, and the late latent stage, during which relapse is very unlikely. Relapse of disease, a consequence of a dysfunction in cellular immunity such as may develop during the last trimester of pregnancy, may occur as long as 4 years after contact, but 75% of cases are seen within the first year. *Late syphilis* refers to the tertiary disease that develops in up to a third of untreated persons. In most cases it involves the vasa vasorum of the aorta, the arteries of the CNS, or both, although late syphilis also may be manifested by the development of a gumma, a rubbery, gray-white, necrotic mass.

Two histologic features that are characteristic but not pathognomonic of the lesions of syphilis occur in all stages of the disease: obliterative endarteritis (concentric endothelial and fibroblastic proliferative thickening; Fig. 39–2) and an inflammatory infiltrate consisting primarily of plasma cells. Microscopically, the primary chancre is characterized by numerous spirochetes and scattered polymorphonuclear leukocytes and macrophages ingesting organisms. Sections of the mucocutaneous lesions of secondary syphilis and of condyloma lata show a perivascular mononuclear cell infiltrate composed mainly of plasma cells and many spirochetes. The gumma consists of a central area of coagulated, necrotic material containing shadowy outlines of underlying tissue (thus differing from frank caseation necrosis) but no vital native or inflammatory cells, surrounded by a rim of plump fibroblasts resembling the epithelioid cells seen in tuberculosis (see Chapter 40), plasma cells, lymphocytes, and small blood vessels narrowed by obliterative endarteritis. Spirochetes are scarce in gummas but when present typically are found in the inflammatory wall.

The rabbit model of syphilis has been used most extensively to study the pathogenesis of the disease. In this model the primary lesion, which histologically resembles the primary lesion that develops in humans, appears to be a manifestation of specific delayed hypersensitivity. Sensitized T lymphocytes attract and activate macrophages, which phagocytose and destroy most but not all of the infecting organisms. Moreover, clearance of spirochetes from infected sites during the second (reactive) stage of infection in rabbits correlates with the appearance of specific antibodies to Treponema pallidum subsp pallidum. The latter may function as opsonins, making organisms more susceptible to phagocytosis by macrophages, but they do not provide complete protection against infection (3,8).

Clinical Manifestations

The classic chancre of *primary syphilis* begins 3 to 90 days (average, 21 days) after contact as a single painless papule at the site of inoculation, most often the external genitalia, but sometimes the cervix, mouth, perianal area, or anal canal. The papule quickly ulcerates, becoming indurated with a smooth base and raised, firm borders. This is accompanied by painless regional lymphadenopathy. No exudate is present unless the lesion becomes secondarily infected. The chancre heals in 1 to 12 weeks (3 to 6 weeks is usual) with little or no scarring, but the lymphadenopathy typically persists. Atypical presentations of primary syphilis also are possible: the primary lesion may not occur; the lesion may not ulcerate, especially if the inoculum is small or the patient has a history of syphilis; or multiple chancres may develop, particularly in persons infected with human immunodeficiency virus (HIV) (9,10).

Secondary syphilis begins 2 to 8 weeks after the appearance of the chancre, which still may be present. Classic macular, maculopapular, papular, or pustular (but not vesicular) skin lesions develop in about 90% of persons with secondary syphilis. Discrete, 3- to 10-mm diameter, pink to red macules usually begin on the trunk and proximal extremities but may involve any body surface, persist for a few days to a few months, often evolve to papules and occasionally to pustules, and may spread to involve the entire body, especially the palms and soles (11). These lesions are less florid, asymmetrically distributed, and more infiltrated during relapses of secondary syphilis, suggesting a more effective host immune response. Involvement of the hair follicles may cause temporary patchy alopecia; and in warm, moist, intertriginous areas the papules enlarge, coalesce, and erode, producing painless, broad, moist, gray-white to erythematous, highly infectious plaques called condyloma lata. Mucous patches, painless, gray, superficial erosions surrounded by a red periphery that are teeming with spirochetes, may develop on mucous membranes.

Constitutional symptoms—malaise, low-grade fever, anorexia, weight loss, pharyngitis, laryngitis, arthralgias, and generalized painless lymphadenopathy, especially involving the epitrochlear nodes—are present in about 70% of cases of secondary syphilis. CNS involvement, characterized by headache, meningismus, and increased cerebrospinal fluid (CSF) protein levels and lymphocyte counts, occurs in 8 to 40% of cases; and 1 to 2% of persons with secondary syphilis develop acute aseptic meningitis. Uncommon manifestations of this stage of the illness include immune complex glomerulonephritis, the nephrotic syndrome, hepatitis (characterized by a markedly elevated alkaline phosphatase level with normal or moderately increased serum bilirubin), proctitis, infiltration or ulceration of the mucosa of the gastrointestinal tract, anterior uveitis, synovitis, osteitis, and periostitis (12–15).

Persons who have *latent syphilis* have a positive specific treponemal antibody test (described later), no clinical manifestations of syphilis, and normal CSF findings. Relapses, usually mucocutaneous, occur only during the early latent stage (first 4 years); however, a person with late latent syphilis may transmit the infection via transfused contaminated blood, and a pregnant woman may infect her fetus in utero during this stage.

Late tertiary syphilis, a slowly progressive inflammatory disease that affects any organ in the body, is manifested clinically as neurosyphilis, cardiovascular syphilis, or gummatous syphilis years after the initial infection. In persons infected with HIV, however, the course of syphilitic infection is accelerated, and neurosyphilis may develop less than 1 year after the primary infection (16,17). *Late neurosyphilis* may be symptomatic or asymptomatic. The latter is diagnosed only by one or more abnormal findings in the CSF (pleocytosis, elevated protein concentration, decreased glucose concentration, or a positive Venereal Disease Research Laboratory [VDRL] test [discussed later]). Of persons with untreated syphilis, 8 to 40% develop asymptomatic neurosyphilis, but because the diagnosis requires lumbar puncture and CSF examination it is difficult to determine how many of these persons become symptomatic. Symptomatic neurosyphilis is divided into two clinical categories, meningovascular and parenchymatous, which correlate with pathologic findings, although they may overlap somewhat.

Meningovascular neurosyphilis usually occurs 5 to 10 years after the onset of disease. It is characterized by endarteritis obliterans affecting the small blood vessels of the meninges, spinal cord, and brain, and subsequent multiple small areas of infarction, manifested clinically as hemiplegia or hemiparesis, focal or generalized seizures, or aphasia. *Parenchymatous neurosyphilis*, during which nerve cells (predominantly those in the cerebral cortex) are destroyed, includes general paresis and tabes dorsalis, usually manifest 15 to 20 years and 25 to 30 years after the onset of disease, respectively. General paresis is characterized by changes in personality (emotional lability, paranoia), affect, sensorium, intellect, insight, and judgment; hyperactive reflexes, slurring of speech, Argyll Robertson pupils (small irregular pupils that accommodate to near vision but do not react to light or painful stimuli), optic atrophy, and tremors of the face, tongue, hands, and legs. The spinal cord damage of tabes dorsalis (demyelination of the posterior columns, dorsal roots, and dorsal root ganglia) causes an ataxic, wide-based gait and footslap, paresthesias, shooting or lightning pains, bladder disturbances, fecal incontinence, impotence, loss of position and vibratory sense, loss of ankle and knee jerk, and loss of deep pain and temperature sensation. Other findings in tabes dorsalis are Romberg's sign (inability to stand with feet together and eyes closed without falling over), Argyll Robertson pupils, and involvement of cranial nerves II through VIII. Trophic degenerative joint disease (Charcot's joints) and traumatic ulcers or sores on the lower extremities and feet today are uncommon. Two other forms of neurosyphilis are syphilitic otitis (asymmetric deafness, tinnitus) and syphilitic eye disease (optic atrophy, asymptomatic progressive vision loss leading to blindness, ptosis) (18,19).

Cardiovascular syphilis is characterized by endarteritis obliterans involving the vasa vasorum of the aorta or other large arteries, such as the temporal artery, resulting in medial necrosis with destruction of elastic tissue and aortitis with subsequent saccular or, occasionally, fusiform aneurysm formation (20). The predilection to involve the ascending aorta causes widening of the aortic ring and narrowing of the mouths of the coronary ostia, which lead to aortic regurgitation and coronary artery stenosis. The transverse portion of the aortic arch is the second most frequently involved area, but the aorta rarely is affected below the renal arteries. About 10% of persons with untreated syphilis, many of whom have neurosyphilis, develop symptomatic syphilitic aortitis, and autopsy examination of persons with untreated neurosyphilis reveals lesions of aortitis in as many as 80% of cases, but in countries where antimicrobial therapy has been successful cardiovascular syphilis is rare (4).

Gummas were the most frequent late complication of syphilis observed in the Oslo study, an extensive report published in 1955 based on 30 to 50 years' observation of 1000 persons with untreated disease, but they rarely are seen today (3). They may be located anywhere, but the most common sites are the skeletal system, the skin, and mucous membranes.

The clinical manifestations of *congenital syphilis* vary with the severity of the infection. Late abortion, stillbirth, neonatal death, neonatal disease, or latent infection may develop, and often the physical examination findings are normal (21–24). Necrotizing funisitis—inflammation of the matrix of the umbilical cord characterized by obliterative endarteritis—is virtually pathognomonic of congenital syphilis and should be suspected when the umbilical cord is swollen and shows red, white, and blue discoloration (25). In the perinatal period (infantile form) the mucocutaneous tissues and bones most often are involved. Rhinitis, which occurs in about 40% of cases, usually is the earliest sign and typically is followed by a diffuse, maculopapular and desquamative rash, most prominent on the palms, the soles, and around the mouth and anus; vesicles and bullae may develop. Generalized osteochondritis and perichondritis, seen in about 55% of cases, may affect all bones, but the nose (saddle nose) and metaphyses of the lower extremities (saber shin or anterior bowing) are involved most often. Anemia and thrombocytopenia are present in about 30% of infants, and liver involvement (Plate VIF) with hepatosplenomegaly and jaundice occurs in about 20% of cases. If death occurs it generally is due to liver failure, pneumonia, or pulmonary hemorrhage. Untreated infants who survive the first 6 to 12 months of life enter a latent period, followed by late manifestations: interstitial keratitis, asymptomatic or symptomatic neurosyphilis, and eighth nerve deafness are most common; other stigmata include recurrent arthropathy and bilateral knee effusions (Clutton's joints); centrally notched, widely spread, peg-shaped upper central incisors (Hutchinson's teeth), frontal bossing and poorly developed maxillas.

Treponema pallidum subspecies pertenue

Yaws, also called frambesia, pian, buba, and bouba, is believed to have existed in Africa since pre-Biblical times (26). It was introduced into the Western Hemisphere in the sixteenth century by African slaves. The pathogen, Treponema pallidum subsp pertenue, was recognized in lesions of yaws shortly after Treponema pallidum subsp pallidum was identified in lesions of syphilis in 1905.

Epidemiology and Pathogenesis

Yaws, a disease of childhood, occurs among rural populations of warm, humid, tropical climates. Most cases are reported from Africa (especially West Africa), Southeast Asia, and Oceania; and in South America, sporadic cases (fewer than 500 per year) occur in focal regions of Colombia, Guyana, Suriname, and French Guiana. In the 1950s an estimated 50 to 100 million persons were infected worldwide, a number reduced to fewer than 2 million by the mid-1970s by mass treatment campaigns (27,28). Since then, a resurgence of the disease has occurred in West Africa, where the prevalence approaches that of the 1950s (29).

Treponema pallidum subsp pertenue is transmitted when traumatized skin contacts infectious exudate from active yaws lesions. Organisms then enter the blood and are transported to bone, lymph nodes, and distant skin sites, where they elicit granulomatous inflammation indistinguishable from that in lesions of syphilis, and endarteritis in late lesions. Spirochetes are numerous in early skin lesions but rare in bone or late skin lesions.

Clinical Manifestations

Three to five weeks after inoculation, cutaneous papules appear, usually on the extremities (particularly the legs); they enlarge and become papillomatous and superficially eroded. The lesions heal spontaneously within 6 months, and weeks to months later a generalized eruption of similar lesions appears. During the next 5 years (the secondary stage) multiple relapses of these skin lesions occur, often accompanied by lymphadenopathy, and periostitis, osteitis, and osteomyelitis, typically involving the fingers, long bones, or paranasal maxillae, may develop. After a latent period of several years the late stage of yaws begins. Cutaneous plaques, ulcers, nodules, and papillomas appear on the hands and feet (including the palms and soles), and gummas develop in the skull, sternum, tibia, or other bones.

Treponema pallidum subspecies endemicum

Endemic syphilis (also called bejel, siti, and dichuchwa), once common in southern Europe, the Middle East, and North Africa, usually in regions with unhygienic and crowded living conditions, now is gradually disappearing (3).

Epidemiology

Endemic syphilis, which currently exists in focal areas of Africa, western Asia, and Australia, predominantly affects children in rural populations where standards of living and personal hygiene are poor (30). It is transmitted by nonsexual body contact or by sharing eating and drinking utensils.

Clinical Manifestations

Most often, no primary lesion is observed, probably owing to the small size and the oral location of the inoculum (31). Secondary lesions include oropharyngeal mucous patches, split papules at the corners of the mouth, condyloma lata, periostitis, and regional lymphadenopathy; and late manifestations are gummas of the skin, nasopharynx, and bones. Cardiovascular and neurologic lesions and congenital disease are rare.

Treponema carateum

Treponema carateum, the agent of pinta (also called carate or mal de pinto) and probably the oldest human treponematosis, first was identified in lesions in 1938 (26).

Epidemiology and Pathogenesis

Pinta is found exclusively in rural areas of Mexico, Central America, and Colombia, predominantly in arid inland regions, and in recent years only a few hundred cases have been reported annually (27). Treponema carateum enters the body during direct contact of broken skin with infectious lesions, multiplies locally, enters the blood and lymphatics, and spreads to distant skin sites.

Clinical Manifestations

The initial skin lesions of pinta appear on the face, neck, chest, extremities, or abdomen about 1 to 3 weeks after inoculation. These small, erythematous, pruritic papules enlarge, coalesce, and in several years, heal with residual hypopigmentation. Secondary lesions, small scaly papules (pintids), appear 3 to 12 months after the initial lesions, usually at the same sites. Occasionally they become brown, gray, or blue, particularly those on the face, and they may recur for up to 10 years. During the late stage of pinta depigmented skin lesions appear, typically on the wrists, elbows, and ankles. Viscera are not involved during any stage of the illness.

Laboratory Diagnosis

Infections caused by the pathogenic treponemes are diagnosed by direct microscopic examination of clinical specimens or by serologic tests. Identification of the species, however, is difficult. These organisms are morphologically identical and immunologically closely related and, therefore, are indistinguishable by these techniques. The treponematoses may be differentiated by infecting different animals in the laboratory (the rabbit for Treponema pallidum subsp pallidum, rabbits or hamsters for Treponema pallidum subsp endemicum and Treponema pallidum subsp pertenue, and the chimpanzee for Treponema carateum), but because animal inoculation is difficult, time consuming, and costly, it is not performed in the clinical laboratory. Therefore, a definitive diagnosis is based on epidemiology and clinical manifestations (discussed earlier).

Direct Microscopic Examination. Darkfield microscopy is the recommended method for direct visualization of treponemes, although phase-contrast microscopy may be used. Gloves should be worn by the examiner collecting the specimen and by laboratory personnel handling the specimen because the exudate is infectious. If multiple lesions are present, the newest one that exudes material should be sampled, because the likelihood of visualizing spirochetes decreases with the age of the lesion and because organisms are difficult to observe in specimens from dry lesions. Specimen collection, transport, and processing are discussed in Chapter 61. The diagnosis is based on observing spirochetes that have the appropriate structure (described earlier) and show characteristic motility—rapid rotation about their longitudinal axis and flexing, bending, and snapping about their full length.

In general, darkfield examination is a sensitive and specific diagnostic test for primary syphilis; however, its sensitivity is reduced by excess debris or red blood cells that obscure the organisms, recent local or systemic antimicrobial therapy, and an inadequate sample. Given these limitations, examination of three specimens is recommended before a negative result is accepted as true (32). In addition, the specificity of the test is lower when exudate from rectal or oral lesions is examined, because nonpathogenic treponemes that are normal flora in these sites appear morphologically similar to Treponema pallidum subsp pallidum by darkfield microscopy. Consequently, spirochetes found in rectal and oral samples must be interpreted with caution. Darkfield microscopy also is useful for demonstrating spirochetes in primary and secondary lesions of yaws, secondary lesions of endemic syphilis, and primary and secondary lesions of pinta.

As an alternative to darkfield examination the exudate from a lesion (collected on a glass slide) may be fixed with acetone and then stained with fluorescein-labeled antibodies specific for Treponema pallidum (currently not available commercially).

Serologic Tests. Two types of serologic tests are used to diagnose infections caused by treponemes: nontreponemal tests detect antibodies against lipoidal antigens formed during the interaction of host tissues with the treponemes, and treponemal tests detect antibodies specific for the Treponema organisms or their components. The *nontreponemal tests* used most frequently are the VDRL test and the rapid plasma reagin (RPR) card test. To perform the VDRL test, purified cardiolipin-lecithin-cholesterol antigen is mixed with heated serum on a glass slide, rotated mechanically, and read microscopically for flocculation. Results are reported as reactive (medium and large clumps), nonreactive (no clumps), or weakly reactive (small clumps). The test may be quantitated by serially diluting the serum. The RPR card method is similar, except that serum is not heated, carbon particles are included in the antigen suspension, and it is read macroscopically. In general, these tests are comparable, and titers are similar for most positive sera; but because some sera show markedly different titers one test should be used to follow the course of the infection in a given individual. Moreover, only the VDRL test should be performed on cerebrospinal fluid (unheated), and results are reported as reactive or nonreactive.

The treponemal tests most commonly used are the fluorescent treponemal antibody–absorption (FTA-ABS) test, the microhemagglutination–Treponema pallidum (MHA-TP) test, and the hemagglutination treponemal test for syphilis (HATTS). Each is approved for use with serum only, not CSF. In the FTA-ABS test heated serum is mixed with sorbent (a sonicate of nonpathogenic Reiter treponemes) to remove nonspecific antibodies and is placed on slides to which Treponema pallidum antigen is fixed. Slides are incubated, stained with fluorescein-labeled antihuman globulin, viewed by fluorescence microscopy, and reported as reactive, nonreactive, or minimally reactive. In the latter case a follow-up specimen should be tested to verify the result. The MHA-TP test is performed by reacting absorbed serum with sensitized (coated with sonicated T. pallidum) sheep erythrocytes in a microtiter plate. If antibodies are present they react with the sensitized cells and produce a uniformly thin mat of agglutinated erythrocytes that covers the entire bottom of the well. If antibodies are absent red blood cells do not agglutinate and settle as a smooth ring or button at the bottom of the well. The HATTS test is similar to the MHA-TP test, except that sonicated T. pallidum is coupled to glutaraldehyde-stabilized turkey erythrocytes. In general, the MHA-TP and HATTS tests are satisfactory substitutes for the FTA-ABS test, they are preferred in most laboratories because they are easier to perform and interpret, and they are more cost effective because they require less technical time. The one potential disadvantage is their lower sensitivity for primary syphilis (32–34).

The VDRL (or RPR) test usually becomes reactive sometime during primary syphilis. The titer rises rapidly, and if the infection is not treated remains elevated during the first year and then slowly falls, reaching low levels in late syphilis and spontaneously reverting to nonreactive in about 25% of cases. After adequate treatment the VDRL titer falls at a rate related to the pretreatment titer and the stage of disease. For example, persons treated within the first 6 months are usually seronegative within a year; those treated later in the infection may not become seronegative for 2 years or longer; and in persons with late syphilis, a state of seronegativity may take 5 years to develop, if it ever does (35–37). The FTA-ABS, MHA-TP, and HATTS generally become reactive in primary syphilis and remain reactive for the persons' lifetime regardless of therapy, though there are a few exceptions: treatment very early may prevent seroreactivity, an occasional person treated in the early stage of disease reverts to being seronegative, and persons with AIDS often become seronegative (33,38). The FTA-ABS result typically is the first to become positive, followed by the microhemagglutination tests and the VDRL (and RPR) shortly thereafter.

The sensitivity of the VDRL (or RPR), MHA-TP, and FTA-ABS tests for diagnosing primary syphilis has ranged from about 60 to 76%, about 73 to 89%, and about 81 to 100%, respectively. In one study sensitivity appeared to be related to the duration of the infection, being least sensitive for infections of less than 30 days' duration and most sensitive for infections of more than 40 days' duration (32,39). The FTA-ABS result rarely is negative when either the VDRL (or RPR) or MHA-TP (or HATTS) test is positive, but it may be positive in as many as 25% of persons with a negative VDRL (or RPR) or a negative MHA-TP (or HATTS) test, and in about 10% of those with primary syphilis who are seronegative by VDRL (and RPR) *and* MHA-TP (and HATTS) tests. As many as 16% of persons with primary syphilis may have a positive VDRL (or RPR) and a negative MHA-TP test, and an equal proportion may have a negative VDRL and a positive MHA-TP (32). For untreated secondary syphilis all serologic tests are 100% sensitive (32,34,39). For symptomatic late syphilis the sensitivity is about 70% for the VDRL (or RPR) test, 94 to 100% for the MHA-TP (or HATTS), and 100% for the FTA-ABS test (32,34).

Biologic false-positive nontreponemal reactions may be transient, occurring in conjunction with a strong immune stimulus such as an acute bacterial or viral infection or immunization, or they may be persistent, associated with drug addiction, chronic infections such as leprosy, aging, hypergammaglobulinemic states, and autoimmune or connective tissue disease, particularly systemic lupus erythematosus. False-positive FTA-ABS and MHA-TP test results have been reported in sick patients, especially in association with autoimmune or connective tissue diseases and drug addiction, but they are rare in healthy persons (32).

Recommended guidelines for using these diagnostic tests to evaluate symptomatic and asymptomatic persons, monitor therapy, assess CSF, and diagnose congenital syphilis are as follows (32): For persons with a primary chancre, darkfield microscopy should be performed (if the test can be interpreted appropriately), and the VDRL (or RPR) test should be done at the initial visit to confirm the diagnosis. The titer should be followed to assess the adequacy of treatment. If the darkfield and the VDRL test results are negative and syphilis is strongly suspected, the VDRL (or RPR) test should be repeated in 1 week and, if negative at that time, again 1 month later. For persons with clinical manifestations of secondary syphilis, the VDRL (or RPR) test should be performed for diagnosis and titers should be followed to assess the adequacy of treatment. Darkfield examination of exudate from cutaneous lesions may be performed to provide an immediate diagnosis. In a person with a negative darkfield examination and a stable, low titer VDRL, results of an MHA-TP (or HATTS) test distinguish a false-positive VDRL result from adequately treated syphilis or latent syphilis.

The VDRL (or RPR) test is preferred for screening asymptomatic persons, and treponemal tests are used to confirm positive VDRL (or RPR) results. In the United States, serologic screening for syphilis is required during pregnancy, a second screen is recommended during the third trimester for high-risk populations, and screening the mother's serum at delivery also is recommended by investigators at the Centers for Disease Control (CDC) for mothers living in areas where the prevalence of syphilis is high (7). Using cord blood for screening should be avoided because such specimens may give either a false-positive or a false-negative result (40). The VDRL (or RPR) test also is used to screen blood donors and persons in groups known to be at high risk. Screening proven contacts of persons with active syphilis may be useful, but because contacts may have incubating syphilis, a stage during which the sensitivity of treponemal and nontreponemal tests is low, a negative screen result does not exclude disease. To prevent further spread of the infection, proven contacts probably should be treated immediately, despite results of serologic screening.

Routine evaluation of the CSF is not necessary for persons with early syphilis, except perhaps those who have AIDS, whose disease may progress more rapidly than usual. In addition, CSF examination is in order for persons with syphilis who have neurologic abnormalities, before re-treatment of those who suffer relapse after treatment, as a baseline measure when "nonpenicillin therapy" is planned, and for all infants suspected of having congenital syphilis (32). A positive CSF VDRL test indicates neurosyphilis, and an elevated white blood cell (WBC) count indicates active disease. Although the CSF VDRL is a very specific indicator of neurosyphilis, it is insensitive, yielding a positive result in only 22 to 69% of persons with active neurosyphilis (41). The CSF VDRL test may remain positive for a long time after adequate therapy and, so, cannot be used to monitor response to treatment. Response is measured by the WBC count, which generally returns to normal within 6 to 12 weeks, and in symptomatic disease by improvement in clinical findings. Normal WBC counts at 6, 12, and 24 months after therapy indicate a high probability of cure. Appropriate interpretation of a negative CSF VDRL result and an elevated CSF WBC count in a person who is seropositive for syphilis is not clear; but given the insensitivity of the CSF VDRL test, asymptomatic neurosyphilis cannot be excluded, and other causes of CNS disease should be considered, especially if the WBC count does not decline as expected.

Recently, new guidelines to define congenital syphilis for reporting have been approved by the Council of State and Territorial Epidemiologists and the CDC, to enable reporting of congenital syphilis based on information available at birth or at the initial investigation (Table 39-1) (7). Screening all mothers at delivery and using these guidelines should identify most cases of congenital syphilis; however, asymptomatic disease in infants born to mothers with incubating syphilis very likely will not be detected, because mother and infant probably will be seronegative at delivery. Because these infants do not always present with signs and symptoms specific for congenital syphilis, performing a serologic test for syphilis on all infants with fever and aseptic meningitis, hepatomegaly, or hematologic abnormalities should be considered, even if previous tests for syphilis were negative (24). In addition, in infants of mothers who have a positive VDRL (or RPR) and were adequately treated in the past, the diagnosis of congenital syphilis due to maternal reinfection may be difficult. If lesions are present, visualizing spirochetes by darkfield examination establishes the diagnosis. A test to detect specific immunoglobulin (Ig) M may be useful, but because currently none is commercially available asymptomatic infants must be followed serially for 3 to 6 months with VDRL (or RPR) tests. Congenital syphilis is diagnosed if the titer increases or stabilizes and does not decline.

In addition to the treponemal and nontreponemal tests discussed, other methods for diagnosis of syphilis have been evaluated. One commercially available enzyme-linked immunosorbent assay (ELISA) appears to be an acceptable alternative to the FTA-ABS test, though data regarding its performance are limited (42,43). ELISA that detects IgM to nontreponemal and treponemal antigens has a potential role in the diagnosis of congenital syphilis, but currently this test is not commercially available (44). Moreover, the polymerase chain reaction may become a valuable tool for detecting Treponema pallidum subsp pallidum directly in clinical specimens (45).

Treatment and Prevention

Penicillin is the antimicrobial agent of choice for syphilis; and tetracycline, chloramphenicol, and ceftriaxone are effective alternatives for persons allergic to penicillin (4). Venereally transmitted syphilis can be prevented by avoiding sexual contact with an infected individual, and condom use should decrease the risk of spread. Congenital syphilis can be prevented by detecting and treating early syphilis in pregnant women.

Yaws, endemic syphilis, and pinta also respond to penicillin. Yaws and pinta can be prevented by treating contacts and persons with latent infection. Effective treatment plus improved socioeconomic conditions can prevent the spread of endemic syphilis (46).

BORRELIA

Borrelia organisms are microaerophilic helical bacteria 5 to 25 μm long and 0.2 to 0.5 μm wide with 4 to 30 coils. They possess an outer envelope or membrane that encloses a coiled protoplasmic cylinder composed of a peptidoglycan layer and the cytoplasmic membrane that surrounds the protoplasmic contents of the cell. Seven to twenty-two axial filaments (periplasmic flagella), responsible for motility, are attached subterminally beneath the outer envelope to opposite ends of the protoplasmic cylinder and extend toward the middle of the cell, where they overlap. Borrelia multiply by binary fission and require long-chain fatty acids for growth. They have an affinity for acid dyes and stain with nearly all analine dyes. Borrelia burgdorferi (the agent of Lyme disease) and the species of Borrelia responsible for relapsing fever are discussed in this chapter.

Table 39-1. Surveillance Case Definition for Congenital Syphilis

For reporting purposes, congenital syphilis includes cases of congenitally acquired syphilis in infants and children as well as syphilitic stillbirths.

A CONFIRMED CASE of congenital syphilis is an infant in whom Treponema pallidum is identified by darkfield microscopy, fluorescent antibody, or other specific stains in specimens from lesions, placenta, umbilical cord, or autopsy material.

A PRESUMPTIVE CASE of congenital syphilis is either of the following:
 A. Any infant whose mother has untreated or inadequately treated* syphilis at delivery, regardless of findings in the infant;
 OR
 B. Any infant or child who has a reactive treponemal test for syphilis and any one of the following:
  1. Any evidence of congenital syphilis on physical examination[†]; or
  2. Any evidence of congenital syphilis on long-bone radiograph; or
  3. Reactive cerebrospinal fluid (CSF) VDRL; or
  4. Elevated CSF cell count or protein (without other cause); or
  5. Quantitative nontreponemal serologic titers which are fourfold higher than the mother's (both drawn at birth); or
  6. Reactive test for FTA-ABS-19S-IgM antibody.

A SYPHILITIC STILLBIRTH is defined as a fetal death in which the mother had untreated or inadequately treated syphilis at delivery of a fetus after a 20-week gestation or of a fetus weighing >500 g.

* Inadequate treatment consists of any nonpenicillin therapy or penicillin given <30 days prior to delivery.
† Signs in an infant (<2 years of age) may include hepatosplenomegaly, characteristic skin rash, condyloma lata, snuffles, jaundice (syphilitic hepatitis), pseudoparalysis, or edema (nephrotic syndrome). Stigmata in an older child may include: interstitial keratitis, nerve deafness, anterior bowing of shins, frontal bossing, mulberry molars, Hutchinson's teeth, saddle nose, rhagades, or Clutton's joints.

(From Centers for Disease Control: Congenital syphilis—New York City, 1986–1988. MMWR, 38: 825, 1989.)

Borrelia burgdorferi

Lyme disease was first recognized in the United States in 1975, when close geographic clustering of what initially was diagnosed as juvenile rheumatoid arthritis occurred during the summer and early fall in Lyme, Connecticut, and was reported to the State Health Department by mothers of the affected children (47). Aspects of the illness, however, had been known under different names in Europe for many years. A migrating annular skin lesion developing at the site of a tick bite, initially called erythema migrans and later named erythema chronicum migrans (ECM) because of its prolonged duration, was reported in a person at the beginning of the century, representing the first lesion that later was related to Lyme disease (48). The association of neurologic manifestations with this skin lesion was reported by Garin and Bujadoux in France in the early 1920s, and about 20 years later Bannwarth described lymphocytic meningitis and neuritis, frequently involving the facial nerve (an entity that became known as lymphocytic meningoradiculoneuritis or Garin-Bujadoux, Bannwarth syndrome), in several persons, a few of whom had experienced a previous skin lesion similar to ECM, though none reported a tick bite (49–51). Lennhoff described spirochete-like organisms in skin specimens from lesions of ECM in 1948 (52). In the 1950s, empiric penicillin therapy was found to be beneficial for ECM and meningitis, and investigators concluded that the entity was caused by a penicillin-sensitive organism transmitted by Ixodes ricinus, the European sheep tick (53–55).

Data from the epidemiologic investigation instigated by the reported cluster of cases of "juvenile rheumatoid arthritis" in the United States showed that the prevalence of the disease was at least 100 times higher than expected and that about 25% of affected persons gave a history of an erythematous skin lesion. This caused investigators to believe the illness was a new entity, which was called Lyme arthritis. Soon, the similarity of the cutaneous lesion to ECM was recognized, and the fact that neurologic and cardiac manifestations, in addition to arthritis, may follow the skin lesion became apparent. The entity was renamed Lyme disease, to indicate multisystem involvement (56). Further studies showed that the distribution of the disease was similar to the distribution of the Ixodes dammini tick, and in 1982 the agent was discovered in the midgut of these ticks by Dr. Willy Burgdorfer, after whom it was named (57).

Borrelia burgdorferi is 18 to 30 μm long and 0.2 to 0.3 μm wide and has 7 to 11 flagella. Its outer envelope consists of glycolipids and proteins, three of which have been recognized by electrophoresis: outer membrane proteins A (31 kd) and B (34 kd), and a 66-kd polypeptide. All isolates examined to date contain four to seven plasmids, of which one (of 49 kilobases) is responsible for the production of outer surface proteins A and B. In addition, strain differences (indicated by plasmid heterogeneity) have been demonstrated among isolates, especially between those from the United States and those from Europe.

Epidemiology

In the eastern and midwestern United States, Borrelia burgdorferi is transmitted to humans by the nymph (or second stage) of the deer tick, Ixodes dammini, during the salivation stage of its feeding period, accounting for transmission between May and July. Ixodes pacificus is the vector along the west coast of the United States; ticks of the Ixodes ricinus complex transmit the organism in Europe; and in China Ixodes persulcatus has been implicated (58–60). Between 10 and 35% of Ixodes dammini ticks in Connecticut, more than 50% of I. dammini ticks on Shelter Island, New York, and only about 2% of Ixodes pacificus ticks in California and Oregon are infected with Borrelia burgdorferi (61–64). The main reservoir of the organism is the white-footed mouse, Peromyscus leucopus, in eastern and central United States; however, Ixodes dammini has been found in many mammals and in birds, suggesting that other reservoirs also may be important (65). In nature, infection with Borrelia burgdorferi is maintained by horizontal transmission from infected nymphal Ixodes dammini ticks to Peromyscus leucopus (66). When a larval Ixodes dammini tick feeds on an infected mouse it becomes infected and then molts into the nymphal stage, which is capable of transmitting the organisms during a blood meal. Moreover, deer, abundant in areas of New England where Lyme disease is endemic, also are important in the life cycle of I. dammini.

National surveillance for Lyme disease in the United States was established by the CDC in 1982, and in January 1991 the disease was declared nationally reportable. Between 1982 and the end of 1989 the annual reported number of cases of Lyme disease increased from about 500 in 1982 to over 8000 in 1990 and nearly doubled each year from 1986 through 1989 (67–69). In 1989 increases in the reported cases occurred in the South Atlantic region and in Ohio, Illinois, Iowa, and Missouri, possibly indicating emerging foci of Lyme disease in the central midwest (70). In 1989 and 1990 transmission of Lyme disease was reported in 46 states (all except Nebraska, Montana, Arizona, and Alaska), but the occurrence of Borrelia burgdorferi in nature has not been documented in all of them (67). During that time, the states reporting the largest numbers of cases were New York, New Jersey, Connecticut, Pennsylvania, Wisconsin, Georgia, California, and Rhode Island (in decreasing order) (Fig. 39–3).

In the United States in 1987 and 1988 age-specific incidence rates were highest for children under 15 years of age and for persons between ages 25 and 44 years, except in the Pacific states, where more cases were reported in the latter age group and proportionately fewer were reported in children. The sex ratio was nearly 1:1. The seasonal distribution of cases differed between regions. In the northeast and north central regions the illness began between May and August in 78% of cases, and in the north central region a significantly higher percentage of cases began in May than in the northeast region. In the Pacific region 46% of cases began between May and August, and most of the remaining cases occurred between September and April.

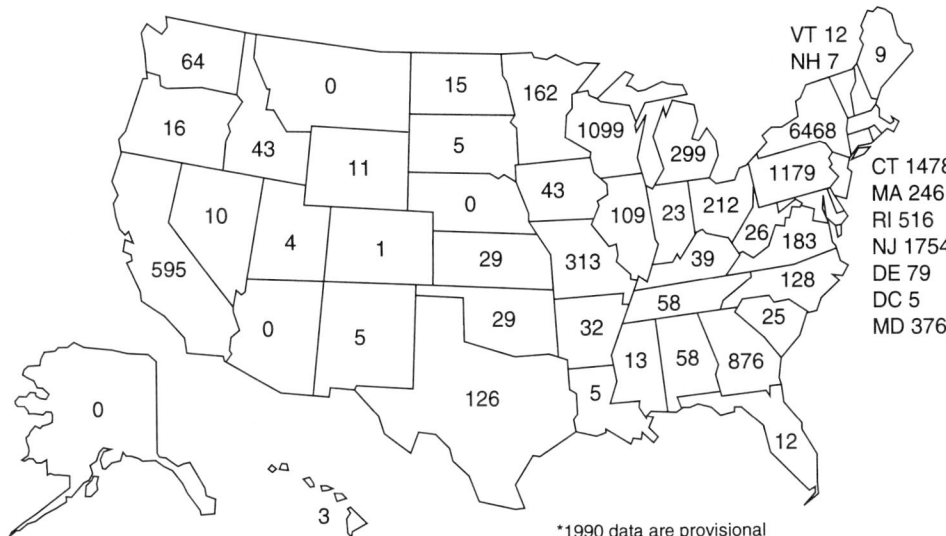

Fig. 39-3. Reported cases of Lyme disease in the United States, 1989-1990 (data from 1990 are provisional). (From Centers for Disease Control: Lyme disease surveillance—United States, 1989-1990. MMWR, 40:417, 1991.)

In addition to being transmitted by a tick bite, Borrelia burgdorferi acquired during pregnancy may cross the placenta, causing congenital infection. One woman who developed Lyme disease during the first trimester and was not treated delivered an infant at 35 weeks' gestation, and within 1 week the infant died of congenital heart disease. Autopsy examination showed B. burgdorferi in the spleen, kidneys, and bone marrow (71). In another study of 19 cases of Lyme disease in pregnant women, five pregnancies had adverse outcomes, including syndactyly, cortical blindness, intrauterine fetal death, prematurity, and rash in the newborn (72). Another woman who developed ECM during the first trimester and received oral penicillin delivered a normal-looking infant at term, who, however, died suddenly 23 hours after birth and B. burgdorferi was found in the infant's brain and liver at autopsy (73).

Pathogenesis and Immunology

Borrelia burgdorferi is injected into the skin by the tick, multiplies locally, enters the blood, and is disseminated to distant sites, including the CNS, synovium, bone, muscle, myocardium, retina, liver, spleen, and other skin sites. While in the skin, B. burgdorferi elicits an inflammatory response composed of lymphocytes and plasma cells. Although the exact pathogenesis of ECM is not known, the host inflammatory response with release of cytokines such as interleukin-1 could be involved (74).

The cellular immune response to infection with Borrelia burgdorferi begins early, before a measurable humoral response. Initially, suppressor T-cell activity is elevated. After the first several weeks mononuclear cells show increased responsiveness to B. burgdorferi antigens and to mitogens, suppressor cell activity is lower than normal, the total IgM level is elevated, and cryoprecipitates and circulating immune complexes are detected (75). An IgM response to a 41-kd endoflagellar antigen occurs early in the disease, peaks in the first 3 to 6 weeks, and may decline over the next several months or may persist for years. An IgG response to the same 41-kd protein begins 4 to 6 weeks after the onset of illness and persists months to years (75). Following the appearance of antibodies to the 41-kd flagellar protein, additional antibodies to multiple constituents of the organism are produced. Localized antibody production in the CNS correlates with CNS infection.

Despite production of specific antibodies in serum and CSF, frequent persistence of clinical disease suggests that these antibodies do not eradicate the organism. However, viable organisms may not be required for disease progression. For example, late or refractory disease may represent an autoimmune phenomenon. The 41-kd flagellar protein shares an antigenic determinant with human tissue found on myelinated peripheral nerve fibers, nerve cells, axons of the CNS, epithelial cells of joint synovia, and heart muscle cells, suggesting that antibodies to the 41-kd endoflagellar immunogen of Borrelia burgdorferi also may be directed against, and stimulated by, similar molecular constituents of human tissues (76). However, because treating the late manifestations of Lyme disease with antimicrobial agents occasionally results in clinical improvement, an autoimmune process probably is not the only mechanism responsible for persistent disease (77,78).

Given that Lyme borreliosis is a multisystem illness with a chronic relapsing course, its pathogenesis very likely is multifactoral. Possible mechanisms of disease include prolonged active infection, immune complex formation due to the persistence of antigenic components from the organism, autoimmunity, or a combination of these. Moreover, the HLA-DR4 and HLA-DR2 class II major histocompatibility genes appear to determine host immune response to Borrelia burgdorferi resulting in chronic arthritis and failure to respond to antimicrobial therapy (79).

Clinical Manifestations

Lyme borreliosis has been divided into three distinct stages—stage 1, ECM; stage 2, neurologic or cardiac involvement; and stage 3, arthritis; however, as the systemic nature of the disease has become better-defined these divisions have become obsolete. More appropriately, Lyme borreliosis is thought of as a progressive, chronic, multisystem, infectious disease.

The earliest and most easily recognized manifestation of infection with Borrelia burgdorferi is ECM. The skin lesion develops in two thirds to three fourths of affected persons 2 days to 4 weeks after a tick bite (only about a third recall a tick bite) and it may be accompanied by malaise, fatigue, arthralgias, myalgias, and fever. A painless, nonpruritic red macule or papule appears at the site of the bite (commonly the groin, thigh, or axilla) and gradually expands in a circular fashion, typically forming a flat lesion 3 to 70 cm in diameter (median, 15 cm), with a bright red outer border and central clearing. The appearance of the lesion, however, varies; confluent erythema and bullseye patterns are common, and central vesicles or necrosis may occur. Hematogenous dissemination of the organisms occurs early in the disease, an event manifest in 10 to 15% of persons by the appearance of one or more secondary annular lesions several days after the initial one. In addition, most persons with disseminated infection develop fever, headache, stiff neck, malaise, migratory musculoskeletal pain, generalized lymphadenopathy, sore throat, and nonproductive cough.

Without treatment, skin lesions fade in 3 to 4 weeks (range, 1 day to 14 months), but subsequent abnormalities may develop in one or more major organ systems (80). Acute neurologic or cardiac involvement occurs in about 20% of infected persons within 4 to 6 weeks of the onset of infection. Bell's (seventh nerve) palsy is the most common neurologic manifestation, but other cranial nerves may be affected, and 5 to 8% of persons develop acute meningitis or meningoencephalitis. Most persons with neurologic manifestations have a lymphocytic pleocytosis in the CSF (about 100 cells per microliter) and an elevated protein concentration, although the CSF may be normal in persons who have only facial palsy. Acute cardiac involvement, recognized in up to 6% of cases, most often is manifested by varying degrees of atrioventricular block. About 60% of those who have cardiac involvement develop myocarditis or pericarditis; congestive heart failure is rare. Hepatitis is common during the acute disseminated phase of the infection but rarely is manifest clinically. As the host immune response develops the number of spirochetes declines, and the chronic phase of the disease begins. Persons may enter a latent period, and like some syphilis patients, some later develop various dermatologic, rheumatologic, cardiac, and neurologic manifestations while others never experience late manifestations.

In North America about half the persons who go untreated develop episodic arthritis, primarily in large joints (especially the knees) within 2 years (sometimes later), and in 10% of these cases the arthritis becomes chronic. Treatment appears to prevent arthritis; and with increasing awareness of the disease and earlier diagnosis and treatment, the prevalence of frank arthritis appears to be declining in the United States and in Europe. Chronic neurologic manifestations—chronic encephalopathy, polyneuropathy and, less often, leukoencephalitis—develop months to years after the initial infection (81).

Species of Borrelia That Cause Relapsing Fever

Relapsing fever, an illness characterized by recurrent episodes of fever and spirochetemia, may be caused by several species of Borrelia. Borrelia recurrentis, transmitted by the human body louse, Pediculus humanus, is responsible for epidemic relapsing fever, and many of the species of Borrelia transmitted by soft ticks of the genus Ornithodoros cause endemic relapsing fever (Table 39–2).

Epidemiology

Relapsing fever occurs worldwide in tropical and temperate climates except for a few areas in the Southwest Pacific such as New Zealand and Australia (82). Humans are the only known reservoir of louse-borne relapsing fever, a disease that predominantly affects persons living under adverse hygienic conditions, and it usually occurs in epidemics associated with catastrophic events, such as

Table 39–2. Features of Borrelia That Cause Tick-Borne Disease in Humans

Species	Arthropod (Ornithodorus) Vector	Animal Reservoir	Geographic Distribution
B. duttonii	O. moubata	Humans	Central, Eastern, and Southern Africa
B. hispanica	O. erraticus (large variety)	Rodents	Spain, Portugal, Morocco, Algeria, Tunisia
B. crocidurae, -merionesi, -microti, -dipodilli	O. erraticus (small variety)	Rodents	Morocco, Libya, Egypt, Iran, Turkey, Senegal, Kenya
B. persica	O. tholozani	Rodents	Area from West China and Kashmir to Iraq and Egypt, former USSR, India
B. caucasica	O. verrucosus	Rodents	Caucasus to Iraq
B. latyschewii	O. tartakowskyi	Rodents	Iran, Central Asia
B. hermsii	O. hermsi	Rodents, chipmunks, tree squirrels	Western United States
B. turicatae	O. turicata	Rodents	Southwestern United States
B. parkeri	O. parkeri	Rodents	Western United States
B. mazzottii	O. talaje	Rodents	Southern United States, Mexico, Central and South America
B. venezuelensis	O. rudis	Rodents	Central and South America

war or famine, that result in overcrowding and dissemination of body lice. During the last large epidemic of relapsing fever, which occurred in North Africa and Europe during World War II, an estimated 50,000 persons died (83). Louse-borne disease no longer exists in the United States except for rare imported cases, but it remains endemic in the highlands of Central and East Africa and the South American Andes (84). The boy louse ingests spirochetes while feeding on a person who is spirochetemic and it remains infective for its lifetime (10 to 60 days). Organisms multiply only in the hemolymph and central ganglion of the louse, and because they do not invade the louse tissues they cannot be transmitted transovarially or by louse saliva or feces. Humans acquire the disease by crushing the louse, releasing infective organisms capable of penetrating intact skin or mucous membranes (85).

Tick-borne relapsing fever, a zoonosis that occurs sporadically worldwide, is transmitted to humans who invade the habitats of the Ornithodoros ticks: warm, humid environments such as caves, decaying wood, rodent burrows, and animal shelters at altitudes of 1500 to 6000 feet. The ticks become infected by feeding on borrelemic rodents and small animals such as chipmunks, squirrels, rabbits, rats, mice, owls, and lizards that serve as natural reservoirs for the species of Borrelia capable of causing the disease (see Table 39–2). In the tick, the spirochetes multiply rapidly and within hours invade all tissues, including salivary glands, excretory organs, and the genital system. Humans acquire the infection when saliva or feces are released from the tick during a blood meal, which often is unnoticed because the ticks feed at night and have a painless bite. Infection also is transmitted transovarially to tick progeny, a mechanism important for perpetuating the organisms, as ticks may survive 15 years without feeding (85). In the United States, between 400 and 500 cases of tick-borne relapsing fever have been reported since 1960, but the disease is under-reported because it is seldom recognized. The largest outbreak, transmitted by Ornithodoros hermsi, affected 62 persons camping for several nights in log cabins on the North Rim of Grand Canyon in Arizona in 1973 (86). The most recent outbreak in Grand Canyon National Park occurred from May through August 1990 and involved almost 20 persons (87).

Pathogenesis and Pathology

During a blood meal, Borrelia organisms are introduced into the blood, where they multiply, producing the signs and symptoms of relapsing fever (described later) when the concentration of organisms reaches 10^6 to 10^8 per milliliter of blood. Organisms do not proliferate at extravascular sites but are sequestered in internal organs during afebrile periods, when circulating spirochetes are killed by phagocytes in the presence of specific antibodies. Relapses occur when the organisms re-emerge, antigenically modified, from sites of sequestration. With successive relapses organisms eventually revert to antigenic types similar to those present during previous relapses, and they are eliminated by specific borreliacidal antibodies, terminating the disease.

Autopsy examination of fatal cases of louse-borne disease has revealed hepatitis and foci of hepatocyte necrosis; miliary abscesses in the spleen; hemorrhages, perivascular inflammation, and focal neuronal degeneration in the CNS; myocarditis; and hemorrhage in the lungs and gastrointestinal tract (83,88).

Clinical Manifestations

The clinical manifestations of louse-borne and tick-borne relapsing fever are similar, although the former typically is a more severe illness associated with a longer incubation period, longer febrile and afebrile intervals, and fewer relapses (Table 39–3). Characteristically, the primary illness begins acutely after an incubation period of 4 to 18 days (mean, 7 to 8 days) with high fever, rigors, severe headache, myalgias, arthralgias, lethargy, photophobia, cough, and abdominal pain, and it ends abruptly in 3 to 6 days. Hepatosplenomegaly and jaundice may develop, especially with louse-borne disease. Neurologic findings—coma, cranial nerve palsies, hemiplegia, meningitis, and seizures—occur in as many as 30% of those with louse-borne disease and fewer than 10% of persons with tick-borne relapsing fever. A truncal petechial, macular or papular rash lasting 1 to 2 days is common at the end of the primary febrile illness, particularly with tick-borne disease. The primary febrile illness may be associated with fatal hypotension and shock; but more often the patient survives and the fever and symptoms recur suddenly in 7 to 10 days, although their duration and intensity decrease progressively with each relapse.

Laboratory Diagnosis

The species of Borrelia that cause relapsing fever can be cultivated in vitro from blood by using a growth medium called Kelly medium, which also has been modified for cultivation of Borrelia burgdorferi from blood, skin, and CSF. Culture requires several weeks, however, and the medium generally is not available in the clinical microbiology laboratory, so alternative approaches to diagnosis are necessary.

Borrelia burgdorferi. Three keys to diagnosis of Lyme disease are clinical suspicion, recognition of the characteristic signs and symptoms, and appropriate tests for antibodies to B. burgdorferi. The clinical case definition of Lyme disease as formulated by investigators at the

Table 39–3. Clinical Features of Relapsing Fever

	Mean Value	
Characteristic	Louse-borne Disease	Tick-borne Disease
Mortality (%)	4–40	2–5
Duration of initial fever (days)	5.5	3
Duration of afebrile period (days)	9	7
Duration of relapses (days)	2	2–3
Relapses (No./range)	1–2/1–5	3/0–13

CDC is as follows: ECM (≥5 cm in diameter), *or* at least one late manifestation (musculoskeletal, nervous, *or* cardiovascular system involvement) *and* laboratory confirmation of infection (67). Laboratory criteria for diagnosis include isolation of B. burgdorferi from a clinical specimen, demonstration of diagnostic levels of IgM and IgG to B. burgdorferi in serum or CSF, or demonstration of a significant change in IgM or IgG titer in paired acute- and convalescent-phase serum samples (67). ECM is diagnostic of early Lyme borreliosis; and for persons who have this lesion, serologic testing is neither necessary nor useful, because at this stage it is associated with a false-negative rate of 50% or more (89,90). Given this high false-negative rate, early Lyme disease is difficult to diagnose in the absence of ECM, when the patient has only a nonspecific flulike syndrome.

Detection of antibodies to Borrelia burgdorferi is the most common commercially available method of diagnosis of Lyme disease; however, problems with serologic tests exist (91). For example, the primary humoral response to infection is directed predominantly against the 41-kd flagellar antigen, which is not species specific and has significant amino acid–sequence homology with flagellar antigens of other bacteria. Thus, many apparently healthy persons have low levels of cross-reacting antibodies. Because the sensitivity of the commercial serologic tests for diagnosis of early Lyme disease is low, a negative result early in the disease does not exclude Lyme borreliosis. Some manufacturers separate IgM and IgG antibody testing to increase sensitivity, but using a combined polyvalent test appears to be at least as sensitive as separate tests and is most cost effective. Moreover, testing currently is not standardized, and the consequence is significant inter- and intralaboratory variation in results (92,93). Therefore, when the antibody test result is negative in a person whose illness is consistent with Lyme disease, repeat testing, preferably by a second laboratory using a different method, is recommended.

Two types of serologic tests are available currently: the indirect immunofluorescent assay (IFA) and ELISA. Each has potential advantages and disadvantages. The IFA involves reacting the test serum with slides coated with Borrelia burgdorferi and then staining with fluorescein-labeled antihuman immunoglobulin. It is ideal for low-volume testing and allows recognition of false-positive reactions due to rheumatic diseases, which typically produce a beaded fluorescent pattern. However, a fluorescence microscope is required, and interpretation is subjective and, therefore, potentially associated with much variability, a problem that is magnified by the variable quality of commercially available slides. The ELISA, in which test serum is incubated in microtiter wells coated with B. burgdorferi antigen, is ideal for high-volume work but may be used for low-volume testing if the kit comes as strip wells. The ELISA results are quantitative and are not influenced by technical subjectivity, but a microtiter plate ELISA reader is required, and different ELISA test kits produce varied results (91,93).

Other methods of diagnosis of Lyme disease currently are being evaluated at large reference laboratories and research institutions. The Western blot test is performed by reacting test serum with antigens of Borrelia burgdorferi subjected to electrophoresis in acrylamide gels and transferred to nitrocellulose paper. The reaction is developed with enzyme- or radioisotope-linked antihuman immunoglobulin, and the resulting bands are analyzed and interpreted. Problems with this test are the lack of standardization and the fact that interpretation of the results may be difficult because healthy persons and hospitalized patients who do not have Lyme disease frequently have IgG bands, and the latter group, IgM bands as well (91). Therefore, limiting the Western blot to diagnostically difficult cases and to those for which false-positive serologic test results are a major concern is recommended until the technique is standardized and criteria for interpretation have been determined. Tests for detection of B. burgdorferi antigens in urine have been developed and are being evaluated; and a probe to detect B. burgdorferi by the polymerase chain reaction has been constructed and tested for sensitivity, but it has not yet been evaluated with clinical specimens (94–96).

Borrelia species That Cause Relapsing Fever. Relapsing fever is diagnosed by demonstrating the organisms in the peripheral blood of febrile persons. Organisms are found by darkfield examination of wet preparations of blood or in thick or thin smears stained with the Giemsa or Wright stain in about 70% of cases, and in a larger percentage if smears are stained with acridine orange and viewed by fluorescence microscopy (processing of the blood specimen is discussed in Chapter 58). Specific antibodies are present in serum, but serologic tests are not commercially available and have limited diagnostic value because of the antigenic variation of the organisms.

Treatment and Prevention

Borrelia burgdorferi. The optimal treatment for Lyme borreliosis has not been established. Oral therapy with penicillin or tetracycline is effective in persons with erythema chronicum migrans and in those with facial palsy and no overt signs of meningitis or other evidence of neurologic involvement. Larger intravenous doses of penicillin or ceftriaxone is standard therapy for persons with other neurologic complications such as meningitis or encephalitis and is effective in most cases of Lyme arthritis (97). Parenteral therapy is recommended for severe cardiac involvement, but oral regimens probably are adequate if only first-degree heart block is present.

Prevention of Lyme disease is a problem in areas where infected ticks are abundant. Persons who live in such areas can take measures: wearing light-colored protective clothing during outdoor activity, spraying pant legs and socks with an insect repellent containing diethyltoluamide or permethrin, and carefully inspecting the body surface and scalp for ticks and removing any promptly. Pets should likewise be examined.

Borrelia species That Cause Relapsing Fever. The treatment of choice for relapsing fever is tetracycline or erythromycin. Tick-borne relapsing fever may be prevented by avoiding the arthropod vector and by preventing rodents from nesting in human shelters in areas where tick-borne relapsing fever is endemic. Insecticides may be used in dwellings, and insect repellents should be applied to clothing. Louse-borne disease may be prevented by good personal hygiene and if necessary, by delousing.

LEPTOSPIRA

Leptospira interrogans is the agent of leptospirosis, an acute generalized infectious disease principally of wild and domestic mammals that is only occasionally transmitted to humans via direct or indirect contact with infected animals. The clinical illness was described in humans by Weil in 1885, and the responsible organism, first seen in sections of kidney tissue in 1907, was successfully cultivated in 1915. Currently, two species of Leptospira are recognized: Leptospira biflexa, found predominantly in fresh surface waters, rarely is associated with human infection and is not discussed further here. Leptospira interrogans, a potential pathogen for humans and other mammals, occurs naturally in many wild and domesticated mammals worldwide. About 180 serologic variants (serovars) of L. interrogans are recognized by microscopic agglutination and agglutinin adsorption tests with serovar-specific antiserum.

Leptospira organisms are tightly coiled, motile spirochetes, 6 to 20 μm long and 0.1 μm wide, with semicircular hooked or bent ends. These organisms are composed of an external sheath surrounding a cylindrical body that is helicoidally wound about two periplasmic flagella inserted subterminally at opposite ends of the body and extending toward the middle of the cell. Leptospires are aerobic and may be cultivated in vitro in medium of pH 6.8 to 7.8 containing 10% serum or serum albumin plus long-chain fatty acids. They stain faintly with aniline dyes and are invisible by light microscopy but are easily demonstrated by darkfield microscopy.

Epidemiology

Leptospirosis is a zoonosis that occurs worldwide. The natural reservoirs of infection are chronically infected rodents and other feral and domestic animals, such as cattle, pigs, and dogs, that carry Leptospira interrogans in their proximal renal tubules and shed the organisms in their urine, contaminating soil, mud, ground water, streams, and rivers. Organisms can survive 3 months or longer in neutral or slightly alkaline water but do not persist in a brackish or acid environment. Humans become infected by direct contact with an infected animal or, more commonly, via indirect contact with water or soil contaminated with infected urine. Organisms enter the body through skin abrasions, through the nasopharyngeal or esophageal mucosal surfaces, or through the eyes. Rats are the most common source of human infection worldwide, but in the United States dogs and livestock are the most important sources, followed by rodents, wild mammals, and cats. Persons at increased risk of infection are those who have occupational exposure (farmers, veterinarians, abbatoir workers, dairymen, swineherds, fish and poultry processors) or recreational exposure (persons who camp near or bathe or swim in infected ponds or streams). Most cases of leptospirosis occur in young men in summer and early fall. In the United States about 50 to 100 cases are reported annually.

Pathogenesis and Pathology

Organisms penetrate abraded skin or intact mucous membranes, enter the circulation, and are disseminated throughout the body, including the CSF and eye, where they may persist for months in the aqueous humor, occasionally causing chronic or recurrent uveitis (98). When the number of organisms reaches a critical level in the blood and tissues, lesions (predominantly damage to the endothelium of small vessels and subsequent local ischemia) and symptoms appear (99). Jaundice results from hepatocellular damage without necrosis. Renal tubular necrosis secondary to hypoxemia or a direct toxic effect of the organisms is responsible for renal failure (99,100). Meningitis probably is caused by an antigen-antibody reaction, because organisms are present in the CSF during the first week of infection, when meningeal signs are absent, but are not found after antibodies are produced and meningitis develops (101). Myalgia may be prominent, but histologic changes in muscle often are minimal and include cytoplasmic vacuoles in myofibrils and a mild infiltrate of neutrophils. Focal hemorrhagic myocarditis, vasculitis, and hemolysis (possibly related to hemolysin produced by some serotypes of Leptospira interrogans) are rare manifestations of leptospirosis.

Clinical Manifestations

Leptospirosis, often a biphasic illness, begins after an incubation period of 7 to 12 days (range, 2 to 20 days) with the septicemic phase, during which organisms can be recovered from blood, CSF, and most tissues. This phase usually lasts 4 to 7 days and is followed by an afebrile interval of 1 to 2 days, and then the immune phase, characterized by the appearance of serum antibodies, meningitis, uveitis, rash, and hepatic and renal damage. During the immune phase, which lasts 4 to 30 days, organisms are found in urine, kidney, and aqueous humor but cannot be recovered from blood or CSF. About 90% of persons ill with leptospirosis have the milder, anicteric form of disease; the remainder have severe disease with jaundice (Weil's disease).

Anicteric leptospirosis begins abruptly, with fever, chills, headache, severe muscle aches, malaise, abdominal pain, nausea, vomiting, prostration, and rarely, circulatory collapse. It persists 4 to 7 days and almost never is fatal. The immune stage may not occur or may be a low-grade illness characterized by fever, headache, mild delirium, nausea, vomiting, abdominal pain, and myalgias lasting 1 to 3 days. Muscle tenderness, conjunctival suffusion, and hepatosplenomegaly are common. A pretibial rash—1- to 5-cm erythematous lesions—occurs in infections caused by serovar autumnalis; this is part of the syndrome called Fort Bragg fever (102). During the second week of illness, some 80 to 90% of persons have CSF pleocytosis (typically fewer than 500 cells per microliter with a mononuclear cell predominance), and half of them have clinical signs of meningitis. Uveitis occurs in about 2% of cases several months after the acute illness, and it may be prolonged.

Weil's disease originally described infections with Leptospira interrogans serotype icterohaemorrhagiae, but it can develop with infection by any serotype. The illness is characterized by impaired renal and hepatic function, hemorrhage, vascular collapse, severe alterations in consciousness, and a 5 to 10% mortality rate (99,101). The serum bilirubin level generally is below 20 mg/dl; alkaline phosphatase activity is moderately elevated; and transaminase values are only slightly increased. Severely jaundiced patients are most likely to develop renal failure, hemorrhage, and cardiovascular collapse. Thrombocytopenia, which correlates with renal failure, occurs in about half of affected persons.

Laboratory Diagnosis

Leptospirosis may be diagnosed by isolating the organisms from blood or CSF collected during the febrile period of the first 7 to 10 days of the illness, or from urine collected after the first week of disease, or by detecting specific antibodies in acute- and convalescent-phase serum specimens. Collection, transport, and processing of specimens for culture are discussed in Part III.

Inoculated cultures are incubated 4 to 6 weeks at 25 to 30° C, in the dark. In semisolid media (see Table 54–4) the leptospires grow in the form of a linear disk located 1 to 3 cm below the surface of the medium, although absence of a disk does not rule them out. Material should be collected from this level weekly and examined by darkfield microscopy. Leptospires are identified by their structure (described earlier) and characteristic motility, which is unique because of the spinning hooked ends. In a liquid medium leptospires move backward and forward, rotating along their longitudinal axis; in a more viscous medium they show serpentine, boring, and flexing movement.

Leptospirosis usually is diagnosed serologically by using pools of bacterial antigens. The macroscopic slide agglutination test, which uses commercially available killed antigens, is most useful for screening; the microscopic agglutination test, which uses live or formalin-treated antigens, is more specific. An indirect hemagglutination test and ELISA that detects IgM antibodies also are available (103,104). Agglutinating antibodies typically appear on day 6 to 12 of the illness, peak by week 3 to 4, then decline to a low level and often persist for years. The humoral response, however, may be suppressed or delayed by antimicrobial therapy, and some persons remain seronegative, principally because the infecting serotype was not represented in the antigen pools. Because cross-reactions are common serologic tests may not accurately identify the infecting serotype.

Treatment and Prevention

Treatment of leptospirosis includes intravenous penicillin or ampicillin, for severe disease, or oral doxycycline, ampicillin, or amoxicillin, for less severe illness, plus general supportive therapy. Preventing leptospirosis is difficult, given the impossibility of eliminating the large animal reservoir of infection. In the United States, vaccinating domestic livestock and pets has reduced the prevalence of infection in some animals; however, renal infection may occur in vaccinated dogs, and infection may be transmitted from adequately immunized dogs to humans (105). Rat control, disinfecting contaminated work areas, and prohibiting swimming in contaminated waters have reduced the prevalence of disease in certain locations.

ANAEROBIC SPIROCHETES

Anaerobic Species of Treponema

The cultivable anaerobic species of Treponema—Treponema vincentii, -denticola, -refringens, -macrodentium, and -oralis—are normal inhabitants of the oral cavity or genital tract of humans and recently have been recognized as an important component of acute necrotizing ulcerative gingivitis (Vincent's gingivitis), a destructive lesion of the gums. To detect these organisms samples of exudate or diseased tissue should be collected; a smear should be prepared from part of the sample, and the remainder should be placed in anaerobic dilution broth. Treponemes may be detected by darkfield examination of samples of the broth or by light microscopic examination of smears of the lesion stained with methylene blue. Culture of the organisms requires inoculating broth or semisolid medium containing growth requirements—serum, thiamine, pyrophosphate, fatty acids (present in rumen fluid), glucose, and pectin—and antimicrobial agents. (A more detailed discussion of culture and isolation techniques can be found in reference 106.) Penicillin and the tetracyclines are effective against all species of Treponema.

Anaerobiospirillum succiniciproducens

Anaerobiospirillum succiniciproducens, a spiral bacterium first identified in the throats and intestines of dogs, may cause bacteremia in humans and has been recovered from the stool of persons with diarrhea, although its role in the causation of gastroenteritis in these cases is not clear (107–111). How human infection with A. succiniciproducens is acquired is not known; but since some persons who have bacteremia have had an intercurrent dental infection, and since the organism has been recovered from diarrheal feces, probable sources are the oral cavity and the gastrointestinal tract. Almost all persons who have A. succiniciproducens bacteremia have an underlying disorder such as alcoholism, atherosclerosis, malignancy, diabetes mellitus, or a recent history of a surgical procedure; and in many the bacteremia is preceded or accompanied by gastrointestinal signs and symptoms, fever, and leukocytosis.

The organism grows in supplemented peptone broth, trypticase soy broth, chopped meat broth, and in broth medium used with the radiometric blood culture system, but it grows poorly in thioglycollate broth (110). In smears of broth cultures stained with the Gram stain, the bacterial cells appear as a mixture of gram-negative spiral shapes and straight rods often showing bipolar staining. Cells of Anaerobiospirillum succiniciproducens are about three times wider and two times longer than cells of Campylobacter jejuni (see Chapter 37), with which it might initially be confused. On chocolate or blood agar, A. succiniciproducens forms moist, spreading colonies 1 to 2 mm in diameter, after incubation at 35° to 37° C in an anaerobic atmosphere for 2 to 3 days. A. succiniciproducens has bipolar tufts of flagella and demonstrates corkscrew motility when visualized by darkfield microscopy. Additional useful identifying features include negative reactions for catalase, oxidase, and indole; production of succinic acid (nonvolatile fatty acid) and acetic acid (volatile fatty acid) from glucose, as demonstrated by gas-liquid chromatography (see Chapter 30); and no growth at 25° or 42° C. In vitro, most isolates tested have been susceptible to carbenicillin, cefoxitin, chloramphenicol, and metronidazole and resistant to vancomycin and clindamycin; however, testing has been limited and different techniques have been used (108,110,111).

SPIRILLUM MINUS

Spirillum minus (formerly Spirillum minor) is one cause of rat-bite fever (the other is Streptobacillus moniliformis, see Chapter 41), predominantly in Japan (where the illness is called soduku) and rarely in the United States (112). The organism, a short, thick, gram-negative, tightly coiled spiral rod, 2 to 5 μm long and about 0.5 μm wide, having two to six spirals and bipolar tufts of flagella that are responsible for its darting motility, has not been cultured on artificial media. Spirillum minus is part of the normal respiratory tract flora of rats and is transmitted to humans via a rat bite or scratch. The bite wound heals spontaneously but in 1 to 4 weeks becomes painful, swollen, and purple. This recurrence is accompanied by regional lymphangitis, lymphadenitis, fever, chills, headache, and malaise. The wound becomes indurated and ulcerates, and a blotchy, erythematous or reddish-brown macular rash appears on the extremities, face, scalp, and trunk, which fades during afebrile intervals. Without specific antimicrobial therapy fever lasts 3 to 4 days and recurs after regular afebrile intervals of 3 to 9 days. Rare complications include endocarditis, myocarditis, hepatitis, and meningitis. The mortality rate is 6 to 10% without treatment (113).

Infection caused by Spirillum minus is diagnosed by microscopic visualization of the organism in exudates from the initial lesion, aspirates of involved lymph nodes, or blood. Wet mounts of exudate and aspirates are examined by darkfield microscopy, and blood films are stained with the Wright or Giemsa stain. The organism also may be detected in mice or guinea pigs inoculated in the laboratory by intraperitoneal injection with lesion material or blood from a person suspected to have rat-bite fever; however, this is not performed in the clinical microbiology laboratory. No specific serologic test is available currently.

Penicillin is the recommended treatment for rat-bite fever caused by Spirillum minus. Bite wounds should be cleaned thoroughly, and tetanus prophylaxis should be given if indicated (see Chapter 30).

REFERENCES

1. Fitzgerald TJ: Treponema. *In* Manual of Clinical Microbiology. 5th ed. Edited by A Balows, et al. Washington, DC, American Society for Microbiology, 1991.
2. Pusey WA: The history and epidemiology of syphilis. Springfield, IL, Charles C Thomas, 1933.
3. Sell S, and Norris SJ: The biology, pathology, and immunology of syphilis. Int Rev Exp Pathol, 24:203, 1983.
4. Tramont EC: Treponema pallidum (syphilis). *In* Principles and Practice of Infectious Diseases. 3rd ed. Edited by GL Mandell, RG Douglas, Jr, and JE Bennett. New York, Churchill Livingstone, 1990.
5. Wilcox RR, and Guthe T: Treponema pallidum. A bibliographical review of the morphology, culture and survival of T. pallidum and associated organisms. Bull WHO, 35(suppl):1, 1966.
6. Centers for Disease Control: Summary of notifiable diseases, United States, 1989. MMWR, 38(54):40, 1990.
7. Centers for Disease Control: Congenital syphilis—New York City, 1986–1988. MMWR, 38:825, 1989.
8. Fitzgerald TJ: Pathogenesis and immunology of Treponema pallidum. Ann Rev Microbiol, 35:29, 1981.
9. Magnuson HJ, et al: Inoculation syphilis in human volunteers. Medicine, 35:33, 1956.
10. Chapel TA: The variability of syphilitic chancres. Sex Transm Dis, 5:68, 1978.
11. Chapel TA: The signs and symptoms of secondary syphilis. Sex Transm Dis, 7:161, 1980.
12. O'Regan S, et al: Treponemal antigens in congenital and acquired syphilic nephritis. Ann Intern Med, 85:325, 1976.
13. Keisler DS, et al: Early syphilis with liver involvement. JAMA, 247:1999, 1982.
14. Ross WH, and Sutton HF: Acquired syphilitic uveitis. Arch Ophthalmol, 98:496, 1980.
15. Hansen K, et al: Bone lesions in early syphilis detected by bone scintigraphy. Br J Vener Dis, 60:265, 1984.
16. Johns DR, Tierney M, and Felsenstein D: Alteration in the natural history of neurosyphilis by concurrent infection with the human immunodeficiency virus. N Engl J Med, 316:1569, 1987.
17. Musher DM, Hamill RJ, and Baughn RE: Effect of human immunodeficiency virus (HIV) infection on the course of syphilis and on the response to treatment. Ann Intern Med, 113:872, 1990.
18. Rothenberg R: Syphilitic hearing loss. South Med J, 72:118, 1979.
19. Wilson WR, and Zoller M: Electronystagmography in congenital and acquired syphilitic otitis. Ann Otol, 90:21, 1981.
20. Jackman JD, and Radolf JD: Cardiovascular syphilis. Am J Med, 87:425, 1989.
21. Ikeda MK, and Jenson HB: Evaluation and treatment of congenital syphilis. J Pediatr, 117:843, 1990.
22. Centers for Disease Control: Guidelines for the prevention and control of congenital syphilis. MMWR, 37(S-1):1, 1988.
23. Chawla V, Pandit PB, and Nkrumah FK: Congenital syphilis in the newborn. Arch Dis Child, 63:1393, 1988.
24. Dorfman DH, and Glaser JH: Congenital syphilis presenting in infants after the newborn period. N Engl J Med, 323:1299, 1990.
25. Fojaco RM, Hensley GT, and Moskowitz L: Congenital syphilis and necrotizing funisitis. JAMA, 261:788, 1989.
26. Hackett CJ: On the origin of the human treponematoses. Bull WHO, 29:7, 1963.

27. Hopkins DR: After smallpox eradication: Yaws? Am J Trop Med Hyg, 25:860, 1976.
28. St. John RK: Yaws in the Americas. Rev Infect Dis, 7(suppl 2):266, 1985.
29. Antal GM, and Causse G: The control of endemic treponematoses. Rev Infect Dis, 7(suppl 2):220, 1985.
30. Csonka G, and Pace J: Endemic nonvenereal treponematosis (bejel) in Saudi Arabia. Rev Infect Dis, 7(suppl 2):260, 1985.
31. Grin EI: Epidemiology and control of endemic syphilis. Report on a Mass Treatment Campaign in Bosnia. WHO Monograph Series No. 11. Geneva, World Health Organization, 1953.
32. Hart G: Syphilis tests in diagnostic and therapeutic decision making. Ann Intern Med, 104:368, 1986.
33. Jaffe HW, Larsen SA, Jones OG, Dans PE: Hemagglutination tests for syphilis antibody. Am J Clin Pathol, 70:230, 1978.
34. Larsen SA, et al: Specificity, sensitivity, and reproducibility among the fluorescent treponemal antibody–absorption test, the microhemagglutination assay for Treponema pallidum antibodies, and the hemagglutination treponemal test for syphilis. J Clin Microbiol, 14:441, 1981.
35. Brown ST, et al: Serological response to syphilis treatment. JAMA, 253:1296, 1985.
36. Fiumara NJ: Treatment of primary and secondary syphilis. Serological response. JAMA, 243:2500, 1980.
37. Fiumara NJ: Serologic responses to treatment of 128 patients with late latent syphilis. Sex Transm Dis, 6:243, 1979.
38. Haas JS, et al: Sensitivity of treponemal tests for detecting prior treated syphilis during human immunodeficiency virus infection. J Infect Dis, 162:862, 1990.
39. Alessi E, and Scioccati L: TPHA test: Experience at the Clinic of Dermatology, University of Milan. Br J Vener Dis, 54:151, 1978.
40. Larsen SA, Hunter EF, and McGrew BD: Syphilis. In Laboratory Methods for the Diagnosis of Sexually Transmitted Diseases. Edited by BE Wentworth and FN Judson. Washington, DC, American Public Health Association, 1984.
41. Schmidt BL, and Luger A: Diagnosis of neurosyphilis by CSF examination. Geneva, World Health Organization, 1980.
42. Moyer NP, Hudson JD, and Hausler WJ, Jr: Evaluation of the Bio-EnzaBead test for syphilis. J Clin Microbiol, 25:619, 1987.
43. Burdash NM, Hinds KK, Finnerty JA, and Manos JP: Evaluation of the syphilis Bio-EnzaBead assay for detection of treponemal antibody. J Clin Microbiol, 25:808, 1987.
44. Pedersen NS, Sheller JP, Ratnam AV, and Hira SK: Enzyme-linked immunosorbent assays for detection of immunoglobulin M to nontreponemal and treponemal antigens for the diagnosis of congenital syphilis. J Clin Microbiol, 27:1835, 1989.
45. Burstain JM, et al: Sensitive detection of Treponema pallidum by using the polymerase chain reaction. J Clin Microbiol, 29:62, 1991.
46. Grin ET, and Guthe T: Evaluation of a previous mass campaign against endemic syphilis in Bosnia and Herzogovina. Br J Vener Dis, 49:1, 1973.
47. Steere AC, et al: Lyme arthritis: An epidemic of oligoarticular arthritis in children and adults in three Connecticut communities. Arthritis Rheum, 20:7, 1977.
48. Afzelius A: Erythema chronicum migrans. Acta Derm Venereol, 2:120, 1921.
49. Garin CH, and Bujadoux M: Paralysie par les tiques. J Med Lyon, 71:765, 1922.
50. Bannwarth A: Chronische lymphocytare Meningitis, entzundliche Polyneuritis und "Rheumatismus" eing Beitrag zum problem "allergic und nervensystem." Arch Psychiatr Nervenkr, 113:284, 1941.
51. Bannwarth A: Zur Klinik und Pathogenese der "chronischen lymphocytare Meningitis." Arch Psychiatr Nervenkr, 117:161, 1944.
52. Lennhoff C: Spirochaetes in aetiogically obscure diseases. Acta Derm Venereol, 28:295, 1948.
53. Hollstrom E: Successful treatment of erythema migrans Azfelius. Acta Derm Venereol, 31:235, 1951.
54. Hollstrom E: Penicillin treatment of erythema migrans Azfelius. Acta Derm Venereol, 38:285, 1958.
55. Binder E, Doepfmer R, and Hornstein P: Experimentelle Ubertrangung des Erythema chronicum migrans: Von Mensch zu Mensch. Hautarzt, 6:494, 1955.
56. Steere AC, et al: Erythema chronicum migrans and Lyme arthritis: The enlarging clinical spectrum. Ann Intern Med, 86:685, 1977.
57. Burgdorfer W, et al: Lyme disease—a tick-borne spirochetosis. Science, 216:1317, 1982.
58. Burgdorfer W, et al: The western black-legged tick, Ixodes pacificus: A vector of Borrelia burgdorferi. Am J Trop Med Hyg, 34:925, 1985.
59. Barbour AG, et al: Isolation of cultivable spirochete from Ixodes ricinus of Switzerland. Curr Microbiol, 8:123, 1983.
60. Ai CX, et al: Clinical manifestations and epidemiological characteristics of Lyme disease in Hailin County, China. Ann NY Acad Sci, 539:302, 1988.
61. Magnarelli LA, et al: Spirochetes in ticks and antibodies to Borrelia burgdorferi in white-tailed deer from Connecticut, New York State, and North Carolina. J Wildlife Dis, 22:178, 1986.
62. Bosler EM, et al: Prevalence of the Lyme disease spirochete in populations of white-tailed deer and white-footed mice. Yale J Biol Med, 57:651, 1984.
63. Ginsberg HS, and Ewing CP: Habital distribution of Ixodes dammini (Acari: Ixodidae) and Lyme disease spirochetes on Fire Island, New York. J Med Entomol, 26:183, 1989.
64. Magnarelli LA, Anderson JF: Ticks and biting insects infected with the etiologic agent of Lyme disease, Borrelia burgdorferi. J Clin Microbiol, 26:1482, 1988.
65. Anderson JF: Mammalian and avian reservoirs for Borrelia burgdorferi. Ann NY Acad Sci, 539:180, 1988.
66. Benach JL, Szczepanski A, and Monco JCG: Biologic features of Borrelia burgdorferi. Lab Med, 21:293, 1990.
67. Centers for Disease Control: Lyme disease surveillance—United States, 1989–1990. MMWR, 40:417, 1991.
68. Ciesielski CA, et al: Lyme disease surveillance in the United States, 1983–1986. Rev Infect Dis, 2:S1435, 1989.
69. Ciesielski CA, et al: The geographic distribution of Lyme disease in the United States. Ann NY Acad Sci, 539:283, 1988.
70. Miller GL, Craven RB, Bailey RE, and Tsai TF: The epidemiology of Lyme disease in the United States 1987–1988. Lab Med, 21:285, 1990.
71. Schlesinger PA, et al: Maternal-fetal transmission of the Lyme disease spirochete, Borrelia burgdorferi. Ann Intern Med, 103:67, 1985.
72. Markowitz LE, et al: Lyme disease in pregnancy. JAMA, 256:3394, 1986.
73. Weber K, et al: Borrelia burgdorferi in a newborn despite oral penicillin for Lyme borreliosis during pregnancy. Pediatr Infect Dis J, 7:286, 1988.
74. Habicht GS, et al: Lyme disease spirochetes induce human and murine interleukin 1 production. J Immunol, 134:3147, 1985.
75. Finn AF, Jr, and Dattwyler RJ: The immunology of Lyme borreliosis. Lab Med, 21:305, 1990.

76. Aberer E, et al: Molecular mimicry and Lyme borreliosis: A shared antigenic determinant between Borrelia burgdorferi and human tissue. Ann Neurol, 26:732, 1989.
77. Steere A, Pachner A, and Malawista S: Neurologic abnormalities of Lyme disease: Successful treatment with high-dose intravenous penicillin. Ann Intern Med, 99:767, 1983.
78. Dattwyler R, Halperin J, and Pass H: Ceftriaxone as effective therapy in refractory Lyme disease. J Infect Dis, 155:1322, 1987.
79. Steere AC, Dwyer E, and Winchester R: Association of chronic arthritis with HLA-DR4 and HLA-DR2 alleles. N Engl J Med, 323:219, 1990.
80. Dattwyler RJ: Lyme borreliosis: An overview of the clinical manifestations. Lab Med, 21:290, 1990.
81. Logigian EL, Kaplin RF, and Steere AC: Chronic neurologic manifestations of Lyme disease. N Engl J Med, 323:1438, 1990.
82. Burgdorfer W: The enlarging spectrum of tick-borne spirochetoses (RR Parker Memorial Address). Rev Infect Dis, 8:932, 1986.
83. Bryceson ADM, et al: Louse-borne relapsing fever. A clinical and laboratory study of 62 cases in Ethiopia and a reconsideration of the literature. Q J Med, 39:129, 1970.
84. Felsenfeld O: The problem of relapsing fever in the Americas. Ind Med, 42:7, 1973.
85. Burgdorfer W: The epidemiology of relapsing fevers. In The Biology of Parasitic Spirochetes. Edited by RC Johnson. New York, Academic Press, 1976.
86. Centers for Disease Control: Relapsing fever. MMWR, 22:242, 1973.
87. Centers for Disease Control: Outbreak of relapsing fever—Grand Canyon National Park, Arizona, 1990. MMWR, 40:296, 1991.
88. Southern PM, Jr, and Sanford JP: Relapsing fever: A clinical and microbiological review. Medicine, 48:129, 1969.
89. Russell H, et al: Enzyme-linked immunosorbent assay and indirect immunofluorescence assay for Lyme disease. J Infect Dis, 149:465, 1984.
90. Shrestha M, Grodzicki RL, and Steere AC: Diagnosing early Lyme disease. Am J Med, 78:235, 1985.
91. Golightly MG, Thomas JA, and Viciana AL: The laboratory diagnosis of Lyme borreliosis. Lab Med, 21:299, 1990.
92. Magnarelli LA: Quality of Lyme disease tests. JAMA, 262:3464, 1989.
93. Schwartz BS, et al: Antibody testing in Lyme disease: A comparison of results in four laboratories. JAMA, 262:3431, 1989.
94. Benach JL, Coleman JI, and Golightly MG: A murine IgM monoclonal antibody binds an antigenic determinant in outer surface protein A, an immunodominant basic protein of Lyme disease spirochete. J Immunol, 140:265, 1988.
95. Bosler EM, and Schulze T: The prevalence and significance of Borrelia burgdorferi in the urine of feral reservoir hosts. Zentralbl Bakteriol Mikrobiol Hyg A, 263:40, 1986.
96. Rosa PA, and Schwan TG: A specific and sensitive assay for the Lyme disease spirochete Borrelia burgdorferi using the polymerase chain reaction. J Infect Dis, 160:1018, 1989.
97. Wormser GP: Treatment of Borrelia burgdorferi infections. Lab Med, 21:316, 1990.
98. Alexander A, et al: Leptospiral uveitis: Report of bacteriologically verified case. AMA Arch Ophthalmol, 48:292, 1952.
99. Arean VM: The pathologic anatomy and pathogenesis of fatal human leptospirosis (Weil's disease). Am J Pathol, 40:393, 1962.
100. Sitprija V: Renal involvement in human leptospirosis. Br Med J, 2:656, 1968.
101. Edwards GA, and Domm BM: Human leptospirosis. Medicine, 39:117, 1960.
102. Gochenour WS, Jr, et al: Leptospiral etiology of Fort Bragg fever. Public Health Rep, 67:811, 1952.
103. Adler B, et al: Detection of specific and antileptospiral immunoglobulins M and G in human serum by solid-phase enzyme-linked immunosorbent assay. J Clin Microbiol, 11:452, 1980.
104. Watt G, et al: Rapid serodiagnosis of leptospirosis: A prospective comparison of the dot enzyme-linked immunosorbent assay and the genus-specific microscopic agglutination test at different stages of illness. J Infect Dis, 157:840, 1988.
105. Feigin RD, et al: Human leptospirosis from immunized dogs. Ann Intern Med, 79:777, 1973.
106. Smibert RM: Anaerobic spirochetes. In Manual of Clinical Microbiology. 5th ed. Edited by A Balows, et al. Washington, DC, American Society for Microbiology, 1991.
107. Davis CP, Cleven D, Brown J, and Balish E: Anaerobiospirillum, a new genus of spiral-shaped bacteria. Int J System Bacteriol, 26:498, 1976.
108. Shlaes DM, Dul MJ, and Lerner PI: Anaerobiospirillum bacteremia. Ann Intern Med, 97:63, 1982.
109. Malnick H, Thomas M, Lotay H, and Robbins M: Anaerobiospirillum species isolated from humans with diarrhoea. J Clin Pathol, 36:1097, 1983.
110. Park CH, et al: Anaerobiospirillum succiniciproducens. Am J Clin Pathol, 85:73, 1986.
111. McNeil MM, Martone WJ, and Dowell VR, Jr: Bacteremia with Anaerobiospirillum succiniciproducens. Rev Infect Dis, 9:737, 1987.
112. Gunning JJ: Rat-bite fevers. In Tropical Medicine. 5th ed. Edited by GW Hunter III, JC Swartzwelder, and DF Clyde. Philadelphia, WB Saunders, 1976.
113. Piot P: Gardnerella, Streptobaccilus, Spirillum, and Calymmatobacterium. In Manual of Clinical Microbiology. 5th ed. Edited by A Balows, et al. Washington, DC, American Society for Microbiology, 1991.

Chapter 40

MYCOBACTERIA

Mycobacteria are acid-fast, alcohol-fast, aerobic, non–spore-forming, slowly growing bacteria with a high lipid content in their cell wall. Many species of Mycobacterium are found in soil, water, food, and several animals, but for a few species—Mycobacterium tuberculosis, Mycobacterium africanum, and Mycobacterium leprae—humans are the primary reservoir. In this chapter the epidemiology, pathogenesis, and clinical manifestations of disease caused by the mycobacteria are discussed for the Mycobacterium tuberculosis complex; the nontuberculous mycobacteria, which are divided into potential pathogens and rarely pathogenic mycobacteria; and Mycobacterium leprae.

MYCOBACTERIUM TUBERCULOSIS COMPLEX

Members of the Mycobacterium tuberculosis complex—Mycobacterium tuberculosis, Mycobacterium bovis, and Mycobacterium africanum, all of which have been referred to as the tubercle bacillus—are the agents of human tuberculosis.

Mycobacterium tuberculosis

Tuberculosis (initially called phthisis or consumption for its wasting effects), became a major problem in the seventeenth and eighteenth centuries, where crowded urban living conditions favored its spread. During that time, it was responsible for about 25% of deaths in adults. In 1865 Francoise Villemin transmitted tuberculosis in the laboratory by injecting diseased human tissue into guinea pigs. In 1882, Koch discovered the tubercle bacillus and formulated criteria ("Koch's postulates") to identify the agent of an infectious disease: (1) The organism is found in the lesions of the disease regularly; (2) the organism can be isolated in pure culture on artificial media; (3) inoculating the culture of the organism into animals in the laboratory produces a similar disease; (4) the organism can be recovered from lesions in the animals.

Epidemiology

Currently, the estimated annual incidence of tuberculosis is 8 to 10 million new cases worldwide, and 2 to 3 million persons die from tuberculosis each year. Most cases and deaths are caused by Mycobacterium tuberculosis. In some parts of Africa, Asia, and Oceania and among immigrants to the United States from Asia during the first year after arrival, the annual incidence may exceed 300 per 100,000 population.

In the United States the number of reported cases of tuberculosis steadily declined, from about 84,300 in 1953, when national reporting of tuberculosis began, to 22,200 in 1985, and the annual risk decreased from 53.0 to 9.3 per 100,000 population (1). Almost 22,800 new cases of tuberculosis were reported to the Centers for Disease Control (CDC) in 1986, the first year since 1953 that the number of cases increased. The number of reported cases declined in 1987 to about 22,500 and in 1988 to about 22,400; however, the observed decline (about 1% in 1987 and only 0.4% in 1988) was less than the average annual decline of almost 7% between 1981 and 1984 (Fig. 40–1) (2). In 1989 the number of reported cases increased almost 5% over the total reported in 1988, and in 1990 the number increased more than 9% over the 1989 total. Among the age groups, the largest increase occurred in the 25- to 44-year-old group. In all age groups the number of cases increased among blacks and Hispanics but decreased among whites, Asians and Pacific Islanders, and American Indians and Alaskan natives. Among metropolitan areas, New York City reported the most marked increase. The failure of the rate of acquisition of new cases of tuberculosis in the United States to continue its downward trend since 1985 is attributed to the epidemic spread of human immunodeficiency virus (HIV), poverty, homelessness, and continued immigration from countries where tuberculosis is prevalent.

Risk factors for tuberculosis in the United States have changed significantly over the past few decades. Fifty years ago the death rate was highest among infants, adolescents, and young adults, but owing to improved living standards and the availability of effective chemotherapy, the death rate declined in younger age groups. Currently, the age-specific risk of tuberculosis is lowest in the 5- to 14-year age group and increases steadily with age. In both sexes and all races, most cases occur in the oldest segment of the population, a circumstance that may be attributed to activation of latent foci of infection and to group living conditions. Elders who live in nursing homes are at substantial risk of acquiring a new infection with Mycobacterium tuberculosis and consequently are at high risk of developing clinical disease (3). The risk of acquiring tuberculosis is high for all racial minorities, especially Hispanics, blacks, American Indians, Alaskan natives, and Asians and Pacific Islanders (4). In the United States in 1987, the number of cases of tuberculosis among non-Hispanic blacks surpassed the number among non-Hispanic whites for the first time, and more than a fifth of cases reported in 1986 and 1987 were among foreign-born persons. In all races males are at greater risk of disease than females.

Mycobacterium tuberculosis is transmitted principally via inhalation of dried residues of small infected droplets (1 to 5 μm in diameter) expelled during coughing, sneezing, or talking, and the most important source of infection is an undiagnosed person with cavitary (and sputum

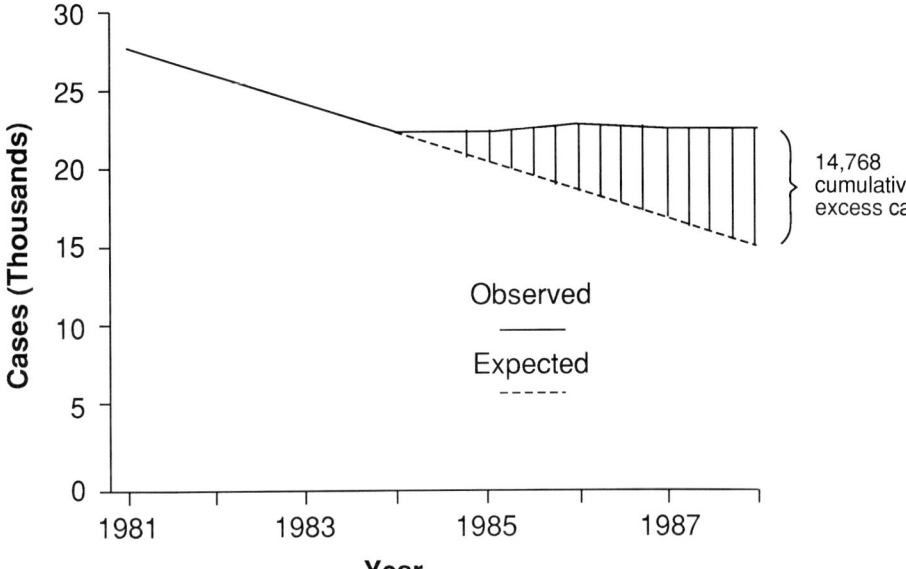

Fig. 40-1. Observed and expected cases of tuberculosis in the United States, 1981–1988. (From Centers for Disease Control: Update: Tuberculosis elimination—United States. MMWR, 39:153, 1990.)

smear positive) tuberculosis. Although the minimum infective dose for humans is unknown, data from cross-infection studies in tuberculosis wards where air quality was monitored suggest that infection may occur after inhaling one or two viable organisms (5). Despite great susceptibility to infection with M. tuberculosis, most infected persons do not develop active disease. The risk of active pulmonary disease is low after a single exposure to the organism, but it increases significantly under conditions of stress or in a confined environment where repeated exposure to the organism occurs. M. tuberculosis also may be transmitted by direct inoculation of abraded skin, an event most likely to occur when laboratory workers handle infected tissues.

Pathogenesis

The specific structures, antigens, and mechanisms responsible for the virulence of Mycobacterium tuberculosis are unknown, but two properties are associated with the ability of virulent strains to produce disease: cord factor and sulfatides. In vitro, cord factor is responsible for the morphologic appearance of M. tuberculosis: serpentine cords consisting of bacilli in close parallel arrangements. This growth pattern correlates with the presence in the bacillus of the glycolipid trehalose-6,6′dimycolate, a substance that when injected into mice in the laboratory inhibits neutrophil migration, elicits granuloma formation, and stimulates protection against virulent infection. Despite these activities in animals, the specific role of cord factor in the pathogenesis of human tuberculosis has not been determined. Sulfatides, peripherally located glycolipids responsible for the neutral red activity associated with virulent M. tuberculosis, inhibit the fusion of secondary lysosomes with phagosomes within the macrophage containing bacilli, possibly promoting intracellular survival of the organism.

The usual host response to infection with Mycobacterium tuberculosis is activation of the cell-mediated immune system. During primary (initial) infection, bacilli are inhaled, reach the alveolar spaces, and are ingested by resident macrophages. These macrophages are incapable of killing the mycobacteria, which multiply intracellularly during the first several days after infection. The infected macrophages migrate to regional tracheobronchial lymph nodes and present the sensitizing antigen(s) to immunocompetent T cells or enter the lymphatics and the blood and travel back to the lungs (primarily the apices) and to distant organs (especially the lymph nodes, kidneys, epiphyseal areas of the long bones, vertebral bodies, and meninges), where bacilli continue to multiply until the cellular immune response is activated. Immunocompetent T cells migrate from regional lymph nodes back to the site of infection in the lung and release chemotactic, migration-inhibitory, and mitogenic cytokines (described in Chapter 2), resulting in recruitment of blood-derived monocytes and lymphocytes, in macrophage and lymphocyte division, and in macrophage activation. The activated macrophages have enhanced microbicidal activity and produce cytokines that stimulate or regulate other components of the immune system, properties that help limit the infection. However, the cytokines (interleukin-1, interferon γ, and tumor necrosis factor) and lytic enzymes released by the macrophages also contribute to the concomitant local tissue destruction. With time, the activated T-cell population declines and is replaced by long-lived memory immune T cells, which protect the host against reinfection with M. tuberculosis and provide some cross-protection against infection with other species of Mycobacterium.

Approximately 90% of initial infections become quiescent once the cellular immune system has been activated, and the symptoms resolve. The lesion heals by fibrosis, and eventually calcifies. In very young or immunocompromised persons incapable of mounting the necessary immune response the primary infection may disseminate, producing miliary disease, or progress and spread by contiguity or erosion into bronchi, resulting in cavitating pul-

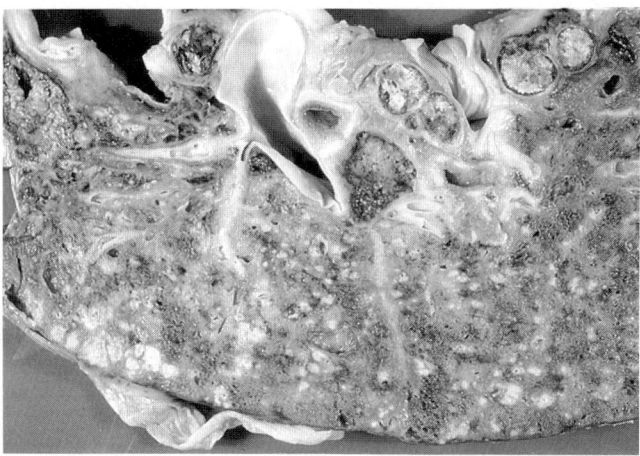

Fig. 40–2. Micrograph of lesions (tubercles) of pulmonary tuberculosis. (Courtesy of Cathy Looby, M.D., Medical College of Pennsylvania.)

monary tuberculosis or large areas of consolidation (tuberculous pneumonia).

Despite the limitation of further mycobacterial multiplication in primary and metastatic foci by the activated macrophages and memory T cells, a residual nidus of infection remains indefinitely in the lung (most frequently in the apex, where oxygen tension is high) and less often in distant sites. Therefore, the potential exists for endogenous infection (reactivation of quiescent foci) to develop during periods of immunosuppression. Most often, these foci of reactivation remain localized and eventually heal by fibrosis; however, if the infection erodes into a bronchiole, drainage of the caseous material transforms the lesion into a cavity, and miliary disease may ensue if organisms enter the lymphatics and blood to seed distant organs. Isolated-organ extrapulmonary tuberculosis also is possible in metastatic foci such as the meninges, kidneys, adrenals, bones, fallopian tubes, and epididymis.

Pathology

The primary focus of pulmonary infection (the Gohn lesion) most often is located subjacent to the pleura in the lower part of the upper lobes or the upper part of the lower lobes of one lung, corresponding to areas of the lung that receive the greatest volume flow of inspired air. Lesions (tubercles) appear as well-circumscribed areas of grayish white consolidation, 1 to 2 cm in diameter, with soft to necrotic centers (Fig. 40–2). Similar-looking tubercles generally are seen in the regional tracheobronchial lymph nodes, and these plus the primary lung lesion are termed the Gohn complex. Microscopically, these lesions are composed of well-circumscribed aggregates of histiocytes, lymphocytes, and epithelioid histiocytes, with or without Langhans' giant cells, surrounded by proliferating fibroblasts (Fig. 40–3). Central caseation necrosis may or may not be present, and organisms may be seen in tissue sections stained with an acid-fast stain. With time, the lesions are replaced by hyalinized fibrous tissue, and eventually they calcify. Cavitary lesions of variable size, most often located in the apices, commonly are traversed by thrombosed arteries. The lesions of miliary tuberculosis—distinct, yellow-white firm areas of consolidation without gross caseation, 1 to several millimeters' diameter—resemble tubercles microscopically.

Clinical Manifestations

Mycobacterium tuberculosis may cause disease in any organ, but in the United States pulmonary tuberculosis

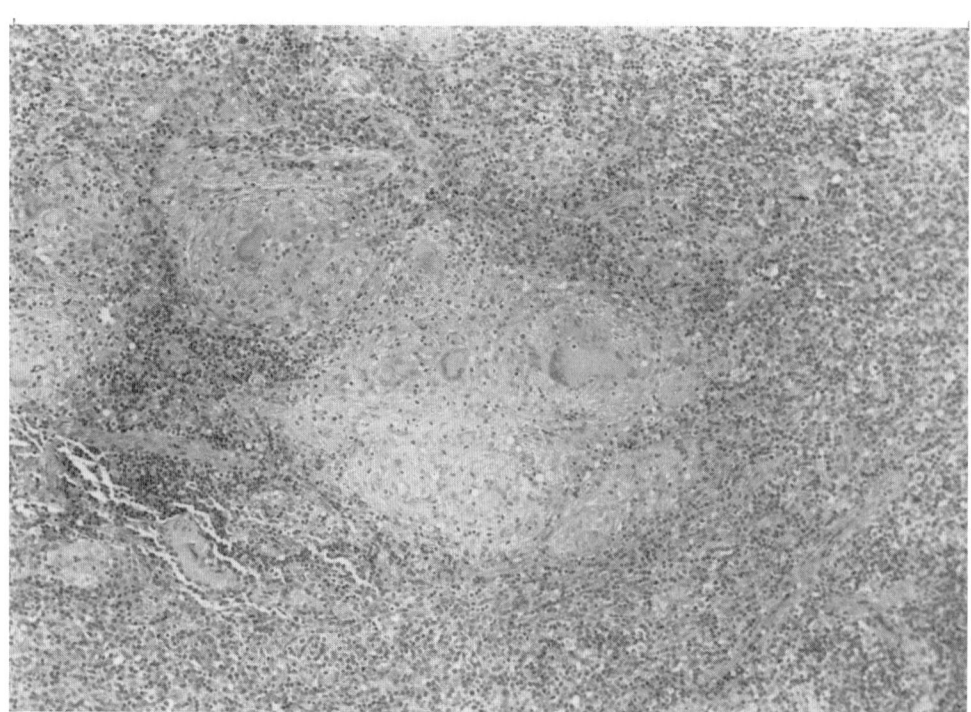

Fig. 40–3. Micrograph of a lymph node shows granulomatous inflammation caused by Mycobacterium tuberculosis (hematoxylin and eosin, ×40).

accounts for about 85% of cases. The manifestations of primary pulmonary disease vary with the age of the patient. Infants and young children most often are symptomatic, exhibiting fever and lassitude. Exuberant hilar or mediastinal lymphadenitis may compress central bronchi, producing cough or local atelectasis, or the infection may drain into a bronchus causing pneumonia. Many adults are asymptomatic; but some experience malaise, fatigue, and low-grade fever. Infrequently, the infection progresses to pneumonia, occasionally with pleural involvement. In most cases the primary lesions heal completely, leaving no evidence of infection except hypersensitivity to tuberculin manifested by a positive skin test reaction (see Laboratory Diagnosis).

Chronic pulmonary tuberculosis in adults usually begins as a focus of pneumonitis surrounding a growing bacterial colony in the subapical posterior aspect of an upper lobe. Anorexia, fever, weight loss, chilly sensations, afternoon remittent fever, and night sweats, followed by cough productive of purulent sputum occur when the population of bacteria reaches a critical size. Mild hemoptysis, due to caseous sloughing or to endobronchial erosion, and chest pain resulting from extension of the inflammatory process to the parietal pleura may develop late in the disease.

Extrapulmonary tuberculosis may be localized, but more often it involves multiple organs; there need not be a concurrent lung infection. Multiple organ tuberculosis, historically a disease of infants and young children, currently predominates among elders and immunocompromised persons, especially those infected with both HIV and Mycobacterium tuberculosis (6–8). The clinical manifestations and laboratory findings associated with extrapulmonary disease are summarized in Table 40–1 (tuberculous meningitis is illustrated in Plate VIIA).

Mycobacterium bovis

An association between tuberculous cervical adenitis (scrofula) in humans and drinking milk from diseased cows was recognized in 1846 (9). Bovine tuberculosis was first transmitted to animals inoculated in the laboratory in 1866, and Robert Koch isolated the tubercle bacillus from human and bovine sources in 1882, a time when 20 to 40% of cattle in many European countries had tuberculosis (10).

Mycobacterium bovis (formerly called Mycobacterium tuberculosis var bovis and Mycobacterium tuberculosis subsp bovis) has one of the broadest host ranges of all known pathogens. It causes disease in domesticated cattle, bison, buffaloes, marsupials, hares, equines, camels, pigs, sheep, goats, deer, antelopes, elephants, cats, dogs, foxes,

Table 40–1. Extrapulmonary Manifestations of Tuberculosis

Site	Clinical Manifestations	Laboratory Findings
Central nervous system		
Meninges*	Acute or chronic meningitis	CSF: 100–500 WBC/µl, ↑ protein, ↓ glucose; AFB smear positive in <40%
Cerebral cortex	Tuberculoma—headache, seizures	
Pericardium	Acute pericarditis (fever, chest pain); chronic pericarditis (cardiovascular compromise)	AFB smear usually negative; culture positive in 25–50%; PPD positive
Skeletal		
Spine	Pain, paralysis of lower extremities	
Peripheral	Pain, arthritis of hip, knee	
Genitourinary tract†		
Renal	Dysuria, flank pain	Gross or microscopic hematuria or pyuria in 90%
Male genital	Tender scrotal mass, draining sinus	Oligospermia
Female genital	Menstrual disorders, abdominal pain	
Gastrointestinal tract		
Oral cavity	Nonhealing ulcer of tongue or oropharynx	
Esophagus	Stricture, tracheoesophageal fistula	
Stomach	Ulcer, diffuse thickening	
Small intestine	Perforation, obstruction, enteroenteric or entercutaneous fistula, hemorrhage, malabsorption	
Large intestine	Abdominal pain, anorexia, diarrhea, obstruction, hemorrhage	
Anus	Ulcer, fistula, abscess	
Liver	Granulomatous hepatitis	Alkaline phosphatase ↑, transaminases normal
Peritoneal cavity	Peritonitis: Insidious onset of fever, abdominal pain, weight loss, anorexia; or acute onset of chills, fever, rebound tenderness, ascites	Peritoneal fluid: 500–2000 WBC/µl (lymphocytes), AFB smear negative, culture positive in 25%; positive PPD in 30–100%
Lymph nodes	Lymphadenitis: Draining cervical or supraclavicular nodes	
Skin	Ulcers, nodules, abscesses	
Larynx	Erythema, ulcers, exophytic masses	

* Tuberculous meningitis is characterized by a basal exudate. Neutrophils may predominate in CSF early, and lymphocytes predominate later. The positive rate of cultures increases if serial specimens are examined.
† Involvement of the male genital tract (prostate, seminal vesicles, epididymis, and testes, in that order) usually is due to spread of infection from the kidney. In females, infection, acquired via hematogenous spread, begins in the fallopian tube and may spread to the ovaries, endometrium and, rarely, the cervix.
Key: CSF, cerebrospinal fluid; WBC, white blood cells; AFB, acid-fast bacilli; PPD, purified protein derivative (skin test).

minks, badgers, moles, ferrets, rats, and primates, including humans (11). The organism may be transmitted from cattle to humans who consume contaminated raw milk or inhale particles from live infected cattle or carcasses; (2) from person to person via respiratory exposure, (3) to cattle exposed to urine from humans who have Mycobacterium bovis urinary tract infections; and (4) from cattle to cattle, probably in respiratory tract secretions. Moreover, M. bovis may be transmitted to cattle from wild animal reservoirs such as the bush-tailed possum in New Zealand, recognized as a major source of bovine tuberculosis, and the badger in Switzerland and Great Britain, possibly but not definitely a source of infection (11).

Between 1900 and 1930 Mycobacterium bovis was isolated from 6 to 30% of persons with tuberculosis in the United States and the United Kingdom (11,12). Declining rates of human tuberculosis caused by M. bovis have been associated with milk pasteurization and with cattle inspection programs such as those initiated in the United States in 1917 (11–13). Since 1950 M. bovis has accounted for fewer than 1% of cases of human tuberculosis in North America, though it continues to cause (occasionally fatal) human disease, most commonly in extrapulmonary sites such as cervical and mesenteric lymph nodes, the intestines, bones, and kidneys (10,14).

Mycobacterium africanum

Mycobacterium africanum, the African tubercle bacillus, first was reported and named in 1968 and 1969 by Castets and coworkers, who recovered the organism from persons in West Africa (15,16). Although M. africanum has most often been isolated from persons in Africa, the worldwide prevalence of infection with this organism is difficult to assess because it is not recognized in many laboratories or is misidentified as Mycobacterium bovis. In a large study conducted in England between 1978 and 1980 Mycobacterium africanum was recovered from about 90 of almost 7250 persons, accounting for 1 to 2% of mycobacterial isolates (17). Approximately a third of the infected persons had African names, another third European names, and the remainder Asian names, although some of the latter had lived in east Africa before moving to England. The modes of transmission, the pathogenesis, and the clinical manifestations of disease caused by M. africanum are the same as those associated with Mycobacterium tuberculosis.

NONTUBERCULOUS MYCOBACTERIA

The species of Mycobacterium other than tubercle bacilli have been called atypical mycobacteria because they differ from the tubercle bacilli; however, the terms "nontuberculous mycobacteria" and "mycobacteria other than tubercle bacilli" (MOTT) are preferred, because these organisms are not atypical, they simple have characteristics distinct from those of Mycobacterium tuberculosis.

One of the earliest classifications of the nontuberculous mycobacteria was proposed by Runyon, who recognized four groups (Table 40–2) (18). The system has limitations. For example, Mycobacterium kansasii most often is a photochromogen but may be a nonphotochromogen

Table 40–2. Runyon's Classification of the Nontuberculous Mycobacteria

Group	Description of Colonies
I. Photochromogens	Not pigmented unless exposed to light (optimally during early growth and with good aeration of surface)
II. Scotochromogens	Pigmented when grown in dark and in light
III. Nonphotochromogens	Not pigmented whether grown in dark or light
IV. Rapid growers	Grow in 7 days or less

or a scotochromogen. Isolates of Mycobacterium avium-intracellulare (MAI), classified in Runyon's group III, may be slightly pigmented, in which case they may be misclassified as a scotochromogen. Moreover, Mycobacterium szulgai is a scotochromogen at 37° C but a photochromogen at 25° C. A clinically relevant classification of the nontuberculous mycobacteria, based on their pathogenicity in humans, is used here. Species of Mycobacterium that frequently are pathogenic include MAI, Mycobacterium scrofulaceum, -kansasii, -fortuitum-chelonae complex, -xenopi, -szulgai, -malmoense, -simiae, -marinum, -haemophilum, and -ulcerans. Species that usually are saprophytes and rarely are pathogens include Mycobacterium gordonae, -asiaticum, -thermoresistible, -terrae-triviale, -nonchromogenicum, -flavescens, -shimoidei, -smegmatis, -neoaurum, and -paratuberculosis.

In general, very little is known about the antigens associated with the virulence of the nontuberculous mycobacteria; however, such antigens presumably are responsible for the persistence of the organisms within the hosts' monocyte/macrophage system. The nature of the immune response elicited in response to infection with these mycobacteria also remains ill-understood.

POTENTIAL PATHOGENS

Mycobacterium avium–Mycobacterium intracellulare

Mycobacterium avium and Mycobacterium intracellulare, initially differentiated on the basis of their virulence in chickens and rabbits, have such similar growth characteristics and biochemical reactions that they often are not distinguished in the clinical microbiology laboratory. Rather, isolates of both species are reported as MAI. The MAI complex contains at least 31 serovars, identified by seroagglutination according to species- or type-specific antigens on the cell surface of strains that form smooth colonies or by thin-layer chromatography, a sensitive procedure that separates the serovars based on the structures of these glycopeptidolipid antigens. The latter technique is especially useful for typing isolates that auto-agglutinate and the occasional stains that form rough colonies.

Epidemiology

MAI complex is the second most frequently isolated species of Mycobacterium in the United States, following Mycobacterium tuberculosis. In 1979 and 1980 M. tuberculosis accounted for approximately 70% of mycobacterial isolates and MAI for about 20% (19). The rates of isolation of MAI were highest in the eastern and western South Central regions and the South and Middle Atlantic regions, and, in contrast to previous years, persons infected with MAI did not reside predominantly in rural areas. Since the epidemic of the acquired immunodeficiency syndrome (AIDS) the percentage of isolates of MAI has increased, equaling or even surpassing the number of isolates of M. tuberculosis in some parts of the country.

The environment is the most important source of human infection and disease caused by MAI. Organisms have been isolated from soil, house dust, water (including domestic tap water supplies), dried plants, and bedding. Evidence suggests that human infection is acquired by inhaling infected aerosols or by consuming contaminated water or food; spread does not occur by direct person-to-person contact (20,21).

In the past pulmonary disease caused by MAI occurred in elderly white men who had an underlying chronic lung disease (chronic obstructive pulmonary disease, tuberculosis, bronchiectasis, pneumoconiosis, bronchogenic carcinoma) or had undergone gastrectomy. Recently, however, pulmonary disease caused by MAI has become more common in persons without predisposing factors, and in one study, among elders disease was more frequent in women than in men (22). Disseminated infection with MAI occurs almost exclusively in association with immunosuppression, and the number of such cases has increased considerably during the epidemic of AIDS. Of the 40 to 50% of persons with AIDS who are either colonized or infected with MAI, almost half develop disseminated disease (23).

In the United States serotypes 4 and 8 of Mycobacterium avium are isolated primarily from blood, indicating a disseminated infection; they are recovered most commonly from persons with AIDS; and the frequency of their recovery appears to vary with geographic location. In one study serotype 4 was the predominant isolate from persons with AIDS in New York City, in all of the eastern states as a region, and in San Francisco; serotype 8 predominated in Los Angeles; and serotypes 4 and 8 were almost evenly distributed in the western states as a region (24). Serotypes of Mycobacterium intracellulare, which accounted for a very small percentage of isolates of MAI from persons with AIDS, were recovered primarily from sputum and infrequently from blood, suggesting that strains of M. intracellulare rarely are associated with disseminated disease in these persons (24,25).

Pathogenesis and Pathology

MAI generally has low virulence and often colonizes a host without causing disease. Risk factors for disease include pre-existing pulmonary damage and cellular immune deficiency such as that associated with AIDS or with steroid therapy.

The histologic findings of lesions caused by MAI vary: caseating granulomas with acid-fast bacilli, indistinguishable from tuberculosis; pulmonary interstitial fibrosis with organizing pneumonia; necrotizing granulomatous vasculitis resembling Wegener's granulomatosis; and, especially in persons with AIDS, aggregates of foamy macrophages containing many intracellular acid-fast bacilli (Plate VIIB). In sections of gastrointestinal lesions stained with hematoxylin and eosin such lesions mimic Whipple's disease (Fig. 40–4).

Clinical Manifestations

Disease caused by MAI has a variety of clinical manifestations. Pulmonary infection may be asymptomatic, or it may progress to an illness resembling pulmonary tuberculosis. Manifestations of disseminated disease in persons

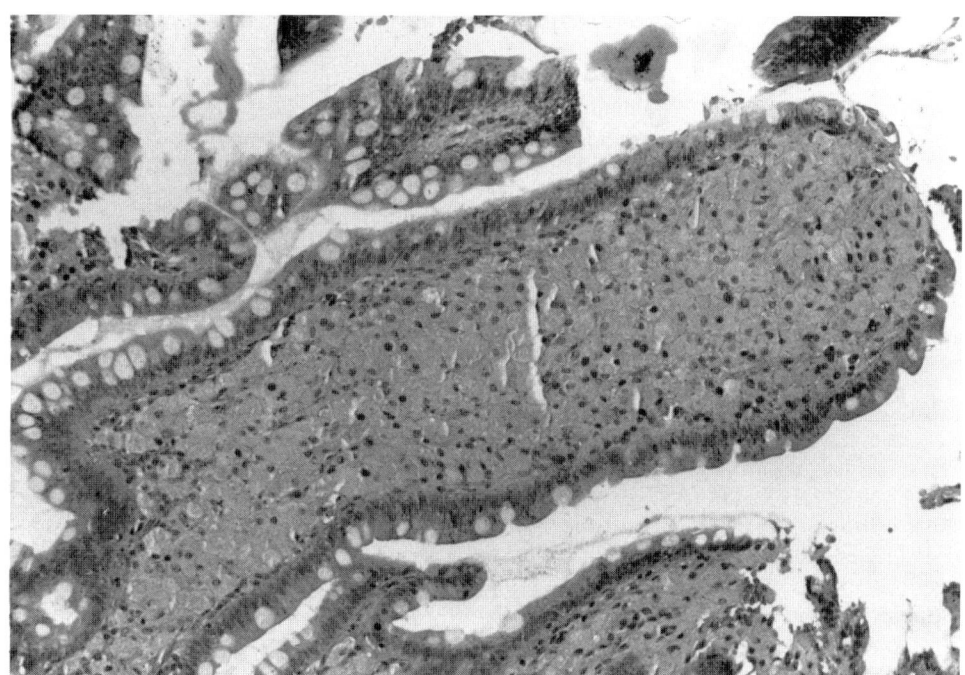

Fig. 40–4. Micrograph of biopsy specimen of the small intestine of a person with AIDS showing an aggregate of foamy macrophages (hematoxylin and eosin, ×157.5). Stool culture grew M. avium-intracellulare.

without AIDS include fever, weight loss, bone pain, lymphadenopathy, hepatosplenomegaly, and skin lesions. In those with AIDS, persistent fever and weight loss are most common; chronic diarrhea, abdominal pain, and extrahepatic obstruction are less common (5,26,27). Cervical lymphadenitis caused by MAI most often affects children, but it also may be seen in adults. Other manifestations of infection with MAI include synovitis, genitourinary tract disease, cutaneous lesions, deep infections of the hand, osteomyelitis, meningitis, ulcers of the colon, and pericarditis (28–36).

Mycobacterium scrofulaceum

Mycobacterium scrofulaceum was named in 1956, after cases of mycobacterial cervical lymphadenitis were reported in children (37). The organism is antigenically similar to MAI; and because occasional isolates identified as M. scrofulaceum by biochemical tests "serotype" as MAI and vice versa, M. scrofulaceum sometimes is classified with MAI as Mycobacterium avium-intracellulare-scrofulaceum complex (MAIS).

Mycobacterium scrofulaceum has been isolated from raw milk and other dairy products, pooled oysters, soil, and water (38). These organisms most commonly cause cervical lymphadenitis in children 1 to 5 years of age, presumably after entering the body via breaks in the skin of the extremities or mucous membranes of the oral cavity. The disease usually is unilateral, involving lymph nodes high in the neck and close to the mandible. Affected children generally appear healthy, are afebrile, and complain of minimal pain and tenderness, if any. As disease progresses the nodes soften and drain, but occasionally they heal by fibrosis and calcification. Extranodal manifestations of infection with M. scrofulaceum include pulmonary disease, disseminated disease, and, rarely, conjunctivitis, osteomyelitis, meningitis, and granulomatous hepatitis (39). Lesions of M. scrofulaceum, characterized by granulomatous inflammation with Langhans' giant cells, various degrees of caseation, and acid-fast bacilli, are histologically indistinguishable from those of Mycobacterium tuberculosis.

Mycobacterium kansasii

Epidemiology

Mycobacterium kansasii, first described in 1953 as the yellow bacillus, accounted for 3% of mycobacterial isolates in the United States in 1979 and 1980 (19,40). Most isolates were clustered in the central states: the distribution formed an inverted T by extending to include Florida and California. States reporting the highest number of isolates included California, Texas, Louisiana, Illinois, and Florida. The natural reservoir of M. kansasii is unknown, but it has been cultured from water samples (38). Pulmonary disease is most common in males 50 to 60 years of age who live in urban areas, among certain occupational groups (miners, welders, sandblasters, painters), and among persons who have pneumoconioses (especially in Europe) or chronic obstructive pulmonary disease. Disseminated disease generally affects persons with impaired cellular immunity. M. kansasii accounts for approximately 10% of mycobacterial isolates from persons with AIDS (principally those in the midwest).

Pathology

The histologic findings of lesions caused by Mycobacterium kansasii vary. Lung and lymph node tissue often show caseating granulomas. Noncaseating granulomas have been seen in synovial tissue, and skin lesions may show granulomas with areas of necrosis or foci of acute and chronic inflammation without well-formed granulomas (39). Acid-fast bacilli are common in lung and lymph node tissue but less common in tissue from other sites.

Clinical Manifestations

The most common manifestation of disease caused by Mycobacterium kansasii is chronic cavitary pulmonary disease, usually involving the upper lobes and rarely associated with pleural effusions and lymphadenopathy. M. kansasii may cause a spectrum of extrapulmonary manifestations: cervical lymphadenitis in children; cutaneous disease resembling pyogenic abscesses, cellulitis, or sporotrichosis (see Chapter 45); musculoskeletal involvement presenting as the carpal tunnel syndrome, synovitis, arthritis, tendinitis and fasciitis, or osteomyelitis; disseminated disease; isolated genitourinary tract disease; and pericarditis (39).

Mycobacterium fortuitum–Mycobacterium chelonae Complex

Mycobacterium fortuitum, once called Mycobacterium ranae, first was described and named in 1938, though the name did not become official until 1972 (41). Mycobacterium chelonae also has been called Mycobacterium friedmannii, Mycobacterium abscessus, Mycobacterium runyonii, and Mycobacterium borstelense. Three biovariants of Mycobacterium fortuitum (Mycobacterium fortuitum biovariant fortuitum, -peregrinum, and an unnamed biovariant designated "third group") and three subspecies of Mycobacterium chelonae (Mycobacterium chelonae subspecies chelonae, -abscessus, and an unnamed subspecies called Mycobacterium chelonae–like organisms) are recognized.

Epidemiology

Mycobacterium fortuitum has been isolated from soil, water, and dust, and Mycobacterium chelonae from soil, water, and sewage. Most persons infected with these organisms give a history of a penetrating injury (trauma or a surgical procedure) that might have been contaminated with soil or water. Outbreaks of infection with M. chelonae have been associated with the administration of diphtheria-pertussis-tetanus-polio vaccine, with histamine injections, with jet injector lidocaine administration, with contaminated water in intermittent peritoneal dialysate, with contaminated hemodialyzers in persons treated with hemodialysis, and with implantation of contaminated porcine heterograft valves (39,42–45).

Pathology

Lesions produced by Mycobacterium fortuitum and Mycobacterium chelonae are characterized histologically by necrosis with minimal caseation, an infiltrate of neutrophils, and granulomas with foreign body or Langhans' giant cells; occasionally lipid-laden macrophages are seen. Clumps of extracellular acid-fast bacilli are found within aggregates of neutrophils in fewer than a third of cases. In lung tissue, foamy macrophages are frequent, a pattern that resembles lipoid pneumonia.

Clinical Manifestations

Infection with Mycobacterium fortuitum and Mycobacterium chelonae results in a spectrum of diseases (38,39). Primary cutaneous disease—localized cellulitis, draining abscesses, or minimally tender nodules—occurs 3 weeks to 12 months (most often 4 to 6 weeks) after a penetrating injury in persons with an intact immune system. Osteomyelitis is an occasional complication, especially after puncture wounds to the feet. Postoperative infections, characterized by failure of the wound to heal or by breakdown of a healed wound with serous drainage in a person who has few systemic symptoms, generally develop 3 weeks to 3 months after the procedure—median sternotomy, augmentation mammaplasty, insertion of a percutaneous catheter, among others (46). Disseminated disease typically occurs in immunocompromised adults, who present with multiple, recurrent skin and soft tissue abscesses; no primary source of infection is evident. Chronic pulmonary disease resembles that caused by Mycobacterium kansasii or MAI, except cavitation is uncommon. Endocarditis involving a prosthetic valve usually becomes manifest 4 to 12 weeks after surgery. Mycobacterium fortuitum and Mycobacterium chelonae are rare causes of keratitis and corneal ulceration after trauma, and of cervical lymphadenitis in all age groups.

Mycobacterium xenopi

Epidemiology

Mycobacterium xenopi, first isolated from a toad and described in 1957, was recognized as a human pathogen in 1965 (38). It has been cultured from both hot- and cold-water taps, from hospital hot-water generators and storage tanks, and from other environmental sources (47). In Great Britain, M. xenopi is found more often in coastal than inland areas, and birds may be a natural reservoir. Most pulmonary infections caused by M. xenopi have been reported from Europe and Great Britain. In the United States it accounted for only 0.2% of mycobacterial isolates reported to the CDC in 1980, and half were reported from Connecticut, Wisconsin, and California (48). Disease has occurred only in adults, predominantly in males. Most persons have pre-existing lung damage or another predisposing condition, such as an extrapulmonary malignancy, alcoholism, diabetes mellitus, or immunosuppressive therapy (49). Nosocomial disease has been reported (50). Disseminated disease is uncommon, and only a few such cases have occurred in persons with AIDS (51–53).

Pathology

Descriptions of the histologic findings of lesions caused by Mycobacterium xenopi are limited but include nonspecific granulation tissue, epithelioid macrophages, Langhans' giant cells, and caseating granulomas containing acid-fast bacilli.

Clinical Manifestations

Pulmonary disease caused by Mycobacterium xenopi may be chronic, subacute, or acute, producing symptoms indistinguishable from those caused by Mycobacterium kansasii or MAI. Extrapulmonary infections due to Mycobacterium xenopi are uncommon and have included osteomyelitis, arthritis, lymphadenitis, and disseminated disease (38,51–53).

Mycobacterium szulgai

Mycobacterium szulgai, first recognized in 1972, is an infrequent human pathogen found worldwide, but its natural reservoir is unknown (54). The most common manifestation of infection is chronic pulmonary disease, predominantly in middle-aged men. The few reported cases of extrapulmonary disease include infections of the olecranon bursa associated with repeated trauma or with cortisone injections, extensive cutaneous disease in persons receiving corticosteroids, osteomyelitis, tenosynovitis with carpal tunnel syndrome, cervical lymphadenitis, and disseminated disease (39). Microscopically, lesions due to M. szulgai show noncaseating granulomas and granulation tissue with or without acid-fast bacilli.

Mycobacterium malmoense

Mycobacterium malmoense was reported as a new species in 1977, but its natural reservoir remains unknown (55). Most cases of human infection have been reported from England, Wales, and Sweden. Mycobacterium malmoense has been isolated in various parts of the United States, but well-documented cases of disease in humans are rare (56). The most common manifestation of infection with M. malmoense is chronic pulmonary disease, typically occurring in middle-aged men who have a pneumoconiosis; two cases of cervical lymphadenitis in children have been described (57).

Mycobacterium simiae

Mycobacterium simiae first was isolated from monkeys imported to Hungary from India in 1965 and was named in 1969 (58,59). In 1971, a "new" species of Mycobacterium isolated from the sputum of persons with pulmonary disease initially was named Mycobacterium habana, but studies later showed that it and Mycobacterium simiae were one organism (60,62). M. simiae is found in monkeys and has been recovered from tap water in hospitals. Rarely a human pathogen, it has been associated with chronic pulmonary disease, osteomyelitis, and disseminated disease (39). Microscopically, lesions show caseating granulomas with acid-fast bacilli.

Mycobacterium marinum

Mycobacterium marinum, previously called Mycobacterium platypoecilus and Mycobacterium balnei, first was described and named in 1926 by Aronson, who was investigating disease of saltwater fish. It was first recognized as a human pathogen in 1951 (63,64). Human infection with Mycobacterium marinum is acquired via trauma to the skin during contact with contaminated nonchlorinated fresh or salt water, trauma not associated with water contact, or contact with water in the absence of antecedent trauma. Typically, a single papulonodular lesion appears 2 to 3 weeks after inoculation, most often on the elbow, knee, foot, toe, or finger, and it often becomes verrucous or ulcerated. Occasionally, cutaneous disease resembles sporotrichosis (see Chapter 45). Rarely, in immunocompromised persons, cutaneous lesions become disseminated (65,66). Extracutaneous manifestations are uncommon but include synovitis, osteomyelitis, and ocular and laryngeal lesions (67–69).

Histologic examination of an early skin lesion shows neutrophil aggregates surrounded by histiocytes. Later, lymphocytes, epithelioid histiocytes, occasional Langhans' giant cells and foci of fibrinoid necrosis are seen; and in lesions present for over 6 months, aggregates of lymphocytes are found in the dermis, often surrounding blood vessels or skin appendages. Acid-fast stains usually show no acid-fast bacilli, but acid-fast bacilli that are longer and broader than bacilli of Mycobacterium tuberculosis and that often show cross-banding may be seen within histiocytes.

Mycobacterium haemophilum

Mycobacterium haemophilum first was described and named in 1978, but it probably was the noncultivable acid-fast bacillus recognized in skin ulcers in 1972 and 1974 (70–72). The organism, unique among the species of Mycobacterium in its growth requirement for hemoglobin or hemin, grows on chocolate agar, 5% sheep blood Columbia agar, Mueller-Hinton agar with Fildes supplement, and Lowenstein-Jensen medium containing 2% ferric ammonium citrate.

Human infections caused by Mycobacterium haemophilum are uncommon; fewer than 50 cases have been reported from Australia, the United States, Europe, and Canada (73–76). Most infected persons have an underlying immunodeficiency such as results from lymphoma, exogenous immunosuppression after organ transplantation, or AIDS, but a few cases of lymphadenitis have been reported in otherwise healthy children. Disease most commonly is manifested as multiple cutaneous nodules, ulcers, or painful swellings, usually involving the extremities, that increase in size and occasionally develop into abscesses and open fistulas that drain purulent material. Microscopically, lesions show foci of necrosis without caseation surrounded by a polymorphous inflammatory infiltrate with occasional Langhans' giant cells in the lower dermis. Acid-fast bacilli frequently are seen singly or in small clusters, often within cells.

Mycobacterium ulcerans

Alsop and Searls first recognized disease caused by Mycobacterium ulcerans as a clinical entity in Bairnsdale, Australia, in the 1930s, although cutaneous ulcers described by Sir Albert Cook in two persons in Uganda in 1897 probably represented the same illness (77,78).

Epidemiology

Infection caused by Mycobacterium ulcerans is endemic in areas of Zaire, Uganda, Nigeria, Ghana, Cameroon, Malaysia, New Guinea, Guyana, Mexico, and Australia that lie between latitudes 25° north and 38° south. Children 5 to 8 years old most frequently are affected, though in one study from Australia the mean age was almost 30 years, and a third of patients were 40 years or older (77). In all endemic areas disease is slightly more common in males. The natural reservoir of the organism and its usual route of transmission to humans are unknown.

Pathology

Acute infection with Mycobacterium ulcerans is characterized by necrosis and edema, especially of adipose tissue, and an infiltrate of lymphocytes, plasma cells, and macrophages. Occasional giant cells may be seen, but not caseating granulomas. Neutrophils are present only if the lesion becomes secondarily infected with other bacteria. Acid-fast bacilli occur in large clusters in areas of necrosis.

Clinical Manifestations

Eponyms for disease due to Mycobacterium ulcerans include Bairnsdale ulcer, for the area in Australia where it was first recognized, and Buruli ulcer or Buruli disease, for the area of Uganda that reports the most cases. The disease begins as one (occasionally multiple) painless, occasionally pruritic boil or subcutaneous lump on an exposed area, most frequently the leg, that may have been the site of previous trauma. After several weeks the lump becomes ulcerated and satellite nodules and ulcers may develop. Lymph nodes usually are not enlarged, and affected persons remain afebrile and without systemic symptoms unless lesions become secondarily infected with bacteria.

RARELY PATHOGENIC MYCOBACTERIA

Mycobacterium gordonae, previously called Mycobacterium aquae or the tap-water bacillus, is recovered from soil and water. It is the most commonly isolated saprophytic species of Mycobacterium, one of the species most frequently encountered in the clinical microbiology laboratory, and rarely a human pathogen. Meningitis associated with ventriculoatrial and ventriculoperitoneal shunts, hepatorenal disease, peritonitis, infection of a prosthetic aortic valve, cutaneous lesions of the hand, and possible pulmonary disease have been reported (79–82). Microscopically, caseating or noncaseating granulomas may be seen; acid-fast bacilli are observed infrequently.

Mycobacterium asiaticum, first isolated from healthy monkeys in 1965 and named and described as a new species in 1971, has rarely been associated with chronic cavitary pulmonary disease (83). Mycobacterium thermoresistible, a rapidly growing Mycobacterium isolated from soil, has the unique ability to grow at 52° C. Three cases of disease in humans have been reported: two pulmonary infections and one cutaneous infection in a recipient of a heart transplant (84,85). Mycobacterium terrae-triviale complex includes Mycobacterium terrae and Mycobacterium triviale. Mycobacterium terrae was first isolated in 1950 from the washings of a radish (hence the name "radish bacillus"), and subsequently it was cultured from soil and other vegetables (86). Infections in humans caused by these organisms have included septic arthritis, synovitis and osteomyelitis, and possibly disseminated disease (87–89).

Primary pulmonary disease caused by Mycobacterium nonchromogenicum, Mycobacterium flavescens, or Mycobacterium shimoidei is rare (90–93). Mycobacterium smegmatis, an organism isolated from the soil, recently has been recognized as a potential human pathogen, causing skin and soft tissue infections (94). One case of human infection—bacteremia in an immunocompromised person with an indwelling Hickman catheter—caused by Mycobacterium neoaurum, a rapidly growing organism isolated from soil, dust, and water, has been reported (95). Mycobacterium paratuberculosis has been implicated as a possible agent of Crohn's disease; however, further research is needed for confirmation (96). Recently, a fatal disseminated infection with a novel, as yet unidentified Mycobacterium was described in a man with AIDS (97).

MYCOBACTERIUM LEPRAE

Mycobacterium leprae, the agent of leprosy (also called Hansen's disease), does not belong to the Mycobacterium tuberculosis complex and, therefore, could be considered one of the nontuberculous mycobacteria. It is discussed separately because it has unique characteristics. Leprosy was common in Europe during the Middle Ages and may have been transported to the western hemisphere by explorers during the fifteenth century. The pathogen was first seen in unstained wet preparations of tissue fluid from the skin of a person with leprosy more than 100 years ago by Hansen, in Norway. M. leprae has not been cultivated, but useful models of infection in animals exist. The mouse foot pad model, developed in 1960, offered a means to quantitate growth of the organism; and in 1971 the nine-banded armadillo was recognized as a susceptible host for M. leprae; thus large quantities of the organism were available for immunologic and microbiologic studies.

Epidemiology

Mycobacterium leprae has been recognized in nearly every part of the world at some time, but its geographic origin is unknown. Of the estimated 10 to 15 million persons in the world who have leprosy, approximately 62% are in Asia and 34% in Africa (98,99). In the United States about 6000 persons have leprosy, most of whom are immigrants, though some are natives of the Gulf Coast states, California, and Hawaii (100–102).

Leprosy predominantly affects humans but also is a natural infection of wild armadillos in Louisiana and Texas, and spontaneous cases have been described in mangabey monkeys (103,104). The mechanism of transmission of Mycobacterium leprae is unknown, but the favored theory is person-to-person spread via aerosolization of organisms from the nose of a person with active lepromatous disease (described later) which then contact the nasal mucosa of another individual (105). Transmission also may occur through intact skin or via penetrating wounds, such as a thorn stick or the bite of an arthropod. Breast milk from lactating women with lepromatous disease contains organisms that may be transmitted to infants, and transplacental transmission of M. leprae is possible. The association between leprosy and contact with armadillos is unclear, but cases of human leprosy following such contact have been reported (106,107). Moreover, the discovery of a naturally occurring leprosy-like disease among armadillos, and the fact that many sporadic cases of leprosy occur in persons who have no known contact with human leprosy, suggest that nonhuman sources of M. leprae may exist (108).

Most persons effectively resist infection with Mycobacterium leprae. Genetic factors may enhance the susceptibility of a person to leprosy or influence the form of disease that develops. For example, persons who have the HLA-DR2 or HLA-DR3 haplotype, or both, may be predisposed to tuberculoid leprosy (described below), and the prevalence of DR2-DQW1 may be greater among persons who have lepromatous leprosy (109–111). Moreover, lepromatous leprosy accounts for 30 to 50% of cases of leprosy among whites and among orientals of Japan, China, and Korea, whereas up to 90% of cases in Africa are tuberculoid (105).

Pathogenesis

Resistance to infection with Mycobacterium leprae depends on the ability of the infected host to mount an effective cell-mediated immune response to M. leprae antigens, as occurs in tuberculoid leprosy. In persons who lack specific cell-mediated immunity to these antigens, continuous multiplication of the organisms within macrophages eventually results in widely disseminated lepromatous leprosy. The defect in cellular immunity, which may involve T-lymphocyte function or the interaction of T lymphocytes with macrophages, appears to be specific for antigens to M. leprae rather than a generalized phenomenon, because persons with lepromatous leprosy have normal ratios of CD4 (helper or inducer) and CD8 (suppressor or cytotoxic) T lymphocytes in the peripheral blood and are not at increased risk of developing cancer or infections with opportunistic pathogens commonly associated with immunocompromised hosts (105). The total number of circulating T lymphocytes is decreased in persons with lepromatous leprosy, but the distribution of circulating CD4 and CD8 cells is not significantly altered. In the skin lesions of lepromatous leprosy the ratio of helper to suppressor T cells is decreased (0.5:1) and T lymphocytes are admixed with macrophages (112–114). The helper-suppressor T-cell ratio in lesions of tuberculoid leprosy remains normal (about 2:1), and helper and suppressor T cells, respectively, are found in the center and in the mantle of the granuloma. The explanation for this difference is not known.

Failure of the macrophages from persons with lepromatous leprosy to kill or inhibit Mycobacterium leprae suggests a possible defect in macrophage function. Production of cytokines that modulate the cellular immune response (see Chapter 2) may be defective, and macrophages may be refractory to activation by interferon γ (105,115). The latter is important because activated macrophages are believed to play a major role in resistance to many obligate and facultative intracellular pathogens. Because M. leprae is an intracellular pathogen, antibodies probably are not involved in resistance to infection, but they may play a role in the pathogenesis of erythema nodosum leprosum reactions by forming antigen-antibody complexes (116).

Clinical Manifestations

The lesions of leprosy, which vary in appearance depending on the immune response of the host to the organism, develop after a 2- to 5-year incubation period. Leprosy always involves peripheral nerves, almost always involves the skin, and frequently involves the mucous membranes. The three cardinal signs of the disease are skin lesions, areas of cutaneous anesthesia, and enlarged peripheral nerves. The system outlined by Ridey and Jopling (presented below) is used most often to classify the spectrum of clinical and histopathologic forms of leprosy determined by the immune response of the host (117).

Indeterminate leprosy, the earliest sign of the disease, is characterized by one or a few hypopigmented skin macules associated with minimal local sensory loss. Microscopically, the lesions show lymphocytes and histiocytes around skin appendages and nerves, resembling chronic dermatitis, and few or no acid-fast bacilli. The disease heals spontaneously in about 75% of affected persons, some cases long remain indeterminate, and some progress to one of the established forms of leprosy.

The polar types of leprosy—lepromatous leprosy, the widespread anergic form of the disease, and tuberculoid leprosy, the localized form—are stable clinically. Lepromatous leprosy is characterized by cutaneous lesions that range from diffuse generalized skin involvement to widespread, symmetrically distributed nodules (lepromas) that contain as many as 10^{10} organisms per gram of tissue. Lesions typically involve the cooler parts of the body surface, such as the anterior third of the eye, the nasal mucosa, and the superficial peripheral nerve trunks, and in advanced disease they are accompanied by sensory loss due to involvement of dermal nerve fibers. Microscopically, lesions show foamy histiocytes containing many acid-fast bacilli, few or no lymphocytes, no significant intraneural inflammation, and many bacilli in nerves, the perineurium, blood vessel walls, and arrector muscles (Fig. 40–5A).

The clinical manifestations of tuberculoid leprosy result

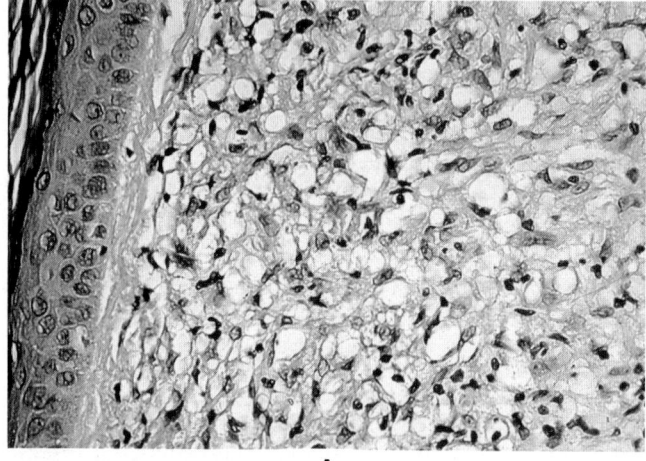

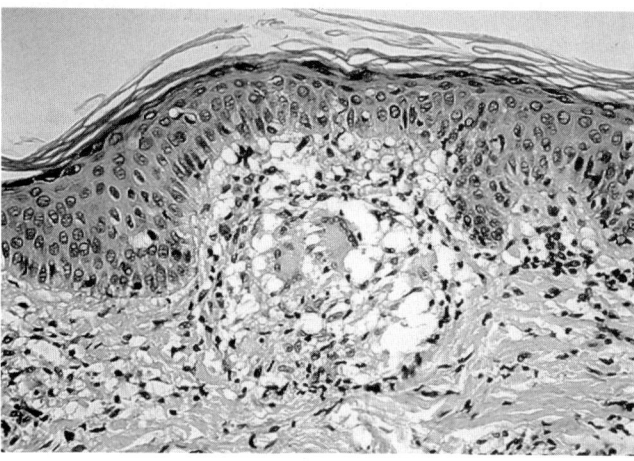

Fig. 40–5. A, Micrograph of a section of a lesion of lepromatous leprosy shows many foamy histocytes in the dermis (hematoxylin and eosin, ×100). B, Section of a lesion of tuberculoid leprosy shows a well-formed granuloma with giant cells in the dermis (hematoxylin and eosin, ×62.5).

from bacterial proliferation plus the host immune response. One or several well-circumscribed anesthetic macules or plaques develop, often accompanied by an enlarged peripheral nerve near the skin lesions. Histologically, lesions demonstrate granulomas composed of epithelioid histiocytes, lymphocytes, and often Langhans' giant cells in the nerves and dermis, extending to involve the basal layer of the epidermis, and few, if any, acid-fast bacilli (Fig. 40–5B).

Borderline leprosy is a clinically unstable condition that encompasses the intermediate types of disease. An individual with borderline leprosy may develop features that more closely resemble tuberculoid disease, a process termed upgrading, or features that resemble lepromatous disease, a process called downgrading. Borderline tuberculoid leprosy resembles tuberculoid disease except that lesions are larger, more numerous, and have less distinct borders; satellite lesions sometimes develop; immune-mediated damage to the peripheral nerves is more widespread and more severe; and microscopically, granulomas do not involve the basal layer of the epidermis and acid-fast bacilli frequently are found in nerves. Borderline lepromatous leprosy resembles polar lepromatous leprosy except that some skin lesions are selectively anesthetic and have more distinct borders; peripheral nerve trunk involvement is more widespread; mucous membranes are involved less extensively; and on histologic examination skin lesions contain more lymphocytes and fewer acid-fact bacilli, though more than a borderline tuberculoid lesion.

About half of leprosy patients experience clinically apparent immune-mediated reactions. Type 1, or reversal reactions, are due to delayed hypersensitivity and typically involve peripheral nerves of persons with borderline to tuberculoid leprosy. These reactions are characterized by edema and erythema in pre-existing lesions and a tendency for the overall disease to upgrade. Type 2, or erythema nodosum leprosum, lesions are manifestations of an Arthus type hypersensitivity reaction characterized by fever and crops of tender, erythematous skin nodules involving any tissue of persons with borderline lepromatous or lepromatous leprosy that contains antigens of Mycobacterium leprae, especially the skin, eyes, joints, and nasal mucosa.

Laboratory Diagnosis

Different methods are used to diagnose infection with mycobacteria. Skin tests generally are not administered or interpreted by laboratory personnel, but because the test is used diagnostically the medical director of the microbiology laboratory may be asked about appropriate administration and interpretation. Therefore, the skin test reagents, their administration, and the interpretation of the test are discussed. Infection with mycobacteria is confirmed by detecting the organism.

Skin Testing

The tuberculin skin test is useful for identifying persons infected with Mycobacterium tuberculosis complex because they develop a hypersensitivity reaction to proteins of the bacilli. The skin test reagent—purified protein derivative (PPD)—is a protein precipitate of old tuberculin (Koch's tuberculin). The large lot of protein produced by Seibert in 1939 was adopted as the biologic activity reference standard (PPD-S). PPD-S should be stored in the refrigerator in the dark, to retain its potency.

The preferred method of skin testing, the Mantoux test, is performed by injecting 0.1 ml of intermediate-strength (5 tuberculin units [TU]) PPD-S intracutaneously. For children, first-strength (1 TU) PPD-S should be used. The reaction is interpreted after 48 to 72 hours by measuring the diameter of induration in millimeters (118); 5 mm or more is a positive result in persons infected with HIV, those who have had recent close contact with someone who has infectious tuberculosis, and those who have chest x-rays consistent with old healed tuberculosis. A reaction of 10 mm or more is positive in persons who do not meet the above criteria but who have other risk factors for tuberculosis, e.g., persons born in Asia, Africa, or Latin America where the prevalence of tuberculosis is high; intravenous drug users; medically underserved, low-income populations (especially racial or ethnic minorities); residents of long-term care facilities; and persons who have a medical condition associated with an increased risk of tuberculosis (e.g., silicosis, gastrectomy, jejunoileal bypass, 10% or more below ideal body weight, chronic renal failure, diabetes mellitus, treatment with large doses of corticosteroids or with other immunosuppressive drugs, and malignancies). A reaction of 15 mm or more is positive in all other persons.

False-positive Mantoux test reactions result from infection with nontuberculous mycobacteria. False-negative reactions may be due to poor technique, such as injecting into the deep layers of the skin, or improper storage of the reagent. If the test is administered appropriately, false-negative reactions are uncommon in relatively healthy persons but occur in up to 20% of persons known to have tuberculosis when they are first tested. Most of these false-negative reactions are attributed to the general illness and revert to positive after 2 to 3 weeks' therapy, when health is restored. Factors that cause a state of general anergy, such as protein malnutrition, concurrent viral infection, sarcoidosis, malignancy (especially lymphoma), immunosuppressive or corticosteroid therapy, or infection with HIV, also may cause a false-negative tuberculin reaction. To detect anergy, skin testing for mumps and candida antigens should be performed simultaneously with the Mantoux test.

In general, the Mantoux test result remains positive as long as viable bacilli persist in quiescent foci. However, with increasing age the reaction may wane below the positive criterion, a phenomenon most common after age 55 years. If this, indeed, happens, the reaction will be boosted (or become positive) if a second test is performed as soon as a week after the first test, a reaction termed the booster effect.

Skin test reagents prepared from species of Mycobacterium other than Mycobacterium tuberculosis include purified protein derivative-A (Mycobacterium avium), PPD-B (Mycobacterium intracellulare), PPD-F (Mycobacterium fortuitum), PPD-G (Mycobacterium scrofulaceum), and PPD-Y (Mycobacterium kansasii). In the United States these reagents at one time were available from the CDC; however this service was discontinued because the antigens were not standardized and the skin reactions were difficult to interpret. In one study of persons with pulmonary disease, skin test profiles of PPD-S and five other mycobacterial antigens "agreed" with the etiologic agent of the infection determined by culture; and in children dual testing with PPD-S and PPD-B has permitted differentiation between tuberculous and nontuberculous lymphadenitis (119–123).

The lepromin test—intradermal injection of lepromin, a heat-killed suspension of Mycobacterium leprae obtained from homogenized human leproma or infected armadillo tissue—is used to establish a person's immune status for M. leprae. The test has prognostic, but not diagnostic, value. Typically, the reaction has two components. The early Fernandez reaction is a delayed hypersensitivity reaction that occurs at 24 to 48 hours in persons with tuberculoid leprosy and in contacts or healthy persons who are sensitized to M. leprae or cross-reacting antigens from other mycobacteria. The late Mitsuda reaction, measured at 21 days, reflects the cell-mediated immune response to M. leprae. It is positive (greater than 5 mm) in persons with tuberculoid leprosy and most of their contacts, and in persons never exposed to M. leprae; intermediate (3 to 5 mm) in persons with borderline disease; and negative (<2 mm) in persons with lepromatous leprosy, indicating no cell-mediated immunity to M. leprae.

Organism Identification

Identification of infection with mycobacteria requires obtaining an appropriate specimen. Specimens recommended for diagnosis are listed in Table 40–3, and their collection, transport, and processing are discussed in Part III. Microbial stains, culture techniques, susceptibility testing, and new methods of detection and identification are reviewed here.

Microbial Stains. In smears stained with the Gram stain, mycobacteria (except Mycobacterium haemophilum, which does not stain by the Gram method) appear as slender, poorly stained, beaded gram-positive bacilli, but sometimes the bacilli do not take up the crystal violet or safranin and appear "gram-neutral" (Gram ghosts) (124). All specimens collected from persons with suspected mycobacterial infection should be examined microscopically for the presence of acid-fast bacilli. If acid-fast bacilli are to be seen more than 10,000 organisms per milliliter of specimen must be present; therefore, a negative result does not rule out the presence of mycobacteria.

Two types of stains detect acid-fast bacilli: carbol fuchsin stains—the classic Ziehl-Neelsen stain (see Appendix, Procedure 4), which requires heating, and the cold Kinyoun's stain (see Appendix, Procedure 5)—and the fluorochromic auramine-rhodamine (see Appendix, Procedure 6) and rhodamine stain. If a fluorescence microscope is available, using a fluorochromic stain to screen smears is recommended, because such stains are more sensitive and easier to read, and smears may be examined at lower magnification (25 and 400×), allowing visualization of more fields in less time. Because cells of the Mycobacterium fortuitum-chelonae complex stain poorly with fluorochromic stains and, so, often are not detected, when these organisms are suspected (for example, in cases of postsurgical wound infections) restaining negative fluorescent smears with the Ziehl-Neelson or Kinyon's stain is recommended to confirm the result. Smears stained with the Ziehl-Neelsen or Kinyon stain should be examined at 800 to 1000× magnification (oil immersion) and reported after viewing 100 fields, according to the guidelines of the American Lung Association (Table 40–4), indicating whether the smear was prepared directly from the specimen or after concentration (see Appendix, Procedure 27, and Chapter 57) (125).

Acid-fast bacilli are purple to red, slightly curved, short or long rods (2 to 8 μm), occasionally beaded or banded (Plate ID). In general the appearance of an acid-fast bacillus does not identify the species of Mycobacterium; however, cells of certain species have features that may be useful diagnostically. For example, cells of Mycobacterium kansasii often appear as cross-barred bacilli larger than Mycobacterium tuberculosis (Plate IE). Cells of MAI typically are pleomorphic, occasionally coccobacillary, and, unique among mycobacteria, stain positively with the periodic acid-Schiff (PAS) stain. Cells of Mycobacterium marinum typically are longer and broader than those of Mycobacterium tuberculosis and often show cross-banding.

Table 40–3. Mycobacterial Infections and Specimens for Diagnosis

Site of Infection	Mycobacterium Species*	Specimens†
Lung	M. tuberculosis, -kansasii, MAI, M. xenopi, -szulgai, -malmoense, -simiae	Sputum, BAL, gastric contents, lung tissue, (pleural fluid)
Lymph node	M. tuberculosis, MAI, M. scrofulaceum	Lymph node aspirate or biopsy
Skin, soft tissue	M. ulcerans, -fortuitum-chelonae, -marinum, -haemophilum	Aspirate or biopsy of lesion
	M. leprae	Smears of nasal secretions and skin slits, biopsy of lesion
Musculoskeletal system	M. tuberculosis, -fortuitum-chelonae, -marinum	Joint fluid, synovium, bone
Nervous system	M. tuberculosis	CSF, brain tissue
	M. leprae	Peripheral nerve biopsy
Genitourinary tract	M. tuberculosis	Urine, involved tissue, kidney, endometrium, fallopian tube, prostate, seminal vesicles, epididymis
Gastrointestinal tract	M. tuberculosis, MAI	Tissue, feces
Peritoneal cavity	M. tuberculosis	Peritoneal biopsy tissue, (peritoneal fluid)
Liver	M. tuberculosis, MAI	Liver tissue
Pericardium	M. tuberculosis	Pericardium, (pericardial fluid)
Several organs	M. tuberculosis, MAI	Blood, bone marrow, involved tissue

* Species listed are those most frequently involved; see text for less common organisms.
† Specimens in parentheses are infrequently positive.
Key: MAI, M. avium-intracellulare complex; BAL, bronchoalveolar lavage; CSF, cerebrospinal fluid.

Table 40–4. Reporting of Smears Stained for Acid-Fast Bacilli

Organisms Observed (No.)	Report
0	Negative
1–2/300 fields	Number seen*
1–9/100 fields	Average no./100 fields
1–9/10 fields	Average no./10 fields
1–9/field	Average no./field
>9/field	>9/field

* Another specimen should be requested.
(Modified from American Thoracic Society: Diagnostic standards and classification of tuberculosis and other mycobacterial diseases. Am Rev Respir Dis, 123:343, 1981.)

Culture. For conventional culture of the mycobacteria two different types of media are available: egg-based media such as Lowenstein-Jensen, American Thoracic Society, Petragnani, and Wallenstein's medium, and clear agar-based media such as Middlebrook 7H10 and Middlebrook 7H11. If conventional culture is the only method used to recover mycobacteria, inoculation of at least one egg-based and one agar-based medium with each specimen is recommended. Of the egg-based media, Lowenstein-Jensen usually is preferred. Petragnani and Wallenstein's medium contain glycerol to support the growth of the nontuberculous mycobacteria and an increased amount of malachite green, which inhibits contaminants, and to some extent the mycobacteria also. Middlebrook 7H11 is the preferred agar medium because it contains 0.1% casein hydrolysate, which improves the recovery rate of isoniazid-resistant strains of Mycobacterium tuberculosis. For specimens contaminated with normal bacterial flora a minimum of one selective medium, such as selective Lowenstein-Jensen, the Gruft modification of Lowenstein-Jensen, or selective 7H11, each containing various concentrations of different antimicrobial agents, also should be inoculated. Sterile body fluids (cerebrospinal fluid, joint fluid, pleural fluid, peritoneal fluid) should be inoculated to solid media and to Dubos albumin or Middlebrook 7H9 broth for enrichment. All cultures should be incubated at 35° to 37°C in 5 to 10% carbon dioxide for 8 weeks. The colony appearance (shown for the most commonly encountered mycobacteria in Plates VIIC–F and VIIIA) and growth characteristics of the cultivable species of Mycobacterium are outlined in Table 40–5.

The time to detection of mycobacteria can be decreased from an average of 17 days by conventional culture to an average of 10 days by using a commercially available radiometric broth culture system (126–128). A special broth medium (one bottle per specimen) is inoculated with digested, decontaminated specimens (see Chapter 57) and with specimens from sterile body sites. To all cultures a mixture of antimicrobial agents (provided by the manufacturer) is added, and bottles are incubated in ambient air at 37°C for 6 to 8 weeks. Bacilli multiply in the broth and utilize metabolites containing carbon-14. The $^{14}CO_2$ released into the atmosphere above the broth in the bottle is measured by an instrument, and a "growth index" is calculated. An index greater than 10 suggests that mycobacteria are present.

When the growth index reaches 50 to 100, a smear of the broth should be stained with an acid-fast stain. If acid-fast bacilli are present, a volume of broth (the volume used varies according to the growth index) is injected into two fresh bottles of medium, one of which contains *p*-nitro-acetyl-amino-β-hydroxypropiophenone (NAP), and both bottles are reincubated and monitored on the instrument daily for 4 to 5 days. An increase in the growth index in the bottle without NAP and no increase in the growth index in the bottle containing NAP indicates the presence of a member of the Mycobacterium tuberculosis complex, because only Mycobacterium tuberculosis, Mycobacterium bovis, and Mycobacterium africanum are susceptible

Table 40–5. Colony Morphology and Growth Characteristics of the Cultivable Species of Mycobacterium

Species	Colony		Growth	
	Morphology	Pigment	Rate*	Temperature (°C)
M. tuberculosis	Rough	N (buff)	Slow	31–37
M. bovis	Rough; thin or transparent	N (colorless to buff)	Slow	37
M. africanum	Rough	N	Slow	37
M. avium-intracellulare	Smooth; small, thin, transparent or large, opaque, domed; ±rough	N; may be lightly pigmented	Slow; up to 8 wk	37 optimal; 25, ±45
M. scrofulaceum	Smooth, globoid	S; light yellow to deep orange	Slow	25–37
M. kansasii	Rough; β-carotene crystals	P (rarely N or S)	Slow	25–37
M. fortuitum-chelonae	Smooth or rough	N (buff)	Rapid	25–40
M. xenopi	Smooth, filamentous extensions	S	Slow	42–43 optimal, 37
M. szulgai	Smooth or rough	S at 37°C; P at 25°C	Slow	25–37
M. malmoense	Smooth, dysgonic	Colorless	Moderate	25–37
M. simiae	Smooth	P†	Slow	37
M. marinum	Wrinkled, shiny; smooth, hemispherical; (rarely) rough, dry	P	Moderate	31–33 optimal
M. haemophilum	Rough; ±smooth	N	Slow	20–32 optimal
M. gordonae	Smooth	S; orange	Slow	25–37
M. asiaticum	ND	P	Slow	25–37
M. thermoresistible	Smooth or rough	P (yellow-orange becoming brown)	Rapid	25–52, (37–45 optimal)
M. terrae-triviale	Smooth (M. terrae) rough (M. triviale)	N	Slow	25–37
M. nonchromogenicum	Intermediate in roughness	N	Slow	25–37
M. flavescens	Smooth	S	Moderate	25–37
M. smegmatis	Rough; ±smooth	N (buff)	Rapid	25–45
M. shimoidei	Rough	N	Slow	37

* Average growth rate on solid medium: slow, 4 to 6 weeks; moderate, 2 to 3 weeks; rapid, 5 to 7 days.
† Pigment production often requires prolonged exposure to light.
Key: N, nonphotochromogen; S, scotochromogen; P, photochromogen (see text); ND, not well described in the literature.

to NAP. A portion of broth medium from positive cultures also should be subcultured to a solid medium, because identification of many mycobacteria requires biochemical testing of isolated colonies. To decrease the time to colony growth, inoculating the original specimen to either Middlebrook 7H11 or Lowenstein-Jensen medium in addition to the broth used with the radiometric culture system is recommended.

A biphasic mycobacterial culture system consisting of a broth medium and agar media on a paddle, similar to the biphasic blood culture system described in Chapter 58, recently became commercially available (129). The broth is inoculated with the specimen, the paddle is attached to the top of the bottle, and the system is incubated 6 to 8 weeks at 35° to 37° C in 5 to 7% carbon dioxide. At regular intervals the broth is subcultured to the media on the paddle by tipping the bottle and allowing the broth to cover the surfaces of the agar.

Identification of the mycobacteria by conventional methods is a time-consuming process based on the growth rate of the isolate, pigment production, and various biochemical reactions (described in detail in references 124 and 130). A simplified approach to identification of the species most commonly encountered in the clinical microbiology laboratory is shown in Figures 40–6, 40–7, 40–8, and 40–9 (131). Commercially available DNA probes provide rapid identification (less than 1 hour) of colonies of Mycobacterium tuberculosis complex, Mycobacterium avium, Mycobacterium intracellulare, and Mycobacterium gordonae (132–135). The probes for Mycobacterium tuberculosis complex, Mycobacterium avium, and Mycobacterium intracellulare also have been used in combination with the radiometric detection system to identify these organisms directly in broth samples from bottles containing acid-fast bacilli, thus significantly shortening the time to identification (136). However, currently the probes cannot be used to detect mycobacteria directly in clinical specimens.

Susceptibility Testing. Currently, susceptibility testing should be performed for all isolates of Mycobacterium tuberculosis, given the recent outbreaks of disease caused by strains resistant to multiple antituberculosis drugs (136a). These outbreaks have occurred in prisons and in hospitals in New York State and in Florida, and most affected persons have been infected with HIV.

Susceptibility testing may be performed on isolates of the nontuberculous mycobacteria, though for some species results do not correlate completely with the clinical response. Isolates of MAI typically are resistant to conventional antituberculosis drugs, so susceptibility to agents such as clofazamine, amikacin, and perhaps ciprofloxacin should be evaluated. Moreover, when testing isolates of MAI, transparent colonies should be selected because organisms that form these colonies are more virulent than those that produce opaque colonies (124). Some infections with Mycobacterium fortuitum and Mycobacterium chelonae respond to surgical drainage or debridement, whereas others require antimicrobial therapy. These organisms also are resistant to the conventional antitubercu-

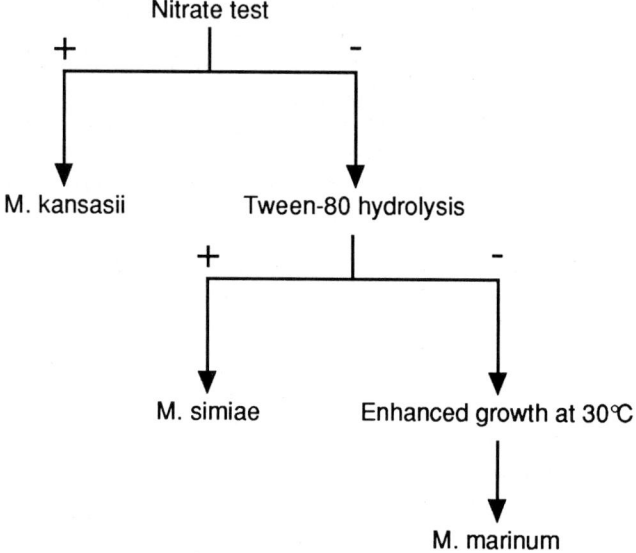

Fig. 40–7. Decision tree for identifying the photochromogenic mycobacteria. (From Roberts GD: Mycobacteria and Nocardia. *In* Laboratory Procedures in Clinical Microbiology. 2nd ed. Edited by JA Washington II. New York, Springer-Verlag, 1985.)

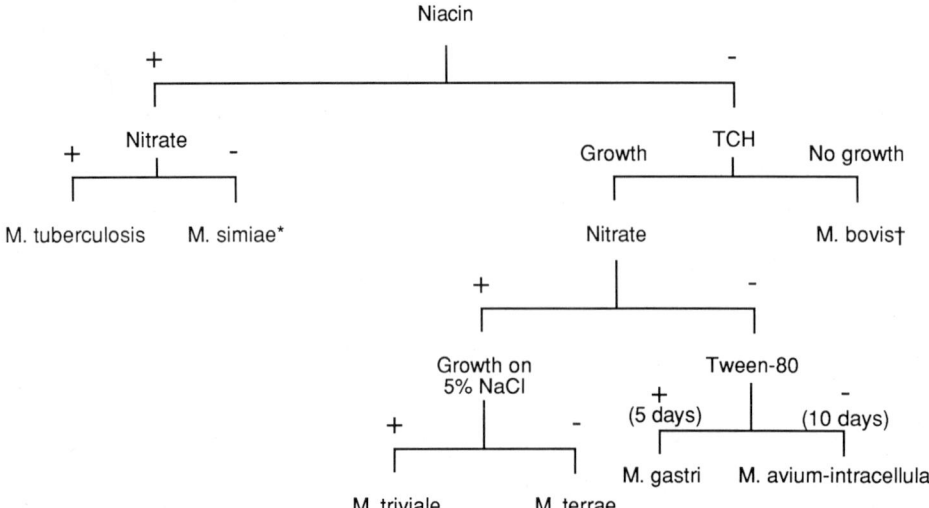

Fig. 40–6. Decision tree for identifying the nonphotochromogenic mycobacteria. Note that M. simiae* usually is a photochromogen, but this feature is unstable and may become apparent only after prolonged exposure to light. Some strains of M. bovis† give a positive niacin reaction.

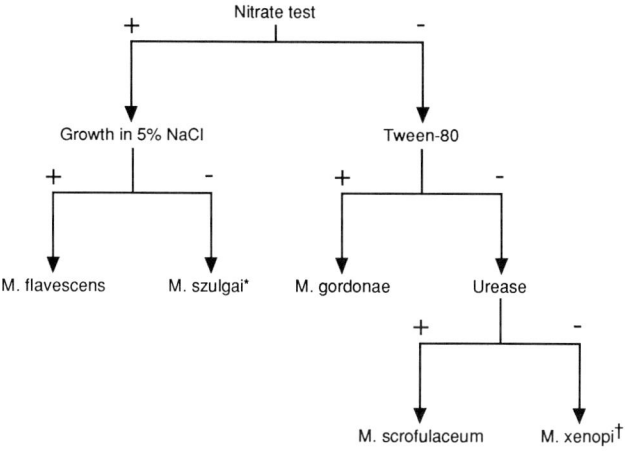

Fig. 40–8. Decision tree for identifying the common scotochromogenic mycobacteria. M. szulgai* is a photochromogen at 25° C and a scotochromogen at 35° C. M. xenopi† grows at 42° C. (From Roberts GD: Mycobacteria and Nocardia. In Laboratory Procedures in Clinical Microbiology. 2nd ed. Edited by JA Washington II. New York, Springer-Verlag, 1985.)

losis drugs, and susceptibility tests for doxycycline, amikacin, erythromycin, cefoxitin, a sulfonamide, and perhaps for imipenem, ciprofloxacin, and tobramycin, should be performed (124).

The proportion method (described in detail in references 123 and 128), a modified agar dilution test, is the conventional method used to evaluate susceptibility of the mycobacteria to typical antituberculosis agents. This technique most commonly is used to test isolates of mycobacteria (indirect susceptibility testing), but it may be modified to directly test specimens known to be positive for acid-fast bacilli by smear. The report should indicate whether the test was direct or indirect, the number of colonies on the control (without drug) quadrant and on each drug quadrant, and the concentration of drug tested. An approximation of the percentage of organisms that are resistant to the drug is calculated with the following formula:

$$\text{Resistance (\%)} = \frac{\text{Colonies on drug quadrant (no.)}}{\text{Colonies on control quadrant (no.)}}$$

Isolates that show greater than 1% resistance are considered resistant to that concentration of drug. Alternative methods of susceptibility testing include broth dilution; radiometric growth detection (approved from Mycobacterium tuberculosis only), and for isolates of the Mycobacterium fortuitum-chelonae complex, agar dilution, disk diffusion, broth microdilution, or agar disk elution may be used (137).

New Methods for Detection and Identification of Mycobacteria. Given the need for a sensitive and specific method that allows rapid detection of mycobacteria, various techniques have been evaluated as potential diagnostic tests. Thin-layer chromatography and gas-liquid chromatography have been used successfully to identify isolates of mycobacteria, but these techniques are labor intensive and require special equipment (138,139). Enzyme-linked immunosorbent assays (ELISA) that detect mycobacterial antigens and antibodies have been evaluated as diagnostic methods for pulmonary and meningeal infections with Mycobacterium tuberculosis; and although the techniques are promising, currently they are research tools only (140,141). Detection of tuberculostearic acid, a structural component of mycobacteria not normally present in human tissues, by gas chromatography and mass spectrometry is a rapid, sensitive, and specific test for diagnosing tuberculosis, but it does not distinguish among the species of Mycobacterium and it requires expensive and complex equipment (142). Preliminary data indicate that gene amplification using the polymerase chain reaction may become a useful method for early and rapid diagnosis of infections with M. tuberculosis and with Mycobacterium leprae (143–145).

Treatment

Chemotherapeutic regimens commonly used to treat infections caused by mycobacteria are listed in Table 40–6. For many of the nontuberculosis mycobacteria the optimal duration of therapy has not been determined, but the times listed in the table have proven successful for some investigators (38,39,146,147).

Prevention

Mycobacterium tuberculosis. Four general strategies for controlling tuberculosis are available (148). (1) Early identification and treatment of persons with infec-

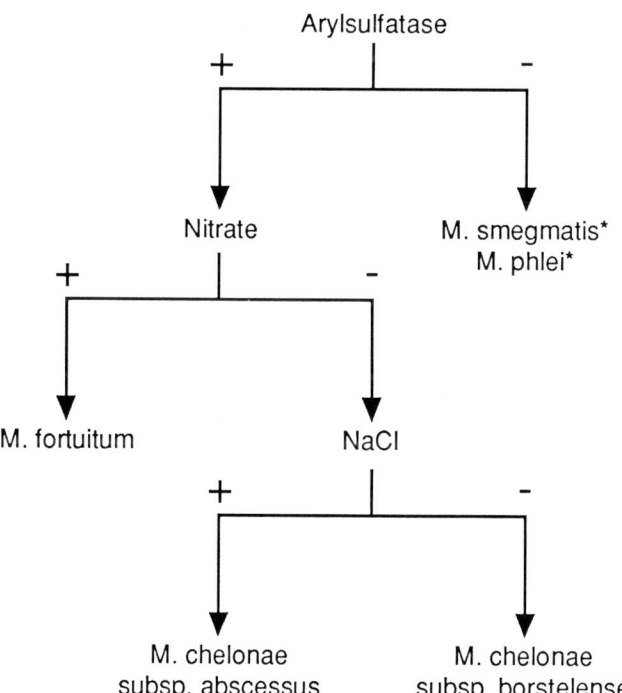

Fig. 40–9. Decision tree for identifying the clinically significant rapidly growing mycobacteria. Asterisk indicates need for additional biochemical testing for differentiation. (From Roberts GD: Mycobacteria and Nocardia. In Laboratory Procedures in Clinical Microbiology. 2nd ed. Edited by JA Washington II. New York, Springer-Verlag, 1985.)

Table 40-6. Chemotherapy for Infections with Pathogenic Myocbacteria

Species	Therapy		
	Surgery	Agents	Duration (mo)*
M. tuberculosis	−	INH, RIF, & PZA†	6
M. avium-intracellulare			
pulmonary	±	INH, RIF, EMB & SM	18–24
disseminated	−	INH, RIF, EMB, SM, & CLF‡	(24–48)
M. scrofulaceum			
lymphadenitis	+	—	
disseminated	−	INH, SM, RIF, & CS	(18–24)
M. kansasii	−	INH, RIF, & EMB	18
M. fortuitum-chelonae	+	AM & either TET, CFX, or RIF	1–2 after clinical response
M. xenopi	±	INH, RIF, & either EMB or SM	(>9)
M. szulgai	−	INH, RIF, & EMB	(18–24)
M. malmoense	±	INH, RIF, & EMB	(≥12)
M. simiae	−	INH, RIF, & EMB	(18–24)
M. marinum	±	RIF alone; RIF & EMB; or TET alone	18; or 1–2 after clinical resolution
M. haemophilium	±	INH, RIF, & EMB	?
M. ulcerans	+	INH & SM; DAP & TET	?
M. leprae	−	DAP, CLF, & RIF	24–36

* Numbers in parentheses have been suggested, but the optimal duration has not been established.
† PZA is given only for the first 2 months. If the person is also infected with HIV, INH is given for a minimum of 1 year. Additional drugs (e.g., SM, EMB) are given for isolates resistant to INH.
‡ Ciprofloxacin and amikacin also may be considered.
Key: INH, isoniazid; RIF, rifampin; PZA, pyrazinamide; EMB, ethambutol; SM, streptomycin; CLF, clofazamine; CS, cycloserine; AM, amikacin; TET; tetracycline; CFX, cefoxitin; DAP, dapsone; ?, unknown, −, not indicated; +, definitely indicated; ±, may be indicated; HIV, human immunodeficiency virus.

tious tuberculosis, the most important and universally applied strategy, cures infected persons and within a few weeks renders them noncontagious. (2) Identifying and treating persons who have noncontagious tuberculosis (extrapulmonary disease, primary pulmonary disease of children, bacteriologically unconfirmed pulmonary disease, and infection with M. tuberculosis that is not yet causing disease) may prevent infectious cases. In countries such as the United States, where the risk of new infection is low, preventing progression of infection to clinical disease is especially useful. (3) Where the risk of transmitting infection is exceptionally high, as in mycobacteriology laboratories, sputum induction cubicles, chest clinic waiting areas, and some homeless shelters, using ventilation and ultraviolet lights to decontaminate air containing infectious droplet nuclei is useful. (4) An attenuated vaccine derived from a strain of Mycobacterium bovis by Calmette and Guerin in France (the BCG vaccine) may be used.

The BCG vaccine was first administered to humans in 1921, and different preparations used in controlled trials conducted before 1955 yielded estimated efficacies of −56% to 80% (149). Fifteen-year follow-up results of a large controlled trial in India begun in 1969 showed that the risk of sputum-positive tuberculosis in persons vaccinated with BCG was no lower than for persons given placebo (150). However, observational studies, which are less reliable than controlled studies, have shown that in vaccinated children younger than 15 years the prevalence of tuberculous meningitis and miliary tuberculosis is 52 to 100% lower than in unvaccinated controls, and that of pulmonary disease 2 to 80% lower (148).

In the United States the BCG vaccine is recommended only for infants and children who have negative tuberculin skin test reactions and who belong to selected population groups (148): (1) those at high risk of intimate and prolonged exposure to untreated or ineffectively treated persons with infectious pulmonary tuberculosis who cannot be removed from the source of exposure and for whom long-term preventive therapy is not possible; (2) those exposed continuously to persons with tuberculosis who have organisms resistant to isoniazid and rifampin; and (3) members of groups whose rate of new infections is greater that 1% per year and for whom the usual surveillance and treatment programs have been attempted but are not feasible. Previously, the BCG vaccine was recommended for health care workers in the United States, because as a group, they experienced high rates of infection. Currently, the recommendation for protection of health care workers is adequate surveillance, which includes periodic tuberculin skin testing and isoniazid preventive therapy for persons who have recently converted from tuberculin skin test negative to positive and for persons who are tuberculin skin test positive and who are close contacts of persons with tuberculosis or have medical conditions such as diabetes, renal failure, or immunosuppression associated with therapy or disease (148).

The BCG vaccine should not be given to immunocompromised persons and should be given with caution to persons at risk of HIV infection. One person with AIDS developed disseminated disease with Mycobacterium bovis after being vaccinated with BCG, and three symptomatic infants infected with HIV developed lymphadenitis with M. bovis after receiving the BCG vaccine (151,152). Disseminated M. bovis disease has not been reported in asymptomatic persons infected with HIV. In populations where the risk of tuberculosis is high, the World Health Organization recommends that the BCG vaccine be given at birth or as soon as possible thereafter to HIV-infected children but not to children with symptomatic HIV infection; and in populations where the risk of tuberculosis is low, the BCG vaccine should not be given to persons known or suspected to be infected with HIV (153).

Mycobacterium leprae. Different approaches to the development of a safe, effective, inexpensive vaccine that provides protection against infection with M. leprae currently are being explored. The BCG vaccine has been used, but results have been inconsistent (154,155). Other possibilities include a killed M. leprae vaccine and a genetically engineered vaccine that incorporates the 18-kd and 35-kd proteins of M. leprae, both of which may be relevant in protection against infection with the organism (105,156–158).

REFERENCES

1. Rieder HL, et al: Tuberculosis in the United States. JAMA, *262*:385, 1989.
2. Centers for Disease Control: Update: Tuberculosis elimination—United States. MMWR, *39*:153, 1990.
3. Stead WW, et al: Tuberculosis as an epidemic and nosocomial infection among the elderly in nursing homes. N Engl J Med, *312*:1483, 1985.
4. Centers for Disease Control: Summary of notifiable diseases, United States, 1990. MMWR, *39*:1, 1990.
5. Des Prez RM, and Heim CR: Mycobacterium tuberculosis. *In* Principles and Practice of Infectious Diseases. 3rd ed. Edited by GL Mandell, RG Doublas, Jr, and JE Bennett. New York, Churchill Livingstone, 1990.
6. Chaisson RE, et al: Tuberculosis in patients with the acquired immunodeficiency syndrome: Clinical features, response to therapy, and survival. Am Rev Respir Dis, *136*:570, 1987.
7. Pitchenik AE, Fertel D, and Block AB: Mycobacterial disease: Epidemiology, diagnosis, treatment, and prevention. Clin Chest Med *9*:425, 1988.
8. Kim JH, Langston AA, and Gallis HA: Miliary tuberculosis: Epidemiology, clinical manifestations, diagnosis, and outcome. Rev Infect Dis, *12*:583, 1990.
9. Moore VA: Bovine Tuberculosis and Its Control. New York, Carpenter, 1913.
10. Francis J: Bovine Tuberculosis. London, Staples, 1947.
11. Grange JM, and Collins CH: Bovine tubercle bacilli and disease in animals and man. Epidem Inf, *92*:221, 1987.
12. Karlson AG, and Carr DT: Tuberculosis caused by Mycobacterium bovis. Ann Intern Med, *73*:979, 1970.
13. Sjoegren I, and Sutherland I: Studies of tuberculosis in man in relation to infection in cattle. Tubercle, *56*:113, 1974.
14. Habib NI, and Warring FC: A fatal case of infection due to Mycobacterium bovis. Am Rev Respir Dis, *93*:804, 1966.
15. Castets M, et al: Les bacilles tuberculeux de type africaine. Rev Tuberc Pneumol, *32*:179, 1968.
16. Castets M, Boisvert H, and Riot N: La variete africaine du tuberculeux humain. Med Afr Noire, *16*:321, 1969.
17. Collins CH, Yates MD, and Grange JM: Subdivision of Mycobacterium into five variants for epidemiological purposes: Methods and nomenclature. J Hyg Camb, *89*:235, 1982.
18. Runyon EH: Anonymous mycobacteria in pulmonary disease. Med Clin North Am, *43*:273, 1959.
19. Good RC: Opportunistic pathogens in the genus Mycobacterium. Ann Rev Microbiol, *39*:347, 1985.
20. Horsburgh CR, and Selik RM: The epidemiology of disseminated nontuberculous mycobacterial infection in the acquired immunodeficiency syndrome (AIDS). Am Rev Respir Dis, *139*:4, 1989.
21. Meissner PS, and Falkinham JO III: Plasmid DNA profiles as epidemiological markers for clinical and environmental isolates of Mycobacterium avium, Mycobacterium intracellulare, and Mycobacterium scrofulaceum. J Infect Dis, *153*:325, 1986.
22. Prince DS: Infection with Mycobacterium avium complex in patients without predisposing conditions. N Engl J Med, *321*:863, 1989.
23. Horsburgh CR, Jr: Mycobacterium avium complex infection in the acquired immunodeficiency syndrome. N Engl J Med, *324*:1332, 1991.
24. Yakrus MA, and Good RC: Geographic distribution, frequency, and specimen source of Mycobacterium avium complex serotypes isolated from patients with acquired immunodeficiency syndrome. J Clin Microbiol, *28*:926, 1990.
25. Guthertz LS, et al: Mycobacterium avium and Mycobacterium intracellulare infections in patients with and without AIDS. J Infect Dis, *160*:1037, 1989.
26. Vincent ME, and Robbins AH: Mycobacterium avium-intracellulare complex enteritis: Pseudo-Whipple disease in AIDS. Am J Roentgenol, *144*:921, 1985.
27. Gillin JS, Urmacher C, West R, and Shike M: Disseminated Mycobacterium avium-intracellulare infection in acquired immunodeficiency syndrome mimicking Whipple's disease. Gastroenterology, *85*:1187, 1983.
28. Lincoln EM, and Gilber LA: Disease in children due to mycobacteria other than Mycobacterium tuberculosis. Am Rev Respir Dis, *105*:683, 1972.
29. Abello VB, Riley HD, Jr, and Rubio T: Atypical mycobacterial infections in children. Scand J Infect Dis, *3*:163, 1971.
30. Sutker WL, Lankford LL and Tompsett R: Granulomatous synovitis: The role of atypical mycobacteria. Rev Infect Dis, *1*:729, 1979.
31. Pergamnet M, Gonzalez R, and Fraley EE: Atypical mycobacteriosis of the urinary tract. A case report of extensive disease caused by the Battey bacillus. JAMA, *229*:816, 1974.
32. Newman H: Renal disease associated with atypical mycobacteria: Battey type. Case report. J Urol, *103*:403, 1970.
33. Soltani K, et al: Cutaneous "MAIS" infectious granuloma [letter]. N Engl J Med, *307*:1456, 1982.
34. Kelly PJ, Karlson AG, Weed LA, and Lipscomb PR: Infection of synovial tissues by mycobacteria other than Mycobacterium tuberculosis. J Bone Joint Surg, *49A*:1521, 1967.
35. Miranda D, Vuletin JC, and Kauffman SL: Disseminated histiocytosis and intestinal malakoplakia: Occurrence due to Mycobacterium intracellulare infection. Arch Pathol Lab Med, *103*:302, 1979.
36. Sanderson TL, et al: Disseminated Mycobacterium avium-intracellulare infection appearing as a panniculitis. Arch Pathol Lab Med, *106*:112, 1982.
37. Prissick FH, and Mason AM: Cervical lymphadenitis in children caused by chromogenic mycobacteria. Can Med Assoc J, *75*:798, 1956.
38. Wolinsky E: Nontuberculous mycobacteria and associated diseases. Am Rev Respir Dis, *119*:107, 1979.
39. Woods GL, and Washington JA II: Mycobacteria other than Mycobacterium tuberculosis: Review of microbiologic and clinical aspects. Rev Infect Dis, *9*:275, 1987.
40. Buhler VB, and Pollak A: Human infection with atypical acid-fast organisms. Am J Clin Pathol, *23*:363, 1953.
41. Runyon EH: Conservation of the specific epithet fortuitum in the name of the organism known as Mycobacterium fortuitum da Costa Cruz. Int J Syst Bacteriol, *22*:50, 1972.

42. Wagner JD, et al: Outbreak of Mycobacterium chelonae infection associated with use of jet injectors. JAMA, 264: 373, 1990.
43. Band JD, et al: Peritonitis due to a Mycobacterium chelonei–like organism associated with intermittent chronic peritoneal dialysis. J Infect Dis, 145:9, 1982.
44. Bolan G, et al: Infections with Mycobacterium chelonei in patients receiving dialysis and using processed hemodialyzers. J Infect Dis, 152:1013, 1985.
45. Laskowski LF, et al: Fastidious mycobacteria grown from porcine prosthetic heart-valve cultures. N Engl J Med, 297: 101, 1977.
46. Wallace RJ Jr, et al: Spectrum of disease due to rapidly growing mycobacteria. Rev Infect Dis, 5:657, 1983.
47. Bullin CH, Tanner EI, and Collins CH: Isolation of Mycobacterium xenopi from water taps. J Hyg (Camb), 68:97, 1970.
48. Good RC, and Snider DE, Jr: Isolation of nontuberculous mycobacteria in the United States. J Infect Dis, 146:829, 1982.
49. Weber J, et al: Pulmonary disease due to Mycobacterium xenopi in a renal allograft recipient: Report of a case and review. Rev Infect Dis, 11:964, 1989.
50. Costrinia AM, et al: Clinical and roentgenographic features of nosocomial pulmonary disease due to Mcyobacterium xenopi. Am Rev Respir Dis, 123:104, 1981.
51. Damsker B, Bottone EJ, and Deligdisch L: Mycobacterium xenopi: Infection in an immunocomprised host. Hum Pathol, 13:866, 1982.
52. Eng RHK, Forrester C, Smith SM, and Sobel H: Mycobacterium xenopi infection in a patient with acquired immunodeficiency syndrome [letter]. Ann Intern Med, 100:461, 1984.
53. Tecson-Tumang FT, and Bright JL: Mycobacterium xenopi and the acquired immunodeficiency syndrome. Chest, 86: 145, 1984.
54. Marks J, Jenkins PA, and Isukamura M: Mycobacterium szulgai—a new pathogen. Tubercle, 53:210, 1972.
55. Schroder KH, and Juhlin I: Mycobacterium malmoense sp. nov. Int J Syst Bacteriol, 27:241, 1977.
56. Warren NG, Body BA, Silcox VA, and Matthews JH: Pulmonary disease due to Mycobacterium malmoense. J Clin Microbiol, 20:245, 1984.
57. Jenkins PA, and Tsukamura M: Infections with Mycobacterium malmoense in England and Wales. Tubercle, 60:71, 1979.
58. Karassova V, Weiszfeiler JG, and Krasznay E: Occurrence of atypical mycobacteria in macacus rhesus. Acta Microbiol Acad Sci Hungar, 12:275, 1965.
59. Weiszfeiler JG: Die atypischen Myobakterien und das Mycobacterium simiae. In: Die Biologie und Variabilitat des Tuberkelbakteriums und die atypischen Myobakterien. Budapest, Akademiae Kiado, 1969.
60. Valdivia A, Mendez JS, and Font ME: Mycobacterium habana: probable neuva especie dentro della microbacterias no classificadas. Boletin de Higiene y Epidemiologia (Habana), 9:65, 1971.
61. Meissner G, and Schroder K-H: Relationship between Mycobacterium simiae and Mycobacterium habana. Am Rev Respir Dis, 111:196, 1975.
62. Weiszfeiler JG, and Karczag E: Synonymy of Mycobacterium simiae Karasseva et al. 1965 and Mycobacterium habana Valdivia et al. 1971. Int J Syst Bacteriol, 26:474, 1976.
63. Aronson JD: Spontaneous tuberculosis in salt water fish. J Infect Dis, 39:315, 1926.
64. Norden A, and Linell F: A new type of pathogenic Mycobacterium. Nature, 168:826, 1951.
65. Gombert ME, et al: Disseminated Mycobacterium marinum infection after renal transplantation. Ann Intern Med, 94: 486, 1981.
66. Sage RE, and Derrington AW: Opportunistic cutaneous Mycobacterium marinum infection mimicking Mycobacterium ulcerans in lymphosarcoma. Med J Aust, 2:434, 1973.
67. Travis WD, et al: The histopathologic spectrum in Mycobacterium marinum infection. Arch Pathol Lab Med, 109: 1109, 1985.
68. Gould WM, McMeekin DR, and Bright RD: Mycobacterium marinum (balnei) infection. Report of a case with cutaneous and laryngeal lesions. Arch Dermatol, 97:159, 1968.
69. Schonherr U, Naumann GOH, Lang GK, and Bialasiewicz AA: Sclerokeratitis caused by Mycobacterium marinum. Am J Ophthamol, 108:607, 1989.
70. Sompolinsky D, Lagziel A, Naveh D, and Yankilevitz T: Mycobacterium haemophilum sp. nov., a new pathogen of humans. Int J Syst Bacteriol, 28:67, 1978.
71. Lomvardias S, and Madge GE: Chaetoconidium and atypical acid-fast bacilli in skin ulcers. Arch Dermatol, 106:875, 1972.
72. Feldman RA, and Hershfield E: Mycobacterial skin infection by an unidentified species. A report of 29 patients. Ann Intern Med, 80:445, 1974.
73. Branger B, et al: Mycobacterium haemophilum– and Mycobacterium xenopi–associated infection in a renal transplant patient. Clin Nephrol, 23:46, 1985.
74. Dawson DJ, Blacklock ZM, and Kane DW: Mycobacterium haemophilum causing lymphadenitis in an otherwise healthy child. Med J Aust, 2:289, 1981.
75. Gouby A, Branger B, Oules R, and Ramuz M: Two cases of Mycobacterium haemophilum infection in a renal dialysis unit. J Med Microbiol, 25:299, 1988.
76. Centers for Disease Control: Mycobacterium haemophilum infection—New York City Metropolitan Area, 1990–1991. MMWR, 40:636, 1991.
77. Lunn HF, et al: Buruli (mycobacterial) ulceration in Uganda (a new focus of Buruli ulcer in Madi District, Uganda). E Afr Med J, 42:275, 1965.
78. Radford AJ: Mycobacterium ulcerans in Australia. Aust NZ J Med, 5:162, 1975.
79. Gonzales EP, Crosby RMN, and Walker SH: Mycobacterium aquae infection in a hydrocephalic child (Mycobacterium aquae meningitis). Pediatrics, 48:974, 1971.
80. Kurnik PB, Padmanabh U, Bonatsos C, and Cynamon MH: Mycobacterium gordonae as a human hepatoperitoneal pathogen, with a review of the literature. Am J Med Sci, 285:45, 1983.
81. Lohr DC, Goeken JA, Doty DB, and Donta ST: Mycobacterium gordonae infection of a prosthetic aortic valve. JAMA, 239:1528, 1978.
82. Shelly WB, and Folkens AT: Mycobacterium gordonae infection of the hand. Arch Dermatol, 120:1064, 1984.
83. Blacklock ZM, Dawson DJ, Kane DW, and McEvoy D: Mycobacterium asiaticum as a potential pulmonary pathogen for humans: A clinical and bacteriologic review of five cases. Am Rev Respir Dis, 127:241, 1983.
84. Weitzman I, Osadcyi D, Corrado ML, and Karp D: Mycobacterium thermoresistible: a new pathogen for humans. J Clin Microbiol, 14:593, 1981.
85. Neeley SP, and Denning DW: Cutaneous Mycobacterium thermoresistible infection in a heart transplant recipient. Rev Infect Dis, 11:608, 1989.
86. Richmond L, and Cummings MM: An evaluation of methods of testing the virulence of acid-fast bacilli. Am Rev Tuberc, 62:632, 1950.

87. DeChairo DC, Kittredge D, Meyers A, and Corrales J: Septic arthritis due to Mycobacterium triviale. Am Rev Respir Dis, 108:1224, 1973.
88. Edwards MS, Huber TW, and Baker CJ: Mycobacterium terrae synovitis and osteomyelitis. Am Rev Respir Dis, 117:161, 1978.
89. Cianciulli FD: The radish bacillus (Mycobacterium terrae): Saprophyte or pathogen? Am Rev Respir Dis, 109:138, 1974.
90. Tsukamura M, Kita N, Otsuka W, and Shimoide H: A study of the taxonomy of the Mycobacterium nonchromogenicum complex and report of six cases of lung infection due to Mycobacterium nonchromogenicum. Microbiol Immunol, 27:219, 1983.
91. Casimir MT, Fainstein V, and Papadopolous N: Cavitary lung infection caused by Mycobacterium flavescens. South Med J, 75:253, 1982.
92. Tsukamura M, Shimoide H, and Schaefer WB: A possible pathogen of Group III mycobacteria. J Gen Microbiol, 88:377, 1975.
93. Wayne LG, et al: First report of the cooperative open-ended study of slowly growing mycobacteria (International Working Group on Mycobacterial Taxonomy). Int J Syst Bacteriol, 31:1, 1981.
94. Wallace RJ, Jr, et al: Human disease due to Mycobacterium smegmatis. J Infect Dis, 158:52, 1988.
95. Davison MB, et al: Bacteremia caused by Mycobacterium neoaurum. J Clin Microbiol, 26:762, 1988.
96. Chiodini RJ: Crohn's disease and the mycobacterioses: A review and comparison of two disease entities. Clin Microbiol Rev, 2:90, 1989.
97. Hirschel B, et al: Fatal infection with a novel, unidentified Mycobacterium in a man with the acquired immunodeficiency syndrome. N Engl J Med, 323:109, 1990.
98. Sansarricq H: Leprosy in the world today. Lepr Rev, 52(suppl. I):15, 1981.
99. Binford CH, Meyers WM, and Walsh GP: Leprosy. JAMA, 247:2283, 1982.
100. Centers for Disease Control: Summary of notifiable diseases, United States—1989. MMWR, 38:1, 1989.
101. Nelson AM, and Meyers WM: Leprosy. American Society of Clinical Pathology Check Sample—Microbiology MB86-6, 29:(6), 1986.
102. Neill MA, Hightower AW, and Broome CV: Leprosy in the United States, 1971–1981. J Infect Dis, 152:1064, 1985.
103. Walsh G, Meyers W, and Binford C: Naturally acquired leprosy in the nine-banded armadillo: A decade of experience 1975–1985. J Leukocyte Biol, 40:645, 1986.
104. Gormus BJ, et al: A second sooty mangabey monkey with naturally acquired leprosy: First reported possible monkey-to-monkey transmission. Int J Lepr, 56:61, 1988.
105. Hastings RC, Gillis TP, Krahenbuhl JL, and Franzblau SG: Leprosy. Clin Microbiol Rev, 1:330, 1988.
106. Lumpkin LR III, Cox GF, and Wolf JE: Leprosy in five armadillo handlers. J Am Acad Dermatol, 9:899, 1983.
107. Thomas DA, et al: Armadillo exposure among Mexican-born patients with lepromatous leprosy. J Infect Dis, 156:990, 1987.
108. Blake LA, West BC, Lary CH, and Todd JR IV: Environmental nonhuman sources of leprosy. Rev Infect Dis, 9:562, 1987.
109. van Eden W, et al: Low T lymphocyte responsiveness to M. leprae antigens in association with HLA-DR3. Clin Exp Immunol, 55:140, 1984.
110. van Eden W, et al: HLA-linked control of predisposition to lepromatous leprosy. J Infect Dis, 151:9, 1985.
111. Scahuf V, et al: Leprosy associated with HLA-DR2 and DQw1 in the population of northern Thailand. Tissue Antigens, 26:243, 1985.
112. Modlin RL, et al: Genetically restricted suppressor T-cell clones derived from lepromatous leprosy lesions. Nature (London), 322:459, 1986.
113. Modlin RL, et al: In situ and in vitro characterization of the cellular immune response in erythema nodosum leprosum. J Immunol, 136:883, 1986.
114. Modlin RL, et al: Suppressor T lymphocytes from lepromatous leprosy skin lesions. J Immunol, 137:2831, 1986.
115. Watson S: Interleukin 1 production by peripheral blood mononuclear cells from leprosy patients. Infect Immun, 45:787, 1984.
116. Bjorvatn B, et al: Immune complexes and complement hypercatabolism in patients with leprosy. Clin Exp Immunol, 26:388, 1976.
117. Ridley DS, and Jopling WH: Classification of leprosy according to immunity: A five group system. Int J Lepr, 34:255, 1964.
118. American Thoracic Society: Diagnostic standards and classification of tuberculosis. Am Rev Respir Dis, 142:725, 1990.
119. Arnold JH, Scott AV, and Spitznagel JK: Specificity of PPD skin tests in childhood tuberculin converters: Comparison with mycobacterial species from tissues and secretions. J Pediatr, 76:512, 1970.
120. Margileth AM: The use of purified protein derivative mycobacterial skin test antigens in children and adolescents: Purified proten derivative skin test results correlated with mycobacterial isolates. Pediatr Infect Dis, 2:225, 1983.
121. Margileth AM, Chandra R, and Altman RP: Chronic lymphadenopathy due to mycobacterial infection. Clinical features, diagnosis, histopathology, and management. Am J Dis Child, 138:917, 1984.
122. Margileth AM: Management of nontuberculous (atypical) mycobacterial infections in children and adolescents. Pediatr Infect Dis, 4:119, 1985.
123. Vandiviere HM, Dillon M, and Melvin IG: Atypical mycobacteria causing pulmonary disease: Rapid diagnosis using skin test profiles. South Med J, 80:5, 1987.
124. Berlin OGW: Mycobacteria. In Bailey and Scott's Diagnostic Microbiology. 8th ed. Edited by EJ Baron and SM Finegold. St. Louis, CV Mosby, 1990.
125. American Thoracic Society: Diagnostic standards and classification of tuberculosis and other mycobacterial diseases. Am Rev Respir Dis, 123:343, 1981.
126. Morgan MA, Horstmeier CD, DeYoung DR, and Roberts GD: Comparison of a radiometric method (BACTEC) and conventional culture media for recovery of mycobacteria from smear-negative specimens. J Clin Microbiol, 18:384, 1983.
127. Park CH, et al: Rapid recovery of mycobacteria from clinical specimens using automated radiometric technic. Am J Clin Pathol, 81:341, 1984.
128. Roberts GD, et al: Evaluation of the BACTEC radiometric method for recovery of mycobacteria and drug susceptibility testing of Mycobacterium tuberculosis from acid-fast smear-positive specimens. J Clin Microbiol, 18:689, 1983.
129. Isenberg HD, et al: Collaborative feasibility study of a biphasic system (Roche Septi-Chek AFB) for rapid detection and isolation of mycobacteria. J Clin Microbiol, 29:1719, 1991.
130. Roberts GD, Koneman EW, and Kim YK: Mycobacterium. In Manual of Clinical Microbiology. 5th ed. Edited A Balows, et al. Washington, DC, American Society for Microbiology, 1991.
131. Roberts GD: Mycobacteria and Nocardia. In Laboratory

Procedures in Clinical Microbiology. 2nd ed. Edited by JA Washington II. New York, Springer-Verlag, 1985.
132. Kiehn TE, and Edwards EF: Rapid identification using a specific DNA probe of Mycobacterium avium complex from patients with acquired immunodeficiency syndrome. J Clin Microbiol, 25:1551, 1987.
133. Drake TA, Hindler JA, Berlin OGW, and Bruckner DA: Rapid identification of Mycobacterium avium complex in culture using DNA probes. J Clin Microbiol, 25:1442, 1987.
134. Walton DT, and Valesco M: Identification of Mycobacterium gordonae from culture by the Gen-Probe rapid diagnostic system: Evaluation of 218 isolates and potential sources of false-negative results. J Clin Microbiol, 29:1850, 1991.
135. Goto M, et al: Evaluation of acridinium-ester labeled DNA probes for identification of Mycobacterium tuberculosis and Mycobacterium avium-intracellulare complex in culture. J Clin Microbiol, 29:2473, 1991.
136. Ellner PD, Kiehn TE, Cammarata R, and Hosmer M: Rapid detection and identification of pathogenic mycobacteria by combining radiometric and nucleic acid probe methods. J Clin Microbiol, 26:1349, 1988.
136a. Edlin BR, et al: An outbreak of multidrug-resistant tuberculosis among hospitalized patients with the acquired immunodeficiency syndrome. N Engl J Med, 326:1514, 1992.
137. Wallace RJ, Jr, Swenson JM, and Silcox VA: The rapidly growing mycobacteria—characterization and susceptibility testing. Antimicrobic Newslett, 2:85, 1985.
138. Brenna PJ, Heifers M, and Ullom BP: Thin-layer chromatography of lipid antigens as a means of identifying nontuberculous mycobacteria. J Clin Microbiol, 15:447, 1981.
139. Tisdall PA, DeYoung DR, Roberts GD, and Anhalt JP: Identification of clinical isolates of mycobacteria with gas-liquid chromatography: A 10-month follow-up study. J Clin Microbiol, 16:400, 1982.
140. Edwards SD, Ferguson LE, and Daniel TM: An ELISA for the serodiagnosis of tuberculosis using a 30,000-Da native antigen of Mycobacterium tuberculosis. J Infect Dis, 162:928, 1990.
141. Watt G, Zaraspe G, Bautista S, and Laughlin LW: Rapid diagnosis of tuberculous meningitis by using an enzyme-linked immunosorbent assay to detect mycobacterial antigen and antibody in cerebrospinal fluid. J Infect Dis, 158:681, 1988.
142. Pang JA, et al: A tuberculostearic acid assay in the diagnosis of sputum smear–negative pulmonary tuberculosis. Ann Intern Med, 111:650, 1989.
143. Pao CC, et al: Detection and identification of Mycobacterium tuberculosis by DNA amplification. J Clin Microbiol, 28:1877, 1990.
144. Sjobring U, Mecklenburg M, Andersen AB, and Miorner H: Polymerase chain reaction for detection of Mycobacterium tuberculosis. J Clin Microbiol, 28:2200, 1990.
145. Plikaytis BB, Gelber RH, and Shinnick TM: Rapid and sensitive detection of Mycobacterium leprae using a nested-primer gene amplification assay. J Clin Microbiol, 28:1913, 1990.
146. American Thoracic Society: Diagnosis and treatment of disease caused by nontuberculosis mycobacteria. Am Rev Respir Dis, 142:940, 1990.
147. Sanders WE, Jr, and Horowitz EA: Other Mycobacterium species. In Principles and Practice of Infectious Diseases. 3rd ed. Edited by GL Mandell, RG Douglas, Jr, and JE Bennett. New York, Churchill Livingstone, 1990.
148. Centers for Disease Control: Use of BCG vaccines in the control of tuberculosis: A joint statement by the ACIP and the Advisory Committee for the Elimination of Tuberculosis. MMWR, 37:663, 1988.
149. Clemens JD, Chuong JJH, and Feinstein AR: The BCG controversy: A methodological and statistical reappraisal. JAMA, 249:2362, 1983.
150. Tripathy SP: Fifteen-year follow-up of the Indian BCG prevention trial. In Proceedings of the XXVIth IUAT World Conference on Tuberculosis and Respiratory Diseases. Edited by International Union Against Tuberculosis. Singapore, Professional Postgraduate Services, International, 1987.
151. Centers for Disease Control: Disseminated Mycobacterium bovis infection from BCG vaccination of a patient with acquired immunodeficiency syndrome. MMWR, 34:227, 1985.
152. Blanche S, et al: Longitudinal study of 18 children with perinatal LAV/HTLV III infection: Attempt at prognostic evaluation. J Pediatr, 109:965, 1986.
153. World Health Organization: Special Programme on AIDS and Expanded Programme on Immunization—joint statement: Consultation on human immunodeficiency virus (HIV) and routine childhood immunization. Wkly Epidemiol Rep, 62:297, 1987.
154. Brown JAK, Stone MM, and Sutherland I: BCG vaccination of children against leprosy in Uganda: Results at the end of second follow-up. Br Med J, 1:24, 1968.
155. Bechelli LM, et al: BCG vaccination of children against leprosy: Seven-year findings of the controlled WHO trial in Burma. Bull WHO, 48:323, 1973.
156. Shepard CC, Walker L, and Van Landingham R: Immunity to Mycobacterium leprae infections induced in mice by BCG vaccination. Infect Immun, 19:391, 1978.
157. Kirchheimer WF, Sanchez RM, and Shannon EJ: Effect of specific vaccine on cell-mediated immunity of armadillos against M. leprae. Int J Lepr, 46:353, 1978.
158. Gill HK, Mustafa AS, and Godal T: In vitro proliferation of lymphocytes from human volunteers vaccinated with armadillo-derived, killed M. leprae. Int J Lepr, 55:30, 1987.

Chapter 41

OTHER GRAM-NEGATIVE BACTERIA

The biochemical and bacteriologic characteristics of the organisms discussed in this chapter have not been defined sufficiently to allow definitive classification. Gardnerella vaginalis has been associated with bacterial vaginosis; Calymmatobacterium granulomatis is the agent of granuloma inguinale; Streptobacillus moniliformis is the agent of Haverhill fever and one cause of rat-bite fever; and Afipia felis is responsible for cat-scratch disease.

GARDNERELLA VAGINALIS

An organism resembling Haemophilus was associated with prostatitis and cervicitis in 1953, and in 1955, Gardner and Dukes identified Haemophilus vaginalis as the pathogen of bacterial vaginosis (also called nonspecific vaginitis) (1,2). The organism was renamed Corynebacterium vaginalis in 1963, because it required neither X or V factor (see Chapter 36) for growth and it occasionally stained gram-positive and formed "Chinese letters," similar to cells of corynebacteria (see Chapter 29). In 1980 it was classified in a new genus, Gardnerella, because genetic studies showed no relationship with other genera (3,4).

Gardnerella vaginalis requires for growth an enriched medium that includes thiamine, riboflavin, niacin, folinic acid, biotin, and two or more purine and pyrimidine bases. It has a unique laminated cell wall typical of neither gram-positive nor gram-negative bacteria and, therefore, has not been placed in a family but is grouped with gram-negative bacteria. The amino acid and fatty acid profiles of the cell wall and cell membrane are typical of gram-positive bacteria, and cell extracts have endotoxic activity similar to that of gram-negative bacteria, but no lipid A (4–6).

Epidemiology and Pathogenesis

The human vagina is the natural reservoir for Gardnerella vaginalis. The organism is found in as many as 70% of women and 14% of girls who have no signs or symptoms of vaginal infection and in almost all women with bacterial vaginosis and in the urethra of most of their male partners. This suggests sexual transmission of the organism (7–9). The role of G. vaginalis in the pathogenesis of bacterial vaginosis is unknown.

Gardnerella vaginalis has pili and in vitro shows hemagglutinating activity and adherence to McCoy cells, factors that may allow it to adhere to vaginal and urinary epithelial cells in vivo (10–12). The organism produces phospholipase A_2, an enzyme that initiates labor by converting amniotic phospholipids to free arachidonic acid, which then converts long-chain fatty acids in the amniotic and chorionic membranes to prostaglandins (13,14). These events could explain the association of bacterial vaginosis with premature rupture of membranes. Moreover, G. vaginalis is resistant to the killing activity of serum (15).

Clinical Manifestations

Gardnerella vaginalis is found with a mixed anaerobic flora in the vagina of almost all women with bacterial vaginosis, a noninvasive condition (hence the term vaginosis rather than vaginitis) characterized by vulvar burning or pruritus and increased volume of malodorous vaginal discharge containing few (if any) neutrophils (16). The organism is an uncommon cause of symptomatic and asymptomatic infections of the urinary tract, principally in women under age 40 years and men with compromised renal function (12,17,18). Gardnerella vaginalis may cause bacteremia, predominantly in women with post partum endometritis, post partum fever, chorioamnionitis, or septic abortion, but also in neonates (12,19,20).

Laboratory Diagnosis

Specimens most often received in the clinical laboratory for detection of Gardnerella vaginalis are vaginal secretions; vaginal, cervical, or urethra swab specimens (two separate swabs are preferred) from women with vaginal discharge; and urethral swab specimens from male sexual partners. Specimen collection, transport, and processing are discussed in Chapter 61. Occasionally G. vaginalis is recovered from urine or from blood. In the latter case, because the sodium polyanetholsulfonate (SPS) used as an anticoagulant in many broth blood culture media inhibits the growth of G. vaginalis, adding 1 to 2% gelatin to the broth, using the lysis-centrifugation method (see Chapter 58), or direct planting of blood onto chocolate agar improves recovery (21).

Bacterial vaginosis is diagnosed presumptively by direct examination of vaginal secretions (see Chapter 61). Culture of Gardnerella vaginalis is not required for diagnosis because the organism may be part of the normal vaginal flora. The presence of clue cells (squamous epithelial cells covered with tiny bacilli) in wet-mount preparations or in smears of vaginal secretions stained with the Gram or Papanicolaou stain (Plate VIIIB) correlates well with the diagnosis of bacterial vaginosis and with detection of G. vaginalis in vaginal fluid. In Gram-stained smears of vaginal discharge of a person with bacterial vaginosis, clue cells are accompanied by many small, gram-negative and gram-variable bacilli, coccobacilli, and some curved, gram-negative bacilli, but no large, gram-positive bacilli (lactobacilli), which typically predominate in smears of vaginal secretions of normal, asymptomatic women. In addition to the presence of clue cells, vaginal discharge from women with bacterial vaginosis has a pH greater than 4.5

and gives off a characteristic fishy odor after the addition of 10% potassium hydroxide (sniff test).

To culture Gardnerella vaginalis from clinical specimens a selective medium such as human blood Tween (HBT), V, or colistin nalidixic acid (CNA) agar (all commercially available) is inoculated. The organism grows poorly on sheep blood agar and does not grow on MacConkey agar. After 48 hours of incubation at 35° C in 5 to 10% carbon dioxide or in a candle jar, colonies of G. vaginalis are convex, opaque, and gray, surrounded by a diffuse zone of β hemolysis on media containing human blood (HBT agar and V agar) and nonhemolytic on CNA agar. A smear of a colony stained with the Gram stain shows small, pleomorphic gram-variable or gram-negative coccobacilli and short bacilli. G. vaginalis is oxidase- and catalase negative and hippurate positive. An isolate from a female genital source may presumptively be called G. vaginalis based on these three test results and the appearance of colonies (including hemolysis on HBT agar or V agar, but not on sheep blood agar) and of cells stained with the Gram stain. Additional results that confirm the identification include indole-negative, positive starch hydrolysis, and fermentation of glucose, maltose, and sucrose but not mannitol. Moreover, G. vaginalis is susceptible to SPS (a commercially available disk is placed on Brucella blood agar inoculated with a lawn of the test organism, yielding a zone at least 12 mm); and by disk-diffusion testing, a zone of inhibition surrounds metronidazole (50 μg disk) and trimethoprim (5 μg disk) but not sulfonamide (1 mg disk) (22,23).

Treatment

Metronidazole is the drug of choice for treating bacterial vaginosis. In vitro most isolates are susceptible to penicillin, ampicillin, vancomycin, clindamycin, gentamicin, carbenicillin, and oxacillin.

CALYMMATOBACTERIUM GRANULOMATIS

Granuloma inguinale (also called donovanosis) probably was described first by McLeod in 1882, and the responsible organism was identified by Donovan in 1905 and called Donovania granulomatis, a name later changed to Calymmatobacterium granulomatis. The organism is an encapsulated gram-negative bacillus, 1.5 μm long and 0.7 μm wide, which in smears prepared from involved tissue appears enclosed in vacuoles within histiocytes, or sometimes within polymorphonuclear leukocytes or plasma cells (24). Its capsular polysaccharide shares some cross-reactive antigens with species of Klebsiella, but a taxonomic relationship between the two organisms has not been established (25).

Epidemiology

Granuloma inguinale is a mildly contagious disease common in New Guinea, India, central Australia, the Caribbean, and many other tropical or subtropical countries, but it is rare in the United States, where fewer than 100 cases are reported annually. The disease probably is transmitted by sexual contact, requiring repeated exposures; however, the role of sexual transmission is controversial because the sexual contacts of many affected persons have no lesions. Rectal lesions in homosexual males are associated with anal intercourse with partners who have penile lesions (26). In one study in New Guinea, lesions were detected in about 4% of children 1 to 4 years of age and in 5% of persons older than 15 years, but not in other age groups, suggesting that young children might be infected by sitting on the laps of parents or relatives who have the disease and that in adults infection is associated with sexual intercourse (27).

Clinical Manifestations and Pathology

The primary lesion of granuloma inguinale begins after an estimated incubation period of 8 to 80 days, as one or more subcutaneous nodules involving the genitalia, and sometimes the inguinal or anal regions. The nodules erode through the skin, producing painless, sharply defined, granulomatous lesions that bleed easily and heal with fibrosis. Inguinal lymphadenopathy often is present, and organisms occasionally spread by hematogenous dissemination to involve bones, joints, and the liver.

Histologic examination of a primary lesion reveals a marked dermal inflammatory infiltrate composed principally of plasma cells and histiocytes in the area of ulceration and pseudoepitheliomatous hyperplasia at the margins. Smears prepared from scrapings of the base of the lesion and stained with the Wright stain show the pathognomonic Donovan body, a large, infected mononuclear endothelial cell, 25 to 90 μm in diameter, with intracytoplasmic vacuoles that contain bacteria. The organisms stain as blue rods with prominent polar granules that impart a safety-pin appearance.

Laboratory Diagnosis

The diagnosis of granuloma inguinale is based on visualizing the characteristic Donovan body in smears prepared from scrapings of an active lesion or from a crushed biopsy specimen of subsurface tissue taken from an area of active granulation and stained with the Wright, Giemsa, or Dieterle stain. Formalin-fixed tissue is less satisfactory because the pathognomonic cells are seen infrequently. Calymmatobacterium granulomatis may be cultivated in vitro from clinical specimens by using media containing growth factors found in egg yolk (described in reference 28), but this is difficult and is not performed in the clinical laboratory.

Treatment

Tetracycline, ampicillin, or trimethoprim-sulfamethoxazole is first-line therapy. Occasionally, however, they fail, in which case gentamicin or chloramphenicol is indicated.

STREPTOBACILLUS MONILIFORMIS

Epidemiology and Pathogenesis

Streptobacillus moniliformis is the agent of Haverhill fever—an illness named after the town in Massachusetts where in 1926 nearly 90 persons were infected by ingesting contaminated raw and unpasteurized milk—and one of the agents of rat-bite fever. It is found worldwide in the respiratory tract of weasels, squirrels, cats, dogs, pigs, ferrets, rats and mice, including laboratory rats and mice. Rat-bite fever is acquired via the bite of a rat, or sometimes another rodent, and Haverhill fever is acquired by ingesting contaminated milk, food, or water. Virulence factors associated with S. moniliformis are unknown; however, the organism spontaneously develops L forms (organisms without cell walls), a feature that could allow it to persist in some sites.

Clinical Manifestations

Rat-bite fever begins abruptly about 10 days (range, 1 to 22 days) after the rat bite, with fever, chills, headache, vomiting, and severe migratory arthralgias and myalgias. Two to four days later, a maculopapular, morbilliform, or petechial rash appears on the palms, soles, and extremities. Asymmetric polyarthritis or septic arthritis, most commonly involving the knees (followed by ankles, elbows, wrists, shoulders, and hips) develops concurrently in about half the cases. Fever usually resolves without antimicrobial therapy in 3 to 5 days, and the remaining symptoms within 2 weeks, but occasionally the fever recurs for weeks or months, and the arthritis may persist as long as 2 years. Haverhill fever is a similar illness, except that vomiting is more severe and pharyngitis is common. Complications of infection with Streptobacillus moniliformis include endocarditis, myocarditis, pericarditis, pneumonia, amnionitis, and abscesses in nearly any organ (29,30).

Laboratory Diagnosis

Infection with Streptobacillus moniliformis is diagnosed by detecting the organism in blood, joint fluid, or purulent material aspirated from an infected wound or an abscess, or by demonstrating specific agglutinins in serum. The laboratory personnel, however, must be notified that infection with S. moniliformis is suspected, because broth and agar media must be supplemented with ascites fluid, blood, or serum to allow growth of the organism. Cultures should be incubated up to 1 week at 35° C in a humidified atmosphere of 5 to 7% carbon dioxide. In thioglycollate broth supplemented with 10 to 30% ascites fluid or serum, S. moniliformis produces puffball-like colonies after 2 to 6 days. On agar, colonies are 1 to 2 mm in diameter, round, smooth, gray, and glistening, and occasionally flat L-form colonies with a fried-egg appearance (resembling colonies of Mycoplasma, see Chapter 27) appear.

Streptobacillus moniliformis is nonmotile and catalase- and oxidase negative. Biochemical characterization requires testing with a basal medium similar to that used for isolation or with cystine trypticase agar supplemented with horse serum. Expected biochemical reactions are described in reference 23. Because S. moniliformis is encountered so rarely in the clinical laboratory, however, suspicious isolates should be sent to a reference laboratory for identification.

An initial agglutination titer of 1:80 or greater or a fourfold rise in titer between acute- and convalescent-phase serum is diagnostic of infection with Streptobacillus moniliformis. Serologic tests are not available commercially, and specimens must be sent to a reference laboratory.

Treatment

Penicillin is the recommended therapy for infections caused by Streptobacillus moniliformis, but for patients who are allergic to this agent tetracycline and streptomycin are effective alternatives. Rodent bite wounds should be cleaned thoroughly, and tetanus prophylaxis should be given if indicated (see Chapter 30).

AFIPIA

Members of the recently described genus Afipia are gram-negative, oxidase-positive, nonfermentative bacilli in the α-2 subgroup of the class Proteobacteria (31). They grow slowly on buffered charcoal-yeast extract agar and in nutrient broth at 25° and 30° C but rarely grow on MacConkey agar. Growth is weak at 35° C and does not occur at 42° C. Organisms are motile via a single flagellum. They are urease positive, nonhemolytic, and give negative reactions for indole and hydrogen sulfide production. Afipia felis, the agent of cat-scratch disease, is reviewed here. The remaining specimens—Afipia clevelandensis, isolated from a tibial biopsy; Afipia broomeae, isolated from sputum; Afipia genospecies 1, isolated from pleural fluid; Afipia genospecies 2, isolated from a bronchial wash specimen; and Afipia genospecies 3, isolated from water—are presumptive human pathogens and are not discussed further here.

Afipia felis (Cat-Scratch Disease Bacillus)

An illness (now known as cat-scratch disease), characterized by regional lymphadenopathy in persons scratched by cats, was recognized by Robert Debre in Paris in the early 1930s (32). Soon thereafter, Hanger and Rose used pus aspirated from an involved lymph node to prepare a skin test antigen that induced a positive intradermal reaction in persons with the infection. The agent of cat-scratch disease was not recognized until 1983, when Wear and colleagues found small, pleomorphic gram-negative bacilli in sections of lymph nodes from persons with the illness (33). The organisms, best visualized with the Warthin-Starry silver stain, were found in capillary walls in areas of hyperplasia and in microabscesses. Sera from some of these persons reacted with these bacteria, which also have been found in primary skin lesions, further supporting their role in the disease (34). More recently, the agent responsible for cat-scratch disease was cultivated on artificial media and further characterized; in 1991 it was named Afipia felis (31,35).

Epidemiology

Cat-scratch disease occurs worldwide with a seasonal pattern in temperate climates, where about 75% of cases occur from September to March (36). About 80% of affected persons are younger than 21 years, 60% are males, 90% have a history of exposure to cats, and 75% have experienced a cat scratch or -bite. Infection is transmitted by direct contact, because most cases follow a scratch, bite, or lick from a young cat; although occasionally dogs, monkeys, and thorns have been implicated as the source of infection. Implicated cats are not ill; they do not react to the skin test antigen; and attempts to recover the pathogen from them have been unsuccessful.

Clinical Manifestations and Pathology

Three to ten days after a cat scratch or contact, a primary skin papule or pustule forms at the inoculation site, though it may not be recognized. Regional lymphadenopathy, the most common clinical feature of cat-scratch disease, usually develops about 2 weeks after contact and persists 2 to 4 months, and occasionally longer. Typically, nodes in the head and neck area are involved, although axillary or, less commonly, epitrochlear, inguinal, or femoral nodes may be. In about half the cases a single lymph node is involved; multiple nodes in the same site are involved in about 20% of cases; and in the remainder lymphadenopathy involves several sites. Most persons appear otherwise well, but low-grade fever lasting several days occurs in about 30% of cases, malaise or fatigue in about 25%, and headache and sore throat in about 10%.

Atypical manifestations of cat-scratch disease include the oculoglandular syndrome of Parinaud, which presents as an ocular granuloma or conjunctivitis with preauricular lymphadenopathy; encephalitis or encephalopathy, usually occurring 1 to 6 weeks after the onset of lymphadenopathy; hepatic granulomas, and osteitis (37,38). In persons with the acquired immunodeficiency syndrome (AIDS) or AIDS-related complex, the disease has presented as disseminated skin lesions, occasionally resembling those of Kaposi's sarcoma and sometimes accompanied by bone involvement, and as disseminated disease involving lymph nodes and one or more organ systems (39–41).

Early in the infection, sections of involved lymph nodes show lymphoid hyperplasia. Scattered granulomas, some containing central necrosis and rare multinucleate giant cells, appear later; and as the disease progresses, stellate areas of necrosis coalesce, forming one or more abscesses (Plate VIIIC), changes also associated with tularemia, lymphogranuloma venereum, brucellosis, and infections caused by fungi and mycobacteria. In early lesions organisms may be demonstrated by staining with the Warthin-Starry silver stain (Plate VIIID) and the Brown-Hopp tissue Gram stain (42).

Laboratory Diagnosis

Currently the diagnosis of cat scratch disease in a person with regional lymphadenopathy is based on the fulfillment of three of the following four criteria: (1) history of contact with an animal, usually a cat or dog, and the presence of a scratch or a dermal or ocular lesion; (2) exclusion of other possible pathogens by culture of exudate aspirated from the node and appropriate serologic tests; (3) a positive skin test reaction for cat-scratch disease; (4) consistent histopathologic changes in sections of a lymph node biopsy specimen (described earlier). Visualization of bacteria in sections of lymph node stained with the Warthin-Starry silver stain or Brown-Hopp tissue Gram stain is useful, but their absence does not exclude the diagnosis because bacteria may not be present in all stages of disease.

Afipia felis can be cultured in the clinical laboratory, but this is not required for diagnosis of cat-scratch disease. The organism grows very slowly on buffered charcoal-yeast extract agar at 30° C and in HeLa cell cultures. Biochemical characteristics listed earlier are discussed in detail in reference 31.

The cat-scratch antigen skin test becomes positive 3 to 4 weeks after the onset of illness in about 90% of persons suspected on clinical grounds of having cat-scratch disease and who have been scratched by or had contact with a cat; however, the test has problems. The skin test antigen is not available commercially and must be prepared from pus aspirated from the lymph node of an infected person; and because a method for assessing the antigen's biologic activity has not been developed, standardization of its potency is difficult. Because the reaction may persist for years a positive result reflects only exposure to the antigen and does not necessarily indicate that the organism is responsible for the current illness.

Treatment and Prevention

The lymphadenopathy of cat-scratch disease is self-limited and resolves spontaneously in several months. Treatment is supportive. Needle aspiration of the lymph node should be performed if suppuration occurs. Occasionally, excisional biopsy is necessary, principally in adults, because of persistent pain or for diagnostic purposes.

The gram-negative bacillus recovered by English and colleagues was susceptible to cefoxitin, cefotaxime, and the aminoglycosides and resistant to penicillin, ampicillin, erythromycin, tetracycline, clindamycin, cephalothin, cefazolin, cefamandole, and chloramphenicol by susceptibility testing in vitro (35). Occasionally, marked clinical improvement is reported in response to therapy with various antimicrobial agents, but currently, a consensus on the need for antimicrobial therapy does not exist, and the optimal antimicrobial regimen, if it is necessary, has not been established.

Preventing cat-scratch disease in persons who keep cats is difficult because animals that carry the organism appear well and probably transmit the bacteria for a short interval. Declawing pet cats may be helpful.

REFERENCES

1. Leopold S: Heretofore undescribed organism isolated from the genitourinary system. US Armed Forces Med J, 4:263, 1953.
2. Gardner HL, and Dukes CD: Haemophilus vaginalis vaginitis. Am J Obstet Gynecol, 69:962, 1955.
3. Zinneman K, and Turner GC: The taxonomic position of "Haemophilus vaginalis" (Corynebacterium vaginale). J Pathol Bacteriol, 35:213, 1963.
4. Greenwood JR, and Pickett MJ: Transfer of Haemophilus vaginalis Gardner and Dukes to a new genus, Gardnerella: G. vaginalis (Gardner and Dukes comb nov). Int J Syst Bacteriol, 30:170, 1980.

5. Harper JJ, and Davis GHG: Cell wall analysis of Gardnerella vaginalis (Haemophilus vaginalis). Int J Syst Bacteriol, *32*: 48, 1982.
6. Csango PA, Hagen N, and Jagars G: Method for isolation of Gardnerella vaginalis (Haemophilus vaginalis): Characterization of isolates by gas chromatography. Acta Pathol Microbiol Immunol Scand [B], *90*:89, 1982.
7. Totten PA, et al: Selective differential human blood bilayer media for isolation of Gardnerella (Haemophilus) vaginalis. J Clin Microbiol, *15*:141, 1982.
8. Hammerschlag MR, et al: Microbiology of the vagina in children: Normal and potentially pathogenic organisms. Pediatrics, *62*:57, 1978.
9. Pheifer TA, et al: Nonspecific vaginitis: Role of Haemophilus vaginalis and treatment with metronidazole. N Engl J Med, *289*:1429, 1978.
10. Boustouller YL, Johnson AP, and Taylor-Robinson D: Pili on Gardnerella vaginalis studies by electron microscopy. J Med Microbiol, *23*:327, 1987.
11. Scott TG, Smyth CJ, and Keane CT: In vitro adhesiveness and biotype of Gardnerella vaginalis strains in relation to the occurrence of clue cells in vaginal discharges. Genitourin Med, *63*:47, 1987.
12. Johnson AP, and Boustouller YL: Extravaginal infection caused by Gardnerella vaginalis. Epidemiol Infect, *98*:131, 1987.
13. Bejar R, et al: Premature labor II. Bacterial sources of phospholipase. Obstet Gynecol, *57*:479, 1981.
14. Gravett MG, et al: Independent associations of bacterial vaginosis and Chlamydia trachomatis infection with adverse pregnancy outcome. JAMA, *256*:1899, 1986.
15. Boustouller YL, and Johnson AP: Resistance of Gardnerella vaginalis to bactericidal activity of human serum. Genitourin Med, *62*:380, 1986.
16. Spiegel CA: Gardnerella vaginalis. *In* Principles and Practice of Infectious Diseases. 3rd ed. Edited by GL Mandell, RG Douglas, Jr, and JE Bennett. New York, Churchill Livingstone, 1990.
17. Josephson S, et al: Gardnerella vaginalis in the urinary tract: Incidence and significance in a hospital population. Obstet Gynecol, *71*:245, 1988.
18. Woolfrey BF, Ireland GK, and Lally RT: Significance of Gardnerella vaginalis in urine cultures. Am J Clin Pathol, *86*:324, 1985.
19. Reimer LG, and Reller LB: Gardnerella vaginalis bacteremia: A review of thirty cases. Obstet Gynecol, *54*:170, 1984.
20. Venkataramani TK, and Rathbun HK: Corynebacterium vaginale (Haemophilus vaginalis) bacteremia: Clinical study of 29 cases. Johns Hopkins Med J, *139*:93, 1976.
21. Reimer LG, and Reller LB: Effect of sodium polyanetholsulfonate and gelatin on the recovery of Gardnerella vaginalis from blood culture media. J Clin Microbiol, *21*:686, 1985.
22. Reimer LG, and Reller LB: Use of a sodium polyanetholsulfonate disk for the identification of Gardnerella vaginalis. J Clin Microbiol, *21*:146, 1985.
23. Piot P: Gardnerella, Streptobacillus, Spirillum minus, and Calymmatobacterium. *In* Manual of Clinical Microbiology 5th ed. Edited by A Balows, et al. Washington, DC, American Society for Microbiology, 1991.
24. Dodson RF, et al: Donovanosis: A morphologic study. J Invest Dermatol, *62*:611, 1974.
25. Kuberski T, Papadimitriou JM, and Phillips P: Ultrastructure of Calymmatobacterium granulomatis in lesions of granuloma inguinale. J Infect Dis, *142*:744, 1980.
26. Marmell M: Donovanosis of the anus in the male. An epidemiologic consideration. Br J Vener Dis, *34*:213, 1958.
27. Zigas V: Medicine from the past—donovanosis project in Goilala (1951–1954). Papau New Guinea Med J, *14*:148, 1971.
28. Goldberg J, Weaver RH, and Packer H: Studies on granuloma inguinale. Bacteriologic behavior of Donovania granulomatis. Am J Syph Gonorr Vener Dis, *37*:60, 1953.
29. Jenkins SG: Rat-bite fever. Clin Microbiol Newslett, *10*:57, 1988.
30. Washburn RG: Streptobacillus moniliformis (rat-bite fever). *In* Principles and Practice of Infectious Diseases. 3rd ed. Edited by GL Mandell, RG Douglas, Jr, and JE Bennett. New York, Churchill Livingstone, 1990.
31. Brenner DJ, et al: Proposal of Afipia gen. nov., with Afipia felis sp. nov. (formerly the cat-scratch disease bacillus), Afipia clevelandensis sp. nov. (formerly the Cleveland Clinic Foundation strain), Afipia broomeae sp. nov., and 3 unnamed genospecies. J Clin Microbiol, *29*:2450, 1991.
32. Debre R, et al: La maladie des griffes de chat. Bull Mem Soc Med Hop (Paris), *66*:76, 1950.
33. Wear DJ, et al: Cat-scratch disease: A bacterial infection. Science, *221*:1403, 1983.
34. Margileth AW, et al: Cat-scratch disease bacteria in skin at the primary inoculation site. JAMA, *252*:928, 1984.
35. English CK, et al: Cat-scratch disease. Isolation and culture of the bacterial agent. JAMA, *259*:1347, 1988.
36. Margileth AM: Cat-scratch disease: A therapeutic dilemma. Vet Clin North Am., *155*:390, 1987.
37. Moriarty RA, and Margileth AM: Cat-scratch disease. Infect Dis Clin North Am, *1*:575, 1987.
38. Carithers HA: Cat-scratch disease: An overview based on a study of 1,200 patients. Am J Dis Child, *139*:1124, 1985.
39. Margileth AM, Wear DJ, and English CK: Systemic cat-scratch disease: Report of 23 patients with prolonged or recurrent severe bacterial infection. J Infect Dis, *155*:390, 1987.
40. Schlossberg D, et al: Culture-proven disseminated cat-scratch disease in acquired immunodeficiency syndrome. Arch Intern Med, *149*:1437, 1989.
41. Koehler JE, LeBoit PE, Egbert BM, and Berger TG: Cutaneous vascular lesions and disseminated cat-scratch disease in patients with the acquired immunodeficiency syndrome (AIDS) and AIDS-related complex. Ann Intern Med, *109*:449, 1988.
42. Miller-Catchpole R, et al: Cat-scratch disease. Identification of bacteria in seven cases of lymphadenitis. Am J Surg Pathol, *10*:276, 1986.

Section III

FUNGI AND ALGAE-LIKE ORGANISMS

Chapter 42

INTRODUCTION TO FUNGI AND ALGAE-LIKE ORGANISMS

Fungi are eukaryotes that possess at least one nucleus surrounded by a nuclear membrane, an endoplasmic reticulum, and mitochondria but lack chlorophyll, a substance found in algae. The fungi are chemotrophic, absorbing nutrients from the environment, especially from decaying organic matter. They grow in two morphologic forms, yeasts and moulds, and reproduce by asexual or sexual processes. In this chapter the taxonomy of the medically important fungi and the classification used in this text are described, structure and reproduction are reviewed briefly, and the laboratory diagnosis and antifungal agents are discussed.

Algae are unicellular organisms similar to fungi, except that most have chlorophyll. Two organisms that resemble algae, Prototheca and Cyanobacterium-like bodies, cause human disease. The structure and reproduction of these organisms are reviewed briefly in Chapter 47, and the laboratory diagnosis of the infections they cause is discussed in this chapter.

Classification of Fungi

The taxonomy of the medically important fungi undergoes constant revision. The following list includes most of the fungi encountered in the clinical laboratory. Names in parentheses refer to asexual (anamorph) forms, and those without parentheses to sexual (teleomorph) forms. When all species in a genus do not have known sexual stages, the genus is listed under the known sexual classification and the asexual one. Some asexual fungi may exhibit more than one sexual appearance and, therefore, have more than one sexual name, and some sexual organisms possess more than one asexual name. Members of the subdivisions Zygomycotina, Ascomycotina, and Basidiomycotina undergo sexual reproduction by forming zygospores, ascospores, and basidiospores (described later), respectively; whereas for fungi in the subdivision Deuteromycotina, or Fungi Imperfecti, a sexual stage does not exist or has not yet been discovered.

Kingdom Myceteae (Fungi)
Division: Amastigomycota
Subdivision: Zygomycotina
Class: Zygomycetes
Order: Mucorales
Representative genera: Absidia, Mucor, Rhizopus, Rhizomucor, Cunninghamella, Saksenaea
Order: Entomophthorales
Representative genera: Basidiobolus, Conidiobolus
Subdivision: Ascomycotina
Class: Ascomycetes
Subclass: Hemiascomycetidae
Order: Endomycetales
Representative genera: Saccharomyces, teleomorphs of some Candida
Subclass: Plectomycetidae
Order: Onygenales
Representative genera: Arthroderma (Trichophyton, Microsporum), Ajellomyces (Blastomyces, Histoplasma)
Order: Eurotiales
Representative genera: (Penicillium), (Aspergillus), (Paecilomyces)
Subdivision: Basidiomycotina
Class: Basidiomycetes
Subclass: Teliomycetidae
Order: Ustilagenales
Representative genera: Filobasidiella (Cryptococcus); Rhodosporidum (Rhodotorula)
Subdivision: Deuteromycotina
Class: Deuteromycetes
Subclass: Blastomycetidae
Order: Cryptococcales
Representative genera: (Rhodotorula), (Cryptococcus), (Candida), (Trichosporon), (Malassezia)
Subclass: Hyphomycetidae
Order: Moniliales

Family: Moniliaceae
Representative genera: (Aspergillus), (Penicillium), (Paracoccidioides), (Sporothrix), (Coccidioides), (Microsporum), (Trichophyton), (Epidermophyton)
Family: Dematiaceae
Representative genera: (Alternaria), (Curvularia), (Drechslera), (Cladosporium), (Phialophora), (Fonsecaea), (Exophiala), (Wangiella), (Bipolaris)
Family: Tuberculariaceae
Representative genera: (Fusarium)

Fungal diseases, called mycoses, often are classified according to the tissue or body site invaded: superficial mycoses affect only the outermost layers of the skin and hair, causing little or no pathologic change; cutaneous mycoses cause destruction of the keratin of skin, hair, and nails but rarely invade deeper tissues; subcutaneous mycoses involve the skin, muscle, and connective tissue immediately below the skin, but deep tissue and organ involvement is rare; and systemic mycoses involve the deep tissues and organs and when the infection is disseminated may invade cutaneous and subcutaneous sites. This type of classification has limitations because some organisms may cause more than one type of infection, depending on the immune status of the host. Therefore, in this book the fungi are separated according to morphologic appearance: yeasts, moulds, and dimorphic organisms. In each chapter, the epidemiology, pathogenesis, and clinical manifestations associated with each of the medically important fungi are discussed individually. Fungi that have not been isolated in the laboratory are reviewed in Chapter 46.

Morphologic Appearance of Fungi

Yeasts. Yeasts are unicellular, spherical to ellipsoid organisms, 3 to 15 μm in diameter, that reproduce by budding, although a few divide by binary fission. Yeasts may produce single or multiple buds, and some produce pseudohyphae, which are buds that elongate, typically do not detach, and may form chains resembling links of sausages with constrictions where the cells attach (pictured in Chapter 43 and Plate VIIIE). Rarely, certain yeasts form true hyphae.

Moulds. Moulds are multicellular organisms that produce filamentous colonies consisting of branching, cylindrical tubules, 2 to 10 μm in diameter, called hyphae. Most hyphae are septate (divided into cells by septa or crosswalls), but one family of fungi, the Zygomycetes, have aseptate hyphae (lacking crosswalls) (pictured in Chapter 44). The mass of intertwined hyphae formed during active growth is called the mycelium. The vegetative mycelium is the food-absorbing portion that grows into the substrate, and the aerial mycelium, composed of reproductive or fertile hyphae, extends above the surface and gives rise to conidia or other reproductive units (described later).

Specific structures formed by the vegetative mycelium (Figs. 42–1 and 42–2) are valuable for identifying certain medically important moulds (see Chapter 44). For example, spirals or coiled hyphae are bedspring-like, helical structures prominent in some strains of Trichophyton mentagrophytes. Nodular organs, enlargements in the mycelium consisting of closely twisted hyphae, are formed by some isolates of Microsporum canis and Trichophyton mentagrophytes. Racquet hyphae, structures formed by several of the dermatophytes, are larger than other hyphae and have a regular enlargement of one end of each segment. A pectinate body, a row of unilateral, short, irregular projections or protuberances formed on one side of a hypha that gives it the appearance of a broken comb, commonly is associated with Microsporum audouinii. Favic chandeliers, structures formed by numerous short, multiple branches appearing at the end of a hypha and resembling the antlers of a buck deer, are characteristic of Trichophyton schoenleinii.

Dimorphic Fungi. Some species of fungi are dimorphic: they grow in more than one form, depending on environmental conditions. The pathogenic fungi that exhibit thermal dimorphism (see Chapter 45) grow as yeasts at 35° to 37° C (body temperature) and as moulds at 25° to 30° C (room temperature). For other dimorphic fungi, morphologic appearance is determined by certain nutrients, carbon dioxide, or the age of the culture.

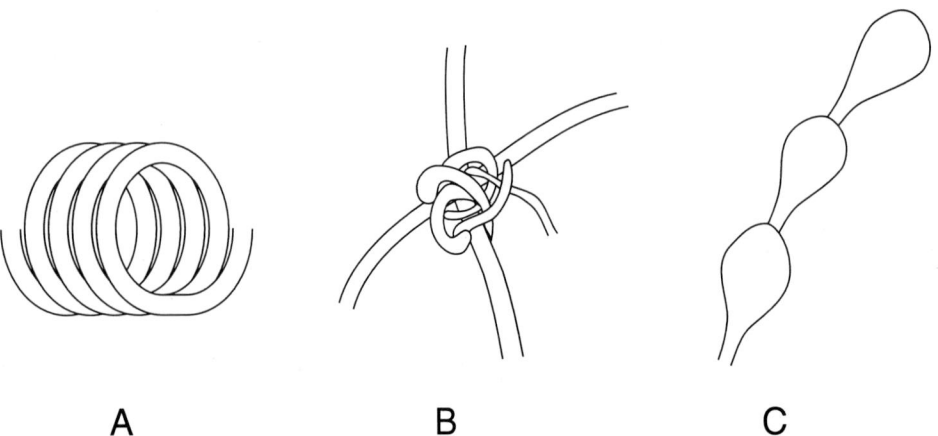

Fig. 42–1. *A*, Diagram of coiled hyphae of Trichophyton mentagrophytes. *B*, Diagram of nodular organs formed by some isolates of Microsporum canis and Trichophyton mentagrophytes. *C*, Diagram of racquet hyphae formed by dermatophytes.

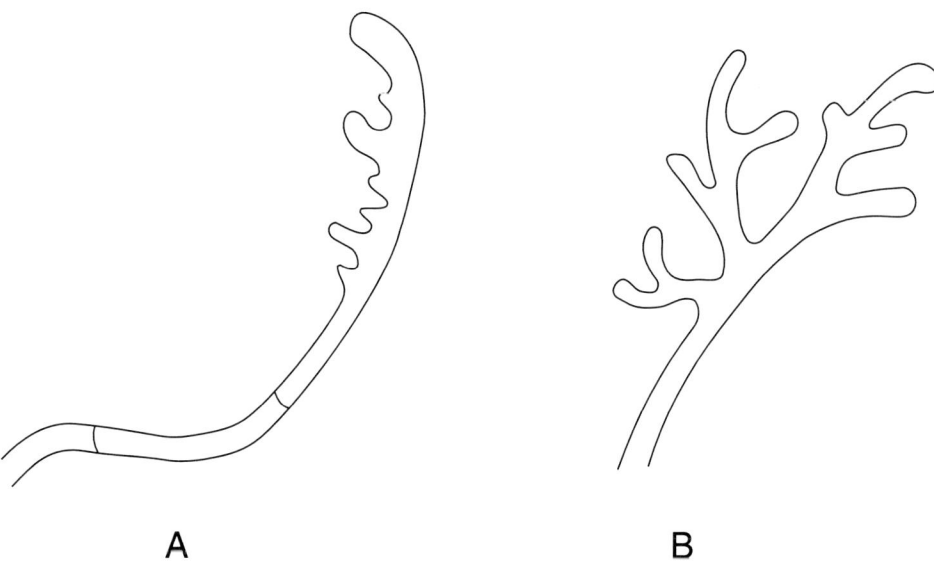

Fig. 42–2. *A*, Diagram of a pectinate body, a structure commonly associated with Microsporum audouinii. *B*, Diagram of favic chandeliers, structures characteristic of Trichophyton schoenleinii.

Fine Structure. A fungal cell consists of a cell wall; a cell membrane; and cytoplasm containing an endoplasmic reticulum, one or more nuclei, nucleoli, storage vacuoles, mitochondria, and other organelles. Some fungi also have an external coating of slime or a more compact capsule composed predominantly of amorphous polysaccharides. The cell wall, composed of 80 to 90% carbohydrate and about 10% protein and glycoprotein, comprises about 90% of the cell's dry weight and provides rigidity, strength, and protection from osmotic lysis. Cell wall polysaccharide polymers such as glucan, mannan, cellulose, and chitin are unique to fungi; the teichoic and muramic acids found in bacterial cell walls (see Chapter 24) are absent. The bilayered cell membrane, similar in structure and composition to those of higher eukaryotes, contains sterols, principally ergosterol and zymosterol, which are essential for viability and are a major site of attack for antifungal agents. The membrane protects the cytoplasm, regulates the intake and secretion of solutes, and facilitates the synthesis of cell wall and capsular material.

Reproduction of Fungi

Asexual Reproduction. Asexual reproduction may occur simply as vegetative growth and expansion of a colony, but the term usually refers to the production of asexual propagules, which may be spores or conidia depending on the mode of production, following mitosis of the parent nucleus. Asexual spores are formed by consecutive cleavages within a saclike structure called a sporangium, whereas conidia are produced free, either by segmentation or by budding of the tips or from the walls of specialized hyphae called conidiogenous cells. There are two types of conidial ontogeny: (1) blastic or budded conidiation, "blowing out" and de novo growth of a part of the hyphal element, and (2) thallic conidiation, in which a part of the preformed hypha is converted into a conidium.

Different types of conidia and spores are described (reviewed in detail in reference 1). Blastoconidia, produced by budding, are formed by yeasts and by some moulds (such as Cladosporium). Phialoconidia, produced by Penicillium and Aspergillus, are formed from a tube- or vase-shaped conidiogenous structure called a phialide, which may exhibit a terminal, cup-shaped collarette (Fig. 42–3) (1). Annelloconidia, observed in cultures of Scopulariopsis, are grown from inside a vase-shaped conidiogenous annellide, which is supported by a simple or branched structure called an annellophore. As each conidium is released from the annellide, a ring of parent outer cell wall material remains behind; thus, the sides of the annellide develop a saw-toothed appearance (see Fig. 42–3).

A macroconidium (or macroaleuriospore) is formed when an entire hyphal element is converted into a multicelled conidium. The microscopic appearance of these structures (see Fig. 42–4) is a useful identifying feature, predominantly for the dermatophytes (see Chapter 44): they may be thick- or thin walled, spiny or smooth, and club-shaped or oval; they may arise on the sides of the hyphae (sessile), or they may be supported by conidiophores; and they may occur individually or in clusters. Microconidia—one-celled, round, oval, or club-shaped structures supported alone or in clusters by a conidiophore—are produced in a similar manner, except that the new conidia remain aseptate.

Chlamydoconidia (Fig. 42–5) are thick-walled conidia at the hyphal tip (terminal), on the sides (sessile), or within the hyphal strand (intercalary) that are formed during unfavorable environmental circumstances and under suitable climatic conditions germinate, producing conidia. Similar-looking chlamydospores produced by such yeasts as Candida albicans, are actually thick-walled vesicles, not conidia, because when mature they do not germinate or produce conidia. Arthroconidia fragment from the hyphae through the septation points, separate within the parent hyphal strand before dispersing, and mature to be thick walled and barrel shaped or rectangular (see Fig. 42–5). Within the hyphae, arthroconidia may form adjacent to each other, as in some species of Tri-

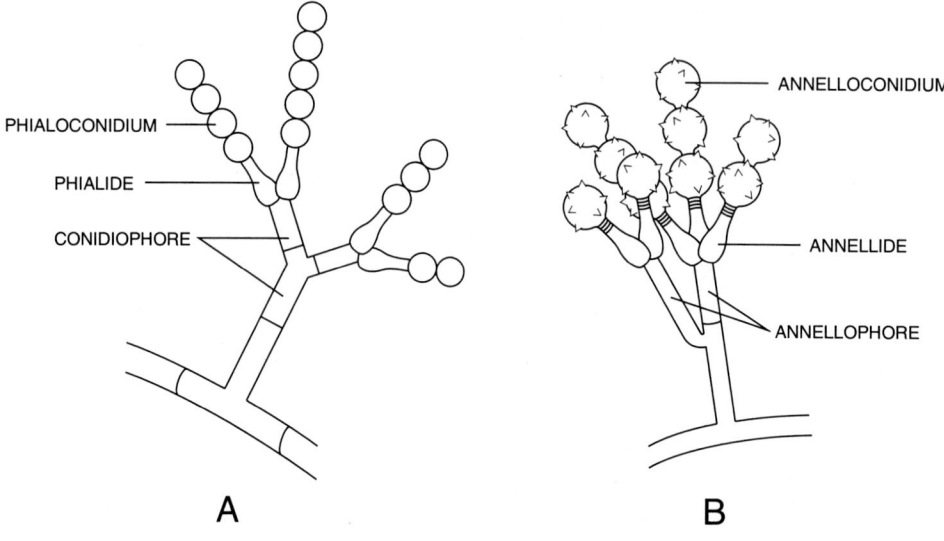

Fig. 42–3. *A,* Diagram of phialoconidia, conidia formed from a tube or vase-shaped conidiogenous structure called a phialide, typical of Aspergillus and Penicillium. *B,* Diagram of annelloconidia—conidia grown from inside a vase-shaped conidiogenous annellide, typical of Scopulariopsis. (From Kern ME: Medical Mycology. A Self-Instructional Text. Philadelphia, FA Davis, 1985.)

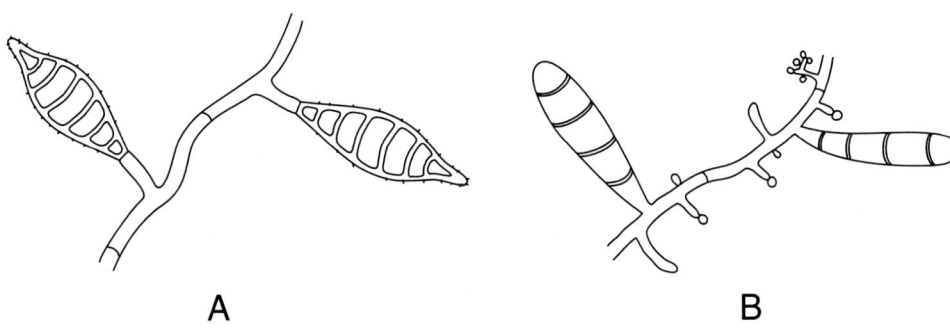

Fig. 42–4. *A,* Diagram of the spiny, thick-walled macroconidia of Microsporum species. *B,* Diagram of the smooth, thin-walled macroconidia and the microconidia of Trichophyton species.

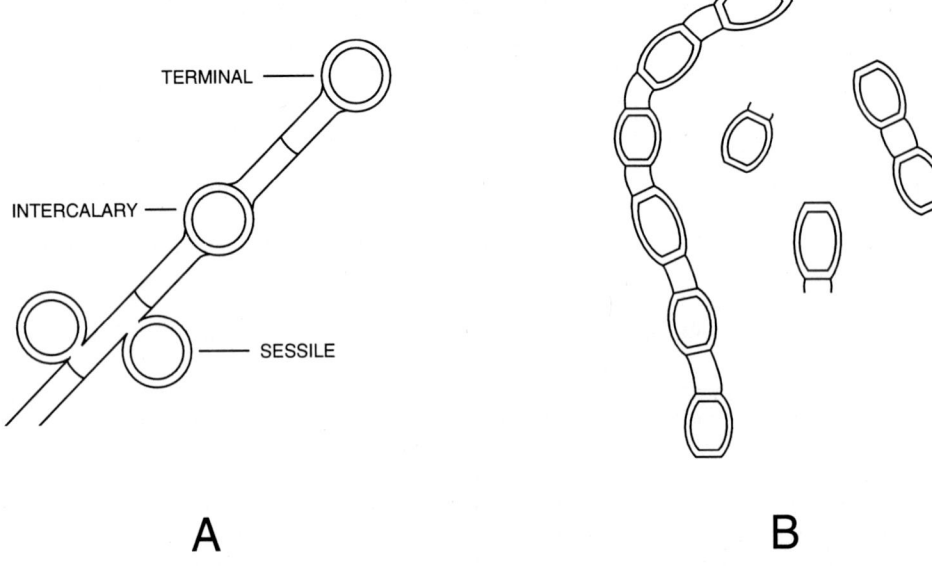

Fig. 42–5. *A,* Diagram of chlamydoconidia, thick-walled conidia formed under unfavorable environmental conditions. (From Kern ME: Medical Mycology. A Self-Instructional Text. Philadelphia, FA Davis, 1985.) *B,* Diagram of arthroconidia, rectangular or barrel-shaped conidia that separate within the parent hyphal strand.

chosporon (Chapter 43), or they may be separated by alternating empty spaces called disjunctor cells, as in Coccidioides immitis (Chapter 45).

Sexual Reproduction. The sexual stage of reproduction, which results in formation of ascospores, basidiospores, or zygospores, is observed infrequently in the clinical laboratory and therefore is reviewed briefly. Ascospore formation is initiated when the nucleus from a male cell (antheridium) passes through a bridge into the female cell (ascogonium) from the same, self-compatible colony or from two colonies of opposite mating types. The male and female nuclei fuse, forming a zygote, and the female cell becomes an ascus. The diploid zygote nucleus divides by meiosis, forming four haploid nuclei that divide by mitosis to form eight nuclei, each of which walls off inside the ascus to form an ascospore. Fungi such as Pseudallescheria boydii (Chapter 44) produce asci within a somatic saclike structure called an ascocarp, which in the medically important fungi is completely enclosed and is termed a cleistothecium.

For fungi that produce basidiospores, such as Filobasidiella neoformans (the sexual stage of Cryptococcus neoformans), two compatible hyphae or yeast cells fuse, forming a binucleate mycelium. The terminal end of the latter enlarges into a club-shaped structure called a basidium, within which the two nuclei fuse to form a zygote. The zygote undergoes meiosis, producing four haploid nuclei, each of which enters into a basidiospore, a small protrusion extending from the end of the basidium. Zygospore formation begins with the fusion of two compatible zygophores, which are arms formed from hyphae within a self-compatible colony or from two colonies of opposite mating types. From this fusion, a thick-walled, protective zygosporangium forms within which a zygospore develops.

Laboratory Diagnosis

Collection of an appropriate specimen and its timely transport to the laboratory are essential for diagnosis of fungal infections (discussed in Part III). Fungi may be recognized in clinical specimens by direct microscopic examination (Table 42–1), or by recovering the organism in culture, and for some fungi serologic testing is useful for diagnosis.

Direct Microscopic Examination. Direct microscopic examination of a clinical specimen is an important diagnostic tool and may provide a diagnosis in less than an hour, whereas culture results usually are not available for several days to several weeks. Various stains or procedures may be used to detect fungal elements and algae-like organisms in clinical samples (see Table 42–1) (2). In a smear stained with the Gram stain (see Appendix, Procedure 3), fungi usually are gram positive; however, cells of Cryptococcus neoformans typically stain weakly (Plate VIIIE), which may be a useful diagnostic feature, particularly when seen in smears of cerebrospinal fluid. The potassium hydroxide (KOH) preparation (see Appendix, Procedure 19) is used primarily for visualizing fungal elements in skin, hair, and nails and in specimens, such as sputum and vaginal secretions, that contain large amounts of cellular material, because KOH dissolves keratin and much of the interfering background debris. Because the background artifacts that are not completely eliminated by KOH may make interpretation of the preparation difficult staining with calcofluor white, a commercially available fluorescent brightener or whitening agent that binds to cellulose and chitin in fungal cell walls and fluoresces with a blue-white color when exposed to ultraviolet radiation, often is preferred. Aqueous solutions of calcofluor white have an absorption spectrum of 300 to 412 nm, with an absorbance maximum of 347 nm; consequently, optimal fluorescence is achieved by using ultraviolet excitation (3). Blue-violet excitation also is acceptable, but microscopes fitted with selective filters for excitation of fluorescein (KP 490 interference filter), which prevent radiation below 490 nm from striking the specimen, cannot be used. Moreover, a mercury vapor lamp rather than a quartz halogen bulb, is recommended, because the low energy output of the latter is not suitable for calcofluor white fluorescence. The India ink stain, used specifically to detect cells of Cryptococcus neoformans (see Chapter 43) in cerebrospinal fluid, no longer is recommended (except for evaluation of specimens from persons with the acquired immunodeficiency syndrome) because it is much less sensitive than the commercially available antigen detection tests (see Chapter 55).

Stains useful for detection of fungi may be performed in areas of the laboratory other than the microbiology section. For example, fungal elements may be seen in tissue sections stained with hematoxylin and eosin, especially when slides are viewed with a fluorescence microscope, because organisms such as Blastomyces,

Table 42–1. Methods for Detection of Fungal Cells in Clinical Specimens by Direct Microscopic Examination

Method	Time (min)	Comments
Gram stain	3	Rapid; detects most fungi; Cryptococcus neoformans may stain weakly.
KOH	5–15	Rapid; background artifacts may be confusing.
Calcofluor white	2	Rapid; fluorescence microscope required; background fluorescence may be a problem; stains Pneumocystis carinii.
Congo red	2	Rapid; cost effective; does not stain bacteria or P. carinii; fluorescence microscope required.
Papanicolaou stain	30	Hyphae may stain weakly.
Methenamine silver	5–10	Rapid; yeast and P. carinii may appear similar.
Periodic acid–Schiff stain	20–30	Artifacts may be confused with yeast cells.
Wright stain	5–10	Useful for diagnosis of disseminated histoplasmosis.
India ink	1	Used to detect C. neoformans in CSF; less sensitive than LA or ELISA.
Mucicarmine stain	60	Stains capsule of C. neoformans.

Key: KOH, potassium hydroxide; CSF, cerebrospinal fluid; LA, latex agglutination; ELISA, enzyme-linked immunoassay.

Cryptococcus, Candida, Aspergillus, Coccidioides, Paracoccidioides, and occasionally Histoplasma brightly autofluoresce and tissue and background material remain dark. Fungi are more easily visualized in tissue sections, imprints, or smears stained with the Gomori methenamine silver or the periodic acid–Schiff stain, in which fungal elements appear black and magenta, respectively. The Congo red stain is a rapid, cost-effective stain for visualizing fungi, although viewing with a fluorescence microscope is necessary (4). The mucicarmine stain may provide a diagnosis of infection with Cryptococcus neoformans, because its capsule stains red (Plate VIIIF) and other yeasts do not. Moreover, disseminated infection with Histoplasma capsulatum may be diagnosed by finding yeast forms (see Chapter 45) inside neutrophils and monocytes in smears of bone marrow and peripheral blood and in imprints of tissue stained with the Wright stain (Fig. 42–6).

Prototheca are detected by many of the procedures used to visualize fungi in clinical samples—the wet mount, KOH preparation, and Gram and silver stains. In wet-mount preparations of fresh, unpreserved stool, Cyanobacterium-like bodies appear as nonrefractile hyaline cysts, 8 to 9 μm in diameter, and under ultraviolet light these organisms autofluoresce, appearing as bright blue circles. Moreover, Cyanobacterium-like bodies stain deep or mottled red or pink with the modified acid-fast stain (see Appendix, Procedure 7).

Culture. In general, two types of culture media, nonselective and selective, are essential for primary recovery of fungi from clinical specimens. Of the available nonselective media, which permit the growth of almost all fungi, inhibitory mold agar and SABHI agar are preferred because they enhance the recovery of some of the more fastidious or slowly growing fungi. Sabouraud's dextrose agar no longer is recommended as a primary recovery medium except when infections with dermatophytes are suspected (see Chapter 44), and then it should contain chloramphenicol and cycloheximide. For optimal recovery of the more fastidious dimorphic fungi such as Blastomyces dermatitidis or Histoplasma capsulatum, using an enriched agar base such as brain-heart infusion supplemented with 5% to 10% sheep blood is recommended (5). If a medium containing blood is used, isolates should be subcultured to a less enriched medium such as Sabouraud's dextrose or potato dextrose agar, on which typical sporulation is most likely to occur.

The second type of medium recommended for primary isolation of fungi is selective for these organisms, containing antimicrobial agents such as penicillin (20 U/ml) plus streptomycin (40 U/ml) or gentamicin (5 μg/ml) plus chloramphenicol (16 μg/ml) to inhibit growth of bacteria. Cycloheximide (0.5 mg/ml) may be added to inhibit the rapidly growing moulds that often overgrow the slower growing dimorphic fungi; however, a medium without cycloheximide also must be used, because this agent inhibits some medically important fungi (such as Cryptococcus neoformans and Aspergillus fumigatus) and the algae-like organisms of the genus Prototheca.

Visual examination of a colony distinguishes yeasts and Prototheca, which produce pasty, opaque, typically cream-colored colonies, 0.5 to 3.0 mm in diameter, often within a few days, from moulds, which form larger filamentous colonies with texture and topography that vary among the different organisms. Yeasts and Prototheca are identified on the basis of specific biochemical tests (see Chapters 43 and 47), whereas the identification of moulds is based on growth rate, inhibition of growth by cycloheximide, colony structure and its microscopic appearance, dimorphism at different incubation temperatures or exoantigen extraction (see Chapter 45), and a few biochemical tests. A general approach to identifying filamentous moulds is presented here, and specific characteristics of the individual organisms are discussed in Chapters 44 and 45.

The growth rate of a mould is a useful identifying feature, but it varies with the concentration of organisms in the clinical specimen, and so, must be used in combination with other characteristics. In general, the dimorphic fungi (see Chapter 45) grow slowly, requiring incubation for 2 to 4 weeks before colonies are visible, although colonies of Sporothrix schenckii, Coccidioides immitis, and occasionally Blastomyces dermatitidis are apparent within 3 to 5 days. Colonies of the Zygomycetes, on the other hand, frequently appear in 24 to 48 hours, and those of other hyaline (having light-colored hyphae and conidia) fungi and some dematiaceous (dark-colored hyphae, conidia, or both) fungi often grow within 1 to 5 days. Moreover, the dimorphic fungi are not inhibited by cycloheximide, whereas most of the rapidly growing moulds will not grow on media that contain cycloheximide.

The appearance of a colony of a filamentous fungus provides useful information, but identification cannot be based on colony structure alone because natural variation among isolates occurs and colony structure varies on different culture media. Certain terms are used to describe fungal colonies. The texture—the height of the aerial hyphae—may be *cottony* or *woolly* (a high, dense aerial mycelium), *velvety* (a low, aerial mycelium resembling velvet), *granular* or *powdery* (flat and crumbly owing to the dense production of conidia), or *glabrous* or *waxy* (a smooth surface characteristic of fungi that do not produce

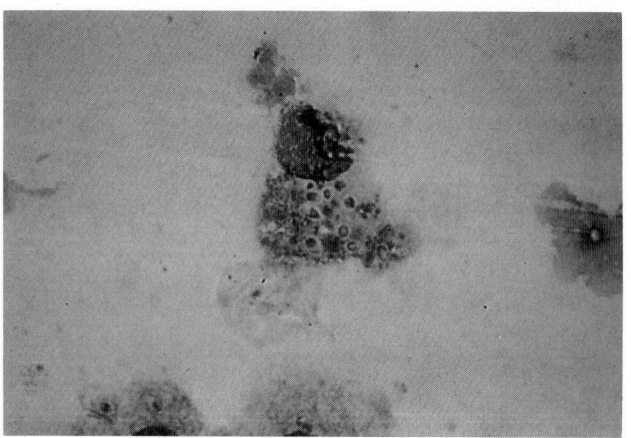

Fig. 42–6. Imprint of a liver biopsy specimen from a patient with disseminated histoplasmosis shows a mononuclear cell filled with yeast forms of the organism (Wright stain, ×320).

an aerial mycelium). Colony topography—the various designs of hills and valleys seen on fungal cultures—may be masked by the aerial hyphae and, so, often is best observed on the reverse side of the colony. Colonies with *rugose* topography have deep furrows radiating irregularly from the center of the culture; those with *umbonate* topography have a button-like central elevation that may be accompanied by rugose furrows around the bottom; those with a *verrucose* topography have a wrinkled, convoluted surface; and *flat* colonies have no hills and valleys. The color of the front and reverse sides of the culture are also important identifying characteristics.

Ultimately, the identification of a mould is based on its microscopic features: the shape, method of production, and arrangement of conidia or spores and the size and appearance of the hyphae, which in general exhibit minimal variation. A fungal isolate may be prepared for microscopic examination in several ways. A tease mount (see Appendix, Procedure 20) can be prepared and examined immediately after the colony has matured on the primary isolation medium, though the rough action of teasing apart hyphae disturbs the juxtaposition of conidia, making it difficult to observe the characteristic conidia or spore arrangements necessary for identification. The Scotch tape preparation (see Appendix, Procedure 21) allows better preservation of the conidia or spore arrangements of the more delicate filamentous fungi, and in most cases permits accurate identification. When a mould cannot be identified by the tease mount or Scotch tape preparation or when permanent slide mounts are desired, the microslide culture technique is recommended (outlined in references 1, 5, 6).

Serodiagnosis of Fungal Diseases. Serologic tests to detect fungal antigens or antibodies to specific antigens occasionally provide evidence that suggests a fungal infection; however, in most cases isolation and identification of the pathogen are necessary for diagnosis. Of the antigen detection tests currently available commercially, only those specific for antigens of Cryptococcus neoformans (latex agglutination tests and an enzyme-linked immunosorbent assay [ELISA]) are reliable for diagnosis (see Chapters 43 and 55). Presently available tests for detection of Candida antigens are neither sensitive nor specific (7,8). ELISA that detects Aspergillus antigens shows promise, but to date this assay has been evaluated only in research laboratories and is not available commercially (9–11).

Tests for detection of antibodies to antigens of the dimorphic fungi are commercially available. An overview of these tests is provided here, and a more detailed discussion is found in Chapter 45. In general, complement fixation and immunodiffusion assays are recommended (though to detect antibodies to Sporothrix schenckii latex agglutination is the only available assay). A complement fixation titer greater than 1:32, even for a single specimen, may be diagnostically significant, whereas lower titers may represent early infection, a cross-reaction, or residual antibodies from a previous infection. Many of the diagnostic antigens used in medical mycology are unpurified mixtures of several antigens, some of which are shared by fungi of different genera or by other microorganisms; therefore, cross-reactions occur. In the United States, concurrent testing for antibodies to Blastomyces, Histoplasma, and Coccidioides allows more accurate interpretation of results than testing for antibodies to a single organism. In addition, a negative serologic test result does not exclude an infection with one of these fungi because immunocompromised persons, and some persons with a systemic infection, may not mount an antibody response. Serologic tests should supplement attempts to recover an organism and should not replace culture.

Antifungal Agents and Susceptibility Testing

Several antifungal agents currently are available to treat fungal infections (Table 42–2), and susceptibility testing of fungal isolates to these agents may be requested to provide information that will allow selection of the best drug or explain an apparent therapeutic failure (12–16). Broth dilution and agar dilution procedures using antifungal agents are similar in design to those described in Chap-

Table 42–2. Antifungal Agents, Their Mode of Action, and Clinical Indications

Agent	Mode of Action	Indications
Amphotericin B	Disrupts integrity of fungal cell membrane	Systemic infections with Histoplasma, Blastomyces, Coccidioides, Cryptococcus, Aspergillus, Candida, and the Zygomycetes
5-Fluorocytosine	Inhibits fungal DNA and RNA synthesis	Systemic infections with Cryptococcus and some species of Candida (in combination with amphotericin B)
Imidazoles and triazoles	Alter structure and permeability of cell membrane by inhibiting ergosterol synthesis	
Clotrimazole		Topical: cutaneous and mucocutaneous infections with Candida and dermatophytes
Miconazole		Topical: as for clotrimazole Parenteral: deep infections with Pseudallescheria
Ketoconazole		Chronic mucocutaneous candidiasis; paracoccidioidomycosis; non–life-threatening, nonmeningeal histoplasmosis and blastomycosis
Fluconazole		Meningitis caused by Cryptococcus neoformans
Itraconazole*		Effective against superficial and cutaneous or mucocutaneous mycoses, blastomycosis, extracutaneous sporotrichosis, paracoccidioidomycosis, histoplasmosis, coccidioidomycosis, chromoblastomycosis, phaeohyphomycosis, and some cases of aspergillosis

* Not currently approved by the Food and Drug Administration for use in the United States.

ter 24 for antibacterial agents. Antifungal susceptibility testing, however, is complicated by the basic properties (solubility, chemical stability, and modes of action) of some of the compounds to be tested, the slow growth of some fungi, and the ability of dimorphic fungi to exist in two forms. Results of antifungal susceptibility tests also are influenced by the composition and pH of the medium, inoculum size, and incubation time and temperature. Moreover, susceptibility testing methods currently are not standardized for fungi. The National Committee for Clinical Laboratory Standards (NCCLS) Subcommittee on Antifungal Susceptibility Tests has made preliminary recommendations for broth macrodilution susceptibility testing for some yeasts (17). Given the lack of standardization and the more involved nature of antifungal susceptibility testing, sending isolates to a reference laboratory where personnel are familiar with the procedures is recommended. A more detailed description of the procedures can be found in references 18 and 19.

In addition to susceptibility testing, bioassays for antifungal agents occasionally are warranted, especially to determine serum levels of 5-fluorocytosine in persons with impaired renal function or when drug toxicity (neutropenia, leukopenia, thrombocytopenia) is suspected. Serum levels of 5-fluorocytosine above 100 to 125 µg/ml are considered potentially toxic (18). Because this test is rarely requested in most clinical laboratories, sending serum samples to an experienced reference laboratory is suggested. A more detailed description of the bioassay is available in reference 18.

REFERENCES

1. Kern ME: Medical Mycology. A Self-Instructional Text. Philadelphia, FA Davis, 1985.
2. Musial CE, Cockerill FR III, and Roberts GD: Fungal infections of the immunocompromised host: Clinical and laboratory aspects. Clin Microbiol Rev, *1*:349, 1988.
3. Harrington BJ, and Hageage GJ: Calcofluor white: Tips for improving its use. Clin Microbiol Newslett, *13*:3, 1991.
4. Slifkin M, and Cumbie R: Congo red as a fluorochrome for the rapid detection of fungi. J Clin Microbiol, *26*:827, 1988.
5. Koneman EW, et al (eds.): Mycology. *In* Color Atlas and Textbook of Diagnostic Microbiology. 3rd ed. Philadelphia, JB Lippincott, 1988.
6. Roberts GD: Laboratory methods in basic mycology. *In* Bailey and Scott's Diagnostic Microbiology. 8th ed. St Louis, CV Mosby, 1990.
7. Ness M, Vaughan WP, and Woods GL: Candida antigen latex test for detection of invasive candidiasis in immunocompromised patients. J Infect Dis, *159*:495, 1989.
8. Escuro RS, et al: Prospective evaluation of a Candida antigen detection test for invasive candidiasis in immunocompromised adult patients with cancer. Am J Med, *87*:621, 1989.
9. Haynes KA, Latge JP, and Rogers TR: Detection of Aspergillus antigens associated with invasive disease. J Clin Microbiol, *28*:2040, 1990.
10. Rogers TR, Haynes KA, and Barnes RA: Value of antigen detection in predicting invasive pulmonary aspergillosis. Lancet, *336*:1210, 1990.
11. Andrews CP, and Weiner MH: Aspergillus antigen detection in bronchoalveolar lavage fluid from patients with invasive aspergillosis and aspergillomas. Am J Med, *73*:372, 1982.
12. Terrell CL, and Hermans PE: Antifungal agents used for deep-seated mycotic infections. Mayo Clin Proc, *62*:1116, 1987.
13. Bossche HV, Willemsens G, and Marichal P: Anti-Candida drugs—the biochemical basis for their activity. Crit Rev Microbiol, *15*:57, 1987.
14. Fromtling RA: Overview of medically important antifungal azole derivatives. Clin Microbiol Rev, *1*:187, 1988.
15. Bodey CP: Azole antifungal agents. Clin Infect Dis, *14*(suppl 1):S161, 1992.
16. Graybill JR: Future directions of antifungal chemotherapy. Clin Infect Dis, *14*(suppl 1):S170, 1992.
17. Pfaller MA, et al: Collaborative investigation of variables in susceptibility testing of yeasts. Antimicrob Agents Chemother, *34*:1648, 1990.
18. Shadomy S, and Pfaller MA: Laboratory studies with antifungal agents: Susceptibility tests and quantitation in body fluids. *In* Manual of Clinical Microbiology. 5th ed. Edited by A Balows, et al. Washington, DC, American Society for Microbiology, 1991.
19. Roberts GD: Fungi. *In* Laboratory Procedures in Clinical Microbiology. 2nd ed. Edited by JA Washington. New York, Springer-Verlag, 1985.

Chapter 43

YEASTS

Yeasts are found in nature in many substrates such as fruits, vegetables, and homemade fermented beverages. The most common human pathogen, Candida albicans, is part of the normal gastrointestinal flora. More than 500 species of yeasts are known, but fewer than 30 are isolated from clinical specimens. In this chapter the yeasts encountered most often in the clinical laboratory—the species of Candida and Cryptococcus neoformans—are discussed in detail. Yeasts that are seen less frequently but may cause invasive disease—Malassezia furfur, Trichosporon beigelii, species of Hansenula, Saccharomyces cerevisiae, Blastoschizomyces capitatus, and Rhodotorula—are reviewed briefly. The group of organisms called "black yeasts" initially grow as unicellular, budding cells, but with age develop a mycelium; these organisms are discussed with the moulds in Chapter 44.

CANDIDA

Candida was identified in oral lesions in the late 1830s and in the early 1860s was recognized as a potential cause of deep-seated infection (1,2). Since the introduction of antimicrobial agents in the 1940s, previously undocumented manifestations of infections caused by Candida have been recognized, and the prevalence of these infections has increased. Today, the species of Candida are the most common causes of systemic fungal infections in immunocompromised persons. More than 150 species of Candida are known, but only Candida albicans (which now includes Candida stellatoidea), Candida tropicalis, Candida krusei, Candida lusitaniae, Candida parapsilosis, Candida kefyr (formerly Candida pseudotropicalis), Candida guilliermondii, and Torulopsis glabrata (an organism included here because it previously was considered a member of the genus Candida) are regarded as medically important (3–9). Candida rugosa, Candida utilis, Candida lipolytica, and Candida zeylanoides are rare human pathogens (10–12).

Epidemiology

Of the species of Candida, Candida albicans most frequently colonizes humans and is part of the normal flora of the oral cavity, gastrointestinal tract, and the female genitourinary tract. Candida tropicalis and Torulopsis glabrata may be part of the normal flora in these same sites but are less common. Candida krusei, Candida guilliermondii, and Candida parapsilosis more often are part of the normal flora of the skin. For all species the colonization rates increase in persons who take cytotoxic drugs that disrupt the gastrointestinal mucosa, broad-spectrum antimicrobial agents that suppress the normal bacterial flora, especially anaerobes, or both.

Diseases caused by the species of Candida are endogenous and develop when normal host defenses are interrupted. For example, alteration of cutaneous or mucosal barriers via intravenous drug use, placement of an indwelling intravascular catheter, burns, a surgical procedure (especially involving the gastrointestinal tract), or drugs or tumors that damage the gastrointestinal tract all are associated with increased risk of disease. Other risk factors include diabetes mellitus, broad-spectrum antimicrobial therapy, pregnancy (especially for Candida vaginitis), corticosteroid administration, neutropenia, cellular immune deficiencies, and the presence of prosthetic devices (heart valves, joints).

Pathogenesis and Pathology

Virulence factors of Candida and host defense mechanisms are involved in the pathogenesis of disease caused by these organisms. In animal models of infection differences in pathogenicity among the species of Candida have been demonstrated: (in decreasing order of virulence) Candida albicans, Candida tropicalis, Candida parapsilosis, Candida kefyr, Candida krusei, and Candida guilliermondii (13). Specific factors that correlate with the ability of these species to produce disease have not been elucidated completely, but fungal components that may contribute to virulence have been identified (14). For example, the adherence of Candida to host epithelial and endothelial cells, a process controlled by adhesins (probably a mannoprotein) on the surface of the fungus that interact with receptors on the host cells, correlates with virulence and is important in the pathogenesis of disease. The cell wall mannan can stimulate or suppress cell-mediated and humoral immune functions, and its oligosaccharide fragments appear to be potent inhibitors of cell-mediated immunity. Several virulence factors have been described specifically for Candida albicans (14,15). Two hydrolytic enzymes, a phospholipase and an acidic carboxyl protease, appear to be involved in fungal attachment to mucosal cells, and the latter probably plays a role in the pathogenesis of Candida vaginitis. Complement receptors may bind and mask opsonic ligands, reducing uptake and killing of the organism by phagocytes. Moreover, the ability to switch phenotype may have a protective role, because the white and opaque yeast phenotypes show differences in sensitivity to the candidacidal activity of neutrophils.

Several host factors protect against disease caused by Candida. The first line of defense is an intact integument. Once organisms invade the dermis or enter the blood, polymorphonuclear leukocytes, monocytes, and eosinophils damage pseudohyphae and ingest and kill yeast cells (16–18). In particular the myeloperoxidase, hydrogen peroxide, or superoxide anion systems of neutrophils and monocytes are responsible for intracellular killing of Candida organisms. The importance of lymphocytes in the host defense against Candida is suggested by the following clinical observations: persons with a defective cell-mediated immune response to Candida antigens are at increased risk of chronic mucocutaneous candidiasis and those with the acquired immunodeficiency syndrome (AIDS) are highly susceptible to mucocutaneous candidiasis. The specific role of the lymphocytes is not completely understood.

In tissues, Candida includes microabscess formation. Initially, polymorphonuclear leukocytes are attracted to the site of infection, followed by histiocytes, epithelioid macrophages, and occasional giant cells, and eventually a granuloma may form. In severely immunocompromised persons the inflammatory response may be minimal or nonexistent, and lesions are composed entirely of aggregates of organisms, with or without tissue necrosis. Generally, both budding yeasts and pseudohyphae are found (Fig. 43–1), and, rarely, true hyphae.

Clinical Manifestations

Infections with Candida may involve the mucocutaneous surfaces or deep organs. Mucosal disease may affect several sites (19–22). Thrush, a condition characterized by white patches on the tongue and other oral mucosal surfaces, is common in persons taking corticosteroids, in persons with cancer, and in those infected with human immunodeficiency virus (HIV). In the gastrointestinal tract, principally the esophagus, Candida may cause ulcers, superficial erosions, or pseudomembrane formation (Fig. 43–2), predominantly in persons with malignancies or those infected with HIV. Candida vaginitis, manifested by vulvar pruritus and a thick, curdlike discharge, most frequently is associated with diabetes mellitus, antimicrobial therapy, or pregnancy.

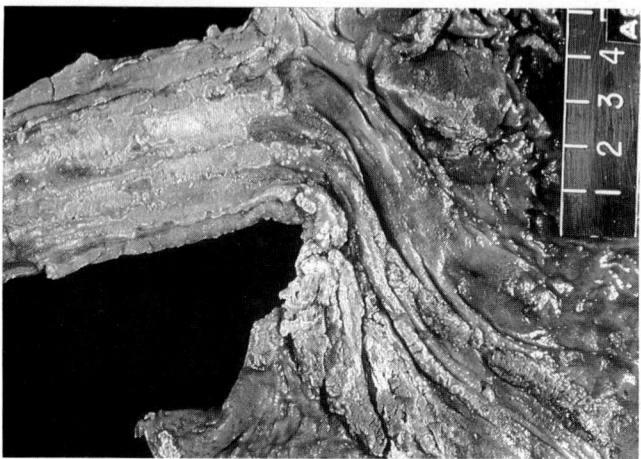

Fig. 43–2. Ulcers and pseudomembranes of Candida esophagitis and gastritis.

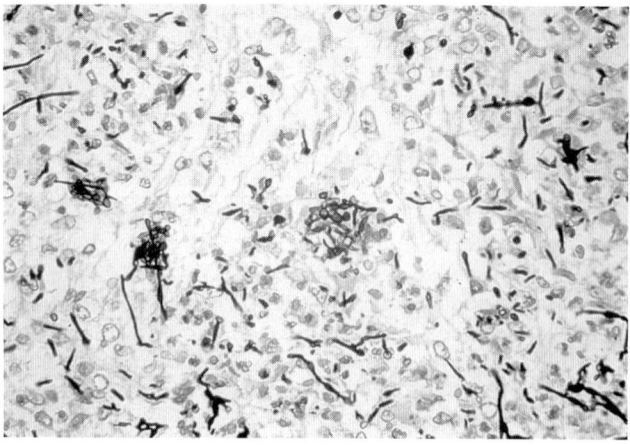

Fig. 43–1. Section of a brain abscess shows budding yeast cells and pseudohyphae of Candida albicans (Gomori's methenamine silver/hematoxylin and eosin, ×128).

Cutaneous manifestations of candidiasis include intertrigo (vesicles and pustules in sites where apposed skin surfaces provide a warm, moist environment), paronychia, (localized inflammation around and under a nail, typically in persons who frequently immerse the hands in water), onychomycosis (infection of the nail itself), and diaper rash (23,24). Chronic mucocutaneous candidiasis is a protracted and persistent infection of the skin, mucous membranes, hair, and nails caused by Candida that occurs in persons who have abnormalities of T-lymphocyte function, of whom about half have an associated endocrine disorder (25,26).

Manifestations of deep organ candidiasis are protean. In the central nervous system the infection may involve the brain parenchyma, producing multiple microabscesses and small macroabscesses, and the meninges, usually as a complication of disseminated disease but occasionally resulting from infection of a ventricular shunt or as a complication of lumbar puncture, trauma, or a neurosurgical procedure (27,28). Candida pneumonia occurs as a local or diffuse process originating from endobronchial inoculation of the lung or, more commonly, as diffuse nodular infiltrates (Fig. 43–3) resulting from hematogenous spread from a distant primary source. In the heart infection with Candida may involve the endocardium, myocardium, or pericardium (29–31). Endocarditis most often affects the aortic or mitral valve, predominantly in persons with one of the following risk factors: underlying valvular heart disease, intravenous drug use, cancer chemotherapy, prosthetic valves, prolonged use of intravascular catheters, or pre-existing bacterial endocarditis. The infection frequently is caused by species other than Candida albicans, and in heroin addicts Candida parapsilosis most commonly is involved (32).

Infection of the urinary tract with Candida may manifest as cystitis, which typically complicates bladder instrumentation, or as pyelonephritis. In the latter situation, yeast organisms generally reach the kidney by hematogenous spread from a distant focus of infection, but they may ascend from a primary infection in the bladder. In the musculoskeletal system Candida may cause osteomyelitis,

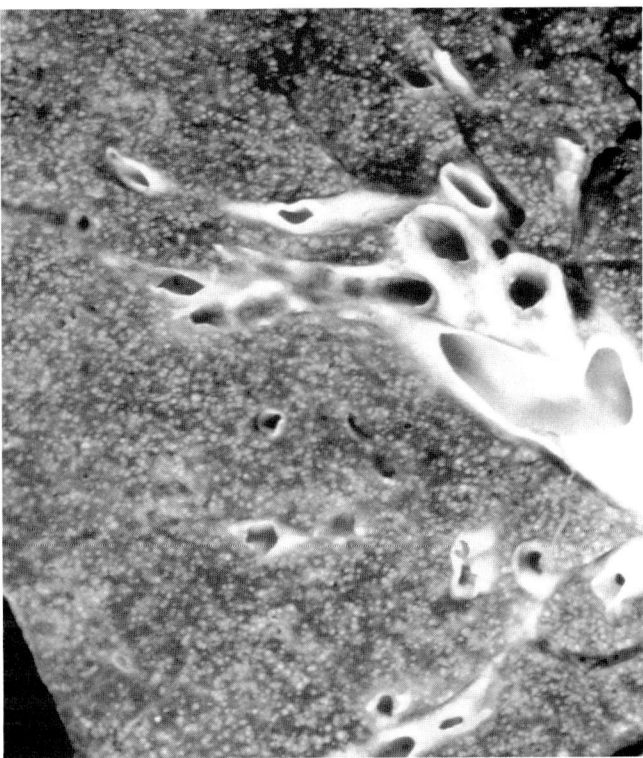

Fig. 43–3. Diffuse nodular infiltrates in the lung of an immunocompromised patient with disseminated candidiasis due to Candida tropicalis.

which most often involves the axial skeleton of adults and the long bones of children, or arthritis, usually a component of disseminated disease. Candida arthritis also may be a complication of trauma, a surgical procedure, intra-articular injection of steroids, or heroin injection, situations in which species other than Candida albicans predominate (33–36).

Intra-abdominal infections caused by Candida include peritonitis, as a complication of peritoneal dialysis, a surgical procedure in the abdomen, or perforation of an abdominal viscus; hepatitis; cholecystitis; or splenic abscess (37–41). In the eye infection with Candida may cause endophthalmitis, which can lead to permanent blindness. Ocular lesions most often result from hematogenous spread and thus serve as an indicator of underlying disseminated disease.

CRYPTOCOCCUS

Cryptococcus neoformans is the only Cryptococcus species of medical importance; human infections caused by other species occasionally have been reported but have not been well-documented (42–44). Four serotypes of Cryptococcus neoformans (designated A through D based on the antigenic specificity of the capsular polysaccharide) have been described, although some strains (called AD) react with antisera to serotypes A and D (45). Serotypes A and D are responsible for most cases of cryptococcosis, but serotypes B and C cause occasional infections, principally in the tropics and subtropics. The sexual form of the organism, a basidiomycete, was recognized in 1975 and named Filobasidiella neoformans. Subsequently, two variants—Filobasidiella neoformans var neoformans (the sexual state of serotypes A and D, called Cryptococcus neoformans var neoformans) and Filobasidiella neoformans var bacillispora (the sexual state of serotypes B and C, called Cryptococcus neoformans var gattii) were identified (46).

Epidemiology

Cryptococcus neoformans, a saprobe in nature, is found worldwide, most commonly associated with the excreta of pigeons, although the birds are not infected (47). Infection with C. neoformans serotypes A and D is believed to be acquired by inhalation of aerosolized organisms, because viable yeast cells smaller than 2 μm in diameter (a size compatible with alveolar deposition) have been recovered in nature from pigeon droppings and soil (48). C. neoformans var gattii has been recovered only from material such as wood, bark, leaves, and debris associated with Eucalyptus camaldulensis trees (49).

Disease caused by Cryptococcus neoformans is most common in males (male-to-female ratio, 3:1), and Caucasians are affected more often than persons of other races. Factors associated with increased risk of disease are corticosteroid administration, lymphoreticular malignancies (especially Hodgkin's disease), sarcoidosis, and infection with HIV; however, in over half the cases no predisposing condition is recognized (50).

Pathogenesis and Pathology

Virulence factors of the fungus and host defense mechanisms are involved in the pathogenesis of disease caused by Cryptococcus neoformans. Its primary virulence factor is its polysaccharide (predominantly glucuronoxylomannan with a minor component of galactoxylomannan) capsule, which inhibits phagocytosis, probably by blocking recognition of the yeast of phagocytes, and may impair leukocyte migration. In vitro, capsular material induces an increase in numbers of suppressor T lymphocytes and the production of macrophage-suppressive lymphokines, events that in vivo could contribute to the depressed chemotaxis and cutaneous anergy observed in persons with cryptococcosis (51–54). Moreover, high concentrations of capsular polysaccharide in serum activate the alternate complement pathway (see Chapter 2), thus depleting serum complement and opsonins (55).

Host immune defenses are important in clearing Cryptococcus neoformans organisms from sites of infection. In mice infected with C. neoformans in the laboratory neutrophils initially clear the organisms, and monocytes predominate later. In vitro, human neutrophils and monocytes ingest and kill cells of C. neoformans via the myeloperoxidase-peroxide-halide mechanism, a process that is enhanced by activating neutrophils with supernatants from stimulated lymphocytes (56,57). Natural killer cells inhibit the growth of C. neoformans in vitro by nonphagocytic mechanisms, but the significance of this activity in clearing organisms acquired naturally via the respiratory route is unknown (58). Antibodies specific for C. neoformans enhance the inhibitory effects of natural killer cells, other effector cells mediate antibody-dependent cell-mediated killing of the fungus, and T lymphocytes may be fungistatic for C. neoformans (59–61).

In tissues, cells of Cryptococcus neoformans multiply, producing little necrosis or organ dysfunction until late in most infections, although tissue damage may occur earlier in infections associated with a large inoculum. The inflammatory response ranges from virtually none to chronic inflammation with macrophages, lymphocytes, foreign body giant cells, and rare polymorphonuclear leukocytes; extensive fibrosis and calcification are uncommon. In the central nervous system a fibrinopurulent exudate typically covers the leptomeninges, particularly at the base of the brain. The infection involves the subarachnoid and the subjacent superficial layers of the brain and spinal cord, producing meningoencephalitis. Frequently, cysts that are composed of clusters of organisms with no accompanying inflammation, which often are large enough to be visualized grossly, form in the superficial layers of the cortex in the depths of the sulci, and occasionally in the deep white matter and the basal ganglia.

Clinical Manifestations

The most common and serious manifestations of infection with Cryptococcus neoformans is meningoencephalitis, which usually begins insidiously over a period of weeks to months but may present as acute disease, especially in persons who take corticosteroids or have a lymphoreticular malignancy. Symptoms include headache, nausea, dizziness, irritability, somnolence, clumsiness, impaired memory and judgment, and behavior changes; if the cranial nerves are involved, decreased visual acuity, diplopia, and facial numbness or weakness may be present. Fever and nuchal rigidity often are absent or minimal; focal sensory or motor findings are rare until late in the disease; and dementia may develop when the brain parenchyma is extensively involved.

Outside the central nervous system infection with Cryptococcus neoformans may involve the lungs, skin, lymph nodes, bones, and many other sites (47,62–65). Pulmonary infection, which may be asymptomatic or manifested by sputum production and dull chest pain, may progress, regress spontaneously, or remain stable for months to years. The skin is involved in some 10% of cases of cryptococcosis; most often with painless lesions of the face or scalp. Other presentations include small papules, pustules, subcutaneous masses, large ulcers, cellulitis, and in persons with AIDS, umbilicated papules resembling molluscum contagiosum (Chapter 4). Bone lesions resembling cold abscesses, similar to those seen in tuberculosis, occur in 5 to 10% of cases.

MALASSEZIA

The genus Malassezia (previously called Pityrosporum) contains at least two species of globose to ellipsoid, unipolar budding yeasts. Malassezia furfur, recovered from normal and diseased human skin, requires long-chain fatty acids for growth. Malassezia pachydermatis, recovered from healthy and diseased skin of several mammals, including dogs, pigs, bears, elephants, and rarely humans, grows on complex media without supplementation with fatty acids (66). These organisms bud repeatedly on a broad base from the same location, forming a "collarette" from which younger buds emerge. Hyphal forms are found on the skin but are rare in culture. Of the two species, Malassezia furfur, the principal human pathogen, is reviewed here. Malassezia pachydermatis rarely is recovered from clinical specimens but is a potential pathogen in infants with risk factors similar to those described later for Malassezia furfur–induced sepsis; this organism is not discussed further here (67).

Epidemiology

Malassezia organisms have been observed on normal and diseased skin and scalp for over a century. In an early study of adults, rates of recovery of Malassezia furfur from the scalp, chest, and back were 74%, 92%, and 100%, respectively, and rates were lower for other sites (68). One study of children showed that those younger than 1 year were not colonized and that the rate of colonization was highest (93%) in 15-year-olds, data suggesting that colonization with M. furfur occurs when the sebaceous glands become active and the concentration of skin lipids increases (69). In recent investigations of hospitalized infants, however, rates of skin colonization by M. furfur have ranged from 32 to 84%, and risk factors for colonization included younger gestational age, housing in a neonatal intensive care unit, longer hospital stay, occlusive dressings, and antimicrobial therapy (66).

Pathogenesis

The pathogenesis of infections caused by Malassezia furfur is not completely understood. Superficial infections are more common in the tropics and may appear after sun exposure, suggesting that the sun may trigger infections; however, the specific stimulus that causes M. furfur to change from a saprophyte to a pathogen is not known. Catheter-related infection is a major problem in premature infants who require catheters for longterm venous access and intravenous lipid therapy, but it may also occur in adults receiving intravenous lipids (70). Catheters may become colonized with M. furfur at the time of surgical placement, by contaminated infusate, by hematogenous seeding from a distant source of infection, or by migration of organisms from the exit site on the skin along the outer catheter wall or from the catheter hub through the lumen, but the exact mechanism is unknown (66). The role of phagocytes, antibodies, and cell-mediated immunity in defense against M. furfur infections have not been evaluated.

Clinical Manifestations

The most common manifestation of infection caused by Malassezia furfur is pityriasis versicolor, a superficial infection of the stratum corneum layer of the epidermis characterized by nonpruritic, painless, hypopigmented or hyperpigmented macules, usually on the trunk or proximal extremities. The organism has also been associated with more symptomatic skin conditions such as seborrheic dermatitis and folliculitis (71). Fungemia with M. furfur occurs almost exclusively in association with long-term administration of intravenous lipids through a central venous catheter but rarely develops in persons without these risk factors (72). Most affected persons have fever, often accompanied by thrombocytopenia, but some are asymptomatic (66). Systemic infections caused by M. furfur—sinusitis, peritonitis, and pulmonary infections—are rare (66,73,74).

OTHER YEASTS

Trichosporon beigelii

Trichosporon beigelii is widely distributed in nature and is a minor component of normal skin flora. It is the agent of white piedra, an asymptomatic superficial infection of the scalp, body, or pubic hair characterized by small, soft, yellow nodules on the hair shafts, that occurs infrequently in tropical and temperate climates. In addition, T. beigelii may cause invasive disease—endophthalmitis, brain abscess, endocarditis, fungemia with accompanying papular red skin lesions, and disseminated disease with multiple organ involvement—in persons with predisposing factors such as neutropenia secondary to cytotoxic chemotherapy, cutaneous wounds or indwelling intravascular catheters, organ transplants, prosthetic heart valves, or intravenous drug use (75,76).

Hansenula species

Though species of Hansenula are rarely human pathogens, most of the cases reported have been caused by Hansenula anomala, which is believed to be part of the normal or transient flora of the human throat and gastrointestinal tract and may be found on plants, fruits, and soil. Infections with H. anomala, including asymptomatic and lethal fungemia, endocarditis, and ventriculitis, have occurred in immunocompromised persons, many of whom were receiving antimicrobial therapy and had an intravascular device in place (77,78). Hansenula polymorpha has been recovered in pure culture from mediastinal lymph nodes of a child with chronic granulomatous disease, and a refractory urinary tract infection with prostatitis caused by Hansenula fabiani was reported in a man with chronic lymphocytic leukemia (79).

Saccharomyces cerevisiae

Saccharomyces cerevisiae (also known as brewers' or bakers' yeast), an asporogenous yeast used in the production of baked goods, beer, and wine and occasionally found in health foods, may colonize the respiratory, gastrointestinal, or urinary tract of persons with underlying chronic disease. This organism is a rare human pathogen but has caused fungemia, endocarditis involving prosthetic valves, pneumonia, and liver and renal abscesses in immunocompromised persons, most of whom were hospitalized for long periods and treated with broad-spectrum antimicrobial agents (80,81).

Blastoschizomyces capitatus

Blastoschizomyces capitatus (formerly Trichosporon capitatum), a fungus characterized by the production of anelloconidia rather than arthroconidia (see Chapter 42), is an uncommon human pathogen that causes disease primarily in immunocompromised persons. In a recent review of infections caused by this organism, Blastoschizomyces capitatus was encountered more frequently in Europe than in the United States (82). The organism has caused pneumonia, splenic abscess, cerebritis, disseminated disease, and endocarditis in association with risk factors similar to those associated with other systemic fungal diseases: immunosuppression due to cytotoxic agents or corticosteroids, underlying malignancy (especially leukemia), and neutropenia.

Rhodotorula species

Species of Rhodotorula, conspicuous in the laboratory by virtue of their production of carotenoid pigment, are normal inhabitants of moist human skin. Invasive disease—fungemia, meningitis—caused by these organisms is rare (83,84).

Laboratory Diagnosis

Specimens required for diagnosis of infections caused by the yeasts are listed in Table 43–1. Specimen collection, transport, and processing are discussed in Part III, but in general, specimens should be delivered promptly to the laboratory, where they should be examined microscopically (by direct wet mount or a stained smear) and planted to culture media or, if processing must be delayed, stored at refrigerator or room temperature, depending on the specimen type.

Cell structure and colony characteristics of the medically important yeasts, identification methods, and serologic tests are discussed in this section. The extent to which isolates of yeasts are identified must be decided by the laboratory director, but identifying all yeasts recovered from sterile body sites—cerebrospinal fluid, blood, body fluids, tissues—to the species level and screening isolates from respiratory secretions for Cryptococcus neoformans is recommended (85).

Cellular Structure and Colony Characteristics

Candida species. In wet-mount or potassium hydroxide (KOH) preparations, stained smears, and tissue sections prepared from clinical specimens, yeast cells of Candida are 3 to 4 μm in diameter, with single buds; pseudohyphae are 5 to 10 μm long, constricted at the ends, and attached like sausage links (see Fig. 43–4). Rarely, true septate hyphae are found, in which case differentiation from Aspergillus is difficult or impossible. Torulopsis glabrata shows only small (2 to 3 μm) budding yeast cells and forms neither pseudohyphae nor hyphae. Species of Candida grow well on most media used specifically to recover fungi (see Chapter 42) and on sheep blood and chocolate agars used for routine bacterial culture, forming cream-colored, glabrous, mucoid or waxy, and smooth or wrinkled colonies after 2 to 3 days (Fig. 43–5).

Cryptococcus neoformans. In tissue sections and direct smears of clinical specimens, yeast cells of C. neoformans vary in size, ranging from 2 to 15 μm in diameter, are usually spherical but may be oval, have single or multi-

Table 43–1. Infections Caused by Yeasts and Specimens for Diagnosis

Infection	Organisms	Specimens
Superficial		
Pityriasis versicolor	Malassezia furfur	Skin scrapings
White piedra	Trichosporon beigelii	Damaged hair
Cutaneous/mucocutaneous		
Thrush	Candida albicans	Diagnosed clinically
Esophagitis	C. albicans	Esophageal brushings, biopsy tissue
Vaginitis	Candida species, Torulopsis glabrata	Vaginal discharge
Paronychia	Candida species	Exudate
Onychomycosis	Candida species	Damaged nail
Skin lesions	Candida species, Cryptococcus neoformans, T. beigelii	Vesicle fluid, exudate, biopsy tissue
Systemic or deep organ involvement		
Meningoencephalitis	C. neoformans, Candida species	Cerebrospinal fluid, brain tissue
Endocarditis	Candida species*	Blood, vegetation, valve tissue
Fungemia	Candida species, T. glabrata, C. neoformans, M. furfur, T. beigelii	Blood, catheter tip
Cystitis	Candida species, T. glabrata	Urine
Pyelonephritis	Candida species	Urine, blood
Osteomyelitis	Candida species, C. neoformans	Bone biopsy
Arthritis	Candida species	Joint fluid, synovial biopsy
Pneumonia	C. neoformans, Candida species	Sputum, tracheal aspirate, transtracheal aspirate, bronchial washings, bronchoalveolar lavage fluid, lung tissue, blood, pleural fluid (if present)
Peritonitis	Candida species, T. glabrata	Peritoneal fluid
Hepatitis	Candida species	Liver tissue

* Species other than C. albicans predominate.

ple buds, and may or may not have an evident capsule; rarely, pseudohyphae are formed. Cells of C. neoformans often stain poorly with the Gram stain (Plate VIIIE), and they are the only yeast cells that stain bright red with the mucicarmine stain (Plate VIIIF). In an India ink preparation of cerebrospinal fluid (CSF) (described in Chapter 55) clear capsules of C. neoformans are easily visualized against a semiopaque background (Fig. 43–6). The overall sensitivity of the India ink test is low, but it may approach 90% in persons with AIDS. Moreover, it is not specific for C. neoformans because other yeasts (some isolates of Rhodotorula, Torulopsis glabrata, and Trichosporon beigelii) occasionally are encapsulated and consequently have a similar appearance, and white blood cells may be confused with yeast cells. Therefore, using the highly sensitive and specific latex agglutination test or enzyme-linked immunosorbent assay (ELISA, discussed later) in place of the India ink preparation is recommended (85,86). Cryptococcus neoformans grows in 1 to 5 days on most mycologic media that do not contain cycloheximide, which is inhibitory. Colonies are smooth and white to tan, becoming mucoid and cream to brown on Sabouraud dextrose agar, but on inhibitory mold agar they are golden yellow and not mucoid.

Malassezia furfur. Direct examination of skin scrapings from a lesion of pityriasis versicolor shows budding yeast cells, 2 to 4 μm in diameter, and short hyphae, which

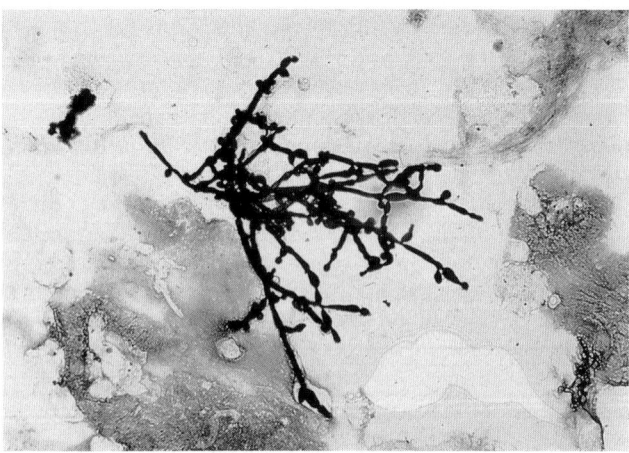

Fig. 43–4. Pseudohyphae of Candida albicans in a bronchoalveolar lavage fluid specimen (Gomori methenamine silver, ×201.6).

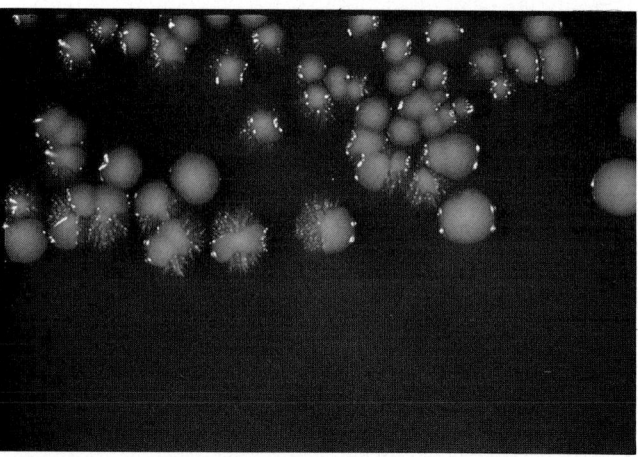

Fig. 43–5. Colonies of Candida albicans on sheep blood agar show characteristic peripheral fringes.

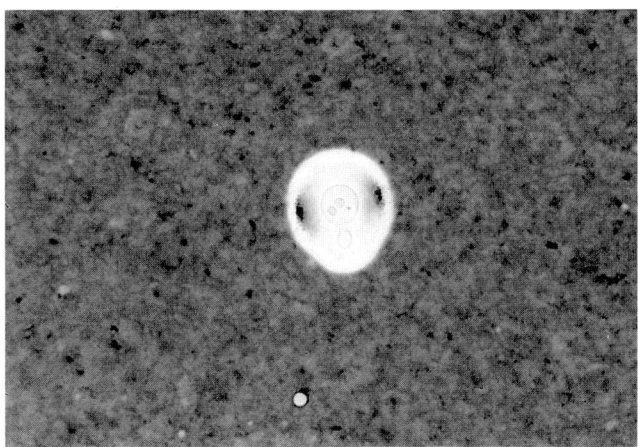

Fig. 43–6. India ink preparation shows an encapsulated, budding yeast cell of Cryptococcus neoformans (×400). (Courtesy of Cathy Soldo, MD, Medical College of Pennsylvania.)

Tests for Identification of Candida albicans. Because C. albicans accounts for about 75% of all yeasts recovered from clinical specimens a test that distinguishes it from other yeasts should be the first step in the identification process. One of the most valuable tests that allows rapid identification of C. albicans is the germ tube test, performed in individual tubes (Appendix, Procedure 22) or 96-well plates. A germ tube is a filamentous extension from a yeast cell that is about half the width and three to four times the length of the cell (Fig. 43–7). Usually, constrictions are not formed at the point of origin from the cell, but C. albicans may form constricted and unconstricted germ tubes. In general, a positive germ tube test result is specific for C. albicans, although rare isolates of Candida tropicalis are germ tube positive. An alternative method for identifying C. albicans is a 90-minute colorimetric test (commercially available) based on the detection of L-proline aminopeptidase and β-galactosaminidase, enzymes only C. albicans produces (88).

Screening Tests for Cryptococcus neoformans. Several tests may be used to screen yeasts isolated from respiratory tract secretions for C. neoformans. One is to test for urease activity, because C. neoformans is one of the few yeasts encountered in the clinical laboratory that hydrolyze urea. A Christensen's urea agar slant (described for Enterobacteriaceae in Chapter 34) is heavily inoculated, incubated in ambient air at 35° C, and read at 4, 24, and 48 hours. Alternatively, urea broth placed in wells of a microtiter plate is inoculated, incubated 4 hours at 37° C, and observed for the production of a pink to purple color, a positive result (85). Isolates yielding a positive result must be further evaluated, because other yeasts—Candida krusei, Trichosporon beigelii, and Rhodotorula—may be urease positive. Another test used to

together are described as resembling spaghetti and meatballs. In smears prepared from blood culture broth and stained with the Gram stain, organisms appear as bottle-shaped, small budding cells, 1 to 2 μm wide by 2 to 4 μm long (Plate IXA). On media typically used to recover fungi, M. furfur grows as tiny, pinpoint colonies, if at all, unless the medium is covered with a thin layer of sterile olive oil, coconut oil, or another lipid source.

Other Yeasts. Direct examination of specimens containing Trichosporon beigelii shows variably-sized budding yeast cells, arthroconidia, pseudohyphae, and occasional true hyphae. The colony characteristics of T. beigelii may be useful for distinguishing isolates that cause invasive disease from those that colonize superficial surfaces (87). Invasive isolates form four distinct colony morphotypes—powdery, rugose, powdery gray, and rugose-gray—which show spontaneous conversions and grow well at 37° C. Isolates from superficial sites form creamy colonies with fuzzy edges, do not demonstrate conversion, and grow poorly at 37° C. The direct microscopic appearance and the colony characteristics of species of Hansenula are very similar to those of Candida, but the former produce ascospores that may be hat shaped, hemispherical, spherical, or shaped like the planet Saturn. Cells of Saccharomyces cerevisiae are oval to spherical, 3 μm by 5 μm, exist as budding cells or short chains, and elongate as rudimentary pseudohyphae. Colonies of Saccharomyces cerevisiae resemble those of Candida. The cellular structure and colony appearance of Blastoschizomyces capitatus are similar to those of Trichosporon beigelii. Cells of Rhodotorula resemble those of Cryptococcus, but the colonies of Rhodotorula are unique, forming a conspicuous carotenoid pigment.

Yeast Identification

The approach to identification of yeasts presented here is discussed in four parts: (1) tests for identification of Candida albicans, (2) screening tests for Cryptococcus neoformans, (3) tests for identification of yeasts other than Candida albicans, and (4) serologic tests.

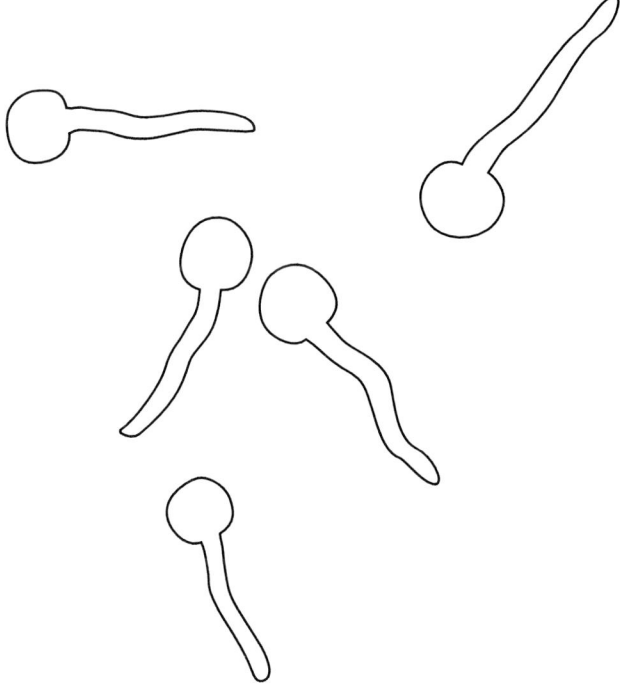

Fig. 43–7. Diagram of germ tubes of Candida albicans.

Table 43–2. Microscopic Appearance of Commonly Encountered Yeasts on Cornmeal-Tween-80 Agar

Yeast	Microscopic Appearance
Candida species	
C. albicans	Chlamydospores occurring singly or in clusters on pseudohyphae; numerous blastoconidia often aggregated in clusters at regular intervals along the pseudohyphae.
C. tropicalis	No chlamydospores; few blastoconidia sparsely distributed along the pseudohyphae without dense clustering
C. parapsilosis	Sagebrush appearance of pseudohyphae; giant hyphae; sparse blastoconidia, occurring singly or in short chains
C. kefyr (pseudotropicalis)	Elongated blastoconidia that dissociate from pseudohyphae and lie in parallel fashion—a "logs-in-stream" arrangement
Torulopsis glabrata	Small, spherical, tightly compact blastoconidia; no pseudohyphae or hyphae
Cryptococcus neoformans	Round to oval, variously-sized blastoconidia, occasionally separated by a capsule; rare pseudohyphae
Trichosporon beigelii	Numerous arthroconidia; pseudohyphae; occasional septate hyphae; blastoconidia may be present, usually in small numbers
Saccharomyces cerevisiae	Large, spherical blastoconidia; occasional rudimentary hyphae

screen isolates for Cryptococcus neoformans is nitrate reduction, performed as described for the Enterobacteriaceae (Chapter 34) or by a rapid method using a cotton swab impregnated with an inorganic nitrate substrate (not commercially available) (85). To perform the latter test, two or three colonies are touched with the swab, which is swirled against the bottom of an empty test tube (to enhance contact of the yeast cells with the cotton fibers) and incubated with the tube at 45° C for 10 minutes. The swab is removed from the tube, two drops each of N-naphthylethylenediamine and sulfanilic acid are added, and the swab is replaced in the tube. The development of a red color indicates a positive result. If no color appears in 10 minutes, zinc dust is added. Then, development of a red color indicates previously unreacted nitrates and a negative result, whereas no color change indicates continuation of the reaction to nitrogen gas and a positive result. C. neoformans is nitrate negative.

Additional screening tests detect the production of phenoloxidase, an enzyme elaborated only by Cryptococcus neoformans that is necessary for the metabolism of 3,4-dihydroxyphenylalanine (dopa) and other phenolic compounds in the pathway of melanine synthesis. Niger seed (or birdseed) agar may be used to detect the enzyme, recognized by growth of brown-pigmented colonies, which occurs only with isolates of C. neoformans. Not all formulations of this medium, however, demonstrate pigment production by all strains of C. neoformans. Therefore, cornmeal-Tween-80 agar containing caffeic acid or a medium or test system containing dopa is recommended for detection of pigment production (85,86). On a medium containing caffeic acid or dopa (commercially available) positive reactions may not be visible for 48 to 72 hours; but if levodopa–ferric citrate disks (commercially available) are used results are available in 6 hours or less (85).

Calling an isolate Cryptococcus neoformans presumptively based on results of all three screening tests is ideal, but all three tests cannot always be done from the primary culture because the inoculum size frequently is limited. Given that phenoloxidase production is the most specific of the three tests for C. neoformans, inoculating a medium containing dopa, cornmeal-Tween-80 agar containing caffeic acid, or niger seed agar and subculturing to isolate the organism is recommended (85). Moreover, if the screening tests yield equivocal results, carbohydrate assimilation tests (discussed below) must be performed.

Identification of Yeasts Other than Candida albicans. The identification of yeasts other than C. albicans (including isolates that yield equivocal results in screening tests for Cryptococcus neoformans) is based on the ability of the organism to utilize various carbohydrates as the sole source of carbon in a chemically defined medium and on the cellular structure of the isolate on cornmeal agar. Carbohydrate utilization profiles are determined by using conventional methods that may require as long as 14 to 28 days for completion (outlined in references 85,86,89), or, more commonly, by using commercially available standardized kit systems (85). Systems containing dehydrated carbohydrate substrates to determine profiles of carbohydrate utilization with or without additional biochemical tests usually provide results in 48 hours, but some systems may require up to 7 days (85,86, 90–93). Recently, systems that utilize chromogenic substrates and provide results in 4 to 24 hours became available commercially, but limited evaluations of these systems indicate that currently they are less accurate than those that require longer incubation (93–96). The cellular structure of several yeasts on cornmeal agar (see Appendix, Procedure 23) is characteristic (Table 43–2), and because this information may differentiate between genera that yield similar biochemical profiles, including cornmeal agar for identification is recommended.

Serologic Tests

Serologic tests for diagnosis of infections with yeasts have been developed to provide a rapid result early in the disease. Those most useful are the latex agglutination test and ELISA (commercially available) that detect capsular polysaccharide antigens of Cryptococcus neoformans. These tests have a sensitivity of 95% or more for diagnosing meningitis caused by C. neoformans when CSF is tested (97,98). The result is positive less frequently with serum than with CSF in cases of meningitis, but it usually is positive with disseminated infections. False-positive latex test results in serum occur in the presence of rheumatoid factor, but they can be eliminated by various treatment methods and reagents (99,100). In CSF, contamination of the sample with surface condensation from agar can cause a false-positive latex result, so the recommended approach is to perform the latex test before culture or on a separate specimen (101). Infection with Trichosporon beigelii also causes false-positive latex test results, but this is an uncommon problem (102).

Another commercially available latex agglutination test is used to detect antigens of Candida in serum. In theory, this type of test could be valuable because diagnosing deep-seated infections with Candida is problematic. Currently available noninvasive methods for diagnosis are unsatisfactory. For example, surveillance cultures do not accurately predict invasive candidiasis, and blood cultures often are negative or become positive late in the infection (103). Thus, it frequently is necessary to perform an invasive procedure to obtain tissue for diagnosis of a patient who already is compromised. In early evaluations the sensitivity and specificity of the Candida antigen test were high; however, data from several later studies indicate that it is not a reliable indicator of invasive candidiasis (104–106).

Treatment

Candida species. Nystatin, clotrimazole, and miconazole are used topically to treat mild to moderate mucocutaneous candidiasis. Ketoconazole, an oral agent, also is effective for mucocutaneous infections, especially in persons with esophagitis. The cornerstone of therapy for disseminated and deep organ infections with Candida is amphotericin B, which may be used in combination with 5-fluorocytosine for rapidly progressing disease, for infections of the central nervous system, and for serious infections caused by species of Candida other than Candida albicans, such as Candida lusitaniae, which appear resistant to amphotericin B by susceptibility testing in vitro (3,6,8). For Candida endocarditis, valve replacement plus amphotericin B is recommended. Intravascular catheters infected with Candida should be removed.

Cryptococcus neoformans. The treatment of choice for meningitis or disseminated infection with C. neoformans is amphotericin B or amphotericin B plus 5-fluorocytosine (65,107). Fluconozole is effective suppressive therapy for persons with AIDS and cryptyococcal meningitis, once the CSF is sterile (108,109).

Malassezia furfur. Pityriasis versicolor may be treated with a topical azole antifungal cream, 2% selenium sulfide lotion, or 20% sodium thiosulfate; although for severe disease, oral ketoconazole or itraconazole is recommended. Fungemia with M. furfur associated with an infected intravascular catheter often responds to removal of the catheter alone; however, infections of deep organs require therapy with amphotericin B.

Other Yeasts. Serious infections caused by Trichosporon, Hansenula, Saccharomyces, Blastoschizomyces, and Rhodotorula are treated with amphotericin B, with or without 5-fluorocytosine.

REFERENCES

1. Langenbeck B: Auffingung von Pilzen aus der Schleimhaut der Speiserohre einer Typhus-Leiche. Neue Not Geb Natur Heilk (Froriep), *12*:145, 1839.
2. Joachim H, and Polayes S: Subacute endocarditis and systemic mycosis (monilia). JAMA, *115*:205, 1940.
3. Edwards JE, Jr: Candida species. *In* Principles and Practice of Infectious Diseases. 3rd ed. Edited by GL Mandell, RG Douglas, Jr, and JE Bennett. New York, Churchill Livingstone, 1990.
4. Wingard JR, Merz WG, and Saral R: Candida tropicalis: A major pathogen in immunocompromised patients. Ann Intern Med, *91*:539, 1979.
5. Bross J, et al: Risk factors for nosocomial candidemia: A case-control study in adults without leukemia. Am J Med, *87*:614, 1989.
6. Blinkhorn RJ, Adelstein D, and Spagnuolo PJ: Emergence of a new opportunistic pathogen, Candida lusitaniae. J Clin Microbiol, *27*:236, 1989.
7. Weems JJ, Jr, et al: Candida parapsilosis fungemia associated with parenteral nutrition and contaminated blood pressure transducers. J Clin Microbiol, *25*:1029, 1987.
8. Hadfield TL, et al: Mycoses caused by Candida lusitaniac. Rev Infect Dis, *9*:1006, 1987.
9. Nguyen VQ, and Penn RL: Candida krusei infectious arthritis. Am J Med, *83*:963, 1987.
10. Alsina A, et al: Catheter-associated Candida utilis fungemia in a patient with acquired immunodeficiency syndrome: Species verification with a molecular probe. J Clin Microbiol, *26*:621, 1988.
11. Levenson D, et al: Candida zeylanoides: Another opportunistic yeast. J Clin Microbiol, *29*:1689, 1991.
12. Walsh TJ, Salkin IF, Dixon DM, and Hurd NJ: Clinical, microbiological, and experimental animal studies of Candida lipolytica. J Clin Microbiol, *27*:927, 1989.
13. Merz WG: Candida albicans strain delineation. Clin Microbiol Rev, *3*:321, 1990.
14. Nelson RD, Shibata N, Podzorski RP, and Herron MJ: Candida mannan: Chemistry, suppression of cell-mediated immunity, and possible mechanisms of action. Clin Microbiol Rev, *4*:1, 1991.
15. de Bernardis F, et al: Evidence for a role for secreted asparatate proteinase of Candida albicans in vulvovaginal candidiasis. J Infect Dis, *161*:1276, 1990.
16. Diamond RD, Clark RA, and Haudenchild CC: Damage to Candida albicans hyphae and pseudohyphae by the myeloperoxidase system and oxidative products of neutrophil metabolism in vivo. J Clin Invest, *66*:908, 1980.
17. Lehrer RI: The fungicidal mechanisms of human monocytes: I. Evidence for myeloperoxidase-linked and myeloperoxidase-independent candidacidal mechanisms. J Clin Invest, *55*:338, 1975.
18. Lehrer RI: Measurement of candidacidal activity of specific leukocyte types in mixed cell populations: II. Normal and chronic granulomatous disease eosinophils. Infect Immun, *3*:800, 1971.
19. Epstein JB, Truelove EL, and Izutau KT: Oral candidiasis, pathogenesis and host defense. Rev Infect Dis, *6*:96, 1984.
20. Eras P, Goldstein MJ, and Sherlock P: Candida infection of the gastrointestinal tract. Medicine, *51*:367, 1972.
21. Trier JS, and Bjorkman DJ: Esophageal, gastric, and intestinal candidiasis. Am J Med, *30*:39, 1984.
22. Kaufman RH (ed): Vulvovaginal candidiasis. A Symposium. J Reprod Med, *31*:639, 1986.
23. Brophy MC, and Dunagin WB: Intertriginous dermatoses. Common puzzling problems. Postgrad Med, *78*:105, 1985.
24. Hay RJ, et al: Candida onychomycosis—an evaluation of the role of Candida species in male disease. Br J Dermatol, *118*:47, 1988.
25. Jorizzo JL: Chronic mucocutaneous candidosis. An update. Arch Dermatol, *118*:963, 1982.
26. Stiehm ER: Chronic cutaneous candidiasis, clinical aspects. *In* UCLA Conference: Severe Candidal Infections: Clinical perspective, immune defense mechanisms, and current concepts of therapy. Ann Intern Med, *89*:91, 1978.
27. Lipton SA, et al: Candidal infection in the central nervous system. Am J Med, *76*:101, 1984.
28. Salaki JS, Louria DB, and Chmel H: Fungal and yeast infec-

tions of the central nervous system. A clinical review. Medicine, 63:108, 1984.
29. Eng RHK, et al: Candida pericarditis. Am J Med, 70:867, 1981.
30. Parker JC, Jr: The potentially lethal problem of cardiac candidosis. Am J Clin Pathol, 73:356, 1980.
31. Ihde DC, et al: Cardiac candidiasis in cancer patients. Cancer, 41:2364, 1978.
32. Odds FC: Candida endocarditis, myocarditis, and other cardiovascular Candida infections. In Candida and Candidosis. A Review and Bibliography. 2nd ed. London, Bailliere Tindall, 1988.
33. Gathe JC, Jr, et al: Candida osteomyelitis. Report of five cases and review of the literature. Am J Med, 82:927, 1987.
34. Simpson MB, Jr, et al: Opportunistic mycotic osteomyelitis: Bone infections due to Aspergillus and Candida species. Medicine, 56:475, 1977.
35. Fainstein V, et al: Septic arthritis due to Candida species in patients with cancer: Report of five cases and review of the literature. Rev Infect Dis, 4:78, 1982.
36. Levine M, Rhehm SJ, and Wilde AH: Infection with Candida albicans of a total knee arthroplasty. Case report and review of the literature. Clin Orthop, 226:235, 1988.
37. Bayer AS, et al: Candida peritonitis. Report of 22 cases and review of the English literature. Am J Med, 61:832, 1976.
38. Solomkin JS, et al: The role of Candida in intraperitoneal infections. Surgery, 88:524, 1980.
39. Thales M, et al: Hepatic candidiasis in cancer patients: The evolving picture of the syndrome. Ann Intern Med, 108:88, 1988.
40. Helton WS, et al: Diagnosis and treatment of splenic fungal abscesses in the immune-suppressed patient. Arch Surg, 121:580, 1986.
41. Irani M, and Truong LD: Candidiasis of the extrahepatic biliary tract. Arch Pathol Lab Med, 110:1087, 1986.
42. Binder LA, Csillaq A, and Toth G: Diffuse infiltration of the lungs associated with Cryptococcus luteolus. Lancet, ii:1043, 1956.
43. Cunha T, and Lusins J: Cryptococcus albidus meningitis. South Med J, 66:1230, 1973.
44. Kamalam A, Yesudian P, and Thambiah AS: Cutaneous infection by Cryptococcus laurentii. Br J Dermatol, 97:221, 1977.
45. Wilson DE, Bennett JE, and Bailey JW: Serologic grouping of Cryptococcus neoformans. Proc Soc Exp Biol Med, 127:820, 1968.
46. Kwon-Chung KJ: A new genus, Filobasidiella, the perfect state of Cryptococcus neoformans. Mycologia, 67:1197, 1975.
47. Littman ML, and Walter JE: Cryptococcosis: Current status. Am J Med, 45:922, 1968.
48. Neilson JB, Fromtling RA, and Bulmer GS: Cryptococcus neoformans: Size range of infectious particles from aerosolized soil. Infect Immun, 17:634, 1977.
49. Ellis DH, and Pfeiffer TJ: Natural habitat of Cryptococcus neoformans var gattii. J Clin Microbiol, 28:1642, 1990.
50. Diamond RD, and Bennett JE: Prognostic factors in cryptococcal meningitis. A study of 111 cases. Ann Intern Med, 80:176, 1974.
51. Bhattacharjee AK, Bennett JE, and Glaudemans CPJ: Capsular polysaccharides of Cryptococcus neoformans. Rev Infect Dis, 6:619, 1984.
52. Henderson DK, Kan VL, and Bennett JE: Tolerance to cryptococcal polysaccharide in cured cryptococcosis patients: Failure of antibody secretion in vitro. Clin Exp Immunol, 65:639, 1986.
53. Drouhet E, and Segretain G: Inhibition de la migration leucocytaire in vitro par un polyoside capsulaire de Torulopsis (Cryptococcus) neoformans. Ann Inst Pasteur, 81:674, 1951.
54. Kozel TR, and Hermerath CA: Binding of cryptococcal polysaccharide to Cryptococcus neoformans. Infect Immun, 43:879, 1984.
55. Macher A, et al: Complement depletion in cryptococcal sepsis. J Immunol, 120:1686, 1978.
56. Diamond RD, Root RK, and Bennett JE: Factors influencing killing of Cryptococcus neoformans by human leukocytes in vitro. J Infect Dis, 125:367, 1972.
57. Kozel TR, Pfrommer GST, and Redelman D: Activated neutrophils exhibit enhanced phagocytosis of Cryptococcus neoformans opsonized with normal human serum. Clin Exp Immunol, 70:238, 1987.
58. Hidore MR, and Murphy JW: Correlation of natural killer cell activity and clearance of Cryptococcus neoformans from mice after adoptive transfer of splenic nylon wool–nonadherent cells. Infect Immun, 51:547, 1986.
59. Nabavi N, and Murphy JW: Antibody-dependent natural killer cell–mediated growth inhibition of Cryptococcus neoformans. Infect Immun, 51:556, 1986.
60. Diamond RD, and Allison AC: Nature of the effector cells responsible for antibody-dependent cell-mediated killing of Cryptococcus neoformans. Infect Immun, 14:716, 1976.
61. Fung PYS, and Murphy JW: In vitro interactions of immune lymphocytes and Cryptococcus neoformans. Infect Immun, 36:1128, 1982.
62. Cameron ML, Bartlett JA, Gallis HA, and Waskin HA: Manifestations of pulmonary cryptococcosis in patients with acquired immunodeficiency syndrome. Rev Infect Dis, 13:64, 1991.
63. Shrader SK, et al: Disseminated cryptococcosis presenting as cellulitis with necrotizing vasculitis. J Clin Microbiol, 24:860, 1986.
64. Perfect JR, Durack DT, and Gallis HA: Cryptococcemia. Medicine, 62:98, 1983.
65. Diamond RD: Cryptococcus neoformans. In Principles and Practice of Infectious Diseases. 3rd ed. Edited by GL Mandell, RG Douglas, Jr, and JE Bennett. New York, Churchill Livingstone, 1990.
66. Marcon MJ, and Powell DA: Epidemiology, diagnosis, and management of Malassezia furfur systemic infection. Diagn Microbiol Infect Dis, 7:161, 1987.
67. Larocco M, Dorenbaum A, Robinson A, and Pickering LK: Recovery of Malassezia pachydermatis from eight infants in a neonatal intensive care nursery: Clinical and laboratory features. Pediatr Infect Dis J, 7:398, 1988.
68. Roberts SOB: Pityrosporum orbiculare: Incidence and distribution on clinically normal skin. Br J Dermatol, 85:264, 1969.
69. Faergemann J, and Fredriksson T: Age incidence of Pityrosporum orbiculare on human skin. Acta Derm Venereol, 60:531, 1980.
70. Dankner WM, Specter SA, Fierer J, and Davis CE: Malassezia fungemia in neonates and adults: Complication of hyperalimentation. Rev Infect Dis, 9:743, 1987.
71. Faergemann J, and Fredriksson T: Tinea versicolor with regard to seborrheic dermatitis. Arch Dermatol, 115:966, 1979.
72. Wurtz RM, and Knospe WN: Malassezia furfur fungemia in a patient without the usual risk factors. Ann Intern Med, 109:432, 1988.
73. Hassall E, Urich T, and Ament ME: Pulmonary embolus and Malassezia pulmonary infection related to urokinase therapy. Pediatrics, 102:722, 1983.
74. Redline RW, Redline SS, Boxerbaum B, and Dahms BB:

Systemic Malassezia furfur infection in patients receiving intralipid therapy. Hum Pathol, *16*:815, 1985.
75. Walling DM, et al: Disseminated infection with Trichosporon beigelii. Rev Infect Dis, *9*:1013, 1987.
76. Ness MJ, et al: Disseminated Trichosporon beigelii infection after orthotopic liver transplantation. Am J Clin Pathol, *92*:119, 1989.
77. Haron E, et al: Hansenula anomala fungemia. Rev Infect Dis, *10*:1182, 1988.
78. Nohinek B, et al: Infective endocarditis of a bicuspid aortic valve caused by Hansenula anomala. Am J Med, *82*:165, 1987.
79. Dooley DP, Beckius ML, McAllister CR, and Jeffrey BS: Prostatitis caused by Hansenula fabianii. J Infect Dis, *161*:1040, 1990.
80. Aucott JN, et al: Invasive infection with Saccharomyces cerevisiae: Report of three cases and review. Rev Infect Dis, *12*:406, 1990.
81. Tawfik OW, Papasian CJ, Dixon AY, and Potter LM: Saccharomyces cerevisiae pneumonia in a patient with acquired immune deficiency syndrome. J Clin Microbiol, *27*:1689, 1989.
82. Martino P, et al: Blastoschizomyces capitatus: An emerging cause of invasive fungal disease in leukemia patients. Rev Infect Dis, *12*:570, 1990.
83. Pien FD, Thompson RL, Deye D, and Roberts GD: Rhodotorula septicemia: Two cases and a review of the literature. Mayo Clin Proc, *55*:258, 1980.
84. Pore RS, and Chen J: Meningitis caused by Rhodotorula. Sabouraudia, *14*:331, 1976.
85. Roberts GD: Laboratory methods in basic mycology. *In* Bailey and Scott's Diagnostic Microbiology. 8th ed. Edited by EJ Baron and SM Finegold. St. Louis, CV Mosby, 1990.
86. Koneman EW, et al (eds): Color Atlas and Textbook of Diagnostic Microbiology. 3rd ed. Philadelphia, JB Lippincott, 1988.
87. Lee JW, et al: Patterns of morphologic variation among isolates of Trichosporon beigelii. J Clin Microbiol, *28*:2823, 1990.
88. Perry JL, Miller GR, and Carr DL: Rapid, colorimetric identification of Candida albicans. J Clin Microbiol, *28*:614, 1990.
89. Warren NG, and Shadomy HJ: Yeasts of medical importance. *In* Manual of Clinical Microbiology. 5th ed. Edited by A Balows, et al. Washington, DC, American Society for Microbiology, 1991.
90. Buesching WJ, Kurek K, and Roberts GD: Evaluation of the modified API 20C system for identification of clinically important yeasts. J Clin Microbiol, *9*:565, 1979.
91. Roberts GD, Wang HS, and Hollick GE: Evaluation of the API 20C microtube system for the identification of clinically important yeasts. J Clin Microbiol, *3*:302, 1976.
92. Bowman PI, and Ahearn DG: Evaluation of the Uni-Yeast-Tek kit for the identification of medically important yeasts. J Clin Microbiol, *2*:354, 1975.
93. Salkin IF, et al: Evaluation of Abbott Quantum IV Yeast Identification system. J Clin Microbiol, *22*:442, 1985.
94. Pfaller MA, et al: Comparison of the Quantum II, API Yeast Ident, and AutoMicrobic systems for identification of clinical yeast isolates. J Clin Microbiol, *26*:2054, 1988.
95. El-Zaatari M, et al: Evaluation of the updated Vitek yeast identification data base. J Clin Microbiol, *28*:1938, 1990.
96. Land GA, et al: Evaluation of the Baxter-MicroScan 4-hour enzyme-based yeast identification system. J Clin Microbiol, *29*:718, 1991.
97. Wu TC, and Koo SY: Comparison of three commercial cryptococcal latex kits for detection of cryptococcal antigen. J Clin Microbiol, *18*:1127, 1983.
98. Gade W, et al: Comparison of the PREMIER cryptococcal antigen enzyme immunoassay and the latex agglutination assay for detection of cryptococcal antigens. J Clin Microbiol, *29*:1616, 1991.
99. Gray LD, and Roberts GD: Experience with the use of pronase to eliminate interference factors in the latex agglutination test for cryptococcal antigen. J Clin Microbiol, *26*:2450, 1988.
100. Hamilton JR, Noble A, Denning DW, and Stevens DA: Performance of Cryptococcus antigen latex agglutination kits on serum and cerebrospinal fluid specimens of AIDS patients before and after pronase treatment. J Clin Microbiol, *29*:333, 1991.
101. Heelan JS, Corpus L, and Kessimian N: False-positive reactions in the latex agglutination test for Cryptococcus neoformans antigen. J Clin Microbiol, *29*:1260, 1991.
102. Melcher GP, et al: Demonstration of a cell wall antigen cross-reacting with cryptococcal polysaccharide in experimental disseminated trichosporonosis. J Clin Microbiol, *29*:192, 1991.
103. Jones JM: Laboratory diagnosis of invasive candidiasis. Clin Microbiol Rev, *3*:32, 1990.
104. Ness MJ, Vaughan WP, and Woods GL: Candida antigen latex test for detection of invasive candidiasis in immunocompromised patients. J Infect Dis, *159*:495, 1989.
105. Escuro BS, et al: Prospective evaluation of a Candida antigen detection test for invasive candidiasis in immunocompromised adult patients with cancer. Am J Med, *87*:621, 1989.
106. Phillips P, et al: Nonvalue of antigen detection immunoassays for diagnosis of candidemia. J Clin Microbiol, *28*:2320, 1990.
107. Dismukes WE, et al: Treatment of cryptococcal meningitis with combination amphotericin B and flucytosine for four as compared with six weeks. N Engl J Med, *317*:334, 1987.
108. Larsen RA, Leal MAE, and Chan LS: Fluconazole compared with amphotericin B plus flucytosine for cryptococcal meningitis in AIDS. Ann Intern Med, *113*:183, 1990.

Chapter 44

MOULDS

The moulds of medical importance are a heterogeneous group of fungi that cause a broad spectrum of diseases. Many are saprobes found worldwide in soil and decaying matter that become pathogens only when host immune defenses are compromised. In this chapter the moulds are separated into four categories—dermatophytes, dermatiaceous fungi, hyaline septate moulds, and zygomycetes—based on the infections they cause, their colony appearance, and microscopic structure.

DERMATOPHYTES

Dermatophytes are keratinophilic moulds, parasites of the nonliving cornified integument that may secrete keratinases, proteolytic enzymes that digest the keratin in epidermis, hair, and nails. Ringworm, one type of dermatophytosis (infection of the skin, hair, or nails by one of the dermatophytes), was the first recognized infectious disease of humans. During the 1800s, ringworm infections were shown to be caused by fungi that could be recovered on artificial media and could produce similar infections in healthy skin. Currently, three genera—Trichophyton, Microsporum, and Epidermophyton—and more than 40 species of dermatophytes are recognized. Species of Trichophyton infect hair, skin, and nails; species of Microsporum infect hair and skin; and Epidermophyton floccosum infects nails and skin. Because these organisms have similar epidemiology and pathogenicity, and because several different species may cause the same disease, the dermatophytes are discussed as a group rather than individually.

Epidemiology

Dermatophytes are grouped into three categories based on habitat and host preference: geophilic (found in soil), zoophilic (found on animals), and anthropophilic (found on humans) (Table 44–1), although many dermatophytes that normally inhabit soil or animals can cause human infections. Many species are found worldwide; as others are restricted geographically (see Table 44–1). Geophilic dermatophytes are infrequent human pathogens, responsible for sporadic infections and occasional outbreaks of disease in exposed workers (gardeners or farm workers), especially in tropical climates (1,2). Of the zoophilic dermatophytes, Trichophyton verrucosum, the cause of cattle ringworm, and Microsporum canis, which causes infections in cats and dogs, are the ones most often responsible for human infections in temperate climates, and M. canis probably is the most common zoophilic dermatophyte infecting humans worldwide. Anthropophilic dermatophytes are the most frequent causes of human dermatophytosis, and in most parts of the world Trichophyton rubrum is the species most commonly implicated.

Dermatophyte infections of the scalp (tinea capitis), a disease primarily of childhood, are rare after puberty but may be seen in elderly women. This age distribution probably is related to the presence of medium-chain fatty acids (C_8–C_{12}) that inhibit dermatophyte growth in sebum of postpubertal persons. In contrast to tinea capitis, dermatophyte infections of the feet (tinea pedis) usually affect adolescents or young adults, and occasionally young children.

Dermatophytes are spread from the soil, animals, or humans by contact with arthrospores (see Chapter 42) that are shed by the primary host with skin scales or hair. Direct contact with an infected person or animal is not necessary. Spread of dermatophytes infecting glabrous skin is especially common in bathing areas or shower rooms, where large numbers of people share common facilities.

Pathogenesis

Susceptibility to infection with the dermatophytes is not universal and appears to be enhanced by moisture, warmth, specific skin chemistry, composition of sebum and perspiration, youth, heavy exposure, and genetic predisposition. Moreover, persons with a cellular immunodeficiency and those with familial endocrinopathies are predisposed to chronic dermatophytosis.

Host and fungal factors probably are involved in restricting dermatophyte infections to cutaneous sites. For example, normal human serum is fungistatic, a property attributed to transferrin, which chelates iron, an essential growth requirement for fungi, and may directly inhibit dermatophyte growth (3). Fungal properties include the affinity of these organisms for keratin and their inhibition at 37° C.

The host immune response to infection with a dermatophyte and subsequent clinical manifestations vary according to the source of the fungus (Table 44–2) (4). Data suggest that T-lymphocyte activation is essential for resolution of the infection (5,6). However, the mechanisms by which T lymphocytes affect recovery are not completely understood. During infection with a dermatophyte, the turnover of epidermal cells is increased, and the immune system may amplify this endogenous epidermal response.

Clinical Manifestations

The typical presentation of dermatophytosis is an annular scaling patch with a raised margin showing a variable degree of inflammation and a less inflamed center, al-

Table 44-1. Dermatophytes That Cause Human Infections and Their Natural Reservoir

Classification	Geographic Distribution	Organisms*
Anthropophilic	Worldwide	E. floccosum, M. audouinii, T. mentagrophytes interdigitale, T. rubrum, T. schoenleinii, T. tonsurans, T. violaceum
	Restricted	M. ferrugineum (Far East, Africa, Asia, Europe); T. concentricum (west Pacific, Malaysia, Assam, Brazil); T. gourvilli (Africa); T. megninii (Europe, Africa); T. soudanense (Africa, Europe)
Zoophilic	Worldwide	M. canis [cats, dogs]; M. gallinae [poultry]; M. nanum [pigs]; M. persicolor [moles]; T. verrucosum [cattle]; T. equinum [horses]; T. mentagrophytes var mentagrophytes [rodents]
	Restricted	T. erinacei [hedgehogs] (Europe, Australia, New Zealand); T. quickaenum [mice] (Europe, Australia); T. simii [monkeys] (India)
Geophilic	Worldwide	M. gypseum, M. fulvum, M. ajelloi, T. terrestre

* Geographic location in parentheses; primary animal reservoir in brackets.

though the clinical appearance varies with the site, the species involved, and the host immune response. Infections with zoophilic dermatophytes typically cause inflammatory lesions that occasionally are large and pustular (kerions); whereas lesions caused by anthropophilic fungi show little inflammation and may become chronic. In per-

Table 44-2. Clinical and Immune-System Features of Acute and Chronic Dermatophytoses

Feature	Acute Infection	Chronic Infection
Etiology	Geophilic or zoophilic species	Anthropophilic species
Inflammation	Severe	Mild
Signs and symptoms	Erythema, vesicles, pruritus, pain	Erythema, scaling, pruritus
Spread of lesions	Usually limited	Often extensive
Duration	Weeks	Months to years
Incidence of skin test reactivity to trichophytin:		
Type I immediate	Low	High
Type IV delayed	High	Low
T-cell responses in vitro:		
To trichophytin	High	Low
To other antigens	Normal	Normal
Incidence of atopy and/or elevated IgE	Normal (8-10%)	High (about 50%)
Response to therapy	Good	Poor
Recurrence	Rare	Frequent

(From Joklik WK, Willett HP, Amos DB, and Wilfert CM (eds): Zinsser Microbiology. 19th ed. Norwalk, CT, Appleton & Lange, 1988.)

sons with defective cell-mediated immunity, dermatophytic lesions usually are less inflammatory but may be pustular and extensive.

The term *tinea* refers to a dermatophytic infection and usually is followed by the Latin description of the involved site. Table 44-3 includes the clinical names of the dermatophytoses, the sites involved, and the most common pathogens. The individual infections are discussed briefly below.

Tinea capitis, an infection of the scalp and hair of children, is characterized by pruritic circular patches of scaling and alopecia (which usually is not permanent) with a variable amount of inflammation. It is common in some urban areas in the United States and Central and South America and in parts of Africa and India but occurs sporadically in Northern Europe. Endemic infections affecting many children are caused by anthropophilic organisms, whereas sporadic disease is associated with zoophilic fungi. Tinea capitis is classified according to the pattern of hair shaft invasion: ectothrix (arthrospores form on the outside of the shaft) and endothrix (arthrospores are present within the hair shaft). Favus, a type of tinea capitis caused by Trichophyton schoenleinii, is characterized by hyphal elements, air bubbles, or tunnels and fat droplets in the hair shaft; the formation of an inflammatory crust, or scutulum, composed of neutrophils and a serous exudate around individual hairs; and the tendency to cause scarring alopecia.

Tinea pedis is an infection of the feet, usually of young adults or teenage children. Typically it is manifested as pruritic cracks in the skin of the lateral interdigital spaces of the foot or the undersurface of the lateral aspects of the toes, but in some cases bullae form and itching is severe. The noninflammatory infections often are chronic or intermittent, whereas when blisters form, the infection usually resolves but may recur months later. Potential complications of tinea pedis include bacterial cellulitis and invasion by the fungus of the toenails (tinea unguinum), causing thickening and discoloration of the nail, or of the skin of the dorsum of the foot and leg. Tinea manuum, a dermatophytic infection of the hand, most commonly involves the palmar surface and resembles noninflammatory tinea pedis.

Tinea corporis—ringworm of the glabrous skin of the trunk, legs, or arms—occurs most frequently in the trop-

Table 44-3. Most Common Pathogens of Dermatophytoses

Disease	Site	Organisms
Tinea capitis	Scalp, hair	T. tonsurans, M. canis
Favus	Scalp, hair	T. schoenleinii
Tinea pedis	Feet	T. rubrum, T. mentagrophytes, E. floccosum
Tinea unguinum	Nail	T. rubrum, T. mentagrophytes, E. floccosom
Tinea manuum	Hand	T. rubrum
Tinea corporis	Trunk, legs, arms	T. rubrum, T. mentagrophytes, M. canis, T. verrucosum, M. gypseum
Tinea cruris	Groin	E. floccosum, T. rubrum
Tinea barbae	Beard	T. verrucosum

ics but may be seen in temperate climates, especially in children. Lesions are single or multiple and may be pruritic. Tinea imbricata, a variant of tinea corporis caused by Trichophyton concentricum, is endemic in the western Pacific, Malaysia, Assam, and parts of the Amazon basin in Brazil. The infection is characterized by concentric rings of scales over large parts of the body that amalgamate to form waves of scaling.

Tinea cruris, a dermatophytic infection of the groin, is seen principally in young adult males but may affect women, especially in the tropics. Tinea barbae is an inflamed, pustular infection of the neck and beard area caused by zoophilic fungi.

The host immune response to infections with dermatophytes may result in secondary rashes, called id reactions, which may be triggered by antifungal therapy. The most common id reaction is an acute vesicular eczema on the hands and feet of persons with inflammatory tinea pedis, and cutaneous cellulitis, characterized by small follicular papules, may occur in persons with inflammatory tinea capitis or tinea corporis. Annular erythema and erythema nodosum are less common id reactions.

DEMATIACEOUS FUNGI

The dematiaceous fungi—those that develop a pale brown to black color in the cell walls of their vegetative cells, conidia, or both and produce darkly pigmented colonies when isolated in the laboratory—are found in soil and vegetative matter worldwide. Those known to cause human disease are listed in Table 44–4. These organisms are associated with three distinct diseases, defined on the basis of clinical, pathologic, and mycologic relationships: chromoblastomycosis, phaeohyphomycosis, and mycetoma, each of which may be caused by several different species. Owing to the importance of these relationships, this group of moulds is discussed with regard to disease rather than the individual organisms.

Chromoblastomycosis

Chromoblastomycosis, a term introduced in the 1920s, is a localized infection of the skin and subcutaneous tissues characterized histologically by the presence of "planate-dividing yeasts" or muriform "sclerotic bodies" (described later). The latter may represent a vegetative form of the infecting fungus phenotypically arrested between the yeast and hyphal stages and formed in response to the acidic conditions produced by the host inflammatory response (7,8). Currently, six moulds are possible agents of chromoblastomycosis (see Table 44–4). Fonsecaea pedrosoi is the most common cause, except in Australia, where Cladosporium carrionii is most prevalent.

Epidemiology

The agents of chromoblastomycosis are found worldwide in soil, decaying vegetation, rotting wood, and forest litter and are transmitted to humans by traumatic implantation through the skin. Chromoblastomycosis occurs throughout the world, but most cases are seen in the tropics and subtropics, especially among poor rural people

Table 44–4. Infections Caused by Dematiaceous Fungi and Representative Organisms

Disease	Pathogens
Chromoblastomycosis	Fonsecaea pedrosoi, Cladosporium carrionii, Fonsecaea compacta, Phialophora verrucosa, Rhinocladiella aquaspersa, Exophiala jeanselmei
Phaeohyphomycosis	
Superficial	
Black piedra	Piedraia hortae
Tinea nigra	Exophiala werneckii
Cutaneous	
Dermatomycosis	Alternaria, Hendersonula toruloidea
Mycotic keratitis	Botryodiplodia theobromae, Curvularia species, Exophiala jeanselmei, Exserohilum rostratum (syn. Drechslera rostrata)
Onychomycosis	Botryodiplodia theobromae, Hendersonula toruloidea, Phyllosticta species
Subcutaneous	Exophiala jeanselmei, Wangiella dermatitidis, Alternaria alternata, Bipolaris spicifera (syn. Drechslera spicifera), Exophiala species, Phialophora species, Phoma species, Scytalidium lignicola, Xylohypha emmonsii, Scedosporium inflatum
Systemic	Bipolaris species, Cladosporium cladosporoides, Curvularia species, Exserohilum rostratum, Dissitimurus exedrus, Exophiala jeanselmei, Wangiella dermatitidis, Xylohypha bantiana, Alternaria alternata, Dactylaria gallopava
Mycetoma	Curvularia species, Phialophora cryanescens, Exophiala jeanselmei

who do not wear shoes and, so, are repeatedly exposed to fungi in the soil. Persons of any age and either sex apparently are susceptible to the disease, but most affected persons are 30 to 50 years of age, and males predominate, except in Venezuela, where males and females work the soil together.

Pathology

Histologically, lesions of chromoblastomycosis show hyperkeratosis, pseudoepitheliomatous hyperplasia, keratolytic microabscesses in the epidermis, and a mixed suppurative and granulomatous inflammatory infiltrate of lymphocytes, neutrophils, monocytes, plasma cells, eosinophils, and occasional Langhans' and foreign body giant cells in the dermis and subcutaneous tissues. In the areas of dermal inflammation the pathognomonic sclerotic bodies—round, thick-walled, muriform (referring to the presence of both vertical and horizontal septa), brown cells 5 to 12 μm in diameter (Fig. 44–1)—are found within macrophages and giant cells or outside cells. Fibrous tissue forms a major component of older lesions.

Clinical Manifestations

Five forms of chromoblastomycosis are described. Nodular lesions are elevated, soft, pink to violaceous, smooth, verrucous, or scaly growths. Tumerous lesions are larger, papillomatous or lobulated masses that may be completely or partially covered by epidermal debris or crusts.

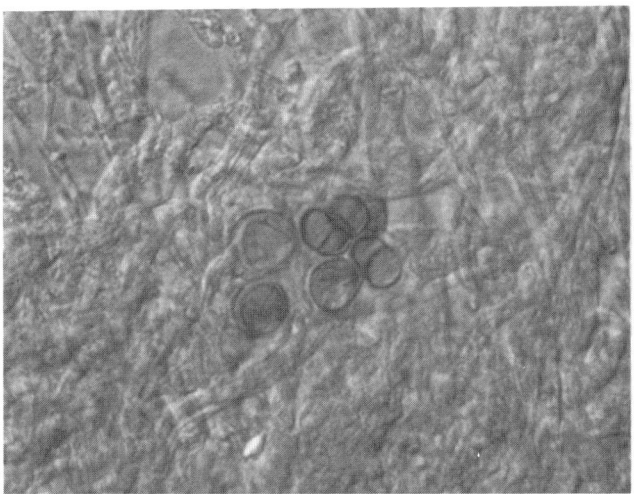

Fig. 44-1. Sclerotic bodies in a lesion of chromoblastomycosis caused by Fonsecaea pedrosoi (potassium hydroxide, ×630). (Courtesy of MR McGinnis, Professor and Vice Chairman, The University of Texas Medical Branch at Galveston.)

Verrucous lesions, often seen along the border of the foot, are hyperkeratotic, resembling a wart. Plaque lesions, the least common type, are flat or slightly elevated, variously sized and shaped, red to violet, and scaly. Cicatricial lesions are annular, arciform, or serpiginous growths that enlarge by expanding centrifugally and heal in their centers by scarring.

Lesions are pruritic and occasionally painful. Secondary bacterial infection or local trauma may cause ulceration. In Central and South America lesions are most common on the lower extremities, whereas in Australia the upper limbs, especially the hands, are usually involved. Satellite lesions may be due to autoinoculation following scratching of the primary lesion or to spread of the organism through the superficial lymphatics. Occasionally, hematogenous spread of infections caused by Fonsecaea pedrosoi to the central nervous system has resulted in cerebral phaeohyphomycosis.

Phaeohyphomycosis

Phaeohyphomycosis, a term coined in 1974 by Ajello, describes a distinct, heterogeneous group of infections caused by fungi that occur in tissue as dematiaceous yeast–like cells, pseudohyphae-like elements, septate hyphae, or a combination of these forms (7,8). These infections may affect any portion of the body, and depending on the site of involvement, phaeohyphomycosis is categorized into four types: superficial, cutaneous, subcutaneous, and systemic. Nearly forty species of dematiaceous fungi, all of which are found worldwide in soil and can be isolated from pine needles, greenhouses, shower curtains, and potting soil, have been recovered from patients who have phaeohyphomycosis; the most common pathogens are listed in Table 44-4. The epidemiology, pathologic findings, and clinical manifestations of phaeohyphomycosis are discussed individually for each of the four types of disease.

Superficial Phaeohyphomycosis. The superficial phaeohyphomycoses include black piedra and tinea nigra. Black piedra is characterized by firmly adherent, black, hard, gritty 1-mm diameter nodules composed of fungus cells on the hairs of the scalp, beard, and mustache. The infection occurs in humid, tropical countries in the Americas and in Indonesia. Piedraia hortae, the pathogen, typically grows superficially around the hair shaft, causing little damage to it, but it can grow within the shaft, weakening the hair and allowing easy breakage. Tinea nigra, manifested by brown to black, asymptomatic macules, typically on the palms or the soles, is most common in children and young adults in tropical areas but may be seen in temperate zones. The pathogens—Exophiala werneckii and Stenella arguata—are found in the stratum corneum and elicit little or no inflammatory response.

Cutaneous Phaeohyphomycosis. The cutaneous phaeohyphomycoses—dermatomycosis, mycotic keratitis, and onychomycosis—are characterized by invasion of keratinized tissue by the infecting fungus (see Table 44-4). The clinical appearance of dermatomycoses caused by the dematiaceous fungi and the host response to the infecting organisms are similar to those of the dermatophytoses. Mycotic keratitis caused by the dematiaceous fungi usually follows implantation of the organism during surgical or other trauma to the eye, and it has been associated with corticosteroid treatment of ocular infections. It begins as a fluffy, gray-white nodule and develops into a painful ulcer, often associated with visual defects. Onychomycosis caused by dematiaceous fungi is characterized by thickening and opacification of the nail plate and associated onycholysis.

Subcutaneous Phaeohyphomycosis. Subcutaneous phaeohyphomycosis, also called phaeomycotic cyst, typically results from traumatic implantation of the fungus (most commonly Exophiala jeanselmei, Wangiella dermatitidis, and species of Bipolaris and Phialophora) into the subcutaneous tissue. Persons with diabetes mellitus may develop lesions at the site of insulin injection; but for many affected persons contact with the soil is the only risk factor. The typical lesion, located at the site of entry of the fungus, is a solitary, discrete, asymptomatic, well-encapsulated subcutaneous mass or nodule that may undergo central necrosis, forming an encapsulated abscess several centimeters in diameter, or ulcerate and extrude pus containing brown-pigmented hyphae or sclerotic cells.

Histologic examination of the lesion shows a central area of necrotic debris and polymorphonuclear leukocytes, surrounded by a mantle of palisading epithelioid macrophages, giant cells, neutrophils, and occasional eosinophils and lymphocytes, and an outer layer of dense collagenous connective tissue. Splinters, slivers, or foreign vegetable matter may be seen in the necrotic tissue; and the fungal elements—parallel strands of brown, septate hyphae 2 to 6 μm in diameter, yeastlike cells, or swollen and distorted cells up to 25 μm in diameter—are found in the wall and in the center of the lesion (Fig. 44-2). The dematiaceous nature of the fungus may not be apparent in sections stained with hematoxylin and eosin but can be demonstrated with a melanin stain.

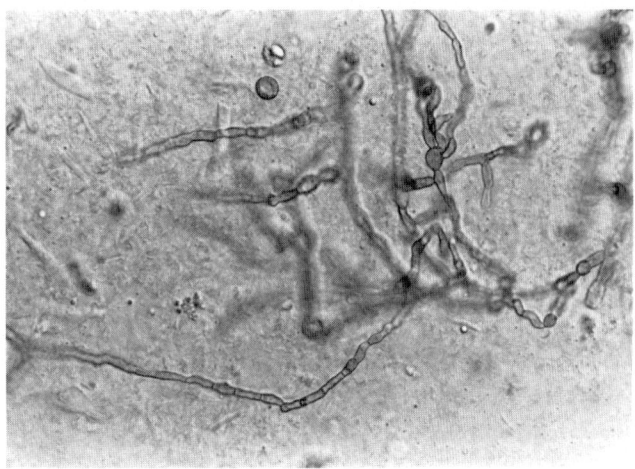

Fig. 44–2. Distorted hyphae of Xylohypha bantiana in aspirate from a brain abscess (potassium hydroxide, ×630). (Courtesy of MR McGinnis, Professor and Vice Chairman, The University of Texas Medical Branch at Galveston.)

Systemic Phaeohyphomycosis. Systemic phaeohyphomycosis, the rarest and most serious type of phaeohyphomycosis, occurs principally in immunocompromised persons (9–12). In most cases the portal of entry is the lungs, whence the fungus disseminates to other internal organs or the sinuses. One of the agents, Xylohypha bantiana (also called Cladosporium bantianum), has a predilection for the brain, especially the cerebral hemispheres and meninges (8). Dissemination of the fungus to other organs, such as liver, spleen, or pancreas, is much less common. Histologically, lesions are characterized by tissue necrosis, invasion of the vasculature by the fungus, granulation tissue, acute inflammation, and, in cases of sinusitis and allergic bronchopulmonary disease, plasma cells and eosinophils.

The clinical manifestations of systemic phaeohyphomycosis depend on the site of infection. Persons with central nervous system (CNS) involvement present with headache, nausea, vomiting, fever, mental confusion, and nuchal rigidity and pain. Those with sinusitis typically have headache, fever, and nasal discharge; polyps may be present. Persons with allergic bronchopulmonary disease have productive cough and bronchospasm. Manifestations of disseminated disease include skin lesions, osteomyelitis, pneumonia, brain abscess, and endocarditis. Moreover, in persons receiving chronic ambulatory peritoneal dialysis, the dematiaceous fungi have caused peritonitis with abdominal pain and fever (12).

Mycetoma

Mycetoma, a localized infection involving cutaneous and subcutaneous tissue, fascia, and bone, is classified by the agent as actinomycotic (caused by an aerobic actinomycete, see Chapter 29) or eumycotic (caused by a fungus) (13). Dematiaceous fungi that have been isolated from mycetomas are listed in Table 44-4.

Epidemiology

Fungi that cause mycetomas are normal inhabitants of soil or plant debris that enter the tissues via traumatic implantation. Mycetoma occurs worldwide between latitudes 15° south and 30° north but is seen most often in northern Africa, southern Asia, and tropical and subtropical zones of the Americas, predominantly in men.

Pathology

Histologically, mycetomas are characterized by localized abscesses that contain a granule or cluster of granules composed of fungal hyphae and aggregates of neutrophils in the dermis and subcutaneous tissues. Surrounding the abscess are palisading epithelioid cells, multinucleate giant cells, plasma cells, lymphocytes, and granulation tissue. Fibrosis is prominent in older lesions.

Clinical Manifestations

Mycetomas are most common on the feet but may involve the hands, arms, head and neck, knees, legs and thighs. The lesion begins several months after traumatic inoculation of the fungus, as a small, firm, painless subcutaneous nodule attached to the skin. It gradually enlarges, and sinuses communicating with the surface of the skin form, through which granules (representing aggregates of fungal cells) up to 2 mm in diameter and of various colors (depending on the organism involved) are discharged. Secondary nodules develop around the initial one, and eventually the organisms spread along fascial planes to adjacent tissue, including bone.

HYALINE SEPTATE MOULDS

The hyaline septate moulds have clear, relatively broad hyphae with uniform, parallel walls and distinct septations. Most are identified on the basis of the structure and arrangements of specialized fruiting bodies, from the surface of which conidia are derived. Of these fungi, species of Aspergillus are the most common human pathogens and are encountered most frequently in the clinical laboratory. Pseudallescheria boydii, Fusarium, Paecilomyces, Penicillium, and Scopulariopsis occasionally or rarely cause human disease.

Aspergillus

The name Aspergillus was used first in 1729 by Micheli, an Italian priest and botanist, who noted that the microscopic appearance of the fungus—a swollen vesicle with radiating chains of conidia—resembled the aspergillum, a church implement used to sprinkle holy water on the congregation (14). The first human infections caused by this fungus were recognized in the 1840s, and the term "aspergillosis" was coined in 1850 to describe these diseases (15). Characterization of the genus began in the early 1900s, but the diversity and importance of aspergillosis was not realized until the early 1950s.

The species of Aspergillus are asexual filamentous fungi that reproduce by means of conidia, although sexual forms of several species have been described. The conidia arise from or are formed in a phialide, which in turn arises directly from the swollen apex of the conidiophore, called the vesicle (uniseriate), or from sterile cells called metulae (biseriate) (Fig. 44–3) (16). Of the nearly 200 species of Aspergillus identified, fewer than 20 have caused

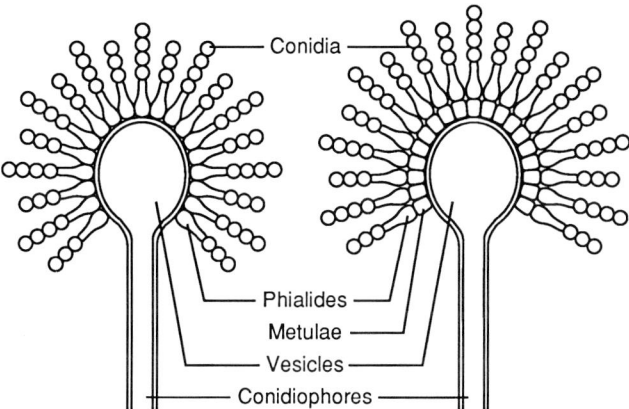

Fig. 44–3. Diagram of the microscopic features of Aspergillus species. (Modified from Raper KB and Fennell DI: The Genus Aspergillus. Baltimore, Williams & Wilkins, 1965.)

human disease. Aspergillus fumigatus is the most common agent of aspergillosis, followed by Aspergillus flavus; other species that have been associated with invasive aspergillosis are listed in Table 44–5 (15).

Epidemiology

Species of Aspergillus, among the most ubiquitous fungi known, are found in soil, water, decaying vegetation, and anywhere there is organic debris. Moreover, these organisms are present in hospital air, which in at least one outbreak was seeded from wood pulp–based fireproofing material (17,18). Aspergillosis usually is acquired by inhaling airborne conidia that are small enough to reach alveoli or enter the paranasal sinuses. Conidia in the air of operating rooms may enter implantation sites of prosthetic cardiac valves or catheters, or the eye during surgical removal of a cataract (19). Moreover, trauma to the eye or, to the skin of immunocompromised persons, may provide a port of entry for the fungus.

Pathogenesis and Pathology

Exposure to conidia of Aspergillus probably is almost universal, but disease is uncommon as it occurs when immune defenses are impaired. Two distinct lines of defense against Aspergillus exist, and both must be breached before the fungus can establish progressive infection (15). Macrophages, which kill conidia, are the first line of defense in aspergillosis, and polymorphonuclear leukocytes, which kill mycelia, constitute the second line. In addition, complement is chemotactic for phagocytic cells and facilitates neutrophil damage to hyphae and monocyte killing of conidia. Factors that predispose to invasive aspergillosis include corticosteroid administration, cytotoxic chemotherapy, recent or concurrent therapy with broad-spectrum antimicrobial agents, leukopenia (fewer than 1000 cells per microliter), acute leukemia in relapse, and acute rejection of a transplanted organ. Persons with hematopoietic and lymphoreticular malignancies are particularly prone to develop invasive disease, probably by virtue of depressed cell-mediated immunity, impaired ability to produce antibodies, and chemotherapy-induced neutropenia. In addition to the role of host defenses in the pathogenesis of aspergillosis, the infecting fungus may produce toxins that affect the course of the disease, though this has not been firmly established (20).

In the lung, hyphae of Aspergillus invade the walls of bronchi and the surrounding parenchyma, producing an acute, necrotizing, pyogenic pneumonitis, often with cavity formation, in persons able to mount an acute inflammatory response. In addition, Aspergillus has a marked tendency to invade blood vessels, causing thrombosis with consequent infarction, hemorrhage, and necrosis, and allowing its dissemination to other tissues. The hyphae of Aspergillus are 3 to 8 μm in diameter, septate (although occasionally septa are rare), and characteristically show repeated, dichotomous branching at an angle of about 45° (Fig. 44–4). Conidia (fruiting heads) usually are not seen in tissues, except in areas exposed to air such as the lung, paranasal sinus, or open wounds (Fig. 44–5). Occasionally the Splendore-Hoeppli phenomenon of eosinophilic halos around hyphae is observed, and granulomas rarely are formed in infections of the paranasal sinus, the orbit, or both.

Table 44–5. Species of Aspergillus Associated with Invasive Disease

Site of Infection	Species of Aspergillus
Pulmonary	A. fumigatus, -flavus, -niger, -nidulans, -terreus, -versicolor, -glaucus group, -amstelodami, -candidus, -carneous, -niveus, -restrictus
Nasal, paranasal, orbital	A. fumigatus, -flavus, -niger, -nidulans, -terreus, -versicolor, -flavipes, -ochraceus, -niveus, -conicus
Cerebral	A. fumigatus, -flavus, -terreus, -versicolor, -glaucus group, -amstelodami, -oryzae, -sydowi, -candidus
Musculoskeletal	A. fumigatus, -terreus, -nidulans, -sydowi
Disseminated	A. fumigatus, -flavus, -niger, -nidulans, -terreus, -versicolor, -glaucus, -niveus, -restrictus, -sydowi, -ustus

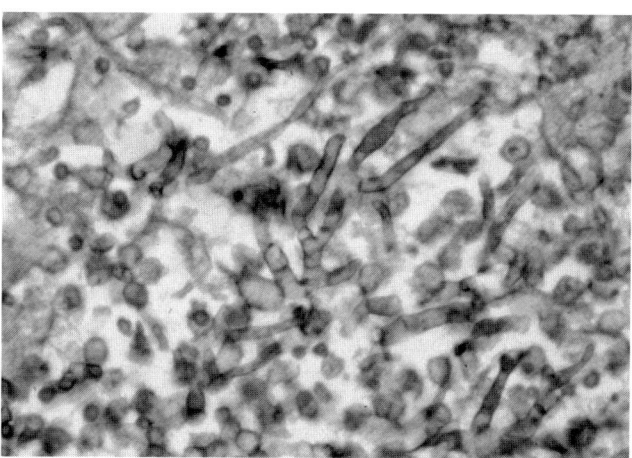

Fig. 44–4. Section of lung from an immunocompromised patient with Aspergillus flavus pneumonia and blood vessel invasion shows septate hyphae (Gomori's methenamine silver, ×320).

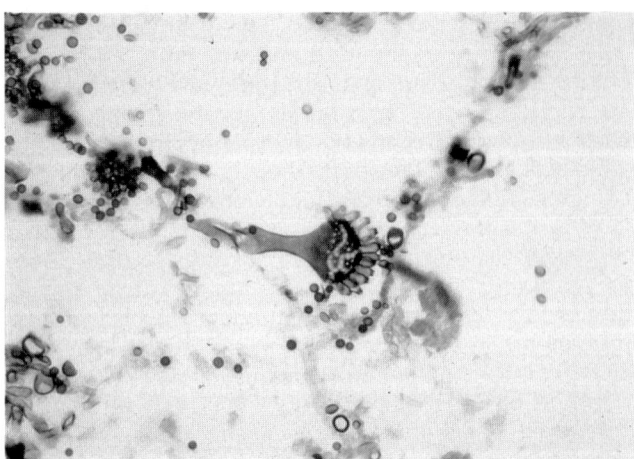

Fig. 44–5. Section of sinus tissue from a recipient of a bone marrow transplant with invasive sinusitis caused by Aspergillus flavus shows a fruiting head (Gomori's methenamine silver, ×205).

Clinical Manifestations

The spectrum of clinical manifestations of infection with Aspergillus ranges from apparently harmless colonization of the respiratory tract in persons with underlying chronic lung disease and impaired mucociliary clearance to fulminant and almost always fatal disseminated disease (21). The most common site of infection is the lung, where Aspergillus may multiply without causing direct tissue damage, a colonization promoted by prolonged use of broad-spectrum antimicrobial agents, corticosteroid administration, malnutrition, or debility. Inhalation of Aspergillus conidia by persons who have tuberculosis, sarcoidosis, histoplasmosis, asthma, chronic bronchitis, bronchiectasis, or other chronic pulmonary disorders may result in the development of a (usually static) fungus ball in pulmonary cavities, cysts, or areas of necrosis. The symptoms and prognosis for this condition are those of the underlying disease, although hemoptysis is common (22). Several hypersensitivity reactions, which depend on the extent of exposure, the species of Aspergillus inhaled, and the genetically predetermined immune responsiveness of the host, have been described: allergic bronchopulmonary aspergillosis, mucoid impaction of the bronchus, eosinophilic pneumonitis, extrinsic allergic pneumonia, and bronchocentric granulomatosis.

Normal children who inhale a very large inoculum of Aspergillus conidia may develop fever, dyspnea, and a miliary infiltrate on chest x-ray within 24 hours (23). These children usually improve spontaneously in 2 to 4 weeks, although metastatic lesions and death have occurred. In immunocompromised persons, especially those with profound and prolonged neutropenia, infection of the respiratory tract with Aspergillus may result in an acute, rapidly progressive pneumonia characterized by fever, dyspnea, and one or more areas of consolidation (Fig. 44-6). The latter frequently are peripheral in location and often become cavitary if bone marrow function returns (15,24). The clinical course usually is fulminant, and death follows in a few weeks. Chronic necrotizing pulmonary aspergillosis is a rarely recognized indolent, cavitating process that

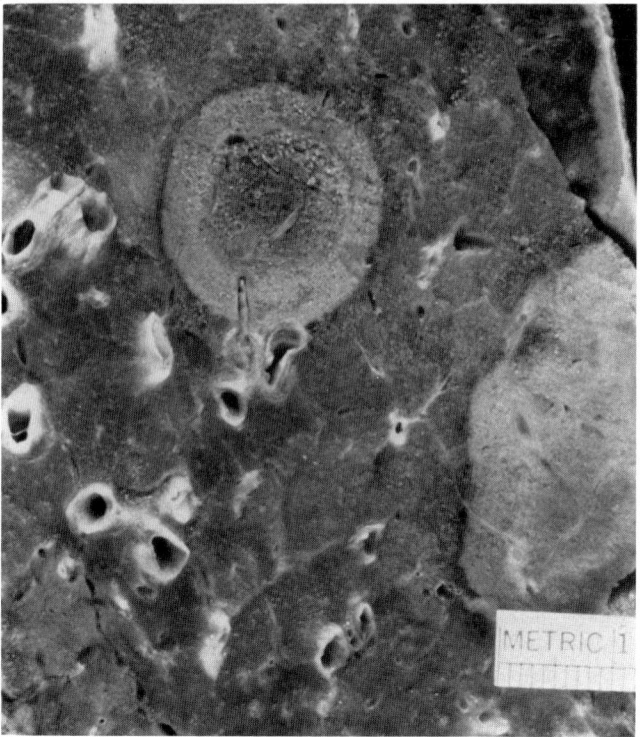

Fig. 44–6. Lung shows well-circumscribed focus of consolidation with central necrosis caused by Aspergillus flavus.

usually occurs in middle-aged persons, often in association with some impairment of host defenses, such as diabetes mellitus or low-dose corticosteroid therapy, and is manifested by fever and productive cough of one to several months' duration (25).

Cutaneous aspergillosis usually is secondary to hematogenous dissemination, a condition characterized by small, red, discrete papules that become pustular and microscopically show microabscesses and centrally necrotic granulomas that contain small colonies of Aspergillus. Cutaneous lesions rarely are primary, in which case the skin is thick, edematous, and purple or ulcerated and covered by a black eschar (15,19,26).

Aspergillus is the most common fungus infecting the nose and paranasal sinuses; and Aspergillus fumigatus is the species most often implicated, except in the Sudan where the infection is endemic and Aspergillus flavus is the usual pathogen (27,28). Two forms of sinus involvement have been described. A benign, infiltrative form that behaves like an Aspergillus fungus ball and does not destroy bone is most common. The invasive form, characterized by invasion of the surrounding bone and orbital tissue by the fungus, may be difficult to diagnose. Symptoms and signs include headache, facial pain, proptosis, visual disturbances, bone pain, local tissue swelling, and occasionally extraocular muscle palsies. Visualization of the involved sinus by sinusotomy reveals greenish black, rubbery, oily material composed of hyphae.

Otomycosis is a benign disease often caused by species of Aspergillus, most commonly Aspergillus niger. Infection of the external canal is a chronic or subacute process characterized by scaling, pruritus, pain, and filling of the canal with cerumen and detritus shed from the cutaneous lining. Rarely, the infection extends into the middle ear cavity, eroding into the mastoid air cells and temporal bone (24).

Ocular infections with Aspergillus include mycotic keratitis, in which fungi from an external source infect the cornea following trauma or superficial disease; endogenous oculomycosis, which results from hematogenous dissemination of a primary focus of infection elsewhere; and extension oculomycosis, which originates from an infection in adjacent tissues. Most ocular infections with Aspergillus occur in immunocompromised persons and result in endophthalmitis (29).

Endocarditis caused by Aspergillus most often involves prosthetic valves, but infections of native valves and of the mural endocardium (Fig. 44–7) have been reported, predominantly in immunocompromised hosts (21,30). From the vegetations, organisms commonly invade the adjacent myocardium, and, typically, embolize to systemic or pulmonary arteries, resulting in foci of infection in the lung, kidney, spleen, and brain. Clinical manifestations of endocarditis are heart failure, conduction disturbances, and evidence of embolic events.

Infection of the central nervous system with Aspergillus, manifested as one or several foci of hemorrhagic necrosis (Fig. 44-8) or, rarely, as meningitis, occurs as a

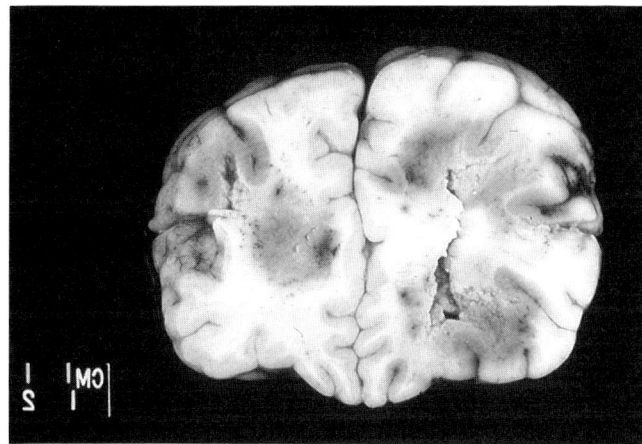

Fig. 44–8. Hemorrhagic intracerebral lesions caused by Aspergillus flavus in a liver transplant recipient with disseminated aspergillosis.

complication of endocarditis or a surgical procedure, as a manifestation of disseminated disease, or, in intravenous drug users, after injection of contaminated material. Signs and symptoms typically are those of a brain abscess.

Disseminated aspergillosis—active infection in two or more noncontiguous sites, most commonly caused by Aspergillus fumigatus or Aspergillus flavus—is a rapidly fulminant, invariably fatal disease almost always seen in persons who take broad-spectrum antimicrobial agents, corticosteroids, cytotoxins, or a combination of these. The lung is the usual target organ; next in frequency are the CNS, kidney, liver, and thyroid gland (15,21,24). The most common terminal event is intracerebral hemorrhage, although death may result from diffuse bilateral pneumonia or massive pulmonary infarction.

Pseudallescheria boydii

Pseudallescheria boydii (previously called Allescheria boydii and Petriellidium boydii) is a saprophyte found in soil, manure, decaying vegetation, polluted streams, and coastal waters in many countries of the world (31). Infection with the fungus is acquired via traumatic inoculation or by the airborne route. The organism is the most common cause of mycetoma (discussed earlier) in the United States. Pseudallescheria boydii also may cause ocular infections and arthritis, both of which usually follow trauma; brain abscesses, which are associated with near drowning in polluted waters, granulocytopenia, cellular immune deficiency, and trauma; sinusitis, endophthalmitis, osteomyelitis, endocarditis, abscesses in the lung and thyroid, and disseminated disease in immunocompromised persons (32–36). Histologically, lesions resemble those of aspergillosis, with tissue necrosis, acute inflammation and branching, and septate hyphae that may demonstrate vascular invasion.

Species of Fusarium

The species of Fusarium, found worldwide in the soil, are important plant pathogens (37). In Russia in 1931, consumption of cereals contaminated with mycotoxin produced by Fusarium sporotrichioides was recognized

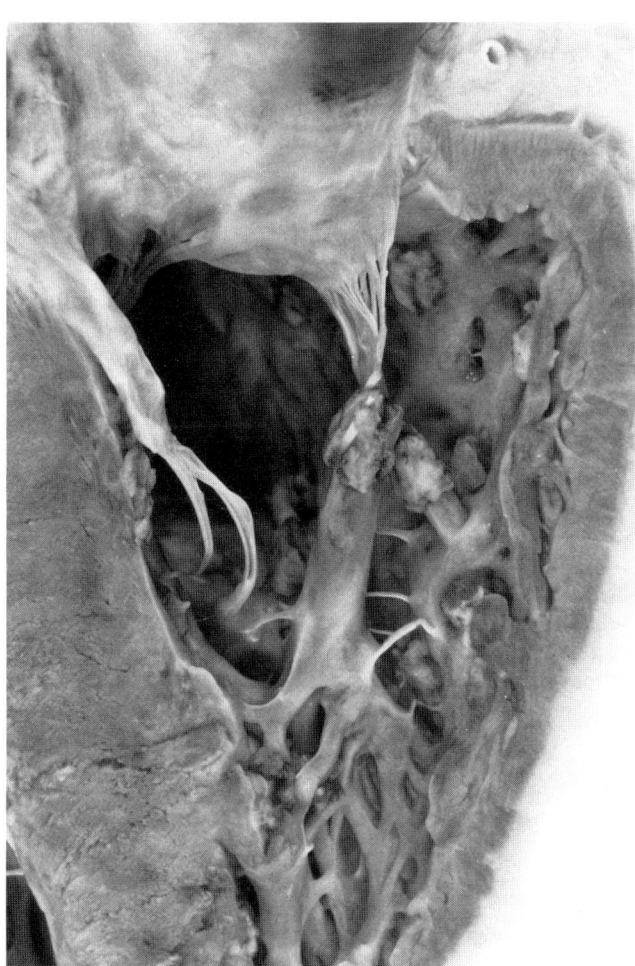

Fig. 44–7. Heart of an AIDS patient involved with mural endocarditis caused by Aspergillus flavus.

as the cause of a systemic illness characterized by gastrointestinal symptoms and weakness that progressed to aplastic anemia and death in those who continued to eat the contaminated grain (38). Other species of Fusarium—Fusarium moniliforme, Fusarium dimerum, Fusarium solani, Fusarium oxysporum, Fusarium chlamydosporum, and Fusarium anthopilum—may cause localized infections of the skin, nails, and cornea. Recently, these organisms have emerged as important pathogens in immunocompromised hosts, causing skin and soft tissue infections, sinusitis, pneumonia, fungemia, invasive infection involving a single organ, or, most commonly, disseminated disease (39–44). Histologically, infection with Fusarium cannot be distinguished from infection with Aspergillus or Pseudallescheria boydii (described earlier).

Other Hyaline Septate Moulds

Paecilomyces has been implicated in endophthalmitis, endocarditis, and skin lesions (45). Penicillium and Scopulariopsis may cause mycotic keratitis, otomycosis, onychomycosis and, rarely, infections of deep organs (46). Penicilliosis, which occurs in debilitated persons after inhaling the conidia of Paecilomyces, Penicillium, or Scopulariopsis, begins as a pulmonary disease but may spread hematogenously to other organs (47).

ZYGOMYCETES

Members of the class Zygomycetes cause zygomycosis, a polymorphic disease with a broad spectrum of clinical manifestations that may be divided arbitrarily into at least six types based on presentation and site of involvement: rhinocerebral, pulmonary, cutaneous, subcutaneous, gastrointestinal, and CNS (discussed later). The Zygomycetes of medical importance are classified in general as follows:

Class: Zygomyctes
Order: Mucorales
Genus: Absidia
Species: Corymbifera
Genus: Mucor
Species: Ramosissimus
Genus: Rhizomucor
Species: Pusillus
Genus: Rhizopus
Species: Arrhizus, microsporus, rhizopodiformis
Genus: Apophysomyces
Species: Elegans
Genus: Cunninghamella
Species: Bertholletiae
Genus: Saksenaea
Species: Vasiformis
Order: Entomophthorales
Genus: Basidiobolus
Species: Ranarum
Genus: Conidiobolus
Species: Coronatus, incongruus

Many members of the order Mucorales produce asexual, nonmotile sporangiospores in closed structures called sporangia, but some form their spores in subdivisions of the sporangia. In nature, but not in routine culture procedures, these organisms undergo sexual reproduction, forming zygospores, which have taxonomic value, by virtue of their ornamentation, suspensor size, color, and ornamental projections, in determining families and genera.

Epidemiology

The Zygomyctes are distributed worldwide. Members of the order Mucorales typically are found in decaying matter. For example, species of Rhizopus frequently are recovered from mouldy bread. Of the members of Mucorales, species of Rhizopus are isolated most frequently from human infections, followed by Rhizomucor; however, disease caused by the less commonly encountered members are clinically indistinguishable from disease caused by members of the former two genera (48–54). Members of the order Entomophthorales are normal inhabitants of the soil throughout the world, but the diseases they cause are most prevalent in Africa, Southeast Asia, Indonesia, and South America and rarely are seen in North America (55,56).

Human infections with the Zygomycetes are acquired from the environment; organisms probably enter the body via inhalation or direct inoculation, but this has not been proven. Nosocomial infections have been traced to contaminated air-conditioning systems and to contaminated bandages (57,58). Most infections occur in persons who are immunocompromised, who have diabetes mellitus, or who have experienced some type of trauma.

Pathogenesis and Pathology

The pathogenesis of zygomycosis is incompletely understood. Much of the current knowledge is derived from the mouse model of infection. Bronchoalveolar macrophages collected from normal mice readily ingest spores of Rhizopus and inhibit their germination; however, bronchoalveolar macrophages harvested from mice with diabetes and from mice treated with corticosteroids do not inhibit spore germination (59,60).

Neutrophils are a prominent component of the host response to infection with the Zygomycetes and are recruited into infected sites by fungus-derived factors and via activation of the alternate pathway of complement (see Chapter 2) (61,62). Normal human serum inhibits the growth of Rhizopus, whereas serum from persons with diabetic ketoacidosis does not, and actually may enhance fungal growth (63,64). Interactions between transferrin, iron molecules, and fungal spores may affect the replication rate of fungal cells, thus explaining, at least in part, the recently recognized association between rhinocerebral mucormycosis and deferoxamine administration (65–67).

Microscopically, infections with the Zygomycetes are characterized by abscess formation, suppurative necrosis, and invasion by the fungus of blood vessel walls and subsequent thrombosis and infarction. Broad, 10 to 25 μm diameter, nonseptate, ribbon-like hyphae (Fig. 44–9), typi-

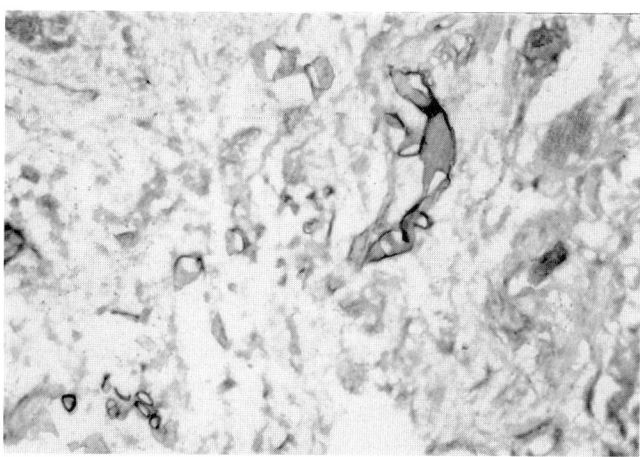

Fig. 44–9. Broad, aseptate hyphae of Zygomycetes (Gomori's methenamine silver, ×256).

cally branching at 90° angles, are present in vessel walls and throughout involved tissues. Rarely, sporangia are seen, primarily in well-aerated nasal and pulmonary tissues (Fig. 44–10).

Clinical Manifestations

The clinical manifestations of zygomycosis are discussed in two parts: those typically associated with infections caused by members of Mucorales—rhinocerebral, pulmonary, cutaneous, gastrointestinal, and CNS involvement—and those associated with the Entomophthorales. The latter infections may be subdivided further, based on the anatomic location of the disease and the genus responsible for the pathologic findings at the involved site, into entomophthoramycosis condiobolae, which typically affects the head and face, and entomophthoramycosis basidiobolae, which causes disease elsewhere in the body, usually the trunk and arms.

Rhinocerebral mucormycosis (most often seen in persons who have diabetes mellitus [especially in the presence of acidosis], in those with leukemia who are neutropenic and are receiving broad-spectrum antimicrobial agents, and those receiving hemodialysis and deferoxamine) almost always present with facial pain or headache, or both (48,68). Fever and evidence of orbital cellulitis are common; and with invasion of the orbit by the fungus, loss of extraocular muscle function can develop. Complications of disease progression include retinal artery thrombosis with loss of vision, cranial nerve dysfunction manifested by ptosis and pupillary dilatation, cerebral abscess, and thrombosis of the cavernous sinus, the internal carotid artery, or both.

Pulmonary mucormycosis, characterized by fever, dyspnea, and hemoptysis, affects immunocompromised persons, especially those who are neutropenic and are receiving broad-spectrum antimicrobial agents and corticosteroids. The chest x-ray shows consolidation or cavity formation, initially involving one segment but progressing to involve multiple contiguous areas in one lung.

Cutaneous mucormycosis may be a primary infection, associated with contaminated elastic bandages, trauma (especially in persons with diabetes mellitus), burn wounds, and rarely intramuscular injections; or secondary hematogeneous spread from a distant site (57,69–72). Affected persons typically present with cellulitis; and with disease progression, muscle may become infected and organisms may invade blood vessels and disseminate to distant sites.

Gastrointestinal mucormycosis is an acute, rapidly fatal disease, mainly of extremely malnourished persons and probably acquired by consuming food contaminated with the organism (73). The stomach, ileum, and colon are

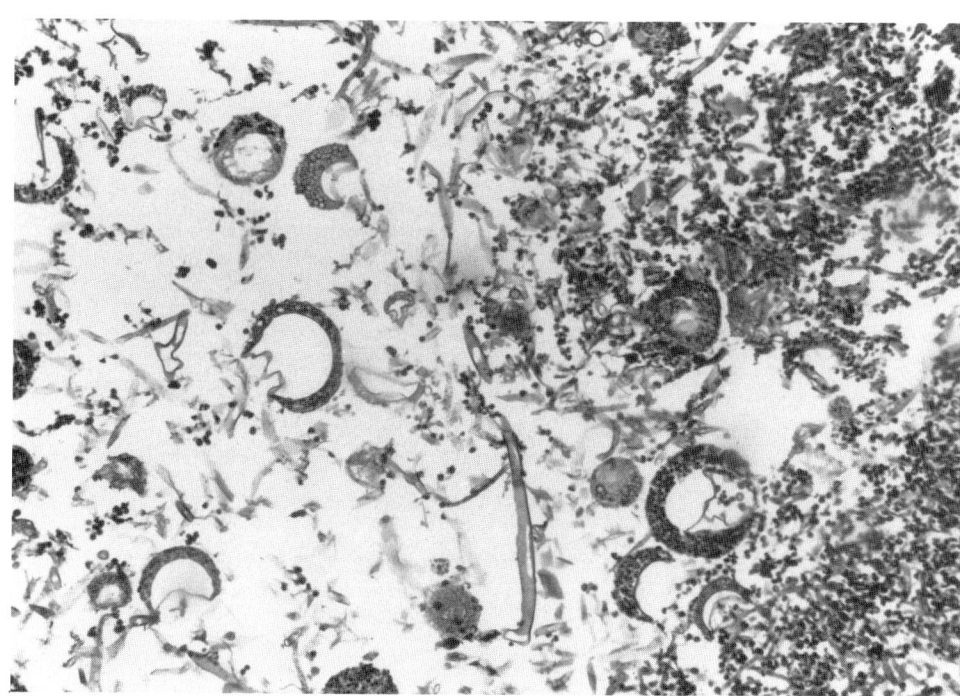

Fig. 44–10. Section of sinus tissue from a patient with rhinocerebral zygomycosis showing Zygomycetes sporangia; culture grew Rhizopus species (hematoxylin and eosin, ×100).

involved most often, but any site may be affected. Symptoms include abdominal pain and distention, nausea, and vomiting, often accompanied by fever and hematochezia.

CNS mucormycosis is a rare form of disease seen in severely debilitated persons; in intravenous drug users, some of whom have the acquired immunodeficiency syndrome (see Chapter 22); and after open head trauma (74–76). Organisms reach the CNS by direct extension from a focus of infection in the nose or paranasal sinuses, via direct implantation at the time of injury, or by injecting contaminated illicit drugs. Symptoms include decreasing consciousness and focal neurologic findings.

Entomophthoramycosis conidiobolae is characterized by swelling of the nose, perinasal tissue, and mouth, accompanied by nasal stuffiness, drainage, and sinus pain. Firm, painless, subcutaneous nodules involve the trunk, arms, legs, buttocks, or rarely, muscle or the gastrointestinal tract (56,77). Disseminated infection with Conidiobolus has been described (78).

Laboratory Diagnosis

Specimens required to diagnose infections caused by moulds are listed in Table 44–6. Specimen collection, transport, and processing are discussed in Part III, but in general all specimens should be transported promptly to the laboratory, where they should be examined microscopically and inoculated to media as soon as possible. If prolonged transport cannot be avoided (for example, if mailing is necessary), antibiotics may be added to the specimen to prevent bacterial overgrowth (see Chapter 54), and specimens should be stored at refrigerator or room temperature; freezing and drying should be avoided. Identification of the medically important moulds is discussed below.

Dermatophytes

Infections caused by the dermatophytes often are diagnosed by their clinical manifestations, regardless of whether septate hyphae can be observed in potassium hydroxide (KOH) preparations of skin scales, hair or nail scrapings. In the case of tinea capitis, examining the affected scalp under a Wood's (long-wavelength) ultraviolet light may be useful because hairs infected with species of Microsporum emit a yellow-green fluorescence. To confirm the diagnosis and identify the pathogen culture is necessary.

Dermatophytes may be divided into two categories based on growth rate. Intermediate growers (mature colonies form in 6 to 10 days) include Epidermophyton floccosum, Trichophyton mentagrophytes, and the species of Microsporum except Microsporum audouinii. Slow growers (mature colonies form in 11 to 21 days) include Microsporum audouinii and the species of Trichophyton except Tricophyton mentagrophytes. The culture and microscopic features useful in identifying the commonly encountered dermatophytes are described in Table 44-7,

Table 44–6. Specimens Required for Diagnosis of Infections Caused by Moulds

Disease	Organisms*	Specimens
Skin infection	Trichophyton spp, Microsporum spp, Epidermophyton, Piedraia, Exophiala werneckii, Alternaria, Aspergillus spp, Zygomycetes, Fusarium spp	Skin scales from periphery of lesion, skin biopsy tissue, aspirated pus
Onychomycosis	Trichophyton spp, Epidermophyton, Botryodiplodia, Hendersonula, Phyllosticta, Fusarium spp	Nail scrapings (from softened material beneath nail plate), nail shavings (obtained after the nail is scraped)
Hair infections	Trichophyton spp, Microsporum spp	Damaged hair; hairs that fluoresce under Wood's lamp
Keratitis	Botryodiplodia, Curvularia spp, Exophiala jeanselmei, Exserohilum, Fusarium spp, Zygomycetes, Pseudallescheria boydii	Corneal scrapings
Subcutaneous infections	Fonsecaea species, Cladosporium, Phialophora spp, Rhinocladiella, Exophiala spp, Wangiella, Alternaria, Bipolaris, Phoma spp, Scytalidium, Xylohypha, Scedosporium, Basidiobolus, Conidiobolus, Pseudallescheria boydii	Scrapings of lesions biopsy tissue, aspirated pus, granules from mycetoma
Sinusitis	Aspergillus spp (Bipolaris spp, Exserohilum spp)	Aspirated pus, infected tissue
Rhinocerebral infections	Zygomycetes (Aspergillus)	Infected tissue, discharge from orbit or nose
Pulmonary infections	Aspergillus spp, Zygomycetes, (Drechslera spp, Bipolaris spp)	Lung tissue, sputum, bronchoalveolar lavage fluid, transbronchial biopsy
External otomycosis	Aspergillus spp, Zygomycetes, (Penicillium, Scopulariopsis)	Scrapings from the auditory canal
Gastrointestinal infections	Zygomycetes	Infected tissue
Central nervous system infection	Aspergillus spp, Zygomycetes, (Pseudallescheria boydii, Xylohypha bantiana)	Infected tissue
Endocarditis	Aspergillus spp, (Pseudallescheria boydii, Paecilomyces)	Infected valve, blood†
Disseminated	Aspergillus spp, Zygomycetes, Fusarium spp	Infected tissue; biopsy specimen from skin lesions, if present; blood, especially for Fusarium

* Organisms in parenthesis involved infrequently.
† Blood cultures almost never positive in Aspergillus endocarditis.

MOULDS

Table 44–7. Diagnostic Features of the Commonly Encountered Dermatophytes

Organism	Colony Morphology	Microscopic Features
Microsporum canis	Granular to fluffy, white to buff surface; bright, lemon yellow apron at periphery; yellow-orange reverse	Thick-walled, spindle-shaped, multiseptate, echinulate macroconidia, some with a curved tip; sparse microconidia laterally attached to hyphae
Microsporum audouinii	Velvety, light tan or buff surface; salmon pink reverse	Rare macroconidia and microconidia; many terminal chlamydospores, favic chandeliers, and pectinate bodies
Microsporum gypseum	Granular, cinnamon-colored surface; light tan reverse	Thick-walled, multiseptate, echinulate macroconidia that are longer and less spindle shaped than those of M. canis and have rounded rather than pointed tips that do not curve
Epidermophyton floccosum	White, floccose surface turning khaki green-brown with age; yellow-brown reverse with folds	No microconidia; large, smooth-walled, clavate macroconidia with two to five cells borne singly or in clusters of two or three
Trichophyton mentagrophytes*	Two colony types: fluffy and granular. White to pink surface; buff to reddish brown reverse; some strains produce red-brown pigment	Many globose microconidia arranged in pine-tree or grape-like clusters; rare thin-walled, smooth, pencil-shaped macroconidia; spiral hyphae in 30% of isolates
Trichophyton rubrum*	Downy or occasionally granular; white, pink, or red surface; wine red to yellow-red reverse	Many tear-shaped microconidia borne laterally and singly from hyphae; rare if any thin-walled, smooth, cigar-shaped macroconidia
Trichophyton tonsurans	Velvety to powdery tan, brown, to creamy red surface with rugal folds and heaped, sunken center; yellow to tan reverse	Rare to absent bizarre-shaped macroconidia; tear- or club-shaped microconidia with flat bottoms that are larger than those of other dermatophytes; occasional balloon forms
Trichophyton schoenleinii†	Waxy, heaped, light yellow to buff surface; colorless to yellow-orange reverse	No macroconidia; favic chandeliers; occasional chlamydoconidia and hyphal swellings
Trichophyton verrucosum	Poor growth on SDA at 30° C; on SDA with yeast extract at 37° C, forms heaped, waxy white to bright yellow colony with nonpigmented to yellow reverse	On SDA, only chlamydoconidia in chains; on thiamine-enriched media, moderate club-shaped microconidia borne along hyphae and rare three- to five-celled macroconidia with elongated rat-tail end

* T. mentagrophytes gives a positive urease test in 2 days and a positive hair penetration test. T. rubrum is urease negative (but may be faintly positive in 7 days) and gives a negative hair penetration test.
† Microconidia are formed on rice grains.
Key: SDA, Sabouraud's dextrose agar.

and examples are illustrated in Plates IXB to IXE and Figures 44-11 to 44-13. In general, species of Microsporum have a predominance of multicelled macroconidia with thick, rough walls and small numbers of oval to elliptical microconidia. Epidermophyton floccosum produces only macroconidia, which typically are club shaped, have three to five cells, and thin, smooth walls. Species of Trichophyton have abundant tear-shaped or oval microconidia and few if any macroconidia that are elongate and pencil shaped, multicelled, and have thin, smooth walls.

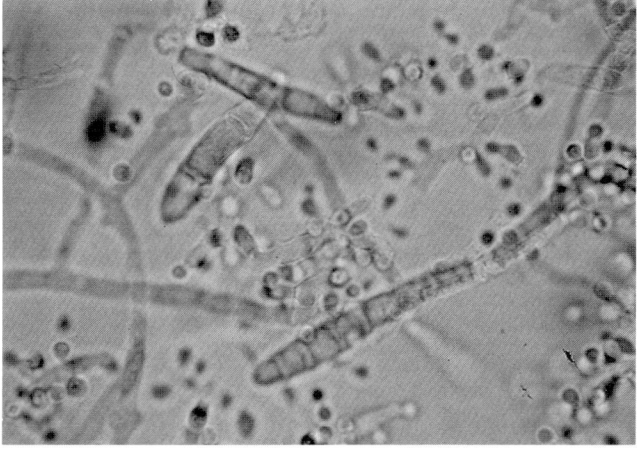

Fig. 44–11. Scotch-tape preparation of a colony of Trichophyton mentagrophytes, shows smooth-walled, pencil-shaped macroconidia and numerous microconidia (lactophenol cotton blue, ×205).

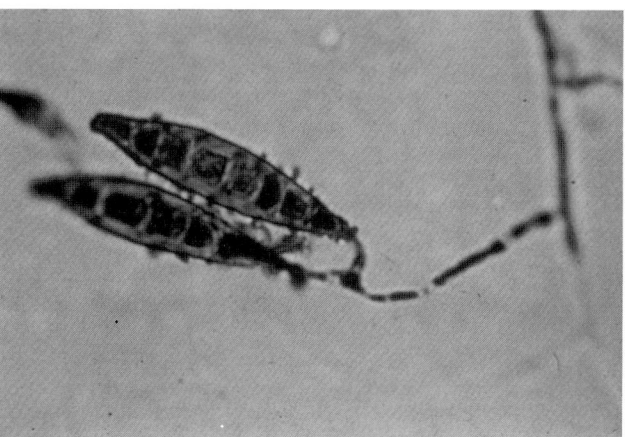

Fig. 44–12. Scotch-tape preparation of a colony of Microsporum canis showing thick-walled, spiny macroconidia (lactophenol cotton blue, ×205).

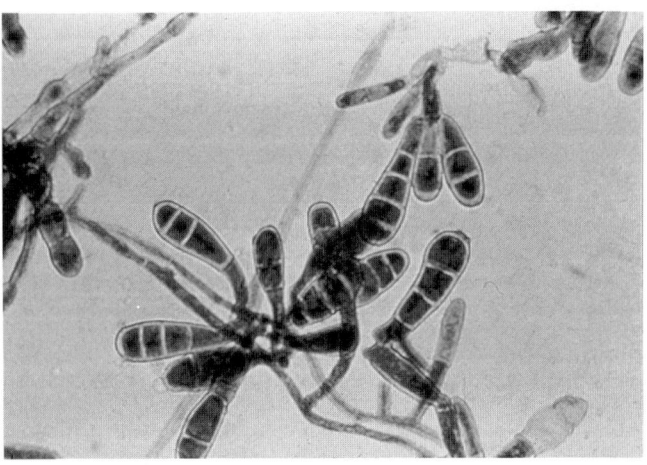

Fig. 44–13. Scotch-tape preparation of a colony of Epidermophyton floccosum shows smooth-walled, club-shaped macroconidia (lactophenol cotton blue, ×205).

Dematiaceous Fungi

Infections with dematiaceous fungi may be diagnosed by observing characteristic brown or black fungal elements in KOH preparations prepared directly from clinical specimens or in formalin-fixed tissue sections stained with hematoxylin and eosin or a melanin stain. For example, the presence of sclerotic bodies—thick walled, muriform, chestnut brown cells, 5 to 12 μm in diameter (see Fig. 44-1)—in aspirates or biopsies of subcutaneous lesions confirms the diagnosis of chromoblastomycosis. Tinea nigra is diagnosed by observing one- and two-celled yeastlike organisms, 1.5 to 5 μm in diameter, and branched, septate pigmented hyphae, 1.5 to 3 μm wide, in KOH preparations of skin scrapings. Black piedra usually is diagnosed clinically, but the organisms, characterized by the production of asci, each containing eight fusiform, single-celled ascospores, can be seen in infected hairs. The diagnosis of phaeohyphomycosis involving nails may require culture, because fungal elements observed in KOH preparations of nail scrapings may be indistinguishable from those of dermatophytes. Potassium hydroxide preparations of specimens from cases of subcutaneous phaeohyphomycosis show irregularly swollen, septate, branched or unbranched, brown hyphae, usually 3 to 4 μm in diameter but occasionally as large as 25 μm, often in conjunction with dematiaceous yeast–like cells that frequently occur in chains. Similar-looking fungal elements also are seen in aspirates or tissue from lesions of systemic phaeohyphomycosis. The diagnosis of mycetoma is based on the presence of typical granules; however, in all of these situations identification of the pathogen requires recovery by culture.

Because many dematiaceous fungi are inhibited by cycloheximide, when infections with these organisms are suspected clinical specimens must be planted onto at least one medium that contains no cycloheximide. In general, the dematiaceous fungi grow slowly, forming dark gray, brown, or black, hairy or velvety colonies with a black reverse after 3 to 4 weeks. Young colonies may be yeastlike in consistency before a mycelium develops, and some dematiaceous fungi form colonies in 1 or 2 weeks. Identification, which is based on differences in the structure, conidiogenesis, and arrangement of microconidia and macroconidia and some biochemical tests, may be difficult. General features of the commonly encountered dematiaceous fungi are outlined in Table 44-8 and illustrated in Figures 44-14 to 44-18; a more comprehensive approach to identification is provided in reference 79.

Table 44–8. Identifying Characteristics of the Dematiaceous Fungi

Organism	Growth Rate (days)	Microscopic Features
Fonsecaea pedrosi	14–21	Four types of conidiation: (1) Septate erect conidiophores; primary conidia at the tip of the conidiophores support one to four secondary conidia, which may produce one to four tertiary conidia (Fonsecaea type). (2) One-celled conidia arising opposite each other at the conidiophore tip (Rhinocladiella type). (3) Branched chains of conidia (Cladosporium type). (4) Flask-shaped phialides with collarettes and balls of phialoconidia
Cladosporium carrionii	14–21	Long or short conidiophores supporting repeatedly branching short chains of elliptical blastoconidia 2–3 μm by 4–7 μm
Phialophora verrucosa	3–7	Flask-shaped phialides with distinct cup-shaped collarette at the apex, bearing clusters of conidia
Exophiala jeanselmei*	5–10	Dark budding yeast initially. With age, annelides on annellophores produce clusters of oval conidia. Collarettes or rings at the apices of the annelides (often visible only under oil immersion) distinguish E. jeanselmei from Wangiella dermatitidis, which lacks a collarette.
Wangiella dermatitidis	5–10	Resembles E. jeanselmei except collarettes are absent
Exophiala werneckii	14–21	Dense dispersion of two-celled, clavate yeast cells separated by a deeply staining septum
Curvularia	3–7	Twisted conidiophores roughened at points of conidial attachments with dark brown, large four- to six-celled, curved or boomerang-shaped macroconidia
Bipolaris	3–7	Conidiophores with bent-knee appearance; dark, thick-walled oblong conidia (8 μm by 26 μm) with three to five septations and barely conspicuous hilum
Drechslera	3–7	Similar to Bipolaris, except conidia are larger (16 μm by 65 μm), and more cylindrical, and hilum is flat
Exserohilum	3–7	Conidiophores with bent-knee appearance; elongate, fusiform conidia (14 μm by 90 μm) with conspicuous, protruding, squared-off hilum
Alternaria	3–7	Chained, dark brown, multicelled macroconidia that contain horizontal and vertical septa and have club-shaped base and tapered apices

* Growth at 42° C and negative nitrate distinguish W. dermatitidis from E. jeanselmei, which does not grow at 42° C and is nitrate positive.

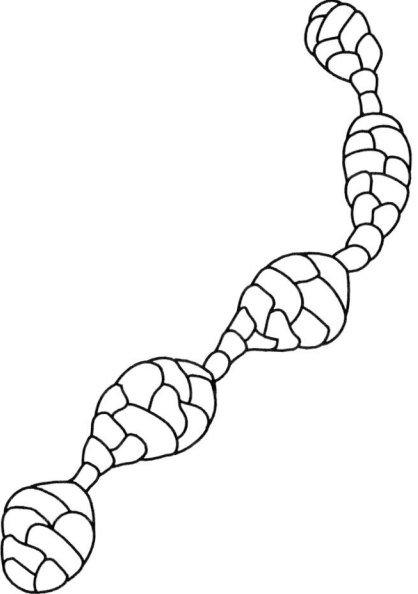

Fig. 44–14. Diagram of the chained, muriform poroconidia of Alternaria, with club-shaped bases, tapered apices, and horizontal and vertical septa.

Hyaline Septate Moulds

Diagnosis of invasive infections caused by the hyaline septate moulds often is difficult, especially early in the illness. These organisms may colonize the upper respiratory tract without producing disease, so a hyaline septate mould recovered from a respiratory tract specimen such as sputum may be a pathogen or a saprophyte. This dilemma has been evaluated most extensively for species of Aspergillus.

Aspergillus species. Invasive aspergillosis is difficult to diagnose early in the disease (80). Data from one study suggest that recovery of Aspergillus fumigatus or Aspergillus flavus from nasal cultures of immunocompromised

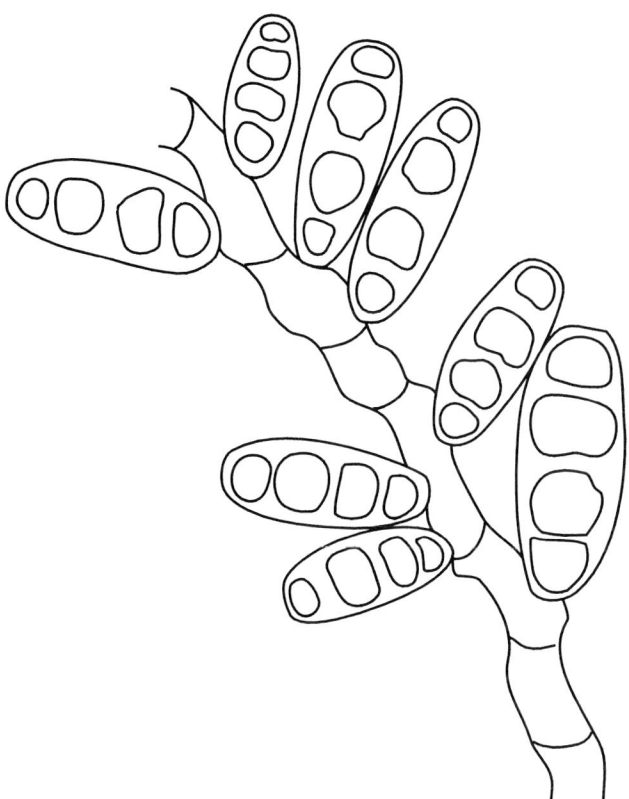

Fig. 44–16. Diagram of the geniculate conidiophore and thick-walled oblong conidia of Bipolaris spicifera.

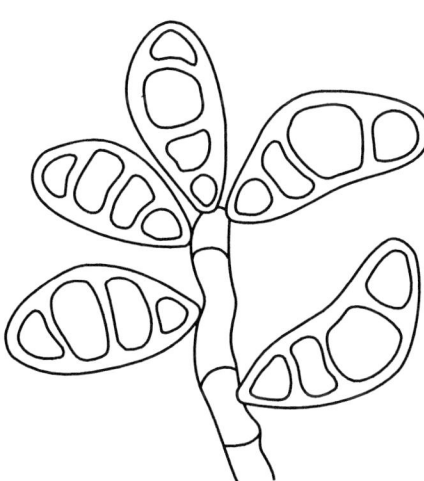

Fig. 44–15. Diagram of boomerang-shaped macroconidia of Curvularia.

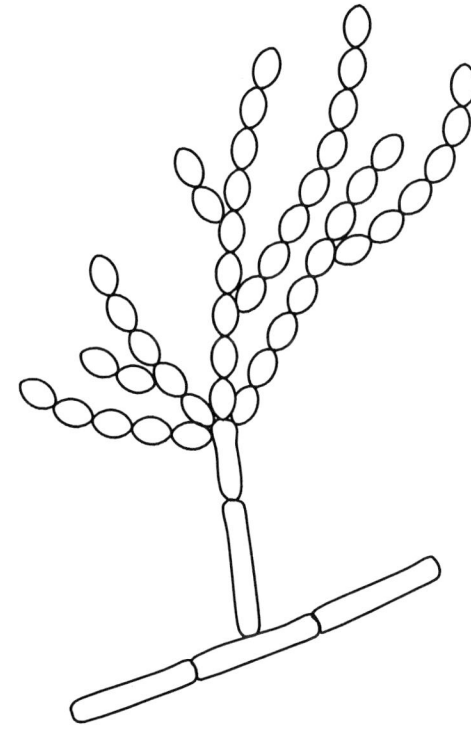

Fig. 44–17. Diagram of the branching chains of blastoconidia of Cladosporium carrionii.

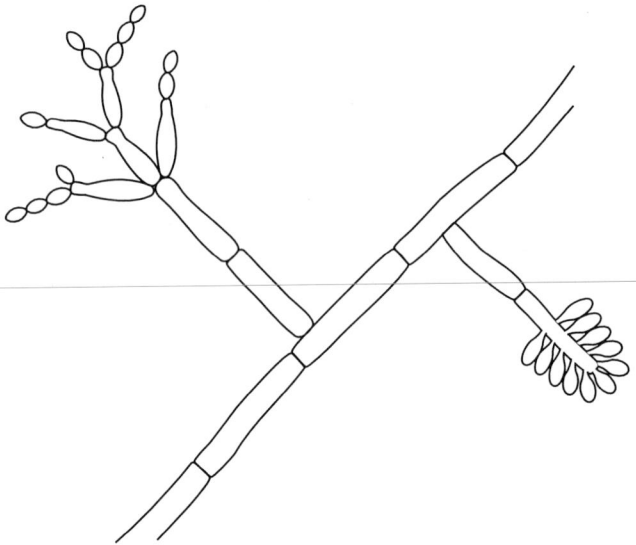

Fig. 44–18. Diagram of the microscopic features of Fonsecaea.

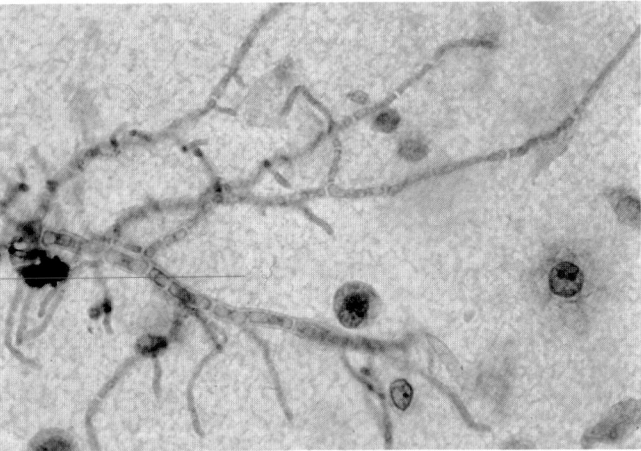

Fig. 44–19. Septate hyphae in Cytospin preparation of bronchoalveolar lavage fluid; culture grew Aspergillus flavus (Papanicolaou stain, ×201.6).

persons correlates with subsequent invasive pulmonary disease; however, a negative nasal culture does not preclude infection with these organisms (81). In an evaluation of sputum cultures collected from persons with leukemia or neutropenia, or both, isolation of Aspergillus fumigatus or Aspergillus flavus was highly predictive of invasive infection (82). In a similar population, observing hyphae in bronchoalveolar lavage specimens had sensitivity of 53% and specificity of 97% as a method for diagnosing Aspergillus pneumonia, whereas cultures of the fluid yielded Aspergillus in only 23% of cases (83).

Frequently, an invasive procedure to obtain involved tissue must be performed to diagnose invasive aspergillosis. This is especially true for Aspergillus endocarditis, because blood cultures almost never yield the organism. Observing septate, branching hyphae in KOH preparations of tissue, in formalin-fixed tissue stained with hematoxylin and eosin or a silver stain, or in cytospin preparations of bronchoalveolar lavage fluid stained with the Papanicolaou (Fig. 44-19) or a silver stain is suggestive of Aspergillus. Unless fruiting heads (see Fig. 44-5) are observed, however, aspergillosis cannot be confirmed because the septate hyphae of other fungi—Pseudallescheria boydii and species of Fusarium, for example—have an identical appearance. Staining tissue with monoclonal antibodies specific for Aspergillus may be useful, but these reagents have been used in a research setting only and are not yet approved for clinical specimens (84). Therefore, in almost all cases the diagnosis of invasive aspergillosis requires isolation of the organism.

The species of Aspergillus grow rapidly, typically producing colonies in 2 to 6 days. Initially colonies are white, and they become pigmented with age. Identification is based on the colony appearance and its microscopic structure. Diagnostic features of the species of Aspergillus most commonly encountered are described in Table 44-9 and illustrated in Plates IXF to IXH and Figures 44-20 to 44-22. Aspergillus differential medium (or Czepek's agar),

specific for Aspergillus flavus, is available, but it is infrequently needed.

Radioimmunoassays and enzyme-linked immunosorbent assays to detect antigens (such as galactomannan) of Aspergillus are potential tools for diagnosing invasive aspergillosis, but currently are not available commercially (84). Immunodiffusion tests that detect antibodies to Aspergillus are available; but their usefulness in immunocompromised hosts (for whom the test would be most valuable) is limited because these persons often do not produce antibodies in response to the infection. When observed in tissue, deposits of oxalic acid, a fermentation product of Aspergillus, especially Aspergillus niger, in conjunction with septate hyphae suggest the diagnosis of invasive aspergillosis (Plate XA). Measuring oxalic acid levels in bronchoalveolar lavage fluid has been suggested as a method to diagnose invasive pulmonary aspergillosis; however, the diagnostic value of the test has not been proven (85).

Pseudallescheria boydii. Infections caused by P. boydii are diagnosed by recovery of the organism from

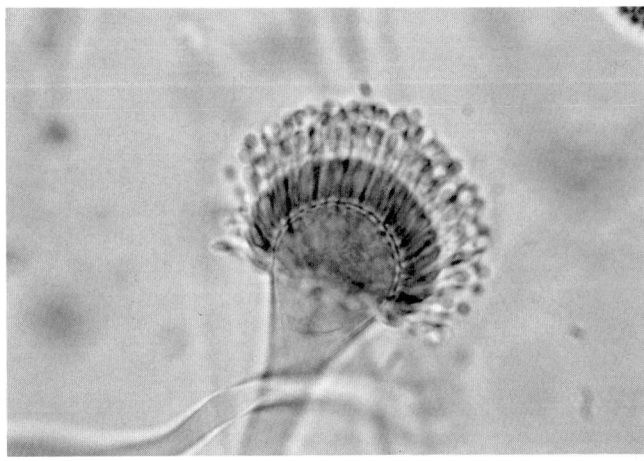

Fig. 44–20. Fruiting head of Aspergillus fumigatus (lactophenol cotton blue, ×256).

MOULDS

Table 44–9. Characteristic Features of the Hyaline Septate Moulds

Organism	Colony Structure	Microscopic Features
Aspergillus fumigatus	Fluffy, granular; blue-green with white apron	Septate hyphae (5–10 μm in diameter); club-shaped vesicle (20–30 μm) with phialides occurring in a single row (uniserate) around the upper half or two thirds of its surface and bearing chains of spherical (2–3 μm) rough-walled conidia
Aspergillus flavus	Fluffy; yellow, yellow-brown, or yellow-green	Septate hyphae (5–10 μm diameter); spherical vesicle (25–45 μm) with phialides occurring in a single or double row (uniserate or biserate) around its entire surface and bearing short chains of globose, smooth to rough-walled conidia (3.5–4.5 μm)
Aspergillus niger	Fluffy; initially white, becoming black with age; light tan to buff reverse	Septate hyphae (5–10 μm in diameter); spherical vesicle (45–75 μm) with phialides occurring in a double row around its entire surface and bearing many brown to black, rough-walled conidia (4–5 μm) that often obscure the structure of the vesicle
Aspergillus terreus	Fluffy; tan to cinnamon	Septate hyphae; hemispherical vesicle (10–16 μm) with phialides in a double row around entire surface and bearing chains of globose to elliptical conidia (2 μm)
Pseudallescheria boydii	Fluffy; white, becoming brownish gray with age, black reverse	Septate hyphae; single-celled elliptical conidia borne singly from tips of long or short conidiophores
Fusarium	Fluffy to cottony; initially white, with age becoming lavender or, less frequently, yellow or green	Septate hyphae; one-celled microconidia in balls; diagnostic two- to five-celled banana-shaped or cylindrical macroconidia; chlamydoconidia are common
Paecilomyces	Powdery, velvety, or cottony; olive tan, occasionally violet or brown	Elongated phialides bearing chains of smooth or rough, hyaline or pigmented oval conidia
Penicillium	Velvety and white, becoming powdery and blue green with white periphery, colorless reverse	Flask-shaped phialides supporting chains of smooth or rough, hyaline to pigmented conidia
Scopulariopsis	Velvety, rugose; light tan or brown with tan reverse	Single, nonbranching anellophores bearing flask-shaped annellides supporting chains of large, lemon-shaped conidia, which become echinulate or spiny with age

involved tissue or, in the case of mycetoma, from aspirated purulent material or granules. Colonies of P. boydii typically appear on media free of cycloheximide, which is inhibitory, after 5 to 10 days. Diagnostic features of the asexual form of the organism (Scedosporium apiospermum) are described in Table 44-9 and illustrated in Plate XB and Figure 44-23. The sexual form, P. boydii, characterized by the production of cleistothecia (saclike structures, 50 to 200 μm in diameter, that contain asci and ascospores), may be induced in the laboratory by culturing on plain water agar.

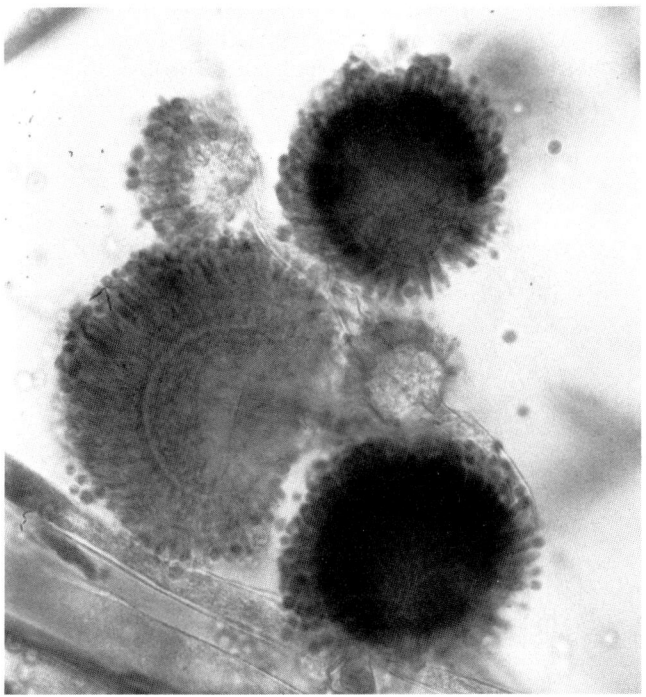

Fig. 44–21. Fruiting head of Aspergillus flavus (lactophenol cotton blue, ×256).

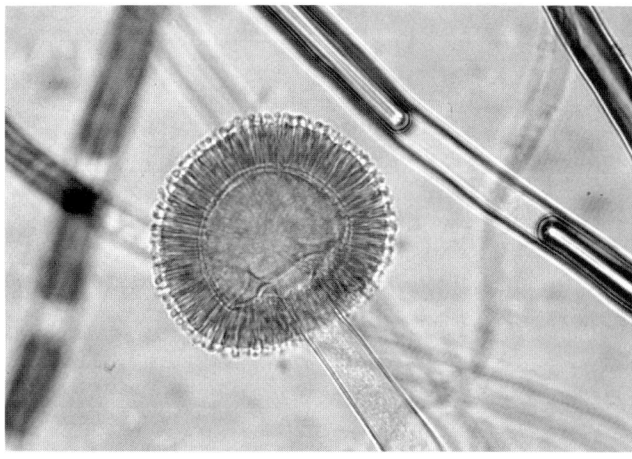

Fig. 44–22. Fruiting head of Aspergillus niger (lactophenol cotton blue, ×256).

***Fusarium* species.** Infections caused by Fusarium are diagnosed by recovering the organism from clinical specimens. In contrast to Aspergillus, in cases of disseminated disease, Fusarium frequently is recovered from blood cultures. The organism grows rapidly, producing visible colonies after 3 to 7 days. Identification is based on the colony appearance (Plate XC) and its microscopic features (Fig. 44-24, see Table 44-9).

Other Hyaline Septate Moulds. Infections caused by Paecilomyces, Penicillium, and Scopulariopsis are diagnosed by repeatedly isolating the organisms in large numbers from clinical specimens. All of these fungi grow rapidly, forming visible colonies in 2 to 5 days. Identification is based on colony appearance and microscopic features (see Table 44-9 and Fig. 44-25).

Zygomycetes

The diagnosis of zygomycosis is based on visualizing large (10- to 30-μm diameter), ribbon-like, aseptate hyphae in potassium hydroxide preparations of exudate or tissue or in tissue sections stained with hematoxylin and eosin (see Fig. 44-9), isolating the fungus from clinical specimens, or both, although culture is necessary to identify the specific organism involved. Rarely, sporangia are observed in tissue sections (see Fig. 44-10).

Members of the Zygomycetes grow rapidly on media that do not contain cycloheximide, which is inhibitory, producing woolly, gray, brown, or gray-black colonies in 1 to 3 days (Plate XD). The most commonly encountered of the Zygomycetes—Rhizopus, Mucor, and Absidia—are differentiated by the microscopic appearance of the colony (Fig. 44-26) (85a). All have aseptate hyphae. Rhizopus has unbranched sporangiophores that support a round, spore-filled sporangium and arise opposite rhizoids (rootlike hyphae connected by stolons) at the nodes. Mucor has single or branching sporangiophores that support round, spore-filled sporangia but has no rhizoids or stolons. With Absidia, branching sporangiophores that support pear-shaped sporangia are found between rhizoid nodes on the stolons.

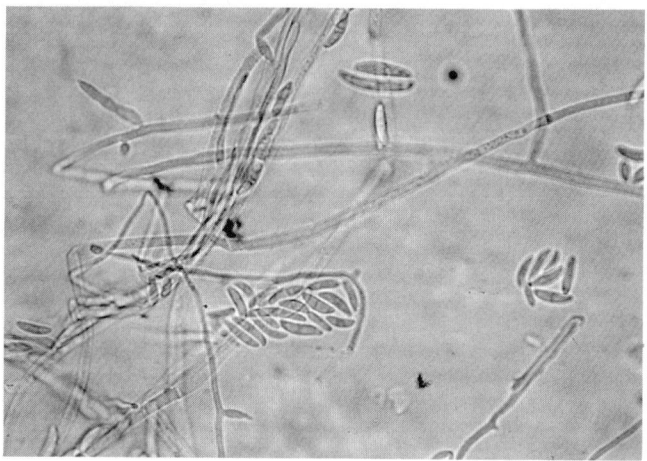

Fig. 44–24. Scotch-tape preparation of a colony of Fusarium shows banana-shaped macroconidia (lactophenol cotton blue, ×156).

Treatment

Dermatophytes. Skin infections caused by dermatophytes are treated with Whitfield's ointment (salicylic and benzoid acid compound), a topical keratinolytic agent, or topical antifungal agents such as clotrimazole and miconazole. Widespread skin infections may be treated with oral ketoconazole or fluconazole (86). Dermatophytic infections of the nails and scalp usually are treated with oral griseofulvin, and itraconazole, a new oral agent currently not approved in the United States, also appears to be effective.

Dematiaceous Fungi. Chromoblastomycosis is difficult to cure. Early in the disease wide and deep excision with subsequent skin grafting often is effective, but most cases are treated with chemotherapeutic agents. Intralesional injection of procaine amphotericin B; 5-fluorocytosine plus ketoconazole, thiabendazole, or amphotericin B; and oral ketoconazole or oral itraconazole, alone or after surgical excision, appear to be effective (8,87). Intra-

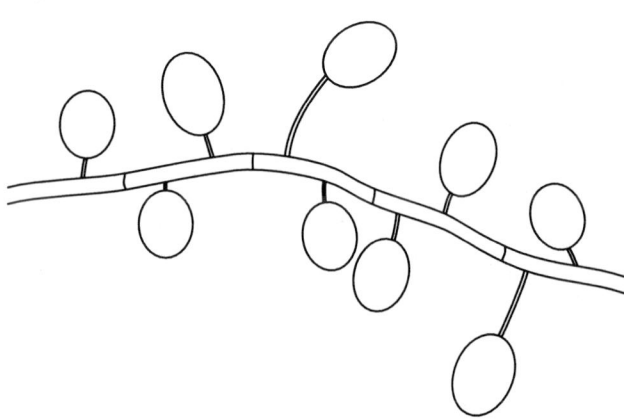

Fig. 44–23. Diagram of the microscopic features of Pseudallescheria boydii showing single pyriform conidia on short conidiophores.

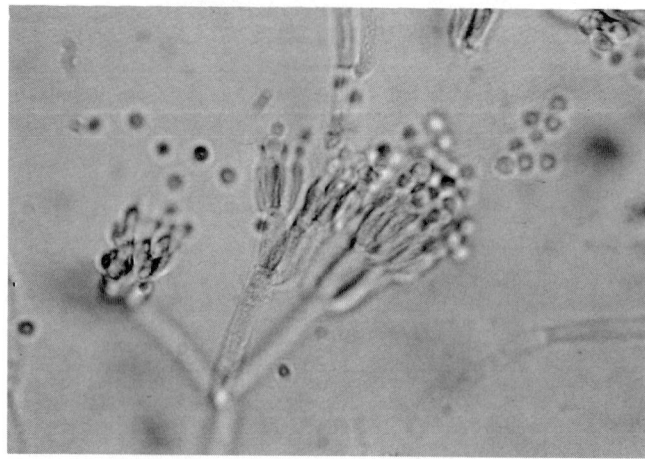

Fig. 44–25. Scotch-tape preparation of a colony of Penicillium shows flask-shaped phialides and chains of smooth conidia (lactophenol cotton blue, ×320).

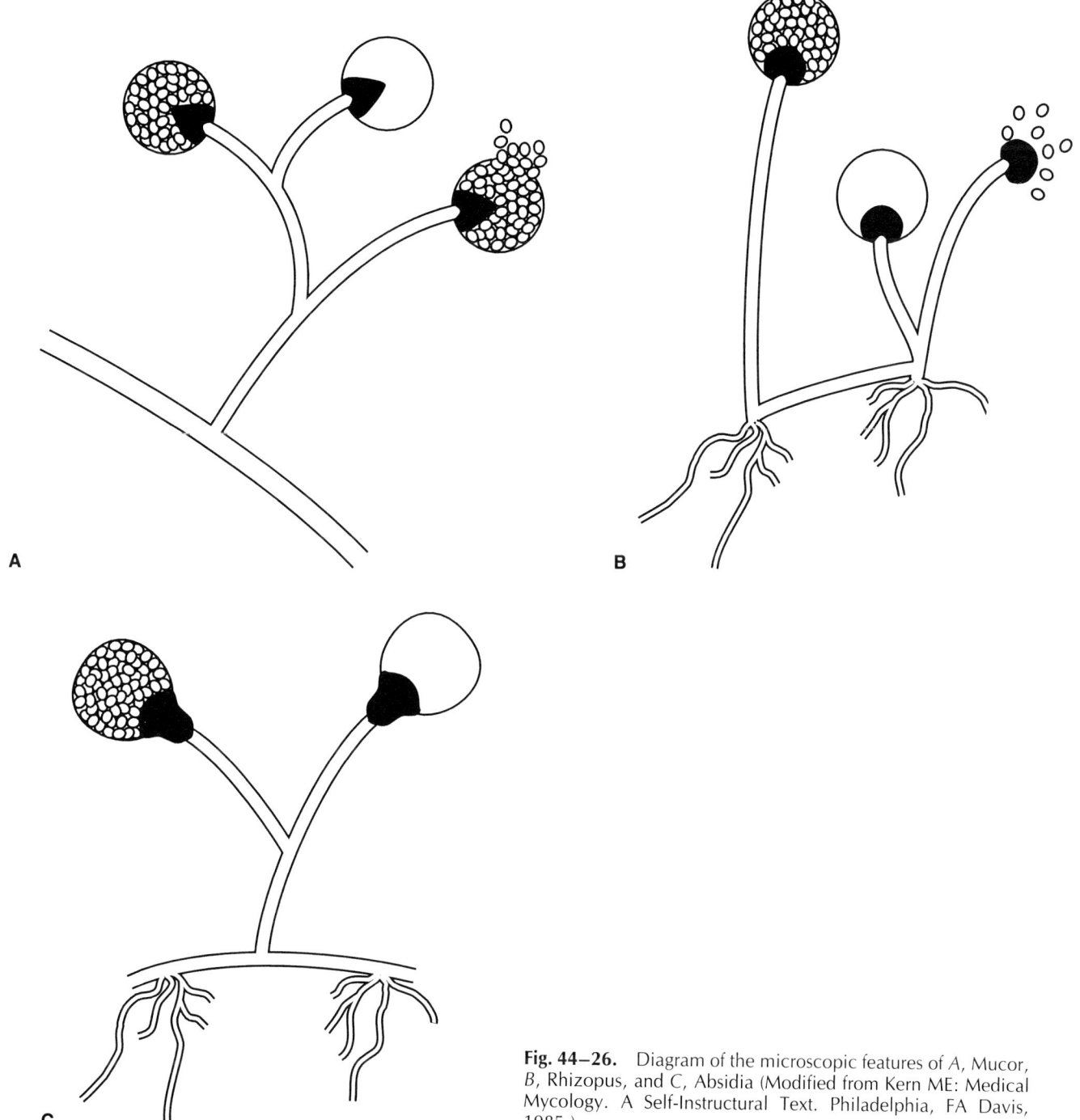

Fig. 44–26. Diagram of the microscopic features of A, Mucor, B, Rhizopus, and C, Absidia (Modified from Kern ME: Medical Mycology. A Self-Instructural Text. Philadelphia, FA Davis, 1985.)

venous amphotericin B alone is not efficacious, and occasionally when 5-fluorocytosine is used alone resistance to the drug develops.

Superficial phaeohyphomycosis may be treated with topical thiabendazole, topical keratinolytic agents such as 4% salicylic acid, mechanical removal of the infected layer of stratum corneum, or oral ketoconazole. Phaeohyphomycosis of the skin and nails may respond to topical antifungal agents such as clotrimazole or to oral ketoconazole or itraconazole (87). Hendersonula toruloidea, which may infect the skin and nails, is resistant to griseofulvin. Natamycin is the agent of choice for corneal phaeohyphomycosis. Subcutaneous phaeohyphomycosis is treated by surgical excision, and ketoconazole or 5-fluorocytosine may be used as adjunctive therapy to prevent recurrence or spread of the infection when the surgical wound is contaminated with fungal elements. Treatment of cerebral phaeohyphomycosis includes surgical excision of the lesion plus intravenous amphotericin B.

Hyaline Septate Moulds. Intravenous amphotericin

B is the drug of choice for invasive aspergillosis. The combination of amphotericin B plus 5-fluorocytosine has been used, but the benefit of adding the latter is unknown. Itraconazole appears to be effective, but more experience is necessary (87,88). Invasive aspergillosis of the brain and paranasal sinuses has been treated successfully with surgical excision. Surgical excision has been used in conjunction with amphotericin B to treat Aspergillus endocarditis, but despite therapy this disease is almost always fatal.

Surgical excision or drainage has been beneficial in the treatment of infections of the lung, sinuses, eye, brain, hand, and foot caused by Pseudallescheria boydii; and amphotericin B plus surgical excision has been successful in treating infections of the brain and sinuses (89). Intravenous amphotericin B without surgical excision is ineffective in cases of P. boydii–induced invasive and noninvasive disease; however, results have been favorable with amphotericin B eye drops and with intra-articular amphotericin B in cases of P. boydii–induced keratitis and arthritis, respectively. Parenteral miconazole appears to be effective in some cases, especially when used in conjunction with surgical débridement to treat subcutaneous infections. Ketoconazole also may be useful, but experience with this agent is limited.

Invasive infections with Fusarium have been treated with intravenous amphotericin B, but not all patients responded clinically. Amphotericin B, likewise, has been used to treat the few cases of invasive disease caused by Paecilomyces, Penicillium, and Scopulariopsis.

Zygomycetes. Invasive infections caused by members of the order Mucorales usually are treated with surgical débridement of necrotic tissue plus amphotericin B, although recently a few cases of infection limited to the central nervous system have been treated successfully with amphotericin B alone. The outcome, dependent on early diagnosis and resolution of predisposing problems, is fatal in as many as 50% of cases. Primary cutaneous infections respond to local débridement and topical amphotericin B. The most effective treatment for subcutaneous infections caused by Conidiobolus or Basidiobolus is unknown, but individual cases have been treated with potassium iodide, trimethoprim-sulfamethoxazole, miconazole, and amphotericin B, and surgical removal of accessible nodules, in addition to medical therapy, also should be considered.

REFERENCES

1. Hay RJ: Dermatophytoses and other superficial mycoses. *In* Principles and Practice of Infectious Diseases. 3rd ed. Edited by GL Mandell, RG Douglas, Jr, and JE Bennett. New York, Churchill Livingstone, 1990.
2. Philpot CM: Geographical distribution of the dermatophytes—a review. J Hyg (Lond), *80*:301, 1978.
3. King RD, et al: Transferrin, iron and dermatophytes 1. Serum dermatophyte inhibitory component definitely identified as unsaturated transferrin. J Lab Clin Med, *86*:204, 1975.
4. Joklik WK, Willett HP, Amos DB, and Wilfert CM (eds): Zinsser Microbiology. 19th ed. Norwalk, CT, Appleton & Lange, 1988.
5. Hay RJ, et al: Immune responses of patients with tinea imbricata. Br J Dermatol, *108*:581, 1983.
6. Jones HE, Reinhardt JH, and Rinaldi MG: Acquired immunity to dermatophytosis. Arch Dermatol, *109*:840, 1974.
7. McGinnis MR: Chromoblastomycosis and phaeohyphomycosis: New concepts, diagnosis, and mycology. J Am Acad Dermatol, *8*:1, 1983.
8. Fader RC, and McGinnis MR: Infections caused by dematiaceous fungi: Chromoblastomycosis and phaeohyphomycosis. Infect Dis Clin North Am, *2*:925, 1988.
9. Terreni AA, et al: Disseminated Dactylaria gallopava infection in a diabetic patient with chronic lymphocytic leukemia of the T-cell type. Am J Clin Pathol, *94*:104, 1990.
10. Wiest PM, et al: Alternaria infection in a patient with acquired immunodeficiency syndrome: Case report and review of invasive Alternaria infections. Rev Infect Dis, *9*:799, 1987.
11. Rinaldi MG, et al: Human Curvularia infections: Report of 5 cases and review of the literature. Diagn Microbiol Infect Dis, *6*:27, 1987.
12. Adam RD, et al: Phaeohyphomycosis caused by the fungal genera Bipolaris and Exserohilum: A report of 9 cases and review of the literature. Medicine, *65*:203, 1986.
13. McGinnis MR, and Fader RC: Mycetoma: A contemporary concept. Infect Dis Clin North Am, *2*:939, 1988.
14. Micheli PA: Nova Plantarum Genera Juxta Tournefortii Methodum Disposita. Florence, Italy, 1729.
15. Rinaldi MG: Invasive aspergilloisis. Rev Infect Dis, *5*:1061, 1983.
16. Raper KB, and Fennell DI: The genus Aspergillus. Baltimore, Williams & Wilkins, 1965.
17. Mullins J, Harvey R, and Seaton A: Sources and incidence of airborne Aspergillus fumigatus (Fres). Clin Allerg, *6*:209, 1976.
18. Aisner J, et al: Aspergillus infection in cancer patients. Association with fireproofing materials in a new hospital. JAMA, *235*:411, 1976.
19. Allo MD, Miller J, Townsend T, and Tan C: Primary cutaneous aspergillosis associated with Hickman intravenous catheters. N Engl J Med, *317*:1105, 1987.
20. Iwata K: Fungal toxins and their role in the etiopathology of fungal infections. *In* Recent Advances in Medical and Veterinary Mycology. Edited by R Iwata. Baltimore, University Park Press, 1977.
21. Bardana EJ, Jr: The clinical spectrum of aspergillosis—Part 2: Classification and description of saprophytic, allergic, and invasive variants of human disease. Crit Rev Clin Lab Sci, *13*:85, 1981.
22. Pena CE: Aspergillosis. *In* Human Infection with Fungi, Actinomycetes, and Algae. Edited by RD Baker. New York, Springer-Verlag, 1971.
23. Bennett JE: Aspergillus species. *In* Principles and Practice of Infectious Diseases. 3rd ed. Edited by GL Mandell, RG Douglas, Jr, and JE Bennett. New York, Churchill Livingstone, 1990.
24. Young RC, et al: Aspergillosis. The spectrum of disease in 98 patients. Medicine, *49*:147, 1970.
25. Binder RE, et al: Chronic necrotizing pulmonary aspergillosis: A discrete clinical entity. Medicine, *61*:109, 1982.
26. Prystowsky SD, et al: Invasive aspergillosis. N Engl J Med, *295*:655, 1976.
27. Zimmerman LE: Fatal fungus infections complicating other diseases. Am J Clin Pathol, *25*:46, 1955.
28. Milosev B, Mahgoub ES, Aal OA, and El Hassan AM: Primary aspergilloma of paranasal sinuses in the Sudan. A review of seventeen cases. Br J Surg, *56*:132, 1969.
29. McGinnis MR: Laboratory Handbook of Medical Mycology. New York, Academic Press, 1980.
30. Woods GL, Wood RP, and Shaw BW, Jr: Aspergillus endocar-

ditis in patients without prior cardiovascular surgery: Report of a case in a liver transplant recipient and review. Rev Infect Dis, *11*:263, 1989.
31. Ajello L: The isolation of Allescheria boydii Shear, an etiologic agent of mycetomas from soil. Am J Trop Med Hyg, *1*: 227, 1952.
32. Berenguer J, Diaz-Mediavilla J, Urra D, and Munoz P: Central nervous system infection caused by Pseudallescheria boydii: Case report and review. Rev Infect Dis, *11*:890, 1989.
33. Travis LB, Roberts GD, and Wilson WR: Clinical significance of Pseudallescheria boydii: A review of 10 years' experience. Mayo Clin Proc, *60*:531, 1985.
34. Winston DJ, Jordan MC, and Rhoses J: Allescheria boydii infections in the immunosuppressed host. Am J Med, *63*: 830, 1977.
35. Davis WA, et al: Disseminated Petriellidium boydii and pacemaker endocarditis. Am J Med, *69*:929, 1980.
36. Elliott ID, Halde C, and Shapiro J: Keratitis and endophthalmitis caused by Petriellidium boydii. Am J Ophthalmol, *178*: 142, 1979.
37. Booth C: The Genus Fusarium. Kew, Surrey, Commonwealth Mycological Institute, 1971.
38. Mayer CF: Endemic panmyelotoxicosis in the Russian grain belt. Part 1. The clinical aspects of alimentary toxic aleukia (ATA): A comprehensive review. Milit Surgeon, *113*:173, 1953.
39. Mohr JA, et al: Fungal endophthalmitis. South Med J, *66*:685, 1973.
40. Cho CT, et al: Fusarium solani infection during treatment for acute leukemia. J Pediatr, *83*:1028, 1973.
41. Veglia KS, Marks VJ, and Danville PA: Fusarium as a pathogen. A case report of Fusarium sepsis and review of the literature. J Am Acad Dermatol, *16*:260, 1987.
42. Young CN, and Meyers AM: Opportunistic fungal infection by Fusarium oxysporum in a renal transplant patient. Sabouraudia, *17*:219, 1979.
43. Zapater RC, and Arrechea A: Mycotic keratitis by Fusarium. A review and report of two cases. Ophthalmologica, *170*:1, 1975.
44. Anaissie E, et al: The emerging role of Fusarium infections in patients with cancer. Medicine, *67*:77, 1988.
45. Kalish SB, et al: Infective endocarditis caused by Paecilomyces varioti. Am J Clin Pathol, *78*:249, 1982.
46. Hall WJ: Penicillium endocarditis following open heart surgery and prosthetic valve insertion. Am Heart J, *87*:501, 1974.
47. Neglia JP, Hurd DD, Ferrieri P, and Snover DC: Invasive Scopulariopsis in the immunocompromised host. Am J Med, *83*:1163, 1987.
48. Sugar AM: Agents of mucormycosis and related species. *In* Principles and Practice of Infectious Diseases. 3rd ed. Edited by GL Mandell, RG Douglas, Jr, and JE Bennett. New York, Churchill Livingstone, 1990.
49. Kwon-Chung KJ, Young RC, and Orlando M: Pulmonary mucormycosis caused by Cunninghamella elegans in a patient with chronic myelogenous leukemia. Am J Clin Pathol, *64*: 544, 1975.
50. Kolbeck PC, et al: Widely disseminated Cunninghamella mucormycosis in an adult renal transplant patient: Case report and review of the literature. Am J Clin Pathol, *83*:747, 1985.
51. Torell H, Cooper BH, and Helgeson NGP: Disseminated Saksenaea vasiformis infection. Am J Clin Pathol, *76*:116, 1981.
52. Hay RJ, et al: Disseminated zygomycosis (mucormycosis) caused by Saksenaea vasiformis. J Infect, *7*:162, 1983.
53. Lawrence RM, et al: Systemic zygomycosis caused by Apophysomyces elegans. J Med Vet Mycol, *24*:57, 1986.
54. Wieden MA, et al: Zygomycosis caused by Apophysomyces elegans. J Clin Microbiol, *22*:522, 1985.
55. Greer DL, and Friedman L: Studies on the genus Basidiobolus with reclassification of the species pathogenic for man. Sabouraudia, *4*:231, 1966.
56. Martinson FD: Clinical epidemiological and therapeutic aspects of entomophthoromycosis. Ann Soc Belg Med Trop, *52*:329, 1972.
57. Gartenberg G, et al: Hospital-acquired mucormycosis (Rhizopus rhizopodiformis) of skin and subcutaneous tissue. Epidemiology, mycology and treatment. N Engl J Med, *299*: 1115, 1978.
58. Dennis JE, et al: Nosocomial Rhizopus infection (zygomycosis) in children. J Pediatr, *96*:824, 1980.
59. Waldorf AR, Ruderman N, and Diamond RD: Specific susceptibility to mucormycosis in murine diabetes and bronchoalveolar macrophage defense against Rhizopus. J Clin Invest, *74*:150, 1984.
60. Waldorf AR, Levitz SM, and Diamond RD: In vivo bronchoalveolar macrophage defense against Rhizopus oryzae and Aspergillus fumigatus. J Infect Dis, *150*:752, 1984.
61. Chinn RYW, and Diamond RD: Generation of chemotactic factors by Rhizopus oryzae in the presence and absence of serum: Relationship to hyphal damage mediated by human neutrophils and effects of hyperglycemia and ketoacidosis. Infect Immun, *38*:1123, 1982.
62. Marx RS, Forsyth KR, and Hentz ZK: Mucorales species activation of a serum leukotactic factor. Infect Immun, *38*:1217, 1982.
63. Gale GR, and Welch A: Studies of opportunistic fungi. I. Inhibition of R. oryze by human sera. Am J Med Sci, *45*:604, 1961.
64. Owens AW, Hacklette MS, and Baker RD: An antifungal factor in human serum. I. Studies of Rhizopus rhizopodiformis. Sabouraudia, *4*:179, 1965.
65. Boelaert JR, Vergauwe PL, and Vandepitte JM: Mucormycosis infection in dialysis patients. Ann Intern Med, *107*: 782, 1987.
66. Windus DW, et al: Fatal Rhizopus infections in hemodialysis patients receiving deferoxamine. Ann Intern Med. *107*:678, 1987.
67. Goodill JJ, and Abuelo JG: Mucormycosis—new risk of deferoxamine therapy in dialysis patients with aluminum or iron overload? N Engl J Med, *317*:34, 1987.
68. Schwartz JN, Donnelly EH, and Klintworth GK: Ocular and orbital phycomycosis. Survey Ophthalmol, *22*:3, 1977.
69. Jain JK, et al: Case report: Localized mucormycosis following intramuscular corticosteroid. Case report and review of the literature. Am J Med Sci, *275*:209, 1978.
70. Wilson CB, et al: Phycomycotic gangrenous cellulitis. A report of two cases and a review of the literature. Arch Surg, *111*:532, 1976.
71. Rabin ER, Lundberg GD, and Mitchell ET: Mucormycosis in severely burned patients. Report of two cases with extensive destruction of the face and nasal cavity. N Engl J Med, *264*:1286, 1961.
72. Meyer RD, et al: Cutaneous lesions in disseminated mucormycosis. JAMA, *225*:737, 1973.
73. Lyon DT, et al: Phycomycosis of the gastrointestinal tract. Am J Gastroenterol, *72*:379, 1979.
74. Ignelzi RJ, and VanderArk GD: Cerebral mucormycosis following open head trauma. Case report. J Neurosurg, *42*:593, 1975.
75. Cuadrado LM, et al: Cerebral mucormycosis in two cases of acquired immunodeficiency syndrome. Arch Neurol, *45*: 109, 1988.

76. Pierce PF, Jr, et al: Zygomycetes brain abscesses in narcotic addicts with serological diagnosis. JAMA, *248*:2881, 1982.
77. Antonelli M, et al: Entomophthoromycosis due to Basidiobolus in Somalia. Trans R Soc Trop Med Hyg, *81*:186, 1987.
78. Busapakum R, et al: Disseminated infection with Conidiobolus incongruus. Sabouraudia, *21*:323, 1983.
79. Larone DH: The identification of dematiaceous fungi. Clin Microbiol Newslett, *11*:145, 1989.
80. Ruutu P, et al: Invasive pulmonary aspergillosis: A diagnostic and therapeutic problem. Scand J Infect Dis, *19*:569, 1987.
81. Aisner J, Murillo J, Schimpff SC, and Steere AC: Invasive aspergillosis in acute leukemia: Correlation with nose cultures and antibiotic use. Ann Intern Med, *90*:4, 1979.
82. Yu VL, Muder RR, and Poorsattar A: Significance of isolation of Aspergillus from the respiratory tract in diagnosis of invasive pulmonary aspergillosis. Am J Med, *81*:249, 1986.
83. Kahn FW, Jones JM, and England DM: The role of bronchoalveolar lavage in the diagnosis of invasive pulmonary aspergillosis. Am J Clin Pathol, *86*:518, 1986.
84. Bennett JE: Rapid diagnosis of candidiasis and aspergillosis. Rev Infect Dis, *9*:398, 1987.
85. Benoit G, et al: Oxalic acid level in bronchoalveolar lavage fluid from patients with invasive pulmonary aspergillosis. Am Rev Respir Dis, *132*:748, 1985.
85a. Kern ME: Medical Mycology. A Self-Instructional Text. Philadelphia, FA Davis, 1985.
86. Montero-Gei F, and Perea A: Therapy with fluconazole for tinea corporis, tinea cruris, and tinea pedis. Clin Infect Dis, *14*(suppl 1):S77, 1992.
87. Graybill JR: Future directions of antifungal chemotherapy. Clin Infect Dis, *14*(suppl 1):S170, 1992.
88. De Beule K, et al: The treatment of aspergillosis and aspergilloma with itraconazole, clinical results of an open international study (1982–1987). Mykoses, *31*:476, 1988.
89. Bennett JE: Miscellaneous fungi. *In* Principles and Practice of Infectious Diseases. 3rd ed. Edited by GL Mandell, RG Douglas, Jr, and JE Bennett. New York, Churchill Livingstone, 1990.

Chapter 45

DIMORPHIC FUNGI

The thermal dimorphic fungi—Blastomyces dermatitidis, Histoplasma capsulatum var capsulatum and -var duboisii, Coccidioides immitis, Paracoccidioides brasiliensis, and Sporothrix schenckii—grow as moulds in nature and on media incubated at room temperature (25° to 30° C) and as yeasts in tissues and on media incubated at 35° to 37° C.

BLASTOMYCES DERMATITIDIS

Blastomyces dermatitidis is the agent of blastomycosis, an illness first described in 1894 by Gilchrist, who initially postulated that it was caused by a protozoan (1). Subsequently, the fungal agent of the illness was established by isolating the organism and transmitting the infection to a dog inoculated in the laboratory (2,3). Blastomycosis originally was believed to be a cutaneous infection, but cases of systemic illness soon were described and the concept that two forms of the disease existed was established: cutaneous, having a port of entry through the skin, and systemic, having a port of entry via the lungs. In the early 1950s Schwartz and Baum showed that the primary route of infection was the lungs and that other manifestations of the disease were secondary to dissemination of the organism (4).

Two serotypes of Blastomyces dermatitidis are recognized by exoantigen analysis of yeast cells: those that possess the A antigen are more common; those deficient in A antigen appear to be most prevalent in Africa (5,6). B. dermatitidis reproduces asexually and sexually, and in the perfect state the organism is called Ajellomyces dermatitidis.

Epidemiology

A complete understanding of the prevalence and epidemiology of blastomycosis has not been possible because of the lack of a reliable skin test and the difficulty of determining the ecologic niche of Blastomyces dermatitidis in nature; however, observations on the occurrence of clinical infection in humans and in dogs, plus data from investigations of epidemics, have provided insight into the disease. In the United States most cases of blastomycosis occur along the Mississippi River Basin and in the southeastern and south central parts of the country. Blastomycosis also occurs in Canada, Latin America, northern South America, Africa, and Israel (7). Exposure to soil is the one common factor in reports of sporadic disease and outbreaks; however, B. dermatitidis rarely has been recovered from nature (8). Data from investigations during which the organism was isolated from the environment in association with studies in vitro indicate that in nature it exists in wooded areas in warm, moist soil rich in organic debris such as decaying vegetation or animal manure and that these favorable growth conditions probably obtain only for short periods (9).

Infection with Blastomyces dermatitidis is believed to occur by inhaling conidia generated during the natural mycelial phase. Rarely, the organism may be transmitted from person to person: vaginal infection acquired from a man with genitourinary blastomycosis and possible intrauterine transmission have been reported (10,11).

Pathogenesis and Pathology

In the lungs, the inhaled conidia of Blastomyces dermatitidis convert to yeast forms, which probably release factors chemotactic for polymorphonuclear leukocytes, the first inflammatory cells at the site of infection. Human neutrophils efficiently phagocytose and kill conidia but not yeast forms of B. dermatitidis, although in vitro the fungicidal activity of neutrophils is enhanced by lymphokine-rich supernatants from immunologically stimulated T lymphocytes (12–15). Macrophages, which appear soon after the neutrophils, play a major role in the phagocytosis and killing of cells of B. dermatitidis. Macrophages from persons recovering from blastomycosis show more inhibition of intracellular growth of B. dermatitidis than macrophages from uninfected persons, and supernatants of antigen-stimulated lymphocytes enhance phagocytosis and intracellular inhibition of growth of B. dermatitidis by alveolar and monocyte-derived macrophages (16).

The characteristic inflammatory response to infection with Blastomyces dermatitidis includes clusters of polymorphonuclear leukocytes and granulomas, usually noncaseating, with epithelioid histiocytes and giant cells, predominantly foreign body type. Early in the disease polymorphonuclear leukocytes predominate, and many organisms—round to subglobose, thick-walled yeast cells, 8 to 15 μm in diameter, typically with *broad-based buds* (Fig. 45–1)—are found. As granulomas form the number of organisms decreases. In immunocompromised persons, large numbers of organisms are seen in tissue, with minimal or no surrounding inflammation; and in immunocompetent persons who develop rapidly progressive and fatal disease the inflammatory response may consist only of neutrophils (17). Disease involving the skin and mucosal surfaces is characterized by prominent pseudoepitheliomatous hyperplasia (that histologically may resemble squamous cell carcinoma) with microabscess formation.

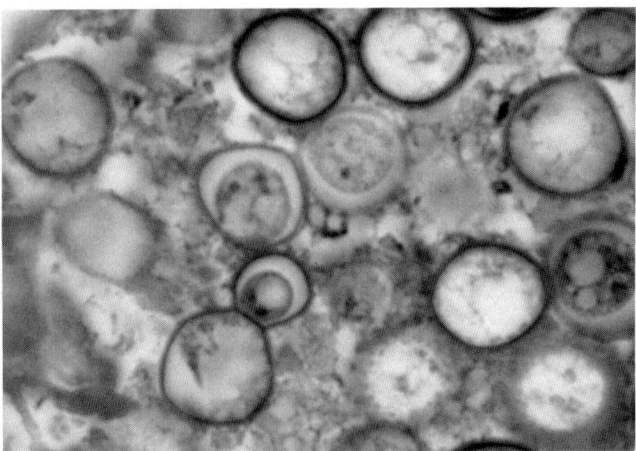

Fig. 45–1. Broad-based bud of Blastomyces dermatitidis in bone marrow of patient with disseminated blastomycosis periodic acid–Schiff (× 400).

Clinical Manifestations

Blastomycosis, a systemic disease with a spectrum of pulmonary and extrapulmonary manifestations, may be classified clinically into acute and chronic (or recurrent) stages. Extrapulmonary disease most commonly involves skin, bone, and the genitourinary tract, although any organ system may be affected; it occurs during the chronic stage of the illness; and it involves multiple organs in about two thirds of infected persons.

Acute pulmonary disease may be asymptomatic, or it may begin abruptly after an incubation period of 30 to 45 days, with myalgias, arthralgias, chills, fever, transient pleuritic pain, and a nonproductive cough that later often becomes productive of purulent sputum. The typical roentgenographic finding is lobar or segmental consolidation, usually involving the lower lobes.

Chronic or recurrent disease is the end point of several pathways: it may result from progression of acute pulmonary disease with or without extrapulmonary involvement; it may develop gradually in the lungs or other sites in a person who has asymptomatic or unrecognized acute disease; or it may represent endogenous reactivation in a person who recovered from symptomatic acute disease. The clinical manifestations of chronic pulmonary disease are those of chronic pneumonia: insidious onset of productive cough, hemoptysis, weight loss, pleuritic chest pain, and low-grade fever. The roentgenographic findings vary: upper lobe nodular infiltrates with or without cavitation are most common, but consolidation and mass lesions may occur.

Skin disease, the most common extrapulmonary manifestation of blastomycosis, occurs in 40 to 80% of cases, usually in conjunction with active pulmonary disease, but it may be the only indication of active disease. Two types of skin lesions occur, sometimes simultaneously. The more characteristic verrucous type, usually involving exposed body areas, typically begins as a papule that gradually becomes elevated and crusted with a serpiginous, swollen, red to violet, abruptly sloping border. Older lesions may show central clearing with scarring and depigmentation. The ulcerative lesion begins as a pustule that rapidly develops into a superficial ulcer with a granulomatous base. Lesions also may involve the mucosa of the mouth, nose, pharynx, and larynx.

Bone is the third most common site of involvement (after lung and skin) of disseminated disease (prevalence, as high as 60% of cases) (7,17). Well-circumscribed osteolytic lesions, most often involving the vertebrae, ribs, skull, and facial and long bones, are typical and may be associated with contiguous soft tissue abscesses and draining sinuses. Arthritis occurs by hematogenous spread or, less frequently, by extension from an adjacent focus of infection in the bone in 3 to 5% of persons with systemic disease. A single joint, most often the knee, ankle, or elbow, is involved. The synovial fluid usually is purulent, and in wet preparations organisms are easily visible. Infection of the genitourinary tract, principally involving the prostate and epididymis, occurs in about one third of infected men. Central nervous system involvement, manifested clinically as an intracranial or spinal mass or as meningitis, develops in 3 to 10% of cases, usually late in the disease (7,17). Meningitis may be difficult to diagnose because smears and cultures of cerebrospinal fluid are positive in only about 50% and about 25% of cases, respectively. Occasionally, blastomycosis involves the liver, spleen, gastrointestinal tract, thyroid, pericardium, adrenal gland, or the eye. In an immunocompromised host blastomycosis often is disseminated when diagnosed, but the clinical presentation and response to therapy usually are similar to those in immunocompetent persons.

HISTOPLASMA CAPSULATUM

Two variants of Histoplasma capsulatum are recognized: Histoplasma capsulatum var capsulatum is found worldwide in temperate zones, and Histoplasma capsulatum var duboisii is found predominantly in Africa but has been reported in Japan (18).

Histoplasma capsulatum var capsulatum

Histoplasma capsulatum var capsulatum is the agent of histoplasmosis, the most common and most extensively studied systemic fungal infection in the United States. The organism was discovered in Panama in 1905 by Darling, who named it Histoplasma capsulatum because he found it in histiocytes. Initially it was believed to be a plasmodium-like protozoan, but it was proven to be an unencapsulated fungus in 1932 (19). Histoplasma capsulatum is the imperfect state of the dimorphic fungus Emmonsiella capsulatum.

Epidemiology

In nature, Histoplasma capsulatum var capsulatum is found in the soil, where its growth is promoted by bird and bat excrement. Birds are not infected, because their high body temperature prohibits replication of the fungus; bats, however, are infected, and their feces may be infectious. H. capsulatum is distributed throughout the temperate climates of the world but is most heavily endemic in the central United States, especially along the Mississippi and Ohio River basins. Blackbird and pigeon roosts, chicken houses, chicken-manure fertilizer, and sites frequented by bats (caves, attics, old buildings, hollow trees) in endemic areas are most likely to be point sources of infection. The organism is acquired by inhalation of airborne microconidia, which are present in increased numbers under dusty, windy conditions. Animal-to-human or human-to-human spread does not occur.

Pathogenesis and Pathology

The pathogenesis and pathologic findings of histoplasmosis are different for the various forms of the disease—acute pulmonary, disseminated, chronic pulmonary, and excessive fibrosis. Acute pulmonary histoplasmosis has been evaluated in animals infected in the laboratory, and a similar process is believed to occur in humans. In animals inhaled conidia of Histoplasma capsulatum reach small bronchioles and alveoli and in 2 to 3 days convert to yeast forms, which are phagocytosed rapidly by macrophages. In nonimmune animals, yeasts proliferate in the cells, and more macrophages, which often become infected, are recruited to the site of infection, forming a small infiltrate. Infected macrophages migrate to mediastinal lymph nodes and other sites in the monocyte/macrophage system, particularly the liver and spleen, where focal infiltrates develop. This continues for about 2 weeks, when the cellular immune system is activated, causing tissue destruction and caseation necrosis at the site of each infiltrate. Activated macrophages demonstrate enhanced fungicidal activity, and the infiltrates become encapsulated and heal by fibrosis and calcification, although yeast cells entrapped in the necrotic tissue persist in calcified nodules. In immune, recently infected animals, the cellular immune response is activated sooner (1 to 2 days after yeast forms appear), allowing minimal proliferation of the organisms and a minimal inflammatory reaction. The factors most important in determining the extent of proliferation of the organism before activation of the cellular immune system—and, therefore, the degree of symptoms—are the inoculum size, which determines the number of infiltrates, and the immune status of the host (19).

Disseminated histoplasmosis occurs in persons with a compromised cellular immune system such as very young children, persons with malignancies of the lymphatic or hematopoietic system, those who take corticosteroids or other immunosuppressive drugs, and those with the acquired immunodeficiency syndrome (AIDS). In these persons yeast cells are phagocytosed, but intracellular killing appears to be deficient, although the specific defect is unknown. Macrophages provide a protective environment and may support intracellular growth of the yeast. The degree of parasitization of the macrophages determines the pathologic changes, the clinical presentation, and the disease course. When parasitization is less marked, focal lesions with tissue necrosis are frequent, but the tissue reaction is minimal when parasitization is extensive and diffuse (Plate XE).

Chronic pulmonary histoplasmosis affects persons with pre-existing emphysema and characteristically involves the apical areas of the lung. Organisms grow only in abnormal pulmonary spaces, where they are found in significant numbers on the necrotic lining of cavities, and, less commonly, in effusions in emphysematous spaces. The typical lesion of early chronic cavitary pulmonary histoplasmosis begins as a segmental area of interstitial pneumonitis characterized histologically by an infiltrate of macrophages, lymphocytes, and scattered plasma cells, foci of necrosis, and few organisms, suggesting that the inflammation occurs in response to antigen rather than to the organisms (19). Over an 8- to 12-week period areas of necrosis heal by fibrosis and contract, and organisms may enter and infect adjacent cavities. The walls of infected bullae thicken and become necrotic, and effusions may develop. Necrosis of the fibrous wall and constant elaboration of new fibrous tissue allow enlargement of the cavity with destruction of adjacent lung tissue.

Histoplasmosis rarely is manifested as excessive fibrosis (i.e., elaboration of fibrous tissue extends far beyond the capsule that develops during the usual healing process). When the excessive fibrosis occurs around a healed primary focus in the lung the lesion is called a histoplasmoma. This is usually a 3- to 4-cm diameter peripheral nodule composed to concentric layers of collagen with clumps of mononuclear cells, principally lymphocytes and young fibroblasts, at the advancing margin. Excessive fibrosis around a healed primary focus in hilar or mediastinal lymph nodes is called mediastinal fibrosis.

Clinical Manifestations

In immunocompetent persons infection with Histoplasma capsulatum usually is asymptomatic; however, symptomatic infection may occur in infants and small children, and an especially heavy inoculum may cause an acute, self-limited influenza-like syndrome in adults. Other manifestations of histoplasmosis represent consequences of recent or remote infection in a host who has some type of abnormality, such as a defective cellular immune system that allows dissemination, structural abnormalities of the lung resulting in chronic pulmonary histoplasmosis, or excessive fibrogenesis during healing with subsequent mediastinal fibrosis or histoplasmoma formation.

Symptomatic primary infection with Histoplasma capsulatum resulting from inhalation of a small to medium-sized inoculum occurs in infants and young children. The illness is manifested by fever and cough, and hilar and mediastinal adenopathy with a small patch or cluster of parenchymal infiltrates are seen on chest roentgenograms. Primary infection following inhalation of a large inoculum begins abruptly after an incubation period of 10 to 23 days, with malaise, headache, chills, fever, and nonproductive cough. A few to many scattered patchy infiltrates, 0.5 to 2 cm, are seen on chest roentgenograms. These gradually heal, leaving small residual nodules that eventually calcify. The infection typically is self-limiting but rarely, in untreated adults, death results from dissemination or acute respiratory failure.

Reinfection acute histoplasmosis differs from primary acute histoplasmosis as follows: A larger inoculum is necessary to produce symptoms. The incubation period is shorter (usually 3 to 7 days), and the illness is less severe. The typical roentgenographic finding is an infiltrate of fine, evenly distributed nodules, 1 to 2 mm in diameter, that clears in about 3 months and does not result in late calcification.

The clinical manifestations of disseminated histoplasmosis may be divided into severe, moderate chronic, and mild chronic disease. Severe disease, characterized by cough, malaise, fever, anorexia, weight loss, nausea, vomiting, diarrhea, and occasionally abdominal pain, occurs predominantly in infants 1 year of age or younger, and occasionally in adults. Interstitial pneumonia is common; hepatosplenomegaly almost always is present; and generalized peripheral lymphadenopathy occurs in as many as 50% of cases. Pancytopenia is usual, and mild alterations of liver function tests are common. If untreated, the illness is fatal in 2 to 10 weeks (average, 5 weeks).

Moderate chronic disseminated disease, characterized predominantly by weight loss, weakness, and intermittent low-grade fever, occurs in adults, and infrequently in children. Hepatosplenomegaly usually is present; hematopoietic disturbances occur in about half the cases; and Addison's disease, meningitis, intestinal ulceration, or endocarditis may develop. If untreated, the illness is fatal in 6 to 12 months. Mild chronic disease, characterized by unexplained weight loss, fatigue, and intermittent low-grade fever lasting a year or more, develops, almost exclusively in adults. The hallmark of the disease, an oropharyngeal ulcer, may cause hoarseness, dysphagia, or a painful lesion on the tongue or gingiva. Mild to moderate enlargement of the liver and spleen occurs in 50 and 30% of cases, respectively, but hematopoietic abnormalities are uncommon.

Symptoms of chronic pulmonary histoplasmosis resemble those of pulmonary tuberculosis (Chapter 40) but are less intense. The illness begins abruptly with malaise, fever, fatigue and mild cough with minimal sputum production; deep, aching chest pain develops in about one third of cases, and occasionally night sweats. The clinical manifestations of histoplasmoma are minimal, and symptoms of mediastinal fibrosis are related to stenosis and obstruction of the adjacent vascular and bronchial structures.

Histoplasma capsulatum var duboisii

Histoplasma capsulatum var duboisii (formerly Histoplasma duboisii) is the agent of a clinically distinct form of histoplasmosis characterized by granulomatous and suppurative lesions primarily involving the skin, soft tissues, and bone and little evidence of pulmonary disease. The organism, a large yeast found in giant cells, first was recognized in the biopsy of a skin lesion of a person in Ghana in 1943 (20). This fungus, culturally identical to Histoplasma capsulatum var capsulatum but resembling Blastomyces dermatitidis in tissue, was named Histoplasma duboisii in 1952 and in 1957 was recognized as a variety of Histoplasma capsulatum.

Epidemiology

Almost all cases of infection with Histoplasma capsulatum var duboisii have occurred in Africa, between the Sahara and the Kalahari desert. Rarely is the organism recovered from the soil, and some infections have been associated with chicken runs and bat-infested caves. The age range of infected persons is 2 to 70 years, though there is a cluster of cases in the second decade; all races are affected, and the male-female ratio is about 2:1 (21,22). The portal of entry of the organism is unknown. It may be the respiratory tract, whence by hematogenous spread the organism reaches a site favorable for proliferation.

Pathology

Histologically, lesions caused by Histoplasma capsulatum var duboisii consist of large aggregates of giant cells, measuring up to 200 μm in diameter, that contain many ovoid, double-contoured, walled yeast cells, 12 to 15 μm in diameter, resembling Blastomyces dermatitidis but lacking the broad-based bud. Scattered neutrophils also may be present, and in lesions that show caseating necrosis extracellular degenerating yeasts may be found. Organisms are rare in fibrotic lesions.

Clinical Manifestations

Infection caused by Histoplasma capsulatum var duboisii may present as a single circumscribed skin lesion, a lesion resembling molluscum contagiosum (see Chapter 4), a subcutaneous granuloma, a lymphocutaneous lesion, or a lesion of bone, without systemic signs (21,22). In other cases, disease is disseminated, involving skin, lymph nodes, bones, and infrequently the intestine and abdominal viscera; is accompanied by fever, weight loss, and anemia; and often is rapidly progressive and fatal.

COCCIDIOIDES IMMITIS

Coccidioides immitis is the pathogen of coccidioidomycosis, an illness initially described by Posada in 1892 in a soldier hospitalized in Buenos Aires with disseminated disease (23). In 1896, Rixford and Gilchrist in San Francisco transmitted the disease to animals inoculated in the laboratory with tissue from an infected person and named the agent Coccidioides (meaning resembling the protozoan Coccidia) immitis (meaning not mild) (24). C. immitis was shown to be a fungus in 1900, and the lung was recognized as the main portal of entry (25). In the 1930s C. immitis was identified as the agent of the self-limited disease San Joaquin Valley fever, and it was recovered from soil at the site of a small epidemic.

Epidemiology

Coccidioides immitis is found only in the western hemisphere. The endemic zone extends from about 40° north, 120° west in northern California to 40° south, 65° west in Argentina, and the most endemic areas are the southwestern United States and the bordering regions of northern Mexico (27). The area of endemicity corresponds to the Lower Sonoran Life Zone, characterized by a semiarid climate with a short, intense rainy season, alkaline soil, and sparse flora.

Coccidioidomycosis is acquired via inhalation of arthrocondria, an event most likely to occur during the dry, windy season when the soil is disturbed. Rarely has acquisition of infection via cutaneous inoculation been reported (28,29). Person-to-person transmission does not occur.

Pathogenesis and Pathology

Arthroconidia of Coccidioides immitis are inhaled and reach the lower airways, eliciting an infiltrate of macrophages and neutrophils, possibly via complement activation and the subsequent generation of chemotactic factors (30,31). Macrophages predominate when arthroconidia convert to spherules, but neutrophils are prominent when spherules rupture. Arthroconidia, endospores, and spherules are resistant to killing by neutrophils; however, macrophages phagocytose and degrade the organism and present antigens to T lymphocytes. The latter thus are stimulated to produce factors that activate the macrophages, enhancing their microbicidal activity and ultimately controlling the infection. Persons who have defective cell-mediated immunity are at increased risk of severe, disseminated disease.

The predominant tissue reaction to infection with Coccidioides immitis is granulomatous inflammation, with or without caseation, although neutrophil aggregates may predominate, and fibrosis often is the main finding in chronic lesions. The characteristic tissue form of C. immitis is the spherule, measuring up to 200 μm in diameter (Fig. 45–2), but careful searching may reveal hyphae in the interior margins of pulmonary cavities, and infrequently in granulomas. Eosinophils are common with disseminated infection and may be present in pulmonary lesions.

Clinical Manifestations

Primary infection with Coccidioides immitis is asymptomatic in about 60% of cases, and in the remainder, symptoms resembling a lower respiratory tract infection or a systemic illness with productive cough, pleuritic chest pain, malaise, fever, chills, night sweats, anorexia, weakness, and arthralgias develops 1 to 3 weeks after exposure. Erythema nodosum or erythema multiforme occurs in fewer than 25% of cases, most often in women. A laboratory abnormality strongly suggestive of the infection is peripheral eosinophilia. In some persons, especially diabetics and immunocompromised hosts, the acute pneumonia progresses to chronic pulmonary disease, characterized by granulomatous lesions and cavities.

In fewer than 1% of cases, Coccidioides immitis disseminates from the lungs to other organs, most often the skin, musculoskeletal system, and meninges. Those at increased risk of disseminated infection are pregnant women, persons exposed to soil containing high concentrations of organisms, those undergoing hemodialysis for chronic renal failure, persons with blood type B or AB, males, neonates, immunocompromised hosts (especially persons receiving corticosteroids, recipients of organ transplants, and those with AIDS, and persons of certain races—blacks, Hispanics, and Filipinos (32).

The most common cutaneous manifestations of disseminated coccidioidomycosis are verrucous granulomas (often on the face), erythematous plaques, and nodules. Bone involvement, typically an irregular lytic lesion, occurs in 40% of persons with disseminated disease, causing bone pain with occasional swelling and redness at the site of infection. Joint infection usually is monarticular, most commonly affecting knee, wrist, or ankle. Meningitis caused by Coccidioides immitis generally occurs within 6 months after the primary infection and may be the first manifestation of the disease. Symptoms and signs are vague: headache, changes in mental status, low-grade fever, weight loss. More than half of affected persons have peripheral eosinophilia, and the cerebrospinal fluid usually shows an elevated protein level, a decreased glucose concentration, and a lymphocytic pleocytosis, although occasionally neutrophils predominate or many eosinophils are seen.

PARACOCCIDIOIDES BRASILIENSIS

Paracoccidioides brasiliensis is the agent of paracoccidioidomycosis (also called South American blastomycosis), the predominant systemic mycosis in Latin America.

Epidemiology

Paracoccidioidomycosis has a restricted geographic distribution, occurring only in the tropical and subtropical forests of Latin America and South America from Mexico (23° north) to Argentina (34° south), though not in the Caribbean Islands and Chile (33). Most cases occur in Brazil and a smaller number in Colombia, Venezuela, and Argentina. Cases have been reported in North America, Europe, and Asia, but the affected persons reported having resided in endemic countries.

The ecologic niche for Paracoccidioides brasiliensis is unknown. Reports of its isolation from soil are rare. However, P. brasiliensis is believed to exist in nature, and infection with the organism probably is acquired by contact with the exogenous source. The route of infection is unknown, but inhalation of conidia is the most accepted theory and traumatic implantation has been suggested (34,35).

Most cases of paracoccidioidomycosis occur in men (male-female ratio, 15:1), especially agricultural workers, aged 30 years or older. The rate of infection as determined by a paracoccidioidin skin test is similar for both

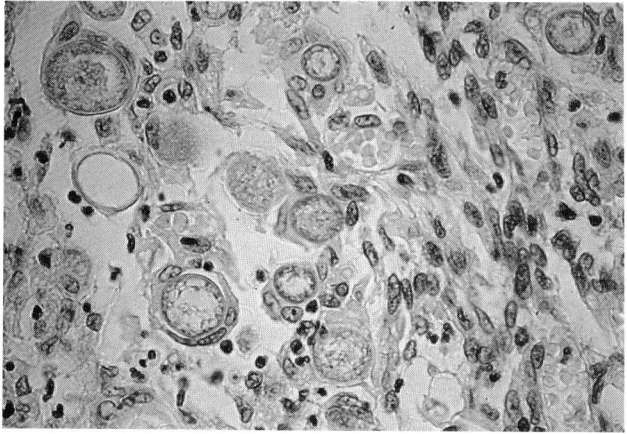

Fig. 45–2. Spherules of Coccidioides immitis in lung tissue (hematoxylin and eosin, × 400).

sexes, and before puberty the prevalence in the sexes is equal. The inhibitory action of estrogens on the mycelium-yeast transition may explain the sex difference in adults (36).

Pathogenesis and Pathology

The cell wall polysaccharides of yeast cells of Paracoccidioides brasiliensis, such as α-glucan, are associated with virulence and the ability to stimulate granuloma formation. The acute, progressive pulmonary infection that occurs in juveniles is a bronchopneumonia characterized by an alveolar exudate composed of neutrophils, multinucleate giant cells, and scattered yeast cells. Chronic progressive pulmonary disease is characterized by interstitial fibrosis, necrotic granulomas often containing diagnostic yeast cells—round-to-oval, variously sized (4 to 40 μm diameter) parent cells surrounded by multiple small buds (2 to 4 μm diameter) resembling a "mariner's wheel" (Fig. 45–3). Extrapulmonary lesions show granulomatous or suppurative and granulomatous inflammation, and lesions involving cutaneous and mucocutaneous surfaces show pseudoepitheliomatous hyperplasia.

Clinical Manifestations

Most initial infections with Paracoccidioides brasiliensis occur in immunocompetent persons and are believed to be subclinical. The organism then becomes quiescent or dormant for an indefinite period, occasionally as long as several decades, or it may resolve, perhaps with scarring. The host's immune defenses determine the clinical form and the severity of the mycosis.

Juvenile paracoccidioidomycosis is an uncommon form of the disease that occurs in persons under 30 years of age and immunosuppressed persons. An acute to subacute progressive infection with a poor prognosis, it is characterized by lymphonodular lesions in the lung and dissemination of the fungus throughout the monocyte/macrophage system. The adult type of paracoccidioidomycosis, a chronic process that develops from a latent infection, has a better prognosis. Lesions may be localized in the lung, or the infection may disseminate to other organs, especially the skin and mucocutaneous tissue, lymph nodes, spleen, liver, and adrenals. Affected persons present with mucosal ulcerations, principally in the mouth and nose; dysphagia and voice changes; cutaneous lesions, most commonly on the face; lymphadenopathy, especially in the cervical area; respiratory manifestations, including shortness of breath, cough productive of purulent or blood-tinged sputum, and chest pain; or a combination of these symptoms and signs, which generally are accompanied by weakness, malaise, fever, and weight loss.

SPOROTHRIX SCHENCKII

Sporothrix schenckii is the pathogen of sporotrichosis, an infection most often manifested as a subcutaneous lesion that arises at the site of minor trauma and spreads proximally along the lymphatics.

Epidemiology

Sporothrix schenckii is found in soil and on living plants and plant debris and is transmitted to humans via minor breaks in the skin that occur during contact with contaminated soil or thorny plants such as roses or sphagnum moss. The disease occurs worldwide, mainly in temperate and tropical zones. Cutaneous sporotrichosis is seen primarily in previously healthy adults under age 30 years who have contact with soil or plants, such as farmers, potters, florists, and gardeners. Extracutaneous sporotrichosis occurs predominantly in males, and about one third of those who have pulmonary disease have a history of alcoholism.

Pathology

Microscopically, lesions of sporotrichosis show a mixed suppurative and granulomatous inflammatory response. Granulomas consist mainly of histiocytes and usually have a central area of microabscess formation. Organisms are difficult to find, even with special stains for fungal elements; but when many sections are examined carefully, single or budding, round, oval, or elongate (cigar-shaped) yeast forms, 2 to 6 μm in diameter, are scattered in the tissues, often in giant cells. In papillomatous skin lesions the epidermis shows hyperkeratosis, parakeratosis, pseudoepitheliomatous hyperplasia, and intraepidermal abscesses, changes similar to those seen with blastomycosis (described earlier). Asteroid bodies—one or more yeast cells surrounded by a stellate, radial corona called Splendore-Hoeppli material that appears brightly eosinophilic in tissue sections stained with hematoxylin and eosin—may be seen in tissues with a mixed inflammatory response, especially within microabscesses, from persons with sporotrichosis in South America, South Africa, Japan, and infrequently in the United States. The asteroid body, however, is not pathognomonic for sporotrichosis; similar-looking eosinophilic material may be deposited around colonies of some bacteria, foreign bodies, and other fungi, including Coccidioides immitis and Aspergillus, and Candida organisms.

Clinical Manifestations

The clinical forms of sporotrichosis may be classified as cutaneous or extracutaneous (37). The most common

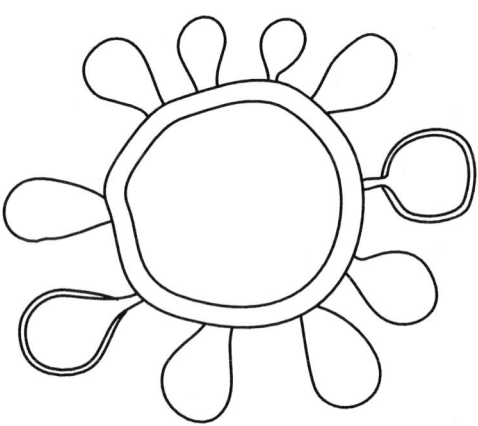

Fig. 45–3. Diagram of a budding yeast cell of Paracoccidioides brasiliensis, which resembles a "mariner's wheel."

presentation of sporotrichosis is the lymphocutaneous form, which begins at the site of inoculation, usually an extremity, after an incubation period of 1 to 12 weeks, as a small, red, painless papule that slowly enlarges, becomes violaceous, ulcerates, and intermittently discharges a small amount of serosanguineous exudate. Later in the disease new lesions appear proximally along the lymphatics draining the area of the primary lesion. Localized cutaneous sporotrichosis, which affects about a third of those who have cutaneous disease, is characterized by ulcerative, verrucous, papillomatous, acneiform, or erythematoid lesions confined to the area of inoculation, such as the face, neck, trunk, or arm, without lymphatic involvement. Rarely, cutaneous lesions of sporotrichosis become disseminated, a form of the disease most commonly seen in immunocompromised persons.

Most cases of extracutaneous sporotrichosis cannot be traced to traumatic inoculation, except ocular disease involving the lids, conjuctiva, lacrimal apparatus, or orbit. Eighty percent of cases of extracutaneous disease involve the bones, the joints, or both, especially knees, ankles, wrists, and elbows. Infection of the lung, an uncommon manifestation of sporotrichosis, occurs predominantly in older men and typically is manifested as an indolent cavitary pneumonitis in one upper lobe, causing productive cough, anorexia, fatigue, and low-grade fever. Very rarely, sporotrichosis involves the central nervous system, an illness manifested by headache and confusion and cerebrospinal fluid abnormalities that include lymphocytic pleocytosis, elevated protein content, and decreased glucose concentration.

Laboratory Diagnosis

Specimens required to diagnose infections caused by the dimorphic fungi are listed in Table 45–1. Specimen collection, transport, and processing are discussed in Part III. The direct microscopic appearance and culture characteristics of the dimorphic fungi are described below and summarized in Table 45–2. In addition to direct visualization and culture of the specimens listed Table 45–1, serum samples for serologic studies may provide information useful in diagnosing infections with Histoplasma capsulatum, Blastomyces dermatitidis, and Coccidioides immitis; limitations of the antibody tests are discussed later.

Blastomyces dermatitidis. Blastomycosis may be diagnosed by observing characteristic organisms in clini-

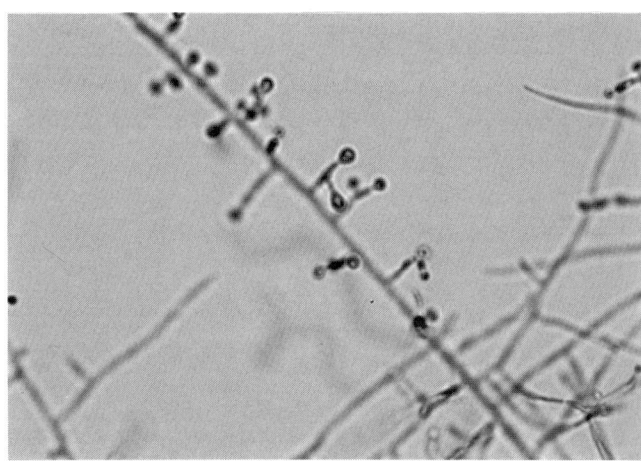

Fig. 45–4. Slide culture of a colony of the mold form of Blastomyces dermatitidis (lactophenol cotton blue, ×40).

cal specimens by direct microscopy. They appear as large, spherical, thick-walled yeast cells 8 to 20 μm in diameter with a single bud connected by a broad-based bud to the parent cell (see Fig. 45–1). At 25° to 30° C, B. dermatitidis grows on media used for fungal isolation in 5 to 30 days as a white to off-white, glabrous or waxy-looking mould (Plate XF) that becomes gray to brown as aerial hyphae develop with age. Microscopically, the mould form of the fungus is characterized by delicate, septate hyphae, 1 to 2 μm in diameter, and most important diagnostically, oval or pyriform single-celled conidia, 2 to 4 μm in diameter, found singly at the tips of short or long conidiophores, resembling lollipops (Fig. 45–4). Although visualizing "lollipops" is suggestive of B. dermatitidis, other moulds—Pseudallescheria boydii, which may be a pathogen (see Chapter 44), and the saprobe Chrysosporium—may have a similar appearance; therefore, identification requires additional testing. P. boydii and Chrysosporium do not grow on media containing cycloheximide and Blastomyces dermatitidis does. This is a useful feature, but the identification is confirmed by demonstrating conversion of the mould to the yeast form, exoantigen testing, or DNA probe analysis.

To demonstrate in vitro conversion of dimorphic fungi from moulds to yeasts, a large inoculum of the mould is transferred to brain-heart infusion agar containing 5 to 10% sheep blood, cysteine-hemoglobin agar, or, if Blasto-

Table 45–1. Specimens Required for Diagnosis of Infections Caused by the Dimorphic Fungi

Infection	Organism*	Specimens
Pneumonia	Histoplasma capsulatum, Coccidioides immitis, Blastomyces dermatitidis, (Sporothrix schenckii, Paracoccidioides brasiliensis)	Sputum, bronchial washings, bronchoalveolar fluid, lung tissue
Cutaneous/subcutaneous	S. schenckii, B. dermatitidis, C. immitis, P. brasiliensis, H. capsulatum var duboisii	Biopsy tissue, exudate
Disseminated disease	H. capsulatum (B. dermatitidis, C. immitis)	Blood, bone marrow
Osteoarticular	B. dermatitidis, S. schenckii, C. immitis	Bone biopsy, joint fluid, synovial biopsy
Mucocutaneous	H. capsulatum, P. brasiliensis (B. dermatitidis)	Biopsy of lesion
Central nervous system	C. immitis, (H. capsulatum, B. dermatitidis, S. schenckii)	Cerebrospinal fluid, brain biopsy

* Organisms in parentheses infrequently cause the infection.

Table 45-2. Characteristic Features of the Dimorphic Fungi

Organism	Direct Microscopic Examination of Clinical Specimens	Growth Rate (days)	Culture Characteristics (25° to 30° C)
Blastomyces dermatitidis	Yeast cells, 8–15 μm, with broad-based buds and double-contoured walls	5–30	Colonies: White, cream, or tan; fluffy to glabrous Microscopic: Septate hyphae, 1–2 μm diameter, with single pyriform conidia on short to long conidiophores
Histoplasma capsulatum	Var capsulatum: small (2–5 μm), oval to spherical budding yeast cells, often within cells of the monocyte/macrophage system Var duboisii: large, 12–15 μm yeast cells	5–30	Colonies: White, cream, tan, or gray; fluffy to glabrous Microscopic: Septate hyphae, 1–2 μm diameter; small pyriform microconidia and large, smooth-walled macroconidia that become tuberculate with age
Coccidioides immitis	Round spherules, 20–200 μm in diameter, containing endospores 2–5 μm in diameter	3–21	Colonies: White, fluffy; may be pigmented (pink, yellow, purple, black) Microscopic: Alternate, barrel-shaped arthroconidia
Paracoccidioides brasiliensis	Yeast cells, 10–40 μm in diameter, surrounded by multiple smaller buds (resembling a mariner's wheel)	21–28	Colonies: Heaped, glabrous with short white aerial hyphae; may turn tan to brown Microscopic: Septate hyphae, 1–2 μm diameter, chlamydospores, few small conidia (3–4 μm diameter)
Sporothrix schenckii	Oval to cigar-shaped yeast cells, rarely visible	3–5	Colonies: Small, white, yeastlike, becoming brown to black, membranous and wrinkled with aerial hyphae Microscopic: Septate hyphae, 1–2 μm diameter; one-celled conidia, 2–5 μm diameter, in "flowerette" or "sleeve" arrangement

myces dermatitidis is suspected, to cottonseed conversion medium. Cultures are incubated at 35° to 37° C for several days and observed for the appearance of yeast-like colonies, which should be examined microscopically by making a tease preparation (see Appendix, Procedure 20). During conversion, colonies initially appear prickly, but eventually waxy and wrinkled, cream to tan colonies of yeasts develop. Microscopic examination of the yeast colonies shows round, thick-walled yeast cells, 6 to 15 μm in diameter, with single buds attached by a broad base (Fig. 45–5), whereas the prickly-looking colonies typically show a combination of hyphae and poorly defined budding yeast forms. The major drawback to conversion in vitro is that prolonged incubation (often several weeks to months) may be required; so, more rapid diagnostic tests—exoantigen detection and nucleic acid probes—have been developed.

The exoantigen test may be used to identify Blastomyces dermatitidis, Histoplasma capsulatum, Coccidioides immitis, and Paracoccidioides brasiliensis. To perform the test, water-soluble, cell-free antigens are extracted from a mature colony of the test isolate on Sabouraud dextrose agar in an aqueous solution of merthiolate for 24 hours. The extract is filtered, concentrated, and tested with homologous antibodies in a double-diffusion agar test system, which is observed for the presence of precipitin bands of identity (Fig. 45–6). Reagents are commercially available, and detailed instructions outlining test performance and interpretation are provided by the manufacturer (38). The presence of an A band identifies an isolate as Blastomyces dermatitidis. Recently, nucleic acid probes for culture confirmation of B. dermatitidis, Histoplasma capsulatum, and Coccidioides immitis became commercially available, and limited data suggest that they are useful for identification.

Fungal serologic testing should include a battery of antigens—those of Blastomyces dermatitidis, Histoplasma capsulatum, and Coccidioides immitis—to simplify interpretation of results, because cross-reactions occur among antigens of these organisms. Complement fixation and immunodiffusion tests should be performed to detect antibodies to Blastomyces dermatitidis. Complement fixation titers of 1:32 or greater indicate active disease, and titers

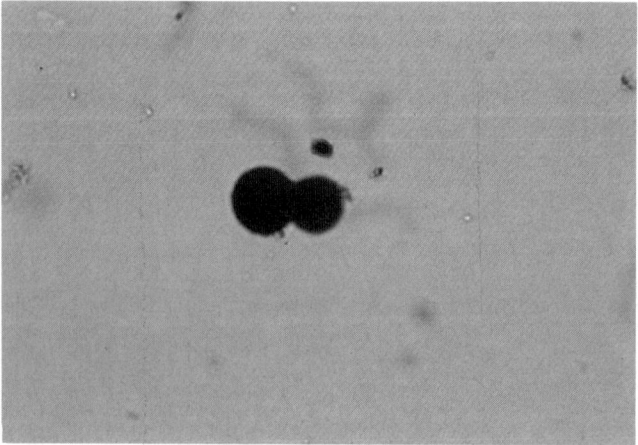

Fig. 45–5. Conversion to yeast with broad-based bud confirms the indentity of the mould shown in Figure 45–4 to be Blastomyces dermatitidis (lactophenol cotton blue, × 400).

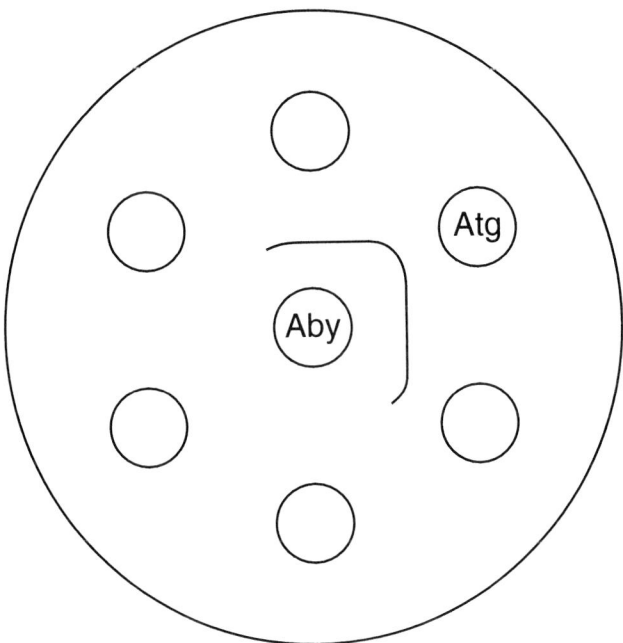

Fig. 45-6. Diagram of the exoantigen test shows lines of identify between antibody (Aby) and antigen (Atg).

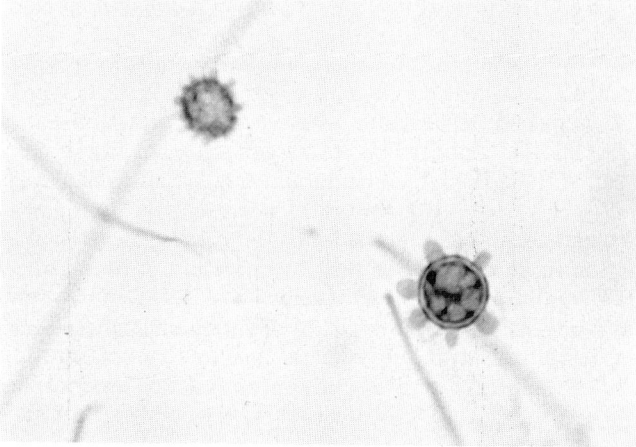

Fig. 45-7. Slide culture of Histoplasma capsulatum shows tuberculate macroconidia of the mold form (lactophenol cotton blue, × 400).

of 1:8 and 1:16 are very suggestive. Cross-reactions caused by infection with Histoplasma capsulatum or Coccidioides immitis occur, but titers usually are lower. The immunodiffusion test for detection of antibodies to the A antigen, which is more sensitive than complement fixation, is positive in about 80% of cases.

Histoplasma capsulatum. Direct microscopic examination of respiratory tract specimens usually is unsatisfactory for detection of H. capsulatum var capsulatum; however, with disseminated disease organisms may be detected in smears of peripheral blood or bone marrow stained with the Wright or Giemsa stain, in which the yeast form appears as small, round to oval cells, 2 to 5 μm in diameter, within mononuclear cells or neutrophils (Plate XIA). Histoplasma capsulatum grows slowly at 25° to 30° C, producing white, cottony colonies (similar to those of Blastomyces dermatitidis, Plate XF) in 2 to 4 weeks or more; from specimens containing large numbers of cells it may be recovered in 1 week or less. Colonies usually turn buff to brown with age, but isolates that produce gray to red colonies have been reported. Microscopic examination of young colonies shows spherical or pyriform, smooth microconidia, 2 to 5 μm in diameter, on the sides of delicate (1 to 2 μm diameter) septate hyphae or attached to short lateral conidiophores; and with age the characteristic and diagnostic large, round or pyriform tuberculate macroconidia (Fig. 45-7), 7 to 15 μm in diameter, appear; although some isolates of Histoplasma capsulatum fail to sporulate. Because Sepedonium, a saprophytic fungus that grows on mushrooms, produces similar-looking tuberculate macroconidia, the identification must be confirmed. This can be accomplished by in vitro conversion of the mould to the yeast form using the procedure discussed earlier for Blastomyces dermatitidis, by demonstrating characteristic H or M bands in the exoantigen test (described earlier), or by nucleic acid hybridization (commercially available). Moreover, most isolates of Sepedonium do not grow on media containing cycloheximide, whereas Histoplasma capsulatum does.

Conversion of the mould to the yeast form often requires several successive transfers at 3- to 5-day intervals. Colonies of yeast are mucoid, membranous, and white, cream, tan, or pink. Microscopic examination shows oval yeast cells, 2 to 5 μm, with single buds attached by narrow necks. The yeast form is not diagnostic alone, but when observed with the mould form, Histoplasma capsulatum is confirmed. Because in vitro conversion is time consuming, the exoantigen test or the nucleic acid probe is recommended.

Direct microscopic examination of pus from skin lesions, abscesses, or draining sinuses of persons infected with Histoplasma capsulatum var duboisii shows large (12 to 15 μm diameter), thick-walled yeast cells with single buds, occasionally attached by a broad base, resembling Blastomyces dermatitidis. The colony morphology of the mould form and its microscopic appearance are identical to those of H. capsulatum var capsulatum. The organism converts easily to the yeast phase: initially it forms small yeast cells, but with time the large, thick-walled cells are produced.

Occasionally, the diagnosis of histoplasmosis is based on results of complement fixation and immunodifusion serologic tests. The complement fixation test using the yeast-form antigen is positive in more than 90% of culturally proven cases of histoplasmosis if sera are evaluated at 2- to 3-week intervals. The test, however, is not specific, because cross-reactions occur with sera from persons with blastomycosis or coccidioidomycosis. Moreover, some persons who have disseminated histoplasmosis fail to produce complement-fixing antibodies. In primary pulmonary histoplasmosis, antibodies to the yeast form usually are detected within 4 weeks after exposure to the fungus. Antibodies to histoplasmin generally develop later and in lower titer, but with chronic disease the histoplasmin titer usually is higher. Complement fixation titers of 1:8 or 1:16 are suspicious of infection with Histoplasma capsulatum, and titers of 1:32 or greater usually indicate active disease. Cross-reactions occur in persons infected with Aspergillus, Blastomyces dermatitidis, or Coccidioides immitis, but titers generally are lower. Repeating the complement fixation test at 2- to 3-week intervals is recommended. A fourfold increase in titer indicates disease progression, and a fourfold decrease, regression.

The immunodiffusion test for detection of precipitins of Histoplasma capsulatum against the H and M protein antigens of histoplasmin is a useful screening procedure or an adjunct in the serologic diagnosis of histoplasmosis. The M band is found in persons with acute or chronic histoplasmosis and in normal sensitized persons after the histoplasmin skin test is administered. It often is the first band to appear and frequently occurs without the H band. The H band is found in the serum of persons with active histoplasmosis. It usually appears later than the M band and disappears earlier, and its disappearance may indicate disease regression. The presence of the M band is considered presumptive evidence of infection with H. capsulatum, but its presence in serum without an H band may be attributed to active disease, inactive disease, or recent administration of the skin test. Serum from about 70% of persons with proven histoplasmosis has M bands, but both M and H bands are found in only about 10% of cases.

Administering the histoplasmin skin test to persons previously exposed to Histoplasma capsulatum causes an increase in the complement-fixing antibody titer, which renders difficult the interpretation of subsequent changes in complement fixation test results. For this reason the skin test is not recommended for persons with suspected active histoplasmosis. If the skin test must be performed, blood for serologic studies should be drawn before or within 2 to 3 days after it is given, because antibodies do not develop that soon.

Methods for diagnosis of histoplasmosis that have been evaluated in research laboratories are enzyme immunoassay for detection of antibodies in serum (recently commercially available) and radioimmunoassay and enzyme-linked immunosorbent assay for detection of a polysaccharide antigen of Histoplasma capsulatum in urine and serum (39–41).

Coccidioides immitis. By direct microscopic examination of sputum, other body fluids and tissue, C. immitis appears as a nonbudding, thick-walled spherule, 20 to 200 μm in diameter (Fig. 45–2), containing granular material or many endospores, 2 to 5 μm in diameter. The latter are released by rupture of the spherule's cell wall, which subsequently appears as an empty and collapsed shell.

Cultures of Coccidioides immitis are a biohazard to laboratory personnel and, so, must be handled in a biological safety cabinet; plates should be sealed with tape. Most commonly, white, delicate, and cobweb-like colonies of C. immitis appear after incubation at 25° to 30° C for 3 to 5 days, but occasionally a more prolonged period is required for growth. Colonies may darken with age, and isolates producing pink, yellow, purple, and black colonies have been reported (42). Microscopic examination of the mould form shows small septate hyphae, often exhibiting right-angled branching and racquet forms. With age, hyphae form rectangular or barrel-shaped arthroconidia, 2 to 4 μm by 3 to 6 μm, that are larger than the hyphae and separated from one another by clear or lighter-staining, nonviable cells, a pattern called alternate arthroconidia (Fig. 45–8). Because the microscopic appearance of other fungi—Arthroderma, Auxarthron, Oidiodendron, and some species of Trichosporon—resembles that of C. immitis, a mould showing alternate arthroconidia must be confirmed as C. immitis by the exoantigen test. In vitro production of endospores by C. immitis may be accomplished using synthetic media, but this is not recommended.

Serologic tests are useful for diagnosis of infection with Coccidioides immitis and for determining prognosis (43). The tube precipitin test detects circulating immunoglobulin (Ig) M specific for C. immitis. It is most useful for diagnosis of early primary infection or exacerbation of existing disease, but it does not provide information about prognosis. Precipitins are detected in serum 1 to 3 weeks after primary infection; occasionally they are detected 6 months after infection. They may reappear if the infection spreads or if relapse occurs and may persist in disseminated disease. Precipitins rarely are found in the cerebrospinal fluid of persons with meningitis caused by C. immitis. The standard tube precipitin assay is performed by combining the test serum with coccidioidin, incubating at 37° C up to 5 days, and observing for a gelatinous button of precipitate, which indicates the presence of tube precipitin antibodies. Tube precipitin antibodies also may be detected by latex particle agglutination, a rapid and sensitive but nonspecific test that must be confirmed by another assay, if positive.

The complement fixation test, which detects IgG antibodies, becomes positive later and stays positive longer than the tube precipitin test. It is most useful for diagnosis of disseminated disease; and because titers parallel the severity of the illness, rising as the disease progresses and declining as the infection clears, the test has prognostic value. A titer of 1:2 or 1:4 usually indicates early, residual, or meningeal coccidioidomycosis, and a titer greater than

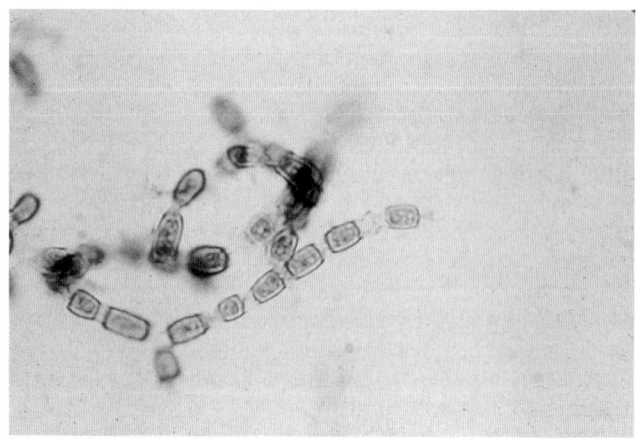

Fig. 45–8. Slide culture of Coccidioides immitis shows alternate arthroconidia of the mold form (lactophenol cotton blue, ×157.5).

1:16 indicates disseminated disease. Persons never infected with Coccidioides immitis, however, may have a low complement fixation titer. Both complement fixation and immunodiffusion tests, therefore, should be performed, and results of the two should agree. Cross-reactions occur in persons infected with Histoplasma capsulatum (but the titer usually is lower), and false-negative results may be seen in persons with solitary pulmonary lesions.

The coccidioidin skin test, which usually detects the earliest immune response to infection, is a valuable screening test. Conversion from a negative to a positive skin test reaction indicates primary infection, and the skin test does not elicit an antibody response in previously sensitized persons. Data from an evaluation of an enzyme-linked immunosorbent assay using spherule-derived antigens indicate that this type of test may allow earlier diagnosis of coccidioidomycosis; such a procedure recently became available commercially (44).

Paracoccidioides brasiliensis. In smears of clinical specimens such as sputum and exudates from mucocutaneous lesions and in tissues, P. brasiliensis appears as a large, round to oval yeast cell, 8 to 40 μm in diameter, with multiple buds, 8 to 15 μm in diameter, surrounding its periphery, resembling a mariner's wheel (see Fig. 45–3). P. brasiliensis grows slowly and in 3 to 4 weeks forms heaped, glabrous, or wrinkled colonies with short white aerial hyphae that often turn tan to brown with age. Microscopically, the mould form shows delicate, septate hyphae, 1 to 2 μm in diameter, numerous chlamydospores, and a few small, delicate globose or pyriform conidia, 3 to 4 μm in diameter arising from the sides of hyphae or on very short conidiophores and resembling those of B. dermatitidis (described earlier). The identification of P. brasiliensis is confirmed by in vitro conversion of the mould to the yeast form on blood-enriched medium or by exoantigen testing. Colonies of the yeast are smooth to cerebriform, cream to tan, and microscopically show yeast cells, 10 to 40 μm in diameter, surrounded by buds attached by a narrow neck.

Sporothrix schenckii. Direct examination of clinical specimens such as exudate from draining cutaneous lesions usually is not useful diagnostically, because characteristic yeast forms of S. schenckii are difficult to find. Small, moist, flat, white, yeastlike colonies of S. schenckii are visible in 3 to 5 days and with age become brown to black, membranous, wrinkled, and matted with aerial hyphae (Plate XIB). Microscopic examination of the mould form shows delicate, septate, branching hyphae bearing one-celled conidia, 2 to 5 μm in diameter, borne bouquet-like in clusters from the tips of single conidiophores ("flowerette" arrangement), and as the culture ages, single-celled, thick-walled black conidia borne along the sides of the hyphae ("sleeve" arrangement) also are seen (Fig. 45–9). Identification is based on in vitro conversion of the mould to the yeast form, a process that usually occurs in 1 to 5 days. At 35° to 37° C colonies of S. schenckii are soft, white to cream colored, and yeastlike and microscopically show singly or multiply budding, spherical, oval, or cigar-shaped yeast cells (Fig. 45–10). A latex agglutination test for detection of antibodies to S.

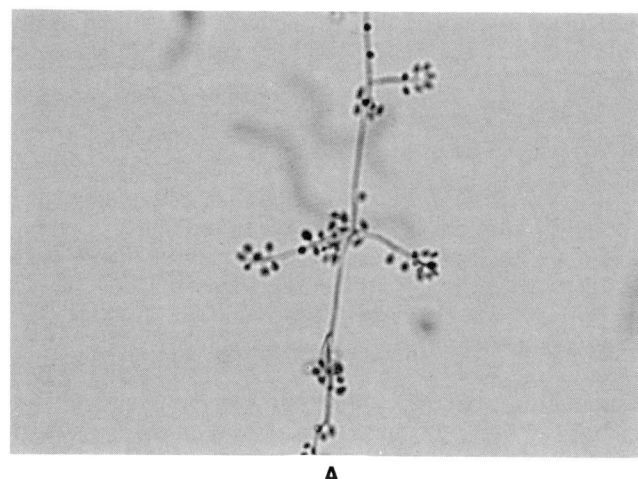

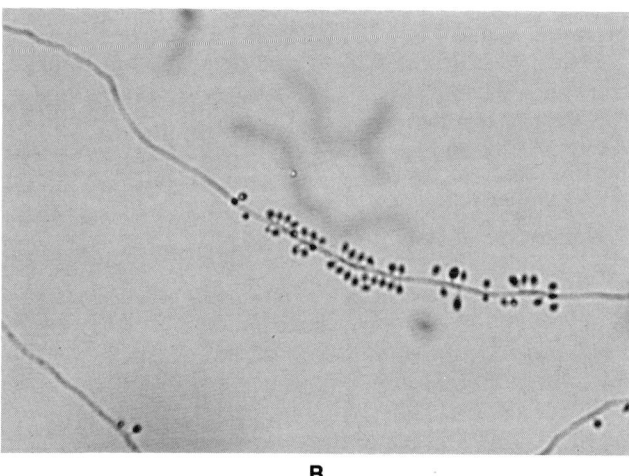

Fig. 45–9. Slide culture of the mold form of Sporothrix schenckii shows, A, "flowerette" and, B, "sleeve" arrangements of conidia (lactophenol cotton blue, × 40).

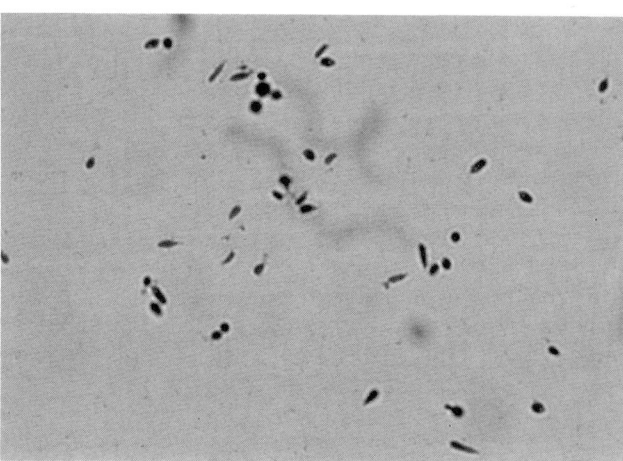

Fig. 45–10. Conversion to yeasts confirms the identity of the mold shown in Figure 45–9 to be Sporothrix schenckii (lactophenol cotton blue, × 40).

schenckii is commercially available but has limited use because the organism grows fairly rapidly and is easy to identify.

Treatment

Blastomyces dermatitidis. Acute pulmonary blastomycosis may resolve without antifungal therapy, but because the disease may recur later at extrapulmonary sites, many clinicians believe that all persons with acute blastomycosis should be treated. For immunocompetent persons with mild to moderate disease, ketoconazole for 6 to 12 months is the treatment of choice; and in case of life-threatening blastomycosis, central nervous system disease, progression of disease during ketoconazole therapy, and ketoconazole intolerance, amphotericin B is given. Itraconazole, a new oral imidazole currently being investigated, appears to be as effective as ketoconazole and may be less toxic (45).

Histoplasma capsulatum. The treatment of histoplasmosis is based on the clinical presentation. Acute histoplasmosis ordinarily does not require specific antifungal therapy. Rest and inactivity shorten the duration of the illness. Prolonged illness in infants and adults should be treated with a short course of amphotericin B, or perhaps ketoconazole. All persons with disseminated histoplasmosis require antifungal therapy. Amphotericin B is the agent of choice for severely ill or immunocompromised persons. For those who do not have endocarditis or meningitis and who are not immunosuppressed, oral ketoconazole for 6 to 12 months is an effective alternative. For persons with chronic pulmonary histoplasmosis, rest and inactivity help alleviate symptoms, but for those with thick-walled cavities, amphotericin B or ketoconazole is recommended. Histoplasmomas do not require therapy but may be removed surgically for diagnostic purposes. No effective treatment for mediastinal fibrosis is known.

Coccidioides immitis. Most persons with primary symptomatic coccidioidomycosis recover without specific antifungal therapy; however, treatment is indicated in the following situations: high complement fixation titer; persistence of symptoms over 6 weeks; extensive, enlarging, or persisting pulmonary disease; persisting precipitins; a negative skin test; debilitation; concurrent disease, such as diabetes mellitus, emphysema, or asthma, that is likely to be adversely affected by the infection; immune impairment. Pregnant women, infants, and members of racial groups predisposed to handle the infection poorly (blacks, Hispanics, Filipinos) also should be treated. All persons with extrapulmonary infection require therapy. Currently, amphotericin B is the drug of choice. Ketoconazole may be an alternative agent in forms of disease other than meningitis, but it has been associated with a high relapse rate (46). Itraconazole currently is being evaluated for nonmeningeal disease (47).

Sporothrix schenckii. Cutaneous sporotrichosis is treated with iodides and extracutaneous infections with amphotericin B, or perhaps itraconazole, although pulmonary disease and meningeal disease are difficult to cure (45).

REFERENCES

1. Gilchrist TC: Protozoan dermatitis. J Cutan Gen Dis, *12*:496, 1894.
2. Gilchrist TC, and Stokes WR: The presence of an oidium in the tissues of a case of pseudo–lupus vulgaris. Johns Hopkins Hosp Rep, 7:129, 1896.
3. Gilchrist TC, and Stokes WR: Case of pseudo–lupus vulgaris caused by blastomycosis. J Exp Med, *3*:53, 1898.
4. Schwartz J, and Baum GL: Blastomycosis. Am J Clin Pathol, *11*:999, 1951.
5. Kaufman L, et al: Detection of two Blastomyces dermatitidis serotypes by exoantigen analysis. J Clin Microbiol, *18*:110, 1983.
6. Turner S, and Kaufman L: Immunodiagnosis of blastomycosis. Semin Respir Infect, *1*:22, 1986.
7. Tenenbaum MJ, Greenspan J, and Kerkering TM: Blastomycosis. Crit Rev Microbiol, *9*:139, 1982.
8. Klein BS, et al: Isolation of Blastomyces dermatitidis in soil associated with a large outbreak of blastomycosis in Wisconsin. N Engl J Med, *314*:529, 1986.
9. Chapman SW: Blastomyces dermatitidis. *In* Principles and Practice of Infectious Diseases. 3rd ed. Edited by GL Mandell, RG Douglas, Jr, and JE Bennett. New York, Churchill Livingstone, 1990.
10. Craig MW, Davey WN, and Green RA: Conjugal blastomycosis. Am Rev Respir Dis, *102*:86, 1970.
11. Watts EA, Gard PD, Jr, and Tuthill SW: First reported case of intrauterine transmission of blastomycosis. Pediatr Infect Dis, *2*:308, 1983.
12. Drutz DJ, and Frey CL: Intracellular and extracellular defenses against Blastomyces dermatitidis conidia and yeasts. J Lab Clin Med, *105*:737, 1985.
13. Schaffner A, et al: In vitro susceptibility of fungi to killing by neutrophil granulocytes discriminate between primary pathogenicity and opportunism. J Clin Invest, 78:511, 1986.
14. Brummer E, Sugar AM, and Stevens DA: Immunological activation of polymorphonuclear neutrophils for fungal killing: Studies with murine cells and Blastomycosis dermatitidis in vitro. J Leukocyte Biol, *36*:505, 1984.
15. Brummer E, Sugar AM, and Stevens DA: Enhanced oxidative burst in immunologically activated, but not elicited, polymorphonuclear leukocytes correlates with fungicidal activity. Infect Immun, *49*:396, 1985.
16. Bradsher RW, Balk RA, and Jacobs RF: Growth inhibition of Blastomyces dermatitidis in alveolar and peripheral macrophages from patients with blastomycosis. Am Rev Respir Dis, *135*:412, 1987.
17. Sarosi GA, and Davies SF: Blastomycosis. Am Rev Respir Dis, *120*:911, 1979.
18. Yamato H, et al: A case of histoplasmosis. Acta Med Okayama, *11*:347, 1957.
19. Goodwin RA, Jr, and des Prez RM: Histoplasmosis. Am Rev Respir Dis, *117*:929, 1978.
20. Duncan JT: A unique form of Histoplasma. Trans R Soc Trop Med Hyg, *40*:364, 1947.
21. Ajello L: Histoplasmosis—a dual entity histoplasmosis capsulati and histoplasmosis duboisii. Igiene Moderna, 79:3, 1983.
22. Cockshott WP, and Lucas AO: Histoplasmosis duboisii. Q J Med, *33*:223, 1964.
23. Posadas A: Un nuovo caso de micosis fungoides con psorospermias. An Circ Med Argent, *15*:585, 1892.
24. Rixford E, and Gilchrist TC: Two cases of protozoan (coccidioidal) infection of the skin and other organs. Johns Hopkins Hosp Rep, *1*:209, 1896.

25. Ophuls W, and Moffitt HC: A new pathogenic mould (formerly described as a protozoan: Coccidioides immitis pyogenes): Preliminary report. Phila Med J, 5:1471, 1900.
26. Dickson EC: "Valley fever" of the San Joaquin Valley and fungus Coccidioides. Calif West Med, 47:151, 1937.
27. Drutz DJ, and Catanzaro A: Coccidioidomycosis. Am Rev Respir Dis, 117:559, 1978.
28. Overholt EL, and Hornick RB: Primary cutaneous coccidioidomycosis. Arch Intern Med, 114:149, 1964.
29. Winn WA: Primary cutaneous coccidioidomycosis. Reevaluation of its potentiality based on a study of three new cases. Arch Dermatol, 92:221, 1965.
30. Savage DC, and Madin SH: Cellular responses in lungs of immunized mice to intranasal infection with Coccidioides immitis. Sabouraudia, 6:94, 1968.
31. Galgiani JN, et al: Complement activation by Coccidioides immitis: In vitro and clinical studies. Infect Immun, 28:944, 1970.
32. Ampel NM, Wieden MA, and Galgiani JN: Coccidioidomycosis: Clinical update. Rev Infect Dis, 11:897, 1989.
33. Restrepo AM: Paracoccidioides brasiliensis. *In* Principles and Practice of Infectious Diseases. 3rd ed. Edited by GL Mandell, RG Douglas, Jr, and JE Bennett. New York, Churchill Livingstone, 1990.
34. Gilardo R, et al: Pathogenesis of paracoccidioidomycosis: A model based on the study of 45 patients. Mycopathology, 58:63, 1976.
35. Franco MF, et al: Paracoccidioidomycosis: A recently proposed classification of its clinical forms. Rev Soc Brasil Med Trop, 20:129, 1987.
36. Restrepo A, et al: Estrogens inhibit mycelium to yeast transformation in the fungus P. brasiliensis: Implications for resistance of females to paracoccidioidomycosis. Infect Immun, 46:346, 1984.
37. Bennett JE: Sporothrix schenckii. *In* Principles and Practice of Infectious Diseases. 3rd ed. Edited by GL Mandell, RG Douglas, Jr, and JE Bennett, New York, Churchill Livingstone, 1990.
38. Roberts GD: Laboratory methods in basic mycology. *In* Bailey and Scott's Diagnostic Micobiology. 8th ed. Edited by EJ Baron and SM Finegold. St. Louis, CV Mosby, 1990.
39. Lambert RS, and George RB: Evaluation of enzyme immunoassay as a rapid screening test for histoplasmosis and blastomycosis. Am Rev Respir Dis, 136:316, 1987.
40. Wheat JL, Kohler RB, and Tewari RP: Diagnosis of disseminated histoplasmosis by detection of Histoplasma capsulatum antigen in serum and urine specimens. N Engl J Med, 314:83, 1986.
41. Zimmerman SE, et al: Comparison of sandwich solid-phase radioimmunoassay and two enzyme-linked immunosorbent assays for detection of Histoplasma capsulatum polysaccharide antigen. J Infect Dis, 160:678, 1989.
42. Huppert M, Sun SH, and Bailey JW: Natural variability in Coccidioides immitis. *In* Coccidioidomycosis. Edited by L Ajello. Tucson, University of Arizona Press, 1967.
43. Pappagianis D, and Zimmer BL: Serology of coccidioidomycosis. Clin Microbiol Rev, 3:247, 1990.
44. Galgiani JN, Grace GM, and Lundergan LL: New serologic tests for early detection of coccidioidomycosis. J Infect Dis, 163:671, 1991.
45. Graybill JR: Future directions of antifungal chemotherapy. Clin Infect Dis, 14(suppl 1):S170, 1992.
46. Galgiani JN: Ketoconazole treatment of coccidioidomycosis. Drugs, 26:355, 1983.
47. Tucker RM, et al: Treatment of mycoses with itraconazole. Ann NY Acad Sci, 544:451, 1988.

Chapter 46

MISCELLANEOUS FUNGI

The fungi discussed in this chapter include the yeastlike organism tentatively named Loboa loboi, which causes the chronic, localized subepidermal infection, lobomycosis, and Rhinosporidium seeberi, the agent of rhinosporidiosis, a chronic localized infection of mucous membranes. Though these organisms have not been cultured and currently remain unclassified, both are believed to be fungi.

LOBOA LOBOI

Lobomycosis was first described in 1931 by Jorge Lobo, who believed the infection was a mild form of paracoccidioidomycosis (see Chapter 45) (1). The disease was known only in humans until the 1970s, when natural infection was discovered in bottle-nosed dolphins (2,3). The pathogen—a multinucleate, spherical, elliptical, or lemon-shaped yeastlike organism, 9 to 10 μm in diameter, tentatively called Loboa loboi—has not yet been cultivated in vitro, so its true taxonomic relationships cannot be determined.

Epidemiology

The ecology of Loboa loboi is unknown. Most of the more than 100 cases of lobomycosis reported have occurred in the Amazon valley of Brazil or in Surinam, with scattered cases in Colombia, Venezuela, French Guiana, Panama, and Costa Rica (4–7). Most affected persons are males who work in agriculture or live in rural areas. Trauma may be the inciting event, but usually no specific incident is remembered. A reported case in a European animal handler following contact with an infected Atlantic dolphin suggests that animal-to-human transmission may occur (8).

Pathology

The typical lesion of lobomycosis is a subepidermal granuloma that does not involve the overlying skin or deep subcutaneous tissue. Histologically, the granuloma is characterized by extensive hyaline fibrosis with scattered histiocytes and giant cells but no necrosis or suppuration. Thick-walled yeast cells, about 10 μm in diameter, in chains are found, principally in giant cells and macrophages, and occasionally outside of cells (Fig. 46–1). Ulceration and minimal acute inflammation may be present in older lesions.

Clinical Manifestations

Lesions typically involve exposed areas such as the ears, legs, arms, and face. They begin as small, painless or slightly pruritic, sharply defined and freely moveable, hard nodules with a smooth surface, resembling keloids, and spread slowly in the dermis over many years. Older lesions become verrucoid and may ulcerate, and the infection may be transferred to other areas of the skin via autoinoculation, as during scratching or subsequent abrasions. Other types of the disease are these: infiltrative, which usually occurs early in the infection; gummatous, in which organisms are located deep in the tissue; and ulcerated, associated with secondary bacterial infection. Systemic involvement does not occur, but in a few cases organisms have been found in adjacent lymph nodes (4).

RHINOSPORIDIUM SEEBERI

Rhinosporidiosis was recognized in the 1890s but was first reported by Seeber in 1900 (9). The agent was named Rhinosporidium seeberi in the early 1920s by Ashworth, who extensively analyzed the organism and its development in tissue, concluding that it was a lower aquatic fungus (10). The organism has not yet been isolated on artificial media, but it has been grown in cell cultures (11).

Epidemiology

Rhinosporidiosis occurs in humans and in animals such as horses, mules, and cows in almost all parts of the world, but most cases have been reported from India and Ceylon, followed by South America, especially Brazil and Argentina (12–14). Most affected persons are 20 to 40 years of age (range, 3 to 90 years) and come from a rural environment. Males account for 70 to 90% of cases, although this varies with age, site of infection, and geographic location. For example, girls and boys are affected equally before puberty, and ocular infections appear to be more common in women. The disease often is associated with work or play in fresh water, and in several cases the infection occurs at the site of a previous injury (15). Ocular infections are more frequent in arid areas and often are associated with dust storms and injury to the eye (16).

Pathology

Nasal lesions of rhinosporidiosis grossly resemble typical nasal polyps but are more dense and lack mucinous cysts. Microscopically, the epithelium usually is hyperplastic but may be thinned focally, and the core of the lesion is composed of vascular, fibromyomatous connective tissue with a mixed inflammatory infiltrate of plasma cells, lymphocytes, histiocytes, neutrophils, and giant cells; occasionally eosinophils are present in large numbers. Microabscesses and foci of hemorrhage are frequent.

MISCELLANEOUS FUNGI

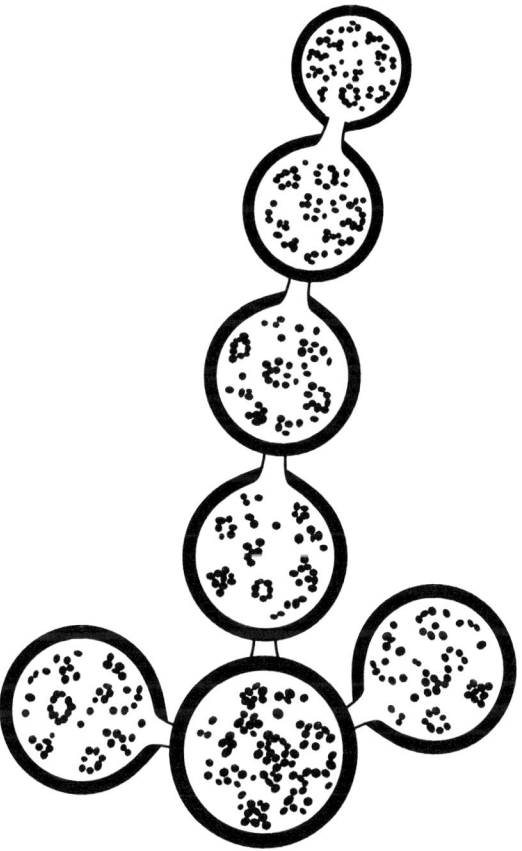

Fig. 46-1. Diagram of yeast cells of Loboa loboi.

Organisms are found in the core, and sometimes in the epithelium. The infecting spore, 6 to 10 μm in diameter with a chitinous wall, clear protoplasm, and vesicular nucleus with a nucleolus, apparently penetrates into the mucosal epithelium and matures in the subepithelial tissue. The organism begins to divide when it reaches 50 μm in size; and when it is 100 μm a layer of cellulose-like material is laid down on the inner surface of the wall of the spherule. When the spherule is 250 to 350 μm in diameter and contains more than 16,000 young spores its pore ruptures and the 7- to 9-μm spores are released into the surrounding connective tissue, which elicits an influx of foreign body giant cells. Organisms (Fig. 46-2) are easily observed in sections of tissue stained with hematoxylin and eosin or silver stain.

Clinical Manifestations

Nasal disease, which accounts for about 70% of cases of rhinosporidiosis, most often involves the mucous membrane of the septum, interior turbinate, and nasal floor, and less often affects middle turbinate, middle meatus, and nasal roof. The first symptom generally is the feeling of a foreign body in the nose, frequently accompanied by mild to intense pruritus and coryza. The lesion develops into a pedunculated polyp, weighing as much as 20 gm, that obstructs the air passages and may cause dyspnea and dysphagia.

Ocular disease accounts for about 15% of cases of rhinosporidiosis. In about 90% of these the palpebral conjunctiva is involved; and in the remainder, the disease affects the bulb, limbus, caruncle, or canthi. The disease, almost always unilateral, is characterized by single, sessile or stalked, moveable, granular growths that enlarge, causing tearing, redness, discharge, photophobia, and eversion of the lid.

The remaining cases of rhinosporidiosis involve the skin or mucous membranes. Painless papules or wartlike growths may involve the scalp, the skin of the abdomen, or other body sites; and pedunculated or polypoid lesions involving the larynx, hard palate, epiglottis, vagina, vulva, uvula, anus, urethra, trachea, and bronchus have been reported (14).

Laboratory Diagnosis

Both lobomycosis and rhinosporidiosis are diagnosed by visualizing characteristic organisms in potassium hydroxide preparations of clinical material obtained by curettage, surgical excision, or biopsy or in formalin-fixed tissue sections. Moreover, spores of Rhinosporidium seeberi may be seen in potassium hydroxide preparations of nasal discharge. Loboa loboi appears as chains of uniform yeast cells, 9 to 10 μm in diameter (range, 7 to 12 μm). In cases of rhinosporidiosis, mature sporangia up to 350 μm in diameter and spores 7 to 9 μm in diameter are seen.

Treatment

Lobomycosis is treated by wide surgical excision of the affected area. Therapy with sulfa drugs, especially sulfadi-

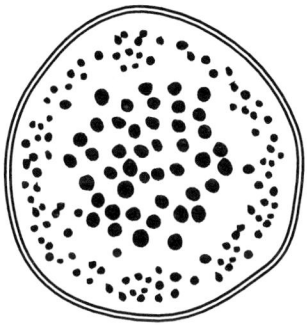

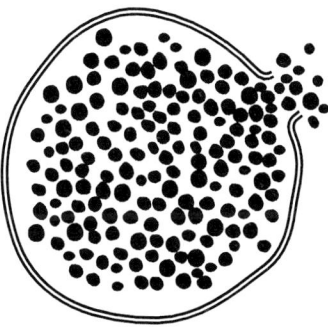

Fig. 46-2. Diagram of cells of Rhinosporidium seeberi.

methoxine, or clofazimine has variable results (17). Rhinosporidiosis also is treated surgically, but recurrences are common.

REFERENCES

1. Lobo J: Um caso de Blastomicose, produzido per uma especie nova, encontrada em Recife. Rev Med Pernambuco, 1:763, 1931.
2. DeVries GA, and Laarman JJ: A case of Lobo's disease in the dolphin Sotalia guianensis. Aquatic Mammals, 1:26, 1973.
3. Bossart GD: Suspected acquired immunodeficiency in a bottle-nosed dolphin (Tursiops truncatus) with chronic active hepatitis and lobomycosis. J Am Vet Med Assoc, 185:1413, 1984.
4. Azulay RD, et al: Keloid blastomycosis (Lobo's disease) with lymphatic involvement: A case report. Int J Dermatol, 15:40, 1976.
5. Jaramillo D, et al: Lobomycosis. Report of the eighth Colombian case and review of the literature. J Cutan Pathol, 3:180, 1976.
6. Lacaz CS, and Rose M: Bibliografia sobre blastomicose salamericana (doenca de Lutz) e blastomicose queloidiforme (duenca de Lobo) (1909–1968). São Paulo, Instituto de Medicina Tropical, 1969.
7. Wiersma JP, and Niemel PLA: Lobo's disease in Surinam patients. Trop Geogr Med, 17:89, 1965.
8. Symmers W St C: A possible case of Lobo's disease acquired in Europe from a bottle-nosed dolphin (Tursiops truncatus). Bull Soc Pathol Exot 76:777, 1983.
9. Wright J: A nasal sporozoon (Rhinosporidium kinealyi). NY Med J, 86:1149, 1907.
10. Ashworth JH: On Rhinosporidium seeberi (Wernicke, 1903) with special reference to its sporulation and affinities. Trans R Soc Edinb, 53:301, 1923.
11. Levy MG, Meuten DJ, and Breitschwerdt EB: Cultivation of Rhinosporidium seeberi in vitro: Interaction with epithelial cells. Science, 234:474, 1986.
12. Grover S: Rhinosporidiosis (epidemiological and clinical study). J Indian Med Assoc, 64:93, 1975.
13. Gupta RL, et al: An epidemiological study of rhinosporidiosis in and around Raipur. Indian J Med Res, 64:1293, 1976.
14. Rippon JW (ed): Rhinosporidiosis. In Medical Mycology. The Pathogenic Fungi and the Pathogenic Actinomycetes. 3rd ed. Philadelphia, WB Saunders, 1988.
15. Karunaratne WAE: Rhinosporidiosis in Man. London, Athlone Press, 1964.
16. Kaye H: A case of rhinosporidiosis on the eye. Br J Ophthalmol, 22:447, 1938.
17. Tapia A, et al: Keloidal blastomycosis (Lobo's disease) in Panama. Int J Dermatol, 17:572, 1978.

Chapter 47

ALGAE-LIKE ORGANISMS

Two organisms that resemble algae are associated with human disease. Species of Prototheca most commonly cause cutaneous lesions and olecranon bursitis. Cyanobacteria (blue-green algae–like organisms) are associated with diarrhea.

PROTOTHECA

Species of Prototheca are achlorophyllous organisms with a life cycle resembling that of the algae of the genus Chlorella. The unicellular form of the organism is a round or ovoid cell about 2 μm in diameter, called an endospore, that enlarges as it grows and reproduces by cleavage of the cytoplasm and cell wall formation. The endospore develops into a distinct multinucleate cluster, 15 to 25 μm in diameter, called the sporangium, that finally releases two to 20 daughter cells, which repeat the reproductive cycle. These organisms are ubiquitous in nature and cause disease in plants and lower animals, but only two species—Prototheca wickerhamii and Prototheca zopfii—cause disease in humans. The first human isolates of a species of Prototheca were recovered in 1930 from the stool of two Puerto Rican patients with tropical sprue (1). The presence of the organisms, however, was coincidental, because these agents have not been recovered from any other persons with sprue or other gastrointestinal diseases. Since the initial recognition of species of Prototheca in human specimens, fewer than 40 cases of disease caused by these organisms have been documented.

Epidemiology

Species of Prototheca are found worldwide in the slime flux of trees, feces of animals, potato skins, streams, ponds, and sewage (2). Infections caused by these organisms have been reported in the United States, Africa, China, Southeast Asia, Australia, New Zealand, and Europe (3–10). In most cases infection is associated with penetrating or nonpenetrating trauma, during which organisms probably are inoculated into tissue. Iatrogenic inoculation of Prototheca wickerhamii has been responsible for peritonitis complicating continuous ambulatory peritoneal dialysis, and rarely, the oral route of exposure may result in infection, especially if a person who has a mucosal injury in the gastrointestinal tract ingests an unusually large inoculum of organisms (3,9).

Pathogenesis and Pathology

The pathogenesis of disease caused by the species of Prototheca is unknown, but the paucity of such cases strongly suggests that direct inoculation of tissue with these low-virulence organisms probably is a prerequisite for disease. Host defenses then affect disease progression and its subsequent response to therapy. The organisms typically elicit a granulomatous response, with histiocytes, lymphocytes, giant cells, and a few neutrophils and eosinophils. Sporangia, 8 to 20 μm in diameter, often with distinct internal divisions representing endospores (Fig. 47–1), are found extracellularly and within giant cells in hematoxylin and eosin–stained sections but are best visualized in sections stained with Gomori methenamine silver or Periodic acid–Schiff stain. In cutaneous infections, the inflammation is located in the dermis and subcutaneous tissue, and the epidermis is hyperkeratotic.

Clinical Manifestations

The predominant manifestations of infections caused by Prototheca are cutaneous lesions and olecranon bursitis. A papule, nodule, ulcer, or drainage from a wound or surgical site most often develops on the extremities or the face and spreads slowly, causing slight tenderness, varying degrees of drainage, and mild inflammation but no adenopathy or systemic symptoms. Olecranon bursitis is manifested by mild tenderness, redness, swelling, and variable fluid accumulation and drainage; adenopathy and systemic symptoms and signs are absent. Prototheca rarely cause a chronic systemic disease associated with jaundice and intestinal symptoms (3,8). Accompanying laboratory abnormalities have included eosinophilia and elevations of liver enzymes, the erythrocyte sedimentation rate, and immunoglobulin levels.

Laboratory Diagnosis

Desirable specimens for diagnosis of infections caused by Prototheca depend on the clinical presentation: skin scrapings or biopsy tissue for cutaneous disease, aspirated fluid or biopsy tissue for olecranon bursitis, and in cases of disseminated disease, involved tissue (for example, liver or gallbladder), blood, and stool specimens should be obtained. Characteristic organisms may be visualized in potassium hydroxide preparations of skin scrapings or tissue and are readily seen in tissue sections (see above). In smears stained with the Gram stain the typical endosporulation of Prototheca is obscured and the organisms resemble nonbudding yeasts such as Blastomyces dermatitidis (Chapter 45) or Cryptococcus neoformans (Chapter 43).

Species of Prototheca grow at 30° to 37° C on sheep blood agar and on fungal media such as Sabouraud's dextrose agar that do not contain cycloheximide, which inhibits growth. Smooth, moist, white to cream-colored, yeastlike colonies typically appear in 48 hours. Wet-

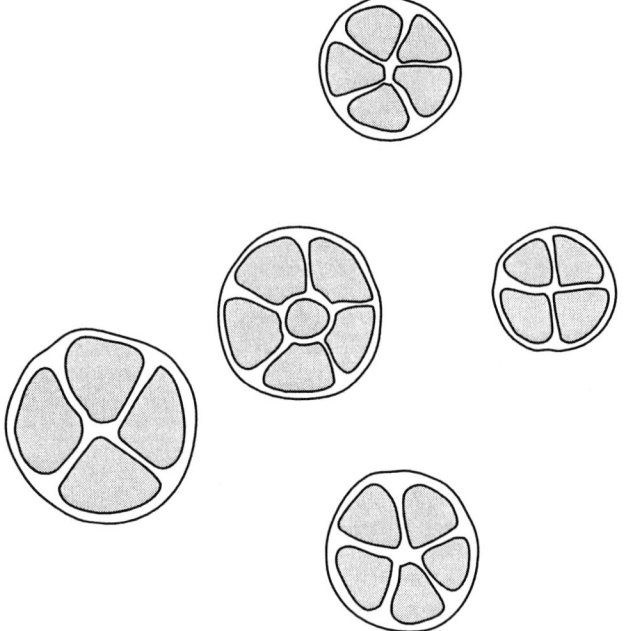

Fig. 47–1. Diagram of Prototheca wickerhamii in tissue.

mount or lactophenol cotton blue preparations show thick-walled sporangia with endospores, typical of Prototheca, and identification is based on sugar assimilation profiles.

Antibodies against Prototheca may be detected in serum of infected persons, and their presence in a person whose stool cultures positive for the organism is presumptive evidence of visceral protothecosis (3). No serologic test is commercially available.

Treatment

Treatment of infections caused by Prototheca has included surgical excision of cutaneous lesions or infected bursae, intrabursal instillation of amphotericin B, intravenous amphotericin B plus tetracycline, ketoconazole, or transfer factor; intravenous amphotericin B alone; and ketoconazole alone.

Cyanobacterium (Blue-Green Algae)–like Organisms

Spherical organisms, appearing as granule-containing cysts, 10 μm in diameter (Fig. 47–2), recently have been identified in stools in association with a syndrome of intermittent, prolonged, watery diarrhea for 2 to 3 weeks, accompanied by anorexia, fatigue, and weight loss. In early reports, affected persons either were immunocompromised or had traveled recently to tropical countries; however, in 1989 and 1990 three outbreaks of this syndrome (one in Chicago and two in Kathmandu, Nepal) occurred in immunocompetent persons, affecting at least 150 persons in all (11–13). In some geographic areas the illness appears to be seasonal: outbreaks occur during periods of increased temperature and rainfall. The implicated organism has been termed a cyanobacterium (blue-green algae)–like body because some of its morphologic and reproductive characteristics are similar to those of the order Chroococcales of cyanobacteria, which are unicellular to multicellular photosynthetic organisms, usually found in water or moist environments; however, the agent does not have all the characteristics of any known cyanobacteria type (12).

Cyanobacteria-like bodies may be visualized in wet-mount preparations of fresh, unpreserved stool, as nonrefractile, hyaline cysts, 8 to 9 μm in diameter. Intact cysts contain a greenish, 6- to 7-μm diameter, spherical mass composed of a hollow cluster of refractile, membrane-bound globules that contain a clear material resembling lipid. In preparations of preserved stool the cyst contents appear as granules that vary in size and shape. Cyanobacteria-like bodies stain deep or mottled red or pink with the modified acid-fast stain, although some do not stain and appear as glassy, membranous cysts. Moreover, these organisms autofluoresce strongly under ultraviolet light, appearing as bright blue circles.

REFERENCES

1. Ashford BK, Ciferri R, and Dalmau LM: New species of Prototheca and variety of same isolated from human intestine. Archiv Protisternkunde, 70:619, 1930.
2. Pore RS, Barnett EA, Barnes WC, Jr, and Walker JD: Prototheca ecology. Mycopathologia, 81:49, 1983.

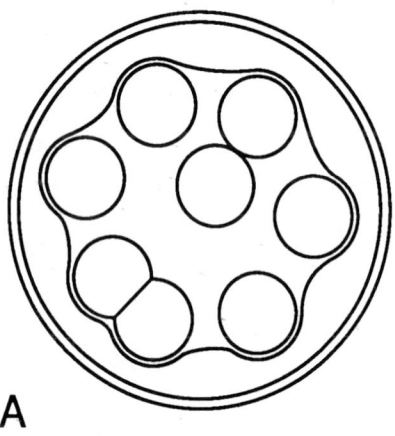
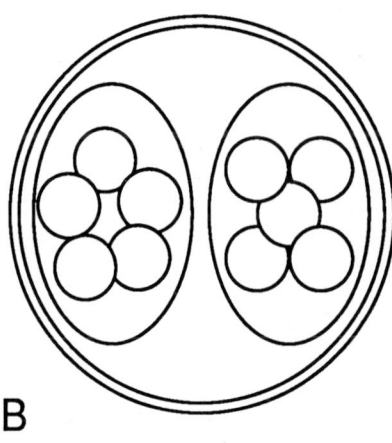

A B

Fig. 47.2. Diagram of Cyanobacterium-like body. *A,* Spherical cyst with internal membranous sac containing refractile globules in freshly passed stool. *B,* Cyst with two intracystic bodies, after 1 week in water. (From Long, EG, et al: Morphologic and staining characteristics of a Cyanobacterium-like organism associated with diarrhea. J Infect Dis, *164:* 199, 1991.)

3. Chan JC, et al: Visceral protothecosis mimicking sclerosing cholangitis in an immunocompetent host: Successful antifungal therapy. Rev Infect Dis, *12*:802, 1990.
4. Pegram PS, et al: Successful ketoconazole treatment of protothecosis with ketoconazole-associated hepatotoxicity. Arch Intern Med, *143*:1802, 1983.
5. Lee W-S, Lagios MD, and Leonards R: Wound infections by Prototheca wickerhamii, a saprophytic alga pathogenic for man. J Clin Microbiol, *2*:62, 1975.
6. Cochran RK, Pierson CI, Sell TL, and Palella T: Protothecal olecranon bursitis: Treatment with intrabursal amphotericin B. Rev Infect Dis, *8*:952, 1986.
7. Sudman MS: Protothecosis—a critical review. Am J Clin Pathol, *61*:10, 1974.
8. Cox GE, Wilson JD, and Brown P: Protothecosis: A case of disseminated algal infection. Lancet, *ii*:379, 1974.
9. O'Connor JP, et al: Algal peritonitis complicating continuous ambulatory peritoneal dialysis. Am J Kidney Dis, *8*:122, 1986.
10. Venezio FR, et al: Progressive cutaneous protothecosis. Am J Clin Pathol, *77*:485, 1982.
11. Long EG, et al: Alga associated with diarrhea in patients with acquired immunodeficiency syndrome and in travelers. J Clin Microbiol, *28*:1101, 1990.
12. Long EG, et al: Morphologic and staining characteristics of a cyanobacterium-like organism associated with diarrhea. J Infect Dis, *164*:199, 1991.
13. Centers for Disease Control: Outbreaks of diarrheal illness associated with cyanobacteria (blue-green algae)–like bodies—Chicago and Nepal, 1989 and 1990. MMWR, *40*:352, 1991.

Section IV

ANIMAL PARASITES

Chapter 48

INTRODUCTION TO ANIMAL PARASITES

In Part II, Section IV of this text, the animal parasites (protozoa, helminths, and arthropods) of humans are reviewed, emphasizing organisms that are recovered and identified in the clinical laboratory. The parasites living in tissues, identified in tissue sections, are mentioned briefly for the sake of completeness (1).

Parasitology deals with animal parasites, organisms that phylogenetically are classified in the animal kingdom. Bacteria, fungi, chlamydia, viruses, exhibit the behavior that fits the definition of parasitism, and thus are also true parasites. From this viewpoint, parasitology is a misnomer born out by the fact that, historically, parasites were the first pathogens observed. Cursory gross examination of a stool sample was sufficient to find a large roundworm or tapeworm, possibly causing the symptoms that the individual was having. Parasitism, then, is a special association between two living organisms: one organism, usually larger, the definitive host, which is inhabited by another, smaller organism, the parasite. This association takes several forms: if no harm occurs to the host the association is termed commensalism; if both parasite and host benefit from the association, it is mutualism; if neither parasite nor host could survive without the other it is symbiosis.

The phenomenon of parasitism follows certain general rules applicable to most situations: The older (in evolutionary terms) the association is between host and parasite, the better the adaptation between them in which case commensalism, mutualism or symbiosis is the rule. The newer the association between host and parasite, the worse are the chances for a good adaptation, and the host suffers some degree of damage, in which case we are dealing with pathogens. The medically important parasites are those pathogens that live *on* (infest) or *in* (infect) humans. In the course of the study of pathogens, however, one encounters similar organisms that are not pathogenic (commensals). Because of the need to distinguish pathogens from commensal organisms, the harmless organisms encountered in humans need to be included in this text.

LIFE CYCLES

The life cycles of animal parasites are generally more complicated than those of bacteria, fungi and others; parasitic protozoa often have several possible hosts in which they develop sometimes, to increase the opportunities to pass from one host to the next. A protozoan may occur in one host and may pass to the next host unchanged to produce a new infection; an example is Trichomonas vaginalis. More often, protozoa have a parasitic stage that evolves into an infective stage, a cyst, which is responsible for transmitting the infection into the new host; an example is Entamoeba histolytica. For still other protozoa vectors, usually arthropods, are responsible for their passage from one host to another, such as Leishmania. Some protozoa have intermediate hosts (the host where the asexual development of the parasite occurs) and a definitive host (where the sexual development takes place), for example, Plasmodium, the agent of human malaria. A mosquito is the definitive host; humans are the intermediate hosts. The reverse is the most common phenomenon, however: the vertebrate is usually the definitive host and the invertebrate the intermediate host (2).

Worms may have even more complicated life cycles. A worm may shed eggs or larvae, which are, or become, infective for another host, for example, Enterobius, Ascaris, or Strongyloides; or a worm may shed an egg or a larva which enters an intermediate host where it evolves to be infective, for example, Taenia or Angiostrongylus. Often, helminths may require more than one intermediate host, making the passage from one host to another even more difficult.

Parasites use humans as their home for adult stages (definitive hosts) and for larval stages (intermediate host). Larval stages usually occur in the tissues, and humans behave as if they were their natural intermediate hosts (cysticercus of Taenia solium), or as an unnatural intermediate host where the parasite grows in a disorganized manner (hydatid cyst of Echinococcus multilocularis); the latter situation usually results in greater damage to the host.

Parasites enter their hosts by many routes. The oral route is the most common and expeditious, but respiratory, dermal, and other routes are also used. Each parasite has its own manner of entering its appropriate host. After a parasite enters the host there is a period between the time of entry and the clinical manifestations of the infection, the incubation period. The duration varies and sometimes is measured in years; the incubation period is different from the prepatent period, which is the period between entry of the parasite and the production of other stages (such as eggs, larvae, or microfilariae). Often, the incubation and the prepatent period are identical. Patent period (or patency) is the entire period during which the parasite produces eggs, larvae, or microfilariae, stages that usually are diagnostic of a particular infection.

DIAGNOSIS

The diagnosis of parasitic infections in the clinical laboratory is based mostly on finding and identifying the parasite or its stages shed in the host such as cysts, eggs, larvae, or microfilariae (3). Often the eggs shed by one parasite are morphologically indistinguishable from those of a related species, and specific identification is not possible (2); only a generic identification should be made.

Most parasites elicit an immune response from the host, the strength of the response usually depends on how much contact with the host tissues takes place. Intestinal parasites (in the lumen) usually elicit little or no response, for example, Enterobius vermicularis. Parasites on the mucosal surface may elicit some form of immunity, such as Giardia lamblia and perhaps Cryptosporidium, because after the first infection has produced disease, subsequent infections generally do not. Parasites in the tissues may also elicit both cellular and humoral immune responses from the host, which are sometimes responsible for modulation of the disease, as in cutaneous leishmania.

The humoral responses are useful because specific antibodies against a parasitic stage hidden in the tissues are detectable, a useful diagnostic technique. This is especially true when obtaining the parasite for diagnosis is difficult or impossible. Metabolic substances produced by the parasite, or body components (antigens), may also be detected with specific tests to determine the presence of a parasite. Most serologic tests used in the parasitology laboratory are expensive, even widely available ones produced by commercial houses, and their use for diagnosis is generally outside the capability of routine clinical diagnostic laboratories. Serologic tests have wider applications in research, especially in the field of seroepidemiology, and most have not been evaluated properly against the standard parasitologic techniques (3).

Serologic diagnosis, such as detection of antibodies in serum, or detection of parasitic antigens in stool samples has been advocated for some intestinal parasites, such as Giardia lamblia. Evaluation of the effectiveness of these tests has always ignored the principle that, when a stool sample is studied under the microscope the microscopist is looking not only for the pathogen suspected by the clinician but for many other pathogens that could explain the clinical picture of the patient. In the laboratory study of samples for parasites is always a search for one of several possibilities, possibilities that the specific serologic test ignores (3).

The principles and the samples required for detection of parasites in different samples are described in Chapters 54 through 64; the morphologic characteristics of the parasites are described in Chapters 49 through 53, together with a discussion on the pathogenicity, the clinical manifestations, and the life cycle of the parasite in question. In Chapters 49 through 53 the discussion of human parasites is organized, grouping the protozoa and helminths by their occurrence either in the intestine or the tissues. No phylogenetic classification was followed in those chapters, but it will be discussed briefly here.

CLASSIFICATION

All the species found in humans as parasites belong to one of three groups of the animal kingdom: protozoa, helminths (worms), and arthropods.

Protozoa

The protozoa of medical importance belong to five groups.

1. Flagellates: Flagellates are characterized by one or more flagella in their body. They belong to several families with many genera and species that parasitize the oral cavity, the intestine, the vagina, and tissues. Many flagellates are commensal; others produce important diseases. Most flagellates have direct life cycles; others use arthropod vectors for passage from one host to the next.

2. Amebae: Amebae are single-celled organisms characterized by locomotion by means of pseudopods. The life cycles are direct, either by passage of a trophozoite to the next host, or more commonly by formation of a cystic stage responsible for transmission. Several genera contain the many species that infect humans, both as nonpathogenic and pathogenic organisms, in the oral cavity, the intestine, and the tissues. In the intestine Entamoeba histolytica is the most important; in the tissues, Acanthamoeba, Leptomyxid, and Naegleria produce important diseases.

3. Apicomplexa: Apicomplexa organisms have intracellular stages at some point in their life cycle. They have sexual development, and many members have life cycles involving intermediate hosts. The Apicomplexa has many families, genera, and species producing some of the most important parasitic infections of humans, such as malaria, trypanosomiasis, and leishmaniasis. Apicomplexa organisms produce important morbidity in persons with acquired immunodeficiency syndrome, because many of the organisms are opportunistic. The main representatives of the Apicomplexa are Cryptosporidium, Isospora, Toxoplasma, Plasmodium, and Babesia.

4. Microspora: Microspora are mostly parasites of invertebrates, though a few occur in vertebrates. They are minute intracellular organisms that form spores. At least one, Enterocytozoon, which occurs in the intestine, will be studied here. Pneumocystis has features akin to those of the Microspora, but also to the fungi, and is classified as inserta sedis (uncertain place). The true nature of Pneumocystis appears to be fungal.

5. Ciliates: Only one species of ciliated organisms is found in humans: Balantidium coli, in the large intestine.

Helminths

The helminths are generally subdivided into roundworms (nematodes) and flatworms (platyhelminths). For general purposes, nematodes are characterized by having a cylindrical body and a body cavity referred to as the pseudocoelom or pseudocele. In turn the platyhelminths are classified in two groups: trematodes and cestodes.

Nematodes

The main groups of nematodes with parasitic forms in humans studied in the following chapters are these:

1. Rhabditida: The Rhabditida are minute forms characterized by a free-living existence; some species have a parasitic phase, for example, Strongyloides stercoralis.
2. Strongylida: Male members of the Strongylida have a bursa at the posterior end, and the organisms are known generally as hookworms. The genera Ancy-

lostoma, Necator, Trichostrongylus, and Angiostrongylus have one or more species that is parasitic in the intestine or the tissues of humans.
3. Oxyurida: Oxyurida has one species that is parasitic in humans, Enterobius vermicularis. Members of this group have an esophagus with a bulb, the eggs embryonate in uterus and often are flattened on one side.
4. Ascaridia: Ascaridia comprises a large group of nematodes parasitic of humans and animals, with many genera and species. They are characterized by three lips with lateral papillae. The superfamily Ascaridoidea, characterized by generally large worms, comprises the genera Ascaris, Toxocara, Anisakis, and others of less importance that parasitize humans.
5. Spirurida: Spirurida account for the largest number of parasitic nematodes of humans. Most require in their life cycle an arthropod intermediate host. The most important group in the Spirurida is the filarial worms, which belong to several genera, for example, Wuchereria, Brugia, Loa, Onchocerca, Dirofilaria and Mansonella, one or more species of which infect humans.
6. Trichuroidea: Trichuroidea has forms parasitic in several organs: intestines, lungs, and other viscera. Three genera, Trichinella, Trichuris, and Capillaria, have species that are parasitic in humans.

Trematodes

The trematodes, or flukes, are flatworms characterized by an unsegmented body measuring a few millimeters to 6 or 8 centimeters. All trematodes are parasitic, and different species inhabit every tissue and organ systems of the human body. The adult worms are hermaphroditic and lay eggs in the tissues or inside the hollow viscera, to be evacuated into the environment. In the environment, the eggs of trematodes are ingested by a snail or release larvae that enter a snail, where some develop to be infective; others require a second host to become infective. Because the snail is always required for development, trematodes are known as snail-transmitted helminths.

Trematodes occur almost worldwide, but their distribution is patchy. Some trematodes produce benign infections; others, infections that are major public health problems in the world, such as schistosomiasis.

The classification of the Trematoda is complicated. For our purposes, the Digenea comprise all the parasitic forms in humans. Members of the Digenea are endoparasites (live inside the body) and are characterized by one or more suckers used for attachment. The genera important in human medicine are Fasciola, Clonorchis, Opisthorchis, Dicrocoelium, Fasciolopsis, Paragonimus, and Schistosoma. The schistosomes, the most important group, are not hermaphroditic; they have two separate sexes.

Cestodes

The cestodes or tapeworms have a head, the scolex, followed by a body, the strobila, composed of segments called proglottids. The size of the strobila varies from a few millimeters to 10 meters, depending on the species. Thus, the number of segments varies from as few as three to several hundreds.

Behind the scolex, tapeworms have a neck region composed of cells that divide continuously to produce new proglottids. The new proglottids are immature at first; as they progress backward (with the formation of new ones), the proglottids become mature: each has a set of female and or male reproductive organs. Mature proglottids begin producing eggs, which usually are stored in the uterus. As the proglottids move toward the posterior end of the worm they become gravid. Some tapeworms lay eggs, but most depend on the proglottids breaking from the strobila to release the eggs. Some groups of tapeworms are characterized by a double set of sexual organs, two male and two female.

The scolex of tapeworms has certain organs for attachment of the parasite. Some have two longitudinal grooves, the bothria. This structure is useful for placing certain tapeworms in the group known as pseudophyllidian. Others have suckers and may also have a rostellum with one or more rows of hooks. These are the cyclophyllidian. The absence or presence of the rostellum, and the number, size, and shape of the hooks are all characteristics used for classification of cestodes.

The classification of cestodes is complicated, mainly because the life cycle of many tapeworms is not known. The medically important genera of the Cyclophyllidea are Taenia, Hymenolepis, Dipylidium, and Echinococcus, and of the Pseudophyllidea, Diphyllobothrium and Spirometra.

REFERENCES

1. Gutierrez Y: Diagnostic Pathology of Parasitic Infections with Clinical Correlations. Philadelphia, Lea & Febiger, 1990.
2. Beaver PC, Jung RC, and Capp EW: Clinical Parasitology. 9th ed. Philadelphia, Lea & Febiger, 1984.
3. Gutierrez Y, and Little MD (eds): Diagnostic of important parasitic diseases. Clin Lab Med, 11:811, 1991.

Chapter 49

INTESTINAL, ORAL, AND VAGINAL PROTOZOA

The protozoa that inhabit the intestine, the oral cavity, and the vagina belong to the flagellates, amebae, ciliates, coccidia (Apicomplexa), and microspora. Different species of each of these groups produce significant morbidity and mortality, both in developed and underdeveloped areas of the world.

The life cycle of protozoa that infect the intestinal, oral, or vaginal cavity is direct (with one exception, Sarcocystis). Most of the intestinal protozoa use the fecal-oral route for transmission, making them common infections in developing areas of the world and in homosexual males in developed areas. Moreover, Cryptosporidium, Isospora, and some members of the Microspora produce opportunistic infections in persons with acquired immunodeficiency syndrome (AIDS).

In general, the diagnosis of infections produced by intestinal protozoa is made with stool samples; those produced by vaginal protozoa, in vaginal and cervical smears. Seldom is a biopsy specimen required for diagnosis of these infections (1), and serologic tests generally have not been fully evaluated or play little role in their diagnosis in the routine laboratory (2,3). For convenience, in this chapter we discuss the common organisms occurring in the intestine and the oral and vaginal cavity, grouped phylogenetically, and stress the species that are pathogenic in humans.

FLAGELLATES

The flagellates of the intestinal, oral, and vaginal cavities are Giardia lamblia, Dientamoeba fragilis, Trichomonas vaginalis, Trichomonas hominis, Trichomonas tenax, Chilomastix mesnili, Enteromonas hominis, and Retortamonas intestinalis. Of these, Giardia lamblia and Trichomonas vaginalis are pathogens; Dientamoeba fragilis is suspected to be a pathogen, and the others are not pathogenic. Knowledge of each one is necessary if accurate identification is to be made in the clinical laboratory (2,3).

Giardia lamblia

Giardia lamblia is the most common parasite in the United States. It was identified in 4% of all stool samples submitted to state health laboratories in 1978 (4), a figure that climbed to about 7% in recent years, indicating an increase in the prevalence of Giardia in the United States. In developing areas of the world Giardia is even more common, with rates of infection of up to 100% in 2-year-olds living in orphanages (5).

Giardia lamblia is easily transmitted, as only a small number of organisms is necessary to produce infection in humans (6). Infants are often affected in endemic areas, where Giardia is the earliest acquired intestinal protozoan infection. Because of the easy transmissibility, outbreaks of giardiasis are common in developed and underdeveloped areas. Outbreaks usually are associated with water systems in municipalities with access to clean water (7) that requires no sedimentation, the first step of water treatment and the one that eliminates the cysts of Giardia. Chlorination does not affect the parasite. The presence of Giardia cysts in municipal water systems has been traced to contamination with feces from beavers and other animals. Giardia has low host specificity, and many animals are commonly infected (7).

The life cycle of Giardia is similar to that of other intestinal protozoans: a flagellated trophozoite (the vegetative form) inhabits the duodenum, where it multiplies by binary fission (Fig. 49–1A). At some point trophozoites develop into cysts that are resistant to the adverse conditions of extracorporeal environment; these stages are capable of producing a new infection when they are ingested by a susceptible host.

The trophozoite (Fig. 49–1B) of Giardia is pear shaped, 10 to 20 μm long, flattened dorsoventrally, with two nuclei on the anterior aspect. On the ventral surface a suction disc occupies the anterior half of the body; it is used to attach to the surface of the epithelial cells of the duodenum. The flagella are paired: two pairs extend laterally, one pair posteriorly, and one pair ventrally. Other structures are less important for diagnostic purposes. The general appearance of the trophozoite of Giardia is that of a symmetric organism with two halves that are mirror images. The cyst of Giardia (Fig. 49–1C) is oval, 8 to 13 μm in largest dimension, with a thin, translucent wall. The organism often is retracted from the wall, leaving a clear space between the cytoplasm of the organism and the wall. In stained preparations the cyst has four nuclei, usually at one of the poles, and remnants of other organelles. Mature cysts have rests of flagella (8).

Infections by Giardia in susceptible hosts usually result in disease. In underdeveloped areas, the symptoms occur mainly in infants and children, who are the susceptible hosts; after the initial bout with the disease, they develop some form of resistance to later infections, which consequently are asymptomatic. In developed countries where the prevalence of the infection is low, persons of all ages are susceptible and the disease is found both in children and adults (1).

The main symptom of giardiasis is diarrhea: bulky, foamy stools with undigested food and a pungent odor. The symptoms may persist, especially in children, sometimes progressing to a spruelike (malabsorption) disease,

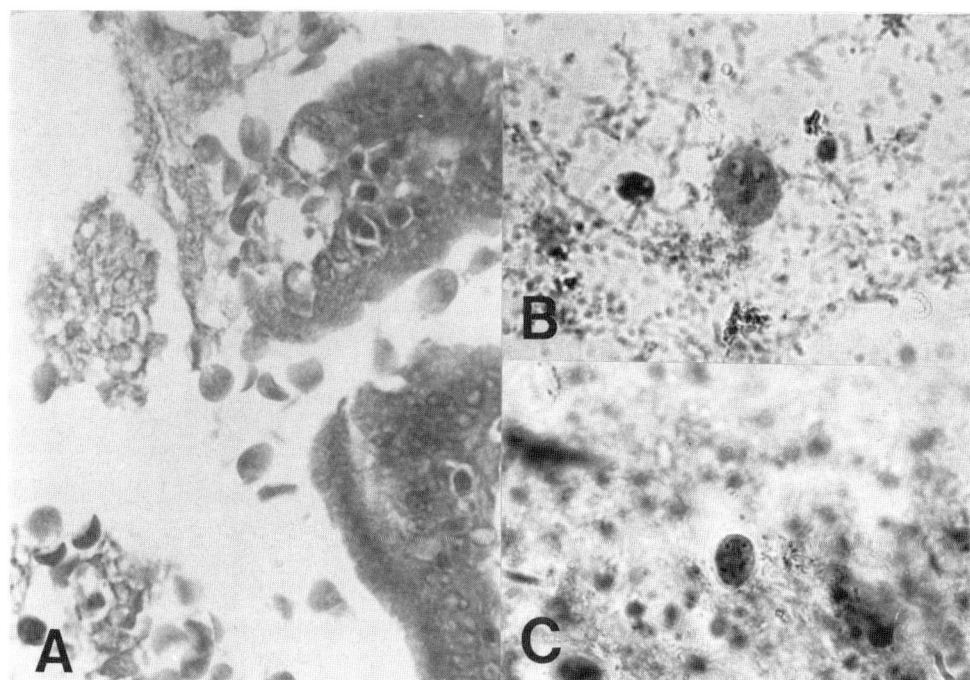

Fig. 49–1. Giardia lamblia. A, Section of duodenum, hematoxylin and eosin stain, shows numerous Giardia trophozoites in the lumen. Different shapes of the organism are due to different sectioning planes (hematoxylin and eosin, ×705). B, trophozoite and C, Cyst in human stool (trichrome, ×1120).

often when an impairment of IgA is associated. In adults, giardiasis often resembles peptic ulcer. The exact mechanism by which Giardia produces symptoms is unknown.

The diagnosis of giardiasis is made by the clinical laboratory on stool samples (2) examined with the microscope both in wet and stained preparations (Chapter 59); trophozoites and cysts are easily detected in wet preparations, because of their characteristic shape. Often, the sample is received in the laboratory with a clinical diagnosis of giardiasis; in these instances, if the parasites are found and identified in wet mounts, it is unnecessary to do other tests. Negative samples should be concentrated (Chapter 59); if negative, they should be stained with trichrome stain for examination and to keep a permanent record in the laboratory (2).

The diagnosis of giardiasis is commonly made on the first stool sample received in the laboratory (9); if the first sample is negative and the clinical impression of giardiasis persists, other stool samples should be taken at intervals of 2 or 3 days and carefully examined (10). If additional stool samples are negative, the procedure should be repeated after 10 to 14 days. Elimination of Giardia cysts is cyclic: periods when no parasites are detectable in the feces alternating with periods of abundant elimination of trophozoites and cysts (11).

The few cases of giardiasis that have been difficult to diagnose have prompted the recommendation—and, in some places, the adoption—of techniques such as the duodenal aspirate and the string test (Chapter 59), but neither has proven superior to a good stool examination (12). Antigen detection in stools using enzyme-linked immunosorbent assay (ELISA) (13), immunofluorescent stain, and indirect immunofluorescent serologic tests also have been described for diagnosis of giardiasis. These tests give good results but are expensive; their value for examination of samples received sporadically for diagnosis of giardiasis remains doubtful (2,14)

Dientamoeba fragilis

Dientamoeba fragilis was classified as a nonpathogenic ameba until 1967, when its flagellate nature was established (15). In recent years a number of reports have tried to establish an association between infections with Dientamoeba and diarrhea (16). The association seems real, but the causal relationship between the parasite and the disease is largely unconfirmed. Dientamoeba has a worldwide distribution, but even in underdeveloped areas the prevalence is not high.

The life cycle of the parasite is unknown (8). In the large intestine of humans Dientamoeba is ameboid, without flagella, 9 to 12 μm, with two nuclei consisting of a thin, invisible nuclear membrane and a cluster of four to eight small chromatin granules (Fig. 49–2). A cystic stage is unknown, and thus often it is said that transmission is through ingestion of trophozoites. The morphology of Dientamoeba in humans is similar to that of some parasitic protozoa of animals. These protozoa have a flagellate stage, and a trophozoite transmitted in nematode eggs (8).

Because of the possible association between infection with Dientamoeba and symptoms in humans, findings of Dientamoeba in stool samples from persons with diarrhea should be reported. Careful differentiation of the parasite from other amebae should be made (3).

Trichomonas vaginalis

Trichomonas vaginalis is a flagellate that occurs naturally in the lumen of the vagina, urethra, and prostate gland. Transmission is through sexual contact, though

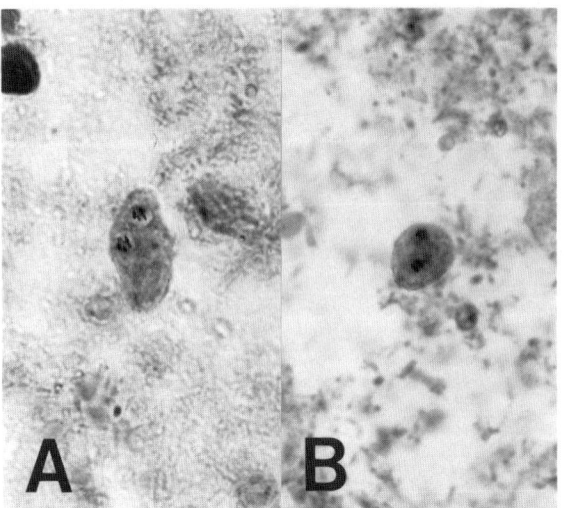

Fig. 49–2. Dientamoeba fragilis trophozoites in human stool (trichrome, ×1120).

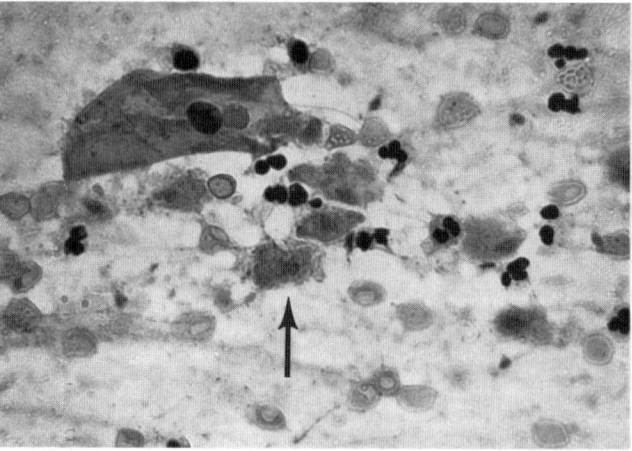

Fig. 49–3. Trichomonas vaginalis in cervical smear. The parasite (*arrow*) looks like a mass with few internal structures, (Papanicolaou stain, ×1120).

other forms of transmission, such as fomites, especially in young girls, have been documented.

Trichomonas vaginalis is a worldwide infection more commonly diagnosed in women; in routine gynecologic practice about 3% of healthy women harbor the parasite. The incubation period of the disease varies between 4 and 28 days, when symptoms of mild to marked vaginitis begin. Sometimes vulvitis is present, with erythema of the inguinal area. A frothy, greenish vaginal discharge, sometimes purulent and abundant, accompanied by dysuria and pruritus, is a common source of consultation. These symptoms are often sufficient for diagnosis and treatment (17).

Trichomoniasis is not recognized as often in men as in women. Men with trichomoniasis have a chronic urethral discharge, nongonococcal, consisting of white, milky fluid, usually lasting 4 weeks or more. The duration of the discharge is characteristic, since 98% of nongonococcal urethritis does not last this long (18).

In both men and women the parasites are found in the discharge, as motile flagellates in fresh preparations. The diagnosis is usually made by the examining physician, or in vaginal smears stained with Papanicolaou stain (Chapter 61) (1). Trichomonas vaginalis organisms in wet smears of cervical mucus are motile and highly refractile. In preparations studied with oil immersion the flagella are in constant motion, the undulating membrane moving at a slower pace than the flagella. In stained preparations the anatomy of the parasite is better observed, especially if stained with iron-hematoxylin. In smears stained with Papanicolaou stain, Trichomonas organisms stain poorly and appear as rounded or oval masses of cytoplasmic material with a faint nucleus (1). Flagella and other structures are not readily visible (Fig. 49–3).

Nonpathogenic flagellates

The nonpathogenic flagellates of the large intestine of humans are Trichomonas hominis, Chilomastix mesnili, Enteromonas hominis, and Retortamonas intestinales. Of these, Trichomonas hominis has no cystic stage and transmission occurs via the trophozoite; the others have cysts in their life cycle. Each of these species of flagellates has a typical morphology, knowledge of which is required to distinguish them from the pathogenic flagellates. These morphologic characteristics are found in standard books of parasitology (8) and are not discussed here.

AMEBAE

The order Amoebida has many organisms classified into many genera; they live as free-living organisms, as parasites, or both. The parasitic amebae of humans inhabit the intestine, the oral cavity, the respiratory tract, and the tissues. Those occurring in the intestine and the oral cavity are discussed here; the others in Chapter 51.

Three genera—Entamoeba, Endolimax, and Iodamoeba—have several species that are parasitic in humans. Most are characterized by a naked protoplast, a distinct nucleus (Fig. 49–4), and a life cycle that generally involves two stages: the trophozoite and the cyst. The genus Entamoeba has several species: Entamoeba histolytica, En-

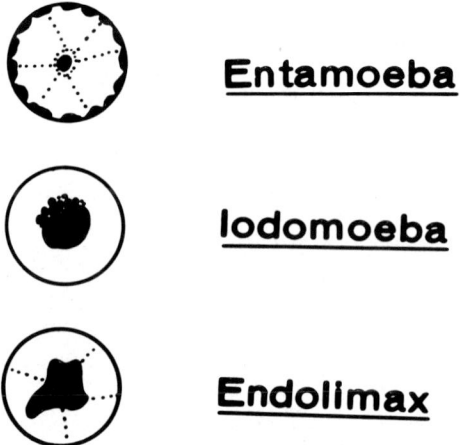

Fig. 49–4. Diagrams of the characteristic nuclear morphology of each genus of Amebae.

tamoeba coli (Fig. 49–5A–D), Entamoeba hartmanni (Fig. 49–5E–H), Entamoeba polecki, and Entamoeba gingivalis. Endolimax and Iodamoeba have only one species each in man: Endolimax nana (Fig. 49–5M–P) and Iodamoeba buetschlii (Fig. 49–5I–L). Of these species, Entamoeba histolytica is the only potential pathogen; Entamoeba gingivalis is the only one that occurs in the oral cavity and the only one that has no cystic stage.

Entamoeba histolytica

Entamoeba histolytica is an inhabitant of the large intestine that is responsible for significant morbidity and mortality worldwide. It has been estimated that in 1981 490 million people were infected with E. histolytica in the world, of whom 36 million developed amebic abscess or colitis, and at least 40,000 died (19). The majority of the infections produced by E. histolytica occur in tropical areas and, to a lesser degree, in the subtropics. In the tropics, prevalence of 50 to 60%, depending upon the socioeconomic status of the community, is not infrequent. In the United States, E. histolytica is endemic, especially in the southeastern part of the country; rates of prevalence are unknown but generally are low. Transmission of the infection is through the fecal-oral route, which explains its higher incidence in lower socioeconomic groups. In developed countries rates of infection among homosexual males (20,21) are similar to those in less developed countries. E. histolytica plays a small role as a pathogen in persons with AIDS. Outbreaks through contaminated water are not unusual.

The life cycle of Entamoeba histolytica is similar to the life cycle of other intestinal amebae of humans: a trophozoite living in the large intestine, usually on the mucous layer of the colon, reproduces by binary fission to maintain large colonies of the parasite. Trophozoites form cysts, probably while transported with the colonic contents, and are evacuated with the feces. In the environment, the cyst is resistant to adverse conditions and initiates a new infection after being ingested by a susceptible host (1).

Entamoeba histolytica is considered a pathogen by some; however, the biologic characteristics of the parasite are those of a commensal ameba that under certain conditions is associated with colitis, but the true nature of such an association is still unknown (1). It is well-established that many persons have asymptomatic E. histolytica infection and pass cysts with formed stools and nonhematophagous trophozoites with semiformed or diarrheal stools. A few persons infected with E. histolytica have mucosal ulcerations that contain amebae, have colitis, and pass hematophagous trophozoites in their stools. It is also well-

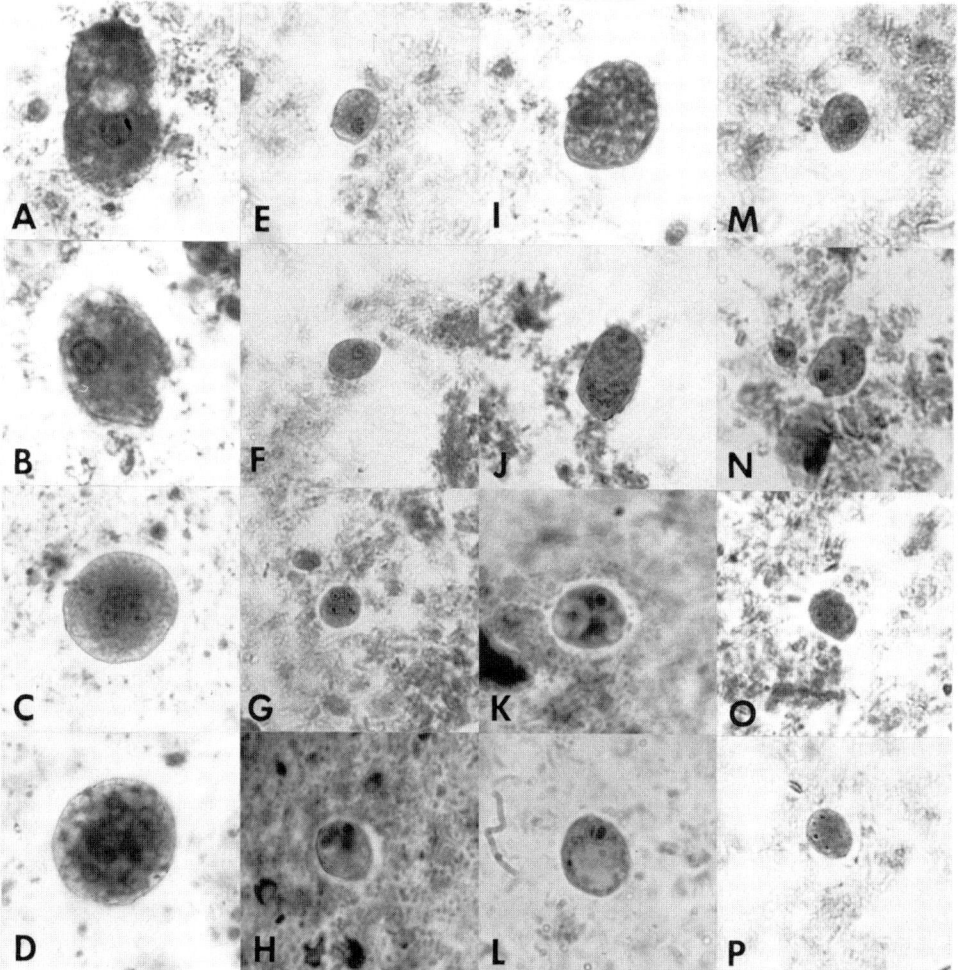

Fig. 49–5. Nonpathogenic ameba trophozoites and cysts in human stool (trichrome stain ×1120). Entamoeba coli trophozoites, A, B, and Cysts, C, D. E. hartmanni trophozoites, E, F, and Cysts, G, H. Iodamoeba buetschlii trophozoites, I, J, and Cysts, K, L. Endolimax nana trophozoites, M, N, and Cysts, O, P.

established that colitis is due to other causes and that finding E. histolytica in some of these persons may be coincidental (1). In general two types of amebiasis are distinguished in humans: intestinal and extraintestinal.

Intestinal amebiasis. The clinical manifestations of intestinal amebiasis vary, probably with the strain of the parasite, the susceptibility of the individual, and the existence in the colon of lesions due to other causes. Most infections with Entamoeba histolytica are asymptomatic, but some people develop symptoms between 1 and 3 weeks after infection, slowly or suddenly; abdominal pain and diarrhea may progress to dysentery, characterized by many liquid bowel movements containing blood and mucus. Abdominal pain and tenderness, especially in the right iliac fossa, as well as enlargement of liver, are common physical findings. Some individuals have a more pronounced and rapid clinical disease with toxic symptoms, perforation, peritonitis, and temperatures of 39 to 40° C. These patients usually have marked ulceration of the colon, and their mortality rate is high in spite of specific therapy (22).

Gross examination of the colon of persons infected with Entamoeba histolytica reveals ulcerations that vary in size from a few millimeters to almost complete destruction of the mucosa and submucosa. Microscopically, the ulcers are superficial at first (Fig. 49–6B), then go deeper, usually

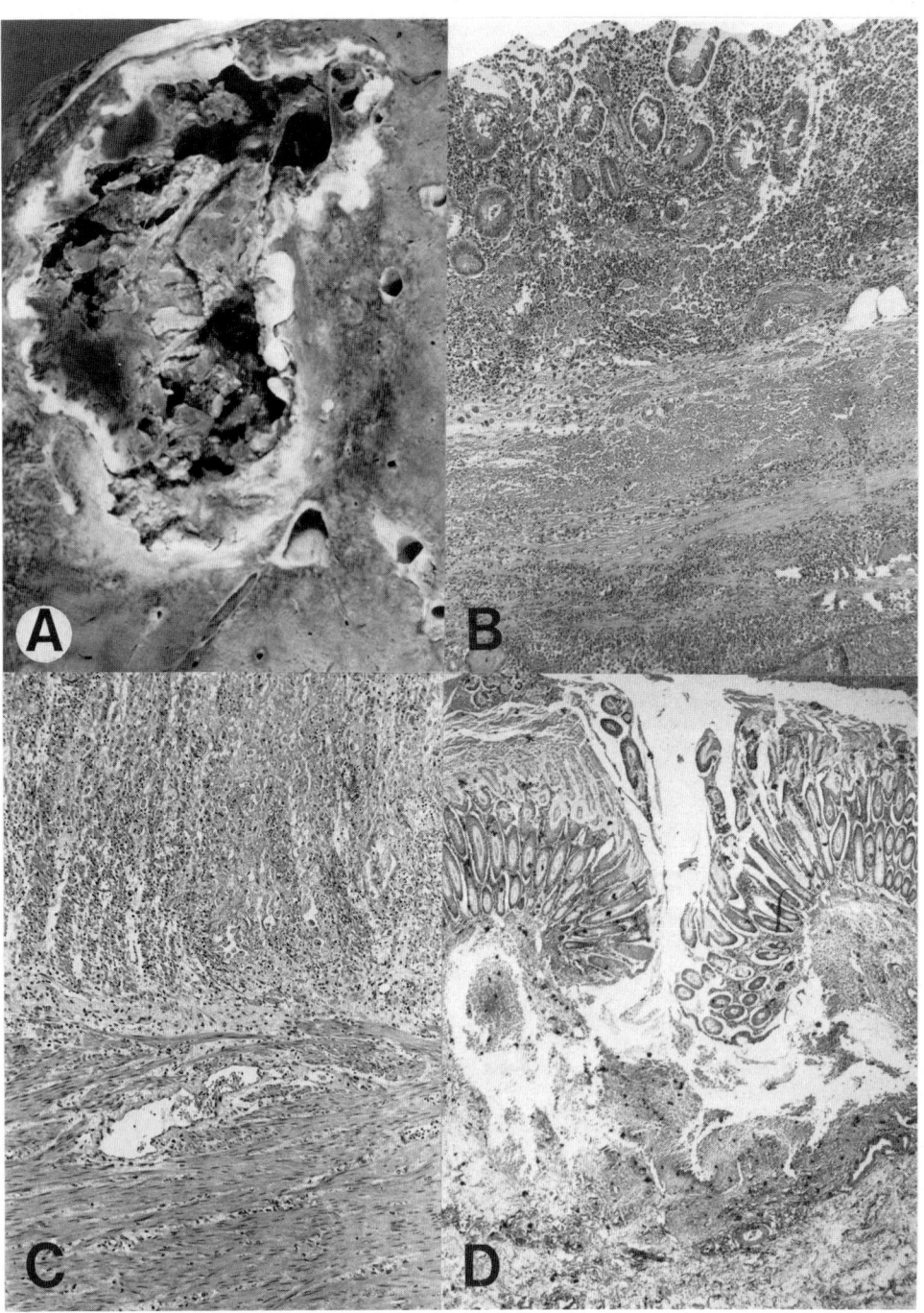

Fig. 49–6. Entamoeba histolytica. *A,* Amebic liver abscess. The central necrotic cavity and thickened wall indicate the abscess has been present for some time. *B,* Section of appendix shows parasites down to the muscular layer (hematoxylin and eosin, ×70). *C,* Marked destruction of the muscle layer. Note the infiltrate (×70). *D,* Typical flask-shape ulceration in colon (×22).

down to the muscle layers (Fig. 49–6D), but in some patients with marked disease the entire colonic wall is infiltrated by parasites and inflammatory cells (Fig. 49–6C), often with perforation and peritonitis. The inflammatory infiltrate consists mainly of polymorphonuclear cells (1).

Extraintestinal amebiasis. From foci in the colonic wall amebae can travel through the vascular system to distant organs to produce abscesses (1). The liver is the main organ affected (Fig. 49–6A), where amebic abscess produces high rates of morbidity and mortality; the abscesses are usually single, more common in the right lobe (6:1), more often in males than in females, and are usually fatal in children younger than 5 years. A person with an amebic liver abscess has right-side upper quadrant pain and tenderness, a palpable liver, and often fever, and appears acutely ill. The diagnosis is sometimes made clinically, and the abscess is often visualized on x-ray films. Confirmation of the diagnosis is done in the laboratory by finding the parasites in aspirated fluid or in biopsy specimens (Chapter 60) (1). Serologic tests produce nonspecific results (3).

The finding of amebic lesions in other organs is a less frequent occurrence, though many organs can be affected, including the brain; the lungs, heart, pleurae, and peritoneal cavity often are involved from extension of an abscess in the liver. Infections in the skin and the genitals are important because the diagnosis can be confirmed on scrapings and smears taken and examined in the clinical laboratory (Fig. 49–7A) (Chapters 61 and 62).

The diagnosis of amebiasis is based on the identification of the parasites in stool samples, smears of cutaneous or cervical lesions, and material aspirated from other organ lesions (3). When these samples are studied either fresh or stained the morphology of the parasites is characteristic. The trophozoites of Entamoeba histolytica have rounded, hyaline pseudopods, are 15 to 25 μm in diameter, and have numerous vacuoles containing bacteria and other debris. The nucleus is 4 to 5 μm in diameter with a membrane with small, uniform granules of chromatin attached to its inner surface. A small, eccentric karyosome is readily visible. In fresh preparations movement is sluggish and unidirectional. This trophozoite is found in the stool of most persons who have no symptoms (Fig. 49–7E); in those with symptoms of amebiasis a hematophagous trophozoite, so named because it has digestive vacuoles with red blood cells, is more common. The hematophagous trophozoites (Fig. 49–7B–D) are up to 50 μm, and display faster directional movement in fresh preparations (3).

The cysts of Entamoeba histolytica are rounded, have a distinct wall and as many as four nuclei, depending on the degree of maturation, nuclei which are identical to the nucleus of the trophozoite. Some cysts have elongated chromatoid bodies with rounded ends (Fig. 49–7G); others may have a large vacuole filled with glycogen (Fig. 49–7F). The cysts are readily seen in fresh preparations with saline as refractile hyaline bodies, and depending upon proper microscopic illumination, the nuclei and chromatoid bodies can be discerned. Wet mounts stained with iodine show these morphologic characteristics better, staining the glycogen vacuole, when present, a deep mahogany. In smears stained with trichome stain the nuclear chromatin stains dark, the chromatoid bodies red, and the vacuole filled with glycogen appears as an empty space (Fig. 49–7F) because the glycogen is dissolved and lost during the staining procedure (3).

CILIATES

The only ciliated organism found in humans in Balantidium coli, which is widely distributed in the tropics and subtropics. Infections are common in certain parts of the world, with prevalence rates of 28% (23). In the United

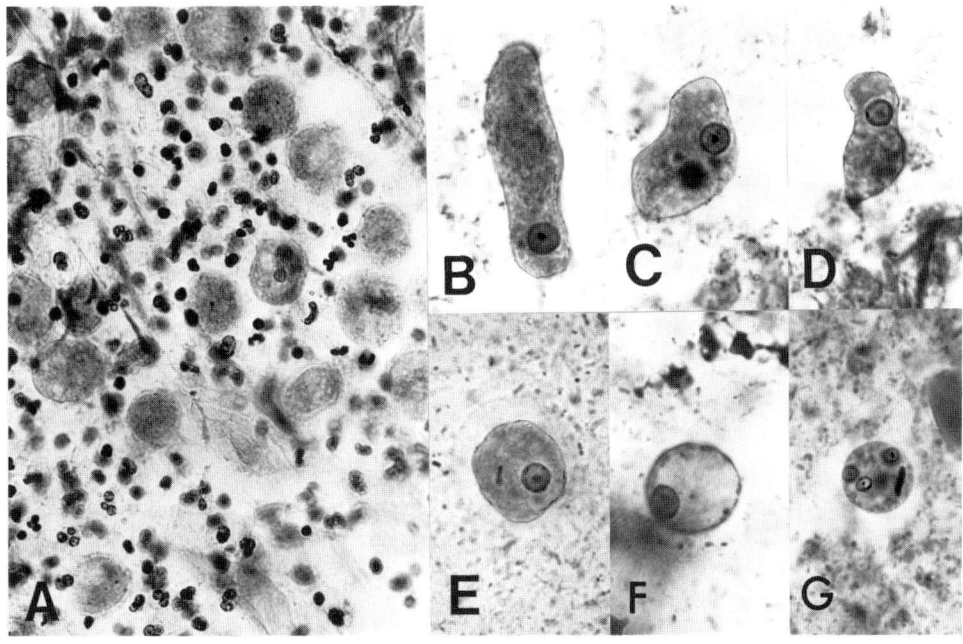

Fig. 49–7. Entamoeba histolytica. *A,* Numerous trophozoites in cervical smear (Papanicolaou stain, ×600). Human stools stained with trichrome exhibit *B–D,* hematophagous trophozoites, *E,* trophozoite in formed stool. (Compare the size of this trophozoite with that of the hematophagous trophozoites); *F,* immature cyst showing a glycogen vacuole; and *G,* mature cyst showing three nuclei and a chromatoid body (×1120).

States Balantidium is seen sporadically, especially in the southern states (24).

The life cycle of Balantidium coli has two stages: a trophozoite and a cyst. The trophozoite (Fig. 49–8B, C) is about 200 μm long and has numerous cilia covering the entire body that move in a wavelike pattern. In the anterior portion the trophozoite has a mouth that is seen as a funnel-like depression. The cytoplasm has a large bean-shaped nucleus (macronucleus) and, next to it, a smaller one (micronucleus). The cyst is spherical with a thick wall, averages 45 to 75 μm in diameter, and contains what resembles a small trophozoite with cilia, macro-, and micronucleus (Fig. 49–8D). The cysts are evacuated with the feces and produce infections in susceptible hosts once they are ingested (1).

Balantidium inhabits the lumen of the large intestine, often producing asymptomatic infections. In a few persons lesions in the mucosa accompanied by symptoms of dysentery may develop, symptoms that are clinically indistinguishable from those produced by Entamoeba histolytica and by other causes of colitis. The symptoms in milder infections are diarrhea and abdominal pain; in the dysenteric form the symptoms are more acute: many bowel movements per day, feces with blood and mucus, abdominal pain, and loss of weight. In a few instances a fulminant form may develop, and in others dissemination of the parasite to the abdominal cavity (due to intestinal perforation) and to other organs has been described (1).

The lesions produced in the colon by Balantidium are usually superficial ulcerations (Fig. 49–8A), but in some instances they extend deep into the submucosa. Microscopically, the ulcer is a shallow one that does not extend beyond the muscle layers. The organisms are easily identified in the ulcers.

The diagnosis of balantidiasis is usually made in stool samples (Chapter 59) examined in the clinical laboratory, where the typical trophozoites and the cysts are found and recognized by their morphologic characteristics (Fig. 49–8B–D).

APICOMPLEXA

The apicomplexan organisms found in the intestine of humans and animals are also known as coccidian, intracellular organisms with dual, asexual and sexual types of multiplication. Our knowledge about the intestinal coccidia of humans (Isospora and Sarcocystis) has been largely revised in recent years, and one new member, Cryptosporidium, has been added to the list of important pathogens.

Cryptosporidium parvum

The first human infections with Cryptosporidium were reported in 1976 in patients with chronic diarrhea (25,26). Since then, Cryptosporidium has been found to be a common agent of acute diarrhea in the general population, and of chronic diarrhea in persons with AIDS, in whom this parasite behaves as an opportunistic pathogen (27). The geographic distribution of Cryptosporidium is worldwide, but figures on its prevalence are lacking. It occurs often in infants in nurseries, where it is easily transmitted through the fecal-oral route.

The life cycle of Cryptosporidium is similar to that of other coccidian parasites. The oocysts are infective when evacuated with the feces; if they are ingested by a susceptible host, they free four sporozoites in the intestine. The sporozoites enter the cells of the intestine and locate in a parasitophorous vacuole in the brush border, where the sporozoites develop asexually to produce merozoites (Fig. 49–9A). The merozoites leave the cell to enter other cells and reinitiate the cycle. Some merozoites develop into male and female gametocytes, which join to produce an oocyst. Two types of oocysts are produced by Cryptosporidium: the thick-walled oocysts (80%), which resist adverse conditions of the environment and thus become

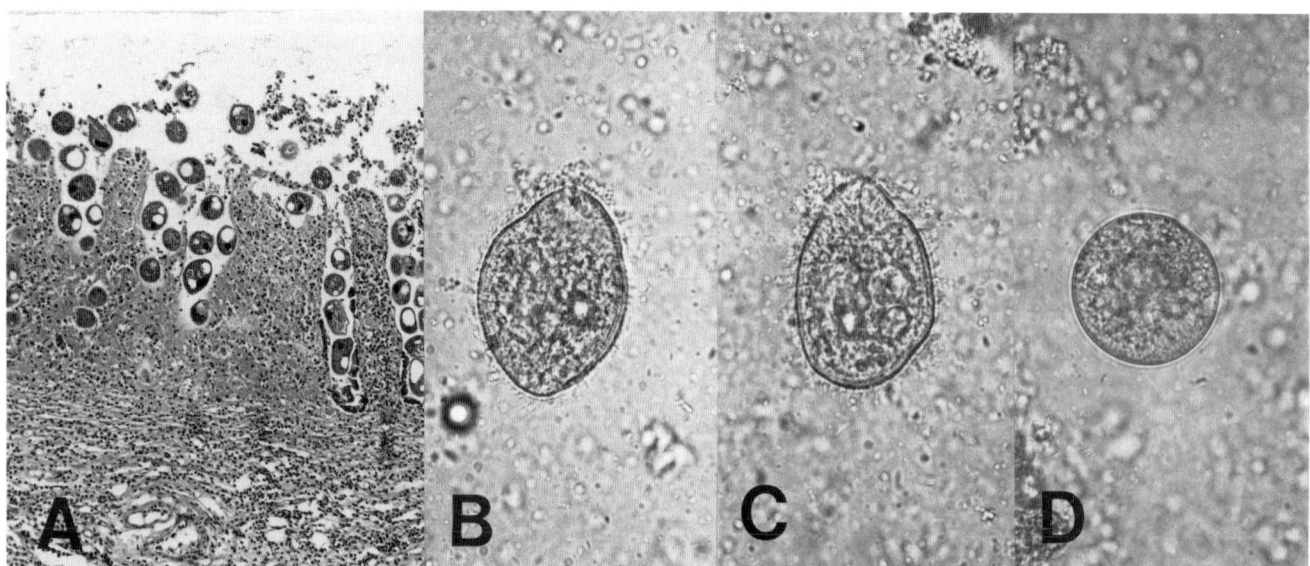

Fig. 49–8. Balantidium coli. A, Section of large intestine shows ulceration and numerous trophozoites in the mucosa (hematoxylin and eosin ×70). In unstained human stool, B, C, trophozoites, and D, a cyst are visible (×450).

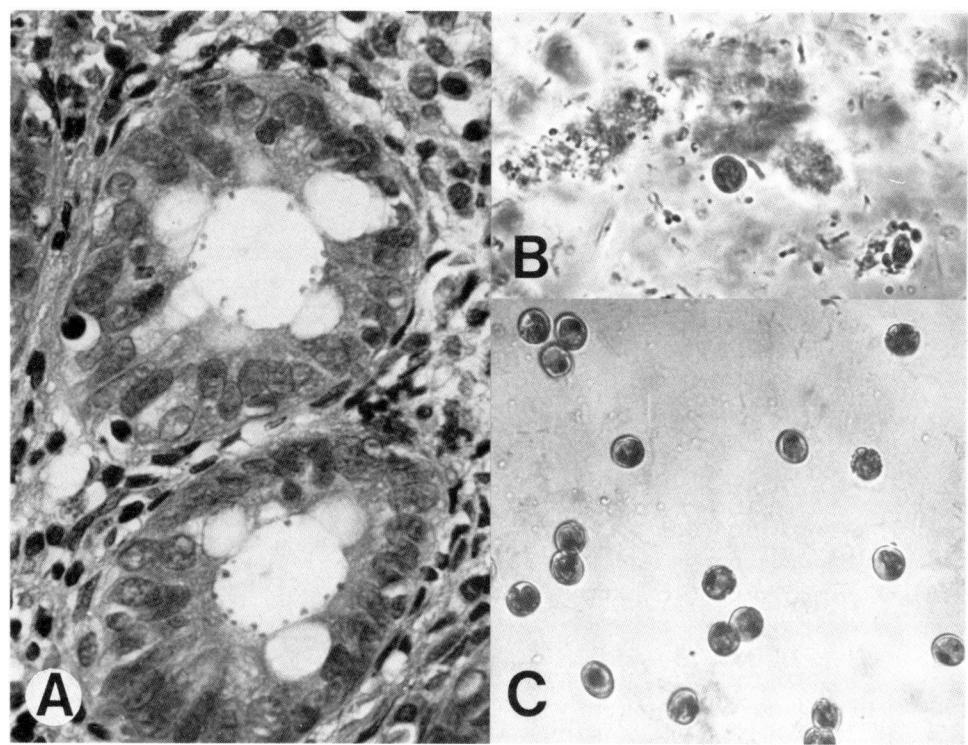

Fig. 49–9. Cryptosporidium. A, Section of rectal mucosa, hematoxylin and eosin stain, shows the parasites on top of the epithelial cells (×705). B, Oocyst in unstained human stool (×1120) and C, oocysts in human stool stained with modified AFB stain (×1120).

the infective stages, and the thin-walled oocysts (20%), which rupture in the intestine and free the sporozoites (autoinfection) to initiate asexual development. This last type of development appears to be unique to Cryptosporidium and is thought to be responsible for the chronicity of the infection in immunodeficient persons (27). The oocysts of Cryptosporidium (Fig. 49–9B, C) are about 4 μm in diameter, which makes their detection in stool samples and in tissues slightly more difficult.

The capacity of Cryptosporidium to produce symptoms is unquestionable, but the mechanism by which these symptoms are produced is unknown. In immunocompetent hosts, Cryptosporidium produces a self-limited infection that lasts about 2 weeks and is characterized by watery diarrhea, abdominal cramps, loss of appetite and of weight, borborygmus, flatulence, and sometimes a slight elevation of temperature (28). These symptoms usually peak 10 to 12 days after onset and are followed by complete resolution. Some persons stop passing the oocysts at the same time the symptoms disappear; others continue excreting oocysts in their feces for an indeterminate period, becoming healthy carriers of the parasite (29). The disease is common among travelers: Cryptosporidium is an important agent of travelers' diarrhea.

In immunodeficient persons the infection persists lifelong, especially because no effective therapy is available for Cryptosporidium; Cryptosporidium is an important cause of chronic diarrhea in persons with AIDS.

The histologic alterations of the intestinal tract of immunocompetent individuals infected with Cryptosporidium are unknown, except for the fact that the parasites are present in the brush border of the enterocytes (Fig. 49–9A). In persons with AIDS the mucosa varies from mostly normal to one with marked distortion of the normal architecture with abundant inflammatory infiltrate of mononuclear cells, crypt abscesses, and increased mitotic index (1).

The diagnosis of Cryptosporidium is made clinically, but it is confirmed in the laboratory by careful examination of the stools (27). The typical oocysts are easily identified in wet saline (Fig. 49–B) and iodine preparations made directly from the stool sample or from the stool concentrate; a modified acid-fast bacillus stain allows easy screening of the smears and recognition of the parasite (Fig. 49–9C) (Chapter 59) (27). Antigen may be detected in stool using an ELISA or an immunofluorescent stain, but this is expensive if the test is performed infrequently.

Isospora belli

Isospora belli has been known for many years as a cause of mild diarrhea worldwide, but it is infrequently diagnosed. In recent years Isospora has played a role as a producer of chronic diarrhea in persons with AIDS, in whom the parasite is an opportunistic infection (30).

Isospora belli occurs worldwide, more in developing countries because its transmission is related to fecal contamination of the environment, unlike Cryptosporidium, which uses the fecal-oral route. The life cycle of Isospora is much like that of Cryptosporidium, with these general exceptions: The parasite is located in the epithelial cells of the small intestine (Fig. 49–10A), not in the brush border; the oocyst is immature (unsporulated) at the time of its evacuation with the feces and requires a period of maturation in the environment; last, the oocyst in feces is 20 to 33 μm by 10 to 19 μm and contains only one sporoblast at the time of evacuation (Fig. 49–10A).

The mechanism by which Isospora produces symp-

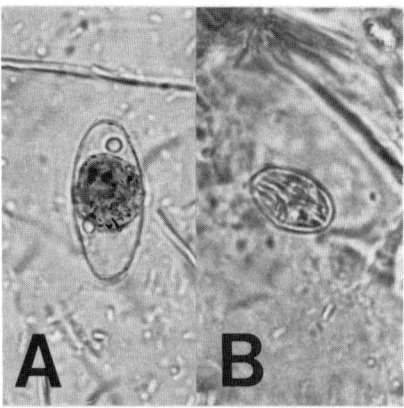

Fig. 49–10. *A*, Isospora belli and *B*, Sarcocystis oocysts in unstained human stools (×705).

toms—and the spectrum of the symptoms in humans—are unknown. It appears that most immunocompetent persons who become infected have no symptoms; others have mild diarrhea with abdominal discomfort and low-grade fever. In immunodeficient hosts Isospora produces chronic diarrhea with markedly increased symptoms, similar to those described above. In addition, steatorrhea similar to that of tropical sprue, enterocolitis, and nonspecific duodenitis may develop in some individuals leading to marked weight loss (31). Interestingly, peripheral eosinophilia of up to 25% may develop, making this coccidium one of the few protozoan infections that produces eosinophilia.

The diagnosis of Isospora is seldom suspected clinically. The parasite is found in stools in the laboratory, where identification of the oocyst (Fig. 49–10A) is easily made by the morphologic characteristics (Chapter 59).

Sarcocystis

The members of the genus Sarcocystis are coccidian parasites closely related to Toxoplasma (Chapter 51) because both have an intermediate host. In the definitive host (a carnivore) Sarcocystis organisms develop in the intestine, while in intermediate hosts they develop in the tissues. Sarcocystis is mostly an asymptomatic infection in humans.

Rates of prevalence for the two Sarcocystis infecting humans—Sarcocystis hominis and Sarcocystis suihominis—are not available, because before 1977 these two species were referred to as Isospora hominis (32,33). Both species have worldwide distribution.

The life cycle of Sarcocystis is initiated with the ingestion of uncooked or undercooked pork (Sarcocystis suihominis) or beef (Sarcocystis hominis). In the muscles of these animals the parasites form cysts (sarcocysts) which contain thousands of small bodies, the merozoites. Merozoites freed in the intestine enter a cell (not yet identified), located below the enterocytes in the lamina propria. Merozoites develop directly in these cells into the sexual gametocytes, which join to produce an oocyst, which develops two sporocysts, each with four sporozoites. The oocysts release the two sporulated (mature) sporocysts, which are evacuated with the feces. The infective sporocysts are ingested by the intermediate hosts, in which complicated asexual development occurs in the endothelial cells of the vessels, and later in the muscles, where they become sarcocysts that are infective for the definitive hosts.

Human infections with Sarcocystis hominis appear to be largely asymptomatic (32); those with Sarcocystis suihominis produce mild diarrhea, vomiting, chills, and fever 6 to 24 hours after infection. In a few patients acute segmental eosinophilic ileitis, necessitating surgical resection, has been described. The histologic appearance of the mucosa of persons with sarcocystosis that produces few or no symptoms is unknown. In patients with eosinophilic enteritis, marked inflammation of all layers of the viscus is characterized by abundant eosinophils, edema, and parasites in the lamina propria (34).

Diagnosis of Sarcocystis is made in the clinical laboratory by identification of the typical sporocysts (Fig. 49–10B). Those of Sarcocystis hominis are 15 by 9 μm and those of Sarcocystis suihominis, 13 by 10 μm (Chapter 59).

MICROSPORA

Microspora are a large group of intracellular parasitic protozoa that cause a wide range of diseases in vertebrates. Members of the Microspora have been found in the tissues of humans, including brain, muscle, respiratory tract mucosa, cornea, and intestine. In the intestine Enterocytozoon bieneusi produces chronic diarrhea accompanied by weight loss in persons with AIDS. These organisms can be detected by light microscopic examination of smears of stool samples or duodenal aspirates stained with a recently described modified trichrome stain (35). The diagnosis, however, usually is made by histologic examination of tissues, so E. bieneusi will not be discussed further here (1).

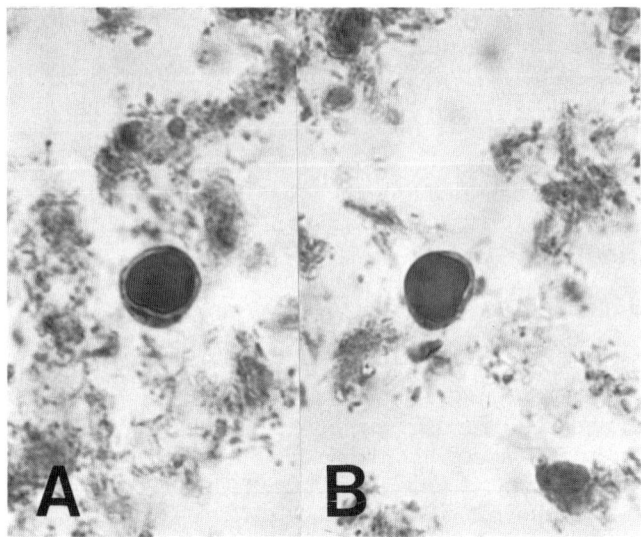

Fig. 49–11. Blastocystis hominis in human stool (trichrome, ×1120).

BLASTOCYSTIS

Blastocystis hominis has been reclassified as a protozoan, but its exact phylogenetic group has yet to be determined (36). For many years, Blastocystis was identified in the feces of humans as a nonpathogenic organism, and therefore, seldom was included in epidemiologic surveys or in clinical laboratory reports. Recently, Blastocystis has been incriminated as a producer of diarrhea (37), but proof of a causal relationship between the organism and the symptoms is still lacking. At present, the presence of Blastocystis (Fig. 49–11) in diarrheal stools (five or more per $400\times$ field) should be reported to the clinician, who should decide whether it is an important finding and whether the patient should be treated.

REFERENCES

1. Gutierrez Y: Diagnostic Pathology of Parasitic Infections with Clinical Correlations. Philadelphia, Lea & Febiger, 1990.
2. Isaac-Renton JL: Laboratory diagnosis of giardiasis. Clin Lab Med, *11*:811, 1991.
3. Proctor EM: Laboratory diagnosis of amebiasis. Clin Lab Med, *11*:829, 1991.
4. Centers for Disease Control: Intestinal Parasite Surveillance. Annual Summary, 1978. Atlanta, Centers for Disease Control, 1979.
5. Dancesco P, and Tintareanu J: Investigation concerning the spread of giardiasis in a children's community. Parasitol Epidemiol Bucharest, *9*:443, 1963.
6. Rendtorff RC: The experimental transmission of human intestinal protozoan parasites. II. Giardia lamblia cysts given in capsules. Am J Hyg, *59*:209, 1954.
7. Lippy EC: Water supply problems associated with a waterborne outbreak of giardiasis. *In* Waterborne Transmission of Giardiasis. Edited by W Jakubowski and JC Hoff. Proceedings of a Symposium. Sept 18–20, 1978. Cincinnati, U.S. Environment Protection Agency, 1979.
8. Beaver PC, Jung RC, and Cupp EW: Clinical Parasitology. 9th ed. Philadelphia, Lea & Febiger, 1984.
9. Montessori GA, and Bischoff L: Searching for parasites in stool: Once is usually enough. Can Med Assoc J, *137*:702, 1987.
10. Garcia LS, and Bruckner DA: Macroscopic and microscopic examination of fecal specimens. *In* Diagnostic Medical Parasitology. New York, Elsevier, 1988.
11. Nash TE, and Keister DB: Differences in excretory-secretory products and surface antigens among 19 isolates of Giardia. J Infect Dis, *152*:1166, 1985.
12. Korman SH, Hais E, and Spira DT: Routine in vitro cultivation of Giardia lamblia by using the string test. J Clin Microbiol, *28*:368, 1990.
13. Ungar BL, Yolken RH, Nash TE, et al: Enzyme-linked immunosorbent assay for the detection of Giardia lamblia in fecal specimens. J Infect Dis, *149*:90, 1984.
14. Nash TE, Herrington DA, and Levine MM: Usefulness of an enzyme-linked immunosorbent assay for detection of Giardia antigen in feces. J Clin Microbiol, *25*:1169, 1987.
15. Camp RR, Mattern CFT, and Honigberg BM: Study of Dientamoeba fragilis. Jepps and Dobell. I. Electron microscopic observations of the binucleate stages. J Protozool, *21*:69, 1974.
16. Turner JA: Giardiasis and infections with Dientamoeba fragilis. Pediatr Clin North Am, *32*:865, 1985.
17. Wolner-Hanssen P, Krieger JN, Sterens CE, et al: Clinical manifestations of vaginal trichomoniasis. JAMA, *261*:571, 1989.
18. Latif AS, Mason PR, and Marowa E. Urethral trichomoniasis in men. Sex Transm Dis, *14*:9, 1987.
19. Walsh JA: Problems in recognition and diagnosis of amebiasis: Estimation of the global magnitude of morbidity and mortality. Rev Infect Dis, *8*:228, 1986.
20. Phillips SC, Mildvan D, Williams DC, et al: Sexual transmission of enteric protozoa and helminths in a venereal disease clinic population. N Engl J Med, *305*:603, 1981.
21. Allason-Jones E, Mindel A, Sargeaunt P, et al: Entamoeba histolytica as a commensal parasite in homosexual men. N Engl J Med, *315*:353, 1986.
22. Wilmot AJ: Clinical Aamoebiasis. London, Blackwell Scientific Publications, 1962.
23. Ewers WH: Parasites of man in Papua-New Guinea. Southeast Asian J Trop Med Public Health, *3*:79, 1972.
24. Arean VM, and Koppisch E. Balantidiasis. A review and report of cases. Am J Pathol, *32*:1089.
25. Nime FA, Burek JD, Page DL, et al: Acute enterocolitis in a human being infected with the protozoan Cryptosporidium. Gastroenterology, *70*:592, 1976.
26. Meisel JL, Perera DR, Meligro C, et al: Overwhelming watery diarrhea associated with Cryptosporidium in an immunosuppressed patient. Gastroenterology. *70*:1156, 1976.
27. Current WL, and Garcia LS: Laboratory diagnosis of cryptosporidiosis. Clin Lab Med, *11*:873, 1991.
28. Wolfson JS, Richter JM, Waldron MA, et al: Cryptosporidiosis in immunocompetent patients. N Engl J Med, *312*:1278, 1985.
29. Jokipii L, Pohjola S, and Jokipii AMM: Cryptosporidium: A frequent finding in patients with gastrointestinal symptoms. Lancet, *2*:358, 1983.
30. De Hovitz JA, Pape JW, Boncy M, et al: Clinical manifestations and therapy of Isospora belli infection in patients with the acquired immunodeficiency syndrome. N Engl J Med, *315*:87, 1986.
31. Brandborg LL, Goldberg SB, and Breidenbach WC: Human coccidiosis—a possible cause of malabsorption. The life cycle in small bowel mucosal biopsies as a diagnostic feature. N Engl J Med, *283*:1306, 1970.
32. Rommel M, and Heydorn AO: Beitrage zum Lebendszyklus der Sarkosporidien. 3. Isospora hominis (Railliet und Lucet, 1891) Wenyon, 1923, eine Dauerform der Sarkosporidien des Rindes und des Schweins. Berl Munch Tierartzl Wochenschr, *85*:143, 1972.
33. Heydorn AO: Bietrage zum Lebenszyklus der Sarkosporidien. IX. Entwicklungszyklus von Sarcocystic suihominis N. spec. Berl Munch Tierartzl Wochenschr, *90*:218, 1977.
34. Bunyaratvej S, Bunyawongwiroz P, and Nitiyanant P: Human intestinal sarcosporidiosis: Report of six cases. Am J Trop Med Hyg, *31*:36, 1982.
35. Weber R, et al: Improved light-microscopical detection of microsporidia spores in stool and duodenal aspirates. N Engl J Med, *326*:161, 1992.
36. Zierdt CH, Rude WS, and Bull BS: Protozoan characteristics of Blastocystis hominis. Am J Clin Pathol, *48*:495, 1967.
37. Sheehan DJ, Raucher BG, and McKitriak JC: Association of Blastocystis hominis with signs and symptoms of human disease. J Clin Microbiol, *24*:548, 1986.

Chapter 50

INTESTINAL HELMINTHS

The helminths inhabitating the intestinal tract of humans belong to several groups: the nematodes (round worms), the trematodes (flukes), and the cestodes (tapeworms), each group represented in humans by one or more genera with one or more species (Chapter 48). The intestinal helminths of humans produce important morbidity and occasionally mortality worldwide, especially in children of underdeveloped areas.

The general life cycles of the intestinal helminths vary from a direct type of development to a more complicated one that involves one or more intermediate hosts. One characteristic of the intestinal helminths is that most of them are recognized in stool samples (Chapter 59), making the diagnosis of these infections relatively easy.

In addition to the helminths that live exclusively in the intestine, others that live in the biliary tract (Clonorchis, Opisthorchis, Fasciola), in the pulmonary parenchyma (Paragonimus), and the blood vessels (Schistosoma) shed their eggs in the feces and thus are also diagnosed in stool samples. In this chapter some of these organisms are briefly mentioned as they relate to diagnosis, but they are discussed in more detail in Chapter 52.

NEMATODES

The intestinal nematodes of humans are characterized by having two sexes; some live in the lumen of the intestine, some are attached to the mucosa, and others live buried in the crypts of the mucosa. One important principle governing most infections with intestinal nematodes is that the number of adult worms in the intestine is generally limited by the number of infective stages acquired, so the symptoms produced are related to the number of worms in the intestine. Because of this it is often important for the laboratory to estimate the worm burden by counting the number of eggs in a milligram of feces (Chapter 59).

Intestinal nematodes occur worldwide; in some areas many persons are infected and some suffer important diseases. In other areas the intestinal nematodes play a minor role as pathogens, but laboratory personnel must nevertheless have knowledge of their biology and of the proper way of diagnosing these infections. The most common intestinal nematodes are examined separately.

Enterobius vermicularis

Enterobius vermicularis, known as pinworm, occurs worldwide and is the most common nematode diagnosed in the United States, mostly among children, though its prevalence is declining (1). The adult worms reside in the lumen of the cecum and large intestine (Fig. 50–1A); the male measures up to 5 mm long by 0.2 mm wide, and the female, up to 13 mm by 0.5 mm wide (2). The female has a pointed posterior end, and both sexes have a cephalic cuticular inflation which makes Enterobius easily recognizable in the laboratory on gross examination.

In the lumen of the intestine the parasites mate, the females become gravid, with many eggs in their uteri, and migrate to the perianal area where they lay their eggs. The eggs embryonate (become infective) in a few hours within the perianal folds and are ready to continue development in a new host. Embryonated eggs that are ingested produce larvae, which develop into adults and lay eggs in about 4 to 6 weeks.

Migration of the female worm in the perianal area produces pruritus, the main clinical manifestation of the infection, leading to continuous scratching. Eosinophilia does not develop because the parasites are not in the tissues. The adult Enterobius female in the perianal area is capable of migrating to the vagina, the uterus, or the peritoneal cavity via the fallopian tubes (3). In the vagina the worms lay eggs, which may be found in the vaginal smear (Fig. 50–1B); in the peritoneal cavity, the worms die, producing granulomas that are found incidentally during abdominal surgery or at autopsy, lesions that are usually diagnosed by the anatomic pathologist. In young girls the female worms may enter the urinary bladder via the urethra, introducing micro-organisms responsible for repeated urinary tract infections (4). In older women other symptoms and lesions have been produced by the migration of adult worms (3).

The diagnosis of enterobiasis is made by the detection of the adults or the eggs in samples from the perianal area (Chapter 59) (Fig. 50–1C). These samples are easily taken following the steps of the cellophane tape technique: briefly applying the sticky side of a 3 by 1 inch piece of cellophane tape to the anus, retrieving the tape, and sticking it onto a glass slide which is sent to the laboratory (Appendix, Procedure 29). Examination of the tape under the microscope reveals the typical eggs, and sometimes the adult worms. The eggs of Enterobius are recognized by their thick, smooth, transparent shell, which often contains a coiled larva. The eggs are oval with one side slightly flattened, and measure 50 to 60 μm by 20 to 30 μm (Fig. 50–1B and C).

Trichuris trichiura

Trichuris trichiura inhabits the large intestine, where it lives attached to the mucosa, sometimes producing significant disease. This nematode occurs worldwide, but is most prevalent in the tropics (up to 90%) (5). Trichuris tends to occur more in school children (6). In the United

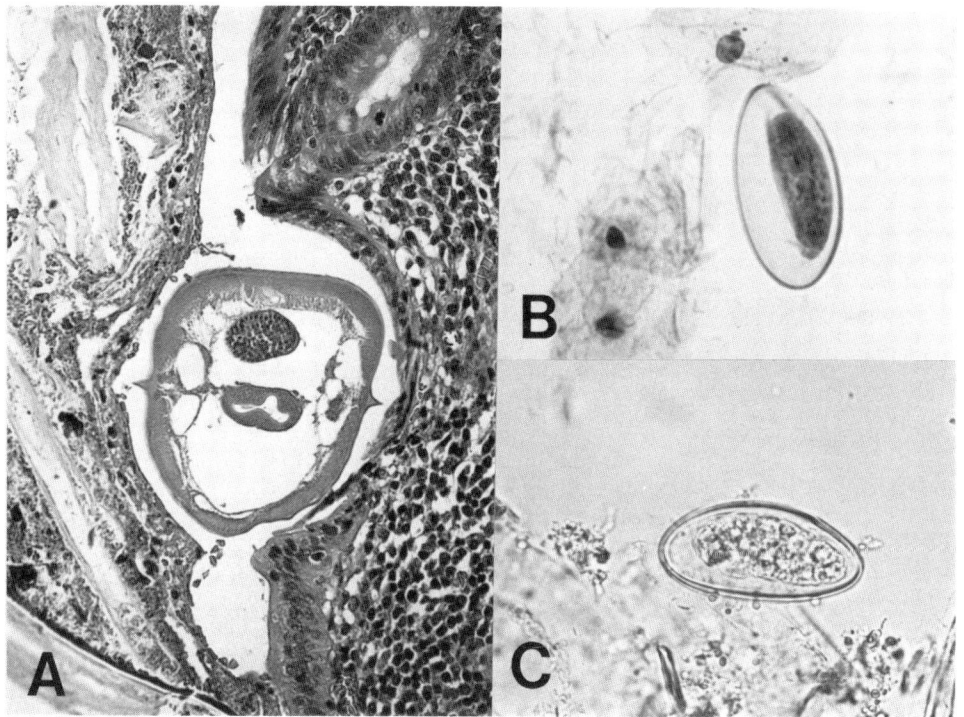

Fig. 50–1. Enterobius vermicularis. A, Cross section of adult worm in the appendix shows the characteristic lateral alae (×280). B, Egg in cervical smear stained with Papanicolaou stain (×600). C, Egg recovered with the cellophane tape technique; a larva is not developed (×600).

States it is a common parasite in the southeastern part of the country.

The life cycle of Trichuris is rather simple. The adult female worms pass eggs, which are evacuated with the feces; in soil the eggs embryonate in 3 to 5 weeks, depending on environmental conditions; after embryonated eggs are ingested by the susceptible host the eggs hatch in the intestine, freeing a larva that travels to the colon, where it penetrates the superficial cells of the mucosa and grows to its full length (Fig. 50–2A) (2).

The worms are about 4 cm long, the anterior part of the body is slender and the posterior is thicker, a configuration that gave this worm the name "whipworm." The anterior slender part of the body is used by the worm to attach to the mucosa (Fig. 50–2A), which attachment occurs early in their development and lasts the entire life of the worm, about 5 years. From this site of attachment the females lay eggs in the intestinal lumen (2).

The clinical manifestations of trichuriasis are related to the number of worms in the colon (6,7), the nutritional status of the host, and the duration of the infection (8). Infections with a small number of worms are well-tolerated; those with a moderate number produce nonspecific symptoms, mainly constipation, lower quadrant pain, indigestion, and weight loss. Large numbers of worms in the colon result in prolonged diarrhea, with blood, mucus, abdominal pain, and loss of weight (7). Some persons have anemia, and fewer than 15% have peripheral eosinophilia. If the infection persists without treatment, growth retardation and anemia are more manifest, and clubbing of the fingers may develop (8–10). In heavy infections, especially in children, manifestations of colitis occur, colitis which is clinically indistinguishable from other forms of colitis (11); rectal prolapse occurs often, showing the worms attached to the mucosa. Especially in children, rectal prolapse is due to chronic straining of the perianal muscles because of the chronic diarrhea.

The mechanism by which Trichuris produces disease in humans is unknown. Grossly, the colon appears hyperemic, edematous, and friable, and has numerous parasites attached, especially in the cecum and ascending colon. Microscopically, the colon shows sections of the anterior portions of the worm within the mucosa (Fig. 50–2A); however, little inflammatory infiltrate is found in most cases (3).

The diagnosis of trichuriasis is made in the laboratory by finding and recognizing the typical eggs in stool samples (Chapter 59). The eggs are about 50 to 54 μm by 22 to 23 μm; they are oval, with two mucus plugs, one at each end, and the shell is mahogany colored (Fig. 50–2B and C). These eggs should be measured, because other species of Trichuris have been described in humans, mainly Trichuris vulpis from dogs (12), eggs which are 70 to 80 μm by 30 to 42 μm. The adult Trichuris worms seldom are submitted to the laboratory for identification. In these cases the typical morphology of Trichuris trichiura should be ascertained.

The Hookworms

The nematodes generally known as hookworms comprise a large group of parasites that infect several organs, and those in the intestine belong to the genera Ancylostoma and Necator. Ancylostoma has two species, Ancylostoma duodenale and Ancylostoma ceylanicum, and Necator, one, Necator americanus, residing in the duodenum and upper jejunum of humans. The larvae of dogs' and cats' hookworms produce zoonotic infections in humans, infections usually confined to the skin and known as cutaneous larva migrans (3).

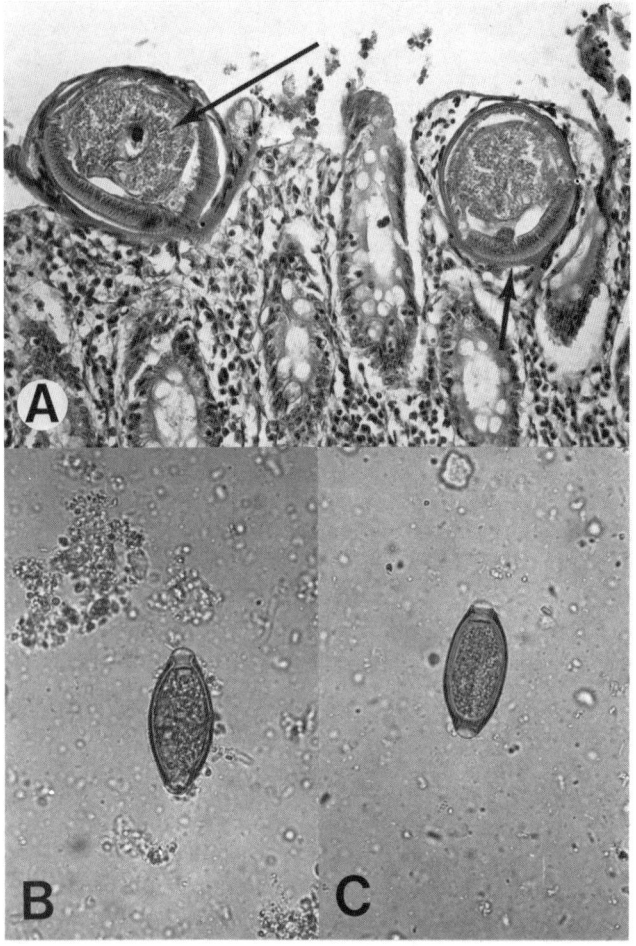

Fig. 50–2. Trichuris trichiura. A, Section of large intestine stained shows two cross sections of the anterior aspect of the worm. The esophagus of the worm (*long arrow*) is at the center and the basilary band (*short arrow*) on the side (hematoxylin and eosin ×220). B, and C, Eggs in unstained human stool (×450).

The geographic distribution of hookworms is mostly tropical and subtropical. Necator americanus predominates in the African and the American continents and Ancylostoma, in southern Europe, northern Africa, parts of the Middle East, Asia and southeast Asia. In these areas, hookworms are responsible for important morbidity, especially among lower socioeconomic groups (5).

Hookworms are soil-transmitted helminths. Adults live attached to the mucosa of the small intestine, by their buccal cavity (Fig. 50–3A). The adults are between 0.7 and 1.3 cm long, depending on the species; the females lay eggs 60 to 76 μm by 35 to 40 μm, with a thin shell containing a mass of cells that appear detached from the shell (Fig. 50–3B). Eggs are evacuated with the feces into the environment, where they develop under proper conditions into infective larvae in about a week. Infective larvae penetrate the skin of a susceptible host and via circulation arrive in the lungs, where the larvae break the capillary vessel to enter the alveolus, migrate upward in the respiratory tree to the epiglottis and pass to the esophagus and intestine, where they grow to adults. Members of the Ancylostoma can develop directly, without passage through the lungs, if larvae are ingested by the host (2).

Hookworms attach to the mucosa using their wide buccal cavity; attachment is temporary because it is used for feeding purposes. A portion of the host's mucosa is sucked into the buccal cavity of the worm and is digested, after which the worm seeks a new position in the intestine and repeats the process (13). Attachment of the worm to the mucosa produces lacerations with bleeding, resulting in anemia, especially if the number of worms in the intestine is large and if the nutritional status of the host is poor (3).

The clinical manifestations of hookworm infection are several. Penetration through the skin of sensitized hosts results in a condition known as "ground itch," a form of cutaneous larva migrans similar to that produced by the hookworms of dogs and cats (3). In the lungs the migrating larvae produce transient pneumonitis known as Loef-

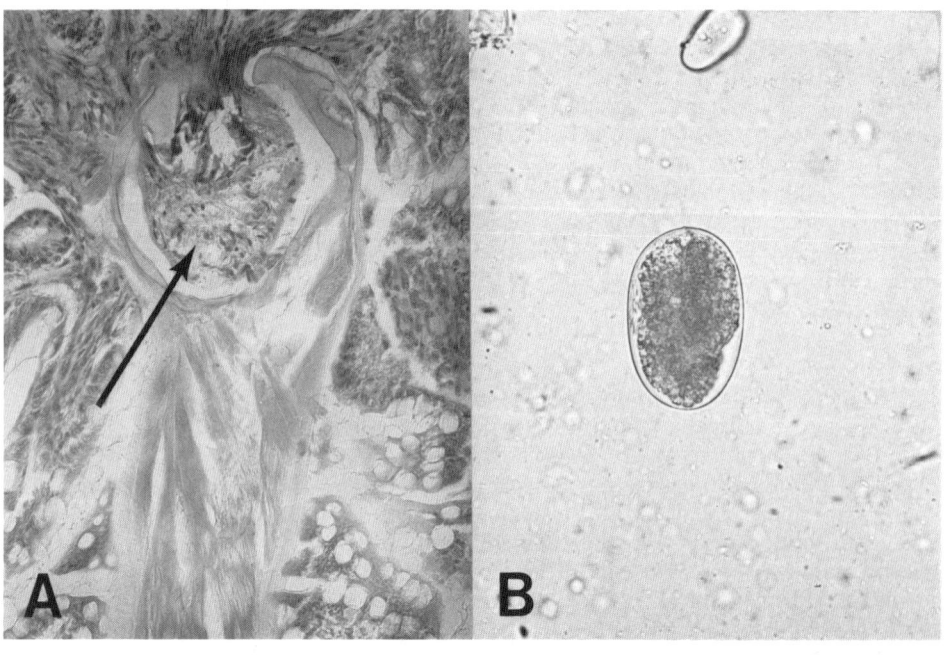

Fig. 50–3. Hookworm. Adult worm attached to the intestinal mucosa. Note portion of mucosa in the buccal cavity of the worm (*arrow*) (hematoxylin and eosin, ×200). (From Gutierrez Y: Diagnostic Pathology of Parasitic Infections with Clinical Correlations. Philadelphia, Lea & Febiger, 1990. B, Egg in stool (×450).

fler's syndrome (see under Ascaris). In the intestine the symptoms are related to the number of worms and the nutritional status of the host. The symptoms are fatigue, nausea, vomiting, and abdominal pain; diarrhea may occur but it is not usual. Sporadic cases, especially in infants, may present with profuse intestinal hemorrhage with fatal consequences. The chronic infection is characterized mainly by a microcytic hypochromic anemia due to chronic blood loss (2,3).

The gross appearance of the intestine in infections with hookworm is focal superficial hemorrhage and worms attached to the mucosa. Microscopically, the changes are nonspecific, varying from mild inflammatory infiltrate to moderate changes of the villi (3).

The diagnosis of hookworm disease is made clinically and is confirmed microscopically by finding in the stools eggs characteristic for the group (Fig. 50–3B). Species identification cannot be based on the morphology of the eggs alone; it is based on the study of adult worms recovered in feces after treatment. The laboratory report should refer only to hookworm eggs, without identifying genus or species, and the report should contain an estimate of the number of eggs per wet-mount preparation (22- by 22-mm cover glass) (Chapter 59). Special care should be placed on differentiating hookworm eggs from Trichostrongylus eggs (see below).

Ascaris lumbricoides

Ascaris lumbricoides is the largest nematode of the intestinal tract of humans, where it inhabits the duodenum and upper part of the jejunum. Infections with Ascaris are common among young children in tropical and, to a lesser extent, in subtropical areas, sometimes producing severe disease. In the United States the largest number of infections are recorded in the southeast, but sporadic cases are observed elsewhere. The prevalence of Ascaris infections in some communities in the tropics is up to 70%, where the epidemiology of Ascaris parallels that of Trichuris. Ascaris is another soil-transmitted helminth.

The adult Ascaris worm lives in the lumen of the small intestine; the female is some 35 cm long and the male is some 31 cm. Eggs laid by the female are evacuated with the feces into the environment, where they embryonate in approximately 3 to 4 weeks. After soil contaminated with infective eggs is ingested, the eggs hatch in the intestine, producing larvae that enter the intestinal wall and, via blood, travel to the liver and lungs. Within the capillary bed of the lungs the larvae require a period of 1 to 2 weeks for maturation, after which they break the capillaries and enter the alveoli to migrate upward in the respiratory tract to the epiglottis and the intestine, to mature into adults (2).

The infection produced by Ascaris in humans has many clinical manifestations. The migration through the lungs produces pneumonitis (Loeffler's syndrome) (14), seen often in endemic areas as outbreaks of pneumonitis when transmission of Ascaris is at its peak, usually during the rainy season. Loeffler's syndrome is a self-limited pneumonitis characterized by fleeting pulmonary infiltrates and peripheral eosinophilia. In most instances the syndrome is related more to sensitization to the parasite than to the number of larvae migrating through the lungs, because a few larvae may elicit pronounced clinical manifestations (15).

The bulk of the clinical manifestations of Ascaris infection are produced by the parasites in the intestine; it is generally divided into manifestations produced by the worms in the intestine and those produced by their migration to other sites.

The intestinal symptoms are variable, depending on the host and the number of worms in the intestine. Heavy infections usually occur in small children and produce abdominal pain, loss of appetite, protuberant abdomen, and general nutritional impairment due to altered absorption of nutrients (16,17). Longterm effects of the poor nutritional status are growth- and mental retardation.

Ectopic Ascaris worms are important because they produce higher morbidity and sometimes death, but the diagnosis of these problems falls within the clinician's and the anatomic pathologist's domain (3). Only when an adult worm is passed in stools or vomited by the patient is the clinical laboratory involved. Ectopic Ascaris are mentioned here briefly for the sake of completeness. Ascaris may migrate from the duodenum into the stomach and to the upper airways, where they may produce cardiopulmonary arrest. Large numbers of worms may dislodge from the duodenum and travel in the intestine to produce intestinal obstruction at the ileocecal valve. Worms may enter the common bile duct and produce obstruction, and they often lodge in the liver, resulting in abscesses. The diverticulum of Meckel and the appendix may be obstructed by an ascarid, with resulting symptoms of appendicitis. After intestinal surgery adult Ascaris may pass through sutures into the peritoneal cavity to produce serious peritonitis (3).

The diagnosis of ascariasis is often made clinically, especially in areas where the disease is common and clinicians are aware of its manifestations. Confirmation of the infection is provided by identification of adult worms recovered from feces or vomitus, usually by the patient, or more often, by finding the typical eggs in stool samples using standard parasitologic techniques in the laboratory. The fertilized eggs excreted in the feces are easily recognizable as light to dark brown, oval structures up to 75 by 60 μm, with an irregular, mamillated exterior layer (Fig. 50–4A, B). Inside this layer, the lipoid layer, with smooth surfaces, and the vitelline layer are visible; inside, the egg cell appears as a dark mass. Sometimes, unfertilized eggs are passed in the feces; they are larger (up to 90 μm) than embryonated eggs, lack a vitelline layer, and contain a mass of disorganized refractile granules (Fig. 50–4C). Estimation of relative numbers of eggs per unit of feces is desirable to assess the clinical importance of the infection and for follow-up treatment (Chapter 59).

The standard fecal smear (Chapter 59) usually contains 2 mg of feces; since a female Ascaris lays 200,000 eggs per day, each standard fecal smear contains about 4 eggs (if 100 g of feces is eliminated each day). This simple calculation shows that finding Ascaris eggs in stools is easy, even if only one pair of worms is present in the intestine; thus

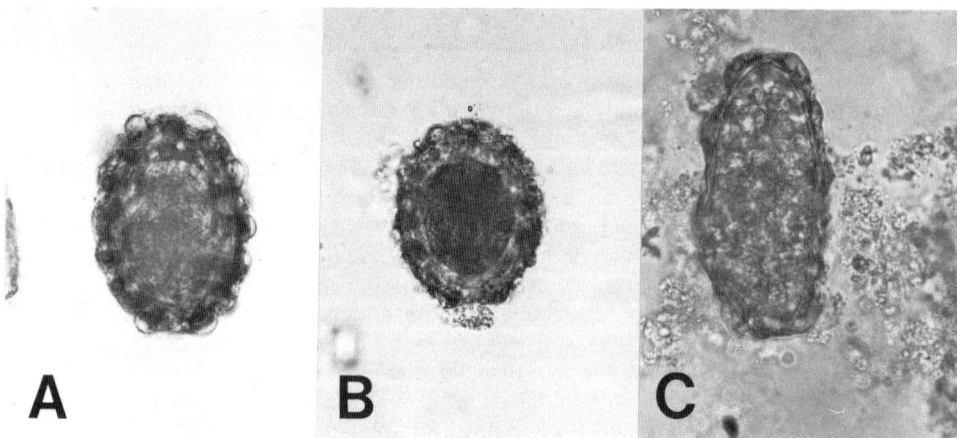

Fig. 50–4. Ascaris eggs in human stools (unstained, ×450).

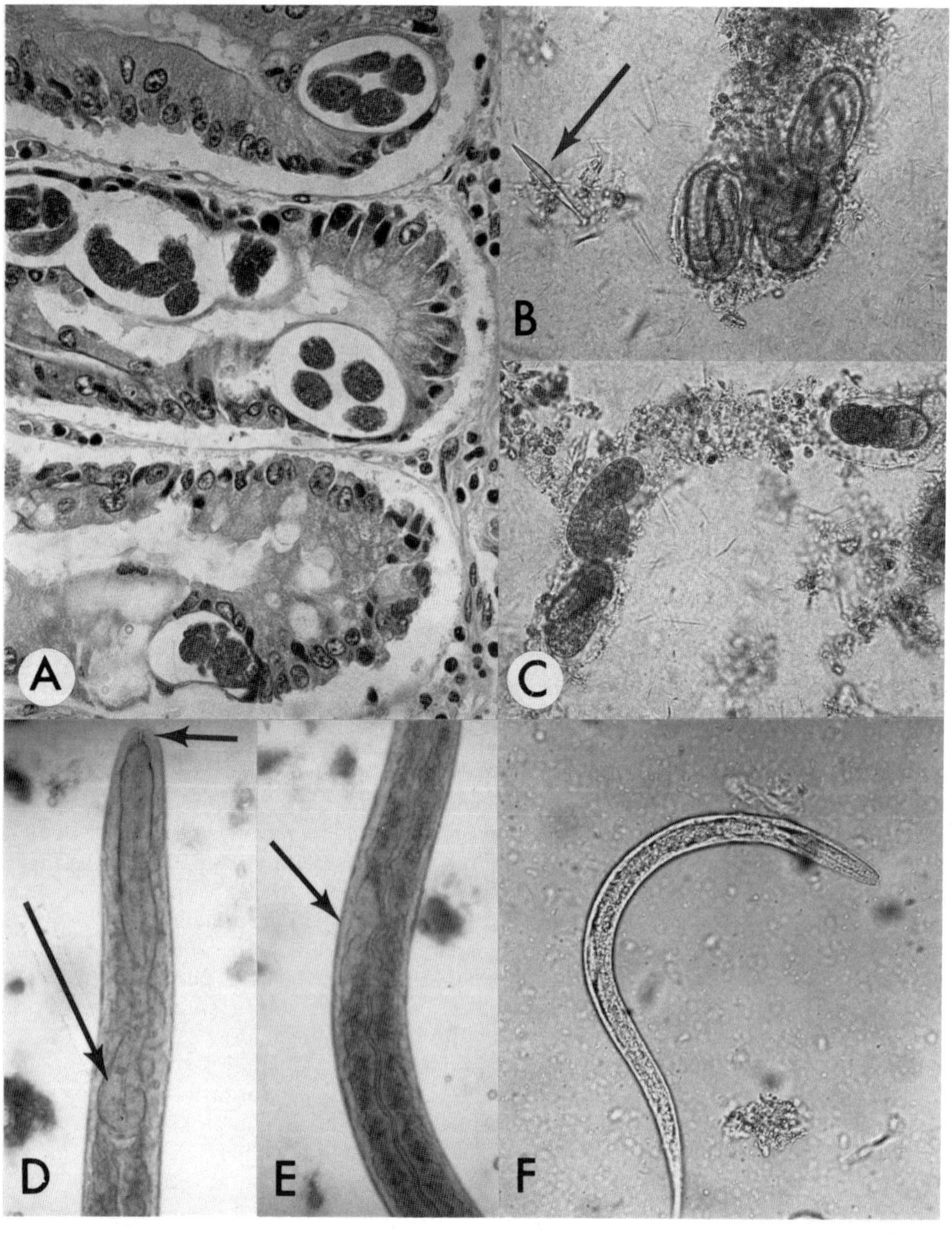

Fig. 50–5. Strongyloides stercoralis. *A,* Developing eggs in the duodenal mucosa (hematoxylin and eosin, ×450). *B,* Eggs and eggs with developed larvae, *C,* were recovered in duodenal scrapings. Note the Charcot-Leyden crystal (*arrow*) indicating eosinophilia (×280). *D–F,* Rhabditoid larvae in human stools stained with iodine: *D,* anterior portion shows the buccal cavity shorter than the diameter of the worm at this level (*short arrow*) and the esophageal bulb (*long arrow*) (×750); *E,* Midbody of larva shows the genital primordium (*arrow* (×750); *F,* whole larva (×400).

diagnosis of Ascaris in stools usually does not require a fecal concentrate.

Strongyloides stercoralis

Strongyloides stercoralis is an important parasite of humans because it produces often fatal infections in hosts who have some forms of immune suppression. The parasite has a worldwide distribution, but is most prevalent in the tropics. Strongyloides is endemic in the United States and cases, or series of cases, are regularly reported. Another species, Strongyloides fuelleborni, found in certain tropical areas, is mentioned briefly.

Strongyloides is a free-living nematode with a parasitic phase in which only the females are parasites of the small intestine of humans and animals. The adult females are as large as 2.7 mm long by 30 to 40 μm wide, living deep in the crypts of the duodenum, where they lay their eggs in the tissues (Fig. 50 5A). The eggs develop rapidly into larvae which migrate to the lumen and are evacuated with the feces. These larvae, known as rhabditoid larvae, have a characteristic shape (see below) and evolve in soil to infective larvae if conditions are optimal. Infective larvae penetrate the skin of susceptible hosts and, via blood, reach the lungs, the tracheobronchial tree and the intestine, where they develop into adult females and begin oviposition (2). Two other forms of development may be followed by Strongyloides. One, in soil, produces under certain conditions a free-living generation of worms, and thus its status of free-living nematode. Second, a more important development occurs when the rhabditoid larvae, travelling down the intestine, transform into infective filariform larvae. Filariform larvae in the intestine are capable of re-entering the intestinal wall, usually at the level of the cecum, to complete the life cycle by migrating through the lungs back to the small intestine. This second phase of development is referred to as autoinfection, and if autoinfection is massive it results in hyperinfection, with important clinical consequences. Autoinfection explains the longevity of the infection with Strongyloides in humans, which in some persons has been estimated to be as long as 40 years (18).

The mechanism by which Strongyloides produces symptoms in humans is unknown. Hyperinfection occurs in persons who receive organ transplants, some tumors of the lymphoid system, prolonged steroid therapy, and malnutrition, but it generally is not associated with infections with the human immunodeficiency virus (3).

The great majority of Strongyloides infections in immunocompetent hosts are asymptomatic. Some persons may complain of diarrhea and may have symptoms of duodenitis. A few may have manifestations that simulate peptic ulcer. In debilitated, immunocompromised hosts with hyperinfection the symptoms are related to the intestinal tract and to the lungs (larvae move through the lungs in great numbers). Diarrhea, abdominal pain, high peripheral eosinophilia, and pneumonitis are common (2,3).

The morphologic changes of the duodenal mucosa in strongyloidiasis are minimal. In hyperinfections, edema and hyperemia are seen in some; the colon shows ulcerations of various sizes. The lungs are heavy, consolidated, and hemorrhagic. Microscopically, adult worms, eggs, and larvae are found in the intestinal wall (Fig. 50–5A), and only larvae in histologic sections of the lung and other organs (3).

The diagnosis of strongyloidiasis is made in the clinical laboratory by identifying the characteristic rhabditoid larvae in the stools (Fig. 50–5F). Direct smears made from stool and from concentrated stools are good for recovery and for identification of the larvae (Chapter 59). The rhabditoid larvae evacuated with the feces are 380 μm long by 20 μm wide, have a muscular esophagus with a well-defined bulb (Fig. 50–5D), and a genital primordium (Fig. 50–5E) located behind the midportion of the body, composed of a group of well-defined cells. The buccal cavity of the larva is shorter than the diameter of the worm at the level of the buccal cavity (Fig. 50–5D). With hyperinfection filariform larvae may be recovered from stool samples collected and examined within a short time of evacuation or in stools fixed soon after evacuation. Filariform larvae are found in body fluids and feces of patients who suffer hyperinfection. They are slender, up to 630 μm long by 16 μm wide, and have a thin esophagus lacking a bulb, occupying about the anterior half of the body of the worm (Fig. 50–6). Rhabditoid larvae in fresh stools transform within 24 hours into filariform larvae, so stools should be examined as soon as possible after arrival to

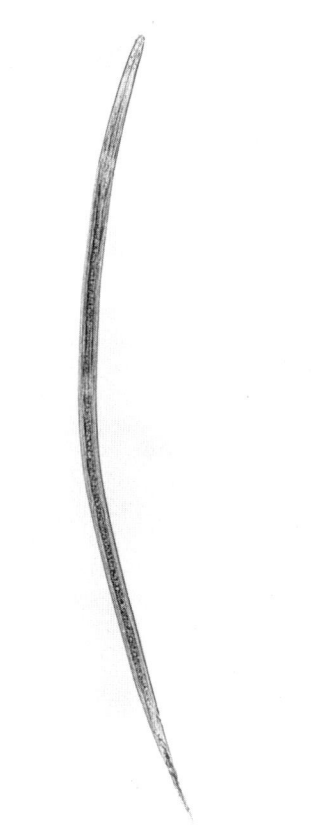

Fig. 50–6. Strongyloides stercoralis filariform larva in culture of human stool (unstained, ×180).

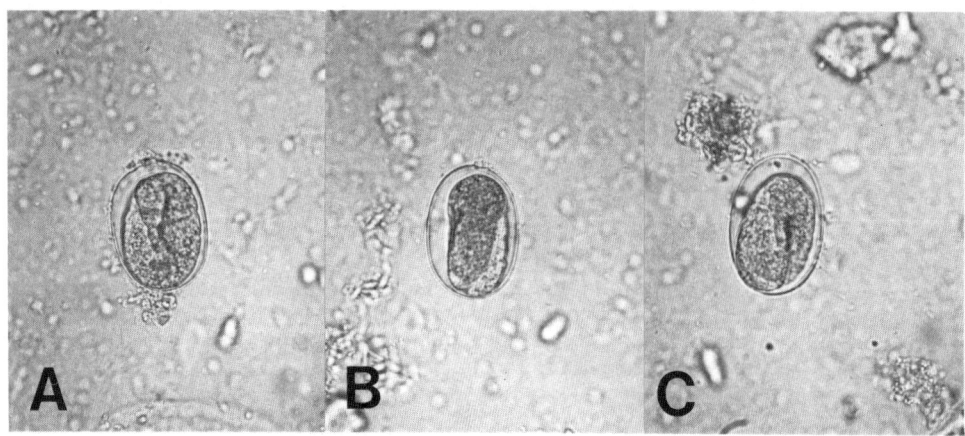

Fig. 50–7. Strongyloides fuelleborni eggs in stools of a native of Papua, New Guinea (unstained, ×450) (Sample courtesy of MD Little, PhD, School of Tropical Medicine and Public Health, Tulane University).

the laboratory. Larvae can also be recovered from sputum samples of persons with hyperinfection (Chapter 57). Other body fluids and tissues may yield similar results, but these samples are usually examined by the anatomic pathologist. Sometimes examination of the duodenal aspirate reveals eggs with developing larvae, larvae, and adults (Fig. 50–5B, C).

Strongyloides fuelleborni. Infections with S. fuelleborni are usually found in certain areas of Africa and New Guinea. The parasite lives in the small intestine, producing in small infants a syndrome known as "swollen belly sickness," consisting of gastrointestinal symptoms, edema, and respiratory distress leading to death (19). The diagnosis is made by finding the typical eggs in the stools, always in the tadpole stage 48 to 54 μm by 32 to 35 μm (Fig. 50–7A–C).

Trichostrongylus

At least nine species of Trichostrongylus produce natural infections in humans in several parts of the world. These nematodes live buried in the mucosa of the small intestine of herbivorous mammals. The eggs are passed with the feces into the environment, where they develop larvae that are freed in soil (pasture) and, if swallowed by an appropriate host, develop to adults in the small intestine. Human infections are common in the Middle East, Australia, Africa, Siberia, Japan, China, and Taiwan, and sporadically worldwide. Rates of prevalence in some endemic areas is up to 40% (20).

The symptoms of trichostrongylosis are not well-known, but abdominal pain, diarrhea, weakness, and profuse eosinophilia have been described in some cases (21). The diagnosis of the infection is made by recognizing the typical eggs in the stools, measuring up to 95 μm in length (Fig. 50–8A, B); the eggs should be differentiated from those of hookworms: Trichostrongylus eggs are larger, have more pointed ends, and a thicker shell that looks like two distinct layers.

Capillaria philippinensis

Capillaria philippinensis is the agent of intestinal capillariasis, a disease first identified in an epidemic in the Philippines, and later as sporadic cases in Japan (22), Thailand, Iran, and Egypt (3). Capillaria is a genus related to Trichinella (Chapters 48 and 52) and Trichuris (see above), and has at least one other species, Capillaria hepatica, that produces infections in the liver of rodents and sometimes in humans (3). In the Philippines, Capillaria philippinensis produces an important infection because of its morbidity, mortality, and because of the large numbers of people affected.

In humans, Capillaria philippinensis lives buried in the glandular epithelium of the lower duodenum, jejunum, and ileum, where the females produce larvae which mature rapidly and re-enter the mucosa to grow to adults (autoinfection) (Fig. 50–9A). Other females lay eggs that are evacuated with the feces to embryonate outside the body in approximately 2 weeks. Embryonated eggs are ingested by freshwater fish, where they develop to infective larvae which, if ingested with the fish (raw), produce the infection in humans (2).

Intestinal capillariasis in the Philippines is mainly a disease of males aged 20 to 50 years. The infection presents acutely, with profuse watery diarrhea that is difficult to control (23). In chronic cases the infection develops to a spruelike syndrome with malabsorption. Other times, the

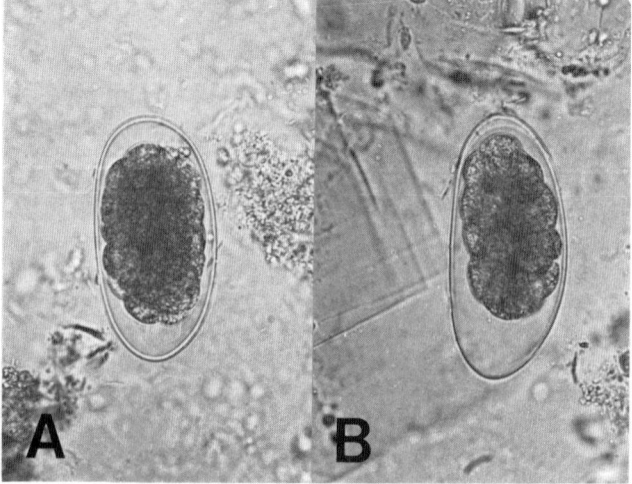

Fig. 50–8. Trichostrongylus eggs in human stool (unstained, ×450). (From Gutierrez Y: Diagnostic Pathology of Parasitic Infections with Clinical Correlations. Philadelphia, Lea & Febiger 1990.)

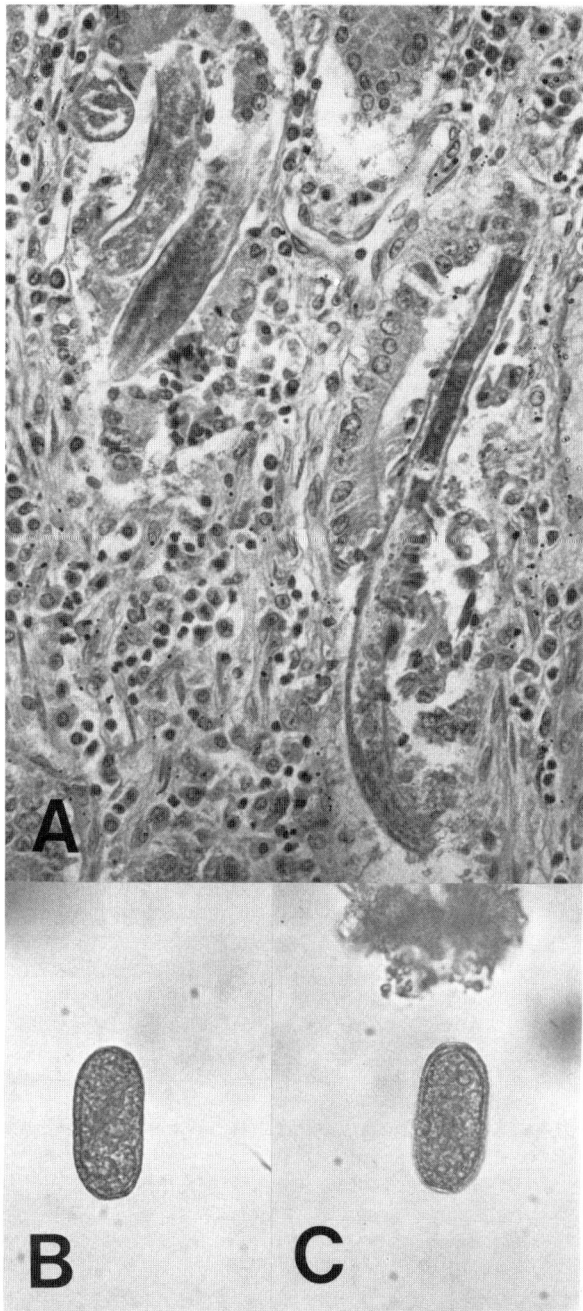

Fig. 50-9. Capillaria philippinensis. A, Adult parasites in small intestine (hematoxylin and eosin, ×350). B, and C, Eggs in human stool (unstained, ×450). (Sample courtesy of JH Cross, PhD, Department of Preventive Medicine and Biometry, Uniformed Services University, Bethesda, Maryland.)

infection results in abdominal pain, anorexia, and slight fever. Blood tests show an increase in white blood cells with eosinophilia. The mechanism by which Capillaria philippinensis produces disease is unknown (24). Microscopically, the small bowel has numerous parasites (males and females) and larvae buried in the crypts, often without eliciting an inflammatory reaction (Fig. 50–9A) (25).

The diagnosis is made by identifying the typical eggs (Fig. 50–9B, C), sometimes larvae, and adult worms in the stools (Chapter 59) (26). The eggs evacuated with the feces resemble somewhat the eggs of Trichuris, but are somewhat smaller (about 36 to 45 μm by 21 μm) with a finely mammelonated shell, giving an irregular appearance.

Anisakis and Pseudoterranova

Anisakis and Pseudoterranova are two genera of ascarid worms parasitic of marine mammals. For practical purposes, the two may be referred to as Anisakis, the infection produced as anisakiasis, and the worms as anisakids (27,28).

The life cycle of anisakids is complicated, but it involves intermediate hosts, the most important being edible marine fish which harbor the infective stage for both marine mammals and humans. In general terms, species of Anisakis have larvae that occur commonly in mackerel and herring; species of Pseudoterranova in cod, pollock, and others.

Human infections with anisakid larvae are common in Japan; they were common in the Netherlands, and are reported sporadically throughout the world, including the United States. The manifestations vary from recovery of worms from the oral cavity while eating or soon after having eaten fish, to expectoration of the larvae, to subacute abdominal symptoms, to "acute abdomen" that necessitates surgical intervention.

Worms recovered by the patient are sometimes referred to the clinical microbiology laboratory for identification (29). Segments of gastrointestinal tract resected at surgery are referred to the surgical pathology laboratory, where the diagnosis is often based on cross-sections of the worm (3).

TREMATODES

The trematodes are a large group of parasitic, usually hermaphroditic, helminths that are flattened dorsoventrally (platyhelminths) and inhabit several organ systems (Chapter 48). The trematodes occurring in the intestine are Fasciolopsis buski, Nanophyetus (Troglotrema) salmincola, several species of heterophyids, and others of less importance. The trematodes occurring outside the intestine are discussed in Chapter 52.

The geographic distribution of the intestinal trematodes is restricted to certain areas of the world where they sometimes produce common infections that result in death, especially in children. In general, all trematodes involve a snail in their life cycle, so trematodes are known as snail-transmitted helminths (Chapter 48).

Fasciolopsis Buski

Fasciolopsis buski produces fasciolopsiasis, a disease sometimes fatal to children. The infection is common in pigs and humans in Southeast Asia, South China, Taiwan, Vietnam, Bangladesh, Thailand, Ossam, Sumatra, and Borneo. In some areas, such as Bangladesh, the prevalence in school children is as high as 39% (2,3).

Fasciolopsis buski, the largest trematode of humans, measures up to 7.5 cm long, 2 cm wide, and 0.3 cm thick (Fig. 50–10A). The body is oval, fleshy, with two distinct

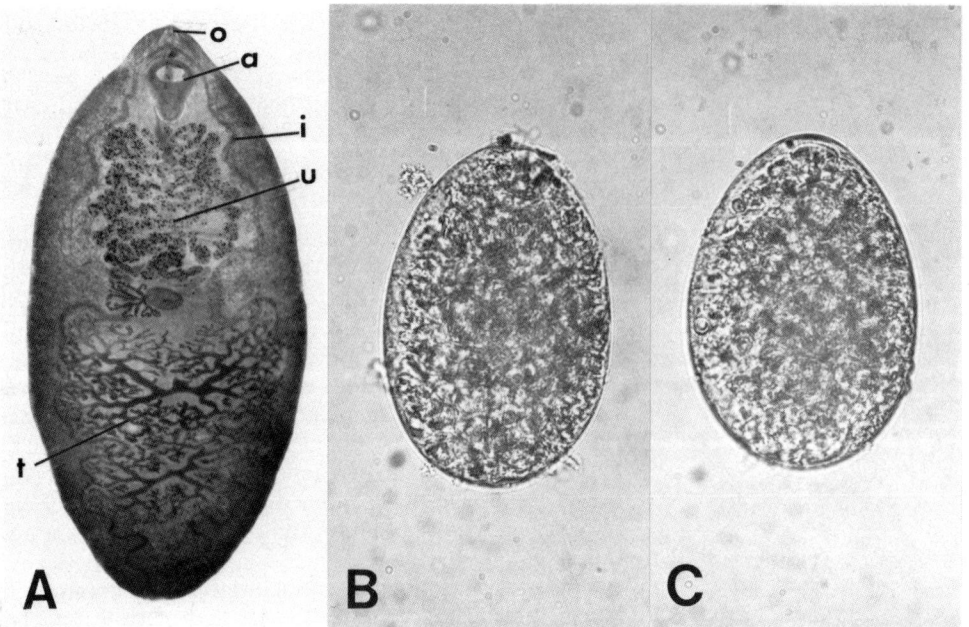

Fig. 50–10. Fasciolopsis buski. A, adult worm (acetocarmine alum, ×2.8). Key: o, oral sucker; a, acetabulum; i, intestine (cecum); u, uterus; t, testes. B, C, Eggs in human stool (unstained, ×450). (From Gutierrez Y: Diagnostic Pathology of Parasitic Infections with Clinical Correlations. Philadelphia, Lea & Febiger, 1990.)

suckers: one, located anteriorly, opens into the mouth of the parasite; the other, the acetabulum, is larger, and slightly posterior to the first one, on the ventral surface, and it serves as the attachment organ for the parasite (Fig. 50–10A). In the small intestine Fasciolopsis worms lay eggs, which are evacuated with the feces and in fresh water embryonate to larvae, which enter a snail (Fig. 50–10B, C). In the snail the parasite undergoes development, which terminates with the production of cercariae that swim to find an appropriate water plant, where they encyst (2). Ingestion of these plants with encysted larvae (metacercariae) produces the infection in susceptible hosts. In the intestine, the larvae abandon their cysts and grow to adults.

It is believed that the symptoms produced by Fasciolopsis in humans are due to the mechanical damage produced on the mucosa by the attachment of the worm and by their metabolic products (30). The infection is more common in 4- to 13-year-olds, and the symptoms are related to the number of worms in the intestine; small numbers are tolerated well, but a heavy worm burden may cause intestinal obstruction. Some persons have diarrhea and abdominal pain, and a few with massive infections die. In chronic infections the main manifestations are chronic diarrhea with electrolyte and protein imbalance, often resulting in anasarca (3).

The diagnosis of the infection is based on finding eggs almost identical to those of Fasciola hepatica (Chapter 52). The eggs have an operculum, are about 130 to 140 μm by 80 to 85 μm, and are unembryonated when passed in the stools (Fig. 50–10B, C).

Nanophyetus salmincola

Nanophyetus (Troglotrema) salmincola is a common intestinal trematode in wild and domestic dogs in Siberia and the Pacific northwest United States, where human infections have been recorded (31). In eastern Siberia prevalence rates of 98% are not uncommon. The life cycle of Nanophyetus is similar to that of Fasciolopsis, with the difference that salmon, rather than aquatic plants, are the second intermediate hosts. The infection is acquired by ingesting raw or undercooked salmon, after which the worms grow in the small intestine. The adult worms are about 0.8 to 1.1 mm long by 0.3 to 0.5 mm wide and live in the intestinal wall of the host.

The symptoms vary from mild gastrointestinal disturbances to diarrhea, nausea, vomiting, weight loss, fatigue, and peripheral eosinophilia of up to 43% (31). The diagnosis is made by identifying the broadly ovoid, operculate, thick-shelled eggs in stool samples. The size of the eggs is 60 to 80 μm by 34 to 50 μm (Fig. 50–11A, B).

Heterophyes heterophyes

Heterophyes heterophyes is only one of more than a dozen similar, small trematodes that inhabit the crypts of the small intestine of humans and animals in the Nile

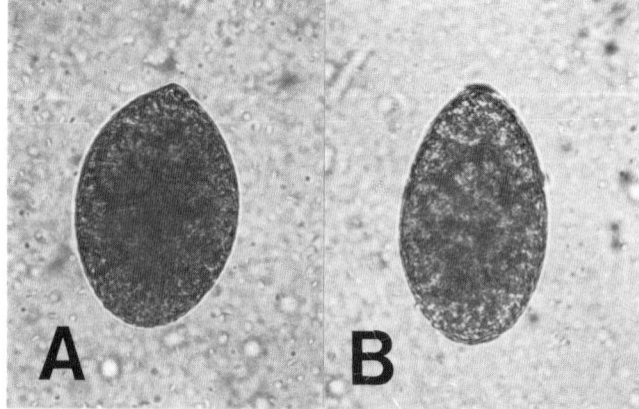

Fig. 50–11. Nanophyetus salmincola eggs in human stool (unstained, ×450). (From Gutierrez Y: Diagnostic Pathology of Parasitic Infections with Clinical Correlations. Philadelphia, Lea & Febiger, 1990.)

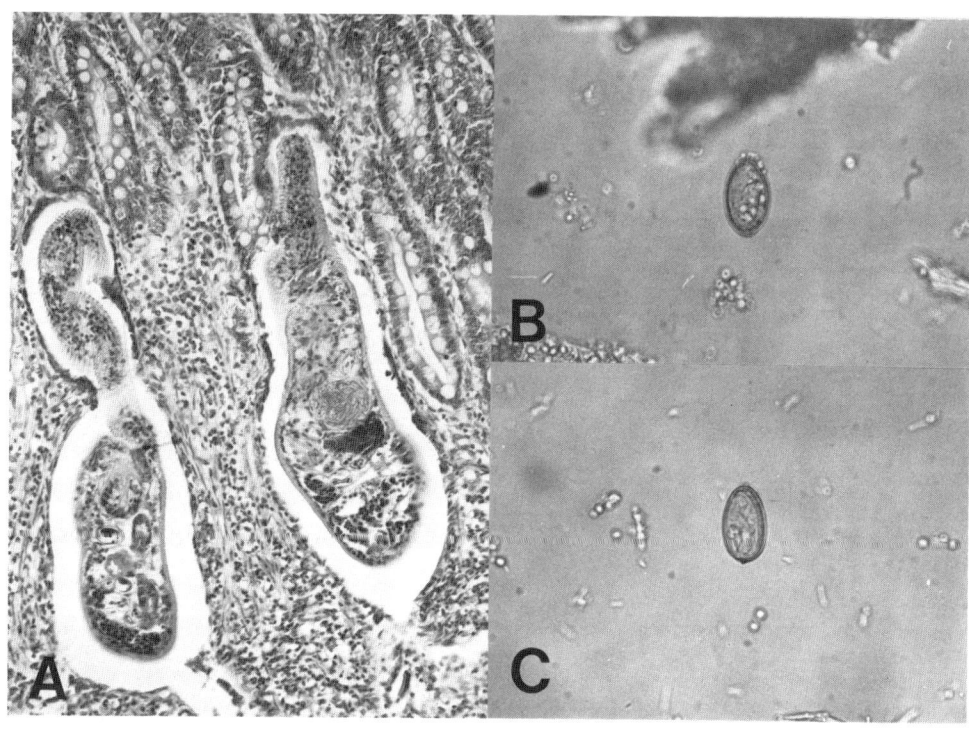

Fig. 50–12. *A*, Note the location of the Heterophyid adult, deep in the crypts of the small intestine, (hematoxylin and eosin, ×280). *B, C,* Eggs in stool (unstained, ×450).

Delta, Turkey, Japan, Korea, China, Taiwan, Philippines, Siberia, and the Balkan countries (2,3). For practical purposes these parasites are grouped here and discussed under H. heterophyes, because they produce similar symptoms. They are referred to here as heterophyids, which as a group generally occur in humans in Southeast Asia and other places.

The parasites, up to 2.5 mm long, lived buried in the crypts of the small intestine (Fig. 50–12A) and have a body that is usually covered with minute spines. Their general shape is that of a delicate flatworm with a large acetabulum at midbody and a uterus filled with eggs in the posterior half of the body. The eggs evacuated with the feces are fully embryonated. After the eggs gain access to water, they hatch. Freed embryos, which enter the snail, then develop into cercariae and finally leave the snail to encyst in several species of fish in brackish water (2).

Most infections with heterophyids are asymptomatic. Some persons with a heavy worm burden may complain of diarrhea and colicky pain, and the stools may contain unusual amounts of mucus. The diagnosis of the infection is made by identifying the eggs in stool samples; the eggs are operculated, 25 to 26 μm by 14 to 16 μm, with a shape common to all species of heterophyids. These eggs are some of the smallest helminth eggs found in the stools of humans (2) (Fig. 50–12B, C).

CESTODES

The general characteristics of cestodes and their classification are outlined in Chapter 48. All adult cestodes are parasitic of the intestinal tract of animals and humans; the larval stages are parasites of tissues in many animals, and in humans produce important diseases because of the morbidity and mortality associated with them. The adult cestodes are platyhelminths composed of a chain of segments of proglottids, usually in different stages of maturation (Fig. 50–13A). Proglottids in the cephalic region are immature (Fig. 50–14A), in the middle of the worm are mature (Fig. 50–14B), and in the posterior region are gravid (Fig. 50–13B). Each segment has both male and female organ systems, and thus, cestodes are hermaphroditic. The life cycles of cestodes vary from a direct cycle involving an egg which moves from a definitive host to another definitive host, without an intermediate host. More complicated cycles require two or more intermediate hosts (2). In this section, a few common intestinal cestodes or tapeworms of humans are discussed; the larval stages are discussed in Chapter 52.

Taenia saginata

Taenia saginata (Taeniarhynchus saginatus), known as the beef tapeworm, occurs in many parts of the world including Africa, Europe, Asia, and Central and South America. In the United States sporadic cases are seen in the general population, but they are more common among Hispanics and other immigrants.

The adult worm lives in the small intestine, where it attains a size of about 6 meters; the body of the adult worm is characterized by a chain of fleshy proglottids (Fig. 50–13A). The scolex (head) of the worm in the anterior end of the body is about 1 mm, quadrate, with four suckers. Beyond the scolex is the neck of the parasite, the region where the growth of the worm occurs: new proglottids, minute at first, form in this region. Proglottids in the anterior part are immature (Fig. 50–14A) but develop as they are pushed caudad by the formation of new ones. At the midportion of the worm the proglottids are roughly square, have well-developed sex organs, and begin form-

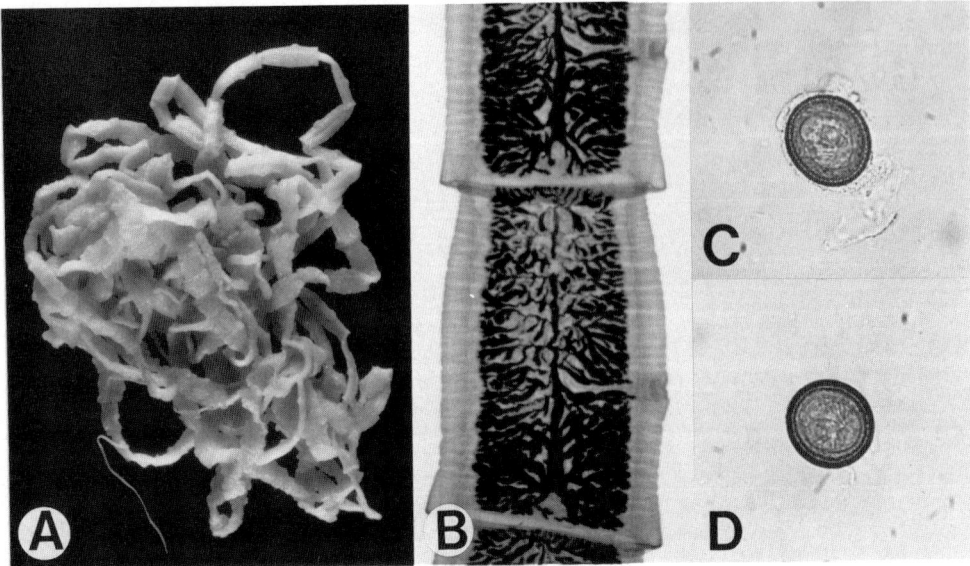

Fig. 50-13. Taenia saginata. *A*, Adult worm. Note the slender anterior end of the worm and the posterior gravid proglottids above. *B*, in the gravid proglottid note the numerous branches of the uterus (acetocarmine alum, ×11). *C, D*, Eggs in human stool (unstained, ×450).

ing eggs, which are stored in the uterus (Fig. 50–14B). In the posterior part of the worm, the proglottids are about 2 cm long by 0.6 cm wide and 0.2 cm thick; the uterus of these proglottids is filled with eggs (gravid). The last proglottid of the chain usually breaks off and frees the eggs, which are evacuated with the feces. Proglottids, often without eggs, are also found in the feces.

The life cycle of Taenia saginata involves cattle, the intermediate host, where the larval stage (cysticercus) develops. Ingestion of eggs, embryonated at the time of evacuation, releases the microscopic embryos in the intestine, embryos which enter the intestinal wall and through the circulation are distributed throughout the body to subcutaneous tissues and muscles of the animal. In these locations the embryos differentiate into larvae, the cysticerci, which measure up to 1 cm in diameter. Cysticerci are composed of a transparent cyst filled with a clear fluid and an invaginated scolex. Ingestion of raw or undercooked beef that contains cysticerci produces the infection in humans. Usually only one worm develops in the intestine.

The symptoms of infection with Taenia saginata are nonspecific, mild, and tolerated well by most persons. Passage of proglottids through the anal sphincter or finding proglottids in clothes or crawling down the leg of the patient is not uncommon. These proglottids are often brought to the laboratory by the patient for identification. The diagnosis of infection often is made on the characteristic proglottids or the eggs found in stools (see below).

Taenia solium

Taenia solium is commonly known as the pork tapeworm because the infection is acquired by eating infected raw or undercooked pork; humans are the only known definitive host of the parasite. T. solium is found commonly in Latin America, North China, India, Pakistan, Manchuria, and Europe (especially among Slavic people). In the United States, it affects mainly the Latin American immigrant population.

The life cycle of Taenia solium is similar to that of Taenia saginata, with the exception that the cysticercus develops in hogs, and thus ingestion of raw or undercooked pork produces the infection (3). The clinical manifestations and the diagnosis of T. solium infection are also simi-

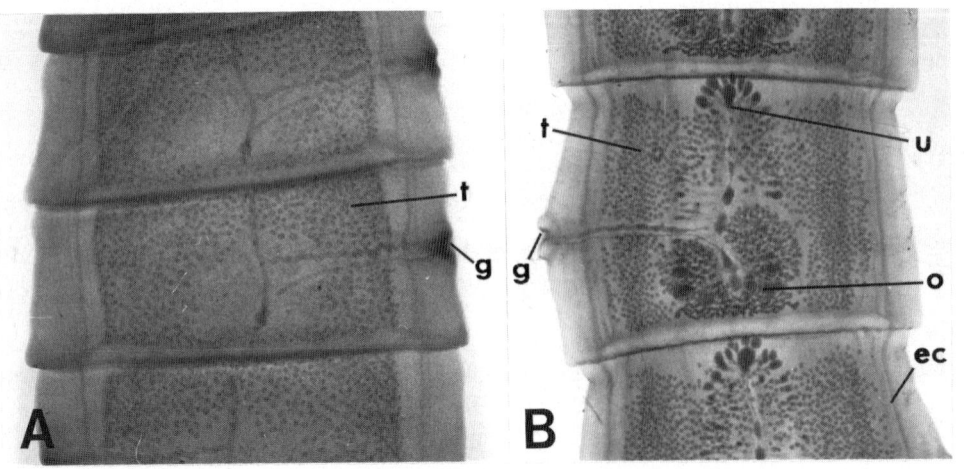

Fig. 50-14. Taenia saginata proglottids (hematoxylin. *A*, Immature, (×22); *B*, mature (×11). Note the immature proglottid is wider than long and the mature one is roughly square. Key: *t*, testis; *o*, ovary; *g*, genital pore; *u*, uterus; *ec*, excretory canals.

INTESTINAL HELMINTHS

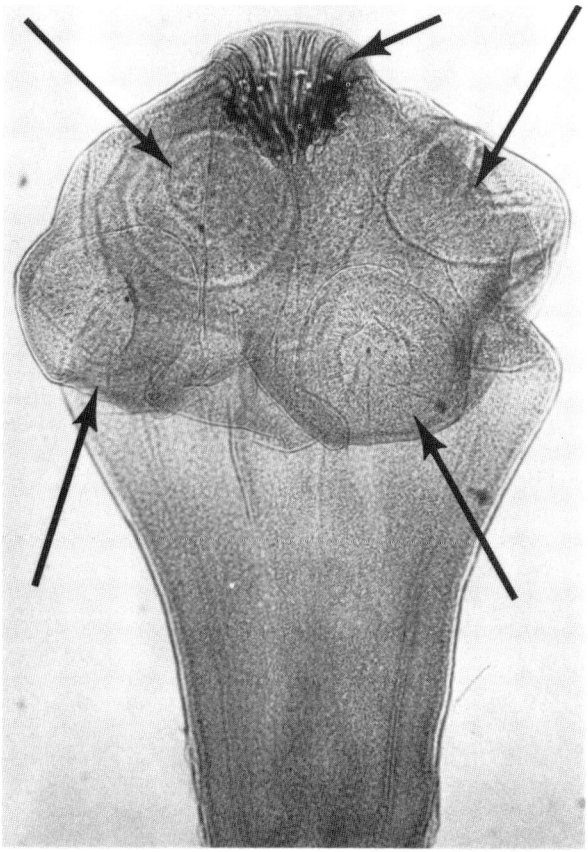

Fig. 50–15. Taenia solium scolex. Note the four suckers (*long arrows*) and the rostellum (*short arrow*) with the hooklets (acetocarmine alum, ×70). (From Gutierrez Y: Diagnostic Pathology of Parasitic Infections with Clinical Correlations. Philadelphia, Lea & Febiger, 1990.)

lar to those of Taenia saginata. However, the medical importance of Taenia solium resides in the fact that its larval stage, the cysticercus, can develop in humans, producing cysticercosis (see Chapter 52). The adult T. solium is between 2 and 7 meters long, is more delicate and slender than Taenia saginata, and the proglottids are rarely found in feces because they disintegrate while moving with the intestinal contents. The scolex of Taenia solium is about 1 mm, quadrate, has four suckers, and in addition, has a rostellum with two rows of hooks (Fig. 50–15) (2).

The diagnosis of Taenia solium and or Taenia saginata is based on the study of proglottids or segments of the strobila evacuated with the feces. Gravid proglottids of Taenia solium usually have a uterus with 7 to 13 lateral branches; Taenia saginata has 15 to 20 branches (Fig. 50–13B). The genital pores, where the male and female sex organs join, of Taenia are located on one side of the strobila. T. saginata has genital pores irregularly alternating on the right and the left of the worm; Taenia solium usually has genital pores regularly alternating between right and left. The eggs are similar in both species: 31 to 43 μm in diameter and composed of a thick shell, with radial striations, containing an embryo with three pairs of small hooks (Fig. 50–13C, D) (2). The best report generated in the laboratory should read as "eggs of Taenia spp."

Hymenolepis

Two species of Hymenolepis produce usually subclinical infections worldwide: Hymenolepis nana and Hymenolepis diminuta; a few individuals infected with Hymenolepis nana may have important symptoms.

Hymenolepis nana. H. nana is the most common tapeworm diagnosed in the United States. The strobila is delicate and up to 32 mm long: thus the common name "dwarf tapeworm" (Fig. 50–16A). The proglottids are wider than long, with a genital pore on the same side of the strobila. The scolex has a rostellum with a row of hooklets. The life cycle of H. nana is dual, with both direct and indirect development. The direct cycle occurs when the embryonated eggs passed in feces are ingested by a susceptible host. The eggs in the intestine release embryos which enter the mucosa of the small intestine and within it develop to infective larvae (cysticercoids); cysticercoids dislodge from the mucosa and grow to adult

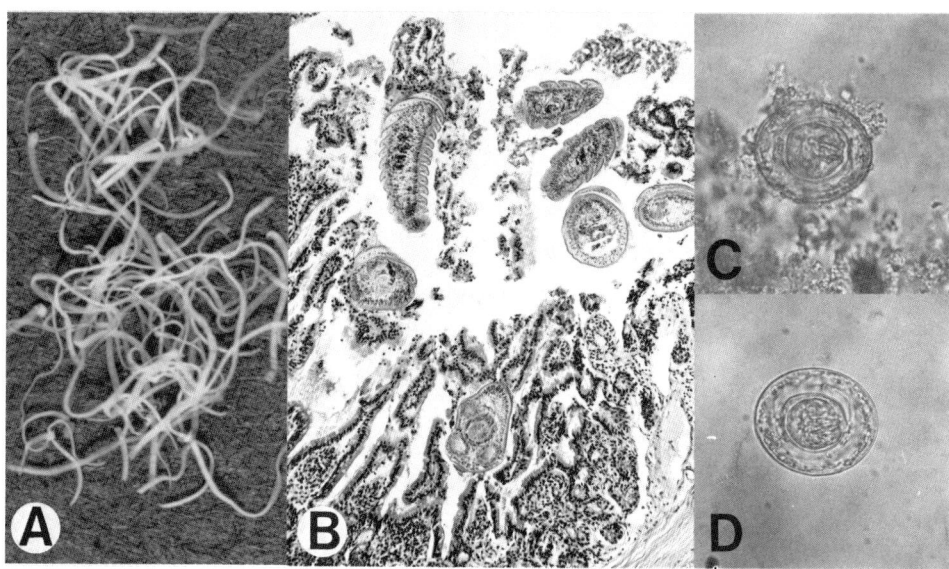

Fig. 50–16. Hymenolepis nana. *A*, Numerous adult specimens recovered from a patient after treatment (unstained, × 2.5). *B*, Sections of adult worm in the intestine of an experimentally infected animal (×110). *C, D*, Eggs in human stool (unstained, × 450).

worms attached to the mucosa (Fig. 50–16B) (32). In the direct type of development the number of adult worms in the intestine correlates with the number of eggs ingested; the development of cysticercoids in the mucosa apparently confers immunity to the host, immunity which does not foster development of more eggs. The result is usually an asymptomatic infection, because only a small number of worms develop.

The indirect cycle is more important medically because it often results in heavy infections (32). The eggs evacuated with the feces are ingested by certain arthropods, the intermediate hosts, where the cysticercoid develops in their tissues. Ingestion of an infected arthropod frees the cysticercoids (usually a few) in the intestine, where they grow to adults in the lumen (no mucosal phase, no immunity). The adult worm soon starts developing eggs, which release embryos that enter the mucosa (internal autoinfection) to develop into cysticercoids, which confer immunity against other embryos developing in the mucosa (32). The cysticercoids return to the lumen and grow to adults, resulting in a large number of worms in the intestine. If the host has some form of immune impairment the cycle could repeat over and over, producing overwhelming infections (32).

Symptoms of Hymenolepis nana infection generally are associated with large numbers of worms and consist of nonspecific diarrhea, abdominal pain, and other manifestations. The infection is diagnosed by recognition of the typical eggs in stool samples (Chapter 59). The eggs are colorless, slightly oval, 30 to 43 μm in largest diameter, with a medium thick shell containing an onchosphere with three pairs of hooklets (Fig. 50–16C, D). The space between the egg shell and the onchosphere is generally narrower than in Hymenolepis diminuta and contains two polar masses from which several filaments arise (2).

Hymenolepis diminuta. H. diminuta, known as the rat tapeworm, is up to 70 cm long, has a well-developed strobila (Fig. 50–17A) and a scolex with four suckers, and a rostellum without hooklets. The proglottids are wider than long and have genital pores on the same side of the strobila. The life cycle is identical to the indirect cycle of Hymenolepis nana, involving an arthropod where the cysticercoid develops without a mucosal phase, and therefore infections consist of one or two adult worms. Infection with Hymenolepis diminuta in humans are accidental (accidental ingestion of arthropods infected with cysticercoids) and occur sporadically worldwide. In the United States infections are seen especially in children, but they are rarely reported in the literature.

The symptoms produced by infection with Hymenolepis diminuta are nonspecific gastrointestinal disturbances. The diagnosis is based on the identification of typical eggs in the stools. The eggs are almost spherical with a diameter of 60 to 86 μm, have a thick shell containing an onchosphere with three pairs of hooklets (Fig. 50–17B, C). The distance between the onchosphere and the shell is greater than in Hymenolepis nana eggs, and the space appears clear and translucent (2).

Dipylidium caninum

Dipylidium caninum is a worldwide parasite of dogs and cats that sporadically produces infections in humans. The life cycle of this tapeworm is similar to that of Hymenolepis diminuta, requiring an arthropod, usually a flea, in which the cysticercoid develops. Accidental ingestion of infected fleas releases the cysticercoid, which grows in the small intestine. The adult worm is about 70 cm long (2).

The scolex of Dipylidium caninum has four suckers and a rostellum with one to seven rows of hooklets. The strobila has characteristic proglottids, barrel-shaped, with a double genital system, one on each side, and thus two genital pores, one on each side of the proglottid (Fig. 50–18B). The uterus of the worm consists of capsules filled with eggs in packs of 8 to 20, which are evacuated with the feces.

The clinical symptoms of dipylidiasis are nonspecific. The diagnosis of the infection is made by finding in the stool proglottids or the typical packets with spherical eggs 24 to 40 μm in diameter (Fig. 50–18A).

Diphyllobothrium

The genus Diphyllobothrium has many species that infect wild animals, especially in temperate zones. Humans have been found to harbor several species of Diphyllobothrium and other related species, the best known being Diphyllobothrium latum. Human infections with Diphyllobothrium are common in Northern Europe, Russia, Central Siberia, Manchuria, and Japan. On the American continent Diphyllobothrium occurs in Chile and in the United States and Canada around the Great Lakes (2). Outbreaks of diphyllobothriasis have been described on the Pacific coast, where they are acquired by consumption of raw salmon (33).

The life cycles of diphyllobothrids are complicated. Adult worms live in the small intestine, where they attain a length of up to 10 meters. The scolex is elongated, has one ventral and one dorsal groove, the bothrids, and lacks

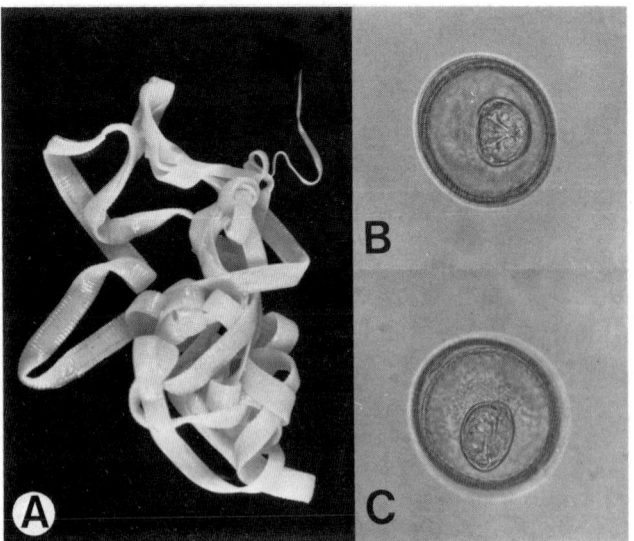

Fig. 50–17. Hymenolepis diminuta. A, Adult worm. B, C, Eggs in human stools (unstained, ×450).

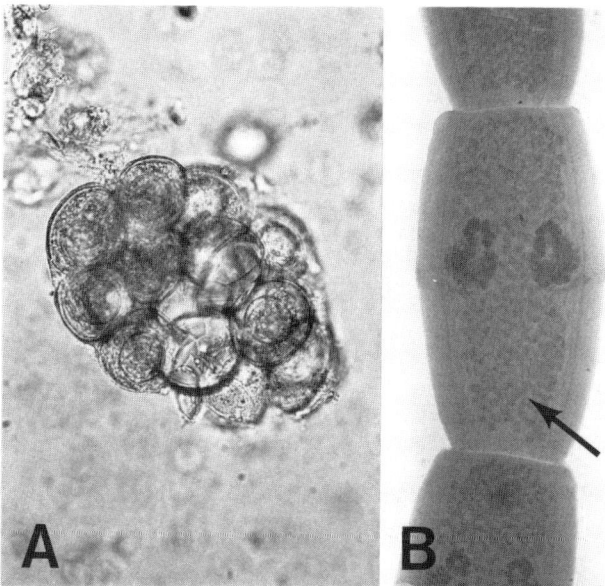

Fig. 50–18. Dipylidium caninum. *A*, Egg packet in human stools (unstained, ×300). *B*, In the proglottid, note the shape of the proglottid, the eggs in uterine cells (*arrow*), and the double genital system, one on each side (aceto-carmine alum, ×22).

a rostellum. The great majority of the proglottids are gravid, because Diphyllobothrium has an opening for oviposition, unlike other tapeworms, which lose the last proglottid to release the eggs (Fig. 50–19A, B). Oviposition is active and accounts for elimination of large numbers of eggs daily (2).

The eggs evacuated with the feces develop in fresh water. After embryonation the egg frees an embryo, which swims until it is ingested by an arthropod, where development to a procercoid larva occurs. Infected arthropods (copepods) are ingested by small fish and small fish by larger fish. In fish, a plerocercoid or Sparganum larva develops, larva which is infective for the definitive hosts, who acquire the infection by eating raw or undercooked infected fish. Freshwater fish are the usual intermediate hosts for Diphyllobothrium; thus the name "fish tapeworm" (2).

The symptoms produced by infection with Diphyllobothrium are often nonspecific. Infected persons often recognize the infection when they evacuate large portions of the strobila. In some cases, especially in northern Europe, infected persons may suffer from megaloblastic anemia (pernicious anemia) due to the competition between the worm and the host for vitamin B_{12}. The vitamin ingested by the host is absorbed by the parasite, resulting in the deficiency, which leads to anemia. Megaloblastic anemia has not been observed in persons with diphyllobothriasis outside northern Europe.

The diagnosis of the infection is made by identifying portions of the parasite evacuated by the patient, but more often by finding the typical eggs in stool samples (Chapter 59). The eggs of Diphyllobothrium are 58 to 76 μm by 40 to 51 μm. They have an operculum, a moderately thick shell, golden brown with a small knob at the opposite end of the operculum, and contain an immature embryo. The eggs alone do not allow identification of the different species that parasitize humans. The laboratory should report "Diphyllobothrium spp eggs" (Fig. 50–19C, D).

REFERENCES

1. Wagner ED, and Eby WC: Pinworm prevalence in California elementary school children, and diagnostic methods. Am J Trop Med Hyg, *32*:998, 1983.

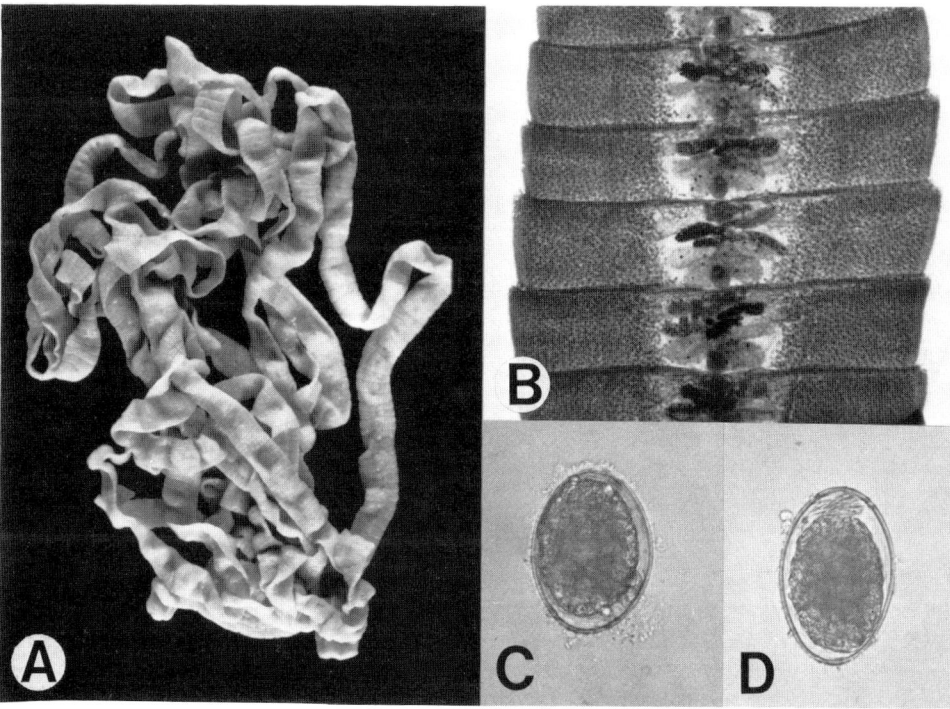

Fig. 50–19. Diphyllobothrium. *A*, Portion of an adult worm passed with the stools. Note width of the proglottids and their uniform size throughout this posterior portion of the worm. *B*, Several proglottids showing the uterus with eggs (*arrow*), (hematoxylin, ×15). *C, D*, Eggs in human stool (unstained, ×450).

2. Beaver PC, Jung RC, and Cupp EW: Clinical Parasitology. 9th ed. Philadelphia, Lea & Febiger, 1984.
3. Gutierrez Y: Diagnostic Pathology of Parasitic Infections with Clinical Correlations. Philadelphia, Lea & Febiger, 1990.
4. Simon RD: Pinworm infestation and urinary tract infection in young girls. Am J Dis Child, 128:21, 1974.
5. WHO: Intestinal Protozoan and Helminthic Infections. Tech Rep Ser No 666. Geneva, World Health Organization, 1981.
6. Bundy DAP: Epidemiological aspects of Trichuris and trichuriasis in Caribbean communities. Trans R Soc Trop Med Hyg, 80:706, 1986.
7. Jung RC, and Beaver PC: Clinical observations on Trichocephalus trichiuris (whipworm) infestation in children. Pediatrics, 8:548, 1951.
8. Gilman RH, Chong YH, Davis C, et al: The adverse consequences of heavy Trichuris infection. Trans R Soc Trop Med Hyg, 77:432, 1983.
9. Kamath KR: Severe infection with Trichuris trichiura in Malaysian children. A clinical study of 30 cases treated with stilbazium iodide. Am J Trop Med Hyg, 22:600, 1973.
10. Bowie MD, Morrison A, and Ireland JD: Clubbing and whipworm infestation. Arch Dis Child, 53:411, 1978.
11. Gilman RH, Davis C, and Fitzgerald F: Heavy Trichuris infection and amoebic dysentery in Orang Asli children. A comparison of the two diseases. Trans R Soc Trop Med Hyg, 70:313, 1976.
12. Wagner ED, and Pena Chavarria A: Observations on "large" Trichuris eggs in man. Proc Helm Soc Wash, 46:135, 1979.
13. Kalkofen UP: Attachment and feeding behavior of Ancylostoma caninum. Z Parasitenk, 33:339, 1970.
14. Loeffler W: Transient lung infiltration with blood eosinophilia. Int Arch Allergy, 8:54, 1956.
15. Vogel H, and Minning W: Beitrage zur klinik der Lungenascariasis und Frage der fluchtigen eosinophilen Lungeninfiltrate. Beitr Klin Turberk, 98:624, 1942.
16. Stephenson LS: The contribution of Ascaris lumbricoides to malnutrition in children. Parasitology, 81:221, 1980.
17. Stephen LS, Crompton DW, Latham MC, et al: Relationships between Ascaris infection and growth of malnourished preschool children in Kenya. Am J Clin Nutr, 33:1165, 1980.
18. Gil GV, and Bell DR: Long-standing tropical infections among former war prisoners of the Japanese. Lancet, 1:958, 1982.
19. Vince JD, Ashford RW, Gratten MJ, et al: Strongyloides species infestation in young infants of Papua New Guinea: Association with generalized edema. Papua New Guinea Med J, 22:120, 1979.
20. Otsuru M: Studies on Trichostrongylus (Nematoda: Trichostrongylidae) of man and animals. Kiseichugaku Zasshi, 11:244, 1962 [In Japanese].
21. Wallace L, Henkin R, and Mathies AW: Trichostrongylus infestation with profound eosinophilia. Ann Intern Med, 45:146, 1956.
22. Nawa K, Imai J-I, Abe T, et al: A case report of intestinal capillariasis—the second case found in Japan. Jpn J Parasitol, 37:113, 1988.
23. Watten RH, Beckner WM, and Cross JH: Clinical studies of capillariasis philippinensis. Trans R Soc Trop Med Hyg, 66:828, 1972.
24. Dauz U, Cabrera BD, and Canlas B Jr: Human intestinal capillariasis. I. Clinical features. Acta Med Philipp, 4:72, 1967.
25. Fresh JW, Cross JH, Reyes V, et al: Necropsy findings in intestinal capillariasis. Am J Trop Med Hyg, 21:169, 1972.
26. Cabrera BD, Canlas B, Jr, and Dauz U: Human intestinal capillariasis. III. Parasitological features and management. Acta Med Philipp, 4:92, 1967.
27. Oshima T: Anisakiasis—is the suchi bar guilty? Parasitol Today, 3:44, 1987.
28. Schantz PM: The dangers of eating raw fish. N Engl J Med, 320:1143, 1989.
29. Little MD: Laboratory diagnosis of worms and miscellaneous specimens. Clin Lab Med, 11:1041, 1991.
30. Rahman KM, Idris MD, and Azad Khan AK: A study on fasciolopsiasis in Bangladesh. J Trop Med Hyg, 84:81, 1981.
31. Eastburn RL, Fritsche TR, and Terhune CA Jr: Human intestinal infection with Nanophyetus salmincola from salmonid fishes. Am J Trop Med Hyg, 36:586, 1987.
32. Heyneman D: Host-parasite resistance patterns—some implications from experimental studies with helminths. Ann N Y Acad Sci, 113:114, 1963.
33. Ruttenberg AJ, Weineger BG, Sorvillo F, et al: Diphyllobothriasis associated with salmon consumption in Pacific coast states. Am J Trop Med Hyg, 33:455, 1984.

Chapter 51

BLOOD AND TISSUE PROTOZOA

Chapter 49 contains a brief review of the groups of protozoa that affect the human gastrointestinal tract, emphasizing that members of the flagellates, amebae, Apicomplexa, and Microspora can be present both in the intestine and the tissues. In this chapter, the species that inhabit the tissues of humans are discussed.

FLAGELLATES

The flagellates of blood and tissues belong to a large family of organisms, the Trypanosomatidae, with two genera—Trypanosoma and Leishmania—which contain many species parasitic in humans, most of which produce morbidity and mortality throughout the tropics and subtropics.

The life cycle of most species of Trypanosomatidae involves two hosts: haematophagous arthropod intermediate host and a vertebrate definitive host. The genus Trypanosoma has species that are parasitic both intra- and extracellularly, while the members of the genus Leishmania are all intracellular parasites. These two genera of flagellates and the diseases they produce are discussed separately.

LEISHMANIA

The leishmaniae are a large group of intracellular protozoa that live in the monocyte/macrophage system, where they multiply by binary fission as aflagellar stages, the amastigotes. Survival of the parasite within the parasitophorous vacuole is accomplished by several mechanisms that inhibit the burst of lysosomal enzymes in the vacuole by the macrophage (1); by modulating the T-cell immune response; and by directing the host's bone marrow to produce immature macrophages. Once the number of intracellular amastigotes reaches a "critical mass," the cell ruptures, freeing the parasites, which are phagocytosed by other macrophages, to continue a new cycle of division. Hematophagous insects of several genera (Phlebotomus, Lutzomia, Psychodopygus), commonly known as sand flies, become infected during a blood meal on a parasitized host; the amastigotes ingested by the fly transform into flagellates (promastigotes) and divide actively in the gut of the insect. The infected fly has masses of flagellates in its gut, which interfere with its feeding, and eventually it regurgitates the promastigotes (infective stages) into a new host to initiate the cycle de novo (2).

Leishmaniae are distributed throughout the tropical and temperate zones, where they produce a variety of diseases, usually in poor, underprivileged persons who carry on a marginal existence. The parasites usually have as their natural host a domestic or a wild animal, and thus leishmaniae are zoonotic and humans are incidental hosts (3). In general, two types of infections are recognized as being produced by leishmaniae: cutaneous and visceral leishmaniasis. Both infections are seen in the United States sporadically; in southern Texas, the cutaneous form is endemic (4,5).

Cutaneous leishmaniasis

Cutaneous leishmaniasis is a group of diseases produced by several species of Leishmania: three species of the Old World—Leishmania tropica, Leishmania major and Leishmania aetiopica—occur in Africa, southern Europe, the Middle East, and parts of Pakistan and Afghanistan; at least seven species of the New World—Leishmania braziliensis, Leishmania guayanensis, Leishmania panamensis, Leishmania mexicana, Leishmania amazonensis, Leishmania venezuelensis, and Leishmania peruviana—occur in different regions of the American continent from southern Texas to southern Brazil (3).

The infection with any of these organisms results in a skin ulcer at the site where the vector bites, usually an exposed part of the body (Fig. 51–1A). In general, the ulcer is painless, evolves in a few days to a few weeks, and generally heals spontaneously after a few weeks or months, depending on the species of Leishmania. Often, lifelong immunity to the species in question develops. The ulcer varies in size, shape, and character, but it frequently consists of loss of the skin in an area up to 6 cm in diameter, often revealing a clean bottom of granulation tissue, or sometimes with secondary bacterial contamination; some persons have dry, crusted ulcers. The borders of the ulcer often are raised and sharply delineated. Usually one ulcer is present, less often more (3,6). On histologic examination the lesions are granulomatous inflammations with numerous histiocytes, lymphocytes, and plasma cells. In areas of ulceration infiltration by polymorphonuclear cells is common. The granulomas vary from poorly formed to well-formed with giant cells. Parasites often are scanty but sometimes numerous (Fig. 51–1C,D).

Infections with Leishmania aethiopica in Africa, and with Leishmania braziliensis, Leishmania guayanensis, and Leishmania panamensis in the New World, may metastasize to the cartilages of the naso-oropharynx, producing a mucocutaneous ulcer characterized by loss of the cartilage with marked disfigurement, and sometimes death if the infection progresses down to the pharynx. This form of the disease is known in some places in Latin American as espundia. Infections with Leishmania aetiopica in Africa and Leishmania mexicana, Leishmania venezuelensis, and Leishmania amazonensis in the New World sometimes result in disseminated disease (diffuse cutaneous leishmani-

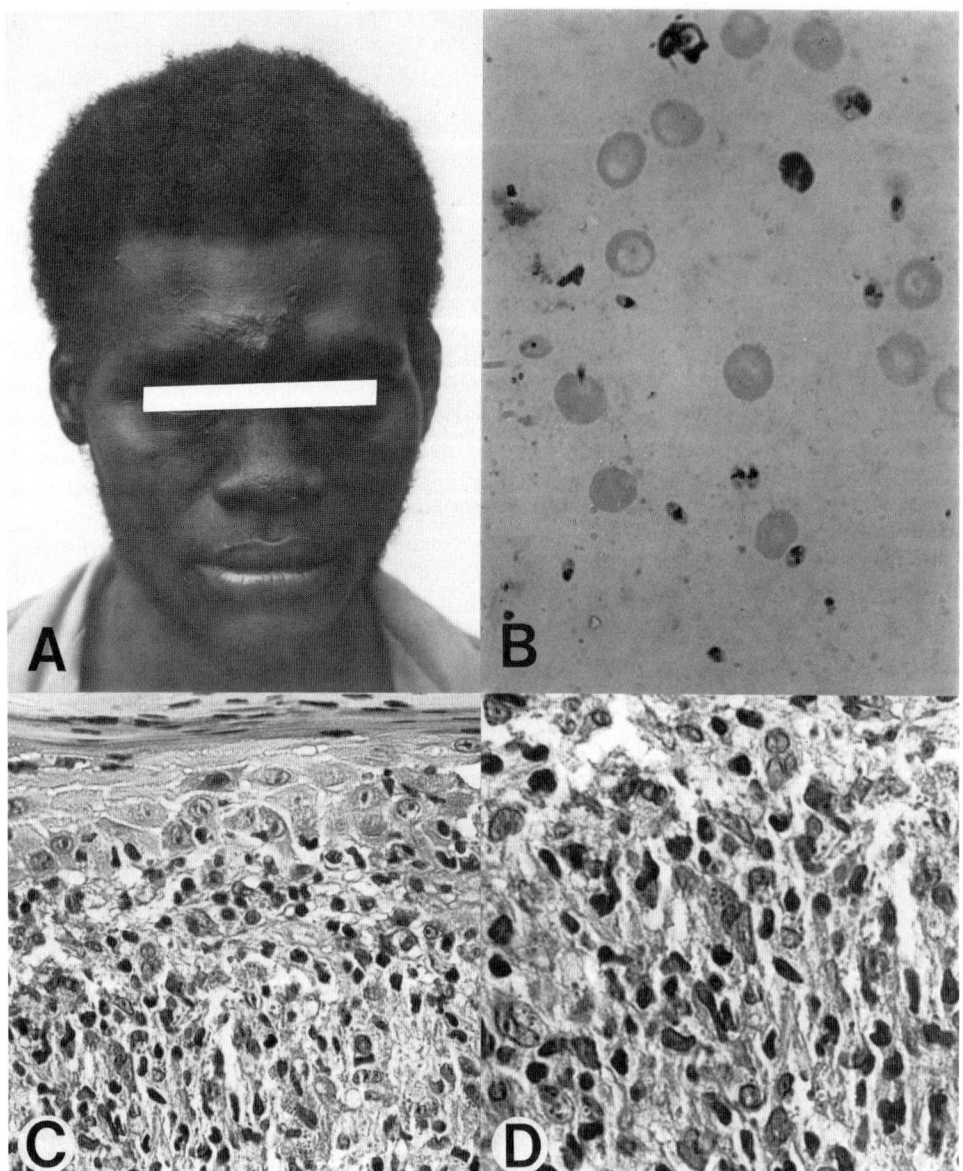

Fig. 51–1. Cutaneous leishmaniasis. A, Gross appearance of skin ulcer. B, Smear of lesion, shows the typical amastigotes (Giemsa ×1120). C, D, Histologic section shows the histiocytic infiltration; some histiocytes contain the parasites in the cytoplasm, seen as small dots, (hematoxylin and eosin, C, ×450; D, ×705).

asis), characterized by numerous subcutaneous nodules composed of large numbers of histiocytes with abundant parasites (Fig. 51–2) and little or no inflammatory reaction. Clinically, a person suffering from diffuse cutaneous Leishmaniasis resembles a patient with lepromatous leprosy, and the circumstances in which diffuse leishmaniasis arises are consistent with anergy, similar to what occurs in leprosy (3).

Regardless of the different manifestations of cutaneous leishmaniasis, the diagnosis often is made clinically, based on the patient's being from or having traveled to an endemic area; more specifically, the patient lives or has been in the habitat where the parasite occurs: the wilderness (7). Leishmaniae are acquired in the city (are urbanized), for example, Leishmania donovani in India (see below).

The diagnosis of leishmaniasis is confined to the clinical laboratory by finding the typical organisms in samples taken from the ulcers, following the guidelines outlined in Chapter 62 (Fig. 62–1 to 4). Smears and imprints stained with Giemsa stain, examined under oil immersion, reveal amastigotes as ovoid organisms, about 4 μm long (half the diameter of a red blood cell). The parasite has a nucleus that stains deep red on the posterior half; a kinetoplast next to the nucleus that also stains red, and an axoneme (a remnant of the flagellum), which usually does not stain with Giemsa stain; the cytoplasm of the parasite stains variably from pale to deep blue (Fig. 51–1B) (6,7).

Amastigotes are three-dimensional objects with the organelles arranged in a specific manner, which gives two main configurations to the parasite, dorsoventral and lateral (Fig. 51–3). These two views, and others produced by other orientations of the parasite, should be kept in mind when examining stained smears if proper identification is to be made. The identification is possible only to the generic level, because the species are classified after isolation of the parasite in cultures, which provide large

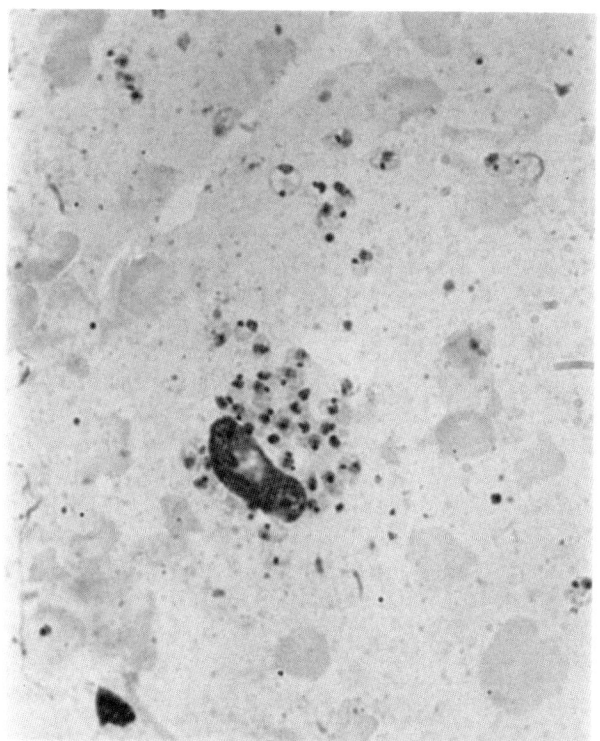

Fig. 51–2. Diffuse cutaneous leishmaniasis, imprint shows abundance of amastigotes, (Giemsa, ×1120).

numbers of organisms for study of their enzymatic patterns (6).

Visceral leishmaniasis

Similar to the cutaneous leishmaniae, visceral leishmaniasis is produced by two species in the Old World: Leishmania donovani and Leishmania infantum, and by Leishmania chagasi in the New World. Leishmania donovani occurs in India, Bangladesh, and China, and is probably

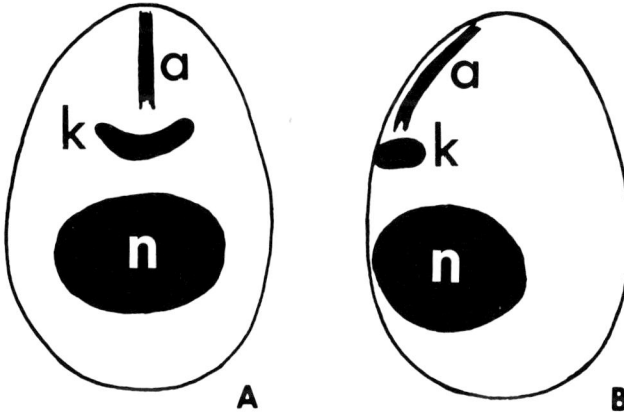

Fig. 51–3. Schematic representation of amastigotes. A, Anteroposterior and B, lateral view. Key a, axoneme; k, kinetoplast; n, nucleus. (From Gutierrez Y: Diagnostic Pathology of Parasitic Infections with Clinical Correlations. Philadelphia, Lea & Febiger, 1990.)

the only species without a reservoir host; therefore, transmission is human-vector-human; Leishmania infantum in the Mediterranean basin, Africa, and the Middle East, and Leishmania chagasi on the American continent (3).

Visceral leishmaniasis is also known as Kala-azar in India; the infection is endemic, but epidemics occur, especially after periods of famine or after natural disasters. The clinical picture is variable; the disease occurs mostly in males, and in the Mediterranean area, India, China, and South America, usually in children of both sexes aged 1 to 4 years. The main symptoms are chronic fever, anorexia, and weight loss, with marked hepato- and splenomegaly. The course of the infection is usually chronic and, if not treated, terminates in death (3).

The diagnosis of visceral leishmaniasis is usually made by the anatomic pathologist in bone marrow smears (Fig. 51–4B,C; Plate XIC) and biopsy specimens of liver (Fig. 51–4A), spleen, or other organs (6,7). If samples are sent to the clinical laboratory the diagnosis is based on similar principles to those used for the cutaneous leishmaniae (Chapter 62) (7).

TRYPANOSOMA

The genus Trypanosoma has several species that infect humans, one of which, Trypanosoma cruzi, has an intracellular phase in its development. Trypanosomes are infections of both animals and humans, especially in the tropical areas, where they cause significant morbidity and mortality (8).

In general, two types of trypanosomiasis are described in humans: the African, produced by two subspecies, Trypanosoma brucei gambiense and Trypanosoma brucei rhodesiense, and the American, produced by Trypanosoma cruzi and Trypanosoma rangeli (2,8).

Trypanosoma brucei gambiense and Trypanosoma brucei rhodesiense

The African trypanosomes are restricted to the tropical belt of Africa, where infections are common. The life cycle of these two species is similar: the vertebrate host has trypomastigotes (flagellates about 25 μm long, with a flagellum, undulating membrane, and a small kinetoplast) in circulating blood, where the parasites reproduce by longitudinal division. The invertebrate intermediate host is a haematophagous fly (the tsetse fly), of the genus Glossina, which acquires the parasite while feeding on an infected host; in the fly the flagellate multiplies in the intestine and develops to infective stages which locate in the fly's salivary glands, whence they are inoculated to the susceptible host to complete the cycle (2,8).

In humans infection with the African trypanosomes produces variable symptoms, depending on the species of the parasite (8). At the site of inoculation (infective bite), a chancre may develop, especially with Trypanosoma brucei rhodesiense infections, more often in outsiders than in those that live in the endemic area. The inoculation chancre begins 2 to 3 days after the infective bite, as a small erythematous and tender swelling, growing to 10 cm in diameter or more in 2 to 3 weeks. The lesion eventually subsides, with desquamation and healing.

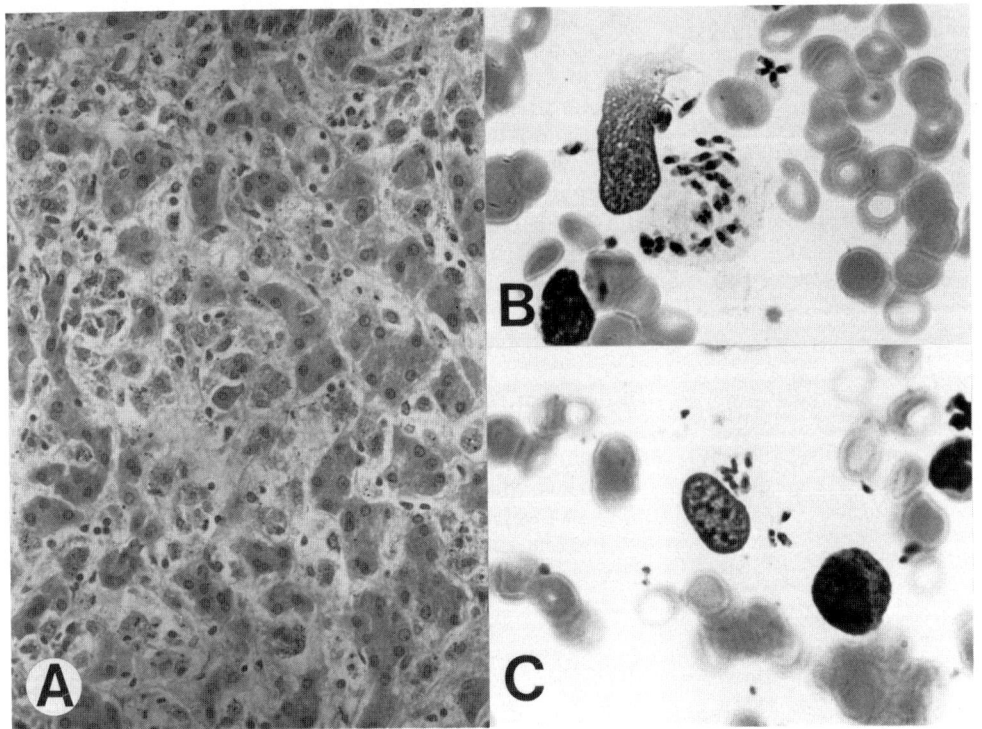

Fig. 51–4. Visceral leishmaniasis. *A*, Section of liver shows numerous macrophages with amastigotes (seen as faint stippling at this magnification) infiltrating the parenchyma (hematoxylin and eosin, ×280). *B, C,* Bone marrow shows typical amastigotes, (Giemsa, ×1120).

After the initial inoculation chancre, infection with Trypanosoma brucei rhodesiense follows an acute course with a rapidly fatal outcome; Trypanosoma brucei gambiense follows a chronic, more protracted course, with severe involvement of the central nervous system. At the beginning, both infections manifest with intermittent fever, owing to cyclic development of trypomastigotes in the blood. Lymphadenopathy is often present in many areas of the body. Infections with Trypanosoma brucei gambiense follow a course similar to that of viral encephalitis, characterized by abnormalities of the cerebrospinal fluid (CSF) (8,9).

The diagnosis of African trypanosomiasis is made clinically and is confirmed in the laboratory by finding the typical trypomastigotes in blood (Plate XID; Chapter 58) or in CSF (Chapter 55). Trypomastigotes from both species are identical, and speciation is not possible on morphologic grounds alone (10).

Trypanosoma cruzi

Trypanosoma cruzi is the agent of Chagas' disease, or American trypanosomiasis, an infection common in Latin America (11). Acute infections have a mortality rate of about 10% in children, while in adults they are silent or produce mild disease. It is estimated that at least 35 million people live under endemic conditions of trypanosomiasis in Latin America, though exact rates of prevalence are not known. The disease has been reported a few times in the United States, and recently has been found in patients who acquired the parasite with transfused blood (11).

The life cycle of Trypanosoma cruzi is different from that of the African trypanosomes in several respects. The trypomastigotes circulate in blood but do not multiply; multiplication occurs inside the cells as amastigotes. The flagellates in blood are ingested by a reduviid bug (kissing bug) of the genera Rhodnius, Triatoma, and others; many species of these genera transmit the infection. The ingested parasites develop in the posterior intestine of the reduviid to produce the infective stages (metacyclic trypomastigotes), which are excreted with the feces of the bug during its next blood meal. Metacyclic trypomastigotes are deposited on the skin, where they find abrasions and enter the tissues; or they may be transported with the fingers to the buccal or the conjunctival mucosae, where they easily gain access to the internal organs. Once inside the flagellates enter any cell, where they transform into amastigotes and divide rapidly until the cell is exhausted. Then they begin transforming into flagellates, the trypomastigotes, which leave the cell to circulate in blood and invade other cells (2,8).

The clinical manifestations of American trypanosomiasis begin usually with mild symptoms; a few persons have an acute course of fever, general malaise, muscle pain, vomiting, and diarrhea. Frequently, the symptoms follow the development of the inoculation chancre, the chagoma. After the initial phase, generalized edema, moderate hepato- and splenomegaly, and cardiac and central nervous system symptoms develop. Cardiac symptoms progress to myocarditis with a relatively high mortality rate, especially in children and persons from nonendemic areas. Following the acute phase, an indeterminate phase of positive serologic findings and electrocardiographic changes ensues, to be followed by a chronic phase of symptoms in many organ systems. These symptoms are related to the mechanical or immune-mediated (12) destruction by the parasite of the effector cells of the parasympathetic system, resulting in alterations of the conduction system of the heart, in achalasia, megaesophagus, megacolon, or other manifestations (6). Women may transmit the parasites to their offspring via the placenta, often resulting in fetal death. Donated blood from any infected individual transmits the infection (11).

Gross and histologic changes related to the infection are found in many organs. Acute Chagas' myocarditis is characterized by marked destruction of the myocardium with abundant mononuclear cell infiltrate, and parasitized cells (Fig. 51–5A). In the chronic phase few or no parasites are found, but small areas of myocarditis may be present. In the brain areas of encephalitis and in the intestine a reduction of the parasympathetic cells are observed (6).

The diagnosis of American trypanosomiasis is made clinically; confirmation is based on finding typical trypomastigotes in blood (Plate XIE; Chapter 58) and body fluids, and amastigotes in sections of biopsy or autopsy tissue (Fig. 51–5A)(6,10). The trypomastigotes of Trypanosoma cruzi in blood are C shaped, about 21 μm long, have an undulating membrane with only two wide folds, and a large kinetoplast in the posterior aspect of the body. The intracellular amastigote is indistinguishable from the amastigotes of leishmaniae. However, as multiplication progresses inside the cell, some amastigotes begin differentiating into flagellar stages, recognized in sections and imprints (Fig. 51–5B,C) as intermediate or developmental stages.

Trypanosoma rangeli

A nonpathogen found in humans in some areas of Latin America, Trypanosoma rangeli has to be distinguished from Trypanosoma cruzi in blood smears (Plate XIF). The body of Trypanosoma rangeli is longer, has more undulations of the membrane, and the kinetoplast is smaller than that of Trypanosoma cruzi.

AMEBAE

The amebae found in tissues belong to several groups of free-living amebae that are parasitic under certain conditions, often producing fatal infections in humans. Naegleria fowleri produces acute encephalitis, and Acanthamoeba and Leptomyxid amebae produce granulomatous diseases. In addition, Entamoeba histolytica, which invades tissues outside the intestinal tract, has already been discussed (Chapter 49).

Naegleria fowleri

Naegleria fowleri is the agent of acute amebic meningoencephalitis, an invariably fatal disease of immunocompetent hosts worldwide. The infection has been recognized in the United States, where cases have been reported in several states, though many more go unreported (13).

Naegleria fowleri is a free-living organism that lives under natural conditions in water and moist soil; small trophozoites multiply by binary fission (Fig. 51–6B). A cystic stage (Fig. 51–6C) develops sometimes, and under certain conditions the trophozoite may develop two temporary flagella, making Naegleria an ameboflagellate (2).

Human infections with Naegleria are accidentally acquired while in contact with water that contains the parasite (most often while swimming in contaminated waters). The parasites are introduced into the nasal cavity, where they gain access to the olfactory mucosa and develop rapidly, producing rhinitis. Soon after, the parasites enter the base of the brain through the cribriform

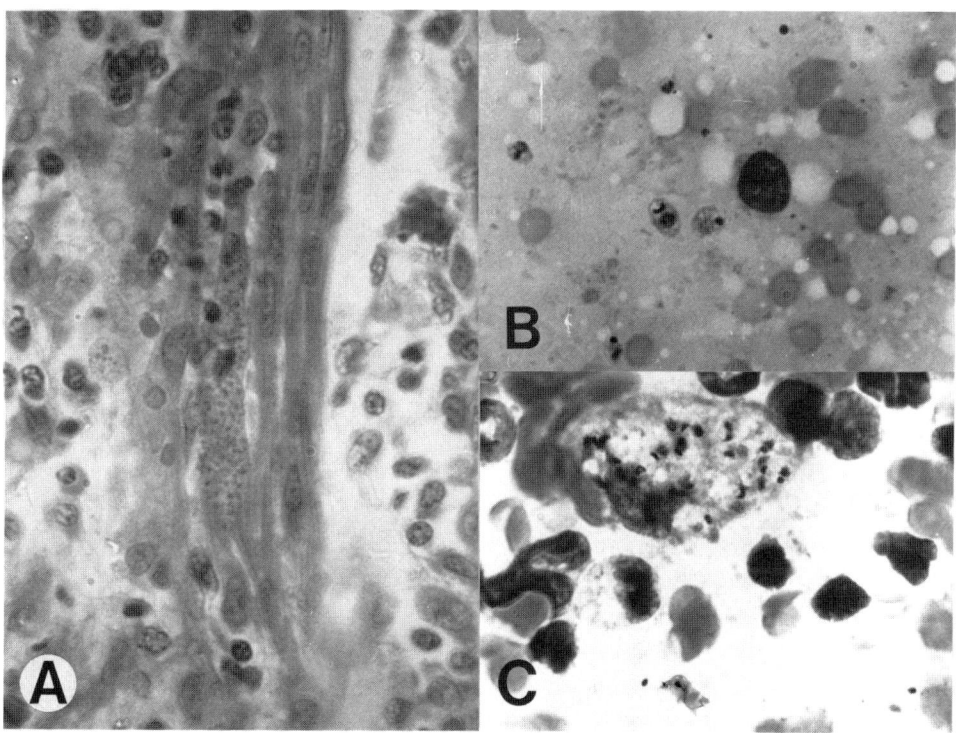

Fig. 51–5. Trypanosoma cruzi. *A*, Section of human heart, shows a cell with amastigotes, (hematoxylin and eosin, ×705). *B*, *C*, Imprints show amastigotes free from the cell (an artifact of the imprint), *B*, and within a cell, *C*, (×1120).

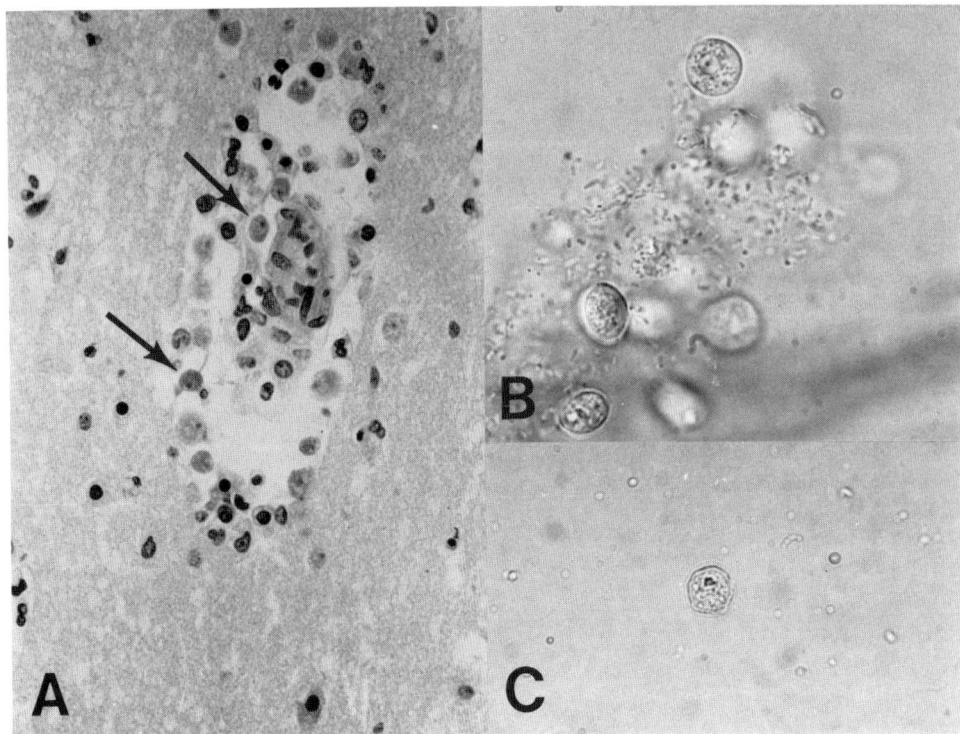

Fig. 51–6. Naegleria fowleri. A, The parasite (*arrows*), in a section of human brain (hematoxylin and eosin, ×450). B, Cysts in culture (unstained, ×1120). C, Trophozoite in culture (unstained, ×1120).

plate, follow the endings of the olfactory nerve, and gain access to the meninges, where they multiply rapidly (Fig. 51–6A). Through the spaces around the blood vessels the parasites enter the brain to form foci of encephalitis. The inflammatory reaction to the amebae is mostly mononuclear, with a few polymorphonuclear cells (6).

The course of the infection is rapid: The first symptoms of headache, slight fever, and malaise begin 2 days after infection; meningeal irritation with signs and symptoms of meningitis and encephalitis soon follow, with a course of progressive deterioration and a fatal outcome about 10 days after the symptoms begin (6,13).

The diagnosis of amebic meningoencephalitis is made in the laboratory, based on detection of the parasite in the CSF (Chapter 55) (14). The diagnosis is made more often in tissues recovered at the autopsy table (6).

Acanthamoeba and Leptomyxid amoeba

Several species of Acanthamoeba and Leptomyxid free-living amebae produce granulomatous amebic encephalitis, and sometimes disseminated infection in immunocompromised hosts; in addition, other infections such as keratitis, otitis media, osteomyelitis, and dermatitis have been described in immunocompetent hosts (13,14). The distribution of Acanthamoeba is worldwide, but the majority of infections have been described in the United States, perhaps because of the interest in the disease (13,15).

The life cycle of Acanthamoeba is similar to that of Naegleria; Acanthamoeba organisms have trophozoites in fresh water or moist soil, about 45 μm or less in diameter, with numerous spinelike projections of the cytoplasm, the acanthopods (Fig. 51–7B). The nucleus has a thin nuclear membrane, and the central karyosome is rounded and large. Surrounding the nucleus are the perinuclear vacuoles. A cystic stage allows the parasite to survive in adverse environmental conditions (Fig. 51–7C); cysts are smaller than trophozoites and consist of an irregular ectocyst (the cyst wall) containing an endocyst morphologically similar to a small trophozoite. Cysts are apparently light, can be carried in the wind, and can enter the respiratory tract to produce infection in humans. The morphologic characteristics of Acanthamoeba do not permit identification of the species, because they appear similar under light microscopy. Speciation of these parasites requires isolation in cultures and special studies (14).

Central Nervous System. In immunocompromised persons Acanthamoeba and Leptomyxid amebae produce a granulomatous amebic encephalitis, and often disseminated disease (13,14). The symptoms are headache, nausea, vomiting, fever, and nuchal rigidity; some patients have symptoms of a space-occupying mass with signs of increased intracranial pressure. Imaging techniques may reveal one or several lesions in the central nervous system, but often the patient dies before the parasites are isolated and identified in the laboratory. Gross examination of the organs reveals lesions in the brain and other parts of the central nervous system, lesions that appear as areas of hemorrhage and necrosis. Microscopically, the main finding in these lesions is parasites that have the characteristic shape of the group (Fig. 51–7A). Both trophozoites and cysts are present (6).

Eye. In the eye Acanthamoeba organisms produce chronic keratitis, often in persons who wear soft contact lenses (16). The disease begins as a corneal ulcer or an abrasion; persons who do not wear contact lenses usually trace the infection to a minor ocular trauma or to washing their eyes with dirty water. The infection usually pro-

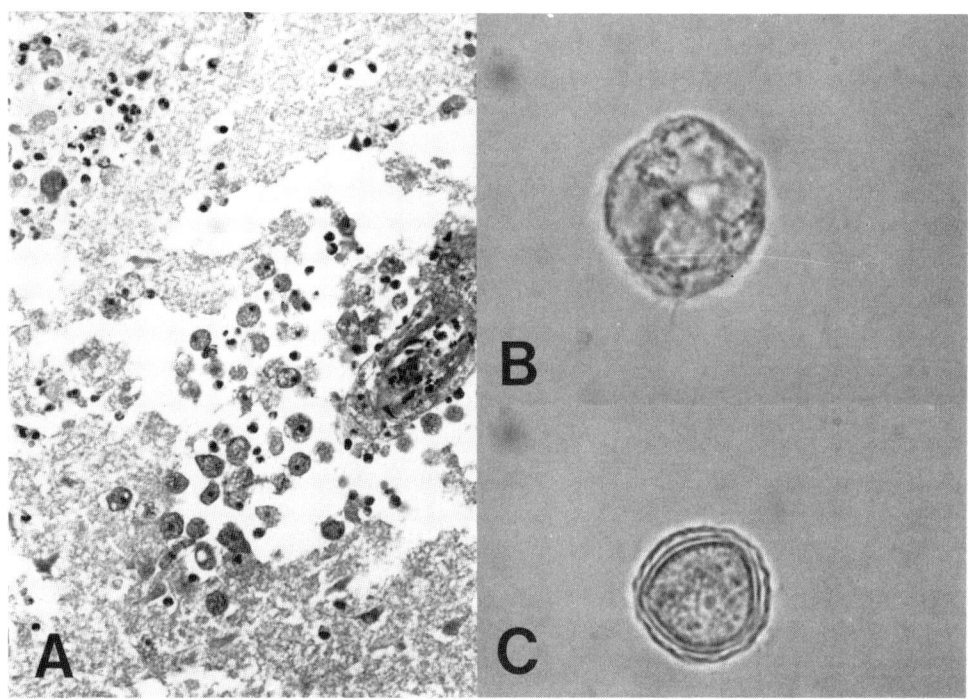

Fig. 51-7. Acanthamoeba spp. A, Numerous trophozoites of Acanthamoeba in a section of human brain (hematoxylin and eosin, ×250). Trophozoite, B, and cyst, C, from culture (unstained, ×1280).

gresses because conventional treatment, if instituted, does not help, and frank keratitis with conjunctivitis and iritis develop, with deterioration of the cornea.

Other Sites. The inner ear, the mandibular bone, and the skin are sites where Acanthamoeba infections may develop (6,14). In these cases, the clinical manifestations are nonspecific, and only a search for the parasites leads to their identification, proper diagnosis, and therapy.

The diagnosis of acanthamoebiasis rarely is made clinically (14). The parasites are identified by their morphologic characteristics in smears (see above), cultures, or biopsy specimens of the affected area (Chapters 55 and 56).

APICOMPLEXA

The Apicomplexa found in tissues belong to three genera: Toxoplasma, Plasmodium, and Babesia. Toxoplasma is rarely found in the microbiology laboratory because samples are infrequently submitted for diagnosis; instead, an anatomic pathologist examining biopsy specimens or tissue recovered at autopsy is more often responsible for the diagnosis of this infection. Plasmodium and Babesia are found in blood parasitizing red blood cells, and the infections they produce—malaria and babesiosis—are diagnosed in the clinical laboratory. Often the diagnosis of malaria is not difficult, but the classification of the different species that parasitize humans is, mainly because workers in the routine clinical laboratory do not handle enough positive specimens each year to become acquainted with the morphologic characteristics of the parasites.

Toxoplasma gondii

Toxoplasma gondii is a coccidian parasite found in cats, where the life cycle occurs in the intestinal cells in a manner similar to that of Cryptosporidium and Isospora (Chapter 49). In humans Toxoplasma occurs in the tissues, where it produces marked morbidity and mortality in immunocompromised hosts. Infections occur worldwide, and Toxoplasma is considered one of the most common infections of humans. Rates of prevalence of antibodies against Toxoplasma vary with the population under study, but in general the rate is high. Moreover, the rates of prevalence are cumulative: the older the population under study the higher the rate. This is important because it indicates that Toxoplasma is acquired on a regular basis by humans and because reactivation of an old (dormant) infection is the most common cause of acute toxoplasmosis in immunocompromised hosts.

The life cycle of Toxoplasma in the cat is initiated by the ingestion of mature (sporulated) infective oocysts in soil. Ingested oocysts release sporozoites in the intestine, oocysts which enter the enterocyte, where they develop asexually to produce merozoites; once the merozoites leave the cell they re-enter other enterocytes to repeat the asexual cycle. Some merozoites develop into sexual stages, male and female, which join to form the oocyst. Oocysts excreted with feces are immature and require maturation in the environment before they become infective to other cats (17).

If mature oocysts are accidentally ingested by animals other than cats (including humans) these animals become intermediate hosts of Toxoplasma and develop the infection in the tissues. The parasites ingested travel from the intestine to the tissues, where they enter the cells actively and develop asexually to form many small bodies known as trophozoites or tachyzoites (Fig. 51-8C,D). Tachyzoites leave the parasitized cells and enter other cells to repeat the asexual cycle, where some of these tachyzoites develop into cystic stages, the bradyzoites. Toxoplasma cysts in tissues (Fig. 51–8B) are forms that when ingested by other hosts are capable of transmitting the infection to these hosts. To summarize: In cats ingestion of cysts or oocysts produces an intestinal infection; in other animals cysts or oocysts produce a tissular infection (17). Therefore, humans become infected with Toxoplasma by ingesting oocysts from the environment passed by cats in their feces or cysts in meat of infected animals, by receiving blood from a person with active infection, or in the womb by passage of organisms from the mother.

Toxoplasma gondii in immunocompetent hosts produces a variety of well-tolerated infections. Most infected persons have a subclinical course, others have a few nonspecific manifestations of short duration, and still others may have lymphadenitis (Fig. 51–8A), which sometimes persists a few weeks, with fever, malaise, and weight loss; or a unilateral ocular infection (granulomatous chorioretinitis). These infections are usually diagnosed clinically, sometimes by study of biopsy specimens.

In immunocompromised hosts, especially those with acquired immunodeficiency syndrome (AIDS), Toxoplasma organisms produce a variety of syndromes because any organ system can be affected, the most important of which is the central nervous system (Fig. 51–8B). The usual presentation of central nervous system toxoplasmosis is that of encephalitis, with headache, disorientation, and drowsiness. If large lesions develop in the brain symptoms of a space-occupying lesion occur, together with symptoms related to the area occupied: in cortical or motor zones, hemiparesis or seizures are common, together with papilledema, decreased mental status, and coma. Involvement of cranial nerves or cord lesions may develop.

Grossly, the lesions in the brain appear as areas of necrosis and hemorrhage, and microscopically the parasites are found especially at the edges of the lesion, where viable tissue is still present (Fig. 51–8B) (6).

In the lungs and the heart significant pneumonitis or myocarditis may develop. Ocular lesions in person with AIDS are characterized by acute necrosis of the retina with sudden loss of vision.

Toxoplasmosis is also acquired in utero, producing fetal morbidity and mortality, especially in areas of the world where the transmission rate is high. The infection is transmitted by the mother to her offspring when the mother suffers the acute infection; thus, it follows that a woman

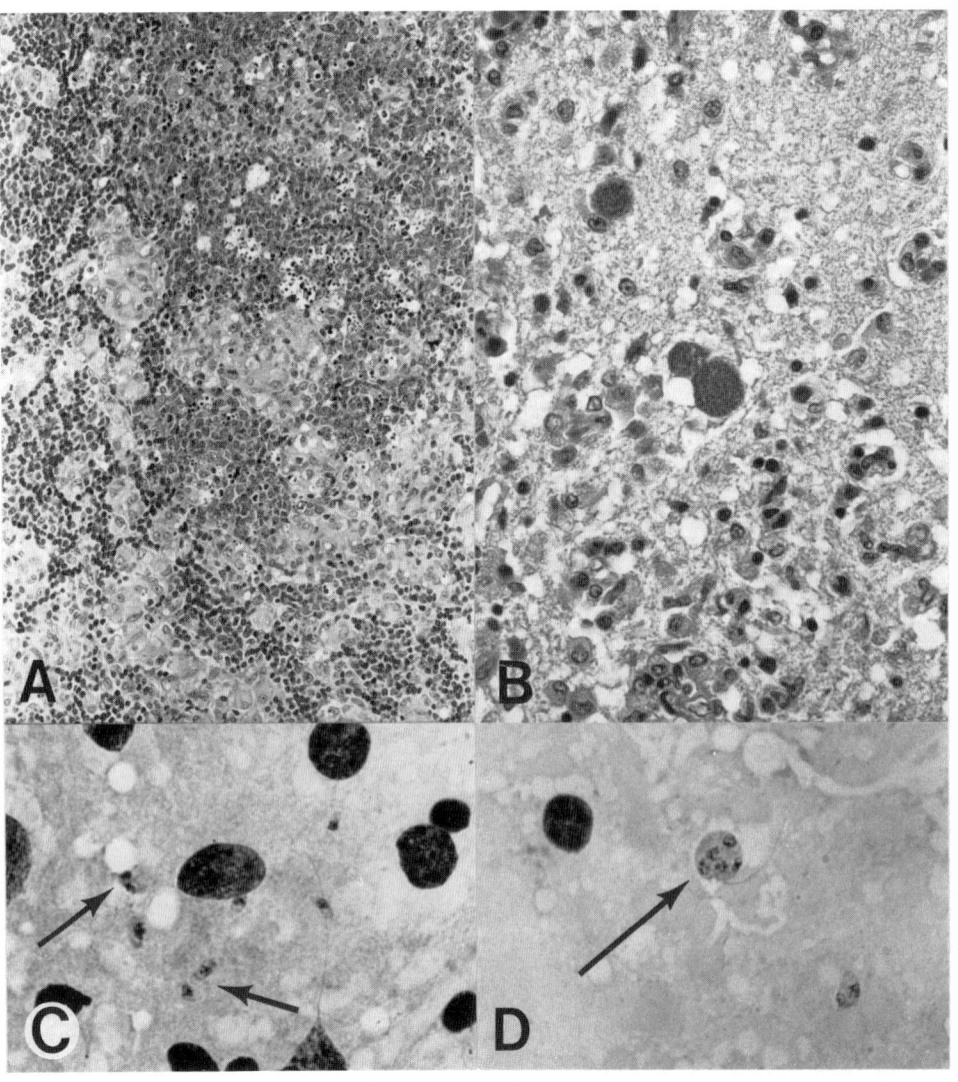

Fig. 51–8. Toxoplasma gondii. *A,* Section of lymph node of immunocompetent human host shows lymphadenitis characterized by numerous histiocytes aggregated as poorly formed granulomas (hematoxylin and eosin, ×180). *B,* Section of human brain shows infiltration by mononuclear cells and three Toxoplasma cysts (hematoxylin and eosin, ×450). *C, D,* (arrows) Brain imprints show tachyzoites free from cells (artifact of the imprint). One group of five tachyzoites are tightly bunched (*long arrow*), (Giemsa, ×1120).

transmits Toxoplasma during one pregnancy only. The manifestation of the infection in the fetus depends on the time at which the parasite is acquired during gestation: if early, the fetus is aborted; if later, premature delivery is the rule; and in both instances, stigmata of a chronic infection are observed in the fetus. Babies born with toxoplasmosis frequently die within 1 or 2 years; those who survive often have marked physical and mental deficits.

In all situations the diagnosis of toxoplasmosis described above is based on clinical observations and roentgenographic studies, and sometimes on serologic tests (18); the confirmation is provided by finding the parasites and identifying them in the clinical laboratory (Chapters 55, 57, 58, and 63). The morphologic features of the tachyzoite and the bradyzoite of Toxoplasma are different in smears and imprints and in tissue sections. In smears and tissue imprints, the tachyzoites have a crescent shape, are 4 to 8 μm long by 2 to 3 μm wide, and if stained with Giemsa stain the cytoplasm stains blue and the nucleus at the center of the parasite stains deep red (Plate XIIA,B). The parasites may be free (Fig. 51–8C,D; an artefact due to rupture of the cells while preparing the smears), or may be intracellular; they appear as a few parasites in the cytoplasm next to the nucleus or filling the entire cytoplasm of the parasitized cells. The latter are known as terminal colonies or pseudocysts. The cysts are about 30 μm in diameter, are spherical, and contain numerous zoites with a morphology similar to that of the trophozoites described above (2,6). In tissue sections one is observing a section of the organism in tissues that have been fixed and have been processed, losing in some instances as much as 51% of their mass, making the parasites more difficult to identify. The identification of Toxoplasma in tissue sections is outside the scope of this discussion (6).

Antibodies against or antigen of Toxoplasma can be determined in serum, plasma, CSF, and eye fluid. Determinations in CSF and eye fluid should be done in parallel with a serum sample. Several tests have been used, such as complement fixation, agglutination (indirect hemagglutination, direct, and latex agglutination), and fluorescent antibody, but they have been largely replaced by the enzyme-linked immunosorbent assay (ELISA). Detection of immunoglobulin (Ig)M antibodies to diagnose acute infection is also carried out with immunofluorescent and ELISA techniques (18). These tests are often performed in reference laboratories, which should be contacted for specifications on how to handle the specimens.

Several commercial kits are available for serologic diagnosis of toxoplasmosis, but these kits have several problems. Proper evaluation of many kits is not available, and the lack of standardization of reporting results makes it impossible to compare results (18).

Plasmodium

Plasmodium is the agent of malaria, one of the most important parasitic infections in the world. It has been estimated that about 200 million new cases of malaria occur each year worldwide, and about 2 million deaths, especially in impoverished Africa (19). The geographic distribution of malaria has changed drastically in the last 50 years, owing to control campaigns undertaken by many governments and agencies throughout the world. Today, the tropics are the main area of endemicity, which extends to the subtropics, especially on the Asian continent (19). Before the control campaigns were undertaken malaria extended well into the Arctic region of Europe, Asia, and the American continent. In the United States malaria has been controlled since 1953, but imported cases occur often, and sometimes outbreaks (reintroduced malaria) have been reported in some areas, owing to local transmission beginning from an imported case (20,21). Four species of Plasmodium are responsible for all the cases of malaria in humans: Plasmodium falciparum, Plasmodium vivax, Plasmodium malariae, and Plasmodium ovale.

The life cycle of Plasmodium is complex, involving a hematophagous mosquito of the genus Anopheles, a genus with many species, capable of transmitting the infection around the world. Transmission of malaria to humans occurs when the infected mosquito (with sporozoites in the salivary glands) bites a susceptible person, into whom the mosquito inoculates the sporozoites. Once the sporozoites are deposited with saliva of the mosquito into the new host the sporozoites travel rapidly via blood to the liver, where they enter the hepatocytes. Depending on the species, one of two forms of development occurs in the liver. (1) All sporozoites of Plasmodium falciparum and Plasmodium malariae develop asexually in the hepatocytes in about 10 to 18 days, to produce merozoites, which leave the hepatocyte to enter the red blood cells. (2) Some sporozoites of Plasmodium vivax and Plasmodium ovale develop to merozoites in the hepatocytes and enter the red blood cells; the rest of the sporozoites remain in the liver, to develop later (exoerythrocytic development), which development is responsible for future relapses of the disease (22).

The merozoites leaving the hepatocytes enter the circulating erythrocytes where they multiply asexually (Fig. 51–9). The erythrocytic multiplication produces merozoites which leave the red blood cell upon its destruction to invade other red blood cells and initiate the multiplication de novo. The interval between entry of a merozoite into the red blood cell and completion of asexual development is 48 hours for Plasmodium falciparum, Plasmodium vivax, and Plasmodium ovale, and 72 hours for Plasmodium malariae (2). Since the malarial attack (the symp-

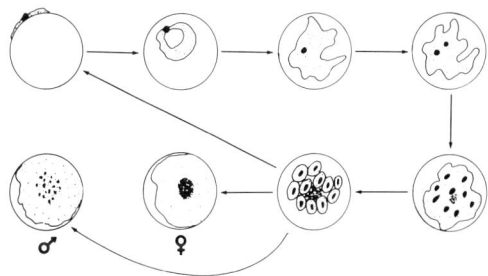

Fig. 51–9. Plasmodium. Schematic drawing of erythrocytic life cycle (schizogony). (From Gutierrez Y: Diagnostic Pathology of Parasitic Infections with Clinical Correlations. Philadelphia, Lea & Febiger, 1990.)

toms) occurs each time asexual development is completed in the erythrocytes, the symptoms repeat each third or each fourth day, depending on the species. Some merozoites in the red blood cells develop into the male and the female gametocytes, the sexual stages ingested by the mosquito, where they join in the stomach to undergo sexual development. The sexual development in the mosquito results in thousands of sporozoites, which locate in the salivary glands, ready to be inoculated into a new host.

The presenting symptoms of malaria are chills and fever, lasting 5 to 8 hours (malarial attack) and, depending on the species, repeating each 48 or 72 hours. During the primary attack (first bout with the infection), the fever may spike daily, until the development of the parasites in the red blood cells synchronizes, followed by the typical attacks at 48 or 72 hours; the attacks become less and less intense, until they spontaneously disappear in about 2 weeks (22). The symptoms can resume at any time for up to $3\frac{1}{2}$ years for Plasmodium vivax, and an uncertain period for Plasmodium ovale, because the stored liver stages reappear in circulation, producing what is known as relapses. Symptoms may reappear also in Plasmodium falciparum for $1\frac{1}{2}$ years after the infection, and in Plasmodium malariae for many years, but these new bouts of the disease are due to forms that remain in circulation in small, indetectable numbers (no liver stages). The name for these bouts of disease in these species is recrudescences.

Malaria in endemic areas is often associated with splenomegaly, and sometimes with anemia, but several other syndromes occur. For practical purposes, malaria should be viewed as two diseases. One disease, produced by Plasmodium vivax, Plasmodium malariae, or Plasmodium ovale, is a benign disease that produces malarial attacks which eventually disappear even without treatment. The other is a disease complex, sometimes fatal, produced by Plasmodium falciparum. Plasmodium falciparum behaves differently from the other plasmodia, because development in the red blood cells occurs while the red cells are sequestered throughout the body in the capillary bed. The parasitized red blood cells sequester about 8 to 12 hours after asexual development begins. Sequestration is directed by the parasite by production of alterations on the red blood cell membrane that are responsible for the attachment onto the endothelial cells of the capillaries (24). In technical terms, schizogony in Plasmodium falciparum occurs in the tissues, and this accounts for the multiple syndromes and for the deaths associated with the infection. The main manifestations of acute Plasmodium falciparum malaria in susceptible persons (children, immigrants from nonendemic to endemic areas) are usually related to the central nervous system and marked by rapid deterioration, shock, coma, and death. Impairment of circulation of blood throughout the tissues correlates with the symptoms of the infection and the demise of the infected person.

The diagnosis of malaria is one important task of the clinical laboratory; it is considered a difficult endeavour, but it is only difficult because of workers' unfamiliarity with the biology of the parasite and because so few samples are received in any given laboratory (23). Classification of the different plasmodia is based on the morphologic characteristics of the parasites during the asexual development in red blood cells, as they appear in well-stained blood smears (2). These morphologic characteristics are changing continuously throughout their development in the erythrocytes. They have to be described accordingly.

First Six Hours. In general, the merozoites leave the liver (or the red blood cells) and enter the red cells to become trophozoites, consisting of a small cytoplasm and a nucleus of a minute granule of chromatin (Fig. 51–10A–H). The trophozoites are about 2 μm, and vary in appearance from an apparently resting, solid body (Fig. 51–10E,G) to a body with a pseudovacuole, giving the appearance of a ring (Fig. 51–10A–D). This trophozoite or ring is similar in all four species. In the next few hours of development some enlargement of the trophozoite is apparent and some may show pseudopods (Fig. 51–10F). The laboratory report at this stage of development should read "Plasmodium spp," because speciation is usually not possible. One exception could be samples with large numbers of parasitized red blood cells (more than 10%), in which case a diagnosis of Plasmodium falciparum is possible (Plate XIIC). In all instances another blood sample

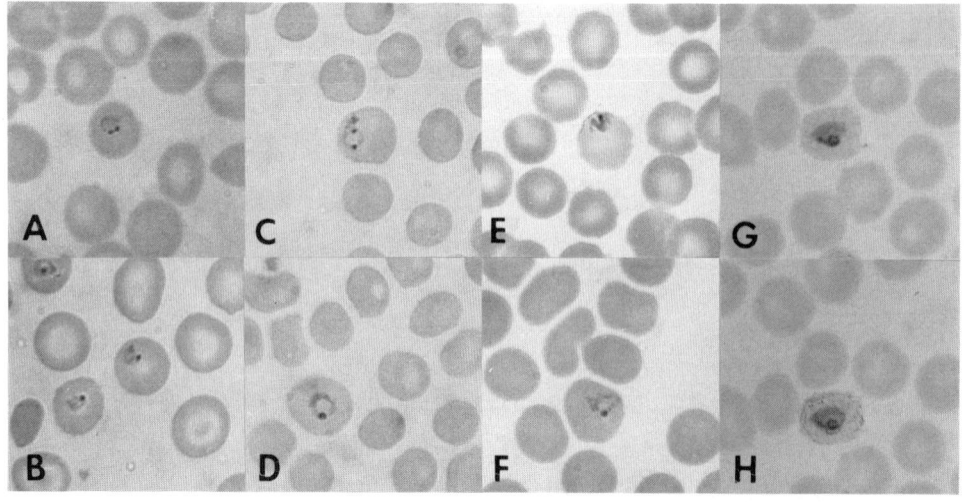

Fig. 51–10. Plasmodium. Morphology in blood smears at the beginning of schizogony. A, B, Plasmodium falciparum; C, D, P. vivax; E, F, P. malariae; G, H, P. ovale (stain shows Schuffner's dots). Note the size of the red blood cells at this stage; the small trophozoites are impossible to speciate at this stage (Wright, ×1120).

taken 6 to 12 hours later should be requested and examined for speciation (see below).

Six to Eighteen Hours. During this time the parasites evolve sufficiently to allow speciation in most cases (Fig. 51–11A–H). The characteristics of each species are as follows:

Plasmodium falciparum has trophozoites less than half the diameter of the red blood cell, and the cell is not enlarged or deformed (Fig. 51–11A,B). The number of parasitized red blood cells could be large, depending on the immune status of the host, but at this time of the cycle the red blood cells parasitized with Plasmodium falciparum begin to sequester themselves, disappearing from the circulation and decreasing their number on the smear. Plasmodium falciparum, especially at the beginning of the infection when the patient has daily spiking fevers, shows two distinct populations of trophozoites in peripheral blood: one small trophozoite (2 μm), the other slightly larger (4 μm) in diameter. These two populations correspond to at least two broods of parasites that mature in circulation at different intervals and are responsible for the daily fevers.

Plasmodium vivax has larger trophozoites with many pseudopods, indicating active movement within the cell (*vivax*, alive). The red blood cell appears enlarged and deformed (Fig. 51–11C,D). Toward the end of this interval schizonts begin appearing (Fig. 51–11D).

Plasmodium malariae has trophozoites with few pseudopods (Fig. 51–11E), sometimes the parasite appears as a resting body, at others in the shape of a band (Fig. 51–11F). The red blood cell is not deformed or enlarged.

Plasmodium ovale is intermediate between Plasmodium malariae and Plasmodium vivax. The vivax-like characteristic is that it enlarges and deforms the red blood cell, making oval about 60% of the parasitized cells (Fig. 51–11G,H); Plate XIIF). The malariae-like characteristic is sluggish movement.

At this time a proper laboratory report should contain speciation of the parasite.

Eighteen to Thirty-six Hours. More growth and differentiation toward completion of schizogony of the parasites have occurred, and the characteristics are more distinctive. In infections with Plasmodium falciparum synchronized to the 48-hour cycle, the blood forms begin to disappear 24 hours after the fever paroxysm because the parasitized red blood cells begin sequestration in the tissues, and it ends at 30 hours. Forms of Plasmodium falciparum present before 24 hours but in small numbers are difficult to speciate. The other plasmodia, even in small numbers, can be speciated, and laboratory reports should name the species. If samples are negative and the clinical diagnosis and the history of the patients are strongly suggestive of malaria other smears taken at later time should be examined. Remember that Plasmodium falciparum could be responsible for the infection but be hidden in the capillary bed.

Plasmodium vivax trophozoites show greater activity, as signaled by the number of pseudopods, which sometimes fill the entire, enlarged red blood cell (Plate XIID). At this interval schizogony is beginning and forms with two or more nuclei begin appearing.

Forms of Plasmodium malariae are usually about half to two thirds the diameter of the red cell; band forms (Plate XIIE) are common in nonenlarged or deformed red blood cells; schizonts are usually not present since the cycle is longer (72 hours) than for the other three species (Fig. 51–11E,F).

Plasmodium ovale organisms at 18 to 36 hours' devel-

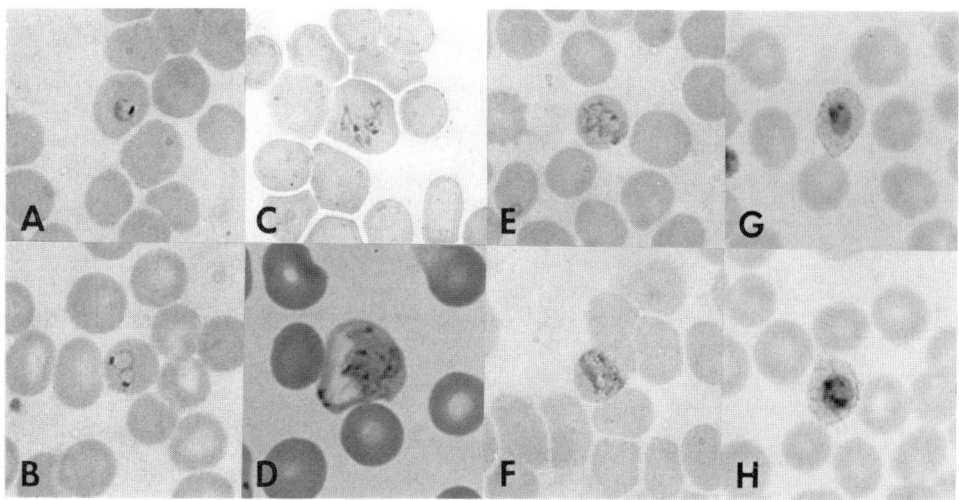

Fig. 51–11. Plasmodium. Morphology in blood smears at midschizogony cycle, Wright stain. A, B, Plasmodium falciparum: note the slight increase in size. Parasitized red blood cell not deformed. Some parasites with two nuclei may be seen, but these forms are beginning to be sequestered in the capillary bed. C, D, P. vivax: note enlargement of the red blood cell and numerous pseudopods of the parasite. Some parasites already have two or more nuclei, the beginning of division. E, F, P. malariae: note the increase in size of the parasite, some are in the characteristic band shape. The parasitized red blood cells are not enlarged. G, H, P. ovale (stain shows Schuffner's dots): note the oval shape of the enlarged parasitized erythrocyte (Wright, ×1120).

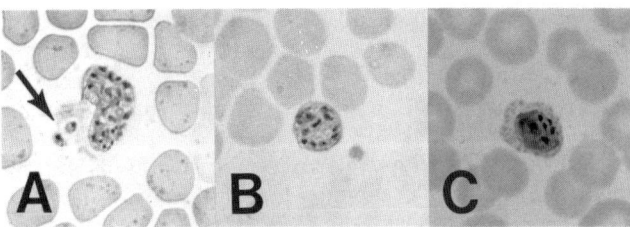

Fig. 51–12. Plasmodium. Morphology in blood smears during last part of schizogony showing mostly mature schizonts. A, Plasmodium vivax: note that the cell is beginning to free the merozoites (arrow). B, P. malariae; C, P. ovale (stain shows Schuffner's dots). P. falciparum is not depicted because it completes its schizogony in the capillary bed (Wright, ×1120).

opment have a large percentage of oval red blood cells. The late trophozoites and young schizonts do not have many pseudopods and are at least half the diameter of the enlarged red blood cell (Fig. 51–11G,H).

Thirty-six to Forty-eight Hours. In Plasmodium vivax and Plasmodium ovale malaria the parasites in the peripheral blood are completing the schizogony, and stages with multiple nuclei, some with merozoites already formed, are seen (Fig. 51–12A–C). Plasmodium malariae (Fig. 51–12B), with a 72-hour schizogony cycle, is behind in its development, requiring another 16 to 24 hours to be at the same stage as Plasmodium vivax (Fig. 51–12A) and Plasmodium ovale (Fig. 51–12C). Mature schizonts of Plasmodium ovale and Plasmodium malariae have eight merozoites (Fig. 51–12B,C); Plasmodium vivax, 12 to 16 (Fig. 51–12A).

Three Weeks or More. The blood smears from patients who have had their primary attack (the bout of the infection following the mosquito's infecting bite characterized by attacks lasting 2 to 3 weeks), and are now experiencing either relapses (from liver stages) or recrudescences (from peripheral blood stages), are different. In these samples, invariably the gametocytes are present (Fig. 51–13A–D), because gametocytes develop deep in the bone marrow and spleen, and take 3 to 4 weeks after the initial infection to appear in circulation. In addition, the other forms as described above are seen, together with the gametocytes.

The gametocytes of Plasmodium falciparum are falciform (Fig. 51–13A; Plate XIIC); often the parasitized red blood cells are not readily stained. The gametocytes of the other three plasmodia are rounded; Plasmodium malariae have small gametocytes filling a nonenlarged or nondeformed red blood cell almost completely (Fig. 51–13C); Plasmodium vivax have large gametocytes in deformed and enlarged red blood cells (Plate XII; Fig. 51–13B); Plasmodium ovale gametocytes are intermediate between the latter two species, within an oval red blood cell (Fig. 51–13D). Gametocytes in blood films should be easily recognized and speciated.

In addition to the gametocytes, the morphology of the parasites is identical to that described above.

Several other morphologic features helpful for speciation of Plasmodium organisms are discussed often; for example, the stippling of the red blood cells, a characteristic useful only when it is present. The absence of stippling on red blood cells is the rule with the modern hematologic stains; to demonstrate stippling requires excellent stain with Giemsa stain and well-prepared buffer solutions.

Malaria is usually suspected clinically, but it requires confirmation in the laboratory. Both thin and thick smears should be prepared and stained (Chapter 58). Sometimes estimation of the percentages of infected red blood cells is requested, to follow response to therapy, especially with Plasmodium falciparum infection. These estimates should be made in samples taken at the same phase of the erythrocyte cycle and need not be complicated: counts in several oil immersion fields of infected and noninfected red blood cells should permit calculation of acceptable estimates of parasitemia.

Babesia

Babesia is a genus with a large number of species of organisms that inhabit red blood cells and produce in animals a disease known as babesiosis. The characteristics of this genus are the lack of production of pigment during their erythrocyte life cycle; the solid, usually pyriform, trophozoites, arranged in pairs or tetrads in the red cell; and the vector, which is a tick rather than a mosquito (2).

Infections with Babesia have been described in several countries, but the most important focus occurs in the United States, in New England. Several species of Babesia affect humans: Babesia microti in New England, where the majority of cases occur; Babesia equi in California, Babesia divergens in Ireland, and Babesia bovis in Yugoslavia, places where sporadic cases have been described, some with fatal consequences, especially in asplenic persons (6).

The asexual life cycle of Babesia involves a vertebrate, where the parasites develop in the erythrocytes, producing only four merozoites, and an invertebrate, a tick, where the sexual development occurs, resulting in the production of sporozoites in the salivary glands.

Infections with Babesia are characterized by gradual

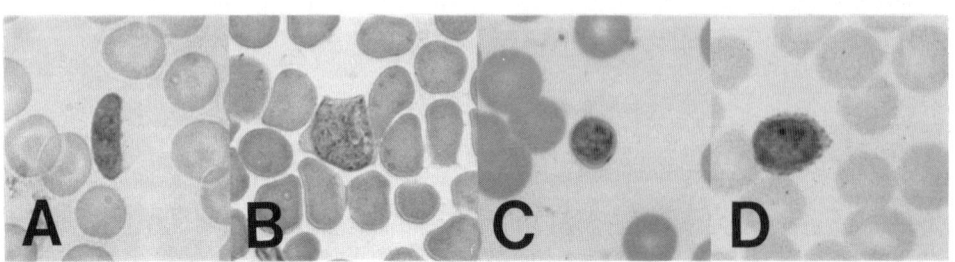

Fig. 51–13. Plasmodium. Morphology in blood smears, after 2 to 3 weeks' infection. All other forms as described above are seen, plus the typical gametocytes of each species. A, Plasmodium falciparum. B, P. vivax; C, P. malariae; D, P. ovale: stain shows Schuffner's dots (Wright, ×1120).

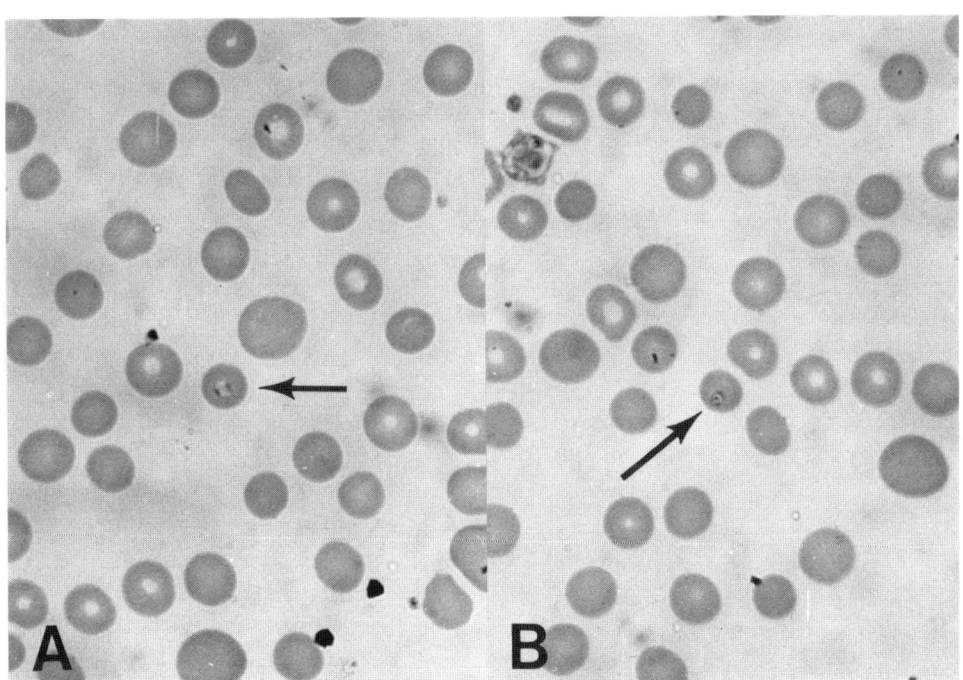

Fig. 51–14. Babesia spp. Human blood: note the small trophozoites (*arrows*), (Wright, ×1120). (Preparation courtesy of SB Taubman, MD, Department of Pathology, Vassar Bros Hospital, Poughkeepsie, NY.)

onset of malaise, anorexia, and fatigue, followed by fever up to 1 week's duration, profuse sweating, and muscle pain. The temperature is between 37.6 and 40.0°C. Splenomegaly may be present. Laboratory tests reveal anemia, sometimes requiring blood transfusions, increased reticulocyte count, and elevated bilirubin value (25).

The diagnosis rarely is made clinically, but the parasites may be recognized and identified in the laboratory in thin and thick blood smears (Fig. 51–14; Chapter 58). The typical trophozoites are less than 2 μm in diameter; the merozoites, seen as tetrads, are of similar size, often arranged as a Maltese cross.

MICROSPORA

Members of the Microspora in tissues have been reported sporadically, in immunosuppressed patients where corneal (26), cerebral, muscular, and nasal infections have been recorded (6). As stated in Chapter 49, the diagnosis is difficult and usually the parasites are detected first in biopsy material. The confirmation of the infection and the speciation are made on electron micrographs (26).

INSERTA SEDIS

One organism, Pneumocystis carinii, is discussed among the Protozoa as inserta sedis because its exact taxonomic position has not been agreed upon (27). Pneumocystis is widely distributed among humans and animals, where it is perhaps the most common parasite, because its prevalence is 100%; only one species is recognized in the genus, Pneumocystis carinii, but it is possible that other species, as yet undescribed, occur.

Pneumocystis is the agent of pneumocystosis in humans, or Pneumocystis carinii pneumonia (PCP), an infection important in immunocompromised hosts, which helped in defining AIDS. The taxonomic position of Pneumocystis has been among the Protozoa, but recent studies suggest that it is a fungus. The known life cycle and the morphologic characteristics of Pneumocystis are not inconsistent with either a fungus or a protozoan (2,6).

The life cycle of Pneumocystis is unknown (28). Two stages in the lower respiratory tract of humans and animals, sometimes in other tissues, have been recognized: the trophozoite and the cyst (Fig. 51–15). Trophozoites

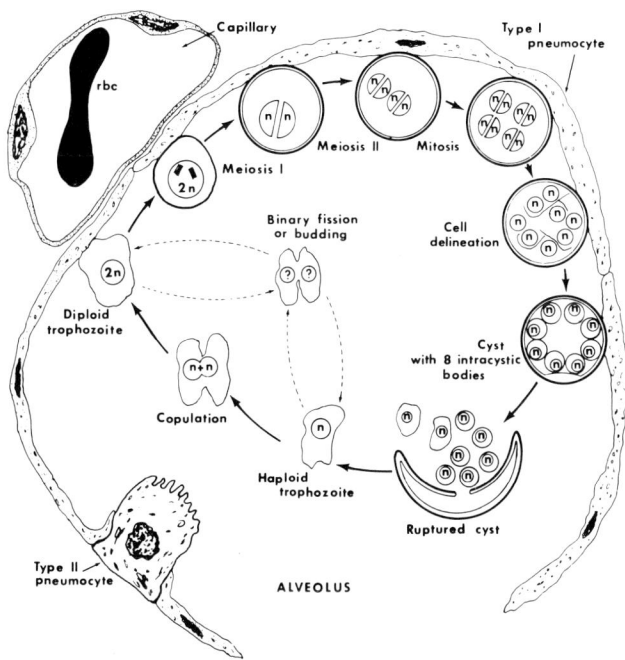

Fig. 51–15. Pneumocystis carinii. Diagram of the known development of Pneumocystis in lung. (From Gutierrez Y: The biology of Pneumocystis carinii. Semin Diag Pathol, 6:203, 1989.)

are firmly attached to type I pneumocytes, where they develop into cystic stages by undergoing meiosis at the same that they form a cyst wall; the mature cyst contains eight hapoid intracystic bodies. The cyst frees the intracystic bodies, which join in the alveolar space (copulation?) to produce a diploid trophozoite, which reinitiates the cycle. In addition, diploid trophozoites also reproduce by binary fission within the alveoli and other tissues (29,30).

The clinical manifestations of Pneumocystis infection have been described in association with terminal cancer, leukemia, steroid therapy, organ transplants, and in debilitated, malnourished infants. Recently, most infections seen are in AIDS patients, for whom Pneumocystis is probably the most important pathogen and the greatest cause of morbidity and mortality (6).

In premature, debilitated infants Pneumocystis was described as producing interstitial plasma cell pneumonia, because of the characteristic plasmacytoid infiltrate of the pulmonary interstitium (31). In persons with AIDS the symptoms of Pneumocystis infection are similar to the symptoms experienced by persons with other forms of immune suppression, but in AIDS they have a more subtle and insidious onset; fulminant presentations are also seen.

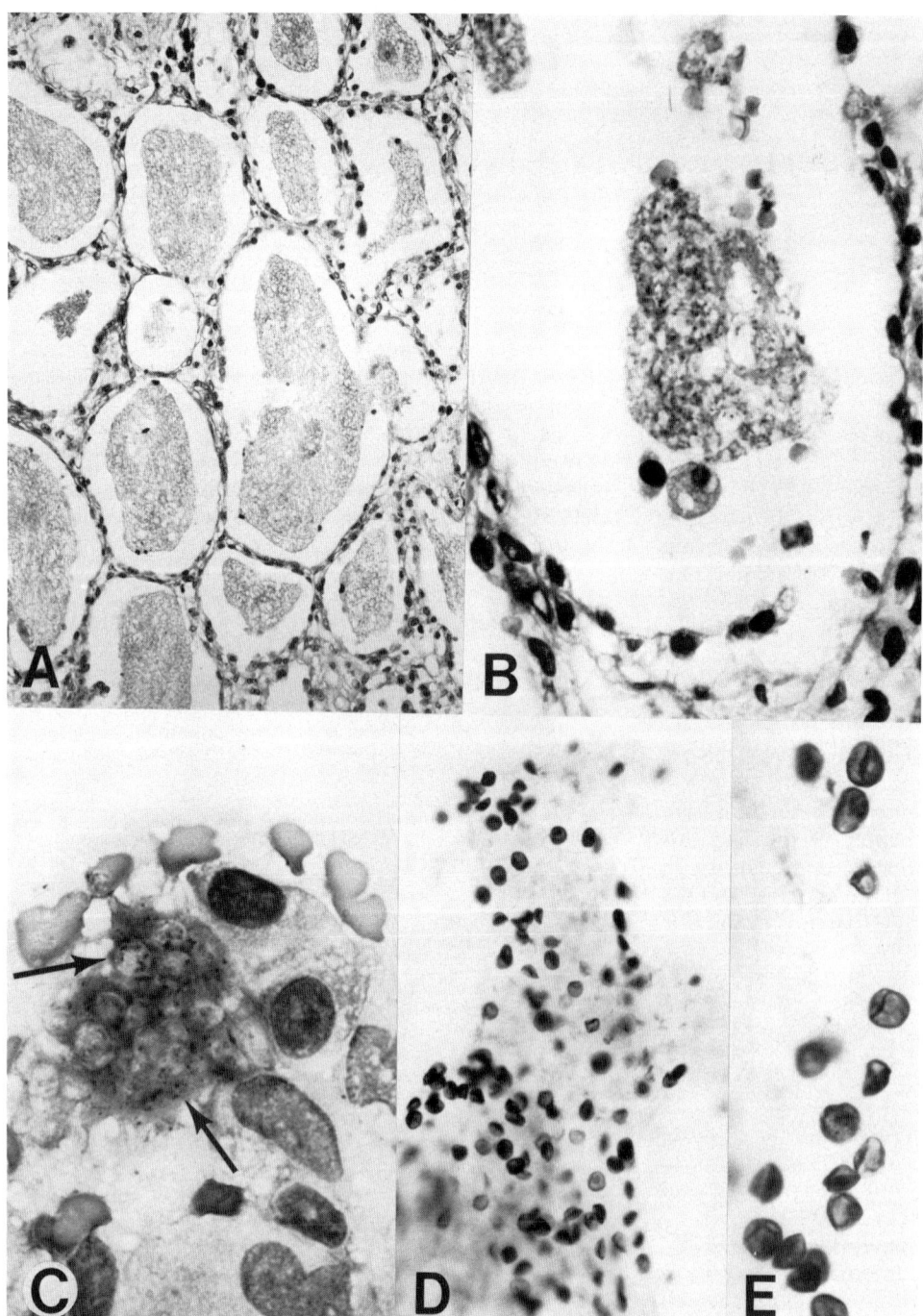

Fig. 51–16. Pneumocystis carinii. A, Low-power view of section of human lung shows the colonies of the parasite in the alveoli (hematoxylin and eosin, ×180). B, Higher magnification, shows the trophozoites with minute nuclei (Giemsa, ×705). C, In imprint note the mass of trophozoites and cysts (arrows), (Giemsa, ×1120)., D, E, Imprint shows cysts (silver; D ×705, E ×120).

At first the cough is dry and nonproductive; it progresses relentlessly until shortness of breath is evident, especially during exertion. Diffuse rales may be heard, mainly at the bases. Untreated infections result rapidly in death, and those who recover after treatment have residual pulmonary function abnormalities as long as 21 months afterward (32).

Dissemination of Pneumocystis to almost any organ outside the lungs has been described (6). The morphologic characteristics of the lungs of patients dying with Pneumocystis infection are a uniform consolidation, with a pale, dry parenchyma on cut section. Sometimes areas of necrosis with cavity formation are seen. Microscopically, the typical colonies of the parasite (see above) fill the alveoli (28).

The diagnosis of pneumocystosis is made clinically, but it is confirmed by the anatomic pathologist in tissue sections recovered by lung biopsy (Fig. 51–16A,B) and samples taken at bronchoscopy (Fig. 51–16C,D); often the diagnosis is made in the clinical laboratory in smears from pulmonary material (Chapter 57) (33). The trophozoites of Pneumocystis carinii are small, ameboid bodies 4 to 5 μm long with a minute nucleus. The cysts are 5 to 6 μm, have a thick wall, and contain the eight intracystic bodies (Fig. 51–16C). In tissue sections the trophozoites and the intracystic bodies stain eosinophilically with hematoxylin and eosin stain, and the nucleus stains basophilically (Fig. 51–16B). In smears stained with Giemsa stain the trophozoites and the intracystic bodies stain blue and the nucleus deep red (Fig. 51–16C). Silver stain stains only the cyst wall darkly, and reveals a small thickening of the cyst wall (Fig. 51–16D,E). The eosinophilic stain of Pneumocystis in tissue sections of lung is responsible for the classic pattern seen filling the entire alveoli and commonly referred to in the literature as an eosinophilic exudate or matrix (Fig. 51–16A). Often it is not realized that this eosinophilic exudate or matrix is a colony of Pneumocystis, containing cysts, cysts in development, and trophozoites (6,28).

REFERENCES

1. Bogdan C, Rollinghoff M, and Solbach W: Evasion strategies of Leishmania parasites. Parasitol Today, 6:183, 1990.
2. Beaver PC, Jung RC, and Cupp EW: Clinical Parasitology. 9th ed. Philadelphia, Lea & Febiger, 1984.
3. WHO: The Leishmaniases. Tech Rep Ser No 701. Geneva, World Health Organization, 1984.
4. Gustafson TL, Reed CM, McGreevy PB, et al: Human cutaneous leishmaniasis acquired in Texas. Am J Trop Med Hyg, 34:58, 1985.
5. Nelson DA, Gustafson TL, and Spielvogel RL: Clinical aspects of cutaneous leishmaniasis acquired in Texas. J Am Acad Dermatol, 12:985, 1985.
6. Gutierrez Y: Diagnostic Pathology of Parasitic Infections with Clinical Correlations. Philadelphia, Lea & Febiger, 1990.
7. Palma G, and Gutierrez Y: Laboratory diagnosis of Leishmania. Clin Lab Med, 11:909, 1991.
8. WHO: The African Trypanosomiasis. Tech Rep Ser No 635. Geneva, World Health Organization, 1979.
9. Pentreath VW: Neurobiology of sleeping sickness. Parasitol Today, 5:111, 1989.
10. Cattand P, and deRaadt P: Laboratory diagnosis of trypanosomiasis. Clin Lab Med, 11:899, 1991.
11. Schmunis GA: Trypanosoma cruzi, the etiologic agent of Chagas' disease: Status in the blood supply in endemic and nonendemic countries. Transfusion, 31:547, 1991.
12. Petry K, and Eisen H: Chagas disease: A model for the study of autoimmune diseases. Parasitol Today, 5:111, 1989.
13. Ma P, Visvesvara GS, Martinez AJ, et al: Naegleria and Acanthamoeba infections: Review. Reviews Infect Dis, 12:490, 1990.
14. Martinez AJ, and Visvesvara GS: Laboratory diagnosis of pathogenic free-living amoebas: Naegleria, Acanthamoeba, and Leptomyxid. Clin Lab Med, 11:861, 1991.
15. Warhurt DC: Pathogenic free-living amoebae. Parasitol Today, 1:24, 1985.
16. Stehr-Green JK, Bailey TM, Brandt FH, et al: Acanthamoeba keratitis in soft contact lens wearers. JAMA, 25:57, 1987.
17. Frenkel JK: Pathophysiology of toxoplasmosis. Parasitol Today, 4:273, 1988.
18. Wilson M, and McAuley JB: Laboratory diagnosis of toxoplasmosis. Clin Lab Med, 11:923, 1991.
19. WHO: The Biology of Malaria Parasites. Tech Rep Ser No 743. Geneva, World Health Organization, 1987.
20. CDC: Outbreak of malaria imported from Kenya. MMWR, 35:567, 1986a.
21. CDC: Plasmodium vivax malaria—San Diego County, California. MMWR, 35:679, 1986b.
22. Oaks SC, Jr, Mitchell VS, and Pearson GW: Malaria. Obstacles and Opportunities. A Report of the Committee for the Study of Malaria Prevention and Control. Washington DC, National Academy Press, 1991.
23. Makler MT, and Gibbins B: Laboratory diagnosis of malaria. Clin Lab Med, 11:941, 1991.
24. Berendt AR, Ferguson DJP, and Newbold CI: Sequestration in Plasmodium falciparum malaria: Sticky cells and sticky problems. Parasitol Today, 6:247, 1990.
25. Carr JM, Emery S, Stone BF, et al: Babesiosis. Diagnostic pitfalls. Am J Clin Pathol, 95:774, 1991.
26. Cali A, Meisler DM, Rutherford I, et al: Corneal microsporidiasis in a patient with AIDS. Am J Trop Med Hyg, 44:463, 1991.
27. Edman JC, Kordes JA, Masur H, et al: Ribosomal RNA sequence shows Pneumocystis carinii to be a member of the fungi. Nature, 334:519, 1988.
28. Gutierrez Y: The biology of Pneumocystis carinii. Semin Diagn Pathol, 6:203, 1989.
29. Matsumoto Y, and Yoshida Y: Sporogony in Pneumocystis carinii: Synaptonemal complexes and meiotic nuclear divisions observed in precysts. J Protozool, 31:420, 1984.
30. Matsumoto Y, and Yoshida Y: Advances in Pneumocystis biology. Parasitol Today, 31:420, 1986.
31. Dutz W: Pneumocystis carinii pneumonia. Pathol Annu, 5:309, 1970.
32. Suffredini AF, Owens GR, Tobin MJ, et al: Long-term prognosis of survivors of Pneumocystis carinii pneumonia. Structural and functional correlates. Chest, 89:229, 1986.
33. Smith JW, and Bartlett MS: Laboratory diagnosis of pneumocystosis. Clin Lab Med, 11:957, 1991.

Chapter 52

BLOOD AND TISSUE HELMINTHS

The helminths inhabiting the tissues belong to the Nematoda, the Trematoda, and the Cestoda (Chapter 48); each group has a large number of representatives in humans, which often produce important morbidity and mortality. These helminths usually have intermediate hosts, where the larval stages develop to become infective before they are transmitted to the new host either by ingestion (Angiostrongylus), by the bite of a hematophagous arthropod (filarial worms), through the skin by active penetration (Schistosomas), or by ingestion of eggs or larvae that subsequently locate in the tissues (cestodes, Toxocara, Trichinella). The cestodes in the tissues (e.g., Cysticercus, Hydatid, Sparganum) behave in humans as if humans were intermediate hosts of the parasite. In general, most infections produced by helminths in human tissues are zoonotic, incidental infections; only a few are exclusively parasites of humans, such as Wuchereria, Onchocerca, and Schistosoma mansoni.

NEMATODES

The nematodes in the tissues of humans are found in almost any tissue or organ, depending upon the species. Some zoonotic nematodes that produce infection in humans reach patency (mature to adults and shed either larvae or eggs); others become larval stages and humans behave as if they were intermediate hosts; still others remain as infective larval stages and humans become paratenic hosts, hosts in which the parasites do not continue their development (see Toxocara). The most important of the tissue nematodes are the filarids, most of which are diagnosed in the clinical laboratory; the others are diagnosed by the anatomic pathologist in biopsy material or in tissues recovered at autopsy.

The Filariae

The filariae are a large group of nematodes that occur in humans and animals worldwide, inhabiting the tissues where they produce embryos known as microfilariae (intermediate stages between eggs and larvae). Filarial worms in humans produce important infections, accounting for much of the morbidity and mortality in certain tropical and subtropical areas of the world.

The life cycle of filarial worms is complicated, but it can be summarized as follows: The adult male and female worms live in the tissues and produce microfilariae, which gain access to the blood or to the skin. From either location, microfilariae are picked up by a haematophagous insect (mosquito, fly) during the insect's bite; in the insect the microfilariae develop to become infective larvae, which eventually locate in the mouth parts of the insect, and enter a new host during the insect's next bite. The infective larvae of filarids begin to develop in the new host, usually in the subcutaneous tissues, then migrate to their corresponding tissue or organ, where they grow to adults and complete the life cycle (1). The following filarids are the most important for the personnel in the clinical laboratory.

Wuchereria bancrofti. Wuchereria bancrofti and certain species of Brugia (see below) are the agents of lymphatic filariasis, one of the most important parasitic infections in the world. It is estimated that 90 million people are infected (1), mainly in central Africa, the Indian subcontinent, southeastern China, southeast Asia, Indonesia, the Pacific Islands, and the Philippines. On the American continent Wuchereria occurs in Brazil, Venezuela, Central America, and some of the Caribbean islands.

The life cycle of Wuchereria is as described above; the insect vectors are mosquitos of the genera Culex, Aedes, Anopheles, and Mansonia, and the parasites inhabit the lymphatics, usually in the lower half of the body. The microfilariae circulate in the blood between 10:00 P.M. and 2:00 A.M. (nocturnal periodicity), an adaptation to the biting habits of the vectors. At other times, they are sequestered in the capillary bed of the lungs (1,2). The adult Wuchereria female is up to 10 cm long and the male up to 4.0 cm. The microfilariae are characteristically sheathed (have a loose, poorly stained cover) with a lack of nuclei at the posterior tip (Fig. 52–1A).

The clinical manifestations of lymphatic filariasis are variable and depend on the endemic area, the susceptibility of the infected individual, and the duration of the infection. In endemic areas the acute symptoms start at about 6 years of age and consist of lymphadenitis and lymphangitis, with fever and malaise. These symptoms repeat two to three times each year, becoming more intense at about 25 years of age. The repetition of these bouts of clinical disease leads to fibrosis and sclerosis of the lymph channels and lymph nodes, resulting in lymphedema, and eventually elephantiasis. Elephantiasis is enlargement, sometimes to grotesque proportions, of the limbs, the scrotum, or the breast, produced by chronic lymphedema (Fig. 52–1B) (1).

Persons who acquire the infection while traveling or while living temporarily in endemic areas, suffer what is known as filariasis without microfilaremia (3). After the infection is acquired, if the individual is removed from the endemic area, bouts of lymphadenitis and lymphangitis similar to those suffered by the person in endemic areas occur; these bouts repeat a few times in a span of about one, to one and one half years after the infection, and disappear without leaving lasting consequences (3,4). Mi-

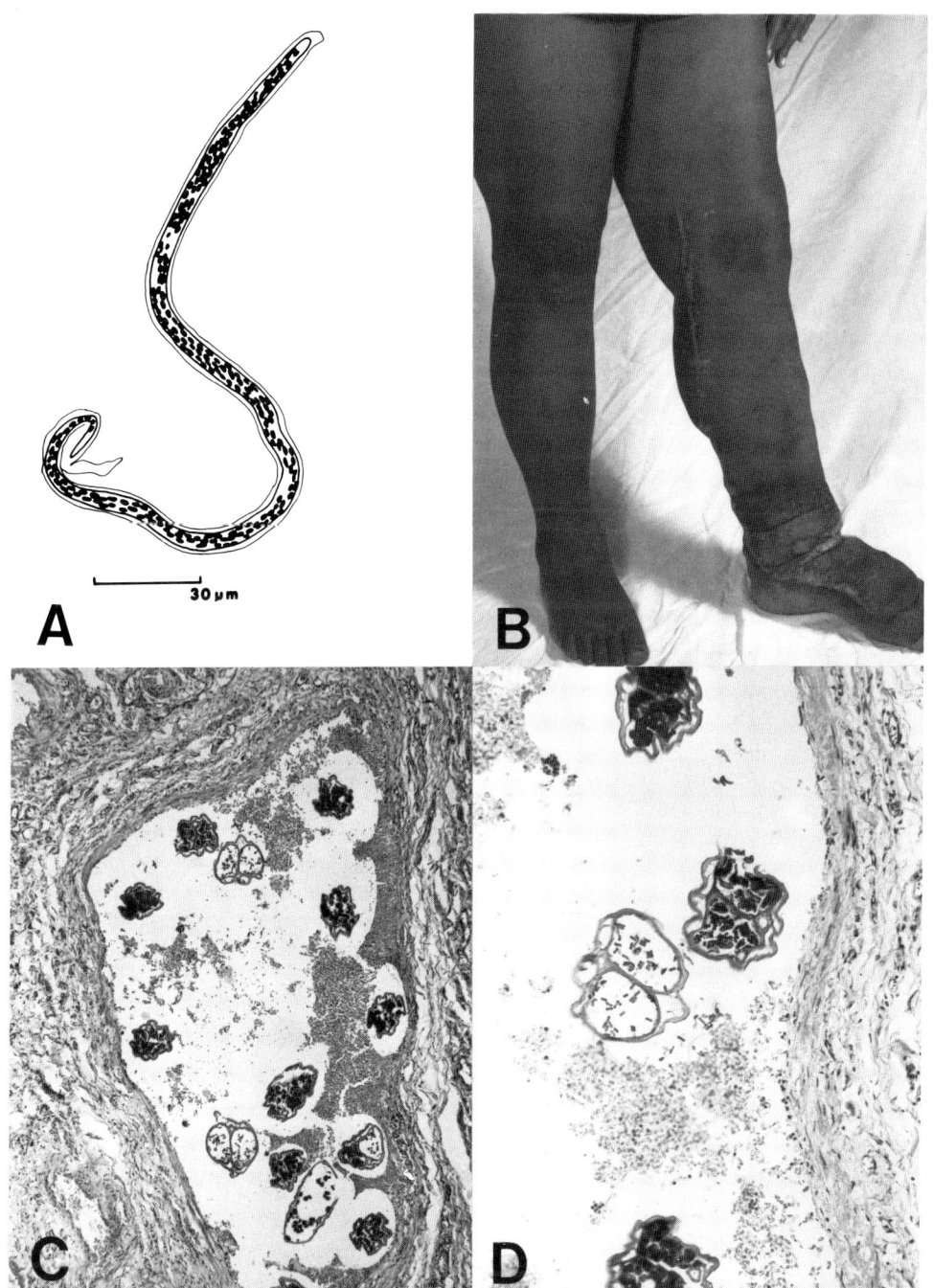

Fig. 52–1. Wuchereria bancrofti. *A*, Scale drawing of microfilaria, from a thick blood smear made from a Knott's concentration, hematoxylin stain. (From Gutierrez Y: Diagnostic Pathology of Parasitic Infections with Clinical Correlations. Philadelphia, Lea & Febiger, 1990.) *B*, Leg involved with elephantiasis. Note the scars produced by previous surgery to correct the tissue enlargement. *C, D*, Tissue sections demonstrate lymphatic channel with multiple cross sections of adult female worm (hematoxylin and eosin; *C* × 55, *D* × 140).

crofilariae are never detected in circulation and the infection becomes self-limited, because the adult filariae worms are destroyed in the tissues. In inhabitants of endemic areas the process is a continuous one: infection, destruction of worms, and reinfections occur throughout their lives. This repeated destruction of parasites in the tissues results in chronic damage to lymphatics, leading to elephantiasis (1–4).

The histologic changes of lymph nodes in filariasis vary with the stage of the disease (Fig. 52–1C, D). Early, granulomas produced by dead worms, leading to focal calcification in enlarged hyperplastic lymph nodes, are frequently seen; inflammation with eosinophils infiltrating the lymph nodes and adjacent tissues is common. Later, total sclerosis with fibrosis of lymph nodes and lymph channels results in lymphedema and fibrosis of subcutaneous tissues. Infiltration with mononuclear cells is common (4).

The diagnosis of lymphatic filariasis is made clinically or histologically, especially in the sporadic cases of filariasis without microfilaremia seen outside endemic areas (4). In advanced cases of elephantiasis the diagnosis is also clinical, but confirmation by the laboratory should be sought, which is based on the identification of the typical microfilariae in blood samples taken at midnight (Chapter 58) (5). The typical microfilaria of Wuchereria bancrofti is between 244 and 296 μm long, has a sheath that stains easily, and the tail is pointed and devoid of nuclei (Fig. 52–1A).

Brugia species. At least two species of Brugia—Brugia malayi and Brugia timori—produce lymphatic filariasis, mostly in southeast Asia (1–4). The life cycle of the parasite is similar to that of Wuchereria, with the exception that Brugia mature to adults in about 2 months rather than the 6 to 8 months required by Wuchereria. The disease Brugia produces is similar to that produced by Wuchereria, and the diagnosis is similarly confirmed in the laboratory using the same techniques (Chapter 58) (5). The sheathed microfilaria of Brugia is between 177 to 230 μm and is characterized by having a small terminal nucleus at the tip of the tail, difficult to stain, and sometimes barely visible (Fig. 52–2A, B).

Onchocerca volvulus. O. volvulus is a filarid of the subcutaneous tissues of humans that produces blindness in a large number of infected persons; the disease is known as river blindness (6). The geographic distribution of Onchocerca is restricted to the river margins of tropical Africa, and on the American continent in small foci in Guatemala, Mexico, Colombia, Ecuador, Brazil, and Venezuela.

The life cycle of Onchocerca is similar to that described above for other filarids, with two exceptions. One, the vector is a fly of the genus Simulium, which requires clear running water to complete its life cycle. Two, the microfilariae occur in the skin of the vertebrate host rather than in the blood (2,6).

The main clinical manifestations of onchocerciasis are subcutaneous nodules, usually hard, mobile, and painless, where the parasites are located within a marked fibrous reaction (Fig. 52–3B)(4). These nodules occur anywhere in the body, but in persons living on the American continent generally they are located in the upper portion of the body, whereas in Africa the nodules are in the lower part of the body (1). The nodules vary from 1 to several centimeters in diameter. Wider manifestations of the infection are due to the microfilariae in the skin, where they die and produce an inflammatory reaction (7). The microfilariae also enter the conjunctiva, the cornea, and the chambers of the eye, where the inflammatory reaction results in blindness (8). Several kinds of chronic dermatitis have been described that are common in the endemic areas; sometimes lymphadenopathy with elephantiasis is observed (9).

The diagnosis of onchocerciasis is made clinically but requires confirmation by proper identification of the microfilariae in samples from the skin (Chapter 62), stained with Giemsa stain (5). The microfilariae are unsheathed, between 315 and 360 μm long with the posterior end free of nuclei (Fig. 52–3A). Rarely, microfilariae are found in blood samples.

Loa loa. Loa loa worms produce subcutaneous infections (Fig. 52–4B) in inhabitants of an area corresponding to the rain forest of central and western Africa, where prevalence rates as high as 61% have been recorded in some places (10). The life cycle of Loa is similar to that described above; the vectors are day-biting flies of the genus Chrysops, so the largest concentration of microfilariae in blood is found at noon (diurnal periodicity) (2).

Loa loa infections are characterized by continuous migration of the adults in the subcutaneous tissues, making the worms visible when they traverse the conjunctiva (eye worms) or palpable under thin skin. The clinical manifestations of loiasis in endemic areas are usually minimal: episodes of localized swellings (Calabar or fugitive swellings), peripheral eosinophilia, and, generally, low levels of microfilaremia. Persons from nonendemic areas who become infected suffer more, with marked swellings. They often have no microfilaremia, have high peripheral eosinophilia, pruritus of the swollen area, and other allergic manifestations (11).

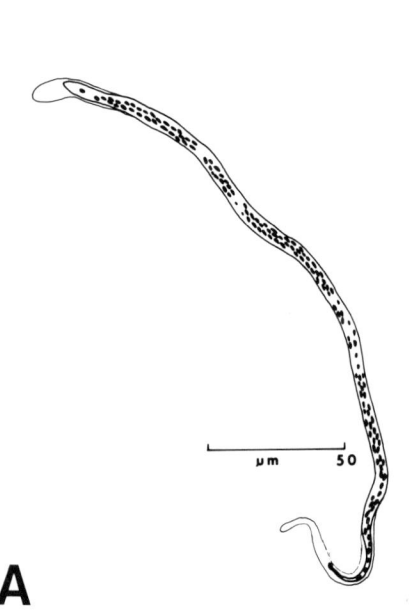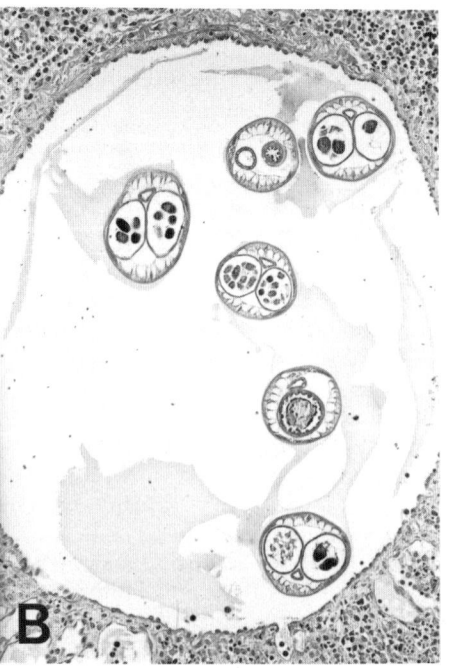

Fig. 52–2. Brugia malayi. *A,* Scale drawing of microfilaria from a thick blood smear made from a Knott's concentration, hematoxylin stain. (From Gutierrez Y: Diagnostic Pathology of Parasitic Infections with Clinical Correlations. Philadelphia, Lea & Febiger, 1990.) *B,* Section of lymphatic, shows adult female worm (hematoxylin, × 140).

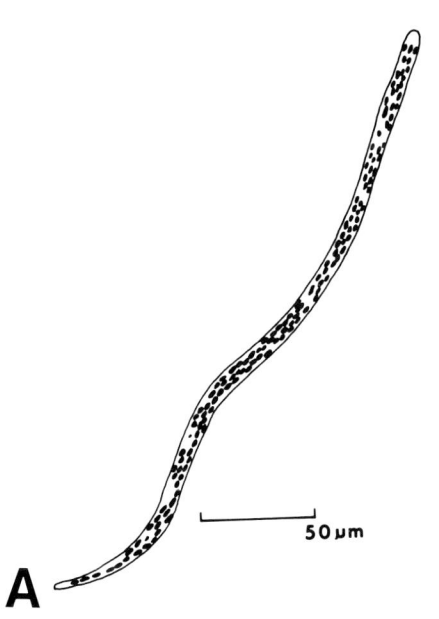

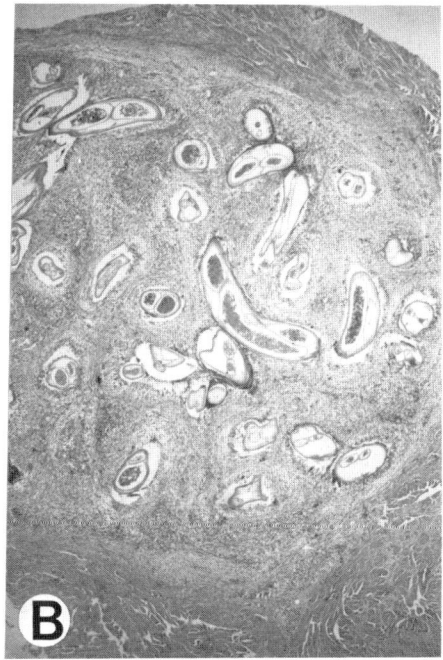

Fig. 52–3. Onchocerca volvulus. A, Scale drawing of microfilaria from a skin snip (Giemsa). (From Gutierrez Y: Diagnostic Pathology of Parasitic Infections with Clinical Correlations. Philadelphia, Lea & Febiger, 1990.) B, Adult worm in nodule section: note dense collagenous tissues surrounding the worm (hematoxylin and eosin, × 22).

The diagnosis of loiasis is made clinically, based on the history of travel to the endemic area and on the clinical presentation. Often, the worm (usually a single one) can be recovered by carefully opening the skin of the inflamed area (4). The recovered parasite should be sent in toto, fresh, to the clinical laboratory for proper identification. Microfilariae may be recovered from blood samples taken at midday and examined in the laboratory (Chapter 58) (5). The characteristic microfilariae have a sheath that does not stain with the usual blood stains; the presence of a sheath is evidenced by the displacement of red blood cells, providing a negative image of the sheath. The terminal nucleus, located at the tip of the rounded tail, is large and stains well. The length is 250 to 300 μm (Fig. 52–4A) (5).

Mansonella species. Three species of Mansonella—Mansonella ozzardi in South and Central America; Mansonella perstans in the tropical areas of South and Central America and Africa; and Mansonella streptocerca in central West Africa—are found in humans, usually producing benign infections. The life cycle of these filarids is similar to that described above for Wuchereria. Small gnats belonging to the genera Culicoides and Simulium serving as vectors (2).

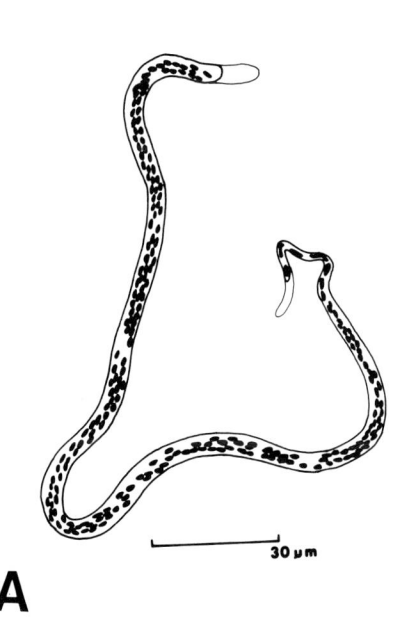

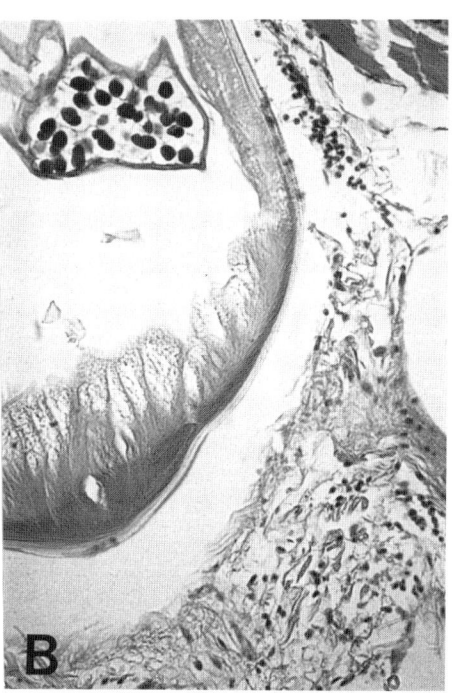

Fig. 52–4. Loa loa. A, Drawing of microfilaria in thin blood smear stained with Wright stain. (From Gutierrez Y: Diagnostic Pathology of Parasitic Infections with Clinical Correlations. Philadelphia, Lea & Febiger, 1990.) B, Cross section of adult worm in subcutaneous swelling (×140). (Preparation courtesy of GRH Kelsall MD, Western Australia. Reported in Charters AD, Welborn TA, and Miller P: Calabar swellings in immigrants in Western Australia. Med J Aust, 1:268, 1972.)

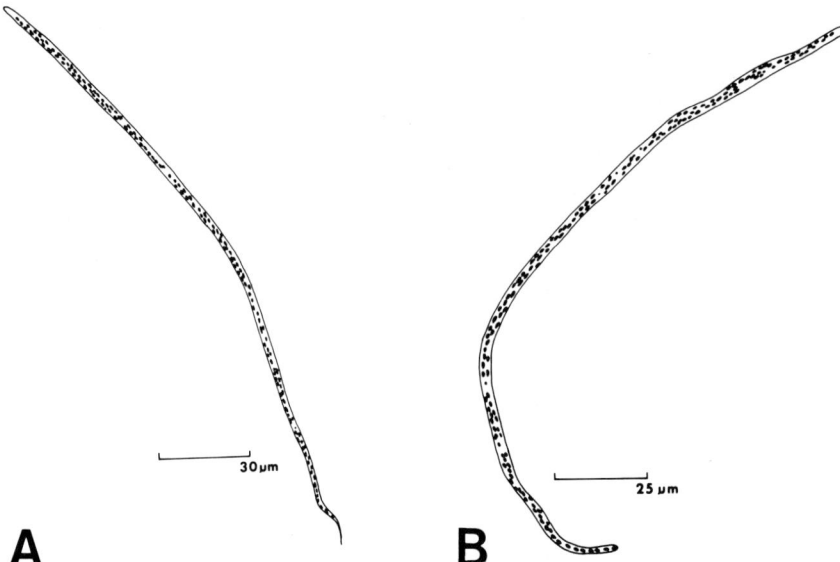

Fig. 52–5. Scale drawings of Mansonella microfilariae from a thick blood smear from Knott's concentration, Giemsa stain: A, M. ozzardi; B, M. pertans. (From Gutierrez Y: Diagnostic Pathology of Parasitic Infections with Clinical Correlations. Philadelphia, Lea & Febiger, 1990.)

The adults of Mansonella ozzardi inhabit the serosal cavities; the microfilariae are found throughout the 24-hour period in blood (Chapter 58) and often are recovered in skin snips (Chapter 62) (Fig. 52–5A).

Mansonella pertans organisms also live in the serosal cavities, but adults have been recovered from lymph nodes, pancreas, kidney, liver, and perirectal tissues. In humans the infections may produce transient swellings and eosinophilia, especially in those who do not live in endemic areas (Fig. 52–5B) (4).

Mansonella streptocerca inhabits the subcutaneous tissues, producing hypopigmentation, urticarial patches and pruritus. The microfilariae are found in skin snips (Chapter 62) (5).

The diagnosis of Mansonella infections is made by the laboratory, usually after identifying the microfilariae in blood or skin snips (Fig. 52–5A and B). These infections are rarely seen in the United States, with the exception of Mansonella ozzardi, which has been found a few times among Haitian immigrants, and rarely in people who have travelled to the endemic areas (5).

Zoonotic filariae. For the sake of completeness the zoonotic filariae, especially those that produce morbidity, are mentioned briefly here, because the diagnosis is made by the anatomic pathologist based on the identification of the worms in the tissues (4,12).

The life cycles of the zoonotic filarids are similar to those described above, usually with different species of mosquitoes as intermediate hosts. Human infections are accidental, and, as a rule, the parasites do not grow to adults, so microfilariae are not produced. The worms die in the tissues, eliciting an inflammatory reaction that is responsible for the symptoms. Three infections produced by zoonotic filariae are recognized. (1) One is pulmonary, produced by Dirofilaria immitis (the dog's heartworm) and characterized by nodules (infarct-like) in the lung (Fig. 52–6A, B). The worms grow in the right heart, die, and embolize, producing the pulmonary lesion (4,13). (2) Another is subcutaneous nodules, produced by Dirofilaria repens in Europe and Asia, Dirofilaria tenuis in the southeastern United States (Fig. 52–6C, D), and others of less importance. These infections are characterized by inflamed subcutaneous nodules, which usually are removed and studied histologically (4,14). (3) Lymphatic infections are produced by Brugia species in the United States, predominantly in the northeastern part of the country, and sporadically in South America. Focal lymphadenitis usually is the presentation; the lymph node is removed and the diagnosis is made on histologic sections (4,12,15).

Trichinella spiralis

Trichinella spiralis is the agent of trichinellosis, an infection that occurs predominantly in subtropical areas. In the United States the infection has been decreasing steadily during the last 40 years, and has become rare, though often it occurs in small clusters of cases (16). The infection is transmitted mostly through the consumption of raw or undercooked pork, but infections acquired from eating contaminated game account for a third of the cases reported each year in the United States.

The life cycle of Trichinella takes place in one host, which is both definitive and intermediate. Infective larvae in the muscles of pigs and other animals are encapsulated (pseudocysts), which after ingestion grow within the mucosal epithelium of the small intestine to adults, male and female. The females lay larvae, which enter the intestinal wall and through the blood vessels and lymphatics gain access to the muscles, where they grow inside the muscle cells (intracellularly) to infective larvae (2).

The symptoms produced by Trichinella infection vary, depending on the phase of the infection. During the intestinal phase, especially in heavy infections, the worms produce malaise, vomiting, diarrhea, nausea, and abdominal cramps (4). The symptoms are often confused with food poisoning. The systemic or tissular phase follows the intestinal phase, as soon as the larvae laid by the adults invade the musculature (Fig. 52–7A, B). Systemic manifestations of fever, muscle pain, and edema of the face (sometimes periorbital) and hands occur, together with generalized

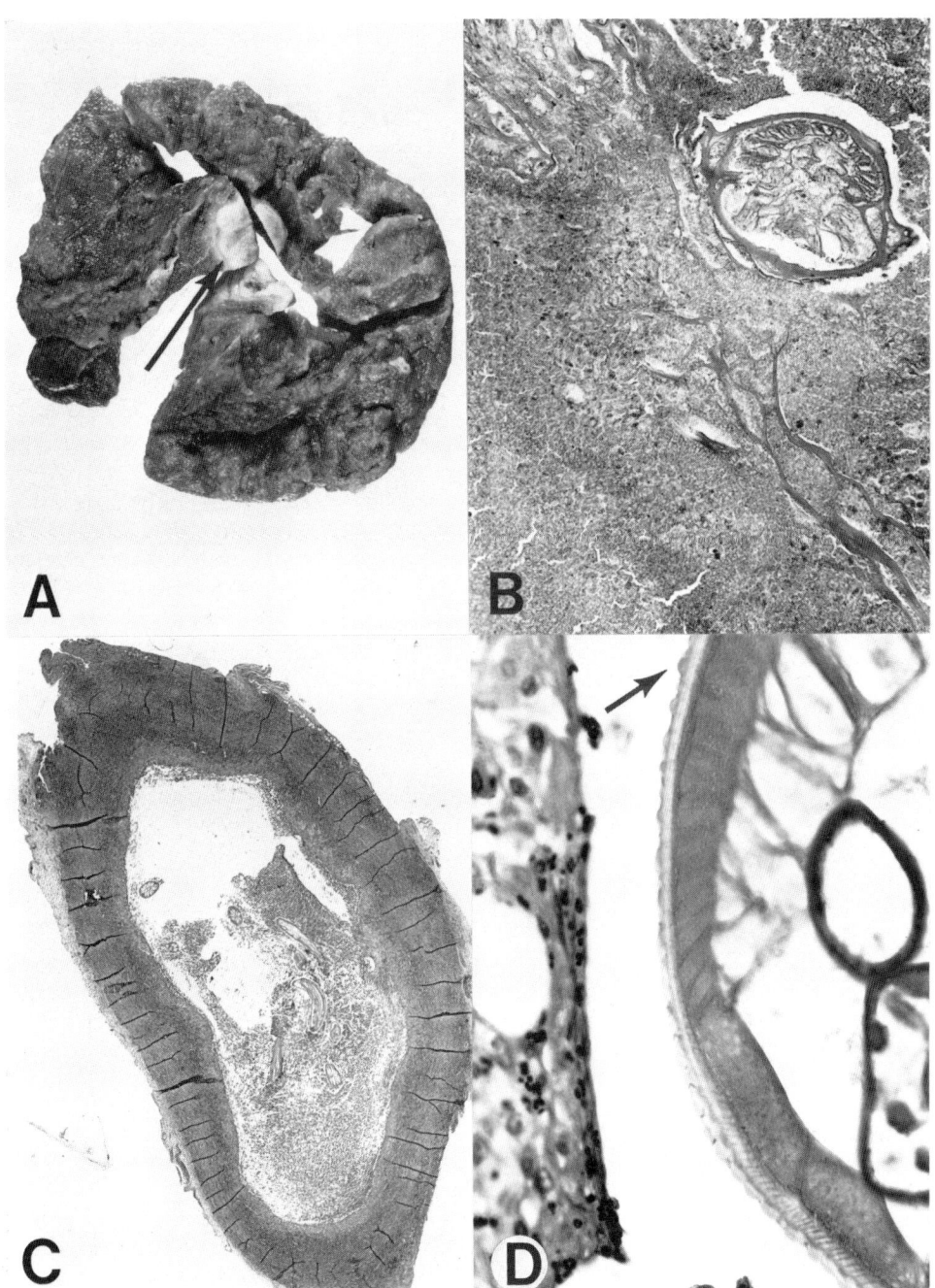

Fig. 52-6. Zoonotic filariae. A, B, Dirofilaria immitis. A, Nodule in a portion of lung removed from an individual with a diagnosis of carcinoma of lungs. Note the necrotic nodule at center (arrow). B, In the microscopic view of a section of nodule note the cross section of the worm and the marked necrosis of both it and surrounding tissues. The worm is in a vessel, the walls not seen here (hematoxylin and eosin, ×146). C, D, Dirofilaria tenuis. C, Low-power micrograph of a histologic section of a subcutaneous nodule. Note the necrotic center containing cross- and oblique sections of the parasite (×9.5). D, Greater magnification shows the characteristic cuticle with the ridges (arrow) (×440).

weakness and high peripheral eosinophilia (4). Eventually, difficulties with eye movement, breathing, chewing, and swallowing develop, sometimes accompanied by central nervous system symptoms (17) and symptoms of myocarditis (18). Death may occur due to the myocarditis or the encephalitis, or both.

The diagnosis is made clinically, but it requires confirmation by the anatomic pathologist in biopsy specimens of skeletal muscle, mainly the deltoid (Fig. 52-7B).

Toxocara species (Visceral Larval Migrans)

Toxocara is a genus comprised of several species related to Ascaris (Chapter 50) that occur in wild and domestic animals, especially dogs and cats, producing zoonotic infections in humans worldwide. Toxocara canis from dogs and Toxocara cati from cats are soil-transmitted infections. Their developmental cycle resembles in most aspects the life cycle of Ascaris. Infections with these nematodes are thus infections of small children who ingest dirt (19).

The adult Toxocara worms live in the small intestine of dogs and cats, where the female lays eggs that are evacuated with the feces. In appropriate soil and under ideal conditions the eggs of Toxocara embryonate (become infective) in 2 to 4 weeks. Embryonated eggs are ingested by the appropriate host, where they hatch and free larvae, which enter the intestinal wall to reach the circulation and travel to the liver and then to the lungs. In the lungs

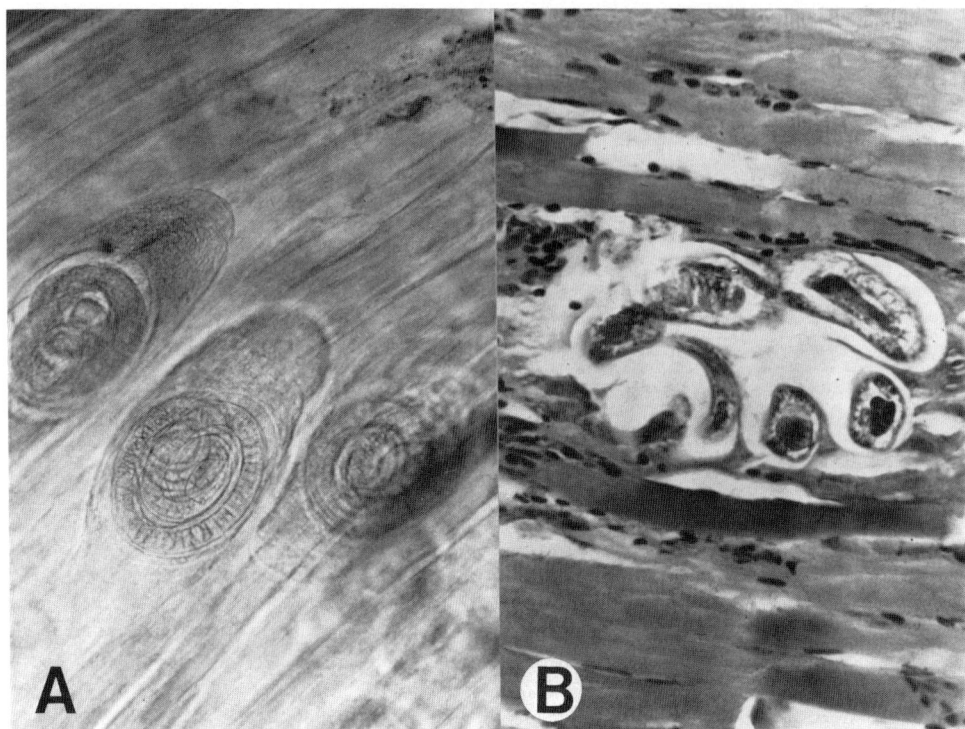

Fig. 52–7. Trichinella spiralis. *A*, Worm in muscle of experimentally infected animal, pressed between two glass slides to show entire cyst, (×120). *B*, Section of deltoid muscle showing sections of the larvae (hematoxylin and eosin, ×300).

the larvae mature somewhat and travel back to the intestine via the respiratory tree, to grow to adults (2). In hosts other than the appropriate ones (abnormal hosts) the ingestion of embryonated eggs produces larvae that migrate to the liver, where they stop their development and persist as infective larvae. Persistence of larvae of Toxocara and other parasites in the tissues, without further development, is a phenomenon known as paratenesis (19). The paratenic host could pass the infection to the definitive hosts (cats and dogs) when it is ingested by these hosts. Humans infected with Toxocara serve as paratenic hosts, and the larvae persist in the tissues, migrating aimlessly (larva migrans), producing lesions (tracks) characterized by an inflammatory response.

The symptoms produced by Toxocara in humans are nonspecific; the patient typically is a 1½- to 4-year-old child, most often 2 years old, who is brought to the physician because of failure to thrive. Physical examination reveals an enlarged liver, high peripheral eosinophilia (up to 80%) with a high white blood cell count (up to 30,000 per microliter), and increased immunoglobulin titers. Results of serologic tests, such as enzyme-linked immunosorbent assay (ELISA) and others, performed in reference laboratories, using Toxocara antigens, are positive. The diagnosis is made clinically, based on this presentation, plus the involvement of other organ systems such as the lungs, the heart, and sometimes the central nervous system.

Liver biopsy is not recommended because the rate of recovery of the parasite in tissues is low. The tissue lesions consist of tracks with marked mononuclear cell and polymorphonuclear infiltrates (Fig. 52–8A); granulomas throughout the liver, with foreign body giant cell reaction, rarely with a larva are observed (Fig. 52–8B). Infiltration by lymphocytes and eosinophils is abundant in the granulomas and throughout the adjacent tissues. Similar lesions are found in every organ studied (4).

Angiostrongylus species

Angiostrongylus are nematodes that inhabit the blood vessels of many animals and have as their intermediate hosts slugs and snails. Angiostrongylus worms occur in several parts of the world, producing severe morbidity and sometimes death. Two species of Angiostrongylus have been recognized in humans: Angiostrongylus cantonensis, which produces eosinophilic meningoencephalitis, and Angiostrongylus costaricensis, which produces abdominal angiostrongyloidiasis.

Angiostrongylus cantonensis. A. cantonensis is a parasite of the pulmonary arteries of rats. The geographic distribution is from the coast of West Africa to southeast Asia, and throughout the islands of the Pacific basin. Infected rats have been found in the United States, Egypt, Cuba, and Puerto Rico (4).

The adult males and females of Angiostrongylus cantonensis live in the pulmonary arteries, where the females lay eggs that embryonate to a larva within the pulmonary parenchyma. The larvae move in the respiratory tree to the epiglottis and into the digestive tract, to be eliminated with the feces; in soil, the larvae are ingested by slugs or snails, the intermediate hosts, where the larvae develop to be infective. Infective larvae ingested by the rodent definitive host migrate from the stomach to the brain, where they develop rapidly, migrate to the meninges (subarachnoid space), and then to the lungs, where they grow to adults in the pulmonary arteries. Humans become infected with A. cantonensis in a similar manner to ro-

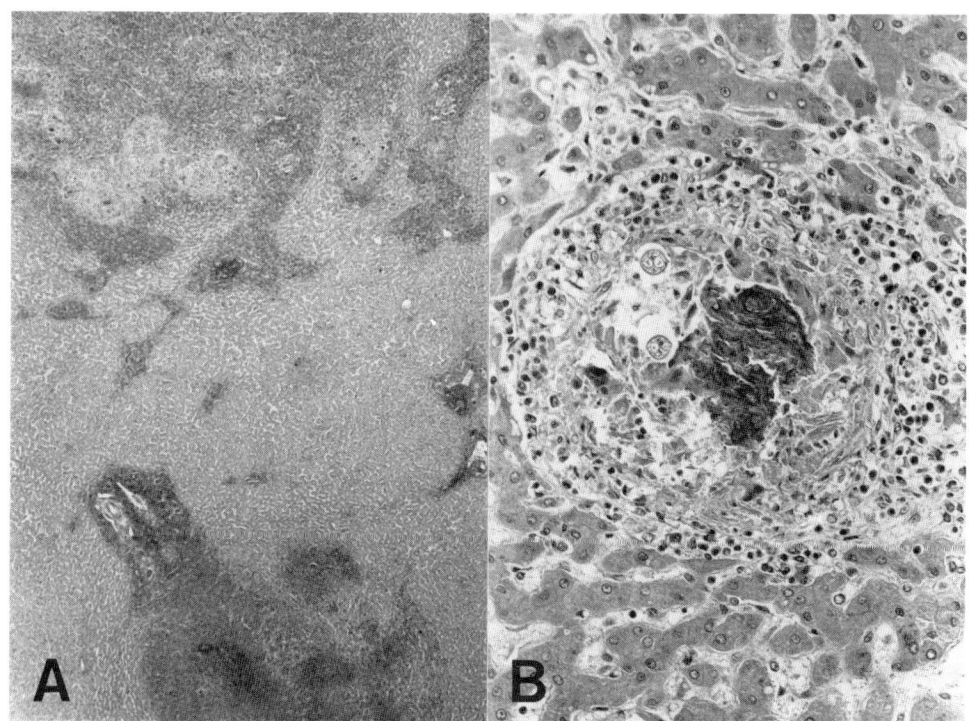

Fig. 52–8. Toxocara canis in tissues. A, Low-power view of a liver section from a 2-year-old child shows marked destruction and inflammation of the parenchyma (hematoxylin and eosin, ×28). B, Higher magnification of a granuloma shows two cross sections of a larva (hematoxylin and eosin, ×220).

dents, by ingesting the larvae with a slug or snail, but more commonly by ingesting larvae shed by the gastropods on vegetables or in water (2).

Humans are abnormal hosts for Angiostrongylus cantonensis, and growth to adults does not take place. The parasites undergo development in the brain and then are lost in their migration to the lungs. The development of A. cantonensis in the brain and the meninges of humans is responsible for the syndrome known as eosinophilic meningoencephalitis (Fig. 52–9A). The prodromal symptoms of eosinophilic meningoencephalitis are vomiting, vague abdominal discomfort, shortness of breath, and occasionally, low fever. The main symptoms are headache, nuchal rigidity, photophobia, vision impairment, and facial paresthesias or paralysis. Other neurologic abnormalities or deficits may be present, that vary with the patient

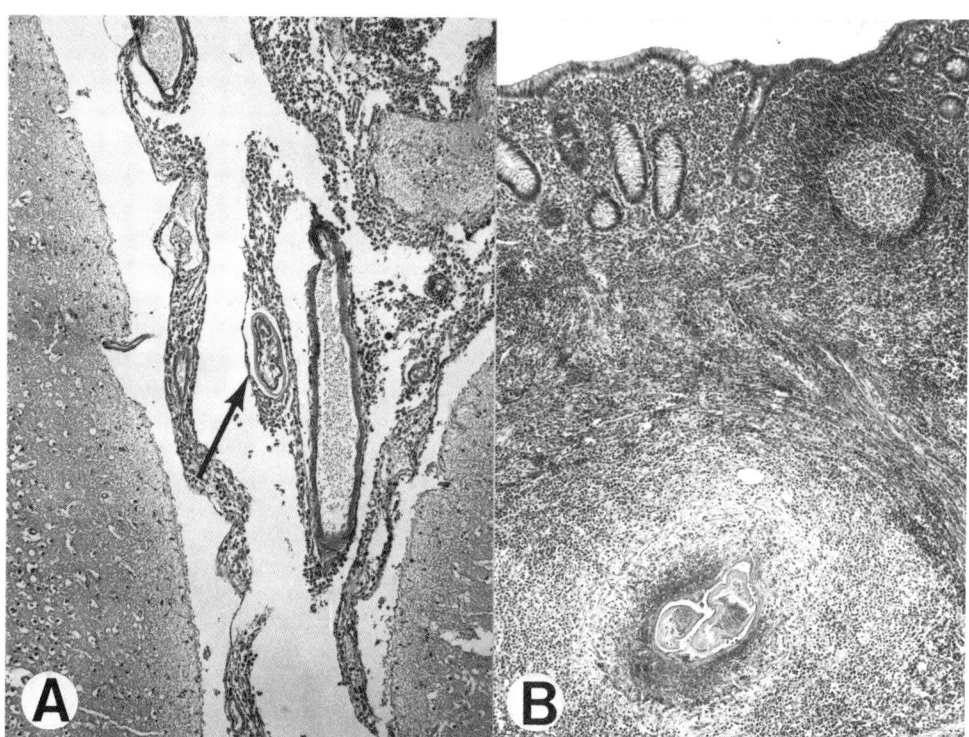

Fig. 52–9. Angiostrongylus in tissue sections. A, A. cantonensis in brain of a person who died of eosinophilic meningitis. Note the inflamed meninges and the cross section of the worm (arrow) (hematoxylin and eosin, ×180). B, A. costaricensis in human appendix. Note cross sections of the worm forming a granuloma; the worm is dead and embolized to the submucosal tissue (×70).

and the extent of involvement. Ocular symptoms are common, and worms have been recovered occasionally from the anterior chamber of the eye (20). In general the infection is benign and self-limiting, but up to 1% mortality has been recorded during some epidemics.

In eosinophilic meningoencephalitis the spinal fluid pressure is mildly elevated; the fluid can be clear, hazy, or cloudy, and may contain as many as 3400 white blood cells per microliter, with eosinophilia of up to 20%; proteins are elevated, and the larvae have been recovered occasionally with the spinal tap (21). Study of brain tissues recovered at autopsy shows slight changes grossly and microscopically. Microscopically the main feature is infiltration of the meninges by abundant eosinophils. The worms are usually visualized either in the brain tissue or (more commonly) in the meninges (4).

The diagnosis of eosinophilic meningoencephalitis is made clinically, based on the presenting symptoms and signs, and on the laboratory tests. If a worm is recovered during the spinal tap, it should be submitted in toto, fresh to the laboratory for examination.

Angiostrongylus costaricensis. A. costaricensis is a parasite of the mesenteric arteries of the cotton rat and the black rat. The known geographic distribution is Central and South America, where most of the cases of abdominal angiostrongyliasis have been reported. In the United States the parasite has been found in cotton rats (4).

The life cycle of Angiostrongylus costaricensis is similar to that of Angiostrongylus cantonensis, except that the infective larvae ingested with the gastropod migrate through the tissues to the branches of the mesenteric artery, where the worms grow to adults and lay eggs in the capillaries of the intestinal wall. The eggs develop larvae, which migrate to the intestinal lumen to be evacuated with the feces of the animal (2).

In humans the location of the adult worm is in the lumen of the arteries irrigating the terminal ileum, appendix, and cecum. The symptoms of the infection are usually abdominal pain in the right iliac fossa, with anorexia, vomiting, diarrhea, constipation, and abdominal rigidity. On palpation the abdominal wall is rigid and painful, and a tumor-like mass may be detected. Temperature is slightly elevated and the great majority of patients have high leukocytosis with eosinophilia of 11 to 61%. Roentgenograms show changes in the terminal ileum, appendix, cecum, and ascending colon. The great majority of patients require surgery (22).

Histologically the removed segment of intestine shows the adult worm in the vessels and a marked granulomatous inflammatory process within the wall of the viscus (Fig. 52–9B). The granulomas may coalesce and elicit marked fibrosis with thickening of the intestinal wall and surrounding structures. Eosinophils are abundant throughout (4,22).

The diagnosis of Angiostrongylus costaricensis is based on the anatomopathologic examination of the removed tissues. The worm, eggs, and larvae are recognized in the tissues and should be identified properly (4). Usually, larvae are not found in the stool samples except in terminally ill patients.

TREMATODES

The trematodes found in the tissues of humans can be placed in three groups, for practical purposes: (1) biliary trematodes—Fasciola sp., Clonorchis sinensis, Opisthorchis species, Amphimerus, and Dicrocoelium; (2) pulmonary trematodes—Paragonimus species; and (3) trematodes of the blood vessels, the schistosomes. All these trematodes in these organs shed eggs, which are evacuated with the sputum, the feces, or the urine, depending on the species.

As stated in Chapter 50, trematodes are platyhelminths that have complicated life cycles involving one or more intermediate hosts, the first being a snail, and thus are referred to as snail-transmitted helminths. The tissue trematodes are widely distributed in tropical and subtropical areas, and some, for example the schistosomes, produce one of the most important parasitic infections in humans. The trematodes of tissues are discussed here.

Biliary Trematodes

Members of two genera of biliary trematodes—Fasciola and Dicrocoelium—occur under natural conditions in cattle, sheep, and goats, animals much used by humans as food. When humans ingest liver from animals that harbor the parasites, the eggs in the parasites are released in the stomach and are evacuated with the feces. These eggs are innocuous, but sometimes are encountered in the clinical laboratory in stool samples; in each instance where Fasciola or Dicrocoelium eggs are identified in a stool sample, the possibility of "spurious parasitism" (false parasitism) should be considered and other samples obtained days apart should be examined. The clinician should be advised to request the second sample after the patient has abstained from eating meat and meat products (4). The other two genera of biliary trematodes—Clonorchis and Opisthorchis—also occur in animals, but generally not ones consumed by humans.

The eggs of the biliary trematodes are found in stool samples, but they were not discussed among the intestinal trematodes because they do not produce lesions in the intestine.

Fasciola. Two species of Fasciola—Fasciola hepatica (Fig. 52–10A) and Fasciola gigantica—are recognized as parasites of cattle, goats, and sheep worldwide. They produce accidental infections in humans, who are unnatural hosts, and therefore, infections with Fasciola are zoonoses (4). The geographic distribution of F. gigantica is more restricted than that of Fasciola hepatica and is confined to certain areas of Africa, the Middle East, and India. Human infection with F. hepatica occurs mainly in Central and South America, Europe, the Middle East, North and South Africa, and Hawaii. The most important areas where infections are regularly encountered in humans are Spain, France, Puerto Rico, Cuba, and Brazil (2).

The adults of Fasciola are hermaphroditic worms that lay eggs in the biliary tree. The eggs are passed to the intestine with the bile and to the environment with the feces; in fresh water, they embryonate and produce larvae, which enter a snail, where they develop to cercariae. Cer-

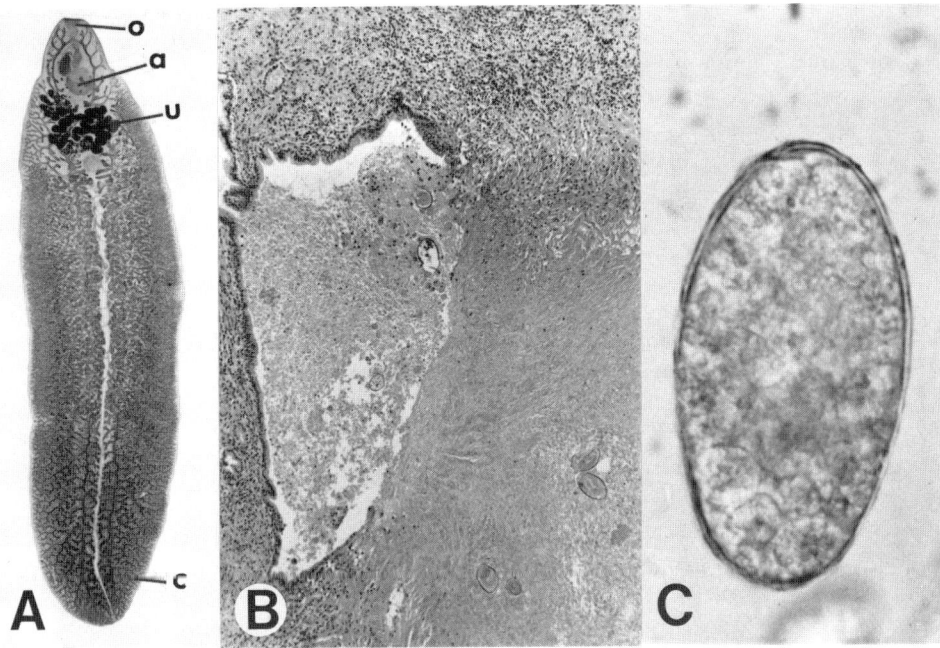

Fig. 52–10. Fasciola hepatica. *A*, Adult worm, Key: o, oral sucker; a, acetabulum; c, cecum; u, uterus aceto-carmine alum, ×3.5). *B*, On section of liver note the partly destroyed bile duct epithelium, the necrosis, and the eggs in the necrotic mass (hematoxylin and eosin, ×55). *C*, Egg in human stool (unstained, ×500).

cariae leave the snail and find a plant, where they encyst; ingestion of cysts by appropriate hosts frees the larvae in the intestine, larvae which penetrate the intestinal wall and drop in the peritoneum to migrate to the liver. After entering the liver the larvae migrate to a bile duct, where they grow to adults (2).

Humans are abnormal hosts for Fasciola, and generally the parasite does not complete the life cycle in these hosts. Young worms usually die, producing abscesses in the biliary system; only a few grow to adults. The consequences are production of symptoms related to the biliary tree. Epigastric or right hypochondrial pain, temperature of 39° to 41° C and sweating are presenting symptoms in some individuals. Allergic manifestations such as urticarial rash, pruritus, and asthma, may occur; anorexia and weight loss often are observed, but eventually, symptoms of chronic obstructive biliary disease predominate (Fig. 52–10B). On examination the liver is enlarged, epigastric pain is exquisite, and laboratory tests show leukocytosis and marked eosinophilia (23). The roentgenographic images, especially those of the biliary tree, and sonograms are useful in diagnosing the infection (4).

The diagnosis is made clinically, especially in endemic areas where clinicians are aware of the infection and its presentation. The laboratory may confirm the presence of Fasciola eggs in the stools, but this does not occur often, because egg production in human infections is low or nonexistent. The eggs of Fasciola are large, ovoid, 130 to 150 μm by 63 to 90 μm, have an operculum, and are immature at the time of evacuation (Fig. 52–10C).

Clonorchis sinensis, and Opisthorchis species. The genera Clonorchis and Opisthorchis have several species that infect animals and humans. The best-known is Clonorchis sinensis, but several species of Opisthorchis also produce infections in humans in several parts of the world. In general these trematodes produce limited morbidity; the great majority of infected persons are asymptomatic.

Clonorchis sinensis occurs in China, Taiwan, Japan, Korea, and Vietnam; Opisthorchis felinus in south central and eastern Europe, the European areas of the former USSR, Turkey, Ukraine, and western Siberia; Opisthorchis viverrini in southeast Asia, and Amphimerus pseudofelinuis (Opisthorchis guayaquilensis) in Ecuador. In the United States these parasites are found especially in immigrants from endemic areas, particularly among Chinese and Vietnamese populations. In the endemic areas of Clonorchis sinensis rates of infection up to 50% are not uncommon (Opisthorchis felinus, 65%; Opisthorchis viverrini, 95%) (4).

The life cycle of Clonorchis and that of Opisthorchis are similar. The eggs are evacuated with the bile to the intestine, and with the feces into the environment, where they are ingested by an aquatic snail, hatch, and develop to cercariae. Cercariae leave the snail and enter a freshwater fish by boring under the scales, and locate in the muscles, where the larvae encyst. Ingestion of raw fish frees the larvae from the cysts in the intestine; they enter the ampulla of Vater and migrate through the common bile duct to the gallbladder and the biliary ducts of the liver, where they grow to adult parasites (Fig. 52–11A) (4).

The symptoms produced by infections with Clonorchis and Opisthorchis are mostly silent. The only indication of the infection is the finding of eggs in the stools. A few persons infected with Clonorchis, especially those who live outside endemic areas, may have malaise, fever to 40° C, slight jaundice, enlargement of the liver, and eosinophilia of up to 88%. Natives may suffer epigastric pain, fever, and vomiting, especially when a new infection (reinfection) is superimposed on an old one (4). Imaging techniques, especially of the biliary tree, may demonstrate the worms, and often biliary obstruction (24).

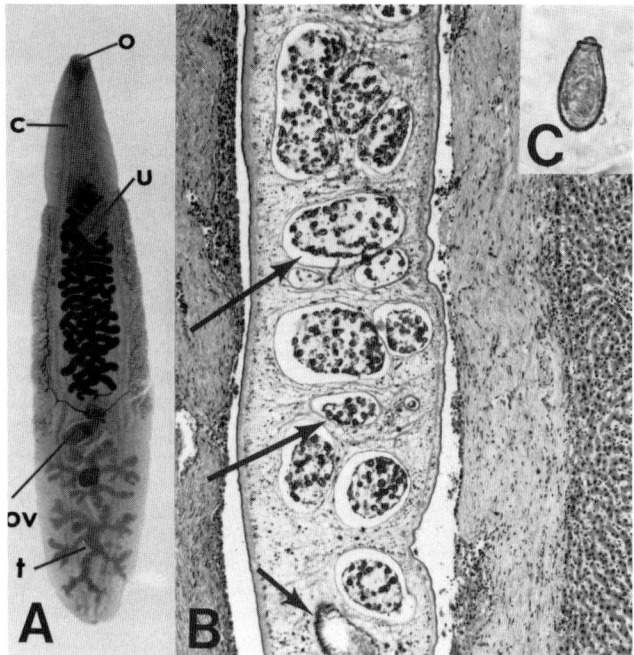

Fig. 52–11. Clonorchis sinensis. *A*, Adult worm, Key: o, oral sucker; c, cecum; u, uterus; ov, ovary; t, testes, aceto-carmine alum, ×9). *B*, Section of liver showing the parasite's cecum (*short arrow*) and several sections through the uterus with eggs (*long arrows*). Note the thickened, fibrotic wall of the bile duct (hematoxylin and eosin, ×70). *C*, Egg in human stool (unstained, ×500).

The main histologic changes associated with infection with Clonorchis and Opisthorchis are inflammation of the bile ducts and proliferation of the epithelium (adenomatous proliferation), with resultant fibrosis of the ducts (Fig. 52–11B) (4). The incidence of cholangiocarcinoma has been reported to be higher in persons infected with these trematodes (25). Moreover, the worms may serve as the nuclei for deposition of bile salts, resulting in an increase of biliary stones (4).

The diagnosis of clonorchiasis and opisthorchiasis is usually made in the clinical laboratory, based on recognition of the eggs in the stools (Chapter 59); the eggs of the different species that parasitize humans are indistinguishable, and therefore, the generic identification should be used in all laboratory reports: eggs of Clonorchis or Opisthorchis. The eggs are 28 to 35 μm by 12 to 19 μm, broadly ovoid with a thick, golden brown shell (Fig. 52–11C). They have a distinct operculum and a knob on the opposite side of the operculum; they are embryonated at the time of evacuation.

Pulmonary trematodes. Trematode infections in the lungs of humans are usually produced by species of the genus Paragonimus, of which Paragonimus westermani is best-known. However, many species of Paragonimus infect humans in different parts of the world, and all of them produce paragonimiasis. Infections with Paragonimus have been reported mainly in Korea, Japan, and Taiwan. Sporadic cases have been found in China, Vietnam, Philippines, Thailand, Malaysia, India, some African countries, Central and South America, and rarely in the United States.

The adult Paragonimus organisms (Fig. 52–12A) live in the lung parenchyma, where the eggs are laid in the tissues and are moved through the bronchi with the mucus and expectorated, but most pass with the mucus into the gastrointestinal tract and are evacuated with the feces. In water, the eggs embryonate, hatch, and release larvae, which enter a snail where they develop to cercariae; cercariae leave the snail and enter some crustaceans (crayfish, crabs) and encyst in their muscles. Ingestion of the raw crustaceans permits the release of the larvae from their cysts, larvae which enter through the intestinal wall to the peritoneal cavity and migrate to the lungs to develop into adults (2).

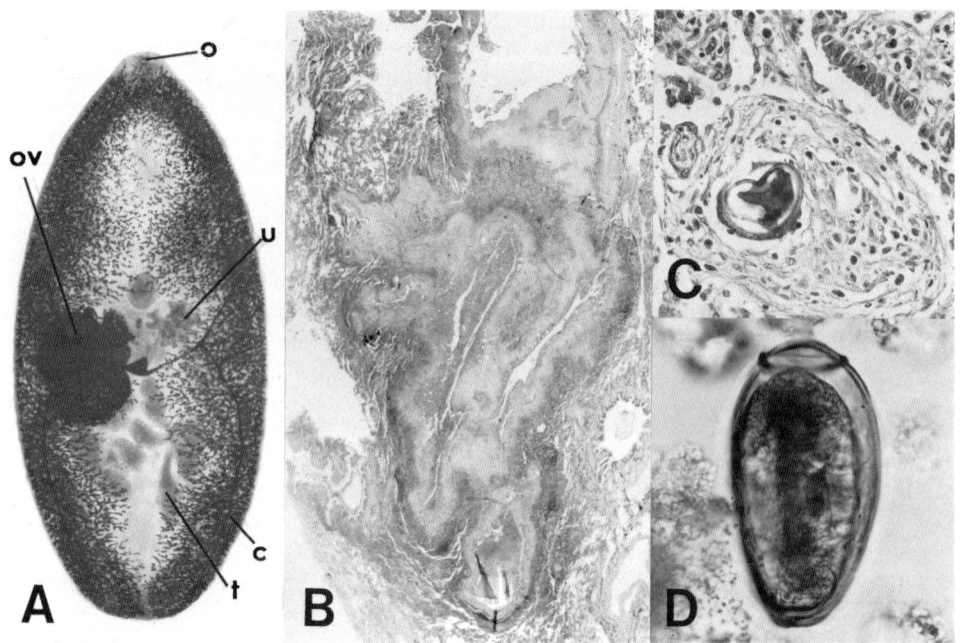

Fig. 52–12. Paragonimus. *A*, Adult Paragonimus organism: o, oral sucker; t, testes; o, ovary; c, cecum, (aceto-carmine alum, ×9). *B*, Low-power view of a lung section shows a large necrotic area where the parasite was lodged (aceto-carmine alum, ×11). *C*, Granuloma in the lung with partly destroyed egg (×450). *D*, Egg in human stool (unstained, ×550).

The clinical symptoms of paragonimiasis are nonspecific, and in general, the infection follows a benign course. The bulk of the infections are found in 10- to 25-year-olds, who usually present with chronic cough and blood-tinged sputum. The infection is chronic, with little impairment of health; peripheral eosinophilia is between 20 and 25%. Heavy infections may cause chest pain, dyspnea, night sweats, and pleural effusions (26). Chest radiographs may show lesions, often cavities resembling chronic cavitary tuberculosis (27). Ectopic location of the worms—in the brain, the subcutaneous tissues, and other organs—is relatively common (4).

In humans the anatomic pathology of paragonimiasis is usually that of a granulomatous inflammation. On cut sections of lung the adult worms may be seen grossly within cavities surrounded by fibrous tissue. More often the cavity is filled with necrotic tissue without a worm, surrounded by indurated pulmonary parenchyma. Microscopically the worms may be seen, but more often, granulomas containing eggs of Paragonimus are present in the wall of the cavity (Fig. 52–12B) (4).

The diagnosis of the infection is clinical, based on the history and the roentgenographic findings. Confirmation is by finding in the stool eggs characteristic of the group (Chapter 59). The eggs of Paragonimus are broadly ovoid, with a golden brown shell. The operculum is distinct, relatively flattened, and at the abopercular end the shell is thickened. The eggs measure about 80 to 118 µm by 48 to 60 µm and are nonembryonated at the time of evacuation (Fig. 52–12C, D).

Trematodes of Blood Vessels

The trematodes of blood vessels, schistosomes, produce a disease known as schistosomiasis or bilharziasis, in many parts of the world. The schistosomes are the only trematodes of humans, with two separate sexes, living in the vessels of the portal or the urinary systems.

The adult Schistosoma male is about 20 mm and the female up to 26 mm long, depending on the species. To the naked eye the male resembles a small nematode, because the lateral aspects of its flattened body are folded toward the midline to form the gynecophorous canal, where the slender, longer female is located. Three species of Schistosoma—Schistosoma mansoni, Schistosoma haematobium, and Schistosoma japonicum—are generally recognized in humans; a fourth species, Schistosoma mekongi, has been implicated in human infections, based on finding the eggs in stools and tissues, but adult worms have not been recovered from humans (2).

The geographic distribution of Schistosoma mansoni is Central Africa, some areas in South America, and some Caribbean islands; Schistosoma haematobium occurs in most of Africa and in the Middle East in smaller foci; Schistosoma japonicum occurs in China, Japan, and the Philippines; and Schistosoma mekongi, in northern Thailand, Laos, and northern Cambodia. These four parasites produce one of the most important parasitic infections of humans, whose estimated prevalence is 200 million cases (28).

The life cycles of all four species of Schistosoma in humans are similar. The adult worms lay eggs in the tissues, eggs which are evacuated with the stools or the urine into the environment. In fresh water the eggs hatch and produce an embryo (miracidium), which enters a snail. The miracidium multiples in the snail to produce hundreds of cercariae, which leave the snail and swim until they come in contact with the skin of an appropriate host. Cercariae actively enter the skin to find the blood vessels, which carry them to the lungs, then to the liver, and finally to the smaller branches of the portal venous system or the urinary bladder venous system, where they grow to adults (Fig. 52–13A) (2).

One interesting aspect of the life cycle of Schistosoma is the passage of eggs from the circulatory system into the lumen of the viscera, where they are located. The eggs of Schistosoma are prone to produce an acute inflammatory response in the tissues, a response that microscopically appears as a microabscess. The production of these microabscesses by the eggs of Schistosoma allows the egg to "move" through the tissues and be extruded into the lumen of the viscera. Eggs are sometimes trapped and destroyed in the tissues, eliciting granuloma formation. Thus, schistosomiasis is classically a granulomatous inflammation of the tissues and viscera (4). In some persons chronic infection with Schistosoma results in deposition of eggs in the liver, because the eggs are carried with the portal blood flow rather than remaining in the viscus wall to be extruded to the lumen of the viscera. Sometimes the eggs reach the lungs to produce similar granulomatous lesions, leading to pulmonary hypertension. In contrast to the eggs, the adult worms elicit no inflammatory reaction in the host (Fig. 52–13A) as long as they remain alive in the vessels. This summary of the events of parasitism of the host by Schistosoma explains the main clinical symptoms and signs of the disease (4).

The clinical manifestations of schistosomiasis vary from person to person, and with the worm burden and the species. In general, Schistosoma mansoni, Schistosoma japonicum, and Schistosoma mekongi produce intestinal and hepatosplenic syndromes, while Schistosoma haematobium produces urinary schistosomiasis, sometimes with hepatosplenic disease.

The skin is the portal of entry for the parasites, and it may show local allergic reactions and signs—edema, urticarial rash, wheals—symptoms that are followed by similar generalized allergic manifestations, corresponding to the migration of the worms through the tissues and that last up to 4 weeks. In the intestine, Schistosoma mansoni and Schistosoma japonicum are located in the colon (Fig. 52–13C & D and 52–14B), whereas Schistosoma haematobium is located mostly in the rectum. The early symptoms of the intestinal invasion consist of diarrhea, sometimes dysenteric; fever, abdominal pain, loss of weight, tenderness of the liver, and marked peripheral eosinophilia. In the absence of reinfection the infection becomes quiescent, but elimination of eggs continues. In the final stages of the infection some persons with hepatosplenic disease have chronic diarrhea because of persistent damage to the intestinal wall.

Involvement of the liver and spleen during the chronic phase of schistosomiasis is silent, but later portal hyper-

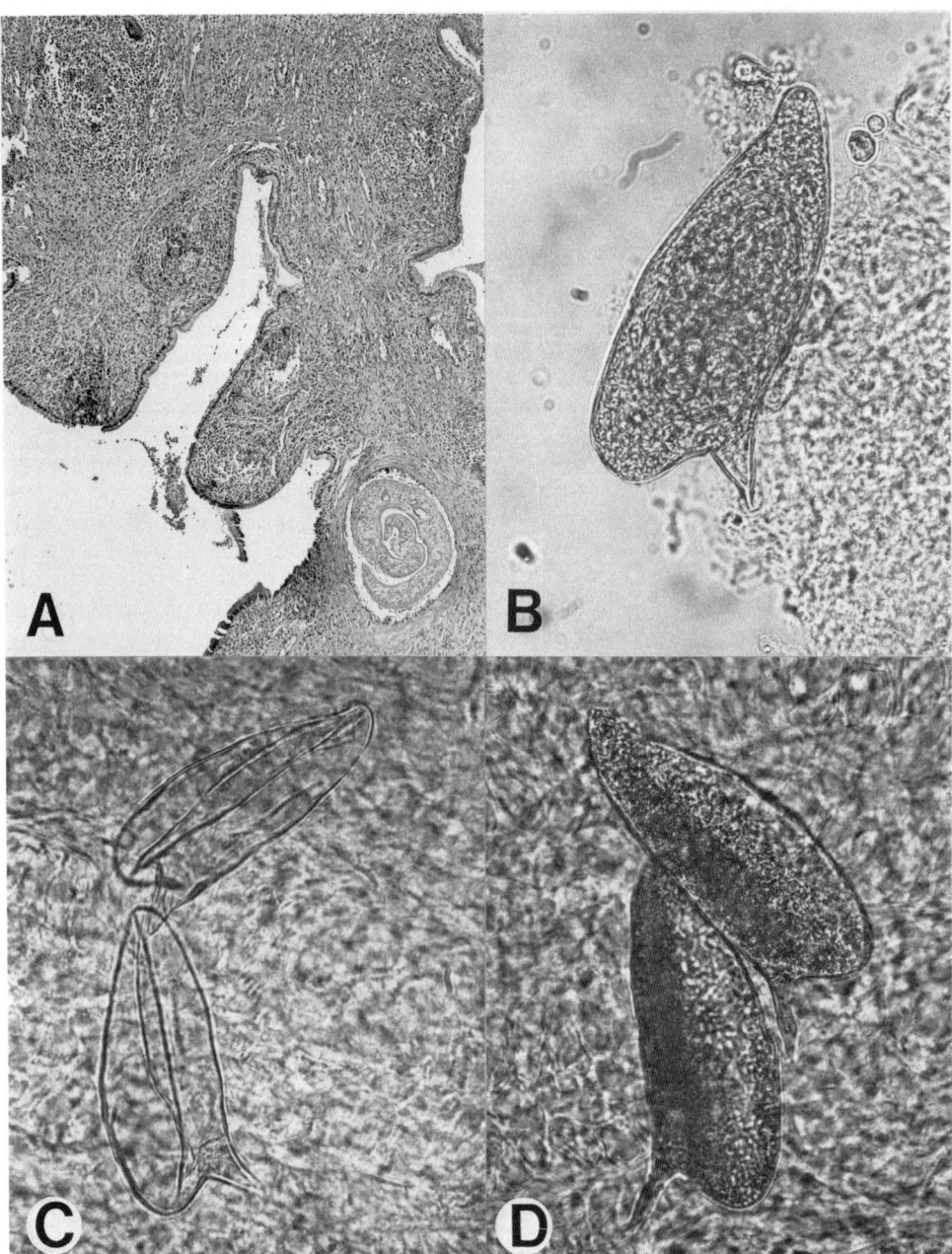

Fig. 52–13. Schistosoma mansoni. *A*, Section of human uterus shows ectopic location of S. mansoni. Note the adult male (female not seen at this level) within a blood vessel (hematoxylin and eosin, ×55). *B*, Egg in human stool (unstained, ×450). *C, D*, Eggs in colonic mucosa. The biopsy specimen was pressed between two glass slides and viewed fresh under the microscope. The eggs are calcified (×450). (Preparation for C and D courtesy of FH Shipkey MD, Department of Pathology, College of Medicine, King Saud University.)

tension is established, with all its signs and symptoms. Persons who have grave hepatosplenic disease are more often infected with Schistosoma japonicum, less frequently with Schistosoma mansoni, and even less with Schistosoma haematobium.

The urinary tract symptoms produced by Schistosoma haematobium are also related to the number of worms, and they begin soon after the parasites locate in the wall of the bladder and other organs of the urinary system (Fig. 52–15B). Microscopic bleeding, and later, blood-tinged urine, is an early sign of the infection. The chronic phase is characterized by different uropathies, obstruction at any level of the ureters being the most common. Often, long-term deposition of eggs, the formation of granulomas, and calcification of eggs (Figs. 52–15A) in the viscus wall are manifested on roentgenograms as calcification of the urinary bladder or other parts of the urinary system.

In schistosomiasis, other organs such as the lungs, the central nervous system, and the genitals may be affected, either because of deposition of eggs carried by the blood flow (lungs), or because of the ectopic location of a pair of worms (central nervous system, peritoneum, skin). These ectopic parasites produce specific syndromes that usually are diagnosed by the anatomic pathologist in tissue sections. The cervix and the vagina are often affected, in which case the eggs are identified in cervical smears stained with Papanicolaou stain (4).

The clinical diagnosis of schistosomiasis is confirmed in the laboratory by studying samples in which the eggs are normally found: the stools and tissue from the intestinal

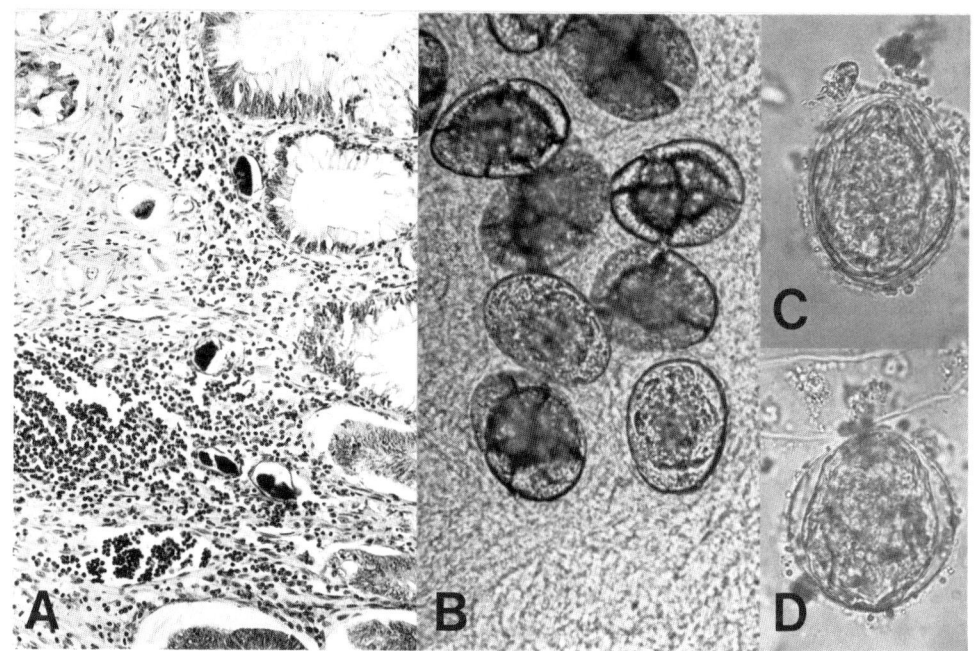

Fig. 52-14. Schistosoma japonicum. A, Section of colon shows calcified eggs, B, Eggs in intestinal submucosa, passed preparation (as in Fig. 52-13), (hematoxylin and eosin × 220). C, D, Eggs in human stools (unstained, × 450).

mucosa (Fig. 52-13C, D; Fig. 52-15B; Chapter 59), or urine and vaginal secretions (Fig. 52-16A-D; Chapter 61). In these samples, recognition of the typical eggs is based on the following characteristics: Schistosoma mansoni eggs are oval, with a prominent lateral spine located toward one of the ends; they have a fully formed miracidium (ciliated embryo) and measure 116 to 180 μm long by 45 to 58 μm wide (Fig. 52-13B). Schistosoma haematobium has similar characteristics, has a terminal spine, and measures 112 to 180 μm by 40 to 70 μm (Fig. 52-15C). Schistosoma japonicum is slightly oval, with a rudimentary lateral spine, difficult to visualize, and is about 75 to 90 μm by 60 to 78 μm (Fig. 52-14C, D). Schistosoma mekongi eggs are morphologically similar to those of Schistosoma japonicum but are only 60 to 70 μm by 52 to 62 μm. The diagnosis of schistosomiasis by the use of immunologic methods is usually beyond the capabilities of the routine clinical laboratory (29).

CESTODES

The cestodes that occur in the tissues of humans are found and identified by the anatomic pathologist, seldom by workers in the clinical parasitology laboratory. The cestodes in tissues are all larvae, and humans serve the same purpose as if they were the natural intermediate hosts. Several larval stages of cestodes are recognized in humans, the most common being the cysticercus of Tae-

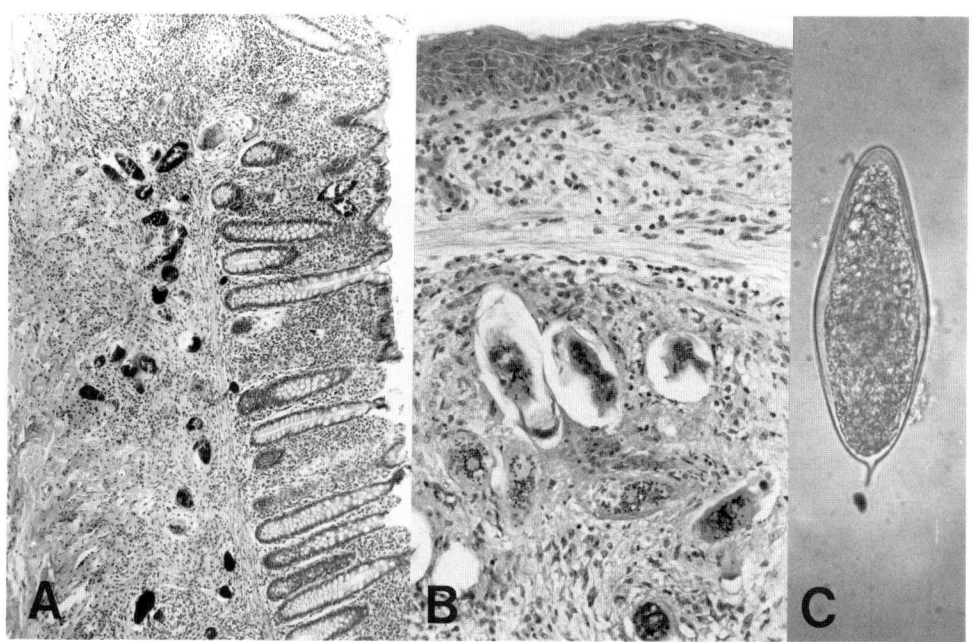

Fig. 52-15. Schistosoma haematobium. A, Section of appendix shows numerous calcified eggs in the mucosa and submucosa (hematoxylin and eosin, ×70). B, Section of urinary bladder with eggs in the submucosa (hematoxylin and eosin ×220). Note scant granuloma formation and squamous metaplasia of the urothelium. C, Eggs in scrapings from urinary bladder (unstained, ×450). Note the egg has no minacidium, only a mass of mineralized debris.

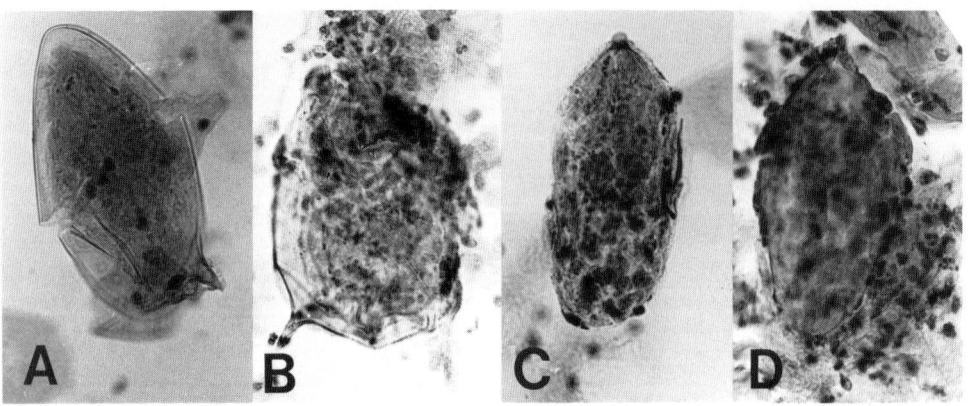

Fig. 52–16. Schistosoma mansoni eggs in cervical smear (Papanicolaou stain, ×450). *A, B,* Eggs with shell showing the typical lateral spine. *C,* Miracidium without the shell; this artifact is created in smearing the material onto the glass slide. *D,* Another egg, covered with cells (granuloma), is difficult to identify.

nium solium, which produces cysticercosis; the hydatid of Echinococcus, which produces hydatidosis; and the plerocercoid or sparganum larva of Spirometra responsible for sparganosis. These infections are reviewed briefly for the sake of completeness.

Cysticercus

The general life cycle of Taenia solium, the agent of teniasis solium and cysticercosis in humans, has already been described (Chapter 50). The eggs of T. solium evacuated with the feces of an infected person are infective to other humans; if humans ingest these eggs, the eggs hatch in the intestine to free an embryo, which enters the intestinal wall to travel via circulation to the tissues, where they grow to cysticercus. A cysticercus is a thin, transparent cyst less than 1.0 cm in diameter, with the head of the worm (scolex) inverted into the cyst. The larva remains viable in the tissues without eliciting an inflammatory reaction for a period of months to years, depending on the host. If the cysticercus dies inflammation may ensue and symptoms result (4).

In human tissues cysticerci may be located throughout the intermuscular and subcutaneous tissues (Fig. 52–17A–C). In general, cysticercosis is a benign infection that results in spontaneous resolution, except when the nervous system, the eye, or another special site is involved. In the central nervous system cysticercosis produces a variety of symptoms, the main ones related to increased intracranial pressure: severe headache, nausea, and vomiting in up to 98% of cases; seizures occur in about 50% of cases. Changes in mental status are frequent manifestations, as are cranial nerve palsies. The main diagnostic tools in neurocysticercosis are the several radiologic imaging techniques, which visualize dead, inflamed cysticerci (4).

Hydatid Cyst

Hydatid disease is produced in humans by each of the four species of Echinococcus: Echinococcus granulosus produces unilocular hydatid disease; Echinococcus multilocularis, alveolar hydatid disease; Echinococcus vogeli, polycystic hydatid disease, and Echinococcus oligarthrus, the newest found in humans, cysts as yet unclassified. By far, the most important Echinococcus of humans is Echinococcus granulosus, because of the number of cases and the extent of the geographic area where it occurs. The

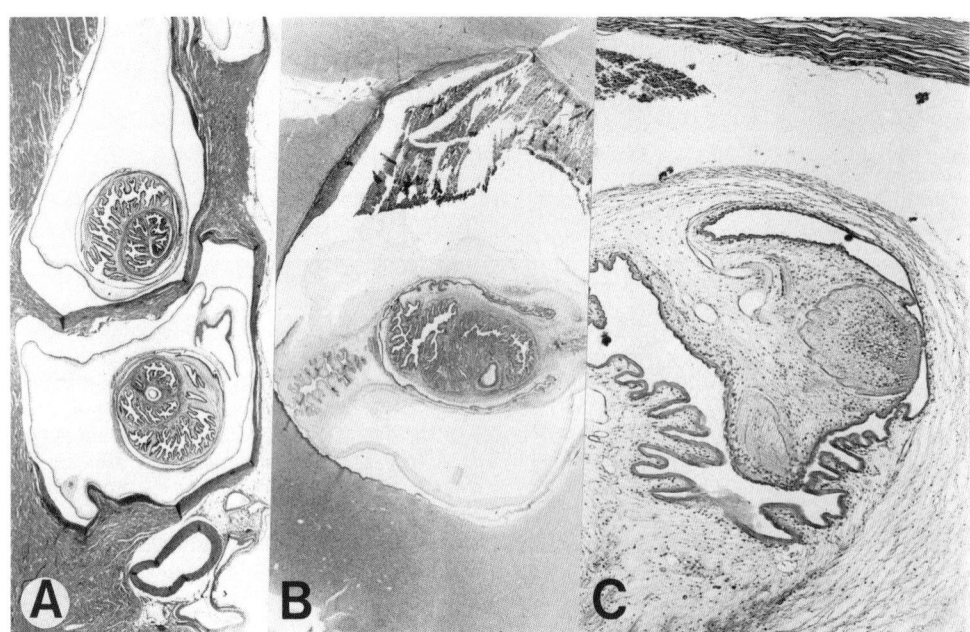

Fig. 52–17. Taenia solium cysticercosis in tissues (hematoxylin and eosin): *A,* muscle (×9); *B,* brain (×9); *C,* detail of cysticercus' scolex.

second is Echinococcus multilocularis, which is more restricted, but causes infections that are regularly fatal (4).

Echinococcus granulosus. The agent of unilocular hydatid disease is widely distributed throughout the world, both in tropical and temperate zones. On the American continent it occurs in Canada, Alaska, parts of the United States, Argentina, Bolivia, Chile, and Uruguay. In Europe it is endemic in most countries; in Africa, usually in the northern and southern parts, as well as in Asia, Australia, and New Zealand (2).

The life cycle involves wild and domestic dogs, in which the adults live in the intestine producing eggs that are evacuated with the feces. The eggs in the environment are ingested by one of several intermediate hosts, such as sheep, goats, cows, pigs, and wild animals such as deer and elk. In the intermediate host the egg hatches in the intestine, and the embryo enters the intestinal wall and travels to the tissues, often the liver, where it grows slowly into a hydatid cyst. A hydatid cyst consists of a fibrous layer, a response of the host to the parasite, followed by a thick lamellated membrane, white and friable, known as the acellular membrane (Fig. 52–18A, B). The acellular

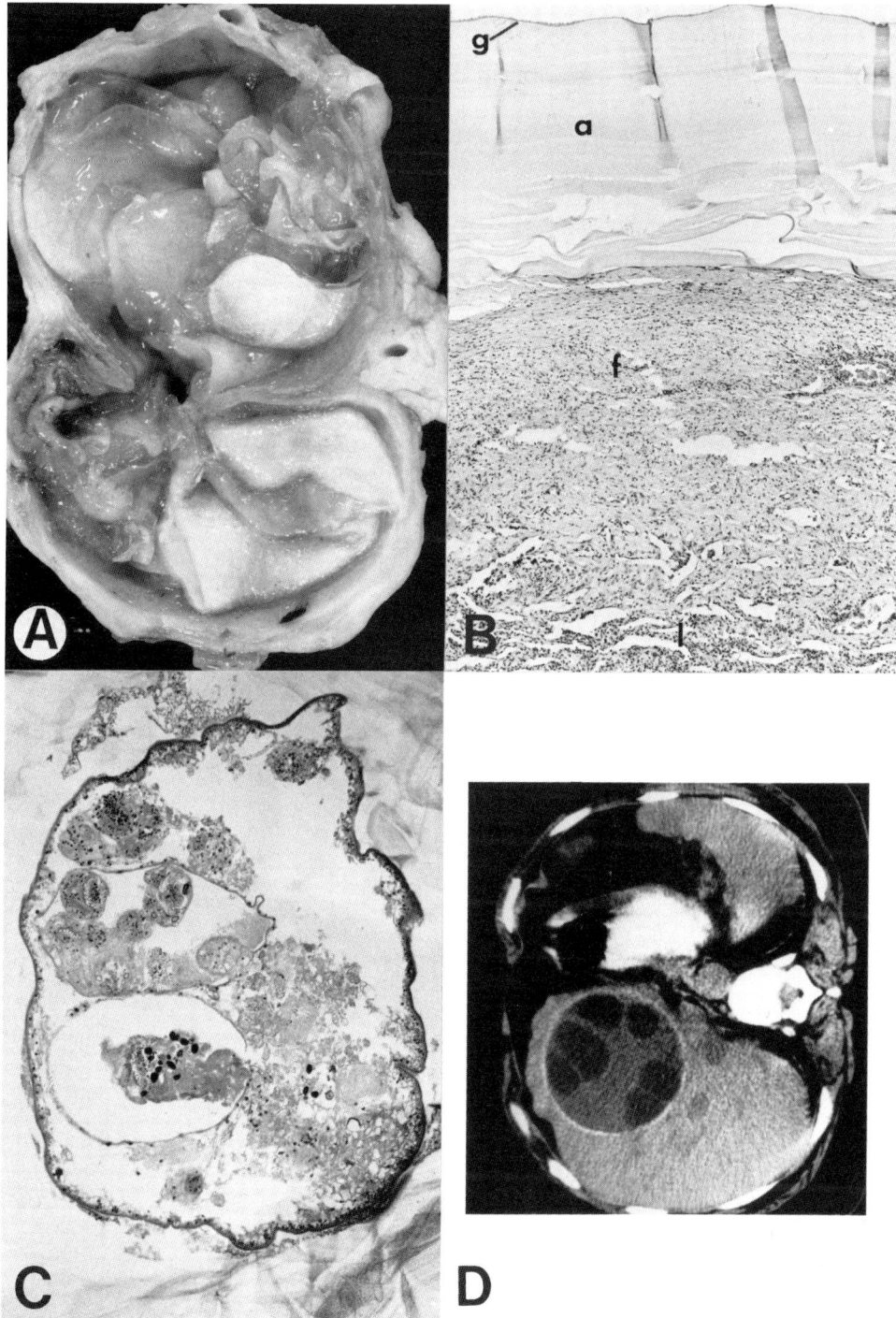

Fig. 52–18. Echinococcus granulosus. A. Cyst of pancreas contains daughter cysts and detached, acellular membrane. B, Section of cyst wall in lung: g, germinal membrane; a, acellular membrane; f, fibrous layer; l, normal lung (×55). C, Small cyst with three brood capsules (×180). D, CT scan shows a large liver cyst and several daughter cysts.

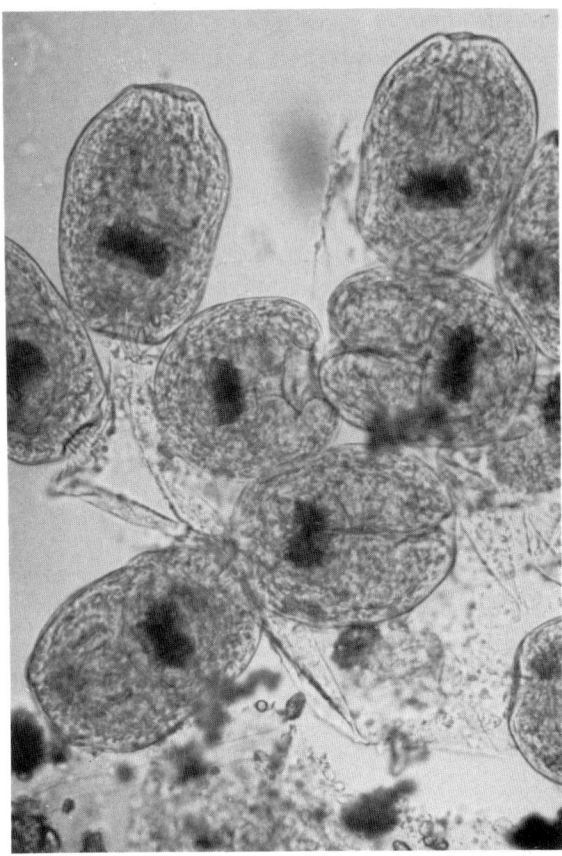

Fig. 52–19. Echinococcus granulosus hydatid sand (unstained, ×250).

52–18C). Brood capsules separate into the fluid to form smaller cysts within the larger mother cyst. Some protoscolices free in the fluid constitute the hydatid sand (Fig. 52–19).

In humans the infection occurs because of accidental ingestion of eggs passed in dog feces; the cysts (usually one) develop in the liver about 75% of the time, followed by the lungs (9%), muscles (5%), and the rest of the organs. Every organ system and tissue is good grounds for the development of a hydatid cyst. The symptoms of hydatid disease are, therefore, variable, depending on the size of the cyst and its location. However, the main presentation is that of a space-occupying lesion that grows for many years (4).

The diagnosis of hydatid cysts is usually made clinically (Fig. 52–18D) and often is confirmed by the anatomic pathologist. Cysts are being sampled more often with fine needles, without deleterious consequences, and the diagnosis is being made in cytologic smears or upon direct examination of the sediment's fluid in wet mounts (Fig. 52–19). Serologic tests have application in diagnosing certain cysts inaccessible to other forms of sampling, but they are not 100% specific. The treatment is usually surgical, but care must be taken to avoid disseminating the infection with spilled fluid in adjacent tissues (4).

Echinococcus multilocularis. The agent of alveolar hydatid disease, E. multilocularis is distributed mostly in the temperate and arctic zones of the northern hemisphere: Alaska on the American continent; parts of Germany, France, Switzerland, and Austria in Europe; the tundra in Russia; northern China, India, and Japan in Asia. Sporadic cases have been reported in some other countries. In the continental United States the parasite occurs in wildlife in the north central portion of the country, where at least one human case has been recorded (30).

The life cycle of Echinococcus multilocularis is similar to that of Echinococcus granulosus. The definitive hosts

membrane is followed by a one-cell-thick membrane attached to its interior surface, the germinal membrane; finally, the cyst is filled with clear fluid. The germinal membrane forms small vesicles, which differentiate into brood capsules with a few protoscolices, the larval stages (Fig.

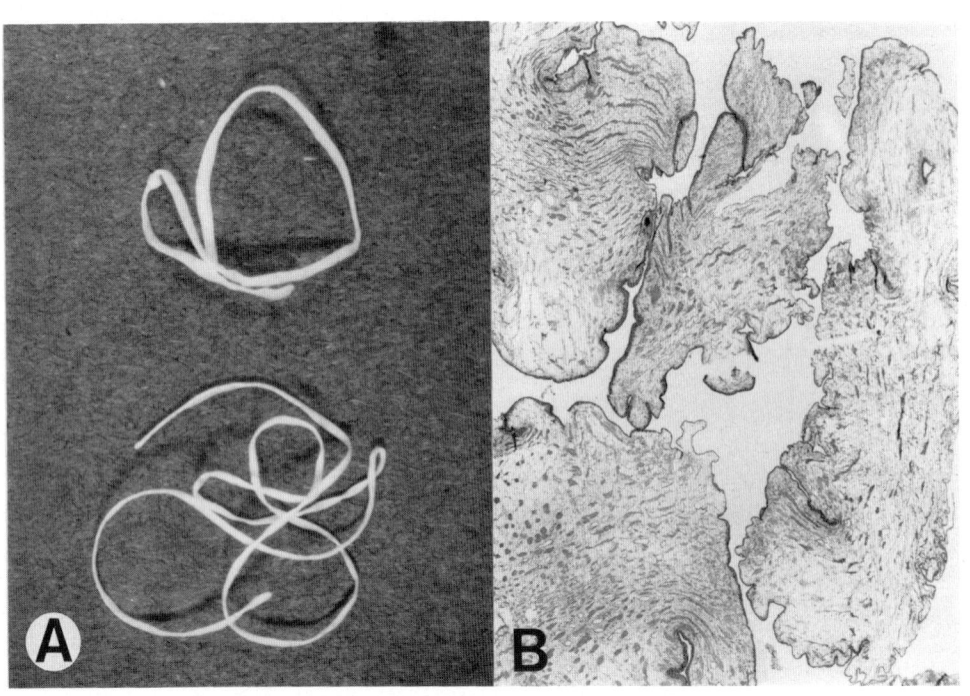

Fig. 52–20. Sparganum. *A*, Gross picture of two spargana recovered from the subcutaneous tissues of a raccoon. (From Gutierrez Y: Diagnostic Pathology of Parasitic Infections with Clinical Correlations. Philadelphia, Lea & Febiger, 1990.) *B*, Section of larva recovered from human tissues. Note the bundles of longitudinal muscles, characteristic of the larva (hematoxylin and eosin, ×22).

are arctic foxes, but domestic dogs can also be infected. The intermediate hosts are small rodents such as the northern vole, mice, shrews, and squirrels. Humans become infected by accidental ingestion of eggs passed in the feces of foxes or dogs, and thus the infections are uncommon (2).

The infection in humans, abnormal hosts for this parasite, are often fatal because the cyst grows in a disorganized manner, invading adjacent and distant tissues (metastases). The cyst always begins in the liver, but metastases to the brain, eye, lungs, and other organs are common. In Europe the great majority of infected persons die within 1 year of diagnosis (31). The cases seen in Alaska follow a similar course, but apparently some people survive the infection, even without treatment (32). The diagnosis is usually made clinically, but it is confirmed on tissues removed surgically or at autopsy.

Sparganum. Sparganosis is a benign infection of the subcutaneous tissues, and less often of the internal organs, produced by the second larval stage of tapeworms of the genus Spirometra (2). Spirometra has a life cycle similar to that of Diphyllobothrium (Chapter 50); the adult worms live in the intestine of dogs and cats, and the second procercoid or sparganum (infective) larva live in snakes, frogs, fish, or other animals (2). Parateneses (see under Visceral Larva Migrans) occurs in Spirometra, the larvae of sparganum passing through different hosts. It is likely that many Sparganum infections acquired in the United States are acquired through the ingestion of raw or undercooked infected pork (33).

Sparganosis occurs in Japan, southeast Asia, and the southeastern part of the United States, and it is sporadically reported in many other countries. The infection is usually benign, producing a subcutaneous nodule that causes no pain until the worm dies (4). Dead worms elicit an inflammatory reaction, the usual cause for consultation and for removal of the worm (Fig. 52–20A). Histologic study of the parasite (Fig. 52–20B), or study of the worm removed in toto, confirms the diagnosis.

REFERENCES

1. WHO: Lymphatic Filariasis. Tech Rep Ser No 702. Geneva, World Health Organization, 1984.
2. Beaver PC, Jung R, and Cupp EW. Clinical Parasitology. 9th ed. Philadelphia, Lea & Febiger, 1984.
3. Beaver PC: Filariasis without microfilaremia. Am J Trop Med Hyg, 10:181, 1970.
4. Gutierrez Y: Diagnostic Pathology of Parasitic Infections with Clinical Correlations. Philadelphia, Lea & Febiger, 1990.
5. Eberhard ML, and Lammie PJ: Laboratory diagnosis of filariasis. Clin Lab Med, 11:977, 1991.
6. WHO: WHO Expert Committee on Onchocerciasis. Third Report. Tech Rep Ser No 752. Geneva, World Health Organization, 1987.
7. Gibson DW, and Connor DH: Onchocercal lymphadenitis: Clinicopathologic study of 34 patients. Trans R Soc Trop Med Hyg, 72:137, 1978.
8. Rodger FC: *In* Onchocerciasis in Zaire. A New Approach to the Problem of River Blindness. Edited by FC Rodger. Oxford, Pergamon Press, 1977.
9. Gibson DW, Heggie C, and Connor DH: Clinical and pathologic aspects of onchocerciasis. Pathol Annu, 15:195, 1980.
10. Ogunba EO: Loaiasis in Ijebu Division, West Nigeria. Trop Geogr Med, 23:194, 1971.
11. Nutman TB, Reese W, Poindexter RW, et al: Immunological correlates of the hyperresponsive syndrome of loiasis in expatriates. Joint Meeting American Society Tropical Medicine Hygine and American Society Parasitologists, 35th Annual Meeting, American Society Tropical Medical Hygine, Denver, Dec 7–11, p. 306, 1986.
12. Gutierrez Y: Diagnostic features of zoonotic filariae in tissue sections. Hum Pathol, 15:514, 1984.
13. Beaver PC, and Orihel TC: Human infection with filariae of animals in the United States. Am J Trop Med Hyg, 14:1010, 1965.
14. Orihel TC, and Beaver PC: Morphology and relationship of Dirofilaria tenuis and Dirofilaria conjunctivae. Am J Trop Med Hyg, 14:1030, 1965.
15. Billups J, Schenken JR, and Beaver PC: Subcutaneous dirofilariasis in Nebraska. Arch Pathol Lab Med, 104:11, 1980.
16. Most H: Trichinosis—preventable yet still with us. N Engl J Med, 298:1178, 1978.
17. Ryczak M, Sorber WA, Kandora TF, et al: Difficulties in diagnosing Trichinella encephalitis. Am J Trop Med Hyg, 36:573, 1987.
18. Metzler MH, Sahgal KK, and Wolff GS: Second-degree atrioventricular block in acute trichinosis. Am J Dis Child, 124:598, 1972.
19. Beaver PC: The nature of visceral larva migrans. J Parasitol, 55:3, 1969.
20. Widagdo, Sunardi, Lokollo DM, et al: Ocular angiostrongyliasis in Semarang, Central Java. Am J Trop Med Hyg, 26:72, 1977.
21. Kuberski T, Bart RD, Briley JM, et al: Recovery of Angiostrongylus cantonensis from cerebrospinal fluid of a child with eosinophilic meningitis. J Clin Microbiol, 9:629, 1979.
22. Loria-Cortex R, and Lobo-Sanahuja JF: Clinical abdominal angiostrongylosis. A study of 116 children with intestinal eosinophilic granuloma caused by Angiostrongylus costaricensis. Am J Trop Med Hyg, 29:538, 1980.
23. Anton Aranda E, Garcia Carasusan M, Celador Almaraz A, et al: Fascioliasis hepatica. Revision de 5 casos. Rev Clin Esp, 176:410, 1985.
24. Choi TK, Wong KP, and Wong J. Cholangiographic appearance in clonorchiasis. Br J Radiol, 57:681, 1984.
25. Vatanasap V, Tangvoraphonkchai V, Titapant V, et al.: A high incidence of liver cancer in Khon Kaen province, Thailand. Southeast Asian J Trop Med Publ Hlth, 21:489, 1990.
26. Romeo DP, and Pollock JJ: Pulmonary paragonimiasis: Diagnostic value of pleural fluid analysis. South Med J, 79:241, 1986.
27. Singcharoen T, and Silprasert W: CT findings in pulmonary paragonimiasis. J Comput Assist Tomogr, 11:1101, 1987.
28. WHO: Epidemiology and control of schistosomiasis. Tech Rep Ser No 643. Geneva, World Health Organization, 1980.
29. Tsang VCW, and Wilkens PP: Immunodiagnosis of schistosomiasis: Screen with FAST-ELISA and confirm with Immunoblot. Clin Lab Med, 11:1029, 1991.
30. Gamble WG, Segal M, Schantz PM, et al: Alveolar hydatid disease in Minnesota: First human case acquired in the contiguous United States. JAMA, 241:904, 1979.
31. Mossiman F: Is alveolar hydatid disease of the liver incurable? Ann Surg, 192:118, 1980.
32. Rausch RL, Wilson JF, Schantz PM, et al: Spontaneous death of Echinococcus multilocularis: Cases diagnosed serologically (by EM_2 ELISA) and clinical significance. Am J Trop Med Hyg, 36:576, 1987.
33. Corkum KC: Sparganosis in some vertebrates of Louisiana and observations on a human infection. J Parasitol, 52:444, 1966.

Chapter 53

ARTHROPODS

Arthropods are important medically because either they are parasites that produce infestations (living on hosts) or infections (living in tissues) or because they serve as vectors of human disease. The latter group is the most important because of the number of diseases they transmit and the numbers of people involved. Among the most important infections transmitted by arthropods are malaria, babesiosis, trypanosomiasis, leishmaniasis, viral encephalitides, filariasis, Lyme disease, and dengue and yellow fever. These infections continue to produce morbidity and mortality in humans and animals, and for most the geographic distribution has changed little, in spite of many efforts to control them. The subject of arthropods as vectors of disease is outside this discussion; some of the many books on medical entomology and parasitology should be consulted if additional knowledge is desired (1,2).

The arthropods that parasitize humans belong to the classes Arachnida and Insecta. Arachnids are characterized by a body divided into two portions, four pairs of legs, and no antennae. Insecta have a head, thorax, and abdomen, three pairs of legs and one pair of antennae, often two pairs of wings, and mouth parts modified for chewing or sucking.

Many species of arthropods in these two classes parasitize humans, some living on the host, for example, louse infestations. Others are capable of invading tissues, for example, some larval stages of flies produce infections known as myiasis. The arthropods studied in this section are mainly those that produce infestations, because they are easily recovered by the infected individual or the examining physician, and are sent to the laboratory for identification. Arthropod infections are diagnosed by the anatomic pathologist in sections of biopsy specimens or tissues recovered at autopsy (3).

ARACHNIDA

Two groups of organisms, commonly known as mites and ticks, are the medically important groups of the Arachnida; many species parasitize humans or serve as vectors of disease.

Mites

The mites are distinguished from ticks by being less than 1 mm in length and having mouth parts (hypostome) without teeth. Mites rarely are submitted to the clinical laboratory for identification, and when this occurs they pose a difficult problem, because identification of mites is difficult even for the taxonomist (acarologist) working with this group of organisms. The medically important mites or groups of mites are these:

Producers of Dermatitis. Several species, for example, Ornithonyssus bacoti and Dermanyssus gallinae, ectoparasites of rats and fowl respectively, attack humans in several parts of the world, including the United States. Cheyletiellid mites, such as Cheyletiella yasguri of dogs, Cheyletiella blakei of cats, and Cheyletiella parasitovorax of rabbits, as well as Trombiculid mites, of which there are several genera with many species, also produce dermatitis, some of them in the United States. Infestations by mites are often diagnosed clinically, and rarely are the mites recovered and sent to the laboratory for study and identification. In each instance a mite is submitted for identification, the help of the specialist should be sought.

Producers of Allergies. Inhaled mites in the dust of homes, buildings, and other structures produce sensitization in some persons. The mites that produce allergies also belong to several genera and species, but they have in common that they live on organic debris shed by humans and animals (desquamated cells, hairs, mucus), or food particles on floors, furniture, and rugs, and are often found in the dust collected by vacuum cleaners. It has been estimated that 4% of the U.S. population manifests some form of allergy to these mites.

Transmitters of Disease. Two important rickettsiae, Rickettsia akari and Rickettsia tsutsugamuchi producing rickettsial pox in the United States and scrub typhus in Japan and southeast Asia, respectively, are transmitted by mites. The natural host for Rickettsia akari is Lyponissoides sanguineous, a mite of domestic rats and mice. The vectors of Rickettsia tsutsugamuchi are species of Leptotrombidium in different areas of southeast Asia.

Infestations of Skin. Demodex folliculorum and Demodex brevis are two species of mites in the skin of the face of every human. Demodex folliculorum inhabits the superficial hair follicles (Fig. 53–1A), while Demodex brevis (Fig. 53–1B) inhabits the deeper sebaceous glands. No disease has been associated with these parasites, though some persons have been reported to suffer from mild pruritus. Demodex are commonly found by the anatomic pathologist studying biopsy specimens of facial skin, especially from the nose, forehead, and adjacent regions (3).

Sarcoptes scabiei. Sarcoptes is the agent of scabies, a dermatitis occurring worldwide characterized by pruritus leading to intense scratching. The infestation is common in the United States and is acquired by close personal contact with individuals who harbor the mites (4).

Clinically, the lesions are small, slightly elevated, reddish tracks on the epidermis (Fig. 53–2A–C). They correspond to tunnels, made by mites feeding on squamous

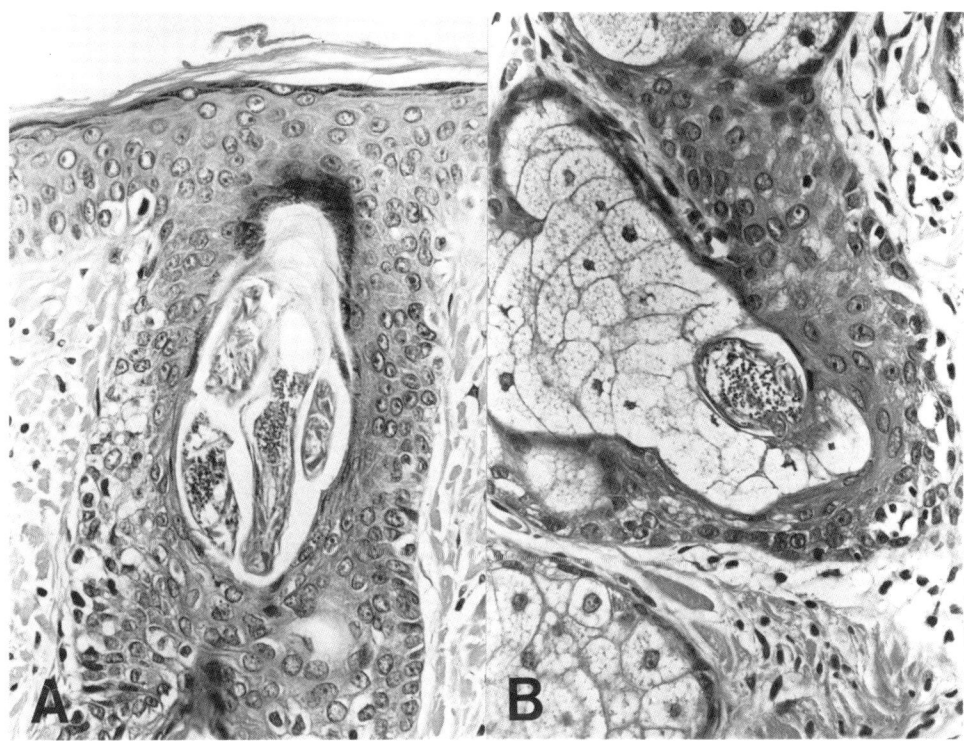

Fig. 53–1. Demodex in human skin sections (hematoxylin and eosin, ×350). Note the specific location of each species: A, D. folliculorum in the hair shaft and B, D. brevis in the sebaceous gland.

cells, where they lay eggs and deposit debris responsible for the pruritus. The continuous scratching produces secondary invasion by bacteria, which is responsible for superimposed infections. In addition, nephritogenic strains of β-hemolytic streptococci commonly infect these persons, resulting often in acute glomerulonephritis (4) (Chapter 28).

The distribution of the lesions produced by Sarcoptes is rather characteristic, usually beginning at the wrist and the interdigital spaces of the fingers, and establishing in the elbows, axillae, groins, breasts, umbilicus, and penis, which are the preferred sites. However, almost any area of skin may become involved.

The infestation in immunosuppressed persons may be opportunistic, with marked dermatitis characterized by abundant desquamation of epidermis in the form of dry scales (Fig. 53–2A,B). This condition, known as Norwegian scabies, is an important dermatosis recognized in persons with acquired immunodeficiency syndrome (5).

The eggs of the mites developing in the burrows (Fig. 53–2B) take about 3 to 5 days to hatch and produce larvae with three pairs of legs, which migrate to the skin surface where they become adults and mate in about a week. After mating, the adults burrow back into the skin to make a tunnel where the female lays one egg at a time.

The diagnosis of scabies is mainly a clinical diagnosis, which rarely is confirmed in the laboratory. The number of mites infesting a given person explains the difficulty in recovering them for identification: more than half of all scabies patients harbor between 1 and 5 female mites; in 20%, 5 to 10 mites are present in the skin; the rest have more than 10 mites (4).

Samples submitted to the laboratory, usually skin scrapings or scales, are observed directly under the microscope to detect mites (Fig. 53–2D) or eggs (Chapter 62).

Ticks

The classification of ticks is difficult and requires special knowledge. Ticks are being submitted more frequently to the laboratory for identification because of the desire to know if a tick found feeding on a person is Ixodes dammini, the vector of Lyme disease. Ticks are ectoparasites adapted exclusively to suck blood from their hosts, usually mammals and birds, but reptiles can also be parasitized. Two groups or families of ticks have all the species important to medicine: the Argasidae and the Ixodidae (2).

The Argasidae are commonly known as soft ticks because they do not have a hard plate (scutelum) on the dorsal aspect (Fig. 53–3). The surface is leathery and expands easily to large proportions during feeding and engorgement. The Argasidae are also characterized by the location of their mouth parts. If the tick is viewed from the dorsal aspect, the mouth parts (capitulum or gnathosoma) are not seen because they are located on the ventral surface, behind the anterior end of the body (Fig. 53–3B).

The Ixodidae are known as hard ticks because they have a plate that covers the entire dorsal surface of the male and the anterior dorsal portion of the female (Fig. 53–4). The capitulum or gnathosoma extends anteriorly and is easily seen from above. The development of ticks involves the eggs, the larvae (with three pairs of legs), and nymphs and adults (with four pairs of legs). Larvae, nymphs, and adults may feed on one host, or each may feed on a different host, a common phenomenon among the Ixodidae. The most common members of the Argasidae in the

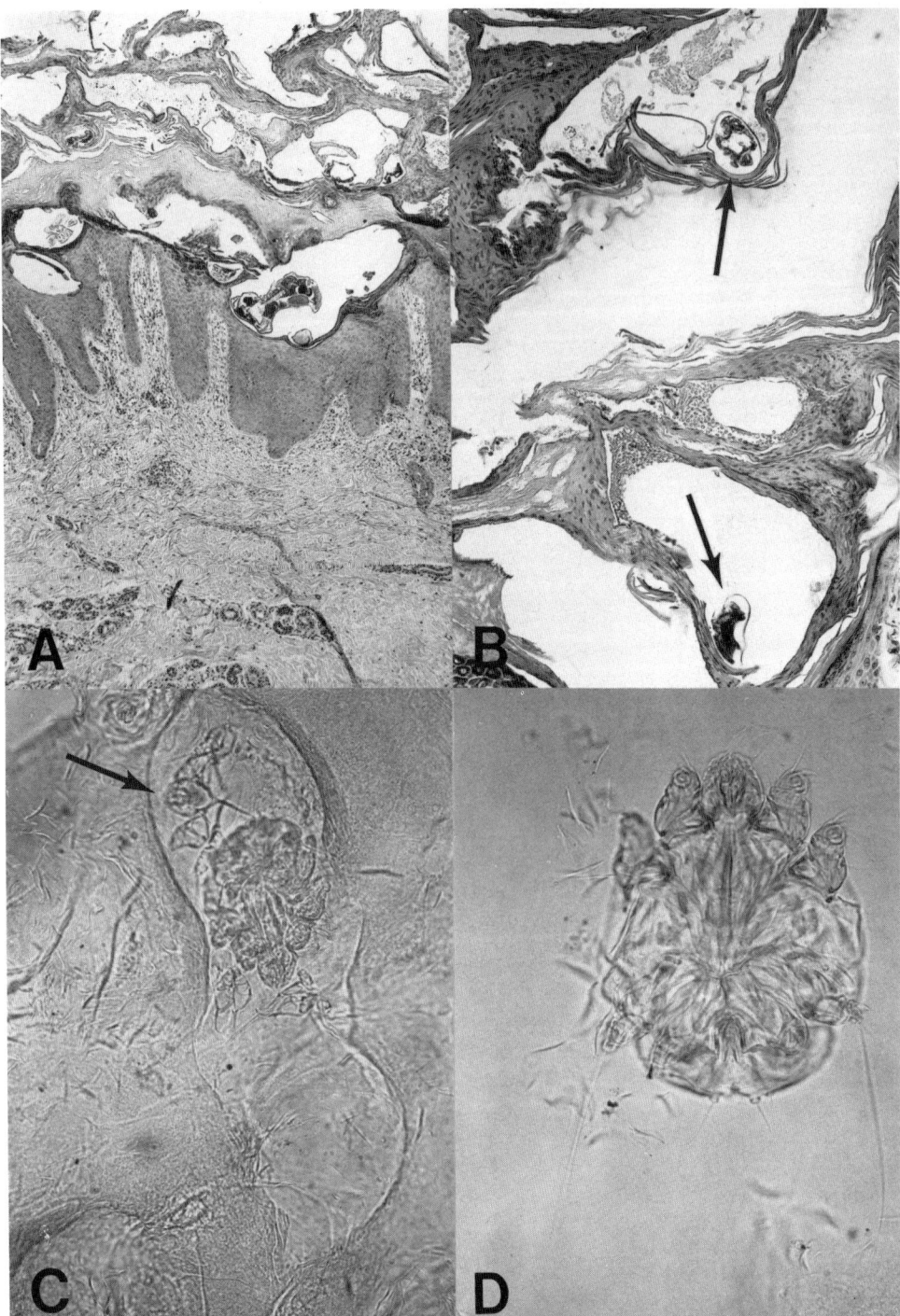

Fig. 53–2. Sarcoptes scabiei. *A, B,* Sections of skin from a patient with Norwegian scabies (hematoxylin and eosin). *A,* Low magnification illustrates the location of the mite and the marked thickening of the epidermis. The spaces are the tunnels borrowed by the mite (×55). *B,* Higher magnification shows eggs in the tunnel (*arrows*) (×140). *C,* Microscopic view of a skin scale, dehydrated, cleaned, and mounted with Permount. Note the tunnel with a molting parasite (molt shown by arrow) (×180). *D,* Adult female (×280).

United States belong to the genera Argas and Ornithodorus; of the Ixodidae to Ixodes, Dermacentor, and Amblyomma.

In general, ticks are important because they transmit different pathogens, among them the rickettsiae of Rocky Mountain spotted fever (Rickettsia rickettsii), boutonneuse fever (Rickettsia conorii), Siberian tick typhus (Rickettsia sibirica), Queensland tick typhus (Rickettsia australis), and Q fever (Coxiella burnetii) (Chapter 26). Ticks also transmit bacterial infections such as relapsing fever (Chapter 39) and tularemia (Chapter 33); viral infections, especially several encephalitides (Chapter 18) and hemorrhagic fever; and protozoan infections, mainly babesiosis (Chapter 51).

The only human disease ticks produce is tick paralysis, a condition occurring worldwide. In the United States tick paralysis is produced by Dermacentor andersoni in the Rocky Mountain states; Dermacentor variabilis in the northeast, and Amblyomma maculatum and Amblyomma americanum in other parts of the country.

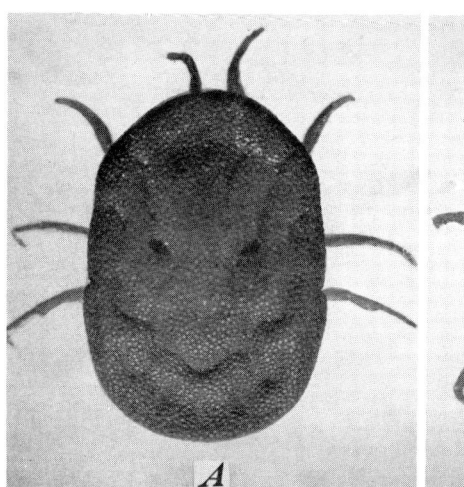
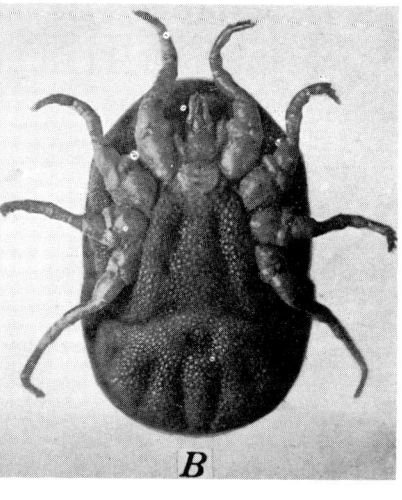

Fig. 53–3. Soft tick, Ornithodoros moubata, female. *A*, Dorsal view. *B*, Ventral view. (From Beaver PC, Jung RC, and Cupp EW: Clinical Parasitology. 9th ed. Philadelphia, Lea & Febiger, 1984.)

The disease is produced by a tick attached anywhere on the body, but especially on the back of the neck. Saliva secreted by the tick contains a toxin that elevates the body's temperature at the same time that ascending flaccid paralysis develops, producing difficulty in swallowing and breathing. Death occurs if the tick is not removed (2).

INSECTA

The class Insecta is a large group of arthropods with many orders. The commonly known lice (Anoplora), fleas (Syphonaptera), and blood-sucking mosquitoes, flies, gnats, and midges (Diptera) have the medically important genera and species. Each of these groups has some few to many species that affect human health, directly or indirectly. For example, lice and fleas produce infestations and transmit certain pathogens, while the mosquitoes are only transmitters of pathogens. Flies are a nuisance and transmit bacteria, protozoa, and helminths, but their larval stages can occur in tissues, producing myiasis (3).

Lice (Anaplora)

Lice are wingless insects about 1 mm long, adapted to suck blood from their hosts. Three species are known to parasitize humans: Pediculus humanus capitis, Pediculus humanus humanus and Phthirius pubis (Fig. 53–5A and B), known respectively as the head, the body, and the pubic louse. Lice have three distinct body segments and the legs have claws adapted to climb hairs and clothing fibers.

The female louse lays eggs 2 days after it reaches sexual maturity, eggs that are "glued" on a hair shaft of the head or neck by head lice; on clothing fibers by body lice, and in pubic or body hair by pubic lice (Fig. 53–5C,D). These eggs are visible to the naked eye as small whitish spots known as nits. The eggs hatch in 4 to 14 days to produce larval stages (nymphs), which molt three times to become adults. The entire cycle is completed in about 4 weeks; adults live about 30 days, during which a female lays about 150 eggs.

Lice are acquired through person to person contact and through contact with clothing from an infected person. The disease, pediculosis, is characterized by dermatitis, with pruritus and scratching, dermatitis that may become complicated by secondary bacterial infections. Head lice are more often found on the back of head, where the dermatitis is more pronounced. Body lice are harbored anywhere in covered areas of the body where they feed,

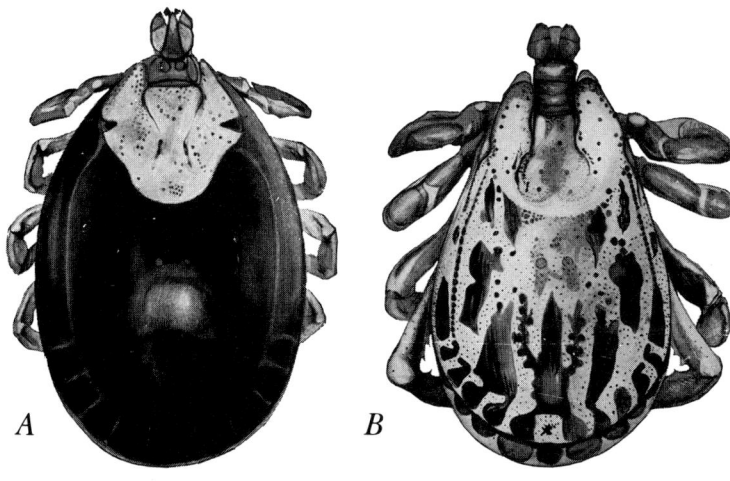

Fig. 53–4. Hard tick, Dermacentor andersoni, dorsal view. *A*, Female. *B*, Male. (From Beaver PC, Jung RC, and Cupp EW: Clinical Parasitology. 9th ed. Philadelphia, Lea & Febiger, 1984.)

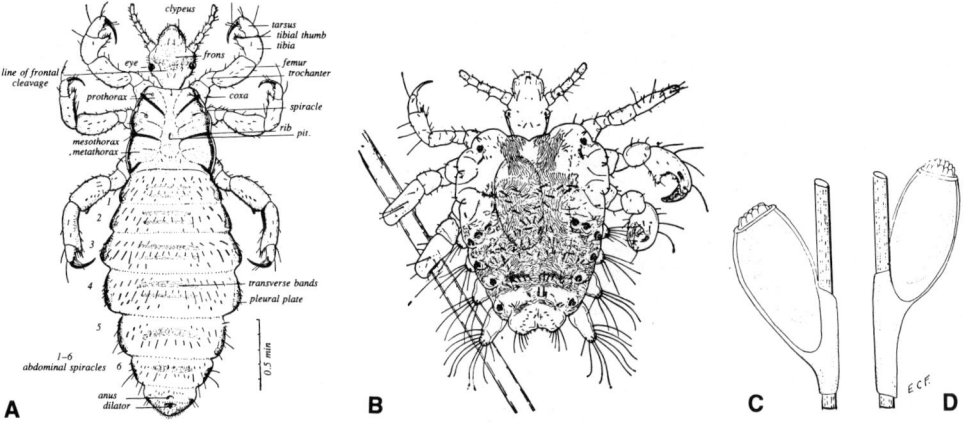

Fig. 53–5. Pediculus. *A*, Pediculus humanus capitis adult male. *B*, Phthirius pubis adult attached to hair. *C*, Egg of P. h. capitis. *D*, Egg of P. pubis (From Beaver PC, Jung RC, and Cupp EW. Clinical Parasitology. 9th ed. Philadelphia, Lea & Febiger, 1984.)

but they spend most of their time on the clothes (4). Pubic lice are found in pubic hairs, but with heavy infestation in the eyebrows as well.

The most important medical role of lice is the different pathogens they transmit: typhus fever (epidemic typhus) produced by Rickettsia prowazekii (Chapter 26); trench fever, and relapsing fever (Chapter 39).

The diagnosis of any of these types of pediculosis is made clinically. The examining physician can easily recover adult lice or nits (Fig. 53–5A–D), upon close examination of the head hairs, the clothing of the individual, or the pubic hair. Often the patient recovers the adult parasites and brings them to the laboratory for identification. Examination and identification of adults, nymphs, or nits confirms the diagnosis. Distinction between head and body lice is difficult on morphologic grounds. For practical purposes the source of the specimens provides the best information because they do not share their environments.

Fleas (Syphonaptera)

Fleas are also wingless insects, widely distributed throughout the world, with several hundreds of species known. They live on blood of humans and animals. It should be noted that fleas are adapted to feed on a given species of vertebrates and rarely feed on others.

The main role of fleas in medicine is the transmission of two diseases: plague (black death, peste) produced by Yersina pestis, and murine or endemic typhus by Rickettsia typhi. The human flea, Pulex irritans (Fig. 53–6), produces a mild dermatitis due to repeated bites. The rat (Xenopsylla cheopis), dog (Ctenocephalides canis), cat (Ctenocephalides felis) flea play little role as human parasites, though the rat flea is the species implicated in transmission of plague and murine typhus to humans.

One species of flea, Tunga penetrans, produces infestation in the glabrous skin of the foot, a disease known as tungiasis (Fig. 53–7A). This disease is common in the tropical communities of Africa and Latin America, where the infection is recognized easily and usually treated by removal of the parasite. In the United States sporadic cases are diagnosed clinically by the dermatologist, sometimes confirmed by the anatomic pathologist in sections of a skin biopsy specimen (Fig. 53–7B) (3).

Blood-Sucking Insects (Diptera)

Mosquitoes. The importance of mosquitoes is in the transmission of pathogens, which produce a number of viral, protozoan, and helminthic infections in humans and animals. Mosquitoes are blood-sucking insects with a slender, delicate body, that require stagnant water for their early development. They occur worldwide, and about 3000 species are recognized. The female is hematophagous because of its need to ingest proteins for the formation of eggs. The mouth parts of the mosquito are long, adapted to sucking blood. Mosquito bites are generally a nuisance because of the allergic reaction produced by the saliva introduced during the bite. In some susceptible persons, the lesions can be marked (Fig. 53–8A,B).

The main viruses transmitted by mosquitoes are togaviruses (Chapter 17), flaviviruses (Chapter 18), and bunyaviruses (Chapter 19). These viral infections are transmit-

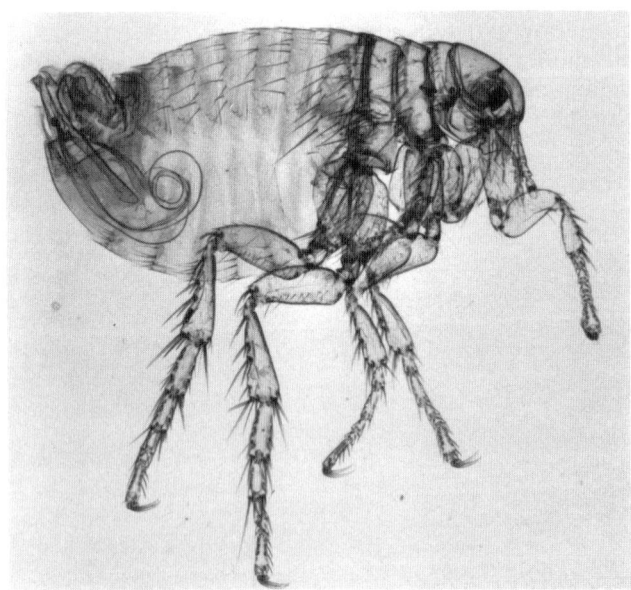

Fig. 53–6. Pulex irritans adult male (×28).

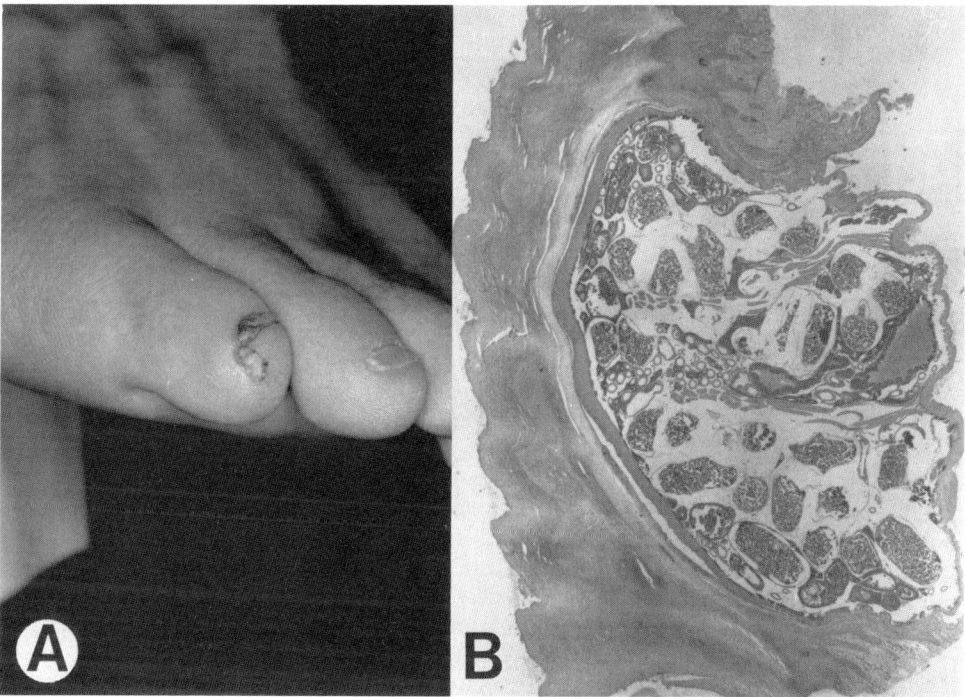

Fig. 53–7. Tunga penetrans. A, Tunga in small toe of a patient. B, Histologic section, hematoxylin and eosin stain. Note the parasite is confined to the epidermis (×22).

ted by numerous species of mosquitoes, different for each region, and too numerous to mention here.

Two important parasitic infections are transmitted by mosquitoes. Human malaria is transmitted by members of the genus Anopheles, of which about 72 species are considered suitable vectors. The other infection is lymphatic filariasis, produced by nematodes of the genus Wuchereria and Brugia (Chapter 52). The genera Aedes, Anopheles, Culex, and Mansonia have many species capable of transmitting these nematodes.

Sandflies. The important sandflies belong to the genera Phlebotomus, Lutzomia, and Psychodopygus, of the family Phlebotominae. In general appearance sandflies resemble mosquitoes, but they generally have more hairs on their bodies. The distribution of sand flies is worldwide and their importance is in the transmission of human diseases.

Both visceral and cutaneous leishmaniasis (Chapter 51) are transmitted by members of Phlebotomus in the Old World and by members of the Lutzomia and Psychodopygus on the American continent. Phlebotomus fever or pappataci fever produced by viruses of the Bunyaviridae (Chapter 19), occurs mainly in the Old World and is transmitted by species of Phlebotomus. Carrion's disease, Oroya fever or verruga peruana produced by Bartonella bacilliformis (Chapter 26) in parts of South America is also transmitted by sandflies.

Gnats. The most important gnats belong to the genus Culicoides, transmitters of filarial worms of the genus Mansonella. Culicoides austeni and Culicoides grahami transmit Mansonella perstans and -streptocerca (Chapter 52) in Africa; Culicoides furens and -phlebotomus transmit Mansonella ozzardi in Central and South America.

Flies. The insects commonly known as flies are important because of the diseases they transmit and because larval stages of some members can invade the tissues of both animals and humans. There are four main groups of flies: (1) Black flies (Simuliidae) are responsible for the

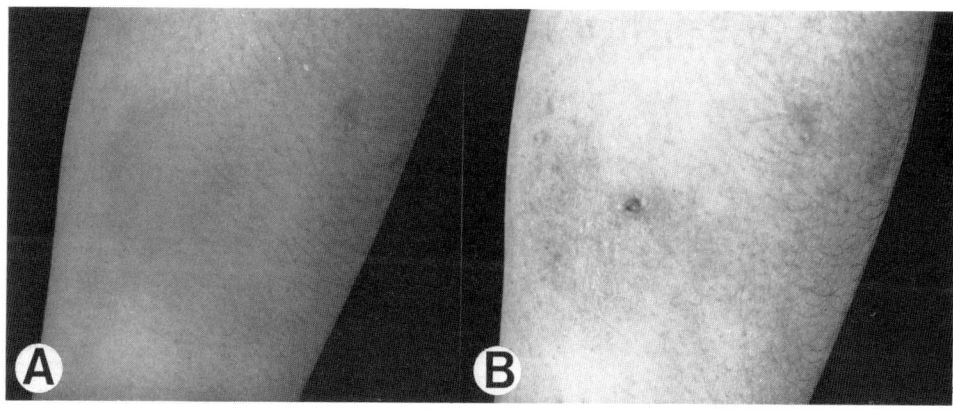

Fig. 53–8. Mosquito bite on an allergic patient. A, Note the large area of erythema 24 hours after the bite. B, Appearance 10 days after the bite.

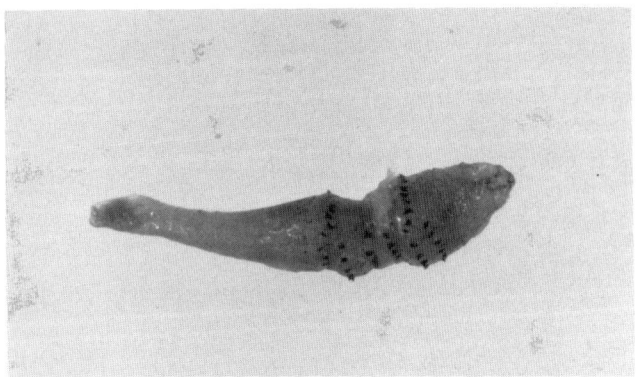

Fig. 53-9. Myiasis. Second-stage larva of Dermatobia hominis removed from a patient. The strangulation is an artifact of removing the larva (×3.5).

transmission of Onchocerca volvulus in Africa and parts of the American continent (Chapter 52). Black flies are minute flies whose development requires clean running water, so their geographic distribution is restricted along rivers. (2) The horse- and deerflies (Tabanidae) are responsible for transmission of Loa loa (Chapter 52) in Central Africa. (3) The blood-sucking flies (Muscidae), of which the genus Glossina is known commonly in Africa as tsetse flies, transmit African trypanosomiasis (Chapter 51). (4) Filth flies and the flies that produce myiasis (Muscidae) are probably the most important group for clinical laboratory workers.

The filth flies are best represented by the housefly (Musca domestica), cosmopolitan and everywhere a nuisance, which serves mainly as a mechanical vector for several pathogens. Most of these organisms produce enteric infections, because of the proclivity of flies to contaminate human food. Salmonella typhi, Salmonella enteritidis, Shigella (Chapter 34), and Vibrio (Chapter 35) are the main enteropathogens; Mycobacterium tuberculosis (Chapter 40), Yersinia pestis (Chapter 34), Bacillus anthracis (Chapter 29), and Brucella abortus (Chapter 33) are some of the nonenteric infectious organisms associated with filth flies.

Flies that produce myiasis belong to several groups whose members have larval stages that invade tissues (3). The main anatomic sites and the circumstances in which myiasis occur in humans are as follows: (1) *Cutaneous myiasis* is a form of larva migrans similar to that produced by hookworms of animals (Chapter 52). It invades the skin, resulting in a furuncle-like lesion where the larva develops and molts several times. The affected person can describe the movements of the parasite. Removal of the larva is the treatment (Fig. 53-9). (2) *Myiasis of wounds, ulcers, and moribund flesh* are produced by fly larvae commonly known as maggots, often brought to the laboratory for identification. They are recovered from wounds or ulcerated tumors exposed to the air, from the nasal cavity of comatose patients, and under other circumstances. The classification of the larvae is difficult, outside the expertise of the microbiology laboratory. (3) *Eyes, intestine, urogenital tract, and other sites* can be invaded by fly larvae, producing different syndromes (3), often by larvae with specific tropisms toward these sites. Recovery of the larvae in toto and study by the specialist often result in generic identification (2,3).

REFERENCES

1. Harwood RF, and James MT: Entomology in Human and Animal Health. 7th ed. New York, Macmillan, 1979.
2. Beaver PC, Jung RC, and Cupp EW: Clinical Parasitology. 9th ed. Philadelphia, Lea & Febiger, 1984.
3. Gutierrez Y: Diagnostic Pathology of Parasitic Infections with Clinical Correlations. Philadelphia, Lea & Febiger, 1990.
4. Orkin M, and Maibach HI: Cutaneous Infestations and Insect Bites. New York, Marcel Dekker, 1985.
5. Glover R, Young L, and Goltz RW: Norwegian scabies in acquired immunodeficiency syndrome: Report of a case resulting in death from associated sepsis. J Am Acad Dermatol, *16*: 396, 1987.

Part III

Specimen Handling and Laboratory Diagnosis, by Organ System

Chapter 54

INTRODUCTION TO SPECIMEN HANDLING AND LABORATORY DIAGNOSIS

In Part III of the text the guidelines for collection, transport, and processing of specimens for detection of infectious agents in the laboratory are set forth. The general principles of processing specimens for detection of viruses, bacteria, fungi and algae, and parasites are reviewed, as well as the requirements for mailing potentially infectious material to a reference laboratory. In following chapters the specific aspects of collection, transport, and processing of specimens from each organ system of the body are discussed in depth.

GENERAL GUIDELINES

In general, the specimens should be voluminous enough to enable performance of the microbiologic studies requested, and they should be obtained from the site of infection with minimal contamination from adjacent tissues and organ secretions. If the volume of the specimen is insufficient, the physician or ward nurse should be notified to request another specimen. If an additional sample cannot be obtained, the first specimen is processed and the report includes a statement indicating that the volume was inadequate. All specimens except stool should be collected in a sterile container and should be labeled with the following information: name and identification number of the person from whom the specimen was collected, the source of the specimen, and the time of collection.

Universal precautions should be followed in handling all specimens. This means that appropriate barriers are used to prevent exposure of skin and mucous membranes to the specimen. Gloves must be worn at all times, and masks, goggles, gowns, or aprons must be worn in situations in which there is risk of splashes or droplet formation. All specimen containers should be opened in a biologic safety cabinet. General guidelines for specimen collection, transport, and processing pertaining to viruses, bacteria, fungi and algae, and parasites are discussed.

Viruses

The likelihood of recovering the agent responsible for most viral infections is greatest early in the acute phase of the illness. If a swab is used to obtain the sample, calcium alginate should be avoided, because it could inactivate herpes simplex virus. Tissues and swab specimens should be placed in a holding medium, of which several are commercially available (Chapter 3). Hanks' balanced salt solution containing 0.5% gelatin and antibiotics (penicillin, 100,000 U/ml; gentamicin, 50 µg/ml; and amphotericin B, 40 mg/ml) is used frequently. Modified Stuart's holding medium, most commonly used for transportation of swab specimens collected for detection of bacteria (discussed later), is satisfactory for specimens collected for virus isolation if they are transported within 4 hours (1,2).

Ideally, specimens collected for virus isolation are delivered immediately to the laboratory, but if delay is unavoidable the specimen should be refrigerated and packed in wet ice for delivery within 12 hours of collection. Never should specimens be left at room temperature or placed in the incubator.

Processing of specimens varies with the detection method used. Currently available techniques for detection of viruses in clinical specimens are discussed in Chapter 3, but cell culture, the reference method, is reviewed briefly here. Nonculture methods are summarized in Table 54–1.

All manipulations of specimens and cell cultures are done in a biologic safety cabinet. All swab specimens are vigorously mixed on a vortex mixer, to release the virions into the transport medium, after which the swab is removed. All specimens should be refrigerated until they are inoculated to the appropriate cell monolayers. Cell cultures are selected for routine use in the clinical laboratory based on their permissiveness to viral replication and the viruses expected to be recovered from different body sites (Table 54–2). To inoculate the cell monolayer, the growth or maintenance medium is removed and 0.2 to 0.3 ml of sample is added. The specimen is adsorbed to the monolayer by incubating the cultures 30 to 60 minutes at 35° to 37° C, after which 1.0 to 1.5 ml of fresh maintenance medium is added. Cultures are reincubated for 2 to 3 weeks, during which monolayers are examined microscopically (at 40× to 100× magnification) two or three times per week for evidence of cell damage induced by virus (cytopathic effect, CPE). Maintenance of inoculated tubes in roller drums decreases the time to virus detection, but if they are unavailable the tubes are placed in stationary racks.

Bacteria

Specimens for recovery of bacteria ideally should be collected before antimicrobial therapy is started and at a time when the likelihood of recovering the suspected pathogen is greatest. Blood specimens should be inoculated immediately into the blood culture system used in the laboratory (Chapter 58). Tissues should be placed on

Table 54–1. Nonculture Methods for Direct Detection of Infectious Agents in Clinical Specimens

Method	Organisms Detected
Fluorescent antibody staining	Viruses: HSV, VZV, CMV, adenovirus, JC virus, parainfluenza viruses, measles virus, RSV, influenza viruses Bacteria: Chlamydia trachomatis, Bordetella pertussis, Legionella species
Enzyme-linked immunosorbent assay	Viruses: HSV, adenoviruses, RSV, rotavirus Bacteria: C. trachomatis, groups A and B Streptococcus, Clostridium difficile (toxin), Neisseria gonorrhoeae Fungi: Cryptococcus neoformans
Latex agglutination	Viruses: Rotavirus Bacteria: Group B Streptococcus, Streptococcus pneumoniae, C. difficile (toxin), Neisseria meningitidis (group B cross-reacts with Escherichia coli), Haemophilus influenzae type b Fungi: C. neoformans
Nucleic acid hybridization	Viruses: Human papillomavirus Bacteria: C. trachomatis, Mycobacterium pneumoniae, Legionella species, N. gonorrhoeae

Key: HSV, herpes simplex virus; VZV, varicella zoster virus; CMV, cytomegalovirus; RSV, respiratory syncytial virus.

moist gauze or covered with a small amount of sterile normal saline solution to prevent drying. For samples collected with a swab, calcium alginate-, Dacron-, or polyester-tipped swabs are recommended; residual fatty acids on cotton swab fibers may inhibit some fastidious bacteria (3). Swabs should be placed into a transport medium or a moist chamber (available commercially), because drying diminishes the recovery of most bacteria except streptococci (4). A commonly used system, available commercially, consists of a plastic tube with a polyester-tipped swab and a small glass ampule containing modified Stuart's holding medium, which is released when the ampule is crushed, providing sufficient moisture for storage at room temperature for up to 72 hours.

Table 54–2. Cell Lines Recommended for Recovery of Viruses from Different Body Sites

Specimen Source	Cell Line*
Respiratory tract†	MRC-5, PMK, A-549, (HEp-2)
Skin, eye (conjunctiva)	MRC-5, A-549, (PMK)
Urine, genital	MRC-5, A-549
Blood	MRC-5
Cerebrospinal fluid, other body fluids	MRC-5, A-549, PMK
Tissue	MRC-5, A-549, PMK
Feces, rectal swab	MRC-5, A-549, PMK, (Graham 293)

* Cell lines in parentheses are added in certain situations: HEp-2 cells for recovery of respiratory syncytial virus from respiratory specimens, November to May; PMK cells for recovery of enteroviruses from skin and eye specimens from June to October in temperate climates; Graham 293 cells to recover enteric adenoviruses from feces and rectal swab specimens.
† Includes throat swab/washing, nasopharyngeal swab/washing, sputum, bronchoalveolar lavage fluid, and lung tissue.
Key: PMK, primary monkey kidney cells.

To recover anaerobic bacteria, aspiration of purulent material with a needle and syringe is ideal. To transport the aspirate, air is expelled from the syringe, the needle is removed, and the syringe is tightly capped. Use of swabs for recovery of anaerobes is discouraged; however, anaerobic transport systems that use swabs are commercially available and they appear to preserve the viability of most anaerobes encountered clinically (4).

Specimens should be transported to the laboratory as soon as possible, but if a delay is unavoidable, urine, sputum, and stool may be refrigerated to prevent overgrowth of normal flora. Cerebrospinal fluid and other body fluids, blood, and specimens collected for recovery of Neisseria gonorrhoeae should be held at room temperature, because refrigeration adversely affects recovery of potential pathogens from these sources.

Each laboratory director should establish criteria for rejecting specimens unsuitable for culture. The following specimens are generally rejected: any specimen received in formalin, 24-hour sputum collections, a single swab submitted with requests for multiple isolations (such as aerobic and anaerobic bacteria, fungi, and mycobacteria), containers from which a portion of the specimen leaked, dried-out culture plates previously inoculated, specimens contaminated with barium, chemical dyes, or oily chemicals, Foley catheters, and duplicate specimens (except blood) received in a 24-hour period (4). In addition, the following specimens should be rejected for anaerobic culture: gastric washings, midstream urine, stool (except for recovery of species of Clostridium associated with gastrointestinal disease [Clostridium difficile and Clostridium perfringens]), oropharyngeal specimens except deep tissue samples obtained during a surgical procedure, sputum, swabs of ileostomy or colostomy sites, and superficial skin specimens.

All respiratory tract specimens and all tissues submitted for detection of bacteria *must be* processed in a biologic safety cabinet. Specimens submitted for recovery of mycobacteria *must be* handled in a biologic safety cabinet and *must be* centrifuged in sealed centrifuge safety cups. Moreover, processing specimens suspected to contain certain bacteria—species of Rickettsia and Coxiella, Bacillus anthracis, Pseudomonas pseudomallei, Francisella tularensis, species of Brucella, and Yersinia pestis—and handling colonies of these bacteria should be done only in a Class II or higher safety cabinet.

In general, processing specimens for detection of bacteria includes preparation of a smear for staining with Gram stain or other stains (see Appendix, Procedure 3 and Chapter 24 for a review of other available stains) for microscopic examination, and inoculation of appropriate media for culture; certain bacteria are reliably detected by nonculture methods (Table 54–1). Methods used to detect bacteria are discussed in detail in Chapter 24, but culture, the method of reference, is reviewed briefly here.

Primary planting media are selected for what pathogens are expected to be found in the specimen submitted. The media listed in Table 54–3 are suggested for primary recovery of common bacterial pathogens from the specimens most frequently received in the laboratory (excluding blood, discussed in Chapter 58). Special media not

Table 54–3. Recommended Primary Planting Media for Recovery of Usual Bacterial Pathogens from Clinical Specimens Other Than Blood

Specimen	Media	Comments
Abscess/pus, tissue	B, MAC, CDC-ANA, Thio	Perform direct Gram stain; grind or homogenize tissue to give a 10 to 20% suspension
Urine	B, MAC	Inoculate with calibrated loop (0.001)
Sputum, tracheal aspirate	B, MAC, CHOC	Screen sputum with Gram stain to determine if acceptable
Throat	B or SSA	Add TM if recovery of Neisseria gonorrhoeae is requested
Stool	MAC, HE, GN broth, CAMPY-B	Subculture GN broth to MAC at 8 to 12 hours
Cervix, urethra	TM	Add CNA or SSA to specimens from cervix if identification of group B Streptococcus requested
Cerebrospinal fluid and other sterile body fluids	B, CHOC, Thio	Centrifuge; Gram stain and culture sediment; may add MAC and CDC-ANA for peritoneal and pleural fluids
Intravascular catheter tip	B	Roll tip on agar surface
Eye	B, CHOC, Thio	
Ear	B, CHOC	Add Thio for tympanocentesis specimens
Nasopharynx	B, CHOC	
Bronchoalveolar lavage fluid	B, MAC, CHOC	Inoculate with calibrated loop (0.001)

Key: B, blood agar; MAC, MacConkey agar, CDC-ANA, CDC formulation of blood agar, enriched to recover anaerobes; Thio, thioglycolate broth; CHOC, chocolate agar; SSA, selective blood agar for groups A and B Streptococcus; TM, Thayer Martin agar (other media for recovery of N. gonorrhoeae may be substituted, see Chapter 31); HE, Hektoen enteric agar; GN broth, gram-negative both; CAMPY-B, Campy blood agar; CNA, Colistin nalidixic acid agar.

Table 54–4. Media and Growth Conditions for Isolation of Fastidious or Slowly Growing Bacteria

Organism	Media	Culture Conditions
Corynebacterium diphtheriae	Cystine tellurite or Tinsdale agar and Loeffler's serum medium	35°–37° C, ambient air, 48 hours
Nocardia spp.	Brain-heart infusion agar or Sabouraud's dextrose agar without chloramphenicol	35°–37° C, 5–7% CO_2, up to 3 weeks
Francisella tularensis	Glucose cystine agar or cystine heart agar containing 5% sheep or rabbit blood	35°–37° C, ambient air, up to 2 weeks
Brucella spp.	Infusion base agar*	35°–37° C, 5–10% CO_2, up to 3 weeks
Bordetella pertussis	Regan-Lowe agar	35°–37° C, humidified atmosphere of ambient air, up to 1 week
Legionella species	Buffered charcoal yeast extract agar containing α-keto-glutarate†	35°–37° C, humidified atmosphere of ambient air, up to 2 weeks
Haemophilus ducreyi	Mueller-Hinton base chocolate agar with 1% IsoVitalex and 3 μg/ml vancomycin and heart infusion base agar with 10% fetal bovine serum and 3 μg/ml vancomycin	35°–37° C, 5–7% CO_2 (or candle jar), up to 1 week
Vibrio species	Thiosulfate citrate–bile salts–sucrose agar and alkaline peptone water	35°–37° C, ambient air, up to 48 hours
Leptospira interrogans	Fletcher's medium or Ellinghausen, McCullough, Johnson, and Harris (EMJH) medium	25°–30° C, dark, ambient air, up to 6 weeks
Mycobacterium spp.	Egg-based medium (Lowenstein-Jensen, the Gruft modification of Lowenstein-Jensen, Wallenstein) plus agar-based medium (Middlebrook 7H10, Mitchison's selective 7H11); or the radiometric broth system; or the biphasic broth-agar paddle system	35°–37° C (plus a set at 30° C for cutaneous specimens), dark, 5–7% CO_2, 6–8 weeks

* Species of Brucella do grow on sheep blood and chocolate agars.
† Also supports growth of F. tularensis.

used routinely but necessary for recovery of certain bacteria are listed in Table 54–4. Species of Chlamydia and Rickettsia (except Rochalimaea quintana) are not recovered on artificial media but are isolated in cell cultures, reviewed earlier in this chapter for viruses and discussed in Chapters 3, 25, and 26.

Most specimens submitted for bacterial culture are inoculated to the surface of the primary planting medium with a swab or an inoculating loop and then are spread into four quadrants with a loop or a straight wire, which is sterilized between each successive quadrant streak (Fig. 54–1). This method of inoculation dilutes the original sample, allowing formation of isolated colonies that can be further evaluated. Micro-organisms have different optimal growth temperatures, but with a few exceptions most bacterial pathogens are isolated from cultures incubated between 35° and 37° C. Specimens submitted for recovery of species of Mycobacterium that cause cutaneous lesions (Mycobacterium marinum, Mycobacterium haemophilum, and Mycobacterium ulcerans), and for recovery of Leptospira interrogans should be incubated at 30° C. Recovery of Campylobacter jejuni is enhanced by incubation at 42° C, and Yersinia enterocolitica grows optimally at room temperature, although most isolates grow slowly at 35° C.

The growth of many bacteria is enhanced by incubation in an atmosphere of 5 to 7% carbon dioxide (CO_2). Specific CO_2 incubators may be purchased; if only an ambient air incubator is available, an atmosphere of increased CO_2 is created by placing inoculated media in a candle jar,

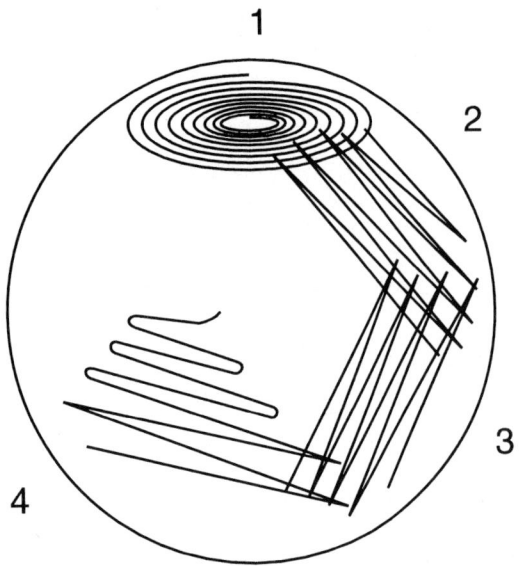

Fig. 54-1. Diagram of four-quadrant streaking on an agar medium for isolation of bacteria from clinical specimens.

which then is placed in the incubator. Species of Campylobacter and Helicobacter require a microaerophilic atmosphere (10% CO_2, 5% oxygen, 85% nitrogen), produced with commercially available gas-generating envelopes used in conjunction with plastic bags or plastic jars, or by evacuating the air and replacing it with the gas in plastic bags or anaerobic jars. Anaerobic bacteria are cultivated by the anaerobic jar technique, in which an anaerobic atmosphere is produced with a disposable hydrogen–carbon dioxide generator, or by evacuation-replacement, plastic bags, or an anaerobic glove box. In all cases, anaerobic conditions should be monitored by including an oxidation-reduction indicator, such as a methylene blue strip (commercially available) that is white when reduced (indicating anaerobiosis) and blue when oxidized (indicating the presence of oxygen).

Primary cultures are incubated and examined at 24 and 48 hours, except agar plates incubated anaerobically, because they should be maintained in anaerobiosis for 48 hours before they are examined. Plates that show no growth at 48 hours are discarded, with these exceptions: Cultures for Campylobacter jejuni and Neisseria gonorrhoeae are held 72 hours before discarding; certain bacteria listed in Table 54–4 need even longer incubation for recovery; tubes of thioglycolate broth should be incubated a minimum of 4 or 5 days.

Fungi and Algae

Specimens collected for detection of fungi and algae should be obtained from the area most likely to be infected and should be transported promptly to the laboratory, because the slow-growing fungi may be overgrown by bacterial and fungal contaminants. If transport is delayed the specimen should be refrigerated, and if it is to be mailed to a reference laboratory, antibiotics are added (50,000 U penicillin plus 100,000 μg streptomycin or 0.2 mg of chloramphenicol per milliliter of specimen). Collecting specimens with a swab should be discouraged because fungi become entrapped in the fibers, adversely affecting their recovery.

All specimens submitted for detection of fungi should be processed in a biologic safety cabinet. Processing includes direct microscopic examination of a saline wet mount, a potassium hydroxide preparation, or a smear stained with the Gram, calcofluor white, Congo red, or Gomori's methenamine silver stain, and inoculation of primary planting media for culture. Methods for detection of fungi are discussed in Chapter 42, but culture, the reference method, is reviewed briefly here.

For optimal recovery of fungi it is recommended that most specimens be inoculated onto enriched media such as inhibitory mold agar or SABHI agar containing antibiotics with and without cycloheximide. Sabouraud's dextrose agar should be used only for specimens suspected to contain a dermatophyte or an alga; brain-heart infusion agar supplemented with 5 to 10% sheep blood should be considered when infection with one of the more fastidious dimorphic fungi is suspected. Ideally, each medium selected should be inoculated with at least 0.5 ml of specimen, but smaller volumes are acceptable. Cultures should be incubated at 25° to 30° C for a minimum of 4 weeks, even if a rapidly growing contaminant mould appears earlier, because a slowly growing pathogen may be present.

Petri dishes or culture tubes may be used for primary recovery of fungi. For laboratories with a low volume of fungal cultures, with personnel who may not be familiar with handling fungi, or with equipment that is less than optimal, the use of large culture tubes (150 by 25 mm) with tight-fitting screw-capped tops is ideal. These tubes are safer to handle, require less storage space and less media than Petri dishes, and are stable longer. However, fewer fungi may be recovered because the surface area is small and organisms become concentrated at the bottom of the slant when tubes are incubated upright. In contrast, laboratories that have a high volume of fungal cultures should use Petri dishes because they provide better aeration and have a larger surface, allowing easier subculturing, recovery, and identification of mixed fungal colonies. A major disadvantage of plates is their potential for dehydration, a problem minimized by using culture dishes with 40 ml of medium (6 to 8 mm depth), taping the lids, placing the plates into lightly sealed plastic wrappers, and using an incubator with a 30 to 40% humidity, which is accomplished by placing a flat pan of water on its bottom shelf.

Parasites

Specimens received in the clinical microbiology laboratory for parasitologic examination can be obtained from every organ system. Only general principles that apply to all samples are given here; more detailed information is discussed under each organ system and each type of specimen.

The most common specimen submitted for detection of parasites is the stool sample, which may be received fresh, especially when both bacteriologic and parasitologic studies are requested, or fixed, a procedure carried out by the patient or the nurse when the sample is collected. Stool samples often are collected in commercially available containers consisting of two vials with fixative, which allow examination by direct microscopy methods, concentration by different techniques, and preparation of smears for staining (Chapter 59).

Samples for parasitologic examination other than stool arrive randomly in the laboratory, in small numbers and when least expected. These samples are the most challenging, and their processing requires a good knowledge of parasitology, because the detection of important or unusual parasites often depends on proper specimen handling. In order of decreasing frequency, these samples are: smears (blood, fluids, scrapings from ulcers, bronchoalveolar lavage fluid, and others), imprints made from biopsy specimens, tissue samples, and finally, parasites (worms and arthropods) and objects resembling parasites. In all these instances the sample received should be processed and studied following strict guidelines.

Smears and imprints, especially those to be stained with the Giemsa stain, must be fixed in absolute methanol (one dip is enough), whereas those to be stained with other stains (e.g., Papanicolaou, methenamine silver) do not require alcohol fixation. Tissue samples (biopsy specimens, autopsy material) should be delivered fresh without delay to the laboratory for processing, following guidelines for each suspected or requested organism.

Parasites and "objects" believed to be parasites are some of the most difficult specimens to handle. They *always* should be sent to the laboratory fresh and processed immediately. The first step is to determine if the sample received is truly a parasite, a free-living organism, or an artefact mistaken for a parasite. If the specimen is a parasite, it is necessary to determine if it is nematode, cestode, trematode, or arthropod, because each is handled differently.

MAILING INFECTIOUS MATERIAL

All specimens suspected to contain a potentially infectious agent, and all cultures of infectious agents that require shipping through the United States Postal Service must be limited to a 40-ml volume and must be packaged according to requirements of the Interstate Shipment of Etiologic Agents code. Cultures of bacteria and fungi should be grown in tubes on solid media. The cap of the primary container (tube or vial) should be sealed with waterproof tape and inserted into a second container (preferably metal), surrounded by sufficient packing material to absorb the entire volume of the culture or specimen if the primary container leaks or breaks. The second container should be capped and placed in a shipping container (made of corrugated fiberboard, cardboard, or Styrofoam) and labeled with an official Etiologic Agents label (available from the Centers for Disease Control). Specimens that must be shipped on dry ice, which is considered a hazardous material, must be marked "Dry ice, frozen medical specimen." The dry ice should be placed outside the second container with the packing material in a way that the container does not become loose inside the outer container as the dry ice evaporates.

REFERENCES

1. Huntoon CJ, House RF, Jr, and Smith TF: Recovery of viruses from three transport media incorporated into culturettes. Arch Pathol Lab Med, *105*:436, 1981.
2. Yeager AS, Morris JE, and Prober CG: Storage and transport of cultures for herpes simplex virus type 2. Am J Clin Pathol, *72*:977, 1979.
3. Pollock MR: Unsaturated fatty acids in cotton plugs. Nature, *161*:853, 1948.
4. Koneman EW, et al (eds): Introduction to medical microbiology. Part 1: Presumptive laboratory diagnosis of infectious diseases. *In*: Color Atlas and Textbook of Diagnostic Microbiology. 3rd ed. Philadelphia, J B Lippincott, 1988.

Chapter 55

CENTRAL NERVOUS SYSTEM

Specimens from the central nervous system (CNS) such as cerebrospinal fluid (CSF), material from abscesses, and brain tissue are among the most important samples received in the clinical microbiology laboratory because of the potentially devastating nature of the infections that involve this part of the body. For example, acute meningitis is a medical emergency associated with a mortality rate of about 30%, a rate that can be lowered if the clinician recognizes the illness early, rapidly determines the most likely pathogens, and institutes appropriate therapy, and if timely identification of the pathogen is achieved (1).

Infectious agents reach the CNS by the blood, the peripheral nerves, or the olfactory tract. Entrance via the blood is the most common mechanism for bacteria, fungi, and parasites, and has been well-documented for some viruses (2,3). Neural pathways are important for rabies, herpes simplex, and varicella-zoster virus, and occasionally, for polioviruses (4–6). In humans entry via the olfactory nerves has been documented only for Naegleria, a free-living amoeba (7).

Pathogens that remain in the subarachnoid space cause meningitis and produce symptoms of meningeal irritation such as headache and stiff neck, plus fever. Organisms that invade the brain parenchyma produce encephalitis, manifested by alterations of consciousness, or one or more abscesses, manifested with focal neurologic signs and often simulating a tumor. Encephalitis may be accompanied by inflammation of the meninges or spinal cord, or both, processes termed meningoencephalitis, encephalomyelitis, and meningoencephalomyelitis, respectively.

CEREBROSPINAL FLUID

CSF, the most common specimen collected from the CNS, most often is obtained to diagnose meningitis, and less frequently viral encephalitis (Table 55–1). Meningitis is divided into three clinical syndromes: acute (less than 24 hours' duration), subacute (1 to 7 days' duration), and chronic (persisting or progressing at least 4 weeks). An acute presentation of infectious meningitis occurs in about 10% of cases and is most likely caused by pyogenic bacteria. Almost all persons with viral meningitis and about three-fourths of those with bacterial meningitis have a subacute presentation (8–10). The rest present with chronic meningitis, most likely produced by one of the following organisms: species of Brucella, Treponema pallidum, Leptospira interrogans, Mycobacterium tuberculosis, species of Candida, Cryptococcus neoformans, Histoplasma capsulatum, or Coccidioides immitis.

The enteroviruses are the agents most often responsible for meningitis, and they should be considered first in the differential diagnosis of meningitis acquired by a child during the late summer or early fall. The organisms most likely to be involved in bacterial meningitis vary with the age of the patient (Table 55–2).

CSF usually is obtained by lumbar spinal puncture, sometimes aspirated from the ventricles, or collected from a shunt, but it always should be submitted to the laboratory in three glass tubes. The first tube is used for cell counts and differential stains; the second, for preparation of smears to stain with the Gram stain or other stains and for culture; the last, to measure protein and glucose, and, if indicated, for special tests such as the cryptococcal antigen, serologic test for syphilis, other serologic studies, and cytology.

Normal CSF looks like water, is sterile, and has a lymphocyte count of 5 cells per milliliter or fewer, a glucose concentration of 45 to 100 mg/dl (about two thirds the level of a simultaneous serum glucose), and a protein concentration of 14 to 45 mg/dl. In acute bacterial meningitis the white blood cell count in the CSF typically ranges from 500 to 20,000 cells per milliliter with a predominance of neutrophils, whereas viral, tuberculous, or fungal meningitis generally is associated with a lymphocytic pleocytosis ranging from 20 to 2000 cells per milliliter, although neutrophils may predominate early in the illness. The CSF glucose concentration is normal in viral meningitis but decreased in bacterial and often in fungal meningitis, and the CSF protein concentration is increased in most forms of infectious meningitis.

CSF should be transported promptly to the laboratory and processed as rapidly as possible. If a brief delay in processing of CSF is unavoidable it should be held at room temperature unless viral culture is requested, in which case a portion (at least 1 ml) is refrigerated for a short time. Specimen processing differs for viruses, bacteria, fungi, and parasites, and so, is discussed separately for each group of organisms.

Viruses

Processing CSF for diagnosis of viral infections involves conventional cell culture or, for some viruses, serologic tests. Of the viruses listed in Table 55–1, enteroviruses are the ones most frequently recovered in the clinical laboratory. Herpes simplex virus, varicella-zoster virus, and cytomegalovirus are rarely isolated from CSF; brain tissue is preferred to detect these agents. Mumps virus is easily recovered in the clinical laboratory, but routine culture of CSF specimens for mumps virus is not done because it is not cost effective; if desired, it must be requested specifically. Inoculating CSF to MRC-5, A549, and

Table 55–1. Infectious Pathogens of the Central Nervous System and Specimens Useful for Diagnosis

Organism	Specimens	Discussion (Chapter)
Viruses		
Herpes simplex virus	CSF, BT	5
Varicella-zoster virus	CSF, BT	5
Cytomegalovirus	CSF, BT	5
JC virus	BT	7
Measles virus	CSF, BT	10
Mumps virus	CSF	10
Enteroviruses	CSF, BT	13
Rabies virus	CSF, BT	16
Togaviruses	CSF, BT	17
Flaviviruses	CSF, BT	18
Bunyaviruses	CSF	19
Lymphocytic choriomeningitis virus	CSF	20
Retroviruses	CSF, BT	22
Creutzfeldt-Jakob disease agent	BT	23
Bacteria		
Staphylococcus aureus	CSF, BA, EA, SE	28
Staphylococcus epidermidis	CSF	28
Group B Streptococcus	CSF	28
Streptococcus pneumoniae	CSF	28
Viridans streptococci	BA, EA, SE	28
Listeria monocytogenes	CSF, BT	29
Nocardia species	BA, BT	29
Actinomyces species	BA, BT	30
Neisseria meningitidis	CSF	31
Flavobacterium meningosepticum	CSF	33
Brucella species	CSF, BT	33
Escherichia coli	CSF, BA, EA, SE	34
Other Enterobacteriaceae	CSF, BA, EA, SE	34
Haemophilus influenzae	CSF	36
Haemophilus species	BA	36
Bacteroides species	BA, EA	38
Other anaerobic gram-negative bacilli	BA, EA	38
Treponema pallidum	CSF	39
Borrelia burgdorferi	CSF	39
Leptospira interrogans	CSF	39
Mycobacterium species	CSF, BA, BT	40
Fungi		
Candida species	CSF, BA, BT	43
Cryptococcus neoformans	CSF, BA, BT	43
Dematiaceous fungi	BA, BT	44
Aspergillus species	BA, BT	44
Pseudallescheria boydii	BA, BT	44
Zygomycetes	BA, BT	44
Histoplasma capsulatum	BA, BT	45
Coccidioides immitis	BA, BT	45
Parasites		
Entamoeba histolytica	BT	49
Trypanosoma gambiense	CSF, BT	51
Trypanosoma rhodesiense	CSF, BT	51
Naegleria fowleri	CSF, BT	51
Acanthamoeba spp.	CSF, BT, BA	51
Toxoplasma gondii	CSF, BT, BA	51
Cysticercus	BT	52

Key: CSF, cerebrospinal fluid; BT, brain tissue; BA, brain abscess material; EA, epidural abscess material; SE, subdural empyema material.

Table 55–2. Common Bacterial Pathogens of Acute Meningitis, by Age of Host

Age	Organisms
≤3 mo	Group B Streptococcus, Escherichia coli, Listeria monocytogenes,* Streptococcus pneumoniae
4 mo–6 yr	Haemophilus influenzae type b
6–45 yr	Neisseria meningitidis
>45 yr	S. pneumoniae, L. monocytogenes, Group B Streptococcus

* May cause meningitis in immunocompromised persons of any age group.

In addition to virus isolation, detection of antibodies in CSF is useful in the diagnosis of certain infections. For example, subacute sclerosing panencephalitis is diagnosed by measuring complement-fixing antibodies specific for measles virus in both CSF and serum. Neurologic disease caused by human T-cell leukemia virus type I (HTLV-I) or by human immunodeficiency virus (HIV) may be diagnosed by demonstrating specific immunoglobulin (Ig) G in CSF (Chapter 22).

Rabies virus, lymphocytic choriomeningitis virus, HTLV-I, and HIV may be isolated from the CSF and tests for specific IgM are useful in diagnosing several viral encephalitides: western equine, eastern equine, Venezuelan equine, St. Louis, Japanese, and LaCrosse. Culture and serologic tests for detection of these viruses, however, are available only in reference laboratories, which should be contacted for specific requirements for handling the specimen.

Bacteria

Processing CSF for diagnosis of bacterial infections differs for each organism or group of organisms and, therefore, is discussed separately for the bacteria detected by routine culture methods and for species of Brucella, Treponema pallidum, Leptospira interrogans, Borrelia burgdorferi, and Mycobacterium tuberculosis.

Bacteria Detected by Routine Culture. Processing CSF for routine bacterial culture includes concentration (if a sufficient volume of CSF, 1 ml or more, is received), preparation of a smear for staining with the Gram stain, and culture. CSF is concentrated by centrifuging the fluid at a minimum of 1500 g for 15 minutes. The supernatant is decanted into a sterile tube, leaving about 0.5 ml of sediment and fluid, which is thoroughly mixed on a vortex mixer, or by forcefully aspirating up and down into a sterile pipette. Alternatively, if 2 ml or more of CSF is received, the fluid may be concentrated by filtering it through a 0.45-μm, sterile, disposable filter, and using the filter for culture (discussed later). Before filtering the specimen, however, about 0.5 ml of CSF is transferred to a sterile tube and processed by centrifugation for preparation of smears to stain with the Gram stain (as previously described) or, preferably, by making a cytocentrifuged preparation (11).

A smear stained with the Gram stain must be done on all CSF specimens. To prepare a smear, 1 drop of sediment (prepared as described earlier) or unspun CSF (for sam-

primary monkey kidney cells (Chapter 54) ensures recovery of the viruses listed above, except some coxsackieviruses that are detected only by inoculation of suckling mice. The specimen is adsorbed, and cultures are incubated as described in Chapter 54. Virus identification is discussed in Chapters 5, 10, and 13.

ples consisting of less than 1 ml) is placed, without spreading, on a sterile or alcohol-wiped microscope slide. After the fluid has dried a second drop is added to the same area and allowed to air dry. The material then is heat-fixed and stained with the Gram or acridine orange stain (Chapter 24).

After the smear is prepared, several drops of sediment are inoculated onto 5% sheep blood and chocolate agars (incubated in an atmosphere of 5 to 7% carbon dioxide or in a candle jar), and into thioglycolate broth (incubated in ambient air). Incubation times and temperatures are described in Chapter 54. For filtered specimens the filter is placed "organism" side down on the surface of chocolate agar and incubated as described above. The filter should be moved with sterile forceps to another location on the agar after 24 hours and 48 hours, to allow detection of colonies forming beneath it. Organism identification is discussed in Part II.

In addition to smears stained with the Gram stain and culture, latex agglutination tests for detection of antigens of group B Streptococcus, Streptococcus pneumoniae, some serotypes of Neisseria meningitidis, Escherichia coli (the K1 capsular antigen cross-reacts with that of Neisseria meningitidis type B), and Haemophilus influenzae type b may be done on the supernatant of a centrifuged specimen, the filtrate of a filtered sample, or the original fluid. These latex tests are most useful in diagnosing partially treated meningitis and in confirming a positive smear stained with the Gram stain. Routine use of these tests should be discouraged, because, compared with smears stained with the Gram stain their sensitivity is not significantly greater and they are much more expensive.

Brucella species. Culture of CSF for isolation of species of Brucella must be specifically requested. The CSF is concentrated as described earlier for routine bacterial culture, and a smear is stained with the Gram stain and examined. Recommended media for inoculation and incubation conditions are outlined in Table 54–4.

Treponema pallidum. The diagnosis of neurosyphilis is based on the following findings in the CSF: pleocytosis, elevated protein concentration, and a positive Venereal Disease Research Laboratory (VDRL) test (CSF VDRL), which currently is the only useful method for detecting antibodies to T. pallidum in the CSF (Chapter 39). The CSF VDRL test is indicated only if the person has a positive serum test result for syphilis (Chapter 39) (12). The specimen should be refrigerated until it is tested.

Borrelia burgdorferi. Borrelia burgdorferi may be isolated from CSF, but this is not done routinely in the clinical laboratory. Therefore, involvement of the CNS by B. burgdorferi usually is diagnosed by detection of specific IgM and IgG in CSF and serum (Chapter 39).

Leptospira interrogans. Leptospira interrogans may be cultured from the CSF during the first few weeks of illness. A special medium is inoculated with a few drops of CSF and incubated as outlined in Table 54–4.

Mycobacterium species. Processing CSF for detection of mycobacteria is indicated only if samples have abnormal cell counts, or glucose or protein values (13). The specimen of CSF is centrifuged 30 minutes at 3000 to 3600 g, the supernatant is decanted, the sediment is thoroughly mixed on a vortex mixer and used for preparation of smears for staining with auramine rhodamine or acid-fast stain (Appendix, Procedures 4–6) and for inoculation of appropriate media (see Table 54–4 and Chapter 40). If the volume of CSF received is insufficient for concentration, the specimen is used directly for smears and culture.

Fungi

Processing of CSF for detection of fungi is similar to the approach described earlier for bacteria detected by routine culture. If 2 ml or more fluid is received, organisms are concentrated by filtration, or for smaller volumes by centrifugation. A cytocentrifuge preparation or a smear of the sediment stained with the Gram stain is examined, and appropriate media are inoculated for culture. For filtered specimens the filter is cut in half with sterile scissors, one half is cultured for bacteria (as described earlier), and the other half for fungi by placing the filter on the surface of brain-heart infusion or SABHI agar without antibiotics. Centrifuged specimens are cultured by placing 1-drop aliquots of the sediment onto several areas of the agar surface. Culture conditions are discussed in Chapter 54.

In addition to smears stained with the Gram stain and culture of CSF rapid tests are available for diagnosis of meningitis produced by Cryptococcus neoformans: the India ink preparation, latex agglutination, and an enzyme-linked immunosorbent assay (ELISA). The latter two are specific for the capsular antigen. The large polysaccharide capsule of C. neoformans is visible in CSF mixed with India ink (1 drop of CSF sediment with 1 drop of India ink, available at art supply stores) on a glass slide, and examining the preparation under high-power magnification for characteristic encapsulated yeast cells (Chapter 43), especially encapsulated budding forms, which are diagnostic. Except in persons with the acquired immunodeficiency syndrome, the sensitivity of the India ink stain is low, so, the cryptococcal latex agglutination test or the ELISA, each highly specific and better than 90% sensitive, is recommended for diagnosis. These commercially available tests can be done on CSF filtrate if the sample was concentrated by filtration, on the supernatant of a centrifuged specimen, or on unspun CSF. False-positive latex agglutination results do occur, owing to introduction of trace amounts of condensation from agar into the test fluid. To avoid this problem the latex test should be done before culture, or better, on a separate sample (14).

Parasites

CSF occasionally is sent to the laboratory for diagnosis of African trypanosomiasis (Trypanosoma gambiense or Trypanosoma rhodesiense), infection with free-living amoebae (Naegleria fowleri, and species of Acanthamoeba), toxoplasmosis, and cysticercosis. The CSF is collected as described and promptly transported at room temperature, without refrigeration or freezing until it is processed, especially for detection of amoebae.

Once the specimen is received in the laboratory it should be processed immediately. Wet preparations consist of a drop of the fluid covered with a cover glass for examination under the microscope with the condenser in a low position to allow visualization of trophozoites. Phase-contrast microscopy is highly recommended because it facilitates finding and identifying the parasites. Wet preparations also should be made after centrifugation of the specimen at 250 g for 10 minutes.

African trypanosomes are seen in direct wet preparations from the CSF and from the sediment, as small flagellates moving actively. Smears prepared from the sediment are stained with Giemsa or Wright stain.

For detection of free-living amoebae the wet smears are prepared in an identical manner and the centrifugation is done after shaking the tube gently, a necessary step because the parasites tend to stick to the wall of the tube. Examination of the wet mounts could reveal trophozoites and flagellates of Naegleria, or trophozoites and cysts of Acanthamoeba (15,16). Identification of the organism is accomplished with stains and cultures (Chapter 51).

Stains of CSF for free-living amoebae are done on smears, using the trichrome, Giemsa, Wright, calcofluor white, or another stain (Appendix, Procedures 24–26). The characteristics of the parasites are discussed in Chapter 51.

Cultures of free-living amoebae from CSF are done on non-nutrient agar plates covered with a suspension of Escherichia coli or Enterobacter aerogenes, after centrifuging the CSF at 250 g for 10 minutes. The supernatant is removed with a sterile pipette; the sediment is mixed with 0.5 ml of saline solution and poured at the center of the plate. Incubation at 37° C and daily examination for 10 days is standard procedure. The plates are examined under a microscope, with 10× objective (15,16).

After these studies are completed the remaining CSF should be frozen and kept for either antibody or antigen determinations, if necessary, procedures done only at a few reference laboratories.

Only rarely has Toxoplasma gondii been found and identified in the CSF—in immunocompromised hosts (17). The procedures for detection of trophozoites (tachizoites) and cysts are centrifugation of the CSF, preparation of smears using the sediment, and staining with Wright or Giemsa stain. The organisms are identified by their morphologic and staining characteristics (Chapter 51).

Diagnosis of cysticercosis by detecting specific antibodies in CSF has been recommended, but no real advantage over detection of antibodies in serum is apparent (18).

ABSCESS AND EMPYEMA MATERIAL

Microbiologic studies of aspirated purulent material are done to identify organisms that cause brain abscesses, subdural empyemas, and epidural abscesses (Table 55–1). Brain abscesses develop by direct extension from a contiguous focus of infection, via hematogenous spread from a distant site of infection, and after surgical or nonsurgical trauma, but in about 20% of cases no focus of infection is identified (19–21). The location of the abscess and the pathogenic organisms depend on the predisposing conditions. Most solitary abscesses originate from an adjacent suppurative focus (22). Otitis media and mastoiditis are associated with abscesses involving the temporal lobe and the cerebellum and are caused by anaerobic and viridans streptococci, Bacteroides fragilis, and members of the Enterobacteriaceae. Infections of the frontal, ethmoid, or sphenoid sinuses predispose to brain abscesses caused by the same bacteria, plus Staphylococcus aureus and species of Haemophilus. Such abscesses usually involve the frontal lobe or, if the sphenoid sinus is involved, the temporal lobe. Dental infections are associated with frontal lobe abscesses caused by species of Fusobacterium, Bacteroides, and Streptococcus.

Hematogenous brain abscesses most frequently originate from a focus of infection in the chest, are located in the territory of distribution of the middle cerebral artery, occur at the junction of the gray and white matter, are poorly encapsulated, usually multiple and multiloculated, and are associated with a high mortality rate (21,23,24). The pathogens vary with the predisposing condition. Abscesses associated with congenital heart disease typically are caused by anaerobic and viridans streptococci and by species of Haemophilus; those associated with lung abscesses, empyema, and bronchiectasis are caused by streptococci, Nocardia asteroides, and species of Fusobacterium, Bacteroides, and Actinomyces. Bacterial endocarditis predisposes to abscesses caused by viridans streptococci and Staphylococcus aureus, and in immunocompromised hosts, fungi, members of the Enterobacteriaceae, or Nocardia asteroides often are involved. Immunocompromised hosts also may develop abscesses produced by protozoa, such as Toxoplasma gondii and species of Acanthamoeba and Leptomixid amoebae. Entamoeba histolytica is a potential pathogen in immunocompetent hosts.

The clinical manifestations of a brain abscess are those of a space-occupying mass: headache, focal neurologic findings (dependent on the location and size of the lesion), a change in mental status, nausea, and vomiting (25). Fever, seizures, nuchal rigidity, and papilledema occur in fewer than half of the cases. If cerebral abscess is suspected or proven lumbar puncture should not be performed because the CSF examination is not diagnostic and the procedure may cause herniation.

Intracranial subdural empyema most frequently results from extension of an infection of the frontal or the ethmoid sinuses, or both, or of the middle ear and mastoid sinus (26). Less often the infection is metastatic, predominantly from the lung, or it follows surgical or nonsurgical trauma. Organisms involved include viridans and microaerophilic streptococci, Staphylococcus aureus, Streptococcus pneumoniae, Haemophilus influenzae, members of the Enterobacteriaceae, and species of Bacteroides. Clinical manifestations include fever, focal headache, vomiting, and stiff neck, and as the infection progresses focal neurologic signs appear and rapidly progress unless therapy is instituted.

The etiology, pathogenesis, and bacteriology of intracranial epidural abscesses are similar to those described earlier for intracranial subdural empyema (27). Initial clinical manifestations are those of sinusitis or otitis, followed by focal neurologic signs and focal or generalized seizures. Acute and chronic spinal epidural abscesses most often result from hematogenous spread from a distant focus or direct extension of vertebral osteomyelitis. Less commonly the infection is caused by penetrating injuries or by extension from a decubitus ulcer or a paraspinal abscess. The abscess most frequently involves the thoracic spine, followed by the lumbar and the cervical spine. Staphylococcus aureus is the most common agent of acute and chronic infections, accounting for 60 to 90% of cases, and viridans and anaerobic streptococci, Escherichia coli, and Pseudomonas aeruginosa also may be involved. Most abscesses evolve through four clinical stages in a few days to a few weeks: (1) focal vertebral pain, (2) root pain, (3) deficits of motor, sensory, or sphincter function, and (4) paralysis.

For all potential pathogens specimen collection and transport are similar. Specimen processing, however, differs for bacteria, fungi, and parasites, and each is discussed separately.

Material is collected surgically from a lesion visualized and located precisely by computed tomographic scanning by aspirating with a needle and syringe guided stereotactically. The needle is removed, the air is expelled, and the syringe is tightly capped and promptly delivered to the laboratory. Alternatively, purulent material may be transferred to an anaerobic transport system.

Bacteria

Routine processing of aspirated purulent material allows detection of most bacterial pathogens except species of Nocardia and Mycobacterium tuberculosis, which are discussed separately.

Bacteria Detected by Routine Culture. Aspirated purulent material should be processed as rapidly as possible (if a brief delay is unavoidable it is held at room temperature). A smear is stained with the Gram stain, and the sample is inoculated to sheep blood and MacConkey agar and thioglycolate broth, which are incubated in ambient air, and to anaerobic blood agar incubated anaerobically. The routine incubation times and temperatures discussed in Chapter 54 are adequate for recovery of most organisms. If the specimen contains "sulfur granules" or if it is suspected that the infection is produced by Actinomyces, anaerobic cultures should be incubated for 2 weeks. If long, thin, branching, beaded, gram-positive bacilli typical of species of Nocardia (see Plate IIIE) are seen in the stained smear, steps should be taken to ensure recovery of these organisms (see below).

Nocardia species. Processing aspirated material for detection of Nocardia involves preparing a smear for staining with the Gram stain and inoculating appropriate media for culture (see Table 54–4). Moreover, if organisms characteristic of Nocardia are visualized in smears stained with the Gram stain, a second smear should be prepared and stained with the modified acid-fast stain (see Appendix, Procedure 7). Nocardia usually survives the decontamination procedure used for recovery of mycobacteria (see below) and can be recovered from specimens submitted for isolation of acid-fast bacilli.

Mycobacterium tuberculosis. Purulent material aspirated from a focal lesion in the CNS should not be contaminated with normal flora and, so, should not require decontamination. A smear of the specimen should be prepared for staining with auramine rhodamine or acid-fast stain, and appropriate media (see Chapter 40 and Table 54–4) should be inoculated directly. However, for specimens that appear contaminated (that are yellow or green or have a foul odor), a smear stained with the Gram stain should be examined; if bacteria are seen the specimen should be decontaminated. To do this the specimen is transferred to a sterile 50-ml centrifuge tube containing 10 ml of sterile, filtered, distilled water; mixed on a vortex mixer, allowed to stand 20 minutes, and processed as a sputum specimen (see Appendix, Procedure 27). Identification of the species of Mycobacterium is discussed in Chapter 40.

Fungi

Processing aspirated purulent material for detection of fungi involves direct microscopic examination and inoculation of appropriate media. Methods available for direct microscopic detection of fungi include the potassium hydroxide preparation (see Appendix, Procedure 19), and smears stained with the Gram, Gomori's methenamine silver, calcofluor white, or Congo red stain (Chapter 42). To isolate fungi, media (brain-heart infusion agar and SABHI agar, with and without antibiotics, see Chapters 42 and 54) are inoculated by placing 1- or 2-drop aliquots of the aspirate onto several areas of the agar surface without streaking. Cultures are incubated as discussed in Chapter 54. Organism identification is reviewed in Part II.

Parasites

Purulent material aspirated from a brain abscess and received for examination in the parasitology laboratory could in immunocompromised hosts yield Toxoplasma gondii or Acanthamoeba, and in others Entamoeba histolytica. Other parasites that produce abscesses or abscess-like lesions in the brain are too rare to mention here.

The sample is examined by preparation of wet mounts for detection of Acanthamoeba and Entamoeba, and smears stained with the Giemsa, Wright, or trichrome stain for Acanthamoeba, Entamoeba, and Toxoplasma. Both wet mounts and stains are performed as previously described. In addition, culture should be carried out for Acanthamoeba.

BRAIN TISSUE

Brain tissue, obtained during a neurosurgical procedure or at autopsy, is useful in the diagnosis of viral encephalitis, progressive multifocal leukoencephalopathy (caused by JC virus), subacute sclerosing panencephalitis (caused by measles virus), HIV encephalopathy, Creutzfeldt-Jakob disease (CJD), and infections caused by several bacteria, fungi, and parasites (see Table 55–1). Specimen collection and transport are the same for all potential pathogens, but specimen processing differs for different groups of organisms and is discussed separately for viruses, bacteria, fungi, and parasites.

As much tissue as possible is obtained, placed in a sterile container, and transported promptly to the laboratory.

Fresh tissue is examined by a pathologist and properly divided for histologic and microbiologic studies.

Viruses

Processing of brain tissue varies for detection of different viruses or groups of them. Rabies virus, the viruses of the equine encephalitides (western, eastern, Venezuelan), St. Louis encephalitis virus, Japanese encephalitis virus, and HIV may be isolated from brain tissue. In addition, antigens of rabies, St. Louis encephalitis, and Japanese encephalitis virus can be detected by immunofluorescence staining of frozen tissue. Isolation and antigen detection tests for identification of these viruses generally are done in a reference laboratory, which should be consulted about requirements of the sample. Processing brain tissue for detection of viruses isolated by routine culture techniques, JC virus and measles virus, and the CJD agent are discussed individually.

Viruses Detected by Routine Isolation. Of the viruses listed in Table 55–1, herpes simplex and varicella-zoster virus, cytomegalovirus, and the enteroviruses are easily recovered in the clinical laboratory. Brain tissue is placed into a viral transport medium such as Hanks' balanced salt solution and is refrigerated for a short time until it is processed. The tissue is homogenized in the transport medium with a sterile tissue grinder or a mortar and pestle to make a 10% to 20% suspension, and is clarified by centrifugation for 15 to 20 minutes at 1500 to 2000 g. The supernatant is handled as described earlier for CSF.

JC Virus and Measles Virus. When progressive multifocal leukoencephalopathy or subacute sclerosing panencephalitis is suspected the pathologist must be alerted, to ensure appropriate processing of the brain tissue. In each case part of the specimen should be fixed in formalin for histologic examination, part should be fixed in glutaraldehyde for electron microscopy, and the remainder should be frozen at −70°C for possible immunofluorescence or nucleic acid hybridization studies.

Cruetzfeldt-Jakob Disease Agent. CJD is diagnosed by demonstrating the characteristic histologic features (see Chapter 23) in a brain biopsy specimen or autopsy tissue. The pathologist must be alerted when tissue is submitted from a patient suspected of having CJD or when CJD is part of the differential diagnosis of a patient examined at autopsy, because special precautions must be taken to prevent transmission (Chapter 23).

Bacteria and Fungi

Processing brain tissue for detection of bacteria and fungi involves the preparation of a 10 to 20% suspension of the tissue in broth by using a sterile tissue grinder or a mortar and pestle. The homogenate is used to prepare smears for direct microscopic examination and for inoculation onto appropriate media, as described earlier for brain abscess material.

Parasites

Brain tissue is received fresh in the laboratory and should be processed promptly if diagnosis of a parasitic infection is requested. The organisms involved are Toxoplasma gondii, Naegleria fowleri, species of Acanthamoeba, and Entamoeba histolytica. Cysticercosis is diagnosed in the surgical pathology laboratory.

The biopsy specimen should be used to prepare imprint smears (touch preparations), which are fixed and stained with Wright, Giemsa, calcofluor white, and trichrome stains. If free-living amoebae are suspected, cultures of small portions of the tissue are standard procedure, following the technique described earlier for CSF. The rest of the tissue should be fixed in 10% formalin and processed for routine histologic examination. If the tissue is submitted with a diagnosis of cyticercosis, imprint smears are unnecessary; the whole specimen should be submitted for processing and sectioning.

REFERENCES

1. McGee ZA, and Baringer JR: Acute meningitis. *In* Principles and Practice of Infectious Diseases. 3rd ed. Edited by GL Mandell, RG Douglas, Jr, and JE Bennett. New York, Churchill Livingstone, 1990.
2. Johnson RT: Viral Infections of the Nervous System. New York, Raven Press, 1982.
3. Mims CA: The Pathogenesis of Infectious Agents. 2nd ed. London, Academic Press, 1982.
4. Murphy FA: Rabies pathogenesis: A brief review. Arch Virol, *54*:279, 1977.
5. Bodian D, and Howe HA: Experimental studies on intraneural spread of poliomyelitis virus. Bull John Hopkins Hosp, *68*:248, 1941.
6. Baringer JR: Herpes simplex virus infection of nervous tissue in animals and man. Prog Med Virol, *20*:1, 1975.
7. Martinez AJ, et al: Experimental Naegleria meningoencephalitis in mice. Penetration of the olfactory mucosal epithelium by Naegleria and pathologic changes produced: A light- and electron microscopic study. Lab Invest, *29*:121, 1973.
8. Carpenter RR, and Petersdorf RG: The clinical spectrum of bacterial meningitis. Am J Med, *33*:262, 1962.
9. Swartz MN, and Dodge PR: Bacterial meningitis: A review of selected aspects. N Engl J Med, *272*:725, 1965.
10. Karandanis D, and Shulman JA: Recent survey of infectious meningitis in adults: Review of laboratory findings in bacterial, tuberculous, and aseptic meningitis. South Med J, *69*: 449, 1976.
11. Shanholtzer CJ, Schaper PJ, and Peterson LR: Concentrated Gram stain smears prepared with a cytospin centrifuge. J Clin Microbiol, *16*:1052, 1982.
12. Albright RE, Jr, et al: Issues in cerebrospinal fluid management. CSF Venereal Disease Research Laboratory Testing. Am J Clin Pathol, *95*:397, 1991.
13. Albright RE, Jr, et al: Issues in cerebrospinal fluid management. Acid-fast bacillus smear and culture. Am J Clin Pathol, *95*:418, 1991.
14. Heelan JS, Corpus L, and Kessimian N: False-positive reactions in the latex agglutination test for Cryptococcus neoformans antigen. J Clin Microbiol, *29*:1260, 1991.
15. Martinez JA: Free-living amoebas: Natural history, prevention, pathology and treatment of disease. Boca Raton, FL, CRC Press, 1985.
16. Martinez JA, and Visvesvara GS: Diagnosis of pathogenic free-living amebas. Clin Lab Med, *11*:861, 1991.
17. Threlkeld MG, Graves AH, and Cobbs CG. Cerebrospinal fluid staining for the diagnosis of toxoplasmosis in patients with acquired immunodeficiency syndrome [Correspondence]. Am J Med, *83*:599, 1987.

18. Richards F, Jr, and Schantz PM: Laboratory diagnosis of cysticercosis. Clin Lab Med, *11*:1011, 1991.
19. Morgan H, Wood M, and Murphy F: Experience with 88 consecutive cases of brain abscess. J Neurosurg, *38*:698, 1973.
20. Samson DS, and Clark K: A current review of brain abscess. Am J Med, *54*:201, 1973.
21. Brewer NS, MacCarty CS, and Wellman WE: Brain abscess: A review of recent experience. Ann Intern Med, *82*:571, 1975.
22. Dacey RG, and Winn HR: Brain abscess and perimeningeal infections. *In* Internal Medicine. Edited by JH Stein, MJ Cline, and WJ Daly. Boston, Little Brown, 1983.
23. Waggener JD: The pathophysiology of bacterial meningitis and cerebral abscesses: An anatomical interpretation. Adv Neurol, *6*:1, 1974.
24. Nielsen H, Glydensted C, and Harmsen A: Cerebral abscess. Aetiology and pathogenesis, symptoms diagnosis and treatment. Acta Neurol Scand, *65*:609, 1982.
25. Wispelwey B, and Scheld WM: Brain abscess. *In* Principles and Practice of Infectious Diseases. 3rd ed. Edited by GL Mandell, RG Douglas, Jr, and JE Bennett. New York, Churchill Livingstone, 1990.
26. Greenlee JE: Subdural empyema. *In* Principles and Practice of Infectious Diseases. 3rd ed. Edited by GL Mandell, RG Douglas, Jr, and JE Bennett. New York, Churchill Livingstone, 1990.
27. Greenlee JE: Epidural abscess. *In* Principles and Practice of Infectious Diseases. 3rd ed. Edited by GL Mandell, RG Douglas, Jr, and JE Bennett. New York, Churchill Livingstone, 1990.

Chapter 56

HEAD AND NECK: EYE, SINUSES, EAR, AND ORAL CAVITY

Specimens collected for diagnosis of infections involving structures of the head and neck include conjunctival scrapings, swab specimens, and tissue; corneal scrapings and biopsy specimens; aspirates from the anterior chamber of the eye, from the vitreous cavity, and from abscesses involving the eye; aspirates of purulent material from the sinuses, ear drainage fluid and fluid obtained by tympanocentesis, aspirates of purulent material and granules from a focus of infection in the oral cavity, and a swab or biopsy specimen of an ulcerative lesion in the oral cavity.

CONJUNCTIVAL SCRAPINGS, SWAB SPECIMENS, AND TISSUE

Conjunctival scrapings, and swab and tissue biopsy specimens are collected to determine the agent of conjunctivitis, the most common ocular disease in the western hemisphere and to diagnose rabies by antigen detection. (1). Clinically, conjunctivitis is manifested by hyperemia, secretions, and edema. Of the many causes of infectious conjunctivitis (Table 56–1), bacteria are the most common agents, and those most frequently implicated are Streptococcus pneumoniae, Staphylococcus aureus, and Staphylococcus epidermidis in adults, and Haemophilus influenzae, Streptococcus pneumoniae, and Staphylococcus aureus in children (2–5). Trachoma, caused by Chlamydia trachomatis, is a leading cause of blindness worldwide (6). Viruses are responsible for about 15 to 20% of cases of acute infectious conjunctivitis, and in the United States most epidemics of viral conjunctivitis are caused by adenoviruses (1,2,4). Rarely, parasites are causes of conjunctivitis.

Collection, Transport and Processing

Specimen collection is similar for all organisms that cause conjunctivitis. Because of the site, the quantity of specimen collected often is insufficient to perform all tests ordered, and the physician should be asked to prioritize requests based on the clinical manifestations and the agents most likely to be involved.

Conjunctival cells are obtained from the superior and inferior tarsal conjunctiva by using a swab moistened with broth or a sterile platinum spatula. Ideally, smears are prepared, and if a bacterial or fungal infection is suspected culture media are inoculated (as described later) directly by the person who collects the sample. Smears should be air-dried and promptly transported, with the inoculated media, to the laboratory. If viral culture is requested a second sample (swab or scrapings) is collected, placed in 2 ml of viral transport medium, and delivered promptly to the laboratory or refrigerated for a short time and then transported on wet ice. If direct preparation of smears and inoculation of media is not possible, swab specimens may be collected. Biopsy specimens of conjunctival lesions are obtained surgically and delivered promptly to the surgical pathology suite. Fresh tissue is examined by a pathologist and divided appropriately for histologic and microbiologic studies.

Specimen processing is different for detection of viruses, bacteria, fungi, and parasites, and is discussed separately for each group of organisms.

Viruses

Processing conjunctival specimens for detection of viruses differs for different viruses or groups of viruses and, therefore, is discussed separately for molluscum contagiosum, the viruses detected by routine isolation techniques, human papillomavirus, and rabies virus.

Molluscum contagiosum. Lesions produced by molluscum contagiosum (Chapter 4) are located along the eyelid margin and are associated with chronic follicular conjunctivitis, possibly caused by the toxic effect of incomplete virions (7). These lesions have a typical appearance, and the diagnosis usually is based on the clinical presentation alone, but it may be confirmed by histologic examination of the tissue. The microscopic appearance of lesions of molluscum contagiosum is described in Chapter 4 (see Fig. 4–1).

Viruses Detected by Routine Isolation. All of the viruses listed in Table 56–1, except molluscum contagiosum and human papillomavirus, are detected by using techniques available routinely in the clinical virology laboratory. Rapid diagnosis may be provided by direct or indirect immunofluresence staining of smears of conjunctival cells with virus-specific antibodies, but culture, the most sensitive method for detecting these viruses, always should be done.

Smears are prepared directly by the person collecting the specimen or from scrapings or swab specimens received in viral transport medium. Swab specimens are thoroughly mixed on a vortex mixer to dislodge the collected cells, and the swab is removed. To prepare smears, 1 ml of the mixed medium from the swab specimen or from the medium containing scrapings is transferred to a separate sterile tube and is centrifuged at 1500 to 2000 g for 15 to 20 minutes. The supernatant is removed, and the sediment is resuspended in 0.5 ml of sterile phosphate-buffered saline. One drop of the suspension is placed inside each of two marked circles on one or more glass slides previously cleaned with alcohol, and the material is allowed to air-dry. Air-dried smears (including those prepared directly) are fixed in acetone for 10 minutes and

Table 56–1. Specimens Useful for Detection of Organisms That Cause Ocular Infections

Organism	Conjunctival Scrapings, Swab	Conjunctival Tissue	Corneal Scrapings, Tissue	Aspirate, Anterior Chamber, Vitreous	Wound Abscess (Posttraumatic or Surgical)	Chapter
Viruses						
Molluscum contagiosum virus		X				4
Herpes simplex virus	X		X	X		5
Varicella-zoster virus	X		X	X		5
Cytomegalovirus				X		5
Adenovirus	X		X			6
Human papillomavirus		X				7
Measles virus	X					10
Influenza virus	X					11
Enteroviruses	X					13
Bacteria						
Staphylococcus aureus	X		X	X	X	28
Staphylococcus epidermidis			X	X	X	28
Streptococcus pneumoniae	X		X	X	X	28
Bacillus cereus			X	X	X	29
Bacillus spp			X	X	X	29
Clostridium spp			X	X	X	30
Propionibacterium acnes	X		X	X	X	30
Peptostreptococcus spp	X		X			30
Neisseria gonorrhoeae	X		X			31
Neisseria meningitidis	X			X		31
Branhamella catarrhalis	X		X			31
Pseudomonas aeruginosa	X		X	X	X	32
Acinetobacter spp	X		X	X	X	32
Moraxella spp	X		X	X	X	32
Francisella tularensis	X					33
Enterobacteriaceae	X		X	X	X	34
Aeromonas spp	X		X			35
Haemophilus influenzae	X			X	X	36
Treponema pallidum	X		X			39
Mycobacterium spp	X		X	X	X	40
Fungi						
Candida species	X		X	X	X	43
Cryptococcus neoformans				X		43
Dematiaceous fungi			X	X	X	44
Aspergillus spp			X	X	X	44
Pseudallescheria boydii			X	X	X	44
Fusarium spp			X	X	X	44
Zygomycetes				X	X	44
Blastomyces dermatitidis				X		45
Histoplasma capsulatum				X		45
Coccidioides immitis				X		45
Sporothrix schenckii	X			X	X	45
Rhinosporidium seeberi		X				46
Protozoa						
Entamoeba histolytica	X	X	X	X	X	49
Acanthamoeba	X	X	X			51
Nosema		X	X			51
Nematodes						
Onchocerca (microfilaria)	X	X	X			52
Loa		X[1]				52
Dirofilaria		X[1]				52
Angiostrongylus cantonensis				X[1]		52
Cestodes						
Cysticercus		X[3]				52
Sparganum					X[2]	52
Echinococcus		X[3]				52
Arthropods						
Maggots	X[1]	X[1]			X[2]	53

Key: [1], Adult or larva; [2] abscess not by surgical procedure or trauma; [3] a cystic structure.

stained with specific antibodies according to the manufacturer's directions. Currently, antibodies specific for herpes simplex virus, varicella-zoster virus, adenovirus, measles virus, and influenza A and B virus are available for direct immunofluorescence, indirect immunofluorescence, or both.

The remaining 1 ml of the specimen is used for culture. To ensure recovery of viruses that cause the conjunctivitis (see Table 56–1), inoculating MRC-5, A549, and primary monkey kidneys cells is recommended (see Table 54–2). Specimens are inoculated and adsorbed, and cultures are incubated as discussed in Chapter 54. Virus identification is discussed in Part II (see Table 56–1 for the appropriate chapter).

Centrifugation culture has been used successfully for detection of herpes simplex virus, varicella-zoster virus, adenovirus, and influenza A and B viruses (8–11). The procedure is similar to that outlined in Procedure 2 in the Appendix for cytomegalovirus, except that the indicator cells are different for adenovirus (A549 cells are preferred) and the influenza viruses (MDCK or monkey kidney cells are used), and the antibodies are specific for the virus being sought.

Human papillomavirus. Lesions produced by human papillomavirus (Chapter 7) have a typical appearance and usually are diagnosed on the basis of the clinical presentation. The diagnosis may be confirmed cytologically by examining smears of cells scraped from a lesion and stained with Papanicolaou stain, or histologically by examining tissue sections of a lesion removed surgically. Human papillomavirus DNA may be detected in scrapings or tissue by nucleic acid hybridization, a technique currently performed in research laboratories, because the commercially available kits detect types of human papillomavirus found principally in genital lesions and, therefore, the kits yield some false-negative results with specimens from ocular lesions.

Rabies virus. Rabies virus antigen may be detected in smears or corneal scrapings by staining with fluorescent antibodies. Antibodies, however, are not available commercially, and the specimen must be sent to a reference laboratory. The person who performs the test should be contacted for requirements for the specimen. In general, the smear should be air-dried and fixed in acetone, but the temperature and duration of fixation vary (12).

Bacteria

Processing conjunctival specimens for routine bacterial culture detects most bacteria listed in Table 56–1; however, certain organisms require special techniques.

Chlamydia trachomatis. Evaluation of conjunctival scrapings or swab specimens is useful for diagnosing endemic trachoma and inclusion conjunctivitis of newborns and adults. Cytologic examination of a smear stained with the Giemsa stain, prepared directly from conjunctival scrapings of a person (especially an infant) with conjunctivitis produced by C. trachomatis, shows an infiltrate of lymphocytes and neutrophils, and epithelial cells with basophilic intracytoplasmic inclusions may be present. If inclusions are found they are diagnostic of C. trachomatis; however, because monoclonal antibodies are available, and are more sensitive and specific, preparations stained with Giemsa are no longer recommended for diagnosis. For optimal results with the direct fluorescent antibody test, the collection kits provided by the manufacturer should be used. The swab is rolled across the surface of a special glass slide, the material is fixed with methanol, and the slide is transported promptly to the laboratory and held at room temperature or refrigerated for a short time. Slides are stained according to the manufacturer's directions and examined with a fluorescence microscope for elementary bodies (Chapter 25 and Plate IIA). Specimens that contain fewer than 10 columnar or metaplastic squamous cells are considered inadequate. Results should be reported as inconclusive (with an explanation), and another specimen should be requested.

Culture, the reference method for detection of Chlamydia trachomatis, should be done when a diagnosis of conjunctivitis caused by C. trachomatis is strongly suspected and the direct fluorescent antibody test is negative. The specimen, collected with a cotton, rayon, or Dacron-tipped swab on a plastic or aluminum shaft, is placed in 2-sucrose phosphate transport medium and delivered promptly to the laboratory or refrigerated for a short time and transported on wet ice. Further specimen processing for culture is outlined in Procedure 8 in the Appendix.

Recently, a membrane immunoassay for detection of Chlamydia trachomatis in clinical specimens became available commercially. The test was evaluated on a limited basis for endocervical swab specimens and yielded reliable results (13).

Bacteria Detected by Routine Culture. For optimal detection of bacteria that cause conjunctivitis, smears are prepared and media are inoculated directly by the person who obtains the sample. Scrapings collected with a sterile platinum spatula are transferred to a glass slide for Gram staining and are inoculated onto sheep blood and chocolate agar (incubated in an atmosphere of 5 to 7% carbon dioxide), into thioglycolate broth (incubated in ambient air) and onto anaerobic blood agar (incubated anaerobically). Incubation times and temperatures are reviewed in Chapter 54. Alternatively, two swab specimens, one of which is placed in an anaerobic transport system, may be collected, delivered promptly to the laboratory, and used to prepare smears and inoculate media as discussed above. Organism identification is discussed in Part II.

Francisella tularensis. Conjunctival specimens are useful for diagnosing the oculoglandular form of tularemia, which accounts for no more than 2% of all cases. Laboratory personnel must be alerted when specimens are collected from a person suspected to have oculoglandular tularemia, for two reasons. First, the laboratory director may choose to send the specimen to a reference laboratory or to a state or other public health laboratory equipped to handle F. tularensis, one of the agents most commonly responsible for laboratory-acquired infections. Second, if the specimen is processed in the clinical laboratory appropriate media must be inoculated to ensure recovery of the organism. Media and culture conditions are outlined in Table 54–4. Identification of F. tularensis is discussed in Chapter 33.

Treponema pallidum. Spirochetes of T. pallidum may be observed in a darkfield preparation of material obtained from the base of a conjunctival ulcer (as described for genital ulcers in Chapter 61), but given the rarity of syphilitic conjunctivitis serologic tests are recommended for its diagnosis (Chapter 39).

Mycobacterium tuberculosis. For optimal detection of M. tuberculosis, an uncommon cause of conjunctivitis, smears are prepared for staining with auramine rhodamine or acid-fast stain (Appendix, Procedures 4–6), and media are inoculated directly at the time the sample is collected. Alternatively, two swab specimens—one for preparation of a smear for staining and the other for culture—may be collected and delivered promptly to the laboratory in appropriate transport devices. Media and culture conditions are outlined in Table 54–4, and discussed in Chapter 40.

Cat-Scratch Disease Bacillus (Afipia felis). A conjunctival biopsy may be useful in diagnosing the form of cat-scratch disease known as the oculoglandular syndrome of Parinaud, consisting of an ocular granuloma or conjunctivitis with preauricular lymphadenopathy. The diagnosis of this disease is one of exclusion and typically requires biopsy and histologic examination of the ocular lesion, an involved lymph node, or both (Chapter 41). The organism may be recovered by culture, but the appropriate techniques have been determined only recently (14). The ocular granuloma is removed surgically and fixed in formalin. Tissue sections stained with hematoxylin, and eosin should be examined for the characteristic granulomas (Chapter 41) and if present, additional sections are stained with the Warthin-Starry stain and examined for the small, pleomorphic cat-scratch disease bacilli.

Fungi

Processing conjunctival specimens for detection of fungi varies and is discussed separately for fungi detected by routine culture (Candida and Sporothrix) and for Rhinosporidium seeberi.

Fungi Detected by Routine Culture. For optimal detection of species of Candida and Sporothrix schenckii in conjunctival specimens smears are prepared for staining with the Gram, calcofluor white, Congo red, or a silver stain. In addition, a medium such as brain-heart infusion, inhibitory mold, or SABHI agar (Chapter 42) is inoculated directly by the person collecting the sample. Culture conditions are reviewed in Chapter 54.

Rhinosporidium seeberi. Infection with R. seeberi produces a painless, localized lesion that eventually becomes a pedunculated mass. Because the organism has not been cultured, the diagnosis is based on histologic examination and finding the typical thick-walled cysts (Chapter 46).

Parasites

Specimens from the conjunctiva infrequently are submitted to the laboratory for diagnosis of parasites. The specimen may be the parasite itself removed from the conjunctiva, for example fly larvae (maggots), nematodes (filarial worms), or trematodes (Philophthalmus), where they produce an inflammation or a sensation of foreign body. Conjunctival scrapings and tissues infrequently may also yield other organisms (see Table 56–1).

Smears prepared with conjunctival scrapings usually are submitted with corneal scrapings for detection of Acanthamoeba (discussed later). However, Entamoeba histolytica and microfilariae of Onchocerca volvulus should be considered as a rare diagnostic possibility in some patients. Conjunctival tissues usually are handled by the anatomic pathologist and good biopsy specimens could yield several protozoa, helminths, or arthropods in tissue sections (15).

Handling the larvae or adult parasites recovered from the conjunctiva and other structures of the eye requires special procedures.

CORNEAL SCRAPINGS AND BIOPSY SPECIMENS

Corneal scrapings and biopsy specimens are useful in determining the agent of keratitis, an inflammation of the cornea manifested by pain, some vision loss, and photophobia. The infection can potentially produce loss of vision and requires immediate attention. Many organisms cause keratitis worldwide (see Table 56–1), and bacteria account for 65 to 90% of cases. In the United States the organisms most frequently implicated are Staphylococcus aureus, Streptococcus pneumoniae, Pseudomonas aeruginosa, and species of Moraxella (16–18).

Collection, Transport, and Processing

Specimen collection is similar for all potential pathogens. Specimen processing in the laboratory is different for each group of organisms. Corneal scrapings are collected with a sterile platinum spatula and are used for smears by directly transferring them to glass slides for staining, and for inoculation to appropriate media for culture (see below). If viral culture is requested scrapings should be placed directly into viral transport media and delivered promptly to the laboratory or refrigerated for a short time and transported on wet ice. Frequently, the conjunctiva and the eyelids of the involved and the uninvolved eye are cultured concurrently, to determine the normal flora, useful in assessing the results of the corneal cultures. When culture of scrapings of a suspicious corneal ulcer fails to yield a pathogen, superficial keratectomy or corneal biopsy specimens may be obtained by the ophthalmologist, an approach especially useful for detection of fungi and Acanthamoeba organisms.

Viruses, Bacteria, and Fungi

The diagnosis of viral keratitis is often based on clinical observations; only occasionally is culture necessary. Processing corneal samples for viruses routinely isolated in the clinical laboratory is similar to that for conjunctival specimens (discussed previously), except that inoculation of primary kidney monkey cells is unnecessary.

Processing corneal scrapings for routine bacterial pathogens, for Treponema pallidum, for species of Mycobacterium, and for fungi is identical to that described earlier for conjunctival specimens. For fungi, a medium without cycloheximide should be included among the media inoculated, because cycloheximide inhibits growth of some of the fungi that cause keratitis.

Parasites

Corneal scrapings for detection of parasites are submitted mainly for the diagnosis of keratitis produced by Acanthamoeba. Ideally, several smears are submitted for staining with Giemsa, calcofluor white, and trichrome stains for microscopic examination and identification of trophozoites and cysts of Acanthamoeba (Chapter 51). Rarely, if ever, are enough corneal scrapings submitted fresh for cultures of Acanthamoeba, which are carried out as described in Chapter 55.

ASPIRATES OF THE ANTERIOR CHAMBER, VITREOUS CAVITY, OR ABSCESSES

Aspirates of fluid from the anterior chamber and vitreous cavity or aspirates of purulent material from wound abscesses due to trauma and dehiscence (postoperative) should be cultured to determine the agent of the infection known as endophthalmitis, which involves the ocular globe and adjacent structures. Signs and symptoms include pain, blurred vision, hyperemia, and edema. Bacteria are the most common agents of endophthalmitis (Table 56–1) and usually cause infections 24 to 48 hours after a surgical procedure involving the eye. The normal flora of the skin and ocular mucous membranes are the usual pathogens (19). Endophthalmitis, however, may follow penetration of objects into the eye, in which case species of Bacillus often are involved, or it may result from hematogenous spread from a distant focus of infection (20–22).

The prevalence of fungal endophthalmitis has increased significantly in the past several years, a trend probably associated with the widespread use of antimicrobial agents, corticosteroids, and other immunosuppressive agents; with the increasing numbers of intravenous drug users, and with hyperalimentation (23–26). Similar to bacterial endophthalmitis, fungal infections may follow a surgical procedure, nonpenetrating ocular trauma, or hematogenous spread from a distant site, but fungal endophthalmitis usually is a more indolent process, becoming manifest several weeks after the initiating event.

Collection, Transport, and Processing

Specimen collection is similar for detection of all potential pathogens. The quantity of specimen received may be insufficient for detection of all possible organisms, and the physician must be contacted to learn about the isolation priorities based on the clinical presentation and the infectious agents most likely to be involved.

To determine what agent is causing postsurgical or traumatic endophthalmitis, samples of aqueous and vitreous fluid are collected by aspiration with a needle and syringe. The needle is removed, the air is expelled, and the syringe is tightly capped and delivered promptly to the laboratory. A portion of the sample should be used for cytologic studies. Purulent material from a wound abscess or from a dehiscence also should be aspirated with a needle and syringe; if an adequate sample cannot be obtained by aspiration, two swabs—one for aerobic culture and one placed in an anaerobic transport system for recovery of anaerobes—should be collected.

Viruses

When isolation of viruses from aqueous and vitreous fluids is requested, a portion of the sample is placed in viral transport medium such as Hanks' balanced salt solution and refrigerated until processed for cell culture. To recover viruses listed in Table 56–1 by conventional cell culture, two tubes of MRC-5 cells or one tube each of MRC-5 and A549 cells should be inoculated. Inoculation, specimen adsorption, and culture conditions are described in Chapter 54. Cultures are incubated 3 to 4 weeks to ensure recovery of cytomegalovirus. In addition to conventional cell culture, centrifugation culture (Appendix, Procedure 2) is recommended for detection of cytomegalovirus. Centrifugation culture has been used successfully for detection of herpes simplex virus, but whether it can replace conventional cell culture is controversial (8,9).

Bacteria

Processing aqueous and vitreous fluids and aspirates or swab specimens of wound abscesses and wound dehiscences for detection of bacteria includes preparing smears for staining and inoculation of media for culture. The steps involved are very similar to those for detecting bacterial pathogens recovered by routine culture and species of Mycobacterium. Smears of the fluids and purulent material (preparation with a cytocentrifuge is preferred for aqueous and vitreous fluids) are stained with Gram stain, and if culture for mycobacteria is requested an additional smear is stained with auramine rhodamine or an acid-fast stain (Appendix, Procedures 4–6). Material from each site is inoculated to media as described earlier for detection of routine bacterial pathogens and Mycobacterium tuberculosis in conjunctival specimens.

Fungi

Processing aqueous and vitreous fluids and specimens from wound abscesses and dehiscenses for fungi includes direct microscopic examination of the material (cytocentrifuged preparations are preferred for aqueous and vitreous fluids) and inoculation to media for culture as described earlier for detecting fungi in conjunctival specimens. A medium without cycloheximide should be included among those inoculated, because cycloheximide inhibits growth of some of the fungi that cause endophthalmitis.

Parasites

Aspirates of the anterior chamber, vitreous cavity, or abscesses, especially abscesses involving the entire ocular globe or sometimes the periorbital tissues, are necessary for diagnosis of rare cases of ocular infection caused by Entamoeba histolytica. The aspirate is used to prepare smears for staining with trichrome and Giemsa stains and for direct microscopic examination.

Abscesses of the orbital cavity more often are produced by larvae of metazoan organisms, such as fly larvae (maggots) and tapeworm larvae (sparganum), some filarids, for example, Dirofilaria repens and Dirofilaria tenuis (sometimes referred to as Dirofilaria conjunctiva), species of Dipetalonema, and some cestode larvae (Cysticercus, hydatid cyst), none of which usually cause inflammation as long as the parasite is alive. A small abscess involving the conjunctiva, the soft tissues around the eye, or the eyelid forms after the parasite dies. In these instances, the lesion appears confined and usually is removed surgically and sent to the surgical pathology laboratory for study (15).

SINUS ASPIRATES

In persons with roentgenographic evidence of sinusitis material is aspirated from the involved sinus to identify the organism responsible for the infection. Acute sinusitis, which usually is a bacterial complication of a viral upper respiratory tract infection, most often affects adults during the fall, winter, and spring (27). Of the organisms that cause sinusitis (Table 56–2), Streptococcus pneumoniae and strains of unencapsulated Haemophilus influenzae account for about half of all cases in adults. In children, Branhamella catarrhalis is recovered almost as often as Haemophilus influenzae (28,29). Fungi account for only a few cases of sinusitis. Acute fungal sinusitis typically develops in immunocompromised persons, chronic fungal sinusitis in immunocompetent ones.

Collection, Transport, and Processing

The collection of specimens is similar for all potential pathogens and is done by puncturing the sinus with a needle or plastic catheter and aspirating material. If free fluid is not obtained, 1 ml of sterile normal saline or Ringer's lactate is instilled into the cavity and aspirated to provide the sample. Processing of specimens is different for detection of viruses, bacteria, fungi, and parasites, and is discussed separately for each group of organisms.

Viruses

Processing aspirated material from the sinuses for detection of viruses includes appropriate transport and cell cultures. Aliquots of the fluid (0.5 to 1 ml is preferred, but the volume varies with the amount collected and the number of tests requested) are placed in viral transport medium such as Hanks' balanced salt solution with antibiotics, and are promptly delivered to the laboratory or refrigerated for a short time and transported on wet ice. To ensure recovery of all viruses listed in Table 56–2, inoculating A549, MRC-5, and primary monkey kidney cells is recommended. Specimens are inoculated into cultures and absorbed and incubated as described in Chapter 54. Virus identification is discussed in Part II.

Centrifugation culture has been used successfully to detect adenovirus and influenza A and B viruses, but because each of these viruses accounts for fewer than 5% of all cases of sinusitis, performing the test on all sinus aspirate specimens is not practical (10,11). Monoclonal antibodies specific for influenza A, influenza B, the parainfluenza viruses, and adenovirus may be used to stain smears prepared from sinus aspirate material (as described earlier for routine detection of viruses in conjunctival specimens); however, because these viruses are responsible for a small number of cases of sinusitis this approach may not be cost effective. Moreover, the sensitivity of these monoclonal antibodies has not been evaluated for this type of specimen.

Bacteria

Processing sinus aspirate material for detection of potential bacterial pathogens involves appropriate transport and concentration of the fluid for preparation of smears for direct microscopic examination and inoculation of media for culture. Optimally, 1 ml of fluid is aspirated, air is expelled from the syringe, the needle is removed, and the syringe is tightly capped (preferably with a rubber cap) and is delivered promptly to the laboratory. The fluid is concentrated by centrifuging at 1500 to 2000 g for 15 to 20 minutes, and the supernatant is removed, leaving about 0.5 ml of fluid with the sediment, which is thoroughly mixed on a vortex mixer or by forcefully aspirating up and down with a sterile pipette. To prepare a smear, 1 drop of mixed sediment is placed (without spreading it) on a sterile or alcohol-wiped microscope slide, is allowed to air-dry, and is heat-fixed and stained with the Gram stain. The sediment is inoculated (in 1- to 2-drop aliquots) onto sheep blood, MacConkey, and chocolate agar (incubated in an atmosphere of 5 to 7% carbon dioxide), into thioglycolate broth (incubated in ambient air), and onto anaerobic blood agar (incubated anaerobically). Incubation times and temperatures are discussed in Chapter 54. Organism identification is discussed in Part II.

Fungi

Processing sinus aspirate material for detection of fungi involves preparing a smear for direct microscopic examination and inoculating media for culture. Ideally, 2 to 5

Table 56–2. Organisms That Cause Sinusitis and are Detected in Sinus Aspirate Material

Organism	Chapter
Viruses	
Adenovirus	6
Parainfluenza viruses	10
Influenza viruses	11
Rhinovirus	13
Bacteria	
Staphylococcus aureus	28
Group A Streptococcus	28
Streptococcus pneumoniae	28
Peptostreptococcus spp	30
Branhamella catarrhalis	31
Pseudomonas aeruginosa	32
Enterobacteriaceae*	34
Haemophilus influenzae	36
Bacteroides spp	38
Other anaerobic gram-negative bacilli	38
Fungi	
Dematiaceous fungi	44
Aspergillus spp	44
Pseudallescheria boydii	44
Zygomycetes	44

* Most commonly Escherichia coli or Klebsiella pneumoniae.

ml of fluid is collected and concentrated (as described for bacteria). A smaller volume is acceptable, but it cannot be concentrated. Smears of fluid or of mixed sediment are prepared as discussed earlier for bacteria and are stained with the Gram stain or with calcofluor white, Congo red, or a silver stain (Chapter 42). Fungal planting media (Chapter 42) such as inhibitory mold agar or SABHI agar with and without cycloheximide, which inhibits growth of some of the potential fungal pathogens, is inoculated by placing 1-drop aliquots onto several areas on the surface of agar plates (without streaking for isolation) or by adding several drops to the surface of media in tubes. Culture conditions are reviewed in Chapter 54. Organism identification is discussed in Part II.

Parasites

The only parasites recovered from the sinuses are fly larvae (maggots), most often from comatose or semicomatose hospital patients. These larvae belong to several genera and species of flies that normally deposit their eggs, sometimes larvae, on wounds, ulcers, or moribund flesh. This occurs even in clean, well-maintained hospital environments, where a stray fly may enter from the outside. Often the larvae are spotted crawling out of the patient's nose. The larvae should be collected and sent to the laboratory in formalin for identification, a task often outside the capabilities of the routine laboratory.

MIDDLE EAR DRAINAGE AND TYMPANOCENTESIS FLUID

Fluid draining from the middle ear—and, less frequently, fluid obtained by needle aspiration of a middle ear effusion (tympanocentesis)—occasionally is submitted to the laboratory for culture to determine the agent of otitis media, a common affliction of children, or of mastoiditis, one of its complications. Because microbiologic studies of effusions of the middle ear in persons with uncomplicated otitis media yield consistently similar results, antimicrobial therapy is given without cultures (30,31). Of the organisms involved (Table 56–3), Streptococcus pneumoniae and Haemophilus influenzae account for more than half of all cases. However, cultures of middle ear fluid are indicated in selected cases: for persons who are critically ill, those who do not respond to antimicrobial therapy in 2 to 3 days and appear toxic, immunocompromised persons, and persons who have evidence of mastoiditis on x-ray examination.

Specimen collection is similar for all potential pathogens. Specimen processing, however, is different for viruses, bacteria, and parasites, and is discussed separately for each.

Collection, Transport, and Processing

The collection of fluid draining from the middle ear requires cleaning the ear canal first, then obtaining fresh pus with a swab as it is exuded from the tympanic membrane. Handling of the swab for detection of different organisms is discussed in the following paragraphs. Collection of a middle ear effusion is done by aspiration with a needle and syringe; the needle is removed, the air is ex-

Table 56–3. Organisms That Cause Otitis Media and Mastoiditis and are Detected in Middle Ear Fluid

Organism	Chapter
Viruses	
Respiratory syncytial virus	10
Influenza viruses	11
Enteroviruses	13
Rhinoviruses	13
Bacteria	
Chlamydia trachomatis	24
Staphylococcus aureus	28
Group A Streptococcus	28
Streptococcus pneumoniae	28
Branhamella catarrhalis	31
Haemophilus influenzae	36
Parasites	
Acanthamoeba spp	51

pelled, and the syringe is tightly capped and promptly delivered to the laboratory.

Viruses

Processing middle ear drainage fluid and fluid collected by tympanocentesis for detection of viruses includes appropriate transport and cell culture. Fluid should be placed in viral transport medium such as Hanks' balanced salt solution and promptly delivered to the laboratory or refrigerated for a short time and transported on wet ice. To ensure recovery of all viruses listed in Table 55–3, inoculating HEp-2, MRC-5, and primary monkey kidney cells is recommended (Chapter 2). Specimens are inoculated and adsorbed and cultures are incubated as described earlier for routine detection of viruses in conjunctival specimens. Virus identification is discussed in Part II. Rapid methods for detection of respiratory syncytial virus (direct immunofluorescence staining, enzyme-linked immunosorbent assays) and influenza A and B viruses (direct immunofluorescence staining, centrifugation culture) in respiratory specimens (Chapter 57) have not been evaluated for use with middle ear fluids.

Bacteria

Processing middle ear fluid differs for isolation of Chlamydia trachomatis and for bacteria recovered by routine culture techniques, as follows.

Chlamydia trachomatis. Acute otitis media produced by C. trachomatis occurs in infants younger than 6 months and is diagnosed by isolating the organism from middle ear fluid (32). The fluid is placed in 2-sucrose-phosphate transport medium and promptly delivered to the laboratory or refrigerated for a short time and transported on wet ice. Further processing of the sample is outlined in Procedure 8 in the Appendix. The rapid methods for detection of C. trachomatis, such as direct immunofluorescent staining, enzyme-linked immunosorbent assay, and nucleic acid hybridization (Chapter 25), are not recommended because they have not been evaluated for middle ear fluids.

Bacteria Detected by Routine Culture. Processing middle ear fluid for detection of routine bacterial pathogens includes preparation of a smear for staining with Gram stain and inoculation of sheep blood and chocolate agar (incubated in an atmosphere of 5 to 7% carbon dioxide) and thioglycolate broth (incubated in ambient air). Incubation times and temperatures are discussed in Chapter 54.

Parasites

Only recently has otitis media produced by species of Acanthamoeba been described. All samples that arrive in the laboratory, especially those from persons whom conventional therapy has failed, should be investigated for Acanthamoeba. Smears for staining with trichrome and calcofluor white and cultures are prepared as described (Chapter 55). In rare instances otitis media may result from the penetration of an arthropod into the ear canal and perforation of the tympanum with abscess formation.

ASPIRATES OF PURULENT MATERIAL, GRANULES, AND TISSUE FROM OROFACIAL INFECTIONS

Aspirates of purulent material, granules, and tissue biopsy specimens are useful for identifying the organisms responsible for orofacial infections such as periodontal abscesses, cervicofacial actinomycosis, ulcerative tonsillitis, and ulcerative gingivitis (Table 56–4). Such specimens must be collected in a way that excludes the normal oral flora, to allow appropriate interpretation of culture results. For infections in closed spaces aspiration of loculated pus with a needle and syringe using an extraoral approach is recommended. To ensure anaerobiosis during transport, air is expelled from the syringe, the needle is removed, and the syringe is tightly capped and promptly delivered to the laboratory. For granules and tissue specimens one portion should be placed in formalin for histologic studies and the remainder should be placed in an anaerobic transport system, delivered promptly to the laboratory, and homogenized with a sterile tissue grinder or a mortar and pestle (preferably in an anaerobic chamber).

Further processing of aspirated pus and homogenates of tissue or granules includes preparing a smear for staining with Gram stain and inoculation of appropriate media: sheep blood and chocolate agars incubated 5 to 7 days at 35° to 37°C in an atmosphere of 5 to 7% carbon dioxide, and anaerobic blood agar and kanamycin-vancomycin laked blood agar incubated anaerobically for 5 to 7 days. To ensure recovery of Actinomyces from granules media should be incubated up to 2 weeks. Techniques necessary for recovery of the anaerobic spirochetes generally are not available in the routine laboratory, but in most cases the organisms are visualized in smears stained with Gram stain and their isolation is not critical for treatment.

Parasites

For the sake of completeness, a rare infection found in some Latin American countries is mentioned here. Cervicofacial abscesses, which usually present as several draining fistulas resembling actinomycosis, can be produced by an ascarid of the genus Lagochilascaris. Examination of the pus on wet mounts reveals the characteristic eggs (Chapter 52).

SWAB AND TISSUE BIOPSY SPECIMENS OF OROPHARYNGEAL ULCERS

Swab and biopsy specimens are useful in determining the infectious agent of oropharyngeal ulcers (Table 56–5). Specimen collection, transport, and processing are different for viruses, bacteria, fungi, and parasites, and are discussed separately for each group.

Collection, Transport, and Processing

Viruses

Samples for isolation of viruses are taken by vigorously scraping the base of the lesion with a Dacron-tipped swab, which then is placed in viral transport medium such as Hanks' balanced salt solution with antibiotics (Chapter 3) and is delivered promptly to the laboratory, or, if not, is refrigerated for a short time and transported on wet ice. In the laboratory, the specimen is vigorously mixed on a vortex mixer and the swab is removed. To ensure recovery of the viruses listed in Table 56–5, inoculating MRC-5 and primary monkey kidney cells is recommended. Also, inoculating A549 cells previously incubated in maintenance medium containing 10^{-5} M dexamethasone for at least 24 hours (Chapter 5 and reference 33) decreases the time for detection of herpes simplex or varicella-zoster virus. Specimens are inoculated and adsorbed and cultures are incubated as described in Chapter 54.

A second swab specimen may be collected and used for preparation of a direct smear by firmly rolling it on a glass slide. The smear may be stained with the Wright stain (Tzanck preparation) or the Papanicolaou stain and examined for cytopathic changes characteristic of herpes sim-

Table 56–4. Organisms Associated with Periodontal Abscesses, Cervicofacial Abscesses, Ulcerative Tonsillitis, and Ulcerative Gingivitis

Organism	Chapter
Actinomyces spp	30
Actinobacillus actinomycetemcomitans	36
Capnocytophaga spp	36
Anaerobic gram-negative bacilli	38
Anaerobic spirochetes	39

Table 56–5. Organisms That Cause Oropharyngeal Ulcers

Organism	Chapter
Viruses	
Herpes simplex virus	5
Varicella-zoster virus	5
Enteroviruses	13
Bacteria	
Treponema pallidum	39
Mycobacterium tuberculosis	40
Fungi	
Histoplasma capsulatum	45
Paracoccidioides brasiliensis	45
Parasites	
Mucocutaneous leishmaniae	51

plex and varicella-zoster viruses. The disadvantages of this method are the low sensitivity and the inability to differentiate the two viruses. Staining with monoclonal antibodies specific for herpes simplex virus and for varicella-zoster virus allows identification of the virus, but negative stain results must be followed by culture.

Bacteria

Processing oropharyngeal specimens for detection of bacteria differs with each organism and is discussed separately for Treponema pallidum and Mycobacterium tuberculosis.

Treponema pallidum. Spirochetes of T. pallidum may be visualized by examination of material from oropharyngeal ulcers under darkfield illumination (as described for genital ulcers in Chapter 61). Differentiation of T. pallidum from nonpathogenic spirochetes, which are part of the normal oral flora, is extremely difficult, and oral syphilis is more reliably diagnosed by serologic tests (Chapter 39).

Mycobacterium tuberculosis. For detection of M. tuberculosis a biopsy specimen from the ulcer margin should be obtained and transported promptly to the laboratory in a sterile container. Fresh tissue should be examined by a pathologist and divided for histologic and microbiologic studies. Processing of tissue for microbiologic studies should be done in a biologic safety cabinet. The tissue is homogenized in a small amount of broth with a sterile tissue grinder or a mortar and pestle and the homogenate is poured through sterile gauze into a 50-ml centrifuge tube. An equal volume of 2% NaOH-N-acetyl-L cystine is added, the solution is mixed thoroughly, and allowed to stand 20 minutes, after which 25 ml of phosphate buffer is added. The sample is mixed and centrifuged at 3000 to 3600 g for 20 minutes. The supernatant is decanted, and the sediment is resuspended in 1 to 2 ml of buffer and used to prepare a smear for auramine rhodamine or acid-fast staining (Appendix, Procedures 4–6) and to inoculate appropriate media (Chapter 40, and Table 54–4).

Fungi

Detection of fungi in oropharyngeal ulcers requires a biopsy specimen from the margin of the ulcer and its prompt transportation to the laboratory in a sterile container. Fresh tissue is examined by a pathologist and is divided for histologic and microbiologic studies. Processing tissue for detection of fungi involves homogenization, direct microscopic examination, and inoculation to appropriate media for culture. The tissue is homogenized as described earlier for Mycobacterium tuberculosis. The homogenate is used to prepare smears for staining with the Gram, calcofluor white, Congo red, or a silver stain, and for inoculation of primary fungal planting media such as brain-heart infusion, agar supplemented with sheep blood, SABHI agar, or inhibitory mold agar, all of which should contain antibiotics (Chapter 42). Conditions for culture are discussed in Chapter 54, and identification of organisms in Chapter 45.

Parasites

Oropharyngeal ulcers sometimes are produced by species of mucocutaneous leishmaniae. These lesions are common in endemic areas, and especially in some countries of Latin America. If an ulcer in the oropharynx is suspected to be of leishmanial origin smears and biopsies should be taken by an otolaryngologist, as outlined in Chapter 62. Handling of the specimen in the laboratory requires preparation of smears for staining with the Giemsa stain and, if necessary, cultures for isolation of the parasite (Chapter 62).

REFERENCES

1. McDonnell PJ, and Green WR: Conjunctivitis. *In* Principles and Practice of Infectious Diseases. 3rd ed. Edited by GL Mandell, RG Douglas, Jr, and JE Bennett. New York, Churchill Livingstone, 1990.
2. Leibowitz HM, et al: Human conjunctivitis. A diagnostic evaluation. Arch Ophthalmol, *94*:1747, 1976.
3. Seal DV, Barrett SP, and McGill JI: Aetiology and treatment of acute bacterial infection of the external eye. Br J Ophthalmol, *66*:357, 1982.
4. Gigliotti F, et al: Etiology of acute conjunctivitis in children. J Pediatr, *98*:531, 1981.
5. Brook I: Anaerobic and aerobic bacterial flora of acute conjunctivitis in children. Arch Ophthalmol, *98*:833, 1980.
6. Schachter J, and Dawson CR: Human Chlamydial Infections. Littleton, MA, PSG Publishing, 1978.
7. Denis J, et al: Fine structure of palpebral molluscum contagiosum and its secondary conjunctival lesions. Graefe Arch Ophthalmol, *208*:207, 1978.
8. Gleaves CA, Wilson DJ, Wold AD, and Smith TF: Detection and serotyping of herpes simplex virus in MRC-5 cells by using centrifugation and monoclonal antibodies 16 h postinoculation. J Clin Microbiol, *21*:29, 1985.
9. Woods GL, and Mills RD: Conventional tube cell culture compared with centrifugal inoculation of MRC-5 cells and staining with monoclonal antibodies for detection of herpes simplex virus in clinical specimens. J Clin Microbiol, *26*:570, 1988.
10. Woods GL, Yamamoto M, and Young A: Detection of adenovirus by rapid 24-well plate centrifugation and conventional cell culture with dexamethasone. J Virol Methods, *20*:109, 1988.
11. Mills RD, Cain KJ, and Woods GL: Detection of influenza virus by centrifugal inoculation of MDCK cells and staining with monoclonal antibodies. J Clin Microbiol, *27*:2505, 1989.
12. Sureau P, Lafon M, and Baer GM: Rhabdoviridae: Rabies and vesicular stomatitis viruses. *In* Laboratory Diagnosis of Infectious Diseases. Principles and Practice. Edited by EH Lennette, P Halonen, and FA Murphy. New York, Springer-Verlag, 1988.
13. Arumainayagam JT, Matthews RS, Uthayakumar S, and Clay JC: Evaluation of a novel solid-phase immunoassay, Clearview Chlamydia, for the rapid detection of Chlamydia trachomatis. J Clin Microbiol, *28*:2813, 1990.
14. Brenner DJ, et al: Proposal of Afipia gen. nov., with Afipia felis sp. nov. (formerly the cat-scratch disease bacillus), Afipia clevelandensis sp. nov. (formerly the Cleveland Clinic Foundation strain), Afipia broomae sp. nov., and three unnamed genospecies. J Clin Microbiol, *29*:2450, 1991.
15. Gutierrez Y: Diagnostic Pathology of Parasitic Infections with Clinical Correlations. Philadelphia, Lea & Febiger, 1990.

16. Asbell P, and Stenson S: Ulcerative keratitis. Survey of 30 years' laboratory experience. Arch Ophthalmol, *100*:77, 1982.
17. Leisegang TJ, and Forster RK: Spectrum of microbial keratitis in south Florida. Am J Ophthalmol, *90*:38, 1980.
18. Jones DB: Polymicrobial keratitis. Trans Am Ophthalmol Soc, *79*:153, 1981.
19. Allen HF, and Mangiaracine AB: Bacterial endophthalmitis after cataract extraction. II. Incidence in 36,000 consecutive operations with special reference to preoperative topical antibiotics. Arch Ophthalmol, *91*:3, 1974.
20. Affeldt JC, et al: Microbial endophthalmitis resulting from ocular trauma. Ophthalmology, *94*:407, 1987.
21. Burns CL: Bilateral endophthalmitis in acute bacterial endocarditis. Am J Ophthalmol, *88*:809, 1979.
22. Hull DS, Patipa M, and Cox F: Metastatic endophthalmitis: A complication of meningococcal meningitis. Ann Ophthalmol, *14*:29, 1982.
23. Doft BH, et al: Endogenous Aspergillus endophthalmitis in drug abusers. Arch Ophthalmol, *98*:859, 1980.
24. Aguilar GL, et al: Candida endophthalmitis after intravenous drug abuse. Arch Ophthalmol, *97*:96, 1979.
25. Dellon AL, Stark WJ, and Chretien PB: Spontaneous resolution of endogenous Candida endophthalmitis complicating intravenous hyperalimentation. Am J Ophthalmol, *79*:648, 1978.
26. Freeman JB, Davis PL, and MacLean LD: Candida endophthalmitis associated with intravenous hyperalimentation. Arch Surg, *108*:237, 1974.
27. Hamory BH, et al: Etiology and antimicrobial therapy of acute maxillary sinusitis. J Infect Dis, *139*:197, 1979.
28. Gwaltney JM, Jr: Sinusitis. *In* Principles and Practice of Infectious Diseases. 3rd ed. Edited by GL Mandell, RG Douglas, Jr, and JE Bennett. New York, Churchill Livingstone, 1990.
29. Wald ER, et al: Acute maxillary sinusitis in children. N Engl J Med, *304*:749, 1981.
30. Klein JO: Otitis externa, otitis media, mastoiditis. *In* Principles and Practice of Infectious Diseases. 3rd ed. Edited by GL Mandell, RG Douglas, Jr, and JE Bennett. New York, Churchill Livingstone, 1990.
31. Bluestone CD, and Klein JO (eds): Otitis Media in Infants and Children. Philadelphia, WB Saunders, 1987.
32. Tipple MA, Beem MO, and Saxon EM: Clinical characteristics of the afebrile pneumonia associated with Chlamydia trachomatis infection in infants less than 6 months of age. Pediatrics, *63*:192, 1979.
33. Woods GL, and Mills RD: Effect of dexamethasone on detection of herpes simplex virus in clinical specimens by conventional cell culture and rapid 24-well plate centrifugation. J Clin Microbiol, *26*:1233, 1988.

Chapter 57

RESPIRATORY TRACT

Specimens from the respiratory tract received in the laboratory for microbiologic studies include nasopharyngeal and nasal specimens, throat specimens, sputum and tracheal aspirates, transtracheal aspirates; bronchial washing, bronchial brush, and bronchoalveolar lavage specimens; fine needle aspirates from the lung, and tissue from transbronchial and open lung biopsy.

NASOPHARYNGEAL AND NASAL SPECIMENS

Nasopharyngeal aspirates, washings, and swab specimens are useful in diagnosing several viral infections, predominantly of the respiratory tract (Table 57–1), but also measles (1). In addition to viral infections, nasopharyngeal specimens are useful in diagnosing pneumonia produced by Chlamydia trachomatis in infants (Chapter 25), diphtheria (Chapter 29), and pertussis (Chapter 33). Specimens from the nose are useful in identifying carriers of Staphylococcus aureus, and in diagnosing ozaena (Klebsiella ozaenae), leprosy (Mycobacterium leprae), rhinosporidiosis (Rhinosporidium seeberi), and mucocutaneous leishmaniasis (Chapters 28, 34, 40, 46, and 51, respectively).

Collection, Transport, and Processing

Collection and transport of nasopharyngeal and nasal specimens is similar for all organisms. Specimen processing differs for different groups of organisms and is discussed separately for viruses, bacteria, fungi, and parasites.

Nasopharyngeal aspirates and washings are superior to swabs for recovery of viruses, but because swabs are more convenient they frequently are submitted. Washings or swab specimens are collected for detection of Chlamydia trachomatis and Bordetella pertussis; a swab is the preferred specimen for Corynebacterium diphtheriae. An aspirate is a sample collected with a plastic tube used to feed premature infants, attached to a 10-ml syringe or a suction catheter with a mucus trap. A wash is obtained with a rubber suction bulb by instilling and withdrawing 3 to 7 ml of sterile phosphate-buffered saline. The collection of nasopharyngeal secretions and cells with a swab involves removal of all mucus from the nasal cavity, after which a small, flexible nasopharyngeal swab is inserted along the nasal septum to the posterior pharynx and rotated several times against the mucosa.

For detection of viruses nasopharyngeal aspirates, washings, and swabs are placed into 2 to 4 ml of appropriate transport medium, with or without antibiotics (veal infusion broth with 0.5% gelatin, Hanks' balanced salt solution, or sucrose phosphate broth, discussed in Chapter 3), and are transported promptly to the laboratory or stored briefly in the refrigerator and packed in ice for transport as soon as possible.

For detection of Chlamydia trachomatis, a nasopharyngeal swab specimen is collected with a Dacron-, rayon- or cotton-tipped swab, avoiding the use of calcium alginate because it may be toxic to the organisms. The swab specimen may be used for culture, for preparation of a smear for direct fluorescent antibody staining, and possibly for an enzyme-linked immunosorbent assay (ELISA) (depending on whether the system is approved for nasopharyngeal specimens). To culture C. trachomatis the swab should be placed in 2-sucrose phosphate medium containing antimicrobial agents and transported to the laboratory as soon as possible or refrigerated for a short time.

For detection of Bordetella pertussis, washings and swab specimens should be plated at the bedside for optimal results. If this is not possible the sample is placed in sterile casamino broth (commercially available), transported promptly to the laboratory, and processed within 1 to 2 hours.

Nasal secretions are collected from the anterior nares with a polyester-tipped swab, are placed in a tube transport system (commercially available), and are promptly delivered to the laboratory. Nasal biopsy specimens for diagnosis of rhinosporidiosis and mucocutaneous leishmaniasis are delivered immediately to the laboratory in a sterile container, where a pathologist should examine the fresh tissue and divide it for histologic and microbiologic studies.

Viruses

The viruses most often sought in nasopharyngeal aspirates, washings, or swab specimens are those associated with respiratory tract illness (Table 57–1). Adenoviruses and enteroviruses may be detected in nasopharyngeal specimens, but throat specimens are preferred. Measles virus also may be detected in a nasopharyngeal specimen, but the diagnosis of measles usually is based on clinical manifestations and is confirmed serologically. Processing specimens for virus detection is discussed for the respiratory viruses and measles virus as a group because the principles and techniques are similar. Coronaviruses (Chapter 12) are found in the nasopharynx, but their detection requires techniques not available in the general clinical virology laboratory, so they are not discussed further here.

All specimens received in the laboratory for virus detection should be processed as rapidly as possible or stored in the refrigerator if a delay is unavoidable. Specimens are processed according to the physician's request and the methods used for virus detection. Techniques currently

Table 57–1. Viruses That Cause Respiratory Disease

Disease	Viruses*
Common cold	Rhinoviruses, coronaviruses, parainfluenza virus, respiratory syncytial virus, influenza viruses, adenoviruses, some enteroviruses
Croup	Parainfluenza virus, respiratory syncytial virus, influenza viruses, adenoviruses, some enteroviruses
Acute bronchitis	Respiratory syncytial virus, parainfluenza viruses, influenza viruses, rhinoviruses
Pneumonia	Influenza viruses, respiratory syncytial virus, parainfluenza viruses, rhinoviruses, measles virus

* Listed in decreasing order of occurrence

available for identifying viruses commonly present in nasopharyngeal specimens are listed in Table 57–2 and discussed in more detail below.

Cell culture is the reference method for detecting the viruses listed in Table 57–2. Isolation of measles virus in cell cultures requires several weeks, but other reliable methods (discussed later) provide rapid results, and cultures are not recommended. Cell lines are selected according to what viruses are likely to be present in the sample; therefore, detection of viruses listed in Table 57–2 is done by inoculation of primary monkey (rhesus or cynomolgus) kidney, HEp-2, and MRC-5 cells (A549 cells may be added if adenovirus is suspected strongly) (Chapter 3 and Table 54–2). Specimens are inoculated and adsorbed and cultures are incubated as described in Chapter 54, with these exceptions: (1) cultures that may contain myxoviruses and rhinoviruses are incubated at 33° C because these viruses grow best at this temperature; (2) for cultures that may contain influenza viruses the maintenance medium added to the primary monkey kidney cell cultures should be free of serum which might contain inhibitors that adversely affect the detection of influenza viruses. Identification of the virus is based on the appearance of the cytopathic changes (Chapter 6, 10, 11, and 13), hemadsorption, and staining of cells from the infected monolayer with specific monoclonal antibodies.

Influenza viruses and respiratory syncytial virus (RSV)

Table 57–2. Methods Used to Detect Viruses in Naropharyngeal Specimens

	Method				
				ELISA	
Virus	Culture	DFA	IFA	Conventional	Membrane
Adenovirus	X		X	X	
Parainfluenza virus	X	X	X		
Measles virus	X		X		
Respiratory syncytial virus	X	X	X	X	X
Influenza A virus	X	X	X		X
Influenza B virus	X	X	X		
Enteroviruses	X				
Rhinovirus	X				

Key: DFA, direct fluorescent antibody staining; IFA, indirect fluorescent antibody staining; ELISA, enzyme immunoassay.

may be detected by centrifugation culture, using shell vials or 24-well plates containing coverslips seeded with indicator cells (HEp-2 cells for RSV and MDCK or monkey kidney cells for influenza viruses) and, after short incubation, staining with monoclonal antibodies specific for each virus. This technique is an economical adjunct to conventional cell culture for detection of the influenza viruses, but for detection of RSV, it appears to be less sensitive than some of the more rapid diagnostic methods (2,3).

The fluorescent antibody technique (direct or indirect) provides rapid detection of viral antigens in infected cells. Smears of nasopharyngeal cells may be prepared directly from a swab specimen by rolling the swab on a glass slide immediately after it is collected. To prepare a smear from nasopharyngeal aspirates, washes, or swab specimens received in transport medium the sample is mixed on a vortex mixer, the swab is removed (if present), and the specimen is centrifuged at 900 g for 10 minutes. The supernatant is removed, and the cell pellet is resuspended in 0.05 to 0.1 ml of sterile phosphate-buffered saline, and 1 drop of the cell suspension is placed on a glass slide. Smears prepared by either method are air-dried, fixed in acetone for 10 minutes, and then stained. The direct immunofluorescence technique using specific antibodies conjugated with fluorescein isothiocyanate (FITC) is more rapid than the two-step indirect method (staining first with unlabeled specific antibodies to the virus and then with FITC-anti-immunoglobulin G). Immunofluorescence is most reliable for detecting RSV (Chapter 10) but also is useful for measles virus (3,4). Data from several studies indicate that the sensitivity of immunofluorescence with commercial reagents for detection of influenza viruses is low, but is higher when the antibodies are prepared in the laboratory of the investigator (3,5).

Conventional ELISA (commercially available) reliably detects RSV within 2 to 3 hours (6–8). Membrane enzyme immunoassays, which provide results in about 30 minutes, are available for detection of RSV and influenza A virus. Studies have shown that the membrane enzyme immunoassay reliably detects RSV, and limited data suggest that the membrane enzyme immunoassay for influenza A virus is a good screening test but does not replace cell culture (9,10).

Each of the methods of detection listed in Table 57–2 has specific advantages and disadvantages (discussed in Chapters 10 and 11), and laboratory directors should select the best tests based on patient population, needs of the medical staff, test reliability, expertise of the laboratory personnel, and cost.

Bacteria

Nasopharyngeal specimens are taken for diagnosis of infections caused by a few bacteria, including Chlamydia trachomatis, Corynebacterium diphtheriae, and Bordetella pertussis. Corynebacterium diphtheriae is more often detected in throat specimens and is discussed later. Carriers of Staphylococcus aureus are identified by detecting the organism in swab specimens from the anterior nares. Klebsiella ozaenae is a rare pathogen that may be found in nasal discharge, and smears of nasal secretions stained with an acid-fast stain are useful in diagnosing leprosy. Processing of nasopharyngeal and nasal specimens differs for different organisms and is discussed separately for Chlamydia trachomatis, Bordetella pertussis, Staphylococcus aureus and Klebsiella ozaenae, and Mycobacterium leprae.

Chlamydia trachomatis. The reference method for detection of C. trachomatis in nasopharyngeal swab specimens is cell culture, which must be requested specifically. If processing is to be done within 48 hours the specimen should be refrigerated, if a longer delay is anticipated it is stored at $-70°$ C. Preparation of specimens for culture is described in the Appendix, Procedure 8.

The direct fluorescent antibody (DFA) test for detection of Chlamydia trachomatis (reagents are available from several manufacturers) gives results within 1 hour. In general the test is less sensitive than culture, though specific data on nasopharyngeal specimens are limited and good practice dictates that if the DFA test is negative another specimen should be collected for culture (11). To perform the DFA test the swab is rolled on a glass slide immediately after the sample is collected and fixed according to the manufacturer's directions. Fixed specimens may be stored at room temperature until they are stained, which should be done within 72 hours of collection using only antibodies approved for nasopharyngeal specimens.

To perform the ELISA specific for Chlamydia trachomatis the swab specimen is placed in the transport medium provided by the manufacturer and transported to the laboratory. The assays generally are completed in 2 to 4 hours, but the specimen may be stored at room temperature for 5 to 7 days before being tested. The sensitivity of these assays for detection of C. trachomatis in nasopharyngeal specimens is about 70 to 80%, so a negative result does not exclude the diagnosis (12).

Bordetella pertussis. Culture is the most sensitive method for detection of B. pertussis, a fastidious organism that requires special media for isolation (13). Currently the recommended medium is Regan-Lowe agar (composed of Oxoid charcoal agar and 10% horse blood and containing cephalexin), instead of the traditional Bordet-Gengou agar (potato infusion agar with 20% sheep blood); conditions for culture are listed in Table 54–4. Specimens that must be shipped to a reference laboratory for culture should be inoculated to Regan-Lowe transport medium. Identification of B. pertussis is discussed in Chapter 33.

In addition to culture a direct fluorescent antibody stain may be used to detect Bordetella pertussis in nasopharyngeal specimens (a detailed procedure is described in reference 14). This technique provides rapid diagnosis but is associated with false-positive and false-negative results (13). To perform the direct fluorescent antibody stain, the casamino acid medium containing the swab or aspirate is incubated at $35°$ C for 1 hour. The medium is mixed, and 1 drop is placed on a glass slide and dried at room temperature. The sample is reapplied three times, after which the slides are heat-fixed and stained with commercially available fluorescein-conjugated antibodies to B. pertussis. Positive and negative controls must be stained concurrently.

Staphylococcus aureus and Klebsiella ozaenae. To identify persons who carry Staphylococcus aureus in their anterior nares a swab specimen is planted onto 5% sheep blood agar, onto agar selective for gram-positive organisms (colistin–nalidixic acid agar or phenylethyl alcohol agar), or onto mannitol-salt agar, a medium selective for staphylococci and helpful in differentiating coagulase-positive from coagulase-negative species. Klebsiella ozaenae is detected in nasal discharge or swab specimens by planting the sample onto sheep blood and MacConkey agars. For both organisms, plates are incubated at $35°$ C in ambient air. Colonies generally appear after 24 hours' incubation. Organism identification is discussed in Chapters 28 and 34.

Mycobacterium leprae. M. leprae cannot yet be recovered in the clinical laboratory. Finding acid-fast bacilli in smears of nasal secretions from a person who has the clinical manifestations of leprosy (Chapter 40) is useful diagnostically, but a full-thickness biopsy specimen from a cutaneous lesion should be examined histologically for staging of the disease.

Fungi

Rhinosporidium seeberi produces a friable, pedunculated mass in the nose or on the conjunctiva. The organism responsible has not been cultured, and the infection is diagnosed by finding typical cysts with a thick wall (Chapter 46) in potassium hydroxide preparations, in smears of nasal secretions stained with a silver stain, or in histologic sections of biopsy specimens.

Parasites

Lesions of the nasal cavity produced by mucocutaneous leishmaniae usually involve the mucosa, cartilage, and sometimes the skin, of the nose. These lesions, which often are metastatic from a focus elsewhere on the skin, are typically granulomatous inflammations that produce ulceration and progressive destruction of the naso-oropharyngeal cartilages. The ulcer is painless, chronic, and affects persons who live or travel in endemic areas (Chapter 51).

The diagnosis of mucocutaneous leishmaniasis often is made clinically, but it should be confirmed by examination of smears, imprints, and biopsy tissue from the ulcer, as discussed in Chapter 62 for the skin samples.

THROAT SPECIMENS

The throat specimens, mainly washings and swab specimens, most often are collected to determine the agent of pharyngitis. Most cases are caused by viruses and occur as a component of the common cold. The viruses most commonly involved are those listed in Table 57–1 plus adenoviruses and some enteroviruses (both detected more frequently in throat than in nasopharyngeal specimens). The most important bacterial cause of pharyngitis is group A Streptococcus, and throat swabs received in the clinical laboratory for routine culture should be evaluated only for this agent. Other bacteria (Table 57–3) are uncommon or rare causes of pharyngitis, and their detection must be requested specifically.

Table 57-3. Organisms Detected by Microbiologic Studies of Throat Specimens

Organism	Chapter
Viruses	
Herpes simplex virus	5
Cytomegalovirus	5
Epstein-Barr virus	5
Adenovirus	6
Mumps virus	10
Influenza A and B viruses	11
Enteroviruses	13
Venezuelan equine encephalitis virus	17
Bacteria	
Chlamydia trachomatis	25
Chlamydia pneumoniae	25
Mycoplasma pneumoniae	27
Group A Streptococcus	28
Corynebacterium diphtheriae	29
Arcanobacterium haemolyticum	29
Neisseria gonorrhoeae	31
Haemophilus influenzae	36
Fusobacterium necrophorum (and other anaerobes)	38

Throat washings and swab specimens also are useful for detection of viruses shed in oral secretions without causing pharyngitis, such as herpes simplex virus (HSV), cytomegalovirus (CMV), Epstein-Barr virus (EBV), mumps virus, some enteroviruses, and Venezuelan equine encephalitis virus. Throat swab specimens may be helpful in determining the agent of epiglottitis, which almost always is caused by Haemophilus influenzae type b but occasionally by Staphylococcus aureus or Streptococcus pneumoniae. Specimen collection is similar for viruses and bacteria, but specimen processing is different and is discussed separately for each group of organisms.

Collection, Transport, and Processing

Throat washings, used primarily for diagnosis of viral infections, are obtained by gargling with 5 ml of viral transport medium such as Hanks' balanced salt solution containing antibiotics. Throat swab specimens are collected by depressing the tongue with a tongue blade, introducing the swab between the tonsillar pillars and behind the uvula without touching the lateral walls of the buccal cavity, and swabbing back and forth across the posterior pharynx.

Swab specimens for detection of viruses should be placed in viral transport media, and those for detection of bacteria should be placed in a tube transport system containing modified Stuart's medium. Throat washings and swab specimens should be delivered promptly to the laboratory, and those collected for virus detection should be refrigerated for a short time if a delay in transport is unavoidable.

Viruses

Several viruses may be detected in throat specimens, but the mere presence of the virus does not in all cases indicate that it is the cause of disease. For example, HSV, CMV, and EBV commonly are found in the saliva of persons who do not have active viral disease, although in some instances, HSV and EBV are associated with pharyngitis. EBV, HSV, and CMV can be recovered from clinical specimens, but isolation of EBV is more complex and is not done in most clinical laboratories. Disease caused by EBV most often is diagnosed serologically, and is not discussed here. Adenoviruses and enteroviruses may be shed in the pharynx months after resolution of an illness, but concurrent detection of the virus in the stool and the throat suggests that it probably is responsible for current symptoms.

Detection of mumps, influenza, or Venezuelan equine encephalitis virus in throat specimens indicates that the virus is responsible for the disease. Mumps virus usually is detected in urine, however, which is the specimen of choice (Chapter 61); influenza viruses are detected most often in nasopharyngeal specimens, and Venezuelan equine encephalitis is diagnosed serologically.

Cell culture is the reference method for detection of the viruses in throat specimens, and their recovery is ensured by inoculation of MRC-5, A549, and primary monkey kidney cells (see Table 54-2). Specimens are inoculated, absorbed, and cultures are incubated as described in Chapter 54. Virus identification is discussed in Chapters 5, 6, and 13.

Centrifugation culture has been used successfully for detection of HSV, CMV, and adenovirus (15-17). Shell vials or 24-well plates containing coverslips seeded with indicator cells (MRC-5 cells for HSV, CMV, and adenovirus; A549 cells for HSV and adenovirus) are inoculated, centrifuged, and incubated 16 hours (for HSV and CMV) to 40 hours (for adenovirus). Coverslips are stained with specific monoclonal antibodies (Appendix, Procedure 2). Centrifugation culture should be performed in addition to conventional cell culture for detection of CMV in throat specimens from immunocompromised persons and from infants suspected to have congenital disease, but it may not be economical for detection of HSV and adenovirus.

Bacteria

Several bacteria are pathogens of the throat (see Table 57-3), but group A Streptococcus is the only organism that should be identified in routine cultures. Identification of other bacteria in Table 57-3 must be requested specifically. Because reagents necessary for detection of Chlamydia pneumoniae are not yet available commercially, and specimens must be sent to a reference laboratory, this agent is not discussed further. The other bacteria listed in Table 57-3 are discussed individually.

Chlamydia trachomatis. Currently, cell culture is the only method available for detection of C. trachomatis in throat specimens. The throat washing or swab specimen should be placed in 2-sucrose-phosphate transport medium and handled as discussed above for nasopharyngeal specimens and as described in the Appendix, Procedure 8.

Mycoplasma pneumoniae. A throat swab is the specimen of choice for culture of M. pneumoniae, though diagnosis of pneumonia produced by M. pneumoniae often is based on clinical manifestations alone or on serologic tests (Chapter 27). For culture the throat swab is inoculated to a diphasic culture medium, several of which are available commercially, or to a vial of SP-4 broth culture medium. Both cultures are incubated at 35° to 37° C for up to 3 weeks. The broth is subcultured to Edward-Hayflick agar when an acid pH shift occurs (when it turns yellow), or on day 7 (reference 14 describes a complete procedure).

Mycoplasma pneumoniae may also be detected in throat swab specimens by using a commercially available RNA-directed DNA probe (18).

Group A Streptococcus. For diagnosis of group A streptococcal pharyngitis a throat swab is planted onto sheep blood agar or, preferably, onto a blood agar plate selective for group A Streptococcus (several are available commercially). Using a selective medium increases the recovery of group A Streptococcus and, by inhibiting the normal flora, decreases the time required to read plates and further evaluate β-hemolytic colonies (19). Plates should be incubated at 35° to 37° C in ambient air or an atmosphere of 5 to 7% carbon dioxide. Identification of group A Streptococcus is discussed in Chapter 28. When a rapid, direct test for group A Streptococcus is requested two throat swab specimens should be collected. If the direct test is positive the second swab may be discarded, but if the direct test is negative the second swab must be cultured, because the sensitivity of direct tests can be as low as 70% (20).

Corynebacterium diphtheriae. For diagnosis of diphtheria, both a nasoparhyngeal and one (or preferably, two) throat swab specimens are collected. Swabs should be transported to the laboratory immediately; if laboratory personnel are not experienced in the recovery and identification of C. diphtheriae the specimens should be sent dry in packets or tubes containing silica gel or other desiccant to a reference laboratory (21).

To process specimens from persons suspected to have diphtheria, two smears are prepared from one of the throat swabs. One smear is stained with Gram stain, necessary to differentiate diphtheria from Vincent's angina (discussed later); the other smear is stained with Loeffler's methylene blue to visualize the deep blue–staining metachromatic granules of species of Corynebacterium. However, Corynebacterium diphtheriae cannot be identified by cellular morphology alone, and cultures must be done. The nasopharyngeal and the throat swab specimens should be planted onto a slant of Loeffler's serum medium and onto a medium containing potassium tellurite (Tinsdale agar, which has a shelf life of 2 to 3 days, or cystine-tellurite blood agar, with a shelf-life of about 1 month). All plates are incubated at 35° C for 24 to 48 hours. Identification of C. diphtheriae is discussed briefly in Chapter 29 and in more detail in references 21 and 22. In addition, a sheep blood agar plate should be inoculated and examined for group A Streptococcus, because the person may have streptococcal pharyngitis or a dual infection with group A Streptococcus and Corynebacterium diphtheriae.

Arcanobacterium haemolyticum. A. haemolyticum grows on sheep blood agar, but because its colonies are small and are surrounded by a very narrow zone of β hemolysis, which may not be apparent after 24 hours' incubation, recognizing it on this medium is difficult. If infection with A. haemolyticum is suspected the throat swabs are inoculated to rabbit blood agar or human blood agar, neither of which routinely is available in most clinical laboratories. On these media the colonies are larger and are surrounded by a wider zone of β hemolysis. Identification of A. haemolyticum is discussed elsewhere (21).

Neisseria gonorrhoeae. For detection of N. gonorrhoeae in the throat, the swab specimen should be transported to the laboratory promptly and inoculated as soon as possible onto a selective medium such as modified Thayer-Martin agar (other acceptable media are discussed in Chapter 31). If a delay in processing is unavoidable the swab should be held at room temperature. N. gonorrhoeae is extremely sensitive to cold, and its recovery is affected adversely by refrigeration. Plates are incubated at 35° to 37° C in an atmosphere of 3 to 7% carbon dioxide for up to 72 hours. Identification of N. gonorrhoeae is discussed in Chapter 31.

Haemophilus influenzae. To diagnose epiglottitis produced by H. influenzae a swab specimen of the epiglottis should be collected by a physician in a setting where intubation of the patient may be performed immediately if necessary. The specimen should be transported promptly to the laboratory and planted onto chocolate agar and sheep blood agar. The plates are incubated at 35° to 37° C in an atmosphere of 5 to 7% carbon dioxide. Identification of H. influenzae is discussed in Chapter 36.

Fusobacterium necrophorum. F. necrophorum and other anaerobes may cause Vincent's angina, an acute necrotizing ulcerative tonsillitis that resembles the pseudomembranes of diphtheria. An illness with this clinical presentation presumptively may be called Vincent's angina based on finding gram-negative, fusiform bacilli and spirochetes in smears prepared from a swab specimen of the ulcerated lesion and stained with the Gram stain. Cultures of the involved area usually are not helpful because many species of anaerobes are present in the oral cavity; however, blood cultures should be collected because the illness commonly is accompanied by sepsis.

SPUTUM AND TRACHEAL ASPIRATES

Microbiologic studies of sputum (expectorated and induced) and tracheal aspirate specimens are done principally to determine the agents of pneumonia. Many organisms infect the lung, producing different diseases (Table 57-4), but the majority of sputum specimens are collected from persons with a clinical diagnosis of acute bacterial pneumonia. Bacterial pneumonia ranks number five as a cause of death in the United States and, in a recent study, was the fourth most common cause of hospitalization among persons aged 65 years and older (23). Pneumonia accounts for 10 to 20% of all nosocomial infections and, among hospitalized patients, is the leading cause of mortality due to infections. Streptococcus pneumoniae remains the most common cause of community-acquired pneumonia, accounting for 25 to 60% of all cases, whereas gram-negative bacilli are responsible for the majority of nosocomial infections (24).

Table 57–4. Pathogens Detected by Microbiologic Studies of Specimens from the Lower Respiratory Tract*

Organism	Chapter
Viruses	
Herpes simplex virus	5
Varicella-zoster virus	5
Cytomegalovirus	5
Adenovirus	6
Parainfluenza viruses	10
Measles virus	10
Respiratory syncytial virus	10
Influenza viruses	11
Bacteria	
Chlamydia species†	26
Mycoplasma pneumoniae	27
Staphylococcus aureus	28
Streptococcus pyogenes	28
Streptococcus pneumoniae	28
Nocardia asteroides	29
Gram-positive anaerobes†	30
Neisseria meningitidis	31
Branhamella catarrhalis	31
Pseudomonas aeruginosa	32
Pseudomonas cepacia	32
Francisella tularensis	33
Legionella spp	33
Klebsiella pneumoniae	34
Enterobacteriaceae, other spp	34
Haemophilus influenzae	36
Gram-negative anaerobes†	38
Mycobacterium tuberculosis	40
Other Mycobacterium spp	40
Fungi	
Candida species	43
Cryptococcus neoformans	43
Aspergillus spp	44
Zygomycetes	44
Blastomyces dermatitidis	45
Histoplasma capsulatum	45
Coccidioides immitis	45
Paracoccidioides brasiliensis	45
Parasites	
Pneumocystis carinii	51
Toxoplasma gondii	51
Nematode larvae	52

* Includes sputum, tracheal aspirates, transtracheal aspirates, bronchial washings, bronchial brush specimens, bronchoalveolar lavage specimens, needle aspirates, transbronchial biopsies, and open lung biopsies.
† Chlamydia species may be detected in lung tissue, and anaerobes may be present in transtracheal aspirates, open lung biopsy tissue, and possibly bronchial brush specimens.

Collection, Transport, and Processing

Collection and transport of sputum and tracheal aspirates are similar for all organisms that cause pneumonia. Specimen processing, however, is different and is discussed separately for viruses, bacteria, fungi, and parasites.

A specimen of expectorated sputum optimally is collected early in the morning before the patient eats. The patient should rinse the mouth with water and then expectorate a specimen, preferably 5 to 10 ml, produced by a deep cough. Persons with nonproductive cough may produce a specimen by breathing aerosolized droplets of a solution of 15% sodium chloride and 10% glycerin for about 10 minutes or until a cough reflex is initiated. Induced sputum specimens are especially useful in diagnosis of infections due to mycobacteria, fungi, and Pneumocystis carinii. Tracheal aspirates represent lower respiratory tract secretions, which in patients with tracheostomies are collected in a Lukens trap. Patients with tracheostomies are colonized rapidly by gram-negative bacteria and other nosocomial pathogens, and because bacteria that colonize the respiratory tract cannot be differentiated from those that cause invasive disease, interpretation of results of routine cultures of tracheal aspirates is difficult. Sputum and tracheal aspirate specimens should be delivered promptly to the laboratory. If a delay in transport is unavoidable specimens may be refrigerated for a short time only.

Viruses

Sputum is not the preferred specimen for diagnosing infections of the lower respiratory tract produced by viruses, but such specimens should not be rejected. Detection of potential viral pathogens in sputum (see Table 57–4) requires cell culture. To process the sputum, a swab is immersed in the specimen and placed into 2 ml of transport medium without serum, such as Hanks' balanced salt solution, with twice the usual amount of antibiotics (Chapter 54). The specimen is mixed on a vortex mixer, inoculated to MRC-5, A549, HEp-2, and primary monkey kidney cell cultures, and adsorbed as described in Chapter 54. Maintenance medium without serum is added to the primary monkey kidney cells because serum may contain substances that inhibit influenza viruses. Cultures are incubated at 33° to 37° C, but 33° C is the optimal temperature for myxoviruses growing in HEp-2 and primary kidney cells. In addition, the centrifugation culture technique for detection of CMV and the influenza viruses (described earlier) is recommended.

Bacteria

Specimens of expectorated sputum received in the laboratory for routine bacteriologic culture should be screened first to determine whether they are representative of lower respiratory tract secretions or of saliva. A smear is prepared from that portion of the specimen consisting of purulent material and is stained with Gram stain. In general, specimens that have more than 10 epithelial cells per low-power field (Fig. 57–1) are considered to have significant contamination with saliva and should be rejected. Specimens with fewer than 25 epithelial cells but more than 25 neutrophils per low-power field probably are acceptable (25). The number of neutrophils usually is not considered when determining specimen quality, because the patient may be neutropenic. Screening expectorated sputum samples for detection of Mycoplasma pneumoniae, species of Legionella, and mycobacteria and screening induced sputum specimens and tracheal aspirates to assess their quality is not required. Processing sputum and tracheal aspirate specimens for detection of different bacteria is discussed separately in the following paragraphs for each organism or group of organisms. Detection of bacteria other than those recovered by routine culture must be requested specifically.

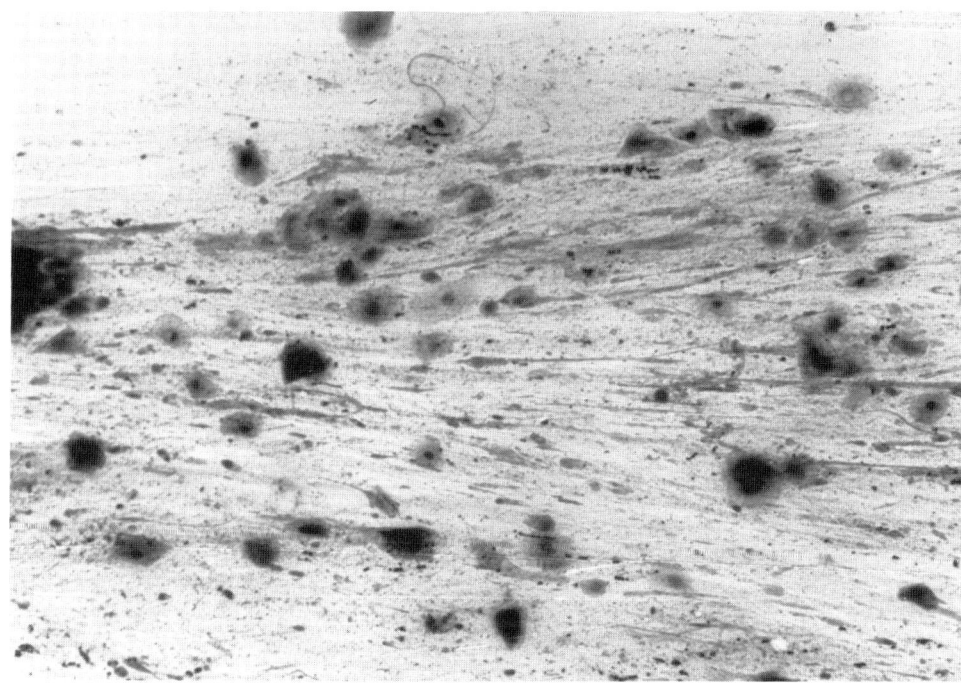

Fig. 57–1. Smear of a sputum considered unacceptable for culture because more than 10 epithelial cells per low-power field are present (Gram stain, ×40).

Mycoplasma pneumoniae. To culture M. pneumoniae from sputum a swab is immersed in the specimen and placed in transport medium with antimicrobial agents (commercially available). Further processing is identical to that described earlier for throat specimens.

Bacteria Detected by Routine Culture. The smears stained with Gram stain prepared from specimens classified as acceptable for culture (discussed above) are examined under oil immersion to determine the relative amounts of organisms. The organisms are estimated as rare, few, moderate, or many, for each kind of bacteria; for example, gram-positive cocci in pairs, chains or clusters, gram-positive bacilli, gram-negative diplococci, and gram-negative bacilli, noting whether or not they are intracellular. Portions of the specimen containing purulent material are inoculated onto sheep blood, MacConkey, and chocolate agar; and it is recommended that specimens from persons with cystic fibrosis also be inoculated onto a commercially available medium selective for Pseudomonas cepacia. Plates incubated at 35° C in an atmosphere of 5 to 7% carbon dioxide are examined after 24 and 48 hours. Organism identification is discussed in Part II.

Media for detection of P. cepacia are incubated at 30°C and held for 4 to 7 days.

Nocardia asteroides. A sputum specimen submitted specifically for recovery of N. asteroides should be screened first to assess its quality (discussed earlier). The smear stained with Gram stain should be examined closely for the presence of long, thin, beaded, branching, gram-positive bacilli typical of Nocardia (Plate IIIE); if such organisms are found a second smear should be prepared and stained with the modified acid-fast stain (Appendix, Procedure 7). Recommended media and culture conditions are outlined in Table 54–4. Inoculation of a second set of plates for incubation at 41° to 45° C is advisable, because N. asteroides grows well at these temperatures and many other bacteria do not. Identification of Nocardia is discussed in Chapter 29.

In many instances cultures for Nocardia are not requested; and because Nocardia usually requires at least 5 to 7 days to grow it would not be detected in a routine culture, which usually is held only 48 hours. Often, typical organisms are seen in the smears stained with Gram stain, alerting laboratory personnel to incubate the plates longer or to inoculate special media (see Table 54–4). If cultures for mycobacteria are requested Nocardia may be detected, because the organism often survives the digestion procedure used to isolate species of Mycobacterium from sputum (described later).

Francisella tularensis. F. tularensis grows on chocolate agar and, therefore, can be recovered by routine bacterial culture of a sputum specimen (discussed earlier), but because it requires prolonged incubation on chocolate agar colonies may not be visible after incubation for 48 hours. If culture for F. tularensis is requested specifically, the specimen should be handled in a biologic safety cabinet and cultured to a medium containing cysteine or cystine. Recommended culture media and growth conditions are outlined in Table 54–4. If the laboratory director prefers that laboratory personnel do not work with infectious material from persons with suspected tularemia, such specimens can be sent to a reference laboratory or to the state health department laboratory.

Legionella species. For optimal detection of species of Legionella, culture and a rapid, direct test (direct fluorescent antibody or nucleic acid hybridization; discussed later) are recommended. Culture is the most sensitive of these methods and should be performed in each case. Sputum specimens and tracheal aspirates submitted for culture of species of Legionella should be diluted 1:10 in a tube of trypticase soy broth containing sterile glass beads and mixed on a vortex mixer or treated with an acid-wash solution (Appendix, Procedure 28) to inhibit overgrowth by the normal bacterial flora. Several drops of the specimen should be inoculated to each of two plates of buffered charcoal yeast extract agar with α-ketoglutarate, one of which should be free of antimicrobial agents. Culture conditions are outlined in Table 54–4. Identification of the species of Legionella is discussed in Chapter 33.

Direct fluorescent antibody staining or nucleic acid hybridization, both of which provide results in several hours, should be used as an adjunct to, but not a replacement for, culture. To perform the direct fluorescent antibody test a smear of the sputum sample is air-dried, heat-fixed, refixed for 10 minutes in 10% neutral buffered formalin, rinsed in distilled water for 1 minute, air-dried, and stained using commercially available antibodies according to the manufacturer's directions. Positive and negative controls should be stained concurrently. Interpretation of the results is discussed in Chapter 33. For nucleic acid hybridization a kit is available commercially, and specimens should be processed according to the manufacturer's directions (26). The sensitivity of the direct fluorescent antibody test and the commercially available DNA probe are similar, so, the method should be selected on the basis of cost effectiveness.

Mycobacterium species. For optimal detection of mycobacteria in sputum, collection of three samples on three separate days is recommended. Sputum and tracheal aspirate specimens must be decontaminated and concentrated to prevent the rapidly growing bacteria in the normal respiratory flora from overgrowing the slowly growing mycobacteria. The N-acetyl-L cysteine–sodium hydroxide method (Appendix, Procedure 27) is used most often for decontamination and concentration; if contamination with gram-negative bacilli (especially Pseudomonas) is a problem, a decontamination procedure using oxalic acid is useful (27). The centrifugal force applied to the specimen influences both the recovery of mycobacteria and the sensitivity of the smears for acid-fast stains (28). For optimal detection centrifugation at 3600 g for 15 minutes or at 2500 g for 20 minutes is recommended (29).

Concentrated sputum and tracheal aspirate specimens should be examined microscopically and inoculated to appropriate culture media. To prepare a smear for staining (with an acid-fast stain or the auramine rhodamine fluorochrome stain, described in Chapter 40 and Procedures 4–6), the sediment is mixed on a vortex mixer, 0.1 to 0.2 ml is aspirated into a Pasteur pipette, and 2 to 3 drops are placed on a glass slide and spread to make a thin, uniform smear. To culture mycobacteria the specimen is inoculated to solid media, a radiometric broth culture system, or a system composed of a broth medium to which a paddle containing solid media is attached for subculturing (Chapter 40). For optimal recovery of mycobacteria with conventional solid media inoculation of three tubes of at least two different media (see Table 54–4) is recommended. Cultures are incubated as described in Table 54–4, and examined weekly for growth. If the radiometric broth culture system is used, 0.4 to 0.5 ml of the specimen is injected into a bottle containing 7H12 medium with added antimicrobial agents. Bottles are incubated in ambient air at 35° to 37° C and tested for carbon dioxide production (according to manufacturer's directions) 3 times per week for 6 weeks. In addition to the broth culture inoculation of one tube of Lowenstein-Jensen medium is recommended. If the biphasic broth-paddle system (commercially available) is selected the broth portion of the system is inoculated, the paddle is attached firmly to the top of the bottle, and the bottle is tipped at regular intervals, allowing the liquid to cover the solid media on the paddle. The system is incubated at 35° to 37° C in ambient air for up to 6 weeks.

Fungi

All specimens submitted for detection of fungi should be handled in a biologic safety cabinet. The quality of the specimens should be determined by screening with smears stained with Gram stain (as described earlier for bacteria). Acceptable expectorated sputum, induced sputum, and tracheal aspirate specimens should be examined microscopically for fungal elements and inoculated to culture media for recovery of fungi. Organisms may be visualized in potassium hydroxide preparations (Appendix, Procedure 19), or in smears stained with the Gram, calcofluor white, or Congo red stain (advantages and disadvantages of these stains are discussed in Chapter 42).

To culture fungi from sputum or from tracheal aspirate specimens several primary planting media are available commercially (Chapters 42 and 54). In general, the following guidelines for media selection are recommended: Media with and without blood enrichment, and with and without cycloheximide should be used; all media should contain antimicrobial agents. In making the selection the laboratory director also should consider cost and the types of fungi usually encountered in the patient population served by the laboratory. Culture conditions are discussed in Chapter 54.

Parasites

The parasites diagnosed in sputum and tracheal aspirates are Pneumocystis carinii, Toxoplasma gondii (Chapter 51) and, rarely, nematode larvae migrating through the lungs on their way to the intestine (Chapter 50).

Pneumocystis carinii. Induced sputum and transtracheal aspirate specimens have been used for diagnosis of pneumocystosis, with mixed results, because with either method it is difficult to collect material washing out of the alveoli (30). In some instances the induced sputum has produced excellent results (31) because of the careful technique used for collection of the sample. In this study (31) more than half the cases of P. carinii pneumonia were diagnosed by examination of the induced sputum. The advantage of this method is the facility with which the sample is collected. Processing and handling of the specimen for diagnosis of pneumocystosis are discussed under bronchoalveolar lavage.

Nematode Larvae. The most important nematode detected in sputum is Strongyloides stercoralis, in persons who have hyperinfection (Chapter 50). Other nematode larvae, such as those of Ascaris lumbricoides in cases of suspected Loeffler's pneumonia and hookworm larvae in cases of the pulmonary phase of cutaneous larva migrans, also can be recovered from sputum (Chapter 50). The sputum sample is delivered to the laboratory, and wet mounts of fresh material are examined under the microscope with low-power magnification. Precise identification of the larvae in question is difficult, best left for the expert in the field; however, if larvae are found in the sputum and the stool, the likely diagnosis is strongyloidiasis.

TRANSTRACHEAL ASPIRATES

A percutaneous transtracheal aspirate is obtained by puncturing the skin and cricothyroid membrane with a needle to create an opening through which a small plastic catheter is inserted into the trachea. Thus, collected secretions are not contaminated by oropharyngeal flora. This technique is especially useful in a patient with severe pneumonia when studies of samples obtained by noninvasive techniques are inconclusive, and for patients with suspected anaerobic pleuropulmonary infection. Transtracheal aspiration, however, cannot be used in patients who are uncooperative, have a bleeding diathesis, or are poorly oxygenated.

Transtracheal aspirates should be transported promptly to the laboratory and processed as rapidly as possible. Pathogens that may be isolated are listed in Table 57–4. Specimen processing is identical to that discussed earlier for sputum, except that screening for its quality is unnecessary, and thioglycolate broth, anaerobic blood agar, and possibly kanamycin-vancomycin laked blood agar also should be inoculated. The latter plates are incubated in an anaerobic atmosphere at 35° to 37° C for 48 hours before being examined, and the broth is incubated 4 to 5 days in ambient air.

BRONCHIAL WASHING, PROTECTED SPECIMEN BRUSH, AND BRONCHOALVEOLAR LAVAGE SPECIMENS

Bronchial washing, protected specimen brush, and bronchoalveolar lavage specimens are useful for diagnosis of pneumonia, especially in ventilated patients and in immunocompromised persons when the pathogen cannot be determined by noninvasive techniques. Bronchial washings are collected by instilling a small amount of sterile physiologic saline into the bronchial tree and withdrawing the fluid. These specimens are contaminated with normal flora of the upper respiratory tract but may provide more useful diagnostic information than sputum culture. For culture of species of Legionella, sputum specimens are preferable to bronchial washings or to bronchoalveolar lavage samples, because the latter are diluted with saline and may contain small amounts of the anesthetic used locally, which inhibits the organism. Processing of bronchial washing specimens is identical to that described earlier for sputum specimens, except that screening smears stained with a Gram stain to determine quality of the specimen is not required.

The protected specimen brush is a small brush that holds 0.01 to 0.001 ml of secretions, placed in a catheter, within a double cannula. The outer cannula has a displaceable polyethylene glycol plug at the tip. To collect a specimen, the cannula is inserted to the desired area, the inner cannula is pushed out, dislodging the protective plug (water soluble), and the brush is extended even farther, beyond the inner cannula. Once the sample is taken, the brush is pulled back into the inner cannula, and both brush and inner cannula are pulled into the outer cannula to prevent contamination of the brush when the catheter is removed.

Specimens collected with a protected specimen brush are used principally for diagnosis of bacterial infections and probably are suitable for aerobic and anaerobic culture. To process the specimen the brush is suspended in 1 ml of broth (for example, thioglycolate broth) or sterile saline, mixed on a vortex mixer, and with an 0.01-ml calibrated inoculating loop the broth is planted onto sheep blood, chocolate, and MacConkey agar, and incubated at 35° to 37° C in an atmosphere of 5 to 7% carbon dioxide. Also, anaerobic blood agar is inoculated for anaerobic incubation. Colony counts greater than 1000 organisms per milliliter of broth (corresponding to 10^6 organisms per milliliter of the original specimen) appear to correlate with infection (32).

A bronchoalveolar lavage specimen, composed of desquamated host cells and secretions from alveolar spaces, is especially useful for detection of viruses, bacteria, fungi, and parasites. Specimen processing is discussed separately for each group of organisms.

Viruses

Processing bronchoalveolar lavage specimens for detection of viruses includes direct microscopic examination and culture. Examination of cytospin preparations stained with Papanicolaou stain allows detection of cytopathic changes, especially useful for diagnosis of pneumonia produced by CMV and HSV (33). Cytospin preparations also may be stained with specific antibodies, a method used mainly for diagnosis of pneumonia caused by CMV (34).

Bronchoalveolar lavage fluid for isolation of viruses is mixed on a vortex mixer and inoculated as described earlier in this chapter for sputum specimens and in Chapter 54. Moreover, centrifugation culture for detection of CMV and the influenza viruses should be performed.

Bacteria

Processing bronchoalveolar lavage specimens for detection of bacteria includes direct microscopic examination and culture. Staining of cytocentrifuge preparations of the fluid with the Gram stain is recommended because visualizing one or more bacteria without squamous epithelial cells per oil immersion field strongly suggests acute pneumonia (35). If requested, cytocentrifuge preparations of fluid also may be stained with specific antibodies to Legionella and with acid-fast stains.

Data indicate that quantitative culture of bronchoalveolar lavage fluid is useful for diagnosis of acute pneumonia caused by routine bacterial pathogens (35,36). The sample is inoculated onto sheep blood, MacConkey, and chocolate agar by using a 0.001-ml calibrated inoculating loop (like that used for urine cultures, Chapter 61). The presence of more than 10^5 colonies per milliliter of lavage fluid correlates with acute bacterial pneumonia, but to recover Nocardia asteroides, Francisella tularensis, or species of Legionella or Mycobacterium the sediment of a centrifuged specimen should be inoculated to appropriate media (as described earlier for detection of these organisms in sputum).

Fungi

Bronchoalveolar lavage specimens submitted for detection of fungi should be examined microscopically and inoculated to appropriate planting media. Organisms may be visualized in a cytospin preparation or in a smear of the sediment of a centrifuged specimen stained with the Gram, calcofluor white, or Congo red stain. For culture, the sediment of a centrifuged specimen should be inoculated onto primary planting media (see guidelines recommended for culture of sputum earlier and Chapters 42 and 54).

Parasites

Samples of bronchial washings, bronchial brush, and bronchoalveolar lavage are used primarily for the diagnosis of pneumocystosis; nematode larvae (see under sputum) and Toxoplasma gondii also can be recovered.

Pneumocystis carinii. The standard sample for diagnosis of pneumonia caused by P. carinii is bronchoalveolar lavage fluid, because more than 90% of the infections are diagnosed by this technique (30). Other samples are less efficient, and open lung biopsy now is reserved predominantly for young children and others for whom a transbronchial procedure is difficult or poorly tolerated. For optimal results the bronchoalveolar lavage should be done in the area of the lung that shows the greatest infiltrate on x-ray films. Random samples, especially in cases with circumscribed lesions, yield poor results.

The specimen should be delivered promptly to the laboratory, and if it is not processed immediately should be refrigerated, except when other microbiologic studies (for example, isolation of cytomegalovirus) are requested from the sample. The specimen is centrifuged at 1200 g for 5 minutes, and smears are prepared from the sediment. A mucolytic agent can be used when the sample has large amounts of mucus, and a lytic agent when it has too many red blood cells (30). The smears should be uniformly thin to allow good staining; imprints should be made from lung biopsy specimens. All smears should be air-dried and fixed in absolute alcohol if the staining procedure requires it. Cytospin preparations are used by some laboratories.

Staining of Pneumocystis carinii for diagnostic purposes has been limited to methenamine silver or one of its many modifications, a practice that often is incomprehensible because methenamine silver stains only the cyst wall. This preference is due, perhaps, to the ease with which the smear can be scanned with low power. Other stains are in use for staining the cyst wall, for example, toluidine blue, modified toluidine blue, cresyl etch violet, Gram-Weigart, and others.

Staining of intracystic bodies and trophozoites is accomplished with Giemsa stain and similar ones. The advantage of these stains is that they stain trophozoites, the largest number of organisms present in a person infected with Pneumocystis carinii, which therefore are easier to detect. P. carinii trophozoites grow in the alveoli in large colonies, erroneously described in the histologic literature as an eosinophilic matrix (37), seen in smears stained with the Giemsa stain as large clumps of organisms staining blue with a minute nucleus. These colonies of organisms are easy to identify under the microscope, but some familiarity with their morphologic characteristics is required.

Other stains based on immunohistochemical methods have been described, especially immunofluorescence and immunoperoxidase, immunostains that are specific and allow easy microscopic scanning of the smear under lower power. The reagents for these staining procedures are available from several manufacturers and their directions should be followed on all steps in processing the sample. Finally, regardless of what stain the laboratory is using, a positive control always must be included.

Toxoplasma gondii. Requests for examination of pulmonary samples for diagnosis of pulmonary toxoplasmosis are rare. T. gondii can be visualized easily in good smears of bronchoalveolar lavage fluid stained with Giemsa stain (38,39).

FINE-NEEDLE ASPIRATES

Percutaneous fine-needle aspiration allows collection of a small amount of material specifically from the involved area of the lung. Given that the volume of the sample collected is small, the clinician should be consulted to establish the priority of requests; the sample is processed accordingly, as described earlier for sputum specimens. Because collecting an aspirate without exposing the sample to air usually is impossible aspirates most often are not acceptable for anaerobic culture.

TRANSBRONCHIAL AND OPEN LUNG BIOPSY SPECIMENS

Transbronchial biopsy specimens are submitted for histologic studies more frequently than for culture. If cultures are ordered, the physician requests must be prioritized, because the specimen generally is small. Impression smears of the tissue are prepared, and the tissue is homogenized in broth to give a 10% suspension (weight to volume) and planted onto the appropriate media (selected according to the request and guidelines presented earlier for sputum specimens).

Open lung biopsy generally is performed when an immunocompromised host has an undiagnosed pulmonary infection. Such specimens should be transported promptly to the laboratory in a sterile container on a piece of moist sterile gauze and processed immediately. A protocol outlining the necessary procedures should be established in the laboratory, to ensure that all tests are performed. The fresh tissue should be examined by a pathologist and divided appropriately for histologic and microbiologic studies (see below).

Viruses

The viruses listed in Table 57-4 are detected in lung tissue by cell culture. The tissue is homogenized in transport medium with a sterile tissue grinder or a mortar and pestle to make a 10% suspension. The suspension is centrifuged at 1500 g for 20 minutes, and the supernatant is used for inoculation of appropriate cell lines (identical to the procedure described earlier for sputum). Centrifugation culture for detection of CMV always should be done; during the influenza season, centrifugation culture for detection of influenza viruses is recommended.

Bacteria

Processing lung tissue for detection of bacteria involves direct microscopic examination and culture. Four to five touch imprints of the specimen should be prepared for staining: Gram stain is used for routine bacteria; auramine rhodamine or an acid-fast stain for mycobacteria (Appendix, Procedures 4–6); the specific fluorescent antibody stain for Legionella (described for sputum earlier), and perhaps a modified acid-fast stain for Nocardia (Appendix, Procedure 7). For culture the tissue is homogenized in broth with a sterile tissue grinder or mortar and pestle to make a 10% suspension and is planted as described earlier for detection of bacteria in sputum, and also to anaerobic blood agar (incubated anaerobically) and to thioglycolate broth (incubated in ambient air). Culture specifically for Francisella tularensis probably is not indicated, although the organism grows on media used to recover Legionella. In addition, culture for Chlamydia trachomatis may be requested, in which case the homogenate should be processed as outlined in the Appendix, Procedure 8.

Fungi

Processing lung tissue for detection of fungi involves direct microscopic examination and culture. Imprints of the lung tissue should be prepared and stained with silver, calcofluor white, or the Congo red stain. The tissue is homogenized as described earlier for bacteria, and is inoculated to appropriate primary planting media (described earlier for sputum).

Parasites

Pulmonary biopsies taken for detection of parasites usually are sent to the surgical pathology laboratory. If they are referred to the clinical laboratory imprints should be made and stained with Giemsa and silver stains. The rest is submitted for histologic processing and examination. The two parasites sought in the imprint preparation are Toxoplasma gondii and Pneumocystis carinii.

REFERENCES

1. Gwalthey JM, Jr: The common cold. *In* Principles and Practice of Infectious Diseases. 3rd ed. Edited by GL Mandell, RG Douglas, Jr, and JE Bennett. New York, Churchill Livingstone, 1990.
2. Mills RD, Cain KJ, and Woods GL: Detection of influenza virus by centrifugal inoculation of MDCK cells and staining with monoclonal antibodies. J Clin Microbiol, *27*:2505, 1989.
3. Johnston SLG, and Siegel CS: Evaluation of direct immunofluorescence, enzyme immunoassay, centrifugation culture, and conventional culture for the detection of respiratory syncytial virus. J Clin Microbiol, *28*:2394, 1990.
4. Minnich LL, Goodenough F, and Ray G: Use of immunofluorescence to identify measles virus infections. J Clin Microbiol, *29*:1148, 1991.
5. Shalit J, McKee PA, Beauchamp H, and Waner JL: Comparison of polyclonal antiserum versus monoclonal antibodies for the rapid diagnosis of influenza A virus infections by immunofluorescence in clinical specimens. J Clin Microbiol, *22*:877, 1985.
6. Masters HB, et al: Comparison of nasopharyngeal washings and swab specimens for diagnosis of respiratory syncytial virus by EIA, FAT, and cell culture. Diagn Microbiol Infect Dis, *8*:101, 1987.
7. Ahluwalia GS, and Hammond GW: Comparison of cell culture and three enzyme-linked immunosorbent assays for the rapid diagnosis of respiratory syncytial virus from nasopharyngeal aspirate and tracheal secretion specimens. Diagn Microbiol Infect Dis, *9*:187, 1988.
8. Halstead DC, Todd S, and Fritch G: Evaluation of five methods for respiratory syncytial virus detection. J Clin Microbiol, *28*:1021, 1990.
9. Swierkosz EM, et al: Evaluation of the Abbott TESTPACK RSV enzyme immunoassay for detection of respiratory syncytial virus in nasopharyngeal swab specimens. J Clin Microbiol, *27*:1151, 1989.
10. Waner JL, et al: Comparison of Directigen FLU-A with viral isolation and direct immunofluorescence for the rapid detection and identification of influenza A virus. J Clin Microbiol, *29*:479, 1991.
11. Paisley JW, et al: Rapid diagnosis of Chlamydia trachomatis in infants by direct immunofluorescence microscopy of nasopharyngeal secretions. J Pediatr, *109*:653, 1986.
12. Hammerschlag MR, Roblin PM, Gelling M, and Worku M: Comparison of two enzyme immunoassays to culture for the diagnosis of chlamydial conjunctivitis and respiratory infections in infants. J Clin Microbiol, *28*:1725, 1990.
13. Friedman RL: Pertussis: The disease and new diagnostic methods. Clin Microbiol Rev, *1*:365, 1988.
14. Baron EJ, and Finegold SM (eds): Bailey and Scott's Diagnostic Microbiology. 8th ed. St. Louis, CV Mosby, 1990.
15. Woods GL, and Mills RD: Conventional tube cell culture compared with centrifugal inoculation of MRC-5 cells and staining with monoclonal antibodies for detection of herpes simplex virus in clinical specimens. J Clin Microbiol, *26*:570, 1988.
16. Woods GL, Young A, Johnson A, and Thiele GM: Detection of cytomegalovirus by 24-well plate centrifugation assay using a monoclonal antibody to an early nuclear antigen and by conventional cell culture. J Virol Methods, *18*:207, 1987.
17. Woods GL, Yamamoto M, and Young A: Detection of adenovirus by rapid 24-well plate centrifugation and conventional cell culture with dexamethasone. J Virol Methods, *20*:109, 1988.
18. Kleemold SRM, Karjalainen JE, and Raty RKH: Rapid diagnosis of Mycoplasma pneumoniae infection: Clinical evaluation of a commercial probe test. J Infect Dis, *162*:70, 1990.
19. Bellon J, Weise B, Verschraegen G, and DeMeyere M: Selective streptococcal agar versus blood agar for detection of group A β-hemolytic streptococci in patients with acute pharyngitis. J Clin Microbiol, *29*:2084, 1991.
20. Bisno AL: Medical progress: Group A streptococcal infections and acute rheumatic fever. N Engl J Med, *325*:783, 1991.
21. Krech T, and Hollis DG: Corynebacterium and related organisms. *In* Manual of Clinical Microbiology. 5th ed. Edited by A Balows, et al. Washington, DC, American Society for Microbiology, 1991.
22. Koneman EW, et al (eds): Color Atlas and Textbook of Diag-

nostic Microbiology. 3rd ed. Philadelphia, JB Lippincott, 1988.
23. Centers for Disease Control: Surveillance of major causes of hospitalization among the elderly. United States, 1988. MMWR, 40(SS-1):7, 1991.
24. Donowitz GR, and Mandell GL: Acute pneumonia. *In* Principles and Practice of Infectious Diseases. 3rd ed. Edited by GL Mandell, RG Douglas, Jr, and JE Bennett. New York, Churchill Livingstone, 1990.
25. Murray PR, and Washington JA II: Microscopic and bacteriologic analysis of expectorated sputum. Mayo Clin Proc, 50:339, 1975.
26. Doebbeling BN, et al: Prospective evaluation of the Gen-Probe assay for detection of Legionellae in respiratory specimens. Eur J Clin Microbiol Infect Dis, 7:748, 1988.
27. Cooper HJ, and Uyei N: Oxalic acid as a reagent for isolating tubercle bacilli and a study of the growth of acid-fast nonpathogens on different mediums with their reactions to chemical reagents. J Lab Clin Med, 15:348, 1930.
28. Rickman TW, and Moyer NP: Increased sensitivity of acid-fast smears. J Clin Microbiol, 11:618, 1980.
29. Ratnam S, and March SB: Effect of relative centrifugal force and centrifugation time on sedimentation of mycobacteria in clinical specimens. J Clin Microbiol, 23:582, 1986.
30. Smith JW, and Bartlett MS: Laboratory diagnosis of pneumocystosis. Clin Lab Med, 11:957, 1991.
31. Bigby TD, Margolskee D, Curtis JL, et al. The usefulness of induced sputum in the diagnosis of patients with the acquired immunodeficiency syndrome. Am Rev Respir Dis, 133:515, 1986.
32. Pollock HM, et al: Diagnosis of bacterial pulmonary infections with quantitative protected catheter cultures obtained during bronchoscopy. J Clin Microbiol, 17:255, 1983.
33. Woods GL, Thompson AB, Rennard SL, and Linder J: Detection of cytomegalovirus in bronchoalveolar lavage specimens: Spin amplification and staining with a monoclonal antibody to the early nuclear antigen for diagnosis of cytomegalovirus pneumonia. Chest, 98:568, 1990.
34. Gleaves CA, and Meyers JD: Rapid detection of cytomegalovirus in bronchoalveolar lavage specimens from marrow transplant patients: Evaluation of a direct fluorescein-conjugated monoclonal antibody reagent. J Virol Methods, 26:345, 1989.
35. Kahn FW, and Jones JM: Diagnosing bacterial respiratory infection by bronchoalveolar lavage. J Infect Dis, 155:862, 1987.
36. Thorpe JE, et al: Bronchoalveolar lavage for diagnosing acute bacterial pneumonia. J Infect Dis, 155:855, 1987.
37. Gutierrez Y: The biology of Pneumocystis carinii. Semin Diagn Pathol, 6:203, 1989.
38. Bendelac A, Laporte JP, Marteau M, et al: Decoverte d'une localisation pulmonaire de Toxoplasma gondii chez in malade immunodeprimee. Nouv Presse Med, 13:1213, 1984.
39. Tourani JM, Israel-Biet D, Venet A, et al. Unusual pulmonary infection in a puzzling presentation of AIDS. Lancet, 1:989, 1985.

Chapter 58

CARDIOVASCULAR AND HEMATOPOIETIC SYSTEMS

Blood is one of the most important specimens received in the laboratory for microbiologic studies. Nearly 200,000 cases of septicemia, confirmed by isolation of the responsible pathogen from blood, occur in the United States each year, and 40 to 50% are fatal (1). Other specimens include intravascular catheter tips, material from endocardial vegetations, endomyocardial biopsy tissue, bone marrow, lymph node tissue and aspirates, and purulent material from splenic abscesses.

BLOOD

Blood samples are collected to detect pathogens in the blood by culture or by microscopic examination of a peripheral smear, reviewed here, and for separation into serum for serologic studies, discussed at the end of this chapter. The ability to detect and identify blood-borne pathogens is one of the most important functions of the microbiology laboratory. Culture of blood is essential for identifying bacteria responsible for bacteremia, sepsis, infections of native and prosthetic valves (Table 58–1), suppurative thrombophlebitis, mycotic aneurysms, and infections of vascular grafts. Blood cultures also are useful for diagnosing some viral infections (Table 58–2) and invasive or disseminated infections caused by certain fungi, especially species of Candida, Cryptococcus neoformans, species of Fusarium, and Histoplasma capsulatum. Parasites are detected in blood by microscopic examination of peripheral smears. In general, blood should be collected for culture before beginning antimicrobial therapy when any of the following findings are present: fever (38° C or greater), hypothermia (36° C or lower), leukocytosis (especially with a leftward shift), granulocytopenia.

Timely detection and accurate identification of organisms in the blood depend on appropriate collection, transport, and processing of the specimen. These steps differ for different groups of organisms and are discussed separately for viruses, bacteria and fungi, and parasites.

Collection, Transport, and Processing

Germane to the detection of all micro-organisms in the blood is the technique of specimen collection. To minimize contamination of blood specimens by skin flora the venipuncture site should be prepared with a bactericidal agent. The skin first should be cleaned with alcohol (70% isopropyl or ethyl alcohol) and then rubbed with a 1 to 2% iodine solution, an iodophor, or chlorhexidine. For maximum antisepsis the area should dry for 1 to 2 minutes prior to venipuncture. Other aspects of specimen collection differ for viruses, bacteria, fungi, and parasites.

Viruses

Blood specimens are useful for diagnosing infections with a limited number of viruses (see Table 58–2). Because viremia usually occurs during the incubation period or the first day or two after symptoms begin, blood should be collected early in the illness. An exception is human immunodeficiency virus (HIV), which is detected nearly continuously in peripheral blood mononuclear cells and plasma of most seropositive persons (2). One blood sample per 24-hour period collected from a peripheral vein or through an intravascular catheter is adequate for virus detection.

Specimen requirements differ for different viruses, as indicated in Table 58–2. All blood samples should be transported to the laboratory for processing as rapidly as possible. If a delay in processing is unavoidable, specimens may be stored overnight at 4° C, except specimens for recovery of HIV, which should be maintained at room temperature.

Of the viruses listed in Table 58–2 only those detected routinely in the clinical virology laboratory—cytomegalovirus (CMV) and the enteroviruses—are discussed. For detection of the remaining viruses the specimens must be sent to a reference laboratory, which should be contacted for specific shipping requirements.

Processing blood specimens for detection of CMV and the enteroviruses involves separating the component most likely to contain the virus and inoculating that fraction to cell monolayers that support viral replication. CMV is recovered most often from neutrophils but may be present in peripheral blood mononuclear cells; thus, for optimal recovery, both neutrophils and mononuclear cells should be cultured (3). The enteroviruses are recovered equally well from leukocytes, primarily mononuclear cells, and from serum (4).

To separate leukocytes, blood with anticoagulants must be collected. Opinions regarding the optimal anticoagulant for recovery of CMV differ. If plasmagel is used to separate leukocytes (described later), sodium heparin is the recommended anticoagulant. Some investigators prefer citrated blood because in one study heparin had an inhibitory effect on some herpesviruses (5). By using plasmagel, both leukocyte populations are separated in one step (6). Briefly, heparinized blood and plasmagel are mixed in a 10-ml tube (four parts blood to one part plasmagel), and the mixture is allowed to settle at room temperature for 45 minutes. The upper layer, containing plasma and leukocytes, is transferred to a second tube and is centrifuged at 200 g for 30 minutes. The plasma is removed, and the cell pellet is washed twice and resuspended in 2 to 3 ml of maintenance medium.

Table 58–1. Organisms Responsible for Infective Endocarditis Involving Native Valves (NVE) and Prosthetic Valves (PVE)

	Prevalence (%)		
		PVE	
Organism	NVE	Early	Late
Viridans streptococci	30–40	<5	25
Other streptococci	15–25	1	<1
Enterococcus spp	5–20	<5	10
Staphylococcus aureus	10–15	15	10
Coagulase-negative staphylococci	<5	35	25
Corynebacterium spp	<1	10	4
Aerobic gram-negative bacilli*	2–15	15	10
Other bacteria†	<5	1	2
Fungi‡	<5	10	5
Culture negative	<5–25	1	5

* Includes Pseudomonas aeruginosa and the Enterobacteriaceae.
† Includes Coxiella burnetii, gram-positive anaerobes, Neisseria gonorrhoeae, species of Brucella, Haemophilus species, Actinobacillus actinomycetemcomitans, Cardiobacterium hominis, Kingella species, Eikenella corrodens, and gram-negative anaerobes.
‡ Predominantly species of Candida and Aspergillus.

Alternatively, a two-step procedure may be used to separate the leukocyte fractions. Mononuclear cells are collected by layering blood in anticoagulant (heparin, citrate, or ethylenediaminotetraacetic acid [EDTA] is acceptable) onto a Lymphoprep or Ficoll Hypaque gradient in a ratio of 2:1. The gradient is centrifuged, the interface containing mononuclear cells is removed and washed, and the cell pellet is resuspended in 2 to 3 ml of maintenance medium. In a second step, the erythrocytes and neutrophils, which sediment below the Ficoll layer, are mixed with dextran in a 2:1 ratio and the mixture is allowed to settle at room temperature for 1 to 2 hours. The neutrophil supernatant is removed, washed, and added to the suspension of mononuclear cells.

To separate serum the blood is collected in a tube without anticoagulant and allowed to clot at 4° C. When a firm clot forms the sample is centrifuged at 2000 g for 10 minutes at 4° C, and the serum is aseptically removed.

Selection of which cell monolayers to inoculate for virus isolation is based on the virus expected to be present. To recover CMV, inoculation of two tubes of MRC-5 cell cultures is recommended. Incubating monolayers in maintenance medium containing 10^{-5}M dexamethasone for a minimum of 24 hours before inoculation increases the rate of detection of CMV and decreases the time for appearance of cytopathic effect (CPE) (7). For recovery of enteroviruses, MRC-5 and primary monkey kidney cells should be inoculated, and the rate of isolation may be increased by also inoculating Buffalo green monkey kidney and human rhabdomyosarcoma cells (8). Serum specimens are inoculated, adsorbed, incubated, and examined for virus-specific cytopathic effect, as described in Chapter 54. For leukocyte suspensions cell monolayers are inoculated with 0.5 ml of specimen, 1.0 ml of maintenance medium is added, and cell cultures are incubated overnight. The cell suspension then is removed, cell monolayers are washed with sterile phosphate-buffered saline, 1.5 ml of maintenance medium is added, and cultures are incubated 2 weeks (for enteroviruses) to 3 weeks (for CMV) and examined two or three times per week for CPE.

In addition to conventional cell culture, centrifugation culture (Appendix, Procedure 2) should be performed when detection of CMV is requested (9,10). Moreover, viremia with CMV may be detected by staining cytospin preparations of leukocytes with monoclonal antibodies against viral matrix antigens, followed by staining with peroxidase-labeled goat antimouse antibodies (11). Leukocytes showing granular staining of the nuclear membrane are positive for CMV.

Bacteria and Fungi

The optimal time to collect blood for cultures when bacteremia or fungemia is suspected is just before the occurrence of a chill, but because this is difficult to predict, most blood cultures are obtained after the onset of fever and chills. Blood is collected with a needle and syringe and, without changing needles, is injected directly into bottles of culture media or other blood culture system (12). The contents of bottles or tubes should be mixed immediately, and the specimen should be transported to the laboratory at room temperature as soon as possible after collection. Specimens never should be refrigerated.

Table 58–2. Specimen Requirements for Optimal Detection of Viruses from Blood*

	Specimen Requirements		
Virus	Type Collected	Fraction Used for Detection	Volume (ml)
Cytomegalovirus	Heparinized blood	Leukocytes	5–10
Enteroviruses	Blood, with or without anticoagulant†	Serum or leukocytes	5–10
Human immunodeficiency virus	Heparinized blood	Mononuclear cells or plasma	30–50
Human herpesvirus-6	Heparinized blood	Mononuclear cells	5–10
Parvovirus B19	Blood without anticoagulant	Serum	5–10
Arthropod-borne viruses‡	Blood, with or without anticoagulant	Leukocytes or homogenized clot	5–10

* All samples are transported at room temperature, except specimens for detection of arthropod-borne viruses are transported at 8° C.
† Heparin, citrate, or EDTA may be used.
‡ Includes viruses of eastern, western, and Venezuelan equine encephalitis, St. Louis and California encephalitis, yellow fever, dengue, and Colorado tick fever.

In adults with bacteremia the number of colony-forming units per milliliter of blood often is small. For example, in one study, one fourth of patients who were bacteremic with Staphylococcus aureus and over half of those with bacteremia due to Escherichia coli or Pseudomonas aeruginosa had colony counts of fewer than one per milliliter of blood (13). Given this low level of bacteremia in adults collection of 20 to 30 ml of blood per culture is recommended strongly (1,14). In infants and children the concentration of micro-organisms is higher, and collection of 1 to 5 ml of blood per culture is satisfactory (15).

Recommendations regarding the number of blood specimens necessary are based on the nature of the bacteremia—transient, intermittent, or continuous. Transient bacteremia follows manipulation of a focus of infection (such as an abscess, a furuncle, or cellulitis), instrumentation of a contaminated mucosal surface (as during dental procedures, cystoscopy, urethral catheterization, suction abortion, or sigmoidoscopy), or a surgical procedure in a contaminated site (such as transurethral resection of the prostate, vaginal hysterectomy, colon resection, and débridement of infected burns). Transient bacteremia also occurs early in the course of many systemic and localized infections such as meningitis, pneumonia, pyogenic arthritis, and osteomyelitis. Typically, intermittent bacteremia is associated with an undrained abscess, whereas continuous bacteremia is the hallmark of intravascular infection such as bacterial endocarditis, mycotic aneurysm, or an infected intravascular catheter. Continuous bacteremia also occurs during the first few weeks of typhoid fever and brucellosis.

Two separate blood cultures are nearly always adequate for isolating pathogens responsible for intravascular infections (16). In one study of persons with intravascular infection, the rates of positivity of the first, first two, and first three blood cultures per septic episode were 80%, 90%, and 99%, respectively (17). Data from another evaluation showed that 91% of all septic episodes were detected by the first blood culture, and the figure increased to 99% with a second culture (18). Therefore, three blood culture specimens in a 24-hour period should be sufficient to detect almost all potential bacterial pathogens (19). The optimal interval between cultures is unknown, but 30 to 60 minutes has been suggested. However, if initiation of antimicrobial therapy is deemed urgent, cultures should be collected before therapy is begun, from separate sites within a few minutes.

Organisms such as the coagulase-negative staphylococci, viridans streptococci, and corynebacteria are frequent blood culture contaminants but also may be true pathogens. Collecting two sets of blood cultures per febrile episode helps distinguish probable pathogens from contaminants, which generally are present in only one bottle of one set of cultures, whereas pathogens typically are recovered from more than one set. Because more than one febrile episode may occur in a 24-hour period, and two sets of cultures should be collected per episode, a maximum of four sets of cultures per day should be allowed.

Most blood specimens for culture are obtained by venipuncture of peripheral veins. Collecting arterial blood does not appear to improve the yield of micro-organisms, and culture of blood collected through an indwelling cannula is associated with increased recovery of presumed contaminants (20,21). Because the latter practice often results in additional cultures and unnecessary antimicrobial therapy, collection of blood for culture through an intravascular catheter is not recommended, except for umbilical artery catheters in infants (22,23). However, quantitative cultures of blood collected through an intravascular catheter may be useful in determining whether the catheter is the site of infection (24).

Processing blood specimens for detection of bacteria and fungi differs for different organisms or groups of organisms, and is discussed separately.

Bacteria Detected by Routine Culture. Because host factors—antibodies, complement, phagocytic white blood cells, and antimicrobial agents—may impede recovery of micro-organisms from blood various approaches have been used to counteract these factors. Diluting the blood specimen in broth medium in a 1:10 ratio provides optimal neutralization of the serum bactericidal activity (1). Incorporating 0.025% sodium polyanetholsulfonate in the blood culture media inhibits phagocytosis and complement activation and inactivates aminoglycosides. Methods used to counteract the presence of antimicrobial agents include adding penicillinases to broth media to inactivate penicillins; using antibiotic-adsorbent resins; and lysing red and white blood cells, concentrating the micro-organisms by filtration or centrifugation, and culturing the concentrate on media free of antibiotics (1).

Several blood culture systems, each with advantages and disadvantages, are available (1,22). Conventional broth culture systems that use nutritionally enriched liquid media recover most bacteria. Tryptic or trypticase soy, supplemented peptone, brain-heart infusion, Columbia, or brucella broth is used to recover aerobes and facultative anaerobes; thioglycolate, Thiol, or anaerobic heart infusion broth is used to isolate of anaerobes. Two bottles should be inoculated, and one should be vented to ensure recovery of aerobes. Both bottles are examined daily for 7 days for evidence of growth, indicated by turbidity, hemolysis, gas production, discrete colonies, or a combination of these. When growth is apparent, a smear of the broth is stained with Gram stain, examined microscopically, and the broth is subcultured to appropriate agar media. Routine subculture of macroscopically negative broths should be performed from the vented bottle 6 to 18 hours after inoculation. Routine subculture of the anaerobic bottle is unnecessary unless the patient is a child, because anaerobic subcultures increase the yield of Haemophilus influenzae, a common childhood pathogen (Chapter 36). Advantages of conventional broth cultures are low cost of materials and a low prevalence of contamination. The major drawback is the time-consuming process of routine subculture.

Using a biphasic system consisting of a conventional blood culture broth bottle with an attached chamber containing agars on a slide obviates routine manual subculture. To subculture this biphasic system the bottle is tipped, allowing the blood-broth mixture to enter the chamber and flow over the agar media. Colonies on the agar medium are used for identification and susceptibility testing. This system is less labor intensive than the conventional system, and, for recovery of aerobic and facultative bacteria and yeasts is comparable to or better than other systems (25). The yield of anaerobes may be higher from conventional broth systems.

The lysis-centrifugation blood culture system consists of a tube containing reagents that inhibit both coagulation and the complement cascade, lyse blood cells, and provide a cushion for the micro-organisms during centrifugation. Blood (6 to 10 ml) is added to the tube, which is inverted several times to prevent clotting, and is transported to the laboratory as soon as possible. Ideally, the specimen is processed immediately; however, processing can be delayed a maximum of 8 hours without adversely affecting recovery of micro-organisms. To process the culture the tube is centrifuged 30 minutes at 3000 g, the supernatant is discarded, and the sediment is mixed on a vortex mixer and planted onto agar media. Special tubes for small-volume samples from infants and young children also are available. Advantages of this system, compared to broth systems, include rapid detection and higher recovery rate of Staphylococcus aureus, some of the Enterobacteriaceae, and fungi; the growth of colonies for direct identification and susceptibility testing, the ability to carry out quantitative cultures, and finally, flexibility, because special media can be inoculated to recover organisms that have specific growth requirements, such as species of Legionella and mycobacteria. However, the system is labor intensive and less likely to detect bacteremia due to Streptococcus pneumoniae, Haemophilus influenzae, or anaerobes, and the risk of contamination is increased.

A few automated blood culture systems are currently available commercially. One relies on infrared detection of carbon dioxide released during metabolism of carbohydrates by micro-organisms (Fig. 58–1). The early model of this system, based on radiometric detection of radioactive carbon dioxide released into the atmosphere above the medium during metabolism of carbon-14–labeled substrates, now is used almost exclusively to detect mycobacteria (Chapter 40). With the infrared detection system two broth culture media in bottles designed specifically for the instrument—one for recovery of aerobes and the other for anaerobes—are inoculated with the blood. During the initial incubation bottles incubed aerobically are agitated on a rotary shaker. At specific intervals the bottles are placed into the monitoring module and automatically moved past a detector, which inserts two needles through a rubber septum on the top of the bottle and draws out a sample for analysis of the gas that has accumulated above the liquid medium. Specimens with readings above a specific threshold or specimens that demonstrate a specified increase in threshold are automatically flagged for smears stained with Gram stain and subculture. Daily reading by the instrument replaces subculture of specimens that have no visual signs of growth. Advantages of this system are

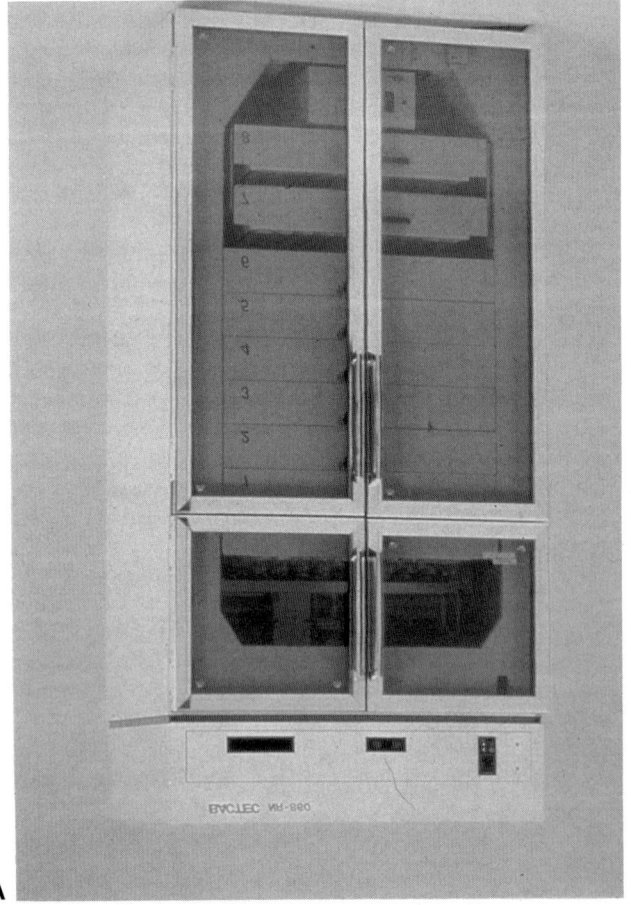
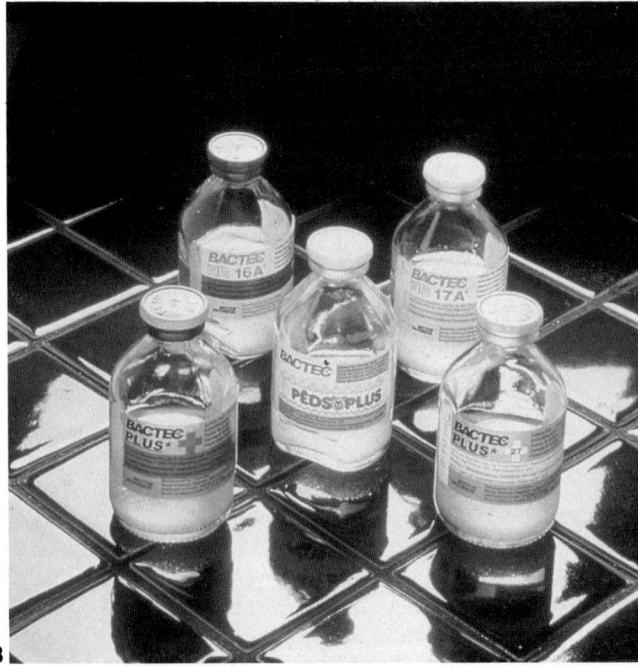

Fig. 58–1. *A*, Fully automated blood culture system that relies on the infrared detection of CO_2. *B*, Available media. (Courtesy of Becton Dickinson Diagnostic Instrument Systems, Sparks, MD.)

automation and the ability to monitor growth without subculture. The major criticism of the system in the past was the cost of handling the recommended 20-ml blood volume per venipuncture, because the maximum blood volume per bottle was 5 ml. However, media that accommodate up to 10 ml of blood have been developed, and data indicate that they allow more rapid and enhanced detection of most bacteria and fungi (26). The presence of resins in these high-volume media obviates the need to use special resin-containing media for persons receiving antimicrobial agents. Moreover, media designed specifically for recovery of organisms from pediatric patients and for recovery of fungi are available (27).

A second automated blood culture system is based on the colorimetric detection of carbon dioxide produced during microbial growth (Fig. 58–2) (28). A carbon dioxide sensor is bonded to the bottom of each blood culture bottle and is separated from the broth medium by a membrane that is impermeable to most ions and to components of media and blood but freely permeable to carbon dioxide. As bacteria multiply, carbon dioxide is released into the broth medium and the pH decreases, causing the sensor to become lighter green and then yellow, a change associated with an increase in reflected red light. Color changes are monitored once every 10 minutes by a colorimetric detector, consisting of a diode that emits red light and a photodiode that absorbs red light.

***Brucella* species.** When brucellosis is suspected, blood should be collected early in the disease. To recover Brucella, one of the systems described earlier, or a vented biphasic (Castaneda) system incubated at 35° C in 5 to 10% carbon dioxide, may be used. All cultures should be incubated 3 to 4 weeks rather than the routine 7 days.

***Borrelia* species.** Infections with species of Borrelia, except Borrelia burgdorferi (the agent of Lyme disease, most commonly diagnosed serologically), are diagnosed by detecting spirochetes in the peripheral blood during febrile periods. Organisms are visualized in wet preparations made by mixing a drop of blood with a drop of sodium citrate and examining it with light or darkfield microscopy, and in thin and thick blood films stained with Wright or Giemsa stains examined by conventional light microscopy. Because spirochetemia may be mild, thick films, prepared by placing a drop of blood on a slide and stirring with a toothpick or applicator stick to evenly spread the blood over a 1-cm area, should be examined first. Dehemoglobinization occurs during staining, making the smear transparent to allow easy recognition of the blue-stained spirochetes. With mild infections microhematocrit concentration enhances spirochete detection (29).

Leptospira interrogans. To isolate L. interrogans from blood, a few drops of fresh or anticoagulated blood collected during the first week of illness are added to each of three or four tubes of leptospiral semisolid culture medium. Recommended media and culture conditions are described in Table 54–4.

***Mycobacterium* species.** Two methods may be used to recover mycobacteria from blood specimens. With the lysis-centrifugation technique, a concentrate is prepared; the sediment is inoculated to Middlebrook 7H10, Lowenstein-Jensen, or both, and the cultures are incubated up to 8 weeks. An alternative, and perhaps more rapid, approach is the commercially available radiometric broth system (Chapter 40). Growth of micro-organisms in the media causes release of radioactive carbon dioxide into the atmosphere above the broth, and an instrument measures the amount of radioactivity present.

Bartonella bacilliformis. B. bacilliformis may be seen in blood smears stained with the Giemsa stain, appearing as red-violet cocci, bacilli, or occasionally as curved or ring forms. To isolate B. bacilliformis the blood is inoculated to brain-heart infusion broth and incubated at room temperature in ambient air.

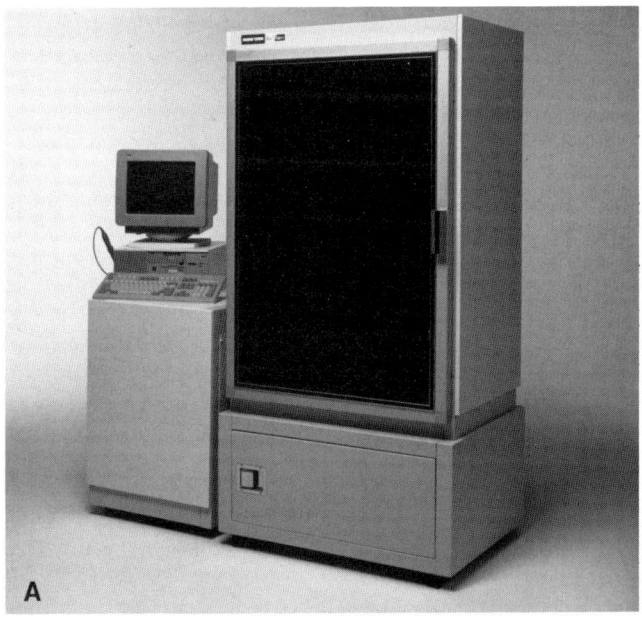
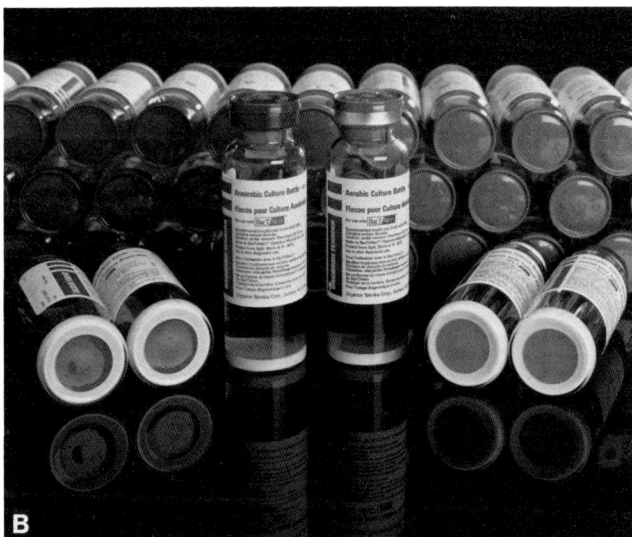

Fig. 58–2. *A*, Fully automated blood culture system that relies on the colorimetric detection of CO_2. *B*, Available media. (Courtesy of Organon Teknika Corporation, Durham, NC.)

Parasites

Blood samples are received in the laboratory for diagnosis of malaria, babesiosis, trypanosomiasis, and some filariases. Occasionally visceral leishmaniasis is diagnosed in peripheral blood samples and, though it has not yet been described, it is expected that Toxoplasma gondii will be reported in blood smears. Blood samples should be collected and received promptly in the laboratory in tubes with anticoagulant. Malaria parasites degenerate rapidly, so samples for its diagnosis should be processed rapidly. Sometimes smears already made are received in the laboratory, but these smears should have been fixed in absolute alcohol soon after they were made. The techniques used in the laboratory for detecting these organisms are the same and, in this section, are discussed in order of the simplest to the most complicated.

Direct Mounts. The simplest preparation from a sample of blood is the direct mount (one drop of blood on a glass slide covered with a cover glass), which should be examined immediately. Direct mounts are excellent when either trypanosomiasis or filariasis is the clinical diagnosis, because the trypomastigotes and the microfilariae easily can be seen moving, often with low or medium power. The definitive diagnosis is made by staining smears and studying the organisms.

Thin Smears. Made as for hematologic work and stained in a similar manner, the thin blood smear is the standard preparation for determining the species of Plasmodium, Babesia, Trypanosoma, and microfilariae. Occasionally it also allows recognition of visceral leishmaniae.

Thin smears for parasitologic work preferably are stained manually with Giemsa stain after fixing the smears. In the clinical laboratory of today, however, automated hematologic staining does just as well. Examination of smears should begin with a quick scan at low power to determine if microfilariae are present. Microfilariae are large organisms (100 to 200 µm), easily seen, usually at the lateral edges of the smear. After they are located, microfilariae should be studied under oil immersion for proper identification (discussed in Chapter 52). After scanning with low power, scanning with a high dry objective is done, searching for trypanosomes. Finally, a careful examination under oil immersion is done to find Plasmodium, Babesia, Trypanosoma and Leishmania, and to identify by the characteristics described in Chapter 51.

Thick Smears. Preparation of thick smears is useful for detection of all parasites mentioned earlier, and is part of the minimum laboratory workup for their diagnosis. A drop of blood is placed on a clean glass slide and, with the corner of another slide, it is gently spread to cover a 1-cm square. The preparation is allowed to dry and without fixation is stained with Giemsa stain, allowing for its dehemoglobinization (Appendix, Procedure 26).

Concentration. For trypanosomiasis, a simple concentration technique is available. The blood sample is centrifuged and the buffy coat is used to make both fresh and thin smears. Other techniques are more research tools and not available to the routine laboratory.

Knott's Concentration. An easy method for diagnosis of filariasis uses 8 ml of 1% formalin and 2 ml of the blood sample. The blood is mixed with the formalin, vigorously shaken until the red blood cells are lysed completely, and centrifuged at 2000 g for 5 minutes. The supernatant is then decanted and the sediment is used to prepare smears, which are allowed to dry and stained with the Giemsa stain or another hematologic stain. The microfilariae usually appear extended because they are fixed by the 1% formalin.

INTRAVASCULAR CATHETER TIPS

Microbiologic study of intravascular catheter tips is done for diagnosis of septicemia related to organisms growing on the catheter, a complication in about 8% of venous cannulations, affecting nearly 25,000 persons in the United States each year (30). Bacteria are responsible for most of these infections, but yeasts occasionally are involved. The infection is diagnosed by the semiquantitative culture method described by Maki and coworkers (30). The catheter is removed, and the terminal 5- to 7-cm segment is placed in a sterile tube and transported immediately to the laboratory, where it is processed as soon as possible. The catheter segment is transferred to the surface of a sheep blood agar plate and, using sterile forceps, rolled back and forth across the surface at least four times. Cultures are incubated up to 72 hours at 35° to 37° C in 5 to 7% carbon dioxide. Organisms recovered in quantities of 15 or more colonies are considered significant.

ENDOCARDIAL VEGETATIONS

Microbiologic studies of endocardial vegetations are performed to identify the pathogen (see Table 58–1). Vegetations obtained at surgery or autopsy should be transported immediately to the laboratory in a sterile container. A pathologist should examine the fresh material and divide the specimen appropriately for histologic and microbiologic studies if separate specimens were not collected.

Processing endocardial vegetations for detection of bacteria and fungi involves preparing a homogenate, used for direct examination and culture. The vegetation fragments are homogenized in a small amount of broth to make a 10 to 20% (weight per volume) suspension. A smear of the homogenate is prepared and stained with Gram stain. When fungal culture is requested, a potassium hydroxide preparation (Appendix, Procedure 19) may be examined, or a separate smear is prepared and stained with Gomori methenamine silver, calcofluor white, or Congo red stains (Chapter 42).

For routine bacterial culture the homogenate is inoculated onto sheep blood and chocolate agar (incubated in 5 to 7% carbon dioxide), into thioglycolate broth (incubated in ambient air), and onto anaerobic blood agar (incubated anaerobically). Incubation times and temperatures are discussed in Chapter 54. When brucellosis is suspected media and growth conditions outlined in Table 54–4 should be used. To recover fungi enriched media (such as brain-heart infusion, SABHI, or inhibitory mold agar), with and without cycloheximide, should be inoculated with 0.5 to 1.0 ml of the suspension and incubated as described in Chapter 54.

ENDOMYOCARDIAL BIOPSIES

Microbiologic studies of endomyocardial biopsy specimens are performed to identify the agent of myocarditis (Table 58–3). Tissue is obtained at surgery and should be delivered immediately to the laboratory in a sterile container. A pathologist should examine the fresh tissue and divide it appropriately for histologic and microbiologic studies if separate samples are not collected. Because the amount of tissue submitted often is small and may be insufficient for all studies requested consultation with the physician is essential to determine which tests should be performed to identify the pathogens most likely responsible for the disease. Specimen processing for detection of viruses, bacteria, fungi, and parasites differs and is discussed for each group of organisms.

Viruses

The enteroviruses are responsible for almost all cases of viral myocarditis. Other viruses (varicella-zoster, cytomegalovirus, Epstein-Barr, adenovirus, hepatitis B, measles, mumps, influenza A and B, rabies, rubella, dengue, yellow fever, lymphocytic choriomeningitis, Argentine and Bolivian hemorrhagic fever, and HIV) are only rarely associated with myocarditis and are not discussed further (31).

Detection of enteroviruses in the clinical virology laboratory requires culture. The biopsy fragments are homogenized in a small amount of viral transport medium (such as Hanks' balanced salt solution) with a sterile tissue grinder or mortar and pestle. The homogenate then is inoculated to appropriate cell monolayers, adsorbed, and incubated as described earlier for blood specimens. Much of the myocardial damage produced by enterovirus is believed to be caused by the host immune response, and when inflammation is prominent, the virus may no longer be detectable by conventional cell culture (32). In the latter situation, however, the viral genome may be identified by nucleic acid hybridization or polymerase chain reaction, techniques currently available in research laboratories (33).

Bacteria

Processing endomyocardial biopsy specimens for detection of bacteria is different for each organism and is discussed separately for Mycoplasma pneumoniae, for organisms detected by routine culture techniques, and for species of Brucella. Myocardial damage associated with diphtheria is caused by the exotoxin produced by Corynebacterium diphtheriae; the organism is not found in endomyocardial biopsy specimens and, therefore, is not discussed further. Myocarditis caused by Chlamydia psittaci, species of Rickettsia, or Borrelia burgdorferi usually is diagnosed serologically, although endomyocardial biopsy specimens may be sent to a reference laboratory for culture of these organisms.

Mycoplasma pneumoniae. Myocarditis produced by M. pneumoniae may be diagnosed serologically or by recovering the organism from endomyocardial biopsy specimens, but culture must be requested specifically. To isolate M. pneumoniae, the tissue fragments are homogenized in a small amount of broth (such as trypticase soy broth), and 0.1 ml of the homogenate is inoculated to a biphasic culture system (several are available commercially). Cultures are incubated at 35° C to 37° C in ambient air for up to 3 weeks. The commercially available nucleic acid probe is approved only for testing respiratory tract samples; its reliability has not been evaluated for other specimens.

Bacteria Detected by Routine Culture. Routine processing of endomyocardial tissue for detection of bacteria involves preparing a homogenate in a small amount of broth, which then is used to make a smear for staining with Gram stain and to inoculate appropriate media for culture—sheep blood and chocolate agar (incubated in an atmosphere of 5 to 7% carbon dioxide), thioglycolate broth (incubated in ambient air), and anaerobic blood agar (incubated anaerobically) are recommended. Incubation temperatures and times are discussed in Chapter 54.

Brucella species. Myocarditis produced by Brucella may be diagnosed serologically or by culture of an endomyocardial biopsy specimen, but culture must be requested specifically. The tissue fragments are homogenized, and the homogenate is used to prepare a smear for Gram stain and for inoculating media for culture. Recommended media and culture conditions are outlined in Table 54–4.

Fungi

Processing endomyocardial biopsy specimens for detection of fungi involves preparing a homogenate for direct microscopic examination and culture. The tissue fragments are homogenized in a small amount of broth. A

Table 58–3. Pathogens Detected by Microbiologic Studies of Endomyocardial Biopsy Specimens

Organism	Chapter
Viruses	
Enteroviruses	13
Bacteria	
Chlamydia psittaci	25
Rickettsia spp	26
Mycoplasma pneumoniae	27
Staphylococcus aureus	28
Group A Streptococcus	28
Corynebacterium diphtheriae	29
Clostridium perfringens	30
Neisseria meningitidis	31
Brucella spp	33
Salmonella spp	34
Borrelia burgdorferi	39
Fungi	
Candida spp	43
Cryptococcus neoformans	43
Aspergillus spp	44
Parasites	
Toxoplasma gondii	51
Trypanosoma cruzi	51

potassium hydroxide preparation (Appendix, Procedure 19) of the tissue suspension may be examined microscopically, or a smear of the homogenate may be stained with the Gomori methenamine silver, calcofluor white, or Congo red stain. To isolate fungi the homogenate is inoculated to an enriched medium such as brain-heart infusion, SABHI, or inhibitory mold agar, with and without cycloheximide, and incubated as described in Chapter 54.

Parasites

Endocardial biopsy specimens have not been used in the microbiology laboratory for diagnosis of parasitic infections. Toxoplasma has been found in sections of biopsy tissue, and perhaps Trypanosoma cruzi also can be detected, but this is outside the scope of this discussion.

BONE MARROW

Microbiologic studies of bone marrow are useful for diagnosing infections with a limited number of viruses, bacteria, fungi, and parasites (Table 58-4). Using sterile technique, bone marrow is aspirated from the posterior iliac crest or the sternum. Separate samples are used for microbiologic studies and to prepare smears for microscopic examination. A core biopsy also should be collected, but the aspirate is preferred for microbiologic studies. Specimen processing differs for the different groups of organisms and, therefore, is discussed separately for viruses, bacteria, fungi, and parasites.

Viruses

Many viral infections are associated with transient anemia, leukopenia, thrombocytopenia, or a combination of these, but the responsible virus usually is not detected in hematopoietic cells. The anemia that accompanies infection with parvovirus B19, however, is caused by replication of the virus within erythroid precursors.

Infections produced by parvovirus B19 (Chapter 8) most frequently are diagnosed serologically but occasionally are suspected when a decrease in erythroid precursors and megaloblastic changes in those present are seen in smears of bone marrow aspirates stained with the Wright or Giemsa stain (34). The virus may be detected in these cells by nucleic acid hybridization or polymerase chain reaction, techniques available in research or reference laboratories, which should be contacted regarding specimen requirements (35).

Bacteria

Processing bone marrow for detection of bacteria should ensure detection of species of Brucella and Mycobacterium, regardless of whether special cultures were ordered, because these are the pathogens most likely to be present. Infection produced by Coxiella burnetii (Chapter 26) may be suspected from observation of histologic changes in a bone marrow biopsy specimen—lipid granulomas, focal necrosis, and histiocytic hemophagocytosis—but the infection generally is confirmed serologically, and is not discussed further here.

To recover bacteria, the aspirated bone marrow material may be inoculated directly into blood culture broth media (discussed earlier), which is incubated for 3 weeks, and into broth or onto solid media for isolation of mycobacteria (Table 54-4 and Chapter 40). Clotted specimens must be homogenized and then inoculated onto sheep blood and chocolate agar, incubated up to 3 weeks at 35° to 37° C in 5 to 7% carbon dioxide for recovery of species of Brucella, and to media used for isolation of mycobacteria.

Fungi

Disseminated infection with Histoplasma capsulatum and, less commonly, with Blastomyces dermatitidis is diagnosed by detecting the organisms in smears of bone marrow aspirate or in core biopsy specimens stained with the Wright or Giemsa stain (Plate XIA). To recover these organisms, unclotted bone marrow or the homogenate prepared from a clotted specimen is inoculated onto enriched primary fungal planting media such as brain-heart infusion agar containing 5% sheep blood and SABHI agar. Histoplasma capsulatum also grows well on buffered charcoal yeast extract agar (primarily used for recovery of Legionella). Cultures are incubated as discussed in Chapter 54. Organism identification is reviewed in Chapter 45.

Parasites

The different species of Leishmania, responsible for visceral leishmaniasis (Chapter 51) are easily detected in bone marrow biopsy specimens; however, such specimens (smears and histologic sections) usually are examined by the anatomic pathologist and rarely are sent directly to the parasitology laboratory. The diagnosis of visceral leishmaniasis is essentially a tissue diagnosis (36).

LYMPH NODE TISSUE AND ASPIRATES

Microbiologic studies of lymph node are useful in determining some of the agents of lymphadenitis (Table 58-5). Other agents that produce lymphadenitis, such as adenovirus, CMV, and herpes simplex, Epstein-Barr, measles, rubella, dengue, Lassa, and human immunodeficiency viruses, and certain bacteria (species of Rickettsia,

Table 58-4. Pathogens Detected by Microbiologic Studies of Bone Marrow

Organism	Chapter
Viruses	
Parvovirus B19	8
Bacteria	
Coxiella burnetii	26
Brucella spp	33
Salmonella spp	34
Mycobacterium spp	40
Fungi	
Blastomyces dermatitidis	45
Histoplasma capsulatum	45
Parasites	
Leishmania donovani	51
Leishmania infantum	51
Leishmania chagasi	51

Table 58-5. Pathogens Detected by Microbiologic Studies of Lymph Node Specimens

Organism	Chapter
Bacteria	
Chlamydia trachomatis (L_1, L_2, L_3)	25
Staphylococcus aureus	28
Group A Streptococcus	28
Pseudomonas pseudomallei	32
Pseudomonas mallei	32
Francisella tularensis	33
Yersinia spp	34
Haemophilus ducreyi	36
Mycobacterium spp	40
Cat-scratch disease bacillus (Afipia felis)	41
Fungi	
Cryptococcus neoformans	43
Histoplasma capsulatum	45
Coccidioides immitis	45
Paracoccidioides brasiliensis	45
Parasites	
Trypanosoma gambiense	51
Trypanosoma rhodesiense	51
Leishmania spp	51

Treponem pallidum, Leptospira interrogans, Spirillum minus, and Streptobacillus moniliformis) are not included in Table 58-5 because they generally are not diagnosed by microbiologic evaluation of the lymph node, and they are not discussed further here. Specimen collection and transport are similar for all organisms listed in Table 58-5. Specimen processing is discussed separately for bacteria, fungi, and parasites.

Collection, Transport, and Processing

Surgically removed lymph nodes are transported immediately to the laboratory in a sterile container. A pathologist should examine the fresh tissue and divide the node appropriately for histologic and microbiologic studies. Material from fluctuant nodes may be aspirated with a needle and syringe. To transport the aspirate, the needle is removed, air is expelled, and the syringe is capped and delivered promptly to the laboratory. Specimen processing differs for detection of different bacteria or groups of bacteria, and is discussed separately for each.

Chlamydia trachomatis. Isolation of C. trachomatis (types L_1, L_2, L_3) from material aspirated from a bubo provides a definitive diagnosis of lymphogranuloma venereum, but cultures are positive in only about one third of suspected cases (37). For optimal recovery of C. trachomatis the aspirate should be processed immediately; if a delay is unavoidable the aspirate material should be transferred to 2-sucrose phosphate transport medium and stored in the refrigerator for up to 48 hours, or at $-70°$C for longer periods. Further processing for culture is described in Procedure 8 in the Appendix.

Bacteria Detected by Routine Culture. Processing lymph node tissue or aspirates involves direct microscopic examination and culture. The tissue is homogenized in a small amount of broth with a sterile tissue grinder or mortar and pestle. A smear of the homogenate or aspirate is prepared for Gram staining, and the specimen is inoculated to sheep blood and chocolate agar (incubated in an atmosphere of 5 to 7% carbon dioxide) and to thioglycolate broth (incubated in ambient air). Recommended incubation temperatures and times are reviewed in Chapter 54.

Francisella tularensis. Cultures for F. tularensis, the agent of tularemia, must be requested specifically. Processing is similar to that described above for routine bacterial isolation, except that media and culture conditions outlined in Table 54-4 should be used. Moreover, a smear (or the entire specimen) may be sent to the Centers for Disease Control (CDC) for fluorescent antibody staining. Investigators at the CDC should be contacted regarding specimen and shipping requirements.

Haemophilus ducreyi. H. ducreyi most often is detected in material collected from genital ulcers but may be recovered from material aspirated from fluctuant inguinal lymph nodes. Specimen processing includes preparing a smear for Gram stain and inoculating appropriate media for culture. Recommended media and culture conditions are outlined in Table 54-4.

Mycobacterium species. Processing lymph node tissue or aspirates for detection of mycobacteria involves direct microscopic examination and culture. The tissue is homogenized. Homogenates and aspirates believed not to be contaminated with other bacteria may be processed without treatment. Smears are prepared for staining with auramine rhodamine or acid-fast stain (Appendix, Procedures 4-6), and the specimen is inoculated to appropriate broth or solid media for culture as outlined in Table 54-4, and discussed in more detail in Chapter 40. Potentially contaminated homogenates are poured through sterile gauze into a 50-ml centrifuge tube, and an equal volume of 2% NaOH-N-acetyl L-cysteine is added. The suspension is mixed and allowed to stand 20 minutes. Phosphate buffer (25 ml) is added, and the suspension is mixed and centrifuged at 3000 to 3600 g for 20 minutes. The supernatant is removed, and the sediment is suspended in 1 to 2 ml of buffer and used to prepare smears and for inoculation of media. Aspirates that may be contaminated are transferred to a 50-ml centrifuge tube containing 10 ml of sterile, filtered distilled water, mixed on a vortex mixer, allowed to stand 20 minutes, and processed as described for sputum (Appendix, Procedure 27).

Cat-Scratch Disease Bacillus (Afipia felis). The diagnosis of cat-scratch disease is based on an appropriate history, failure to recover other pathogens from pus aspirated from an involved lymph node, and a lymph node biopsy histologically consistent with cat-scratch lymphadenitis (Chapter 41). The organism may be cultured, but appropriate techniques have been determined only recently, and recovery of the organism is not necessary for diagnosis (38).

Fungi

Processing lymph node tissue or aspirates for detection of fungi involves homogenization of the tissue, direct microscopic examination, and culture. Direct examination methods include the potassium hydroxide preparation (Appendix, Procedure 19) and staining of smears with the

Gomori methenamine silver, calcofluor white, or Congo red stain. To recover fungi the homogenate or aspirate is inoculated to an enriched medium such as brain-heart infusion agar containing 5% sheep blood, SABHI agar, or inhibitory mold agar, and incubated as discussed in Chapter 54.

Parasites

Lymph node aspirates are used for diagnosis of African trypanosomiasis and cutaneous leishmaniasis. In both infections lymphadenopathy develops; in African trypanosomiasis, it is usually in the posterior anterolateral triangle of the neck (Winterbottom's sign), and in cutaneous leishmaniasis, along the lymph channels draining the area of the ulcer. Often the pattern shown by the enlarged lymph nodes resembles sporotrichosis (Chapter 45).

Enlarged lymph nodes are aspirated with a syringe and a needle, and the material is used for preparation of smears. All smears should be fixed and stained with the Giemsa stain for microscopic examination. The typical trypomastigotes in trypanosomiasis and amastigotes in leishmaniasis are recognized easily (Chapter 51).

SPLEEN ABSCESS MATERIAL

Abscesses of the spleen are uncommon, most frequently occurring via hematogenous spread from a distant focus of infection, from direct extension of a contiguous site, from infected traumatic hematomas, or from infected infarcts in persons with sickle cell hemoglobinopathy. Splenic abscesses associated with bacteremia usually are multiple and most often are caused by Staphylococcus aureus and viridans streptococci. Members of the Enterobacteriaceae, especially species of Salmonella, anaerobes, and in immunocompromised persons species of Candida, may be involved (39–41). In persons with the acquired immunodeficiency syndrome, Mycobacterium tuberculosis is a possible pathogen (42). Clinical manifestations of splenic abscess include tenderness, left side upper quadrant pain referred to the left shoulder, and fever, but signs and symptoms may be absent in persons with many small abscesses.

Microbiologic studies of purulent material aspirated from a radiographically identified abscess are necessary to determine the cause. Material is aspirated with a needle and syringe, the needle is removed, and the syringe is tightly capped and transported immediately to the laboratory.

Specimen processing includes preparing a smear for Gram stain and inoculation of appropriate media for culture: sheep blood and MacConkey agar and thioglycolate broth, incubated in ambient air, and anaerobic blood agar, incubated anaerobically, are recommended. Incubation temperatures and times are described in Chapter 54. To detect mycobacteria, a smear is stained with auramine rhodamine or an acid-fast stain (Appendix, Procedures 4–6), and the material is inoculated to appropriate broth or solid media (see Table 54–4 and Chapter 40). When fungal culture is requested and when yeasts are seen in smears stained with Gram stain, primary fungal planting media such as inhibitory mold agar and SABHI agar containing antibiotics should be inoculated and incubated as discussed in Chapter 54.

SERUM FOR SEROLOGIC TESTING

Infections caused by many organisms typically are diagnosed by detecting specific immunoglobulins in serum (Table 58–6). For several organisms, a test to detect immunoglobulin (Ig)M is available, and a single serum sample often is adequate. However, for others, specific IgG must be measured simultaneously in acute- and convalescent-phase samples (collected 2 to 3 weeks apart), and a four-fold rise or fall in titer is consistent with recent infection.

To obtain serum, blood is collected without anticoagulant and allowed to clot at 4° C. When a firm clot forms, the specimen is centrifuged at 2000 g for 10 minutes at

Table 58–6. Infectious Pathogens Typically Diagnosed Serologically

Organism	Chapter
Viruses	
Epstein-Barr virus	5
Human herpesvirus-6	5
Parvovirus B19	8
Hepatitis B virus	9
Delta agent	9
Mumps virus	10
Measles virus	10
Hepatitis A virus	13
Colorado tick fever virus	14
Eastern equine encephalitis virus	17
Western equine encephalitis virus	17
Venezuelan equine encephalitis virus	17
Rubella virus	17
Dengue virus	18
Yellow fever virus	18
St. Louis encephalitis virus	18
Japanese encephalitis virus	18
California encephalitis viruses	19
Rift Valley fever virus	19
Hantaan virus	19
Crimean-Congo hemorrhagic fever virus	19
Lymphocytic choriomeningitis virus	20
Lassa virus	20
Junin virus	20
Machupo virus	20
Filoviruses	21
Human T-cell leukemia virus type I & II	22
Human immunodeficiency virus type 1 & 2	22
Hepatitis C virus	23
Bacteria	
Chlamydia trachomatis (L_2, L_2, L_3)	25
Chlamydia psittaci	25
Chlamydia pneumoniae	25
Rickettsia spp	26
Mycoplasma pneumoniae	27
Francisella tularensis	33
Brucella spp	33
Treponema pallidum	39
Leptospira interrogans	39

4° C, and the serum is aseptically transferred to a sterile tube. If the sample is not tested immediately it may be stored in the refrigerator for a few days or at −20° C or below for longer periods. Acute- and convalescent-phase samples always should be tested together.

REFERENCES

1. Washington JA II, and Ilstrup DM: Blood cultures: Issues and controversies. Rev Infect Dis, 8:792, 1986.
2. Feorino PM, et al: Transfusion-associated acquired immunodeficiency syndrome. Evidence for persistent infection in blood donors. N Engl J Med, 312:1293, 1985.
3. Howell CJ, Miller MJ, and Martin WJ: Comparison of rates of virus isolation from leukocyte populations separated from blood by conventional and Ficoll-Paque/Macrodex methods. J Clin Microbiol, 10:533, 1979.
4. Prather SJ, Dagan R, Jenista JA, and Menegus MA: The isolation of enteroviruses from blood: A comparison of four processing methods. J Med Virol, 14:221, 1984.
5. Nahmias AJ, and Kibrick S: Inhibitory effect of heparin on herpes simplex virus. J Bacteriol, 87:1060, 1964.
6. Woods GL, and Proffitt MR: Comparison of plasmagel with LeucoPREP™-Macrodex methods for separation of leukocytes for virus isolation. Diagn Microbiol Infect Dis, 8:126, 1987.
7. Thiele GM, and Woods GL: The effect of dexamethasone on detection of cytomegalovirus in tissue culture and by immunofluorescence. J Virol Methods, 22:319, 1988.
8. Dagan R, and Menegus MA: A combination of four cell types for rapid detection of enteroviruses in clinical specimens. J Med Virol, 19:219, 1986.
9. Woods GL, Young A, Johnson A, and Thiele GM: Detection of cytomegalovirus by 24-well plate centrifugation assay using a monoclonal antibody to an early nuclear antigen and by conventional cell culture. J Virol Methods, 18:207, 1987.
10. Woods GL, and Thiele GM: Rapid detection of cytomegalovirus by 24-well plate centrifugation with the use of a monoclonal antibody to an early nuclear antigen. Am J Clin Pathol, 91:695, 1989.
11. Van Der Bij W, et al: Rapid immunodiagnosis of active cytomegalovirus infection by monoclonal antibody staining of blood leukocytes. J Med Virol, 25:179, 1988.
12. Krumholz HM, Cummings S, and York M: Blood culture phlebotomy: Switching needles does not prevent contamination. Ann Intern Med, 113:290, 1990.
13. Henry NK, et al: Microbiological and clinical evaluation of the ISOLATOR lysis-centrifugation blood culture tube. J Clin Microbiol, 17:864, 1983.
14. Ilstrup DM, and Washington JA II: The importance of volume of blood cultured in the detection of bacteremia and fungemia. Diagn Microbiol Infect Dis, 1:107, 1983.
15. Dietzman DE, Fisher GW, and Shoenknecht FD: Neonatal Escherichia coli septicemia—bacterial counts in blood. J Pediatr, 85:128, 1974.
16. Werner AS, Cobbs CG, Kaye D, and Hook EW: Studies on the bacteremia of bacterial endocarditis. JAMA, 202:199, 1967.
17. Washington JA II: Blood cultures: Principles and techniques. Mayo Clin Proc, 50:91, 1975.
18. Weinstein MP, Reller LB, Murphy JR, and Lichtenstein KA: The clinical significance of positive blood cultures: A comprehensive analysis of 500 episodes of bacteremia and fungemia in adults. I. Laboratory and epidemiologic observations. Rev Infect Dis, 5:35, 1983.
19. Aronson MD, and Dor DH: Blood cultures. Ann Intern Med, 106:246, 1987.
20. Vaisanen IT, Michelsen T, Valtonen V, and Makelainen A: Comparison of arterial and venous blood samples for the diagnosis of bacteremia in critically ill patients. Crit Care Med, 13:664, 1985.
21. Bryant JK, and Strand CL: Reliability of blood cultures collected from intravascular catheter vs venipuncture. Am J Clin Pathol, 88:113, 1987.
22. Reller LR, Murray PR, and MacLowry JD: Cumitech IA, Blood cultures II. Edited by JA Washington II. Washington, DC, American Society for Microbiology, 1982.
23. Cowett RM, et al: Reliability of bacterial culture of blood obtained from an umbilical artery catheter. J Pediatr, 88:1035, 1976.
24. Wing EJ, Norden CW, Shadduck RK, and Winkelstein A: Use of quantitative bacteriologic techniques to diagnose catheter-related sepsis. Arch Intern Med, 139:482, 1979.
25. Murray PR, Spizzo AW, and Niles AC: Clinical comparison of the recoveries of bloodstream pathogens in Septi-Chek brain-heart infusion broth with saponin, Septi-Chek tryptic soy broth, and the Isolator lysis-centrifugation system. J Clin Microbiol, 29:901, 1991.
26. Weinstein MP, et al: Controlled evaluation of BACTEC plus 26 and Roche Septi-Chek aerobic blood culture bottles. J Clin Microbiol, 29:879, 1991.
27. Morello JA, Matushek SM, Dunne WH, and Hinds DB: Performance of a BACTEC nonradiometric medium for pediatric blood cultures. J Clin Microbiol, 29:359, 1991.
28. Thorpe TC, et al: BacT/Alert: An automated colorimetric microbial detection system. J Clin Microbiol, 28:1605, 1990.
29. Goldschmid JM, and Mahomed K: The use of the microhematocrit technic for the recovery of Borrelia duttonii from the blood. Am J Clin Pathol, 58:165, 1972.
30. Maki DG, Weise CE, and Sarafin HW: A semiquantitative culture method for identifying intravenous catheter–related infection. N Engl J Med, 296:1305, 1977.
31. Savoia MC, and Oxman MN: Myocarditis, pericarditis and mediastinitis. In Principles and Practice of Infectious Diseases. 3rd ed. Edited by GL Mandell, RG Douglas, Jr, and JE Bennett. New York, Churchill Livingstone, 1990.
32. Weinstein C, and Fenoglio JJ: Myocarditis. Hum Pathol, 18:613, 1987.
33. Chapman NH, Tracey S, Gaunt CJ, and Fortmueller U: Molecular detection and identification of enteroviruses using enzymatic amplification and nucleic acid hybridization. J Clin Microbiol, 28:843, 1990.
34. Frickhofen N, et al: Persistent B19 parvovirus infection in patients infected with human immunodeficiency virus type 1 (HIV-1): A treatable cause of anemia. Ann Intern Med, 113:926, 1990.
35. Kurtzman G, et al: Pure red-cell aplasia of 10 years' duration due to persistent parvovirus B19 infection and its cure with immunoglobulin therapy. N Engl J Med, 321:519, 1989.
36. Gutierrez Y: Diagnostic Pathology of Parasitic Infections with Clinical Correlations. Philadelphia, Lea & Febiger, 1990.
37. Bowie WR, and Holmes KK: Chlamydia trachomatis (trachoma, perinatal infections, lymphogranuloma venereum, and other genital infections). In Principles and Practice of Infectious Diseases. 3rd ed. Edited by GL Mandell, RG Douglas, Jr, and JE Bennett. New York, Churchill Livingstone, 1990.
38. Brenner DJ, et al: Proposal of Afipia gen. nov., with Afipia felis sp. nov. (formerly the cat scratch disease bacillus),

Afipia clevelandensis sp. nov. (formerly the Cleveland Clinic Foundation strain), Afipia broomeae sp. nov., and three unnamed genospecies. J Clin Microbiol, 29:2450, 1991.

39. Nelken N, et al: Changing clinical spectrum of splenic abscess. A multicenter study and review of the literature. Am J Surg, 154:27, 1987.

40. Chun CH, et al: Splenic abscess. Medicine, 59:50, 1980.

41. Haron E, et al: Hepatic candidiasis: An increasing problem in immunocompromised patients. Am J Med, 83:17, 1987.

42. Khalil T, et al: Splenic tuberculous abscess in patients positive for human immunodeficiency virus: Report of two cases and review. Clin Infect Dis, 14:1265, 1992.

Chapter 59

GASTROINTESTINAL TRACT

Specimens from the gastrointestinal tract collected for microbiologic studies include esophageal brushings, gastric contents, duodenal aspirates, stool and rectal swab specimens, and tissue from the esophagus, stomach, duodenum, small intestine, colon, rectum, and anus.

ESOPHAGEAL BRUSHINGS

Esophageal samples are useful in determining the agent of esophagitis, an infection almost always of immunocompromised hosts. Symptoms are odynophagia, retrosternal pain, nausea, anorexia, and weight loss. Potential pathogens include herpes simplex virus (HSV), cytomegalovirus (CMV), and species of Candida. Esophagitis caused by HSV typically is characterized by multiple, deep ulcers, and that caused by CMV by many large, shallow ulcers, although single lesions occur. Candidal esophagitis is associated with diffuse ulcerations and friable, cheesy plaques, crating a cobblestone appearance on the esophageal mucosa. These patterns, however, are not diagnostic, and the cause of the esophagitis must be confirmed by histologic and microbiologic studies.

Collection, Transport, and Processing

Esophageal brushings are obtained during endoscopic examination. Smears are prepared for staining with the Papanicolaou stain, then the brush is placed in sterile physiologic saline and promptly transported to the laboratory. Specimen processing is different for detection of viruses and fungi and is discussed separately for each group of organisms.

Viruses

Cytopathic changes induced by viruses may be observed in preparations stained with the Papanicolaou stain, but cell culture is the most sensitive method for virus detection. All samples submitted for virus isolation should be refrigerated until they are inoculated to cell monolayers.

The cell lines for culture are selected for the viruses most likely to be present in the specimen (see Chapters 3 and 54). Because HSV and CMV are the most common causes of esophagitis, inoculation of MRC-5 cells or MRC-5 and A549 cells is recommended. To decrease the time to detection of cytopathic effect (CPE) produced by these viruses the cell monolayers are incubated in maintenance medium with 10^{-5} M dexamethasone for at least 24 hours before inoculation (1,2). Specimen inoculation, absorption, and culture conditions are discussed in Chapter 54. The cell monolayers are examined microscopically for specific viral CPE two or three times per week for 3 weeks. Identification of HSV and CMV is discussed in Chapter 5.

The centrifugation-culture technique has been used successfully for detection of HSV and CMV (Appendix, Procedure 2) (1,3). For detection of HSV the value of the technique is controversial, and it is recommended that laboratory directors evaluate the test in their own laboratories (1,4). For detection of CMV, the use of this technique to supplement conventional cell culture is strongly recommended because the time for detection is shortened significantly (2,3).

Fungi

Esophagitis produced by Candida may be diagnosed by examining smears of esophageal brush specimens stained with the Gram or Papanicolaou stain. The most sensitive diagnostic test—and the one required for identification—is culture. The specimen is inoculated onto primary culture media (see Chapter 42) such as inhibitory mold agar or SABHI agar with antibiotics. Culture conditions are reviewed in Chapter 54.

GASTRIC CONTENTS

Gastric contents (vomitus) may be submitted during the investigation of an outbreak of short-incubation (1 to 6 hours) food-borne disease. The illness is characterized by nausea, vomiting, diarrhea, and abdominal pain, and begins 1 to 6 hours after ingestion of food contaminated with preformed toxin produced by Staphylococcus aureus or Bacillus cereus. Gastric lavage specimens, which contain sputum swallowed during sleep, occasionally are collected to confirm the diagnosis of pulmonary tuberculosis in persons who are unable to produce sputum, for example, children younger than 3 years of age, persons who are senile, and those who are not ambulatory. The collection, transport, and processing of the specimen are discussed separately for bacteria associated with short-incubation food poisoning and for species of Mycobacterium.

Collection, Transport, and Processing

Bacteria Associated with Short-Incubation Food Poisoning. For investigation of an outbreak of short-incubation food-borne disease, vomitus and stool specimens (discussed later) should be obtained from affected persons. Vomitus is collected in a sterile container, transported promptly to the laboratory on wet ice, and stored in the refrigerator.

Processing gastric contents for detection of Staphylococcus aureus and Bacillus cereus includes preparation and examination of smears stained with the Gram stain. Because Staphylococcus aureus and Bacillus cereus can be present normally in food, quantitative cultures must be performed. A series of dilutions (10^{-1}, 10^{-2}, 10^{-3}, 10^{-4}, and 10^{-5}) of the samples is prepared in buffered gelatin diluent, and 0.1 ml of the undiluted specimen and of each of the dilutions is planted onto colistin–nalidixic acid or phenylethyl alcohol blood agar (selective for gram-positive organisms). In addition, to demonstrate endospore production by B. cereus, 1 ml of the original specimen is mixed with 1 ml of absolute ethanol, and the mixture is allowed to stand at room temperature for 1 hour. Dilutions of the mixture are prepared as described above, and 0.1 ml of each dilution and of the undiluted mixture is planted onto sheep blood agar. All plates are incubated 18 to 24 hours at 35° to 37° C in ambient air, and the colonies are counted. Identification of Staphylococcus aureus and Bacillus cereus is discussed in Chapters 28 and 29, respectively. The presence of at least 10^5 colony-forming units of Staphylococcus aureus or Bacillus cereus organisms per gram of specimen has potential significance, especially if found in samples from the majority of affected persons. Isolates from different persons may be typed to determine if they are identical, and the original specimens may be assessed for enterotoxins of Staphylococcus aureus, but these tests are usually done in a reference laboratory.

Mycobacterium species. Gastric secretions obtained by lavage are collected from hospitalized patients; the procedure cannot be performed in the office or in the clinic. Optimally, three specimens, taken on three consecutive days, are collected at the patient's bedside before the patient arises. With the patient sitting, a Levine collection tube is inserted through a nostril, and the patient swallows the tube, aided by small sips of filtered water. When the tube is in the stomach a syringe is attached to the end and 5 ml of filtered distilled water is introduced through it. About 20 to 25 ml of gastric secretions is withdrawn and slowly expelled into a 50-ml conical collection tube. The Levine tube is slowly withdrawn, and any excess fluid is added to the collection tube, which is tightly capped and delivered immediately to the laboratory.

Gastric lavage specimens should be processed immediately, but if a delay is unavoidable, 10% sodium bicarbonate should be added until the pH of the sample (measured with pH paper) is normal; then the sample is refrigerated until it is processed. If more than 10 ml of secretions is collected the specimen is centrifuged at 3000 g for 20 to 30 minutes, the supernatant is decanted, and the sediment is processed as described for sputum (Appendix, Procedure 27).

DUODENAL ASPIRATE SPECIMENS

Duodenal samples sometimes are received in the laboratory for detection of two parasites: Giardia lamblia and Strongyloides stercoralis, normal inhabitants of the duodenum.

Collection, Transport, and Processing

Duodenal aspirates taken with a nasogastric tube or during endoscopic examination should be placed in clean containers and sent to the laboratory promptly for examination.

Giardia lamblia. The diagnosis of giardiasis generally is made by examination of stool samples (described later). A duodenal sample received in the laboratory should be used to make wet mounts (1 drop of saline solution and 1 drop of the sample are placed on a glass slide, mixed with an applicator stick, and covered with a cover glass), for examination under the microscope. Because only trophozoites of Giardia are found in the duodenum, concentration and staining with iodine is not necessary. Examination of duodenal samples obtained by invasive procedures (nasogastric intubation and endoscopic examination) for detection of Giardia have not been more reliable than examination of stool; thus, collecting these samples for the sole purpose of diagnosing giardiasis is not recommended (5).

A string may be used to collect small duodenal samples for examination. Before breakfast the patient swallows a gelatin capsule containing a weight attached to a string of nylon. A loop of the string pulled from the gelatin capsule is taped to the patient's cheek, and after 4 hours or more the line is retrieved and sent to the laboratory. Samples from the small intestine are bile stained; small fragments of mucus are stripped from the line and are examined microscopically, as described earlier. The string test, however, offers no advantage over stool examination (6).

Strongyloides stercoralis. Strongyloides sometimes is detected in wet-mount preparations made from duodenal samples received in the laboratory. Larvae usually are found, but if parts of duodenal mucosa are retrieved, eggs, eggs with larvae, and adult females often are present. The diagnosis of strongyloidiasis is made by examining stool samples; use of invasive techniques for recovery of material for the sole purpose of detecting S. stercoralis is emphatically discouraged.

STOOL AND RECTAL SWAB SPECIMENS

Stool, and in some cases rectal swab, specimens are useful for determining the agent of infectious diarrhea, which worldwide is second only to cardiovascular diseases as a cause of death (7). Those at greatest risk of mortality from diarrhea and enteric infections are infants and small children living in underdeveloped countries where crowding and poor sanitation are common (8–10). Stool and rectal swab specimens are useful for confirming the diagnosis of botulism or diagnosing infections caused by adenoviruses (primarily upper respiratory tract), enteroviruses (aseptic meningitis, myopericarditis, pleurodynia, and various rashes), and some sexually transmitted pathogens (Table 59–1). Stool or rectal swab specimens generally are not submitted to diagnose fungal infections; however, in immunocompromised hosts surveillance cultures may be used to identify persons colonized by yeasts. In these instances stool or rectal swab specimens are inoculated onto primary fungal media containing antimicrobial agents (see Chapter 42). In addition, stool samples are preferred for diagnosis of infections with intestinal protozoa and helminths, and in some instances with helminths of the respiratory and biliary tracts (Table 59–2).

Table 59–1. Viruses and Bacteria Detected in Stool and Rectal Swab Specimens

Organism	Specimen	Chapter
Viruses		
Adenovirus	S, RS	6
Enteroviruses	S, RS	13
Rotavirus	S, RS	14
Calicivirus	S	15
Astrovirus	S	23
Norwalk virus	S	23
Norwalk-like virus	S	23
Bacteria		
Chlamydia trachomatis	RS	25
Staphylococcus aureus	S	28
Listeria monocytogenes	S	29
Bacillus cereus	S	29
Clostridium botulinum*	S	30
Clostridium difficile*	S, RS (C)	30
Clostridium perfringens*	S, RS (C)	30
Neisseria gonorrhoeae	RS	31
Escherichia coli	S, RS	34
Shigella spp	S, RS	34
Salmonella spp	S, RS	34
Yersinia enterocolitica	S, RS	34
Vibrio spp	S, RS	35
Aeromonas spp	S, RS	35
Plesiomonas shigelloides	S, RS	35
Campylobacter spp	S, RS	37
Mycobacterium spp	S, RS	40

* The organism, its toxin, or both may be detected.
Key: S, stool; RS, rectal swab; RS (C), rectal swab is acceptable for culture of the organism only.

Collection, Transport, and Processing

Collection, transport, and processing of these specimens, different for viruses, bacteria, and parasites, are discussed separately for each group.

Viruses

Stool is preferred for detection of adenoviruses, enteroviruses, and the viruses responsible for gastroenteritis; however, for some agents a rectal swab specimen is acceptable (see Table 59–1). Stool specimens should be collected in a clean container with a tight lid. If feces cannot be obtained, a swab is inserted beyond the anal sphincter, rotated, withdrawn, and placed in viral transport medium (such as Hanks' balanced salt solution) containing antimicrobial agents. Either specimen should be delivered promptly to the laboratory; otherwise, it should be refrigerated for a short time and transported on wet ice. If the specimen must be mailed to a reference laboratory it should be stored at $-70°$ C and shipped on dry ice.

Processing specimens for detection of adenoviruses and enteroviruses, which are identified by routine isolation techniques, differs from those used for detection of rotavirus and most other viruses associated with gastroenteritis.

Viruses Detected by Routine Isolation. To isolate viruses from stool a 5 to 10% suspension of the stool is prepared in Hanks' balanced salt solution, mixed at high speed on a vortex mixer for about 1 minute, and clarified by centrifugation at 2000 g for 15 minutes. Rectal swab specimens received in transport medium are mixed on a vortex mixer, the swab is removed, and the medium is clarified by centrifugation. To recover adenoviruses and enteroviruses, A549, MRC-5, and primary monkey kidney cells are inoculated, and to isolate the enteric adenoviruses, Grahm 293 cells should be added (11). The supernatant of the clarified specimen is inoculated and adsorbed, and cultures are incubated as described in Chapter 54. Virus identification is discussed in Chapters 6 and 13.

Viruses Associated with Gastroenteritis. Rotaviruses are responsible for most cases of viral gastroenteritis and are the only viruses associated with gastroenteritis that are detected in many clinical virology laboratories. Most commonly, rotavirus is detected by enzyme-linked immunosorbent assay (several kits are commercially avail-

Table 59–2. Protozoa and Helminths Diagnosed in Stool Specimens

Organism	Chapter
Protozoa	
Giardia lamblia	49
Dientamoeba fragilis	49
Trichomonas hominis	49
Chilomastix mesnili	49
Entamoeba histolytica	49
Entamoeba coli	49
Entamoeba hartmanni	49
Entamoeba polecki	49
Iodamoeba buetschlii	49
Endolimax nana	49
Cryptosporidium	49
Isospora belli	49
Sarcocystis suihominis	49
Sarcocystis hominis	49
Balantidium coli	49
Nematodes	
Strongyloides stercoralis	50
Strongyloides fuelleborni	50
Hookworms	50
Ternidens deminutus	50
Trichostrongylus spp	50
Ascaris lumbricoides	50
Trichuris trichiura	50
Capillaria philippinensis	50
Trematodes	
Fasciolopsis buski	50
Heterophyes heterophyes	50
Nanophyetus salmincola	50
Echinostoma spp	50
Plagiorchis spp	50
Spelotrema brevicaeca	50
Episthmiun caninum	50
Paragonimus spp	51
Fasciola hepatica	51
Fasciola gigantica	51
Clonorchis sinensis	51
Opistorchis felinus	51
Opistorchis viverrini	51
Amphimerus pseudofelinus	51
Dicrocoelim dendriticum	51
Dicrocoelim hospes	51
Shistosoma mansoni	51
Schistosoma japonicum	51
Schistosoma mekongi	51
Schistosoma haematobium	51
Cestodes	
Taeniorhynchus saginatus	50
Taenia solium	50
Diphyllobothrium spp	50
Hymenolepis nana	50
Hymenolepis diminuta	50
Dipillidium caninum	50

able). Latex agglutination kits also are available, but they appear to be less sensitive (12). Specimens are processed according to the manufacturer's directions.

Direct examination of stool specimens by electron microscopy is the reference method for detection of rotavirus and is the only method for detection of caliciviruses, astroviruses, the Norwalk virus, and Norwalk-like viruses. To visualize virus particles by electron microscopy the stool sample is negatively stained with phosphotungstic acid.

Bacteria

Stool is preferred for detection of bacteria responsible for infectious diarrhea, but for some organisms a rectal swab specimen is an acceptable alternative (see Table 59–1). Stool specimens should be collected in a clean container with a tight lid, and the specimen should not be contaminated with urine, barium, or toilet paper. Rectal swab specimens are obtained as described earlier for viruses and are placed in a tube transport system containing modified Stuart's medium (commercially available) to prevent drying. Stool and rectal swabs should be transported promptly to the laboratory and processed as soon as possible, because the drop in pH that occurs as the stool cools may inhibit growth of many Shigella and some species of Salmonella. If a delay in processing is unavoidable, or if the specimen must be mailed to a reference laboratory, adding a preservative such as 0.03 M phosphate buffer mixed with an equal volume of glycerol is recommended.

Rectal swab specimens submitted for detection of Chlamydia trachomatis are placed in 2-sucrose phosphate transport medium and transported promptly to the laboratory, or are refrigerated for a short time. Rectal swab specimens collected to diagnose gonorrhea are placed in a tube containing modified Stuart's medium and transported promptly to the laboratory, where they are immediately inoculated to appropriate media (described later) or, if a brief delay is unavoidable, held at room temperature until they are processed.

The processing of stool or rectal swab specimens for detection of bacteria is based on the organism or group of organisms expected to be present. Shigella, Salmonella, and Campylobacter jejuni typically are sought in a routine culture of stool or rectal swab. Detection of other possible pathogens should be specifically requested. The possible pathogens include: Chlamydia trachomatis, the bacteria associated with short- and long-incubation food poisoning, Listeria monocytogenes, Clostridium botulinum, Clostridium difficile, Clostridium perfringens, Neisseria gonorrhoeae, Escherichia coli, Yersinia enterocolitica, Vibrio, Aeromonas, Pleisiomonas shigelloides, other species of Campylobacter, and Mycobacterium.

Chlamydia trachomatis.
C. trachomatis may be detected in rectal swab specimens by cell culture (the reference method), direct immunofluorescence, or enzyme-linked immunosorbent assay (ELISA). When sexual abuse is being investigated cell culture must be performed. For culture the specimen is processed as outlined in Procedure 8 in the Appendix. For nonculture methods approved for testing rectal swab specimens, collection kits are available from several manufacturers (see urethral swab specimens in Chapter 61).

Bacteria Associated with Short-Incubation and Long-Incubation Food Poisoning.
Stool specimens collected from persons with short-incubation food poisoning should be evaluated for Staphylococcus aureus and Bacillus cereus, as described earlier for gastric contents. Specimens from persons with long-incubation food poisoning are processed similarly for detection of B. cereus, and additional media are inoculated and incubated anaerobically as described later for detection of Clostridium perfringens.

Listeria monocytogenes.
Culture of stool for recovery of L. monocytogenes is done primarily for epidemiologic purposes and is best accomplished by cold enrichment. The specimen is mixed in tryptose broth and then is kept refrigerated up to 3 months. Subcultures to sheep blood agar or to colistin–nalidixic acid agar are made weekly for 4 weeks and then monthly for 2 months. Organism identification is discussed in Chapter 29.

Clostridium botulinum.
The clinical diagnoses of food-borne botulism and infant botulism may be confirmed by detecting botulinal toxin, C. botulinum, or both in feces. Optimally, 25 to 50 ml of stool, 15 to 20 ml of serum, and a sample of the suspected food should be collected. Most clinical laboratories are not properly equipped to process specimens from persons suspected to have botulism. In the United States when a case of botulism is identified, investigators at the Centers for Disease Control (CDC) should be notified to ensure appropriate diagnosis, treatment, and investigation of the potential outbreak.

Clostridium difficile.
Diseases associated with C. difficile, such as pseudomembranous colitis and antibiotic-associated diarrhea, are caused by the toxins produced by the organism (Chapter 30) and are diagnosed by demonstrating the toxins in a passed fecal specimen or in a sample of lumen contents obtained by colonoscopy. The reference method for detection of the cytotoxin is the cell culture assay. About 25 g (25 to 50 ml) of liquid stool should be collected in a clean, wide-mouthed container and transported promptly to the laboratory. The sample should be processed within 2 hours or stored in the refrigerator. To extract the toxin the stool specimen is clarified by centrifugation at 2000 g for 20 minutes or 10,000 g for 10 minutes and filtered through a 0.45-μm membrane filter. Serial dilutions are prepared and inoculated to cell monolayers.

Alternatively, toxin may be detected in stool samples by commercially available ELISA. This technique appears to be almost as sensitive as cell culture, provides results within a few hours, and does not require centrifugation and filtration (13,14). A latex agglutination test is available but does not give reliable results (15).

For epidemiologic studies, Clostridium difficile may be isolated from stool or from rectal swab specimens placed in an anaerobic transport system for optimal recovery. Because many bacteria are present in stool, procedures must be used that select C. difficile. The stool is diluted (1:200 is suggested) in buffered gelatin diluent, and both undiluted and diluted samples are inoculated to a medium selective for C. difficile, such as cycloserine-cefoxitin-fructose agar (CCFA), and are incubated anaerobically for 48 hours. Alternatively, C. difficile may be isolated by using the alcohol spore selection procedure. Between 0.5 and 1 ml of stool is mixed with an equal volume of absolute ethanol, and after 1 hour at room temperature both treated and untreated samples are planted onto a selective medium such as CCFA and incubated anaerobically. Organism identification is discussed in Chapter 30.

Clostridium perfringens. C. perfringens is one of the causes of long-incubation food poisoning, which is characterized by cramping abdominal pain and diarrhea, usually within 7 to 15 hours of eating contaminated food. It also may cause antibiotic-associated diarrhea, typically in hospitalized elderly patients, or enteritis necroticans (Chapter 30). To diagnose food poisoning caused by C. perfringens quantitative anaerobic culture of a stool specimen that was transported in an anaerobic transport collection system is performed. Ethanol-treated and untreated fecal material is diluted as described earlier under Gastric Contents for detection of bacteria associated with short-incubation food poisoning. Sheep blood and phenylethyl alcohol–blood agar plates are inoculated and incubated anaerobically for 48 hours. Identification of C. perfringens is discussed in Chapter 30. A spore count of 10^5 or more per gram of stool may be significant, especially if demonstrated in samples from the majority of affected persons. Isolates from several persons may be typed to determine if they are identical, and the toxin may be detected in the original stool specimen, but these tests usually are performed in reference laboratories. Similar criteria are used to diagnose diarrhea produced by C. perfringens during antibiotic therapy.

Neisseria gonorrhoeae. Swab specimens submitted for detection of N. gonorrhoeae should be inoculated as promptly as possible onto a selective medium such as modified Thayer-Martin (other acceptable media are listed in Chapter 31) and incubated at 35° to 37° C in atmosphere of 5 to 7% carbon dioxide or in a candle jar for up to 72 hours. Identification of N. gonorrhoeae is discussed in Chapter 31.

Escherichia coli. In cases of hemorrhagic colitis, tests for detection of verotoxin-producing (or enterohemorrhagic) E. coli (EHEC) must be requested specifically. The stool specimen is inoculated onto sorbitol-MacConkey agar (containing 1% D-sorbitol instead of lactose), a medium that differentiates strains of EHEC, which do not ferment sorbitol, from other E. coli, almost all of which do. Plates are incubated 18 to 24 hours at 35° to 37° C in ambient air, and clear colonies (indicating that sorbitol was not utilized) that are identified as E. coli are serotyped as discussed in Chapter 34. In addition to screening on sorbitol-MacConkey agar, the stool filtrate (prepared as described earlier for detection of Clostridium difficile toxin) is tested for toxin production in Vero cells (described in reference 16). Tests for detection of enterotoxigenic, enteroinvasive, enteroadherent, and enteroaggregative strains of Escherichia coli (see Chapter 34) generally are performed only in reference laboratories, and these laboratories should be contacted regarding specimen handling.

Bacteria Detected by Routine Culture. Stool and rectal swab specimens received in the laboratory for routine culture should be processed to allow recovery of species of Shigella and Salmonella and the thermophilic species of Campylobacter (Campylobacter jejuni, -coli, and -lari). In institutions where Aeromonas is recovered frequently the laboratory director may wish to include sheep blood agar or specific media for isolation of Aeromonas (discussed later) in the routine setup. Media used for isolation of Shigella and Salmonella are listed in Table 59–3 (ingredients for media most often used are described in Chapter 24); for optimal recovery of these organisms, one medium from each group should be inoculated, except for the highly selective media, which generally are used for epidemiologic studies of outbreaks of disease caused by Salmonella typhi. The use of Salmonella-Shigella agar is discouraged because the growth of some isolates of Shigella sonnei is inhibited (17). Enrichment broth must be used for rectal swab specimens but may not be necessary for stool samples; its use should be evaluated by the medical director in each institution to ensure good patient care and cost efficiency. Plates are incubated 18 to 24 hours at 35° to 37° C in ambient air, and the enrichment broth is incubated under identical conditions for 4 to 8 hours and then subcultured to a medium of moderate or intermediate selectivity. Clear colonies (lactose-negative), colonies with a black center (hydrogen sulfide–positive), or both could be either Shigella or Salmonella and need further evaluation. Screening such isolates with Kliger's iron agar, lysine iron agar, and urea agar for identification is cost effective. Isolates that yield reactions consistent with species of Salmonella or Shigella (Table 59–4) must be identified using a commercially available system or additional conventional media, and those confirmed to be Salmonella or Shigella must be serotyped and reported to the state health department.

Recovery of the thermophilic species of Campylobacter requires inoculation of a selective medium, most commonly Campy-BAP (described in Chapter 24). Alternatively, the sample is filtered using a 0.65-μm pore size cellulose acetate filter, and the filtrate is planted onto Brucella sheep blood agar or chocolate agar. Media are

Table 59–3. Media Used to Recover Shigella and Salmonella From Stool and Rectal Swab Specimens

Purpose	Media
Moderately selective	MacConkey agar, eosin-methylene blue agar
Intermediately selective	Hektoen enteric agar, xylose-lysine-desoxycholate agar, desoxycholate citrate agar, Salmonella-Shigella agar
Highly selective	Bismuth sulfate agar, brilliant green agar
Enrichment	Selenite F broth, GN broth, tetrathionate broth

Table 59-4. Screening Tests to Identify Salmonella and Shigella in Stool Specimens

Organism	Expected Reactions		
	KIA*	LIA*	Urea
Salmonella (most serotypes)	K/A, H$_2$S, gas	K/K, H$_2$S	—
Salmonella typhi	K/A, H$_2$S	K/K, H$_2$S	—
Salmonella paratyphi A	K/A, gas	K/A	—
Shigella spp	K/A†	K/A	—

* Reaction of slant/reaction of butt
† Rare isolates produce gas from glucose
Key: KIA, Kligler's iron agar; LIA, lysine iron agar; K, alkaline; A, acid; —, negative

incubated in a microaerophilic atmosphere at 42° C for 48 to 72 hours. The necessary atmosphere is created by using gas-generating envelopes (commercially available) in conjunction with plastic bags or plastic jars or by evacuation and replacement in plastic bags or anaerobic jars with an atmosphere of 10% carbon dioxide, 5% oxygen, and 85% nitrogen. Identification of these organisms is discussed in Chapter 37.

Yersinia enterocolitica. Gastroenteritis caused by Y. enterocolitica is uncommon in most parts of the United States, so culture of all stool or rectal swabs on a medium specific for this pathogen is not cost effective. When isolation of Y. enterocolitica is requested, CIN (cefsulodin, irgasan, novobiocin) agar is inoculated and incubated at room temperature for 48 hours. Bright pink colonies with a red center, typical of Y. enterocolitica, are identified using a commercially available kit system or conventional biochemical media (see Chapter 34). Yersinia enterocolitica also can be recovered by altering the protocol described earlier for "routine culture" of stool and rectal swab specimens as follows: The MacConkey plate is incubated at 35° C for the first 24 hours and then at room temperature for 24 hours. Colonies of Y. enterocolitica are purple and pinhead in size.

Vibrio species. Species of Vibrio frequently grow on the media used for isolation of Salmonella and Shigella; however, for optimal recovery of Vibrio cholerae and other species of Vibrio from stool and rectal swab specimens, thiosulfate-citrate–bile salts–sucrose (TCBS) agar and alkaline peptone water (for enrichment) are inoculated. The agar and broth media are incubated in ambient air at 35° to 37° C. Plates are examined at 24 and 48 hours. The broth is incubated about 12 hours and then is subcultured to TCBS agar and incubated under identical conditions up to 48 hours. Identification of the vibrios is discussed in Chapter 35.

Aeromonas species. Species of Aeromonas grow on the media used routinely for recovery of Salmonella and Shigella (described earlier), but because many isolates of Aeromonas ferment lactose and sucrose the colonies do not appear sufficiently distinct to be recognized on these media. To ensure recovery of Aeromonas from stool and rectal swab specimens the culture should be requested specifically and the specimen should be inoculated onto CIN agar (containing 4 mg/L of cefsulodin, rather than the usual 15 mg/L) or onto sheep blood agar with ampicillin (10 mg/L). Plates are incubated at 25° to 30° C in ambient air for up to 48 hours. Identification of species of Aeromonas is discussed in Chapter 35.

Plesiomonas shigelloides. P. shigelloides grows on most media used routinely for recovery of Salmonella and Shigella from stool or rectal swab specimens, but eosin–methylene blue, brilliant green, and Salmonella-Shigella agar inhibit the growth of some isolates. Because as many as 30% of isolates of P. shigelloides ferment lactose, their colonies do not appear sufficiently distinct to be recognized on these media, and screening all colonies for Plesiomonas is not cost effective. Therefore, culture of stool and rectal swab specimens for P. shigelloides must be requested specifically. Inoculation of the selective-differential medium inositol–brilliant green–bile salts agar, on which P. shigelloides usually forms white to pink colonies, has been recommended but is not required (18). Identification of P. shigelloides is discussed in Chapter 35.

Campylobacter species. The nonthermophilic species of Campylobacter associated with gastrointestinal disease—Campylobacter cinaedi, Campylobacter fennelliae, Campylobacter hyointestinalis—grow best in a microaerophilic environment at 37° C. To isolated these agents, a stool filtrate, prepared by passing the specimen through a cellulose acetate filter of 0.65 to 0.8 μm pore size, is inoculated to a selective agar (such as Campy-BAP) and a nonselective agar (such as sheep blood or chocolate agar) and the plates are incubated up to 72 hours at 37° C in a microaerophilic atmosphere (created as previously discussed for thermophilic campylobacters) (19).

Mycobacterium species. Stool specimens usually are submitted for isolation of Mycobacterium avium-intracellulare, but Mycobacterium tuberculosis and other species of Mycobacterium also may be recovered. To process the specimen, 1 to 2 g of formed stool or 5 ml of liquid stool is placed in a 50-ml centrifuge tube, and sterile filtered distilled water is added to give a volume of 10 ml. The suspension is mixed on a vortex mixer and filtered through gauze, after which 10 ml of 2% NaOH-N-acetyl L-cysteine is added. The mixture is allowed to stand at room temperature for 45 to 60 minutes, and 25 ml of phosphate buffer is added. The suspension is mixed and clarified by centrifugation at 2000 g for 20 minutes. The supernatant is decanted, and the sediment is used to prepare slides for staining with auramine rhodamine or an acid-fast stain (Appendix, Procedures 4–6) and to inoculate media (discussed in Chapters 40 and 54, Table 54–4).

Parasites

In the clinical laboratory the backbone of diagnostic parasitology is examination of stool samples for the detection of parasitic protozoa and helminth eggs or larvae. Perianal samples collected with the cellophane tape technique are used for recovery and identification of Enterobius vermicularis (Appendix, Procedure 29). Laboratories that perform tests for detection of parasites should have adequate facilities for handling stool samples, and a good microscope with a calibrated scale to measure the organisms. Staining of fecal smears also is required if identification of intestinal protozoa is to be made.

Collection, Transport, and Processing

Collection of fecal specimens for parasitologic examination is usually done by the patient, and on a few occasions by the physician (during a rectal examination or during proctoscopy) or the nurse at the bedside.

The specimen can be collected without fixative and transported to the laboratory if both bacterial and parasitologic studies are requested. The fresh stool (without fixative) should be placed into a clean, dry, wide-mouthed container. Stool should not be collected from the toilet bowl; it should not be contaminated with urine or other substances such as mineral or castor oil or antidiarrheal compounds, and it should not contain recently administered radiologic contrast medium. Once collected the sample should be delivered to the laboratory immediately, where the bacteriologic studies are done first; then the sample is given to the personnel performing tests for detection of parasites for study within 30 to 60 minutes after its collection. Any delays result in degeneration of trophozoites of Entamoeba histolytica, the only parasite for which examination of fresh specimens may be desirable (20). Fresh specimens should be handled with caution in the laboratory, according to body substance isolation guidelines. Because of the possibility of laboratory-acquired infections the use of fresh specimens for parasitologic examination has been questioned.

If the fecal sample is used only for parasitologic analysis, it can be collected and fixed at the time of collection. The sample is delivered to the laboratory at the individual's convenience, and examined when there is time. Several kits commercially available for collection and transport of fecal samples carry detailed instructions (some in several languages) of the technique used in collection and fixation of the sample. The vials can be obtained in special containers, approved by the U.S. Postal Service, for transport through the mail. Commercially available collection kits usually consist of two vials, one with fixative (formalin) for trophozoites and cysts, and the other with fixative (Schaudinn's solution) plus polyvinyl alcohol (PVA) for preparation of smears for staining.

The question of how many fecal specimens are required to identify all persons with intestinal protozoa or helminths is still without a definitive answer. For diagnosis of amoeba it has been recommended that a minimum of three specimens should be collected on different days and examined (21). In one study the rate of detection of protozoal and helminthic infections was less than 100% when one or two stool specimens were examined (22). For cost containment the clinician should request examination of only one specimen, because about 90% of all infections are diagnosed in the first sample (23). If a parasite is not detected in the first sample, a second or a third one should be requested. Two or more specimens collected on different days and received in the laboratory at the same time should be pooled and evaluated as one (24). Stool examination for parasites in patients who have been hospitalized more than 3 days is inappropriate (25).

Once the fecal sample is received in the laboratory for parasitologic examination, it is studied by standard procedures that detect most parasites listed in Table 59–2. If a specific request is made, or if the laboratory personnel suspect that the parasite being sought is Cryptosporidium, Strongyloides, or Schistosoma, special procedures should be carried out (described later) if these parasites are not detected in the routine workup.

Routine Examination of Stool Samples for Parasites. The routine examination of stool samples for parasites consists of preparation of saline solution and of iodine (Lugol)-stained wet mounts. This is followed by concentration of cysts and helminth eggs, and finally by preparation of smears for staining with the trichrome stain. The wet preparations should be made and examined before concentration and staining. If a diagnosis is secured with the examination of the wet mounts (for example, the clinical diagnosis is giardiasis and one finds Giardia in the saline wet mount), the other tests should not be necessary.

The standard fecal smear, which has about 2 mg of feces, is made from a fresh fecal sample as follows: a drop of saline solution is placed on a clear glass slide; with an applicator stick, a small amount of feces is picked up and with circular movements is mixed thoroughly with the drop of saline solution on the glass slide, until enough sample is dissolved, and the mixture is covered with a 22-mm square coverglass. A good wet smear prepared as described should allow reading of small print through the smear. The smear stained with iodine is prepared in exactly the same manner. Both the saline solution and the iodine solution wet preparations can be made on the same glass slide, at the same time, mixing the feces with the saline solution first, and then with the iodine solution. The saline solution smear shows trophozoites and cysts of protozoa, plus all the helminth eggs and larvae. The smear stained with iodine does not show trophozoites, because, unless the sample previously has been fixed, they are destroyed by the iodine. The main advantage of the iodione stain is that some morphologic characteristics of cysts are better visualized, allowing them to be identified. The saline solution shows movement of trophozoites, which is useful for their identification. Preparation of wet mounts from formalin-fixed material is simple: the contents are mixed well and one drop is placed directly onto the glass slide and onto a drop of iodine solution.

Examination of the saline solution smear usually is carried out with medium power (10× objective) at first. Beginning at the left upper corner of the cover slide, the slide is moved horizontally to the right edge of the cover slide, then moved down one field and moved horizontally from the right to the left. The operation is repeated until the entire 22-mm square coverglass is examined. All helminth eggs or larvae and all protozoan cysts, seen as birefringent small objects, should be noted. The eggs of Ascaris, hookworms, and Trichuris should be counted in the entire 22-mm square coverglass. More than 100 ascaris eggs per smear represents a heavy infection, fewer than 25 a light infection, and intermediate numbers a moderate infection. More than 25 hookworm or Trichuris eggs represents heavy infection; fewer than 5 light infections. After examination with a medium-power objective is completed, the slide is examined with high-power objective to detect and identify protozoa by searching randomly for about 5 to 10 minutes per preparation.

The concentration technique is particularly useful because it allows enrichment of samples with few organisms. Several techniques for concentrating parasites have been described, but the ideal method for routine evaluation is the formalin ether concentration. Formalin ether concentration, made safer by the use of ethyl acetate rather than diethyl ether, is excellent for laboratories that process large numbers of stool samples. Concentration can be done on both fresh and fixed specimens, and commercially available kits that allow standardization of the technique can be purchased (Appendix, Procedure 30).

The permanently stained fecal smear for diagnosis of infection with intestinal protozoa is considered the standard of good practice for North American clinical laboratories, but this is not so in other countries, and especially in the Third World, because of lack of facilities or funds. Stains are made on smears prepared with a small paint brush wetted slightly in saline solution, and are fixed in Schaudinn's solution before they are dried. Smears are also made from samples received fixed in polyvinyl alcohol, using a wooden applicator stick to pick up drops of the sample and place them on clean glass slides, making sure that the film touches the long edges of the glass slide and occupies about half the slide. If the film does not touch the long edges of the slide the film will fall off during staining. After the film is completely dry at room temperature it is ready for staining (Appendix, Procedure 25).

Certain intestinal parasites may require special techniques for detection. These techniques are performed after the routine fecal examination, described earlier, fails to demonstrate these parasites and if they have been requested specifically.

Cryptosporidium. Several techniques have been suggested for detection of oocyts of Cryptosporidium, including the flotation of oocysts in Sheather's sugar solution, zinc sulfate, or saturated sodium chloride. Formalin–ethyl acetate also concentrates oocysts of Cryptosporidium, and some workers have found no differences among these techniques. The other technique used is the modified acid-fast stain or modified Kinyoun cold technique, because trichrome and other stains used for fecal smears are not acceptable for the identification of oocysts of Cryptosporidium (Appendix, Procedure 31).

Strongyloides stercoralis. On rare occasions concentration of larvae in fresh stools with the use of the Baerman technique is necessary (Appendix, Procedure 32).

Schistosoma species. Eggs of Schistosoma sometimes are detected better if a thick fecal smear (Kato technique) or concentration by sedimentation is done (Appendix, Procedure 33).

TISSUES

Tissues collected during an endoscopic or a surgical procedure or at autopsy are useful for determining the cause of a lesion in the gastrointestinal tract. Organisms likely to be detected vary according to the site involved (Table 59–5). Specimen collection is similar for all organisms: the surgeon, endoscopist, or pathologist obtains an adequate sample of the lesion using aseptic technique. Transport and processing of the specimen differ for detection of viruses, bacteria, fungi, and parasites and are discussed separately for each group.

Viruses

Transport and processing of gastrointestinal tissue for identification of viruses such as HSV and CMV, which are detected by routine isolation techniques, are different from those used for human papillomavirus and are discussed separately.

Viruses Detected by Routine Isolation. Tissue collected for routine virus isolation is placed in viral transport medium, such as Hanks' balanced salt solution (Chapter 3), and is promptly delivered to the laboratory or is refrigerated for a short time and transported on wet ice. The tissue is homogenized in the transport medium by using a sterile tissue grinder or a mortar and pestle to make a 10 to 20% suspension, which is mixed on a vortex mixer and clarified by centrifugation at 1500 to 2000 g for 15 to 20 minutes. To ensure recovery of HSV and CMV, the supernatant is inoculated to appropriate cell monolayers and processed as described earlier for esophageal brushings. Moreover, as previously discussed, centrifugation-culture, in addition to conventional cell culture, is recommended for detection of CMV, a technique that also can be used to detect HSV.

Human papillomavirus. To detect human papillomavirus the tissues should be placed in the transport medium provided in the commercially available nucleic acid hybridization kit, transported promptly to the laboratory, and stored in the refrigerator until tested.

Bacteria

Transport and processing of tissue from the gastrointestinal tract for detection of bacteria differ for each organism and are discussed separately.

Table 59–5. Pathogens Detected in Tissues from Different Sites in the Gastrointestinal Tract

Organism	Site	Chapter
Herpes simplex virus	E, S, D, SI, C, R, A	5
Cytomegalovirus	E, S, D, SI, C, R, A	5
Human papillomavirus	R, A	7
Clostridium difficile	C, R	30
Actinomyces spp	C	30
Pseudomonas aeruginosa	SI, C	32
Shigella spp	C	34
Salmonella spp	SI, C	34
Yersinia enterocolitica	SI	34
Campylobacter spp	C	37
Helicobacter pylori	S, D	37
Candida spp	E, S, D, SI, C, R, A	43
Zygomycetes	E, S, SI, C	44
Histoplasma capsulatum	E, S, SI, C	45
Paracoccidioides brasiliensis	E, S, SI, C	45

Key: E, esophagus; S, stomach; D, duodenum; SI, small intestine (especially the ileum); C, colon; R, rectum; A, anus.

Clostridium difficile. Biopsies collected for diagnosis of disease caused by C. difficile should be divided into two equal parts. Half of the sample is transported promptly to the laboratory in a sterile container and is evaluated for the presence of toxin. The tissue is placed in diluent, mixed on a vortex mixer, and clarified by centrifugation at 2000 g for 20 minutes: the supernatant is assayed as described earlier for stool specimens. The other half of the sample is placed in an anaerobic transport system for culture and, ideally, is processed in an anaerobic chamber, where the tissue is homogenized using a sterile tissue grinder or mortar and pestle without exposing it to air. A smear stained with the Gram stain is prepared, and the suspension is inoculated to selective and nonselective media (as described earlier for stool and rectal swab specimens) and to chopped meat broth. If an anaerobic chamber is not available the tissue may be processed as rapidly as possible in a biologic safety cabinet.

Actinomyces species. For detection of Actinomyces the tissue should be placed in an anaerobic transport system and delivered promptly to the laboratory. Optimally, the sample is processed in an anaerobic chamber, but rapid processing in air probably will not prevent the recovery of Actinomyces because most species are aerotolerant. The tissue is homogenized in a small amount of broth with a sterile tissue grinder or a mortar and pestle. A smear is stained with the Gram stain, the homogenate is inoculated to anaerobic blood agar and to chopped meat or thioglycolate broth, and the cultures are incubated anaerobically at 35° to 37° C for up to 14 days. Identification of Actinomyces is discussed in Chapter 30.

Pseudomonas aeruginosa. Tissue obtained from persons suspected to have disease caused by P. aeruginosa (typhilitis and perirectal abscess, see Chapter 32) should be transported promptly to the laboratory in a sterile container and homogenized in a small amount of broth. The suspension is used for preparation of a smear for the Gram stain and for inoculation to sheep blood and MacConkey agar and thioglycolate broth (all incubated in ambient air). Incubation times and temperatures are described in Chapter 54.

Shigella and Salmonella species. Tissue collected from a person with an illness suspected to be caused by Shigella or Salmonella should be transported to the laboratory and homogenized as described above for Pseudomonas aeruginosa. The homogenate is used to prepare a smear for stain with the Gram stain and for inoculation onto MacConkey and Hektoen agars and into GN broth (or alternate media listed in Table 59–3). Culture conditions are identical to those described earlier for detection of these organisms in stool and rectal swab specimens.

Yersinia enterocolitica. Culture for Y. enterocolitica must be requested specifically. The tissue is transported and homogenized as described earlier for Pseudomonas aeruginosa, and the homogenate is used to prepare a smear for stain with the Gram stain and to inoculate MacConkey and CIN agars (described earlier for stool and rectal swab specimens), which are incubated at room temperature. The remainder of the homogenate is placed in the refrigerator for cold enrichment and is subcultured to MacConkey agar (incubated at room temperature) weekly for 4 weeks or until Yersinia enterocolitica is recovered.

Campylobacter species. To detect species of Campylobacter the biopsy should be transported and homogenized as described earlier for Pseudomonas aeruginosa. The homogenate is passed through a cellulose acetate filter of 0.65 to 0.8 μm pore size, the filtrate is used to prepare a smear for stain with Gram stain and is inoculated to Campy-BAP and chocolate agar, which are incubated up to 72 hours at 37° C in a microaerophilic atmosphere (as described earlier for detecting Campylobacter jejuni in stool specimens).

Helicobacter pylori. Gastric or duodenal biopsy specimens collected for detection of H. pylori should be transported in a sterile container to the laboratory immediately; but if a delay is unavoidable the specimen should be refrigerated in isotonic saline or in a 20% glucose solution for a short time. An imprint of a tissue fragment, prepared by rinsing the tissue in dextrose phosphate broth, blotting it on sterile gauze or filter paper, and gently pressing it onto the surface of a sterile glass slide, should be stained with Gram stain. The tissue fragments then are homogenized and inoculated to sheep blood, chocolate, or Thayer Martin agar plates and incubated at 35° to 37° C in a microaerophilic atmosphere for up to 1 week (26). A portion of the homogenate may be inoculated directly to urea broth and incubated up to 24 hours in ambient air. Identification of H. pylori is discussed in Chapter 37.

Mycobacterium species. Tissue from the gastrointestinal tract submitted for culture of mycobacteria should be transported to the laboratory in a sterile container and homogenized with a sterile tissue grinder or a mortar and pestle. The homogenate is poured through sterile gauze into a 50-ml centrifuge tube, and an equal volume of 2% NaOH-*N*-acetyl-L cysteine is added and mixed. The suspension is allowed to stand at room temperature 20 minutes, then 25 ml of phosphate buffer is added, mixed, and centrifuged at 2000 to 3000 g for 20 minutes. The supernatant is decanted, and the sediment is resuspended in 1 to 2 ml of buffer and used to prepare smears for staining with auramine rhodamine or acid-fast stain (Appendix, Procedures 4–6) and to inoculate appropriate media (see Chapter 40 Table 54–4).

Fungi

To detect fungi in gastrointestinal biopsy tissue the specimen should be transported promptly in a sterile container to the laboratory, where it is homogenized in broth using a sterile tissue grinder, a mortar and pestle, or a Stomacher, or by mincing with sterile scissors. A potassium hydroxide preparation of the homogenate (Appendix, Procedure 19), or a smear stained with calcofluor white, Congo red, Gomori's methenamine silver, or the Gram stain, is examined under the microscope. Ideally, 1 ml of the homogenate is inoculated onto primary fungal culture media, such as brain-heart infusion agar, inhibitory mold agar, or SABHI agar, containing antibiotics (discussed in detail in Chapter 42), but the volume inoculated depends on the original sample size. Culture conditions are described in Chapter 54.

Parasites

Tissues from the gastrointestinal tract are seldom received in the laboratory for detection of parasites. If tissues are taken during an endoscopic or a surgical procedure or at autopsy they generally are sent to the surgical pathology laboratory for histologic evaluation.

The only situation in which tissues are sent to the clinical laboratory is for diagnosis of infection with Schistosoma. Usually a biopsy of colonic or urinary bladder mucosa is taken and divided into two portions: half for the anatomic pathologist and half for the parasitology laboratory. The tissue fragment should be fresh, without fixative, and delivered promptly to the laboratory, where it is placed between two glass slides. After steady pressure on the upper slide the tissue should be disrupted and flattened enough to allow examination under the microscope. Eggs of Schistosoma are generally large enough to allow visualization under a low-power objective (Chapter 52).

REFERENCES

1. Woods GL, and Mills R: Effect of dexamethasone on detection of herpes simplex virus in clinical specimens by conventional cell culture and rapid 24-well plate centrifugation. J Clin Microbiol, 26:1233, 1988.
2. Thiele GM, and Woods GL: The effect of dexamethasone on detection of cytomegalovirus in tissue culture and by immunofluorescence. J Virol Methods, 22:319, 1988.
3. Woods GL, Young A, Johnson A, and Thiele GM: Detection of cytomegalovirus by 24-well plate centrifugation assay using a monoclonal antibody to an early nuclear antigen. J Virol Methods, 18:207, 1987.
4. Gleaves CA, Wilson DJ, Wold AD, and Smith TF: Detection and serotyping of herpes simplex virus in MRC-5 cells by use of centrifugation and monoclonal antibodies 16 h postinoculation. J Clin Microbiol, 21:29, 1985.
5. Goka AK, et al: The relative merits of faecal and duodenal juice microscopy in the diagnosis of giardiasis. Roy Soc Trop Med Hyg, 84:66, 1990.
6. Korman SH, Hais E, and Spira DT: Routine in vitro cultivation of Giardia lamblia using the string test. J Clin Microbiol, 29:368, 1990.
7. World Health Organization: WHO reports decry neglect of world health problems. ASM News, 56:358, 1990.
8. Walsh JA, and Warren KW: Selective primary health care: An interim strategy for disease control in developing countries. N Engl J Med, 301:967, 1979.
9. Guerrant RL: Principles and syndromes of enteric infection. In Principles and Practice of Infectious Diseases. 3rd ed. Edited by GL Mandell, RG Douglas, Jr, and JE Bennett. New York, Churchill Livingstone, 1990.
10. Guerrant RL, and McAuliffe JF: Special problems in developing countries. In Infectious Diarrhea. Edited by SL Gorbach. Boston, Blackwell Scientific, 1986.
11. Takiff HE, Straws SE, and Garon CF: Propagation and in vitro studies of previously noncultivable enteric adenoviruses in 293 cells. Lancet, ii:832, 1981.
12. Christensen ML: Human viral gastroenteritis. Clin Microbiol Rev, 2:51, 1989.
13. Gilligan P, et al: Evaluation of the PREMIER Clostridium difficile toxin A (CdTA) enzyme immunoassay (EIA) (Abstract 1192). In Program and Abstracts of the 30th Interscience Conference of Antimicrobial Agents and Chemotherapy. Washington, DC, American Society for Microbiology, 1990.
14. Degirolami PC, et al: Multicenter evaluation of a new EIA for detection of C. difficile toxin A. J Clin Microbiol, 30:1085, 1992.
15. Lyverly DM, Krivan HC, and Wilkins TC: Clostridium difficile: Its disease and toxins. Clin Microbiol Rev, 1:1, 1988.
16. Karmali MA: Infection by verocytotoxin-producing Escherichia coli. Clin Microbiol Rev, 2:15, 1989.
17. Koneman EW, et al (eds): The Enterobacteriaceae. In Color Atlas and Textbook of Diagnostic Microbiology. 3rd ed. Philadelphia, JB Lippincott, 1988.
18. Clark RB, and Janda JM: Plesiomonas and human disease. Clin Microbiol Newslett, 13:49, 1991.
19. Tenover FC, and Gebhart CJ: Isolation and identification of Campylobacter species. Clin Microbiol Newslett, 10:81, 1988.
20. Proctor EM: Laboratory diagnosis of amebiasis. Clin Lab Med, 11:829, 1991.
21. American Society of Parasitologists: Subcommittee on Laboratory Standards, Committee on Education. Procedures suggested for use in examination of clinical specimens for parasitic infections. J Parasitol, 673:959, 1977.
22. Thompson RB, Haas RA, and Thompson JH: Intestinal parasites: The necessity of examining multiple stool specimens. Mayo Clin Proc, 59:641, 1984.
23. Montessori GA, and Bischoff L: Searching for parasites in stool: Once is usually enough. CMAJ, 137:702, 1987.
24. Peters CS, et al: Cost containment of formalin-preserved stool specimens for ova and parasites from outpatients. J Clin Microbiol, 26:1584, 1988.
25. Siegel DL, Edelstein PH, and Nachamkin I: Inappropriate testing for diarrheal diseases in the hospital. JAMA, 263:979, 1990.
26. Edmonds P, Kassman N, Judd RL, and Rudert CS: Clinical and microbiologic features of Campylobacter pylori–associated gastric ulcers in humans. Clin Microbiol Newslett, 10:97, 1988.

Chapter 60

LIVER, BILIARY TRACT, AND PANCREAS

Specimens collected to determine the cause of infections involving the liver, biliary tract, and pancreas include purulent material aspirated from an abscess, bile, and liver tissue. Serum, useful in diagnosing hepatitis caused by several viruses and bacteria, is discussed in Chapter 58.

ABSCESS MATERIAL

Abscesses of the liver may be caused by bacteria, fungi, or parasites (Table 60–1). Organisms reach the liver via the biliary tract; the portal system, originating from an intra-abdominal infection such as appendicitis, diverticulitis, amoebiasis, or inflammatory bowel disease; direct extension of a contiguous infection; via the hepatic artery from a distant focus of infection; penetrating surgical or nonsurgical wounds, and, occasionally, no source of infection is identified.

Pyogenic abscess of the liver can occur at any age but are most common after 40 years and are rare in children (1). Typically, the right lobe is involved with a single abscess. The infection frequently is polymicrobial, and viridans streptococci, members of the Enterobacteriaceae, and anaerobes are the most common isolates (1,2). The most frequent symptoms are fever, chills, and abdominal pain.

Multiple microabscesses in the liver may be part of a systemic infection caused by species of Candida, or the process may be localized to the liver and spleen, usually in association with hematopoietic malignancy, especially leukemia, and granulocytopenia (3,4). Symptoms are similar to those described for pyogenic abscesses.

Most abscesses of the pancreas occur as a complication of pancreatitis, but they may develop as a complication of endoscopic retrograde cholangiopancreatography, a penetrating peptic ulcer, or a secondary infection of a pancreatic pseudocyst (5). As many as 50% of abscesses are polymicrobial, and members of the Enterobacteriaceae, enterococci, viridans streptococci, and anaerobes are frequently involved (5–8). Common clinical manifestations include fever, abdominal pain that may radiate to the back, nausea, and vomiting.

Collection, Tranport, and Processing

To identify the organisms responsible for abscesses of the liver or pancreas, pus is aseptically aspirated with a needle and syringe. To transport the specimen the air is expelled, the needle is removed, and the syringe is tightly capped (preferably with a rubber cap) and delivered promptly to the laboratory. Because specimen processing is different for detection of bacteria, fungi, and parasites, each group is discussed separately.

Bacteria

Methods used to process aspirated purulent material for detection of bacteria differ for different groups of bacteria and are discussed separately for those detected by routine culture and for species of Mycobacterium.

Bacteria Detected by Routine Culture. Routine processing of aspirated pus involves preparation of a smear for Gram staining and inoculation of media for culture. Sheep blood agar, MacConkey agar and thioglycolate broth (incubated aerobically), and anaerobic blood agar (incubated anaerobically) are recommended. Adding kanamycin-vancomycin laked blood agar (incubated anaerobically), selective for species of Bacteroides, may be helpful. Incubation temperatures and times discussed in Chapter 54 allow recovery of most pathogens, though if granules are present or if detection of Actinomyces is requested specifically the anaerobic blood agar plate and the broth should be incubated as long as 2 weeks.

Mycobacterium species. Purulent material aspirated from an abscess of the liver or pancreas should not be contaminated with normal flora and, therefore, should not require decontamination before culture. A smear should be prepared for auramine rhodamine or acid-fast staining (Appendix, Procedures 4–6), and appropriate media (Table 54–4, and discussed in Chapter 40) are inoculated directly. However, if specimens appear to be contaminated (for example, those that are yellow, green, or foul smelling) a smear stained with the Gram stain should be examined, and if bacteria are present the material should be decontaminated by transferring it to a sterile 50-ml centrifuge tube and adding 10 ml of sterile, filtered distilled water. The mixture is mixed on a vortex mixer, allowed to stand 20 minutes, and processed as a sputum specimen (Appendix, Procedure 27). Organism identification is discussed in Chapter 40.

Fungi

Processing aspirated purulent material material for detection of fungi involves direct microscopic examination and inoculation of appropriate planting media. Methods available for direct examination include the Gram stain, the potassium hydroxide preparation (Appendix, Procedure 19), and Gomori's methenamine silver, calcofluor white, and Congo red stains (described in Chapter 42). To isolate fungi, media (such as brain-heart infusion agar and SABHI agar with and without antibiotics, discussed in Chapters 42 and 54) are inoculated by placing 1- to 2-

Table 60-1. Organisms That Cause Abscesses of the Liver and Pancreas

Organism	Chapter
Bacteria	
Staphylococcus aureus	28
Viridans streptococci	28
Enterococcus spp	28
Actinomyces spp	30
Enterobacteriaceae*	34
Bacteroides spp	38
Fusobacterium spp	38
Mycobacterium tuberculosis	40
Fungi	
Candida spp	43
Parasites	
Entamoeba histolytica	49
Balantidium coli	49

* Of the Enterobacteriaceae, Escherichia coli is involved most frequently.

Table 60-2. Specimens Useful for Diagnosis of Organisms That Cause Hepatitis

Organism	Type of Infection	Specimen Liver	Specimen Serum	Chapter
Viruses				
Herpes simplex virus	A	X		5
Varicella-zoster virus	A	X		5
Cytomegalovirus	A, G	X		5
Epstein-Barr virus	A		X	5
Adenovirus	A	X		6
Hepatitis B virus	A		X	9
δ agent	A		X	9
Enteroviruses	A	X		13
Hepatitis A virus	A		X	13
Yellow fever virus	A	X	X	18
Lassa virus	A	X	X	20
Filovirus	A	X		21
Hepatitis C virus	A		X	23
Hepatitis E virus*	A		X	23
Bacteria				
Coxiella burnetii	G		X	26
Listeria monocytogenes	G	X		29
Nocardia spp	G	X		29
Francisella tularensis	G	X	X	33
Brucella spp	G	X	X	33
Salmonella spp	G	X		34
Treponema pallidum	A, G	X	X	39
Leptospira interrogans	A		X	39
Mycobacterium spp	G	X		40
Cat-scratch disease bacillus (Afipia felis)	G	X		41
Fungi				
Candida spp	G	X		43
Histoplasma capsulatum	G	X		45
Coccidioides immitis	G	X		45

* Hepatitis E also is diagnosed by detecting virus particles in stool by electron microscopy
Key: A, acute hepatitis; G, granulomatous hepatitis.

drop aliquots of the aspirated material onto several areas of the agar surface without streaking for isolation or by placing several drops on the surface of media in tubes. Culture conditions are described in Chapter 54, and organism identification is reviewed in Part II.

Parasites

Entamoeba histolytica is the only parasite that produces liver abscesses, a difficult diagnostic problem, especially outside endemic areas. Material from a liver abscess collected for microbiologic examination should be examined grossly in the laboratory. The typical amoebic abscess is not purulent, has a brown appearance, like that of liquefied liver, and a sweet smell. Such material should be examined for trophozoites of E. histolytica in smears stained with the trichrome stain. Cultures for bacteria should be negative.

If the clinician suspects Entamoeba histolytica as the etiologic agent before the abscess is aspirated, small amounts (about 5 to 10 ml) of the abscess material should be aspirated and placed in separate containers. Examination for trophozoites of E. histolytica is carried out on the last sample taken, as described earlier. The other containers can be discarded if they are not needed for other tests in microbiology.

Only rarely has Balantidium coli produced abscesses of the liver; Ascaris lumbricoides migrating through the common bile duct may lodge in the liver and also produce an abscess. In both instances making the diagnosis is difficult if not impossible.

BILE

Microbiologic studies of bile are useful in identifying the organisms causing acute cholecystitis (which almost always is associated with gallstones impacted in the common duct) and complications of the infection limited to the gallbladder (9). The organisms present often are the normal bowel flora (see Table 2-1): members of the Enterobacteriaceae, enterococci, and species of Bacteroides, Clostridium, and Fusobacterium. Potential complications include empyema or gangrene of the gallbladder, emphysematous cholecystitis; pericholecystic, intra-abdominal, or hepatic abscess; peritonitis, cholangitis, and bacteremia.

Bile is collected by aspiration with a needle and syringe. To transport the sample the air is expelled, the needle is removed, and the syringe is tightly capped and delivered promptly to the laboratory. Specimen processing for detection of bacterial pathogens is identical to that previously described for routine processing of abscess material.

Aspirated bile received in the laboratory could be examined, if warranted, for eggs of Clonorchis, Opisthorchis, and Fasciola, trematodes that normally inhabit the biliary tree. Clonorchis and Opisthorchis are very common in some geographic areas (Chapter 52), and although usually asymptomatic, in some cases can produce biliary obstruction and cholangitis. Infection with Fasciola, which produces chronic cholangitis, is more difficult to diagnose.

Examination of bile for trematode eggs is carried out as for stool samples (Chapter 59). Direct and concentration smears should be examined under the microscope to find and identify the characteristic eggs (Chapter 52).

LIVER TISSUE

Microbiologic studies of liver tissue obtained by biopsy or at autopsy are useful for determining the agents of acute hepatitis and granulomatous hepatitis. Acute infectious hepatitis is a syndrome, most commonly caused by one of the hepatitis viruses but occasionally by other viruses or, less frequently, by bacteria (see Table 60–2), characterized by malaise, weakness, anorexia, intermittent nausea, vomiting, and right-side upper quadrant pain, followed by jaundice and dark urine. Abnormal laboratory findings include marked elevations in aminotransferase values, mild elevations in alkaline phosphatase and lactic dehydrogenase, and a variably elevated bilirubin (involving both direct and indirect fractions). Infections caused by hepatitis B virus, the δ agent, hepatitis A virus, hepatitis C virus, Epstein-Barr virus, Leptospira interrogans, and Treponema pallidum are diagnosed serologically, and hepatitis caused by hepatitis E virus is diagnosed serologically (research only) or by detection of virus particles in stool by electron microscopy. These organisms are not discussed further here. Diagnosis of yellow fever, lassa fever, and infections produced by filoviruses requires tests not available in the clinical laboratory; samples must be sent to a specialized reference center, which should be contacted for specimen requirements.

Granulomatous hepatitis, a diagnosis based on finding granulomas in the liver (Fig. 60–1), is a misnomer, because with rare exceptions the lesion does not represent a true hepatitis (meaning necrosis and inflammation of liver tissue) and hepatocellular dysfunction is rare (10). Hepatic granulomas are associated with a broad spectrum of infections (see Table 60–2). A discussion of the noninfectious diseases that may cause granulomatous hepatitis is found in reference 10. Of the potential infectious agents Mycobacterium tuberculosis is the most common cause, accounting for up to 50% of cases of granulomatous hepatitis in some series (10). Infections caused by Coxiella burnetii and Treponema pallidum are diagnosed serologically and not discussed further here.

Collection, Transport, and Processing

Liver tissue should be placed in a sterile container and transported immediately to the laboratory. Fresh tissue is examined by a pathologist and divided appropriately for histologic and microbiologic studies. Specimen processing is discussed separately for viruses, bacteria, fungi, and parasites.

Viruses

Liver tissue to be processed for virus isolation should be placed in viral transport medium, such as Hanks' balanced salt solution, and refrigerated until it is processed. The tissue is homogenized in the transport medium with a sterile tissue grinder or mortar and pestle to give a 10 to 20% (weight per volume) suspension, which is clarified by 15 to 20 minutes' centrifugation at 1500 to 2000 g. The supernatant then is used to inoculate cell cultures; MRC-5, A549, and primary monkey kidney cells are recommended to ensure recovery of herpes simplex virus (HSV), varicella-zoster virus, cytomegalovirus (CMV), adenovirus, and the enteroviruses. The specimen is inoculated and adsorbed and the cultures are incubated as described in Chapter 54. When infection with CMV is suspected cultures should be incubated for up to 3 weeks; otherwise, incubation for 2 weeks is adequate. Virus identification is discussed in Part II of the text.

Centrifugation-culture has been used successfully for detection of HSV, CMV, and adenovirus in clinical specimens (11–14). The technique is outlined for CMV in the

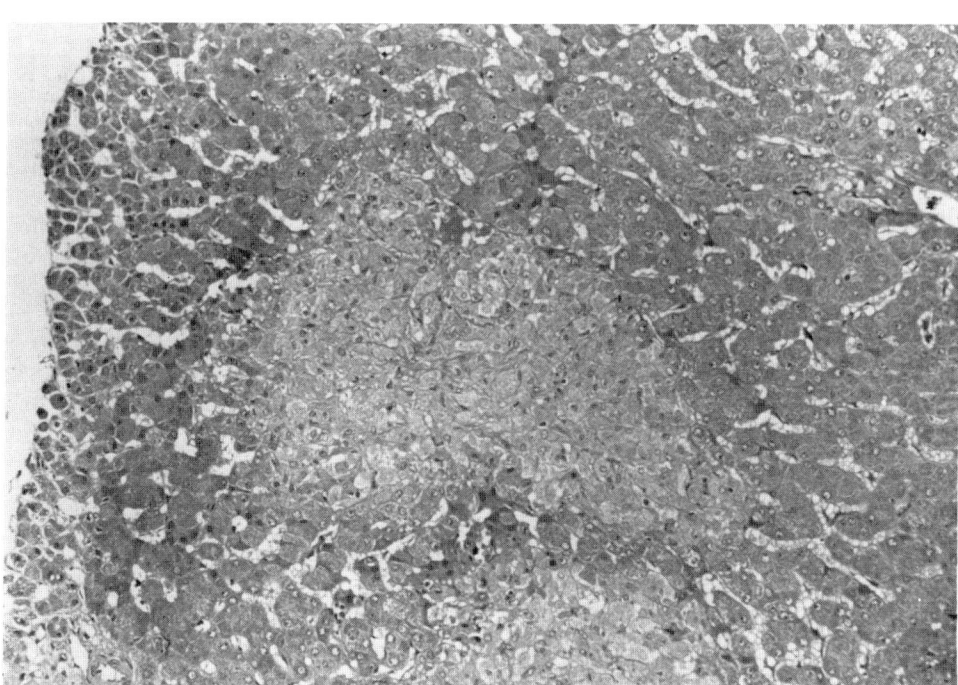

Fig. 60–1. Needle biopsy specimen of liver from an AIDS patient shows granulomas composed predominantly of foamy macrophages (hematoxylin and eosin, ×40). Culture grew Mycobacterium avium-intracellulare.

Appendix, Procedure 2, and is similar for the other viruses, except that different antibodies are used— and for adenovirus different indicator cells (A549 cells). Using centrifugation-culture to supplement conventional cell culture is strongly recommended for detection of CMV because the cytopathic effect it produces often is not apparent for 2 to 4 weeks (occasionally longer). The role of centrifugation-culture in detecting HSV is controversial and should be evaluated in the individual laboratory (11,12). Given that adenovirus is an uncommon cause of hepatitis, centrifugation-culture for detection of this virus in liver tissue is not economical.

Bacteria

Processing liver tissue for detection of bacteria involves preparing a homogenate in a small amount of broth, as described earlier for viruses, a procedure that should be performed in a biologic safety cabinet. Further handling of the sample differs for different organisms and is reviewed individually for each agent.

Listeria monocytogenes. To detect L. monocytogenes, an uncommon cause of granulomatous hepatitis, the homogenate is used to prepare a smear for staining with Gram stain, and for inoculation of media for culture. Listeria monocytogenes is not fastidious, but occasionally its recovery from tissue is difficult. Therefore, to ensure recovery, an enhancement technique is recommended (15). The homogenate is inoculated to each of two tubes of infusion broth; one is incubated at 35° C, the other is stored in the refrigerator. After 24 hours, the 35° C broth culture is subcultured to sheep blood agar, which is incubated with the original culture at 35° to 37° C in an atmosphere of 5 to 7% carbon dioxide or in a candle jar for a minimum of 48 hours. If L. monocytogenes is not recovered from the subcultures at 35° C, the broth initially stored in the refrigerator is subcultured at weekly intervals, as described above, for at least 1 month.

Nocardia species. Culture for Nocardia must be requested specifically, although these organisms are recovered by methods used to isolate mycobacteria (discussed later). The homogenate is used to prepare a smear for staining with Gram stain and for inoculation of media for culture. Moreover, if long, thin, beaded, branching, gram-positive bacilli typical of Nocardia are observed (Plate IIIE) in the smear stained with Gram stain, a second smear should be stained with a modified acid-fast stain (Appendix, Procedure 7). Recommended media and culture conditions are outlined in Table 54–4.

Francisella tularensis. F. tularensis, the agent of tularemia, is an uncommon cause of granulomatous hepatitis. The organism may be recovered from liver tissue, but the infection is diagnosed more frequently by serologic methods. Culture for F. tularensis must be requested specifically, because for optimal recovery special media must be inoculated. Moreover, F. tularensis is among the most common causes of infections acquired in the laboratory, and the laboratory director may prefer to send these specimens to a reference laboratory or to a state or public health laboratory equipped to handle the organism. To process the specimen, the homogenate is used to make a smear for Gram staining and for inoculation of media for culture, as outlined in Table 54–4.

Brucella species. Species of Brucella, which may cause granulomatous hepatitis, can be recovered from liver tissue, but more often the infection is diagnosed by serologic methods. Culture for Brucella must be requested specifically, because prolonged incubation is required for its recovery. To process the specimen the homogenate is used to make a smear for staining with Gram stain and for inoculation of media for culture, as outlined in Table 54–4.

Salmonella species. To detect species of Salmonella, the homogenate is used to prepare a smear for staining with Gram stain and for inoculation of media for culture; sheep blood and MacConkey agars and thioglycolate broth, all incubated in ambient air, are recommended. Incubation times and temperatures are reviewed in Chapter 54.

Mycobacterium species. To process liver tissue for detection of mycobacteria the homogenate is used to prepare a smear for auramine rhodamine or acid-fast staining (Appendix, Procedures 4–6) and for inoculation of media for culture, as outlined in Table 54–4 and discussed in Chapter 40.

Cat-Scratch Disease Bacillus (Afipia felis). The cat-scratch disease bacillus is detected by staining involved tissue with the Warthin-Starry stain (Plate VIIIC) or with the Brown-Hopp tissue Gram stain (see Chapter 41). The organism can be cultured on artificial media, but this is not required for diagnosis (16,17).

Fungi

Processing liver tissue for detection of fungi, which should be performed in a biologic safety cabinet, involves preparing a homogenate, as previously described. The suspension is used to make smears for direct microscopic examination and for inoculation of media for culture. Fungi may be visualized directly by using the potassium hydroxide preparation (Appendix, Procedure 19) or by staining with the Gram, Gomori methenamine silver, calcofluor white, or Congo red stain (Chapter 42). Primary planting media, such as brain-heart infusion agar, inhibitory mold agar, or SABHI agar (plates or tubes), are inoculated (1 ml of sample per medium is optimal but smaller volumes are acceptable). Culture conditions are described in Chapter 54, and organism identification is reviewed in Part II.

Parasites

Liver tissue per se almost never is processed for diagnosis of parasitic infections in the microbiology laboratory. Tissue collected for this purpose usually is sent to the surgical pathology laboratory, where it is processed and studied histologically. Several parasites are found in the liver, but their histologic diagnosis is outside the scope of this discussion (18).

Unusually, fluid from a cystic lesion of the liver is sent to the microbiology laboratory for diagnosis of a hydatid cyst. The typical hydatid cyst fluid is as clear as distilled water, with some gross particles that upon staining of the fluid sediment rapidly. These "particles," hydatid sand, correspond to the protoscolices of the parasite. If aspirated with a Pasteur pipette, placed on a clear glass slide (wet preparation), cover slipped, and examined under the microscope, the protoscolices are identified easily (see Fig. 52–19).

REFERENCES

1. Land MA, Moinuddin M, and Bisno AL: Pyogenic liver abscess: Changing epidemiology and prognosis. South Med J, 78:1426, 1985.
2. McDonald MI, et al: Single and multiple pyogenic liver abscesses. Medicine, 63:291, 1984.
3. Haron E, et al: Hepatic candidiasis: An increasing problem in immunocompromised patients. Am J Med, 83:17, 1987.
4. Thaler M, et al: Hepatic candidiasis in cancer patients: The evolving picture of the syndrome. Ann Intern Med, 108:88, 1988.
5. Hurley JE, and Vargish T: Early diagnosis and outcome of pancreatic abscesses in pancreatitis. Am Surgeon, 53:29, 1987.
6. Altemeier WA, and Alexander JW: Pancreatic abscess. A study of 32 cases. Arch Surg, 87:80, 1963.
7. Aranha GU, Prinz RA, and Greenlee HB: Pancreatic abscess: An unresolved surgical problem. Am J Surg, 144:534, 1982.
8. Shi ECP, Yeo BW, and Ham JM: Pancreatic abscesses. Br J Surg, 71:689, 1984.
9. Berk JE, and Zinbers AS: Acute cholecystitis: Medical aspects. In Gastroenterology. 4th ed. Edited by JE Berk, et al. Philadelphia, WB Saunders, 1985.
10. Harrington PT, et al: Granulomatous hepatitis. Rev Infect Dis, 4:638, 1982.
11. Woods GL, and Mills RD: Conventional tube cell culture compared with centrifugal inoculation of MRC-5 cells and staining with monoclonal antibodies for detection of herpes simplex virus in clinical specimens. J Clin Microbiol, 26:570, 1988.
12. Gleaves CA, Wilson DJ, Wold AD, and Smith TF: Detection and serotyping of herpes simplex virus in MRC-5 cells by use of centrifugation and monoclonal antibodies 16 h post-inoculation. J Clin Microbiol, 21:29, 1985.
13. Woods GL, and Thiele GM: Rapid detection of cytomegalovirus by 24-well plate centrifugation using a monoclonal antibody to an early nuclear antigen. Am J Clin Pathol, 91:695, 1989.
14. Woods GL, Yamamoto M, and Young A: Detection of adenovirus by rapid 24-well plate centrifugation and conventional cell culture with dexamethasone. J Virol Methods, 20:109, 1988.
15. Baron EJ, and Finegold SM (eds): Bailey and Scott's Diagnostic Microbiology. 8th ed. St. Louis, CV Mosby, 1990.
16. English CK, et al: Cat scratch disease. Isolation and culture of the bacterial agent. JAMA, 259:1347, 1988.
17. Brenner DJ, et al: Proposal of Afipia gen. nov., with Afipia felis sp. nov. (formerly the cat scratch disease bacillus), Afipia clevelandensis sp. nov. (formerly the Cleveland Clinic Foundation strain), Afipia broomea sp. nov. and three unnamed genospecies. J Clin Microbiol, 29:2450, 1991.
18. Gutierrez Y: Diagnostic Pathology of Parasitic Infections with Clinical Correlations. Philadelphia, Lea & Febiger, 1990.

Chapter 61

GENITOURINARY TRACT

Specimens from the genitourinary tract received in the laboratory for microbiologic studies include urine, needle aspirates of the kidney, vaginal secretions or swab specimens, urethral and endocervical swab specimens, vesicle fluid or swab specimens, material from ulcers, endometrial tissue or swab specimens, aspirates from the peritoneal cul de sac, abscess material, amniotic fluid, and products of conception.

URINE

Urine specimens are collected to identify the agent of acute pyelonephritis, cystitis, urethritis, and acute and chronic prostatitis, and to diagnose some viral infections that are not specifically associated with urinary tract symptoms, such as infections caused by cytomegalovirus (CMV) (especially in infants and immunocompromised adults) and mumps. Organisms enter the urinary tract via the urethra or the circulatory system. Infection with gram-negative bacilli generally occurs via the urethra (ascending pathway), whereas Staphylococcus aureus, Mycobacterium tuberculosis, and Candida typically are blood-borne pathogens. It is thought that bacteria reach the prostate via the blood, by ascending from the urethra, by lymphatic spread from the rectum, or via reflux of infected urine, but the exact mechanism is unknown.

Infection of the urinary tract occurs at all ages, but the prevalence varies with sex, age, and predisposing factors. Infection is more common in females than males, except in infants and among persons with indwelling catheters. The male-female ratio of infection is 4:1 among infants, 1:15 among preschool-age children, 1:30 or greater among older children and young adults, 1:2 among elders, and 1:1 for catheter-related infections (1).

The incidence of urinary tract infections (UTI) in infants up to 6 months is about 2 cases per 1000 live births (2,3). An estimated 10 to 20% of females experience a UTI sometime during their life; the prevalence of bacteriuria is about 1% in schoolgirls, 1 to 3% in young, nonpregnant women, 4 to 7% during pregnancy, and up to 20% among elderly women (4). Factors associated with increased risk of infection are sexual intercourse and the use of a diaphragm (5,6). In males bacteriuria is uncommon between infancy and about age 60 years, when prostatic obstruction and instrumentation are the major causes of infection (7). The risk of infections associated with catheters is 1% for ambulatory persons, 10% for hospital patients after one brief catheterization, 20% for persons with an indwelling catheter draining into a closed system for 5 or more days, and 100% if an open drainage system is used (8,9).

Symptoms of UTI vary with age and the site of involvement. In children under 2 years of age the main symptoms are failure to thrive, vomiting, and fever. Manifestations of bacterial infections of the lower urinary tract in older children and adults include frequency, dysuria, and urgency. Infections of the urinary bladder caused by adenovirus, herpes simplex virus, and BK virus typically cause hemorrhagic cystitis. Classically, upper UTI is manifested by fever, occasionally with chills and flank pain, frequently accompanied by lower tract symptoms; however, symptoms vary considerably in adults and children. Among elders UTI is often asymptomatic.

Acute and chronic bacterial prostatis are two distinct and unrelated syndromes, although the organisms most commonly involved in both are gram-negative bacilli, especially Escherichia coli (10). Symptoms of acute prostatitis include fever, perineal and back pain, frequency, urgency, and dysuria. Chronic prostatitis may be asymptomatic or may manifest as perineal discomfort and low back pain with periodic symptoms of lower UTI (described earlier). The diagnosis of acute infection is based on clinical manifestations plus culture of a midstream urine sample. Accurate diagnosis of chronic prostatitis requires simultaneous quantitative cultures (described later) of samples of urethral urine, midstream urine, prostatic secretions expressed by massage or ejaculated (semen), and urine voided after massage. A colony count in prostatic secretions, semen, or post-massage urine that is 10 times greater than the count in urethral or midstream urine samples is diagnostic of chronic prostatitis (11).

Collection, Transport, and Processing

Pathogens detected in urine samples are listed in Table 61–1. Urine collection and transport are similar for all groups of organisms. Specimen processing, however, is different for different organisms and is discussed separately for viruses, bacteria, fungi, and parasites.

Acceptable methods of urine collection include midstream clean catch (preferably a first voided morning specimen), catheterization, and suprapubic aspiration. In general, 24-hour urine specimens should be rejected, except when detection of Schistosoma haematobium is requested specifically. Most often urine samples are collected by obtaining the midstream flow of a clean-catch specimen, a procedure that must be performed properly for accurate interpretation of results, especially in women. The periurethral area and perineum first must be cleansed with soapy sterile gauze pads in a front-to-back motion, rinsed with a moistened sterile gauze pad, and dried with a dry sterile gauze pad. For males cleansing the genital area may not improve the detection of bacteriuria significantly and may not be necessary (12). While voiding

Table 61–1. Pathogens Detected in Urine Specimens

Organism	Chapter
Viruses	
Herpes simplex virus	5
Cytomegalovirus	5
Adenovirus	6
BK virus	7
Mumps virus	10
Bacteria	
Chlamydia trachomatis	25
Staphylococcus aureus	28
Staphylococcus epidermidis	28
Staphylococcus saprophyticus	28
Group B Streptococcus	28
Enterococcus spp	28
Neisseria gonorrhoeae	31
Pseudomonas aeruginosa	32
Enterobacteriaceae	34
Leptospira interrogans	39
Mycobacterium tuberculosis	40
Fungi	
Yeasts	43
Parasites	
Trichomonas vaginalis	51
Schistosoma haematobium	52

women should hold the labia apart and men who are not circumcised should hold back the foreskin. The first few milliliters of urine are passed into the toilet bowl or a bedpan, to flush out bacteria that normally colonize the urethra, and the midstream portion is collected in a sterile container with a wide mouth and tightly fitting lid.

Catheterization carries the risk of inducing a nosocomial infection and so should be reserved for persons who are unable to produce a midstream sample; for example, those with altered sensorium and those unable to void because of neurologic or urologic reasons. Using strict aseptic technique the catheter is inserted into the urethra, the first few milliliters of urine passed are discarded to clear organisms that may have entered the tip of the catheter during placement, and the midportion of the sample is obtained for culture. Urine may be collected from an indwelling catheter by aspirating with a 28-gauge needle and syringe through the rubber connector between the catheter and the collecting tubing, taking care to first disinfect the puncture site. Urine should not be collected from catheter bags, and Foley catheter tips should not be accepted for culture because they almost always are contaminated with urethral organisms.

Suprapubic aspiration is used principally for neonates and small children, but it may be done safely in adults. The procedure requires a full bladder; the overlying skin is disinfected, the bladder is punctured above the symphysis pubis with a 22-gauge needle on a syringe, and about 10 ml of urine is aspirated.

All urine specimens should be transported promptly to the laboratory and should be processed within a few hours after collection. If a delay in transport or processing cannot be avoided, specimens may be refrigerated for up to 24 hours. Collection kits containing preservatives to keep the bacterial population stable for 24 hours at room temperature are commercially available, but they offer no advantage over refrigeration.

Viruses

Processing urine specimens for detection of viruses involves cell culture. Infections with CMV and with BK virus may be diagnosed by finding the characteristic cytopathic changes in preparations of urine stained with Papanicolaou stain (see Chapters 5 and 7), which probably is the method by which most infections with BK virus are detected. For optimal recovery of viruses from urine antibiotics (100 U/ml of penicillin, 50 µg/ml of gentamicin, and 40 µg/ml of amphotericin B) should be added to the sample when it is received in the laboratory, to minimize bacterial contamination of cell cultures. Cell lines are selected for inoculation based on the viruses most commonly isolated (discussed in Chapters 3 and 54). In urine CMV is detected most frequently, followed by adenovirus and herpes simplex virus (HSV). Therefore, all urine specimens should be inoculated to MRC-5 cells, and specimens containing blood also should be inoculated to A549 cells. Incubation of MRC-5 cells in maintenance medium containing 10^{-5} M dexamethasone for a minimum of 24 hours before inoculation decreases the time to detection of CMV and HSV (13,14). BK virus may be recovered in MRC-5 cells, but this virus frequently is not recognized because it produces a nonspecific cytopathic effect. Routine culture of all urine specimens for mumps virus, which requires inoculation of primary monkey kidney cells and hemadsorption, is not economical and must be requested specifically. Specimens are inoculated and adsorbed and cultures are incubated as described in Chapter 54. Virus identification is discussed in Part II.

Centrifugation-culture has been used successfully to detect all of the viruses listed in Table 61–1 except mumps virus, and it should be performed routinely to detect CMV in urine specimens (see Appendix, Procedure 2) (14–16). Centrifugation-culture for detection of adenovirus and BK virus may be indicated in specific situations, such as for immunocompromised persons with hemorrhagic cystitis.

Bacteria

Urine specimens submitted for detection of bacterial pathogens are processed according to the organism or group of organisms being sought, and each is discussed separately.

Chlamydia trachomatis. Urine specimens are useful for diagnosis of C. trachomatis urethritis in males, using an enzyme-linked immunosorbent assay (ELISA, commercially available). Such samples are processed according to the manufacturer's directions.

Bacteria Detected by Routine Culture. In healthy humans the urinary tract above the urethra is sterile, but the urethra normally is colonized with many different bacteria (Chapter 2, Table 2–1), and urine specimens collected by a noninvasive method (such as the clean-catch, midstream specimen) become contaminated as they are passed. In most clinical laboratories commensal bacteria are differentiated from potential pathogens by quantitative cultures of urine, a procedure initially promoted by Kass (17). Originally, growth of 10^5 or more colony-forming units (cfu) of bacteria per milliliter of urine was considered highly indicative of infection, but this criterion has been modified for different situations. For example, in young, sexually active women with the acute urethral syndrome (dysuria, frequency, and urgency), as few as 10^2 cfu/ml is considered significant in association with pyuria (18). UTI associated with fewer than 10^5 cfu/ml may occur in infants and children, males, persons who are catheterized, persons previously treated with antimicrobial agents, those who consume large amounts of liquid (which dilutes urine), those who have symptoms and concurrent pyuria, persons with urinary obstruction, and persons with pyelonephritis acquired from hematogenous spread (especially infections due to yeast or Staphylococcus aureus) (1,19). Consequently, proper interpretation of urine culture results requires communication between clinicians and pathologists or clinical microbiologists.

Quantitative culture of a urine specimen is done by inoculation of appropriate media with a measured amount of urine, most often with a plastic or wire calibrated loop (available commercially) designed to deliver a known volume. Inoculation of MacConkey and 5% sheep blood agar allows detection of most pathogens, but a medium selective for gram-positive organisms (colistin–nalidixic acid or phenylethyl alcohol agar) may be substituted for the sheep blood agar to enhance discrimination. An 0.001-ml loop is used to inoculate all urine specimens, except those collected from women suspected to have acute urethral syndrome and suprapubic aspirates, both of which should be inoculated with an 0.01-ml loop. The appropriate loop is inserted vertically into the well-mixed urine sample, and the loopful of urine removed is spread over the surface of the agar plate as illustrated in Figure 61–1 (the standard quadrant streaking, described in Chapter 54, also is acceptable). Without reflaming, the loop is inserted again vertically into the urine, and the sample removed is inoculated to a second plate. Plates are incubated at 35° to 37° C in ambient air and examined for growth after incubation for 24 hours and at 48 hours.

To determine the number of micro-organisms per milliliter of the original specimen, the number of colonies (on the blood agar plate) is counted and multiplied by 1000 if the 0.001-ml loop was used or by 100 if the 0.01-ml loop was used. Growth of three or more species in a clean-catch midstream urine specimen usually is considered to indicate contamination. In such cases, the organisms are minimally characterized (for example, coagulase-negative staphylococci or lactose-positive gram-negative bacilli) and enumerated, but susceptibility testing is not done. One or two isolates present in numbers greater than 10,000 in a clean-catch midstream sample should be identified and antimicrobial susceptibility testing should be performed. Organisms present in numbers less than 10,000 are not evaluated further, with the following exceptions: A pure culture of Staphylococcus aureus is considered significant in any number, and susceptibility testing should be carried out. Growth of 10^2 to 10^4 cfu/ml may be significant in catheter-related infections. In symptomatic males, growth of 10^3 cfu/ml or greater is consistent with infection, and the organism should be identified, but susceptibility testing is done only if specifically requested. All organisms isolated from suprapubic aspirates are identified and susceptibility testing is performed. One isolate growing in numbers of 100 or greater from a woman suspected to have acute urethral syndrome should be identified if pyuria is present, and susceptibility testing should be done if specifically requested.

More than half the urine specimens submitted to the clinical laboratory for culture yield no growth or have bacterial counts below levels considered clinically significant. Screening tests that quickly identify urine samples that yield "negative" results on culture have been developed in an attempt to provide rapid results, eliminate negative specimens, and allow more time for positive specimens, thus improving efficiency and cost. In general, these rapid screens correlate well with culture when 10^5 cfu/ml or greater is used as the reference, but they compare less favorably in the presence of lower colony counts (1). Other issues to consider regarding the use of a bacteriuria screen are the ability to detect pyuria, an important finding when evaluating UTI, and the cost.

Staining with the Gram stain is one of the most rapid, reliable, and economic screening methods. Finding one or more organisms per oil immersion field in a smear prepared from an uncentrifuged specimen correlates well with bacteriuria at 10^5 cfu/ml or greater, but its sensitivity decreases when compared with lower colony counts (1). Moreover, examination of smears stained with the Gram stain is tedious and time consuming. Commercially available dipstick tests that combine nitrate reductase (an enzyme present in gram-negative bacilli that cause UTI) and leukocyte esterase (an enzyme produced by neutrophils) are rapid, inexpensive, and simple to perform, but are not sensitive enough for use as a single screen for UTI (1).

Of the automated urine screening methods the colorimetric filtration system provides rapid results and detects more than 90% of all positive samples (including those that contain white blood cells and only 10^2 cfu/ml), but they may yield false-negative results with enterococci and Pseudomonas aeruginosa (1). Urine is forced through a filter paper, which retains cells (including bacteria and leukocytes). A stain then is passed through the filter, and

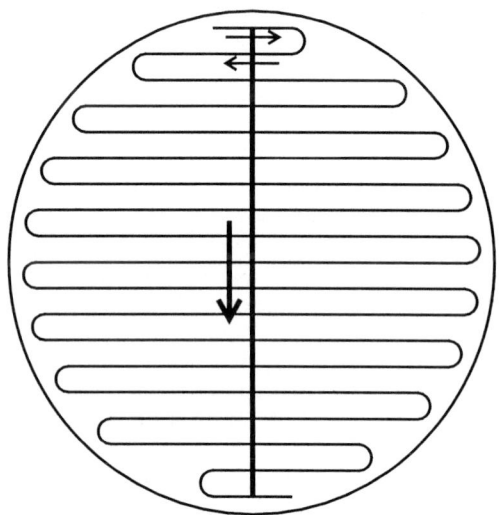

Fig. 61–1. Technique for inoculating urine onto agar plates.

the intensity of the resulting color correlates with the number of particles that adhered to the filter. The filter paper is read manually or with a photometer, which compares the color to a standard.

Bioluminescent systems are automated urine screens based on the enzymatic bioluminescence (light-producing) reaction of adenosine triphosphate (ATP, present in all living cells) with luciferin and luciferase, and the reaction is measured by a luminometer. By selectively releasing ATP from bacteria alone, the number of colony-forming units in a urine sample may be estimated. This technique provides relatively rapid results and compares favorably with culture at a level of 10^5 cfu/ml or greater, but it requires an incubation step and purchase of an instrument.

Automated photometry systems detect bacteriuria by measuring changes in light transmission through a broth medium inoculated with the urine sample. Growth of bacteria causes the medium to become turbid, usually in 2 to 3 hours, but negative results cannot be reported before 5 to 13 hours. These systems compare favorably with culture at a level of 10^5 cfu/ml or greater, and they have the capability of identifying the organism and of antimicrobial susceptibility testing. Disadvantages of currently available photometry systems are the need for incubation and the cost of the instrument.

Each laboratory director should review the volume of urine cultures processed and the proportion of positive specimens to determine whether a urine screen is beneficial. If the efficiency of the laboratory can be improved, system selection should be based on the population tested and the cost.

Neisseria gonorrhoeae. N. gonorrhoeae occasionally is isolated on 5% sheep blood agar and, therefore, potentially could be recovered from a urine sample by routine culture (described earlier). If culture for N. gonorrhoeae is requested specifically, inoculation of chocolate agar with an 0.01-ml loop and incubation in an atmosphere of 5 to 7% carbon dioxide for up to 72 hours is preferred.

Leptospira interrogans. L. interrogans, the agent of leptospirosis, may be detected in urine after the first week of illness and for several months thereafter. Urine should be processed as soon as possible after collection, because acidity may harm the organism. One or two drops of undiluted urine, and urine diluted 1:10 in broth, are inoculated to 5 ml of Fletcher's medium or Ellinghausen, McCullough, Johnson, and Harris (EMJH) medium (commercially available) containing 200 µg/ml of 5-fluorouracil. Cultures are incubated at 25° to 30° C in the dark for up to 6 weeks. Organism identification is discussed in Chapter 39.

Mycobacterium tuberculosis. For optimal recovery of M. tuberculosis early morning–voided urine specimens should be submitted daily for at least 3 days; 24-hour urine specimens should not be accepted. The specimen is divided and poured into two to four 50-ml centrifuge tubes and centrifuged at 3000 to 3600 g for 30 minutes. The supernatant is decanted, leaving about 2 ml of sediment per tube. The tubes are mixed on a vortex mixer, the sediments are combined, and, if necessary, distilled water is added to make a volume of 10 ml. This concentrate is decontaminated with N-aetyl-L-cysteine sodium hydroxide (Appendix, Procedure 27) and then used to prepare a smear for staining with auramine-rhodamine or an acid-fast stain (Appendix, Procedures 4–6) and for inoculation of media for culture (Table 54–4, and Chapter 40).

Fungi

Yeasts may be recovered from urine on the media planted for routine bacterial culture, but if isolation of fungi is requested the sediment of a centrifuged urine specimen should be planted onto media such as inhibitory mold or SABHI agar containing antibacterial agents (Chapter 42) to ensure recovery of fungi, because urine often is contaminated with bacteria (20). Cultures are incubated at 25° to 30° C for up to 4 weeks. Identification of fungi is discussed in Part II.

Parasites

Two parasitic infections can be diagnosed by examination of urine samples. One is infection with Trichomonas vaginalis, which may be diagnosed by microscopic examination of wet preparations of urine sediments. The other is infection with Schistosoma haematobium, the agent of urinary schistosomiasis (Chapter 52).

Examination of urine for the diagnosis of schistosomiasis is best done on specimens collected over a 24-hour period or on the entire first volume of urine voided in the morning. The specimen should be delivered to the laboratory in a clean container, where it is transferred into another container to sediment undisturbed for 1 or 2 hours. The supernatant is discarded, the last 50 to 100 ml of urine is saved, centrifuged at 1500 g for 2 to 5 minutes, decanted, and the sediment is used for preparation of wet mounts. Examination under the microscope reveals the characteristic eggs (Chapter 52).

NEEDLE ASPIRATES OF THE KIDNEY

Percutaneous needle aspiration, performed with ultrasound or computed tomographic guidance, is useful for diagnosis and treatment of intrarenal and perinephric abscesses. Intrarenal abscess occurs as a complication of bacteremia or acute pyelonephritis, whereas perinephric abscess most often is secondary to obstruction of an infected kidney or calyx, but it may be a complication of bacteremia. The organisms usually involved are gram-negative enteric bacilli (when the process is secondary to obstruction of an infected kidney) or Staphylococcus aureus (when the abscess is secondary to bacteremia).

Purulent material should be collected in a sterile syringe. The needle is removed, the air is expelled, and the syringe is tightly capped and transported to the laboratory as rapidly as possible. A smear stained with Gram stain is prepared and examined, and the specimen should be inoculated to 5% sheep blood and MacConkey agars and thioglycolate broth (all incubated in ambient air) and to anaerobic blood agar (incubated anaerobically). Incubation times and temperatures are discussed in Chapter 54.

VAGINAL SECRETIONS OR SWAB SPECIMENS

Vaginal secretions are useful for determining the agent of vulvovaginitis, a common syndrome diagnosed in more than 25% of women attending sexually transmitted disease clinics and in identifying carriers of group B Streptococcus. Symptoms of vulvovaginitis include vaginal discharge, odor, pruritus, and irritation. In postpubescent females the most common causes are Gardnerella vaginalis, which with species of Mobiluncus has been associated with nonspecific vaginosis (so named because the condition is not invasive), species of Candida (predominantly Candida albicans), and Trichomonas vaginalis.

Gardnerella vaginalis is identified in about 40 to 60% of women attending sexually transmitted disease clinics for treatment of other infections, and approximately two thirds of these women are asymptomatic (21,22). Species of Candida, the most common cause of symptomatic vaginal discharge, often are part of the normal vaginal flora and may be cultured from about 20% of asymptomatic women and almost 40% of women with symptoms of vulvovaginitis (23). Risk factors associated with vulvovaginal candidiasis include glucosuria, diabetes mellitus, pregnancy, obesity, and use of antimicrobial agents, corticosteroids, or immunosuppressants. Trichomonas vaginalis accounts for about one fourth of clinically significant vaginal infections in the United States (23). Risk factors associated with acquisition of the infection are increased frequency of sexual activity and multiple sexual partners.

In prepubescent girls Chlamydia trachomatis and Neisseria gonorrhoeae also are agents of vulvovaginitis, an infection that may be associated with sexual abuse. Different tests required to detect these organisms are discussed separately.

In postpubescent females examination of a wet-mount preparation is the most valuable diagnostic test and may be performed by the attending physician. To prepare a wet mount a swab of the discharge is gently agitated in a tube containing about 1 ml of normal saline, and 1 drop of the suspension is placed on a glass slide. Alternatively, 1 drop of saline is placed on a slide and mixed with a loopful of vaginal material. A coverslip is applied, and the preparation is warmed gently by passing it through a flame or holding it over an incandescent light bulb. The slide is examined under low- and high-power magnification for the presence of "clue cells" (epithelial cells covered with small coccobacillary bacteria), consistent with the diagnosis of nonspecific vaginosis; pseudohyphae, suggestive of vaginal candidiasis; or motile Trichomonas. These organisms also can be seen in smears stained with the Papanicolaou stain (Chapters 41, 43, and 49).

In addition to the wet mount, determination of the vaginal pH and the "whiff test," performed by adding 10% potassium hydroxide (KOH) to a drop of vaginal discharge placed on a slide or on the speculum, are useful diagnostic tests. The vaginal pH usually is normal (about 4.5) with vulvovaginal candidiasis but is above 4.5 with nonspecific vaginosis or trichomoniasis. A positive whiff test—generation of a pungent, fishy odor—primarily is associated with nonspecific vaginosis but occasionally occurs with trichomoniasis.

In most cases, these tests are sufficient to identify the agent of vulvovaginitis. However, Gardnerella vaginalis, Candida, and Trichomonas vaginalis may be isolated from vaginal secretions if specifically requested. To culture Gardnerella vaginalis the specimen is inoculated onto human blood Tween agar (commercially available) or colistin–nalidixic acid agar, and either medium is incubated in an atmosphere of 5 to 7% carbon dioxide or in a candle jar for 48 hours. Organism identification is discussed in Chapter 41. To recover Candida the specimens should be inoculated onto sheep blood or colistin–nalidixic acid agar or onto a primary fungal medium such as inhibitory mold or brain-heart infusion agar with antibiotics and incubated at 25° to 30° C up to a week. Cultures for Trichomonas vaginalis are not recommended because the organisms are easily detected in wet preparations or smears stained with the Papanicolaou stain.

Chlamydia trachomatis. C. trachomatis may be detected by culture, the reference method, or by rapid, nonculture techniques, but culture should be used when the patient is a prepubescent girl as sexual abuse may be an issue. To collect the specimen, vaginal secretions should be removed with a swab, then a second swab (Dacron-, rayon-, or cotton-tipped on a plastic stick, Chapter 25) is inserted into the vagina and rotated against the mucosa for 10 to 15 seconds. The swab is placed in 2-sucrose phosphate transport medium, transported promptly to the laboratory, and stored in the refrigerator if processing is to be done within 48 hours or at $-70°$ C if later. A method for culture of C. trachomatis is presented in the Appendix, Procedure 8.

Neisseria gonorrhoeae. Diagnosis of gonococcal vulvovaginitis in a prepubescent girl requires culture. A swab specimen of vaginal secretions is transported to the laboratory in a tube containing modified Stuart's or Amies charcoal medium and held at room temperature until it is inoculated to an appropriate planting medium. Alternatively, the swab is immediately inoculated to modified Thayer-Martin medium (or another medium selective for N. gonorrhoeae, Chapter 31) by rolling it across the agar surface in a "Z" pattern with constant turning to expose all surfaces to the medium. The plate should be transported promptly to the laboratory or stored in a candle jar, preferably in an incubator at 35° to 37° C. If the specimen must be sent to a reference laboratory a transport system that consists of growth medium (commercially available) should be used (24–26). When the plate is received in the laboratory it should be streaked and incubated up to 72 hours at 35° to 37° C in an atmosphere of 5 to 7% carbon dioxide or in a candle jar. Organism identification is discussed in Chapter 31.

Group B Streptococcus. Vaginal specimens collected for detection of group B Streptococcus should be transported to the laboratory in a tube containing modified Stuart's medium (available commercially) and held at room temperature or in the refrigerator until they are processed. To isolate group B Streptococcus, colistin–nalidixic acid agar (selective for gram-positive organisms) or a medium selective for groups A and B Streptococcus is inoculated and incubated at 35° to 37° C in ambient air for up to 48 hours. Organism identification is discussed in Chapter 28.

Kits for rapid detection of group B streptococcal antigen are available commercially. The swabs are placed in the extraction medium provided by the manufacturer and processed according to manufacturer's directions. Because tests for antigen detection may yield false-negative results when small numbers of organisms are present, collection of two swab specimens is recommended, one for detection of antigen, the other for culture if the antigen test result is negative (27).

Parasites

Wet mounts of vaginal secretions, described previously, are used for diagnosis of trichomoniasis. In endemic areas of schistosomiasis, especially that produced by Schistosoma haematobium, wet mounts of vaginal secretions may be used for diagnosis of chronic granulomatous cervicitis. Direct examination of the sample reveals the characteristic Schistosoma eggs. Tissue sections usually show the nature of the lesion (ulcer, polyp, or plaque).

Other parasites found in the vagina usually are detected in smears stained with the Papanicolaou stain, in the cytology laboratory.

URETHRAL SWAB SPECIMENS

Urethral swab specimens are collected to determine the agent of urethritis and to identify persons infected with HSV or human papillomavirus (HPV). Most cases of urethritis are caused by Neisseria gonorrhoeae or Chlamydia trachomatis (28). Trichomonas vaginalis, HSV, and Ureaplasma urealyticum are infrequently pathogenic. Specimen collection and processing are discussed separately for each of these organisms.

Herpes simplex virus. To collect a urethral swab specimen for detection of HSV, a narrow-diameter Dacron swab is inserted 3 to 4 cm into the anterior urethra and rotated gently for 10 to 15 seconds. The swab is placed immediately into appropriate viral transport medium (such as Hanks' balanced salt solution, discussed in Chapter 3) and transported promptly to the laboratory or refrigerated for a short time and then transported on wet ice. In the laboratory the specimen should be refrigerated until it is processed.

Cell culture is required for optimal detection of HSV in a urethral swab specimen. Several cell lines are sensitive to HSV, including A549, MRC-5, mink lung, and primary rabbit kidney cells. Selection of the cell line should be based on quality (if seeded cell culture tubes are purchased), on cost, and on the ability of the laboratory personnel to interpret cytopathic effect. Incubating the monolayer in maintenance medium containing 10^{-5} M dexamethasone for at least 24 hours before inoculation with a specimen decreases the time for detection of the cytopathic effect produced by HSV (14). Inoculation, adsorption, and culture conditions are described in Chapter 54. Monolayers inoculated with genital specimens submitted specifically for detection of HSV should be examined microscopically for cytopathic effect daily for up to 7 days. Virus identification is discussed in Chapter 5.

The centrifugation-culture technique (shell vials or 24-well plates) may be used for detection of HSV in clinical specimens, but its use as a replacement for conventional cell culture is controversial (4,29). Given the conflicting data laboratory directors should evaluate centrifugation-culture in their own laboratories and make a decision regarding its use based on their findings. The principles of the test are the same as those outlined for CMV in Procedure 2 in the Appendix, except that coverslips are stained with monoclonal antibodies to HSV.

Human papillomavirus. HPV may be detected in epithelial cells from the urethra using nucleic acid hybridization, commercially available. To collect the specimen, a urogenital swab is inserted 3 to 4 cm into the anterior urethra and gently rotated for 10 to 15 seconds. The swab is placed in the transport medium provided with the kit, transported to the laboratory, and refrigerated until the test is performed.

Chlamydia trachomatis. C. trachomatis may be detected in urethral swab specimens by culture, direct immunofluorescence using monoclonal antibodies, enzyme immunoassay, or nucleic acid hybridization (discussed in Chapter 25). To collect the specimen, any discharge in the urethra first is removed with a swab, then a Dacron-, rayon-, or cotton-tipped urogenital swab on a plastic stick or wire is inserted 3 to 4 cm into the anterior urethra and gently rotated for 10 to 15 seconds. If culture is ordered the swab is placed immediately into 2-sucrose phosphate medium and transported promptly to the laboratory or refrigerated for a short time as discussed earlier for vaginal secretions.

For optimal detection of Chlamydia trachomatis by direct immunofluorescence, the collection kit provided by he manufacturer should be used. The swab is rolled over the surface of a special glass slide, and the material is immediately fixed with the fixative (methanol or acetone) provided with the kit. Slides are stored at room temperature until they are stained. Collection kits also are provided by the companies that manufacture enzyme immunossays and nucleic acid probes. Swabs are placed immediately into the transport medium provided and are stored at room temperature until testing is performed (within 5 days).

Ureaplasma urealyticum. Detection of U. urealyticum requires culture. A swab specimen, collected as previously described for Chlamydia trachomatis, is placed in an appropriate transport medium, such as modified Stuart's, 2-sucrose phosphate (used for C. trachomatis), or trypticase soy broth with 0.5% albumin and 400 U/ml penicillin, and transported promptly to the laboratory. Specimens may be refrigerated up to 24 hours, but they should be frozen at $-70°$ C in a medium containing protein if a longer delay is unavoidable. For culture, the specimen is mixed on a vortex mixer, 0.1 ml of the medium is inoculated to appropriate agar, broth, or a biphasic system (described in Chapter 27), and cultures are incubated 2 to 3 weeks at $35°$ to $37°$ C in an atmosphere of 5 to 7% carbon dioxide.

Neisseria gonorrhoeae. In males gonorrhea may be diagnosed presumptively by detecting intracellular gram-negative diplococci in a smear of urethral discharge, prepared by rolling exudate collected with a swab over the surface of a glass slide to cover an area of about 1 cm^2, and stained with the Gram stain. A definitive diagnosis requires detecting the organism by culture or nucleic acid hybridization (commercially available). For culture, a swab specimen collected as discussed earlier for Chlamydia trachomatis (cotton swabs should be avoided), is transported to the laboratory in a tube containing modified Stuart's or Aimes charcoal medium. The specimen is held at room temperature until planted, or, better, it is planted immediately and processed as described earlier for vaginal secretions. To detect Neisseria gonorrhoeae by nucleic acid hybridization the swab specimen is placed in the transport medium provided by the manufacturer and stored at room temperature until it is tested (within 5 days). Chlamydia trachomatis may be detected in the same swab specimen by nucleic acid hybridization (using the kit provided by the same manufacturer).

Trichomonas vaginalis. T. vaginalis is considered an infrequent cause of urethritis in men, but the situation is little studied. Trichomonas produces prostatitis and nongonococcal urethritis with discharge consisting of white, milky fluid of 4 or more weeks' duration. Fewer than 2% of cases of nongonococcal urethritis caused by organisms other than T. vaginalis last this long. Examination of wet preparations of urethral secretions reveals the motile trophozoites of Trichomonas. In men, prostatic secretions yield similar results.

ENDOCERVICAL SWAB SPECIMENS

Endocervical swab specimens are collected to determine the agent of cervicitis and to identify persons infected with human papillomavirus (Table 61–2). Group B Streptococcus may be detected in endocervical cultures, but a vaginal specimen is preferred (described earlier). Mucopurulent cervicitis, characterized by mucopus (a yellow exudate on the exocervix), is the counterpart of urethritis, and the same organisms are responsible for both infections.

Collection, Transport, and Processing

Specimen collection is the same for all of these organisms and is discussed for these agents as a group. Specimen transport (including appropriate transport media, if necessary) and processing for detection of HSV, HPV, Chlamydia trachomatis, Ureaplasma urealyticum, Neisseria gonorrhoeae, and Trichomonas vaginalis are the same as described earlier for urethral swab specimens.

Endocervical specimens are collected after the cervix is visualized with the aid of a speculum moistened only with warm water (lubricants may contain antibacterial agents). The cervix first is cleaned with a swab, then the tip of a second swab is inserted a few millimeters into the cervical canal, rotated firmly for 15 to 30 seconds to ensure collection of endocervical cells, and removed without touching the walls of the vagina or the vaginal secretions. A Dacron- or polyester-tipped swab with a plastic shaft is recommended. Cotton swabs may contain fatty acids that inhibit growth of Neisseria gonorrhoeae, and should be avoided. Alternatively, a small, nylon-bristled brush may be used for women who are not pregnant, to ensure collection of cellular material necessary for detection of viruses and Chlamydia trachomatis, but bleeding and some discomfort may occur (30).

VESICLE FLUID OR SWAB SPECIMENS

Vesicular lesions on the glans penis, vulva, perineum, buttocks, or cervix are sampled to confirm infection caused by HSV. The vesicle fluid, containing desquamated cells infected with the virus, is aspirated with a 27-gauge needle on a tuberculin syringe; if only a small vesicle is present it is unroofed and the base of the ulcer is firmly scraped with a Dacron (polyester) swab to assure collec-

Table 61–2. Specimens Useful for Diagnosis of Infectious Agents in the Genital Tract

Organism	Specimen	Chapter
Herpes simplex virus	Urethral swab, endocervical swab, vesicle fluid or swab, ulcer swab, amniotic fluid, products of conception	5
Human papillomavirus	Urethral swab, endocervical swab	7
Chlamydia trachomatis	Vaginal swab, urethral swab, endocervical swab, ulcer swab, endometrial tissue or swab	25
Ureaplasma urealyticum	Urethral swab, endocervical swab, products of conception	27
Mycoplasma hominis	Products of conception	27
Group B Streptococcus	Vaginal swab, endocervical swab, endometrial tissue or swab, cul de sac aspirate, tubo-ovarian abscess material, amniotic fluid, products of conception	28
Enterococcus spp	Endometrial tissue or swab, cul de sac aspirate, tubo-ovarian abscess material	28
Listeria monocytogenes	Products of conception	29
Anaerobes	Endometrial tissue or swab, cul de sac aspirate, material from Bartholin's gland or tubo-ovarian abscess	30, 38
Neisseria gonorrhoeae	Vaginal secretions, urethral swab, endocervical swab, endometrial tissue or swab, cul de sac aspirate; material from Bartholin's gland, tubo-ovarian abscess, or abscess of the epididymis; amniotic fluid, products of conception	31
Enterobacteriaceae	Endometrial tissue or swab, cul de sac aspirate; material from Bartholin's gland, tubo-ovarian abscess or abscess of the testis or epididymis; amniotic fluid, products of conception	34
Haemophilus ducreyi	Ulcer material	36
Treponema pallidum	Ulcer material	39
Gardnerella vaginalis	Vaginal secretions	41
Calymmatobacterium granulomatis	Ulcer material	41
Candida species	Vaginal secretions	43
Trichomonas vaginalis	Vaginal secretions, urethral swab, endocervical swab	51
Schistosoma haematobium	Urine, biopsies of bladder	52

tion of cells. Vesicle fluid and swab specimens should be placed in an appropriate transport medium and processed for conventional cell culture or for centrifugation-culture as described earlier for urethral swab specimens.

HSV also may be detected directly in clinical specimens, but the methods available currently—direct staining of smears and ELISA—are less sensitive than culture and, if results are negative should be followed by culture (31,32). To make a smear, the roof of a vesicle is removed, the base of the ulcer is scraped firmly with a tongue depressor or a Dacron swab, cells are spread on a glass slide, and the material is fixed in acetone. The smear may be stained with the Papanicolaou stain for detection of typical cytopathic changes (see Fig. 5–2), a test that does not distinguish herpes simplex from varicella-zoster virus, or with specific monoclonal antibodies. To perform the ELISA the ulcer base is scraped firmly with a Dacron swab, which is immediately placed in the collection medium provided by the manufacturer.

ULCER MATERIAL

Material from genital ulcers is collected to diagnose sexually transmitted diseases. As many as 10% of persons who present to sexually transmitted disease clinics in the United States have genital ulcers, which in about two thirds of cases are caused by HSV or Treponema pallidum (33). Genital ulcers are more prevalent in developing countries, where Haemophilus ducreyi, Treponema pallidum, and Calymmatobacterium granulomatis are the most common agents. Chlamydia trachomatis (serogroups L_1, L_2, L_3) also should be considered in the differential diagnosis. Specimen collection, transport, and processing are discussed separately for each of these agents.

Herpes simplex virus. Collection, transport, and processing of material from ulcerative lesions for detection of HSV are identical to those discussed earlier for swab specimens from vesicles. In general, both the sensitivity of the direct tests previously described and recovery of the virus are lower with ulcerative lesions.

Chlamydia trachomatis (L_1, L_2, L_3). Serogroups L_1, L_2, and L_3 of C. trachomatis may be detected by cell culture in a biopsy specimen of the ulcerated lesion or in cellular material collected by first removing any exudate from the lesion and then firmly rotating a swab (Dacron-, rayon-, or cotton-tipped on a plastic stick) against its base. Specimen transport and processing are the same as discussed earlier for vaginal secretions.

Haemophilus ducreyi. If infection with H. ducreyi is suspected, material from the base of the ulcer is collected on two cotton or Dacron swabs, transported in modified Stuart's medium to the laboratory, and held at room temperature until they are processed. With one swab a smear is prepared and stained with the Gram stain. Observing many, small, pleomorphic gram-negative bacilli and coccobacilli arranged in chains and groups is suggestive of H. ducreyi. Culture, however, is more sensitive and is necessary for confirmation. The second swab is inoculated onto special media and incubated as outlined in Table 54–4. Organism identification is discussed in Chapter 36.

Treponema pallidum. T. pallidum may be detected in genital or other lesions, but the infections usually are diagnosed serologically. Gloves should be worn when examining lesions of suspected syphilis and when handling specimens obtained from those lesions. To collect the specimen, the surface of the lesion (if multiple lesions are present, the youngest should be selected) is cleaned with saline and blotted dry, and any crusts are removed. The lesion is superficially abraded until slight bleeding occurs, and gentle pressure is applied to its base. The clear serum exudate from the subsurface is collected by touching the fluid with a glass slide or by using a capillary pipette and transferring the fluid to a glass slide. A coverslip is placed on the fluid, and the specimen is examined immediately by darkfield microscopy. Alternatively, lesion material is aspirated with a 26-gauge needle inserted at the base, after which a drop of saline is drawn into the needle. The material then is expressed onto a glass slide, covered with a coverglass, and examined immediately by darkfield microscopy. The spirochetes of T. pallidum are 10 to 13 μm by about 0.15 μm, have a regular tight coil, and are pointed at the ends.

Calymmatobacterium granulomatis. For optimal detection of C. granulomatis subsurface tissue from an area of active granulation is biopsied, and fresh tissue is transported to the laboratory in a sterile, dry container or in one containing a small amount of sterile saline without preservatives. Smears are prepared from a crushed piece of the tissue and stained with the Giemsa or Dieterle stain. The diagnosis is based on finding characteristic, encapsulated C. granulomatis organisms within macrophages (Chapter 41).

ENDOMETRIAL TISSUE OR SWAB SPECIMENS

Endometrial biopsy tissue or swab specimens are useful for determining the agent of pelvic inflammatory disease and postpartum and postoperative endometritis. For optimal collection of a swab specimen the swab is inserted through a catheter with a narrow bore that is introduced into the cervical canal to decrease the likelihood of contaminating the specimen with secretions in the endocervix and vagina. Organisms that may be detected include Chlamydia trachomatis, Neisseria gonorrhoeae, group B Streptococcus, enterococci, anaerobic gram-positive cocci, Enterobacteriaceae, and anaerobic gram-negative bacilli.

To ensure detection of these pathogens, several tissue fragments or several swab specimens should be collected. One tissue fragment or swab specimen should be placed in 2-sucrose phosphate transport medium for detection of Chlamydia trachomatis and handled as described earlier for vaginal secretions, except that the tissue fragment must be homogenized with a sterile tissue grinder or mortar and pestle before inoculation. A second swab specimen should be transported to the laboratory in a tube system containing modified Stuart's transport medium and processed for isolation of Neisseria gonorrhoeae as discussed earlier for vaginal secretions. The final swab specimen or tissue fragment should be placed in an anaerobic transport system and transported promptly to the laboratory, where it is held at room temperature until inoculated to appropriate planting media; sheep blood, chocolate, and MacConkey agar (incubated in an atmosphere of 5 to 7% carbon dioxide), thioglycolate broth (incubated in ambient air), and anaerobic blood agar (incubated anaerobically) are recommended. Incubation times and temperatures are discussed in Chapter 54. If the material submitted is insufficient for all of these above tests, the attending physician must be consulted to prioritize the requests.

CUL DE SAC ASPIRATE

Secretions or exudate aspirated from the cul de sac is useful in identifying the pathogen of pelvic inflammatory disease. The sample is collected with a needle and syringe. The needle is removed, the air is expelled, and the syringe is tightly capped, transported promptly to the laboratory, and held at room temperature until it is processed. A smear stained with the Gram stain is examined, and the specimen is inoculated to appropriate culture media for recovery of Neisseria gonorrhoeae (as described for vaginal secretions), and facultative and anaerobic bacteria (as described for endometrial specimens).

ABSCESS MATERIAL

Purulent material is evaluated to determine what organisms are responsible for abscesses involving Bartholin's gland, the fallopian tubes and ovaries, and the testes and epididymides. The specimen should be collected with a needle and syringe and transported and processed as described above for cul de sac aspirates.

AMNIOTIC FLUID

Amniotic fluid is evaluated to identify potential viral or bacterial pathogens. The specimen is collected with a needle and syringe by the physician. The needle is removed, the air is expelled, and the syringe is tightly capped and transported promptly to the laboratory. Specimen processing to detect viruses and bacteria is different and is discussed separately for each group of organisms.

Viruses

Viruses found in amniotic fluid (see Table 61–2) are detected by cell culture. The specimen should be stored in the refrigerator until it is inoculated to appropriate cell monolayers—MRC-5, A549 and primary monkey kidney cells are recommended (Chapters 3 and 54). The fluid is inoculated and adsorbed, and cultures are incubated as described in Chapter 54. In addition to conventional cell culture, centrifugation-culture may be done for detection of CMV (Appendix, Procedure 2).

Bacteria

Amniotic fluid submitted for bacterial culture is held at room temperature until it is processed. A smear stained with the Gram stain is prepared and examined, and culture media are inoculated; sheep blood, MacConkey, and chocolate agar (incubated in an atmosphere of 5 to 7% carbon dioxide), thiglycolate broth (incubated in ambient air), and anaerobic blood agar (incubated anaerobically) are recommended. Incubation times and temperatures are reviewed in Chapter 54.

PRODUCTS OF CONCEPTION

Products of conception are evaluated to determine the cause of fetal infection or fetal death. Placental tissue or fragments of aborted fetal tissue may be submitted for detection of viruses, bacteria, or both (Table 61–2). Specimen transport and processing are different for detection of viruses and bacteria and are discussed separately for each group of organisms.

Viruses

To detect viruses, placental tissue or aborted fetal tissue is placed in viral transport medium (such as Hanks' balanced salt solution) containing antimicrobial agents (Chapter 3) and transported promptly to the laboratory or refrigerated for a short time and transported on wet ice as soon as possible. In the laboratory the tissue is homogenized in the transport medium with a sterile tissue grinder or a mortar and pestle to make a 10 to 20% (weight to volume) suspension, which is centrifuged at 1000 to 2000 g for 15 to 20 minutes. The supernatant is inoculated to MCR-5, A549, and primary monkey kidney cells, adsorbed, and cultures are incubated as described in Chapter 54.

Bacteria

Tissue for bacterial culture should be placed in a sterile container and transported promptly to the laboratory. A pathologist should examine the fresh tissue and divide the specimen appropriately for histologic and microbiologic studies. The sample for culture is homogenized in a small amount of thioglycolate broth as described above for viruses. A smear stained with the Gram stain is prepared and examined, and the homogenate is inoculated to appropriate culture media—sheep blood, MacConkey, and chocolate agars (incubated in an atmosphere of 5 to 7% carbon dioxide) and thioglycolate broth (incubated in ambient air). Incubation times and temperatures are discussed in Chapter 54.

Special culture conditions are necessary if recovery of Mycoplasma hominis, Ureaplasma urealyticum, or Listeria monocytogenes is requested. To isolate Ureaplasma urealyticum and Mycoplasma hominis the suspension is inoculated to appropriate agar, broth, or a biphasic medium (Chapter 27), and cultures are incubated at 35° to 37° C in an atmosphere of 5 to 7% carbon dioxide for 2 to 3 weeks. To ensure recovery of Listeria monocytogenes the homogenate is inoculated to two flasks of infusion broth. One flask is incubated at 35° C for 24 hours and then subcultured to sheep blood agar, which is incubated in an atmosphere of 5 to 7% carbon dioxide for at least 48 hours. The second flask is refrigerated at 4° C and subcultured to sheep blood agar (incubated as above), weekly for at least 1 month if L. monocytogenes is not recovered from the first flask and its subculture.

REFERENCES

1. Pezzlo M: Detection of urinary tract infections by rapid methods. Rev Clin Microbiol, *1*:268, 1988.
2. Boineau FG, and Lewy JE: Urinary tract infection in children: An overview. Pediatr Ann, *4*:515, 1975.
3. McCracken GH: Diagnosis and management of acute urinary tract infections in infants and children. Pediatr Infect Dis, *6*:107, 1987.
4. Sobel JD, and Kaye D: Urinary tract infections. *In* Principles and Practice of Infectious Disease. 3rd ed. Edited by GL Mandell, RG Douglas, Jr, and JE Bennett. New York, Churchill Livingstone, 1990.
5. Strom BL, et al: Sexual activity, contraceptive use and other risk factors for symptomatic and asymptomatic bacteriuria. Ann Intern Med, *107*:816, 1987.
6. Gillespie L: The diaphragm: An accomplice in recurrent urinary tract infections. Urology, *24*:25, 1984.
7. Kaye D: Urinary tract infection in the elderly. Bull NY Acad Med, *56*:209, 1980.
8. Turck M, Goffe B, and Petersdorf RG: The urethral catheter and urinary tract infection. J Urol, *88*:834, 1962.
9. Garibaldi RA, Burke JP, Dickman ML, and Smith CB: Factors predisposing to bacteriuria during indwelling urethral catheterization. N Engl J Med, *291*:215, 1974.
10. Meares EM: Prostatitis: A review. Urol Clin North Am, *2*:3, 1975.
11. Meares EM, and Stamey TA: Bacteriologic localization patterns in bacterial prostatitis and urethritis. Invest Urol, *5*:492, 1968.
12. Lipsky BA, Innuni TS, Plorde JJ, and Berger RE: Is the clean-catch midstream void procedure necessary for obtaining urine culture specimens from men? Am J Med, *76*:257, 1984.
13. Thiele GM, and Woods GL: The effect of dexamethasone on detection of cytomegalovirus in tissue culture and by immunofluorescence. J Virol Methods, *22*:319, 1988.
14. Woods GL, and Mills R: Effect of dexamethasone on detection of herpes simplex virus in clinical specimens by conventional cell culture and rapid 24-well plate centrifugation. J Clin Microbiol, *26*:1233, 1988.
15. Woods GL, Young A, Johnson A, and Thiele GM: Detection of cytomegalovirus by 24-well plate centrifugation assay using a monoclonal antibody to an early nuclear antigen. J Virol Methods, *18*:207, 1987.
16. Woods GL, Yamamoto M, and Young A: Detection of adenovirus by rapid 24-well plate centrifugation and conventional cell culture with dexamethasone. J Virol Methods, *20*:109, 1988.
17. Kass EH: Asymptomatic infections of the urinary tract. Trans Assoc Am Physicians, *69*:56, 1956.
18. Stamm WE, et al: Diagnosis of coliform infection in acute dysuric women. N Engl J Med, *307*:463, 1982.
19. Baron EJ, and Finegold SM (eds): Microorganisms encountered in the urinary tract. *In* Bailey and Scott's Diagnostic Microbiology. 8th ed. St. Louis, CV Mosby, 1990.
20. Roberts GD: Laboratory methods in basic mycology. *In* Bailey and Scott's Diagnostic Microbiology. 8th ed. Edited by EJ Baron and SM Finegold. St. Louis, CV Mosby, 1990.
21. Embree J, Caliando JJ, and McCormack WM: Nonspecific vaginitis among women attending a sexually transmitted disease clinic. Sex Transm Dis, *11*:81, 1984.
22. Hill LH, Ruparella H, and Embil JA: Nonspecific vaginitis and other genital infections in three clinic populations. Sex Transm Dis, *10*:114, 1983.
23. Osborne NF, Grubin L, and Pratson L: Vaginitis in sexually active women: Relationship to nine sexually transmitted organisms. Am J Obstet Gynecol, *142*:962, 1982.
24. Deveaux DL, et al: Comparison of the Gono Pak System with the candle extinction jar for recovery of Neisseria gonorrhoeae. J Clin Microbiol, *25*:571, 1987.
25. Holston JL, Jr, Hosty JR, and Martin JE, Jr: Evaluation of the bag-CO_2 generating tablet method for isolation of Neisseria gonorrhoeae. Am J Clin Pathol, *62*:558, 1974.
26. Martin JE, Jr, and Jackson RL: A biological environmental chamber for the culture of Neisseria gonorrhoeae. J Am Vener Dis Assoc, *2*:28, 1985.
27. Kontnick CM, and Edberg SC: Direct detection of group B streptococci from vaginal specimens compared with quantitative culture. J Clin Microbiol, *28*:336, 1990.
28. Hook EW, and Holmes KK: Gonococcal infections. Ann Intern Med, *102*:229, 1985.
29. Gleaves CA, Wilson DJ, Wold AD, and Smith TF: Detection and serotyping of herpes simplex virus in MRC-5 cells by use of centrifugation and monoclonal antibodies 16 h postinoculation. J Clin Microbiol, *21*:29, 1985.
30. Kellogg JA, Seiple JW, and Levisky JS: Efficacy of duplicate genital specimens and repeated testing for confirming positive results for Chlamydiazyme detection of Chlamydia trachomatis antigen. J Clin Microbiol, *27*:1218, 1989.
31. Moseby RC, et al: Comparison of viral isolation, direct immunofluorescence and indirect immunoperoxidase techniques for detection of genital herpes simplex virus infection. J Infect Dis, *143*:913, 1981.
32. Zimmerman SJ, et al: Evaluation of a visual, rapid, membrane enzyme immunoassay for the detection of herpes simplex virus antigen. J Clin Microbiol, *29*:842, 1991.
33. Kraus SJ: Genital ulcer adenopathy syndrome: *In* Sexually Transmitted Diseases. Edited by KK Holmes, et al. New York, McGraw-Hill, 1984.

Chapter 62

SKIN, ADNEXA, AND SUBCUTANEOUS TISSUES

Specimens collected for identification of organisms responsible for infections of the skin, adnexa, and subcutaneous tissues include hair, nails, skin scrapings, fluid and swab specimens from vesicles, bullae, and pustules; aspirates from cellulitis; aspirates and swab specimens from ulcers, wound infections and abscesses; smears from skin slits, and biopsy specimens from lesions.

HAIR

Hair usually is collected for diagnosis of infections with dermatophytes, commonly called tinea capitis (several species of Trichophyton and Microsporum infect hair, Chapter 44). Trichosporon beigelii and Piedraia hortae (Chapters 43 and 44, respectively) also infect hair and are detected by the same methods used for detection of dermatophytes. Superficial infections caused by Trichosporon beigelii and Piedraia hortae, however, often are diagnosed on the basis of clinical manifestations alone. Infections with Pediculus capitis are diagnosed clinically, but occasionally infected hair or adult Pediculus lice are received in the laboratory for study.

Collection, Transport, and Processing

Damaged hairs or hairs shown to be infected by Wood's lamp examination (Chapter 44) are removed by plucking with forceps, placed in a sterile Petri dish or paper envelope, and delivered to the laboratory. If delay in transport is unavoidable, the specimen is held at room temperature, not refrigerated. In the laboratory a potassium hydroxide preparation of a few hairs is examined microsopically (Appendix, Procedure 19), and the remaining hairs are inoculated to Sabouraud dextrose agar containing antibiotics and cycloheximide to prevent overgrowth by other bacteria and rapidly growing saprophytic fungi. Culture conditions are described in Chapter 54, and identification of the fungi in Chapters 43 and 44.

Hairs from persons infected with Pediculus, and adult lice are examined directly under the microscope. Mounted on a glass slide, both hairs and adult lice may be made easier to examine if a drop of formalin is used. In hairs identification of the characteristic eggs ("nits") is easy.

NAILS

Nail specimens most frequently are collected for identification of the pathogen of onychomycosis. Potential pathogens include species of Candida (Chapter 43) and several moulds—species of Trichophyton, Epidermophyton floccosum, the dematiaceous fungi, and species of Fusarium (Chapter 44).

Collection, Transport, and Processing

Specimen collection, transport, and processing to detect all of these fungi are identical. Softened material from the nail bed beneath the nail plate should be sampled. Alternatively, the superficial portions of the nail are scraped off and subsurface material, where the infecting organism is most likely to be found, is obtained with a scalpel blade. Specimen transport and processing are as described for hair specimens.

SKIN SCRAPINGS

Skin scrapings are useful in diagnosing superficial and cutaneous infections caused by fungi and species of Prototheca (Table 62–1). Scrapings may be collected to confirm the diagnosis of erythrasma, a superficial infection caused by Corynebacterium minutissimum, usually diagnosed by clinical presentation and Wood's lamp examination alone (Chapter 29). Rarely, skin scrapings are collected for diagnosis of scabies, especially the Norwegian type (Chapter 53), and some subcutaneous filariae with microfilariae residing in the skin, for example, Onchocerca volvulus and Mansonella streptocerca.

Collection, Transport, and Processing

To collect skin scrapings, the peripheral margin of the lesion is gently scraped with the side of a scalpel blade or the edge of a glass slide. The specimen is transported as described earlier for hair.

To detect Corynebacterium minutissimum, a smear of the sample is stained with Gram stain, and scrapings are inoculated onto sheep blood agar or a medium selective for gram-positive bacteria such as colistin-nalidixic acid agar. Culture conditions are described in Chapter 54. Specimen processing for detection of fungi and algae is identical to that described earlier for hair, except that Sabouraud dextrose agar containing antibiotics (but not cycloheximide which inhibits growth of Prototheca) also should be inoculated.

Skin scales for diagnosis of scabies are placed on a glass slide with a drop of a clearing agent such as glycerol, xylene, immersion oil, or histologic mounting medium. The preparation is covered with a cover glass and examined under low power, searching for the adult female mites, eggs, and larvae. In cases of Norwegian scabies in immunocompromised hosts the diagnosis is easy because numerous mites are present. In usual cases of scabies the diagnosis is made clinically, because searching for mites is fruitless. It is estimated that the average patient suffering from scabies harbors only 1 to 5 mites.

Skin samples for diagnosis of infection with Onchocerca

Table 62–1. Pathogens Detected by Microbiologic Studies of Skin Scrapings

Organism	Chapter
Bacteria	
Corynebacterium minutissimum	29
Fungi	
Candida spp	43
Malassezia furfur	43
Trichosporon beigelii	43
Trichophyton spp	44
Microsporum spp	44
Epidermophyton floccosum	44
Dematiaceous fungi	44
Algae	
Prototheca species	47

Table 62–2. Pathogens Detected by Microbiologic Studies of Fluid or Swab Specimens from Vesicles, Bullae, or Pustules

Organism	Chapter
Viruses	
Herpes simplex virus	5
Varicella-zoster virus	5
B virus	5
Enteroviruses	13
Bacteria	
Staphylococcus aureus	28
Group A Streptococcus	28
Clostridium spp	30
Neisseria gonorrhoeae	31
Pseudomonas aeruginosa	32
Enterobacteriaceae	34
Vibrio vulnificus	35
Fungi	
Candida spp	43
Malassezia furfur	43
Trichosporon beigelii	43
Microsporum spp	44
Epidermophyton floccosum	44

volvulus and other filariae are referred to as skin snips. Because a fresh sample is required specimens must be collected at the location where they are to be examined. A hypodermic needle is used to "lift" the skin slightly. The tip of the needle is gently pushed into the epidermis (and inserted no more than 0.3 mm), the needle is raised to lift the skin slightly, and with a surgical blade, the skin under the tip of the needle is cut. No bleeding should occur, and the piece of skin recovered should not be larger than a small pinhead. This operation is repeated several times on adjacent skin, the samples are placed on a glass slide with a drop of saline solution, and with a pair of needles (one in each hand), the skin is teased out. The preparation is covered with a coverslip and examined under the microscope. Under low and medium power microfilariae are seen as small, elongated, motile organisms.

Final specific identification is made by staining the microfilariae. Additional samples are taken for this purpose, or if possible the original one is uncovered, dried, fixed, and stained (Chapter 52).

FLUID AND SWAB SPECIMENS FROM VESICLES, BULLAE, AND PUSTULES

Infections with several viruses, bacteria, and fungi may cause cutaneous vesicles, bullae, and pustules (Table 62–2). Microbiologic studies of fluid or swab specimens obtained from these lesions are useful for identifying the responsible pathogen. Specimen collection and transport are similar for all organisms listed in the table, but specimen processing is different for detection of viruses, bacteria, and fungi, and is discussed separately for each group of organisms.

Collection, Transport, and Processing

Fluid may be collected from a vesicle or bulla by aspirating with a needle and syringe. For transport, the needle is removed, air is expelled, and the syringe is tightly capped and promptly delivered to the laboratory. Vesicles and bullae also may be sampled by unroofing the lesion and vigorously rubbing the base with a swab. Pustules are similarly sampled with a swab after removing any crusted material. Swabs made from calcium alginate, which may inactivate herpes simplex virus (HSV), should be avoided. A minimum of two swab specimens should be collected: one for culture, the other for preparation of smears for staining. If detection of more than one group of organisms (for example, viruses and bacteria, or bacteria and fungi) is requested, at least three swab specimens is optimal. For a suspected viral infection, the collector of the specimen should prepare a smear at the bedside by rolling the entire surface of the swab over a glass slide and allowing the material to air dry.

All swabs may be placed in tube transport systems containing modified Stuart's medium (commercially available). If recovery of viruses is requested placing one swab in viral transport medium such as Hanks' balanced salt solution is recommended, and if anaerobic culture is ordered one swab must be placed in an anaerobic transport device. Smears and swab specimens should be transported promptly to the laboratory.

Viruses

Processing specimens from vesicles or pustules for detection of viruses involves cell culture; and for varicella-zoster virus (VZV) and possibly HSV examination of stained smears is helpful. Specimens for culture are refrigerated briefly until they are processed. Vesicle fluid collected in a syringe is placed in viral transport medium, and swab specimens received in viral transport medium are vigorously mixed on a vortex mixer, and the swab is removed.

To ensure recovery of all viruses listed in Table 62–2, inoculating MRC-5 and primary monkey kidney cells is recommended, and adding A549 cells incubated in maintenance medium containing 10^{-5} M dexamethasone for at least 24 hours decreases the time for detection of herpes simplex virus (1). Specimens are inoculated and adsorbed, and cultures are incubated as described in Chapter 54. HSV may be detected by centrifugation-culture, but using this technique to replace conventional cell culture is controversial (2,3). The procedure is similar to that outlined for cytomegalovirus in Procedure 2 in the Appendix, except that monolayers are stained with HSV-specific antibodies.

A smear of cells obtained from a vesicle or pustule and stained with the Wright stain (Tzanck preparation), may show cytopathic changes consistent with HSV and VZV. However, the sensitivity of this test is low, especially for pustular and crusted lesions, and it does not distinguish infection with HSV from infection with VZV, so other stains are preferred. For example, staining smears with monoclonal antibodies to VZV, a very labile virus that may not survive transport to the laboratory, is more sensitive than cell culture for cutaneous lesions (4). Smears also may be stained with monoclonal antibodies to HSV, but this method is less sensitive than cell culture for detecting HSV.

A membrane enzyme–linked immunosorbent assay for direct detection of HSV in clinical specimens is available commercially (5). Clinical evaluations of the test are limited and have focused principally on genital specimens.

Bacteria

Processing specimens from vesicles, bullae, and pustules for detection of bacteria involves preparation of a smear for staining with the Gram stain and inoculation of appropriate media for culture. For routine culture sheep blood and MacConkey agars are inoculated and incubated in ambient air, as described in Chapter 54. Culture for Neisseria gonorrhoeae and for anaerobes must be requested specifically. To recover N. gonorrhoeae, modified Thayer Martin agar (or other selective medium, discussed in Chapter 31) is inoculated and incubated up to 72 hours at 35° to 37° C in an atmosphere of 5 to 7% carbon dioxide. For anaerobic culture anaerobic blood agar is inoculated (with a swab transported in an anaerobic system) and incubated as described in Chapter 54.

Fungi

Processing specimens from vesicles, bullae, and pustules for detection of fungi involves preparing a smear for direct microscopic examination and inoculating appropriate media for culture. For direct visualization a potassium hydroxide preparation (Appendix, Procedure 19) may be examined, or a smear may be stained with the Gram, Gomori methenamine silver, calcofluor white, or Congo red stain (Chapter 42). Specimens are inoculated onto Sabouraud's dextrose agar containing antibiotics, with and without cycloheximide, and cultures are incubated as described in Chapter 54.

ASPIRATES FROM CELLULITIS

Microbiologic studies of aspirates obtained with a needle and syringe from the point of maximum inflammation of an area of cellulitis (commonly the center rather than the leading edge) may identify the organism responsible for the process (Table 62–3). More often, however, these specimens fail to recover the pathogen. To transport the specimen the needle is removed, and the syringe is tightly capped and promptly delivered to the laboratory.

Table 62–3. Pathogens Detected by Microbiologic Studies of Aspirates from Cellulitis

Organism	Chapter
Staphylococcus aureus	28
Groups A, B, C, and G Streptococcus	28
Erysipelothrix rhusiopathiae	29
Peptostreptococcus spp	30
Enterobacteriaceae	34
Virbrio vulnificus	35
Aeromonas spp	35
Haemophilus influenzae	36
Anaerobic gram-negative bacilli	38

Processing the aspirate for detection of bacteria involves preparation of a smear stained with the Gram stain for microscopic examination and inoculation of media for culture. Inoculation of chocolate agar (incubated in an atmosphere of 5 to 7% carbon dioxide), anaerobic blood agar (incubated anaerobically), and thioglycolate broth (incubated in ambient air) allows recovery of all known pathogens. Incubation temperatures and times are described in Chapter 54.

ASPIRATES AND SWAB SPECIMENS FROM CUTANEOUS ULCERS

Microbiologic studies of aspirates and swab specimens obtained from cutaneous ulcers are useful for identifying the pathogen (Table 62–4). Lesions may be primary (for example, those caused by viruses, Bacillus anthracis, Corynebacterium diphtheriae, Francisella tularensis, Pseudom-

Table 62–4. Pathogens Detected by Microbiologic Studies of Specimens from Primary and Secondary Cutaneous Ulcers

Organism	Chapter
PRIMARY	
Virus	
Herpes simplex virus	5
Varicella-zoster virus	5
Bacteria	
Bacillus anthracis	29
Corynebacterium diphtheriae	29
Pseudomonas aeruginosa	32
Francisella tularensis	33
Mycobacterium spp	40
Fungi	
Cryptococcus neoformans	43
Dematiaceous fungi	44
Blastomyces dermatitidis	45
Sporothrix schenckii	45
Parasites	
Entamoeba histolytica	49
Trypanosomes (inoculation chancre)	51
Acanthamoeba spp	51
SECONDARY	
Bacteria	
Staphylococcus aureus	28
Group B Streptococcus	28
Enterococcus spp	28
Pseudomonas aeruginosa	32
Enterobacteriaceae	34
Anaerobic gram-negative bacilli	38

onas aeruginosa, species of Mycobacterium, fungi, and several parasitic protozoa). Decubitus ulcers may become secondarily colonized or infected with several aerobic and anaerobic bacteria.

Collection, Transport, and Processing

Collection, transport, and processing of swab specimens obtained from cutaneous ulcers for detection of viruses are identical to procedures described for vesicles and pustules. Handling of specimens obtained from cutaneous ulcers differs for different bacteria, fungi, and parasites and is discussed separately for each of the organisms that cause primary lesions and for the bacteria associated with chronic ulcers.

Bacteria

Bacillus anthracis. B. anthracis causes anthrax, a rare disease in the United States limited to persons who work with raw imported wool and other animal products contaminated with spores of B. anthracis. Cutaneous anthrax is a painless lesion that begins as a papule but becomes vesicular, then hemorrhagic, necrotic, and covered with an eschar. For optimal diagnosis, two swab specimens of vesicular exudate material are collected, one for culture, the other for preparation of smears for staining with the Gram stain and with fluorescent antibodies (the latter should be performed in a reference laboratory). Owing to the hazardous nature of B. anthracis, sending specimens from persons with suspected anthrax to a reference laboratory merits consideration. If specimens are processed in the clinical laboratory they must be handled in a biologic safety cabinet. The swab for culture is inoculated onto sheep blood agar, which is incubated in ambient air as described in Chapter 54. Identification of B. anthracis is discussed briefly in Chapter 29 and in references 6 and 7.

Corynebacterium diphtheriae. C. diphtheriae is the cause of cutaneous diphtheria, an ulcerative lesion covered with a layer of necrotic debris resembling a membrane. For optimal diagnosis, a smear for staining with methylene blue is prepared from material collected from the edge of the membrane, and two swab specimens from the membrane are collected. One swab is used for routine bacterial culture (see below under Pseudomonas aeruginosa) and the other for inoculation of media selective for C. diphtheriae (see Table 54–4). Identification of C. diphtheriae is discussed briefly in Chapter 29 and in more detail in references 7 and 8.

Pseudomonas aeruginosa. Ecthyma gangrenosum (Chapter 32) is an ulcerative cutaneous lesion that almost always occurs during bacteremia with P. aeruginosa but rarely during bacteremia with other gram-negative bacilli; therefore, material from the lesion should be cultured to identify the agent (9). Ideally, two swab specimens (transported in a tube system containing modified Stuart's medium) are collected from the ulcer base. One swab is used to prepare a smear for staining with the Gram stain, the other, to inoculate media for culture—sheep blood and MacConkey agars (incubated in ambient air). Incubation temperatures and times are discussed in Chapter 54.

Francisella tularensis. F. tularensis is the cause of tularemia. The diagnosis of the ulceroglandular form of the disease requires the collection of two swab specimens from material at the base of the ulcer. One is processed for routine bacterial culture (see above under Pseudomonas aeruginosa), and one is processed specifically for detection of F. tularensis or is sent to a reference laboratory. Media and culture conditions recommended for recovery of F. tularensis are outlined in Table 54–4, and identification is discussed in Chapter 33.

Mycobacterium species. Species of Mycobacterium that may be isolated from cutaneous ulcers include Mycobacterium tuberculosis, Mycobacterium avium-intracellulare, Mycobacterium kansasii, Mycobacterium fortuitum-chelonae, Mycobacterium marinum, Mycobacterium haemophilum, and Mycobacterium ulcerans. Exudate aspirated with a needle and syringe is optimal for recovery of mycobacteria. To transport the aspirate, the needle is removed, and the syringe is tightly capped and delivered promptly to the laboratory. Exudate collected on a swab and transported in modified Stuart's medium is acceptable, but swab specimens for culture of mycobacteria should be discouraged because the organisms become entrapped in the fibers of the swab and are difficult to dislodge. Specimens may be refrigerated for a short time until they are processed.

Processing of specimens obtained from cutaneous ulcers for detection of mycobacteria involves decontamination, concentration, and using the sediment for preparation of a smear for staining with the auramine rhodamine or an acid-fast stain (Appendix, Procedures 4–6) and inoculation of media for culture. The swab or aspirate is transferred to a sterile 50-ml centrifuge tube containing 10 ml of sterile, filtered distilled water, vigorously mixed on a vortex mixer, and allowed to stand 20 minutes. The swab, if present, is removed, and the specimen is decontaminated with 2% NaOH-N-acetyl-L cysteine and concentrated as outlined in Procedure 27 in the Appendix. Media that may be inoculated for culture of mycobacteria are listed in Table 54–4 and discussed in Chapter 40. To ensure recovery of all mycobacteria associated with cutaneous lesions two sets of media should be inoculated. One set is incubated at 30° and one at 37° C (Mycobacterium haemophilum, -marinum, and -ulcerans grow only at the lower temperature).

Bacteria Infecting Chronic Ulcers. Many aerobic, facultative, and anaerobic bacteria colonize chronic skin ulcers such as deucbitus ulcers and chronic foot ulcers in persons with diabetes. To identify the organisms responsible, cultures of deep tissues or a deep aspirate of purulent material collected with a needle and syringe provide the most useful bacteriologic information. To transport the aspirated pus, air is expelled, the needle is removed, and the syringe is tightly capped and promptly delivered to the laboratory. Processing the specimen involves preparing a smear for staining with the Gram stain and for inoculation of media such as sheep blood and MacConkey agar (incubated in ambient air) and anaerobic blood and kanamycin-vancomycin laked blood agar (incubated anaerobically). Incubation temperatures and times are discussed in Chapter 54.

Fungi

An aspirate of the exudate from the active margin of an ulcer (transported as described earlier for bacteria) is optimal for detection of fungi. A swab specimen of the exudate (transported in a tube transport system containing modified Stuart's medium) is acceptable, but this practice should be discouraged. Processing the specimen for detection of fungi involves preparing a smear for direct microscopic examination and inoculation of appropriate media for culture. Methods of direct examination include the potassium hydroxide preparation (Appendix, Procedure 19) and the stains previously listed for specimens from vesicles and pustules. Enriched fungal media such as brain-heart infusion, inhibitory mold, or SABHI agar containing antibiotics and cycloheximide should be inoculated and incubated as described in Chapter 54. Organism identification is discussed in Chapters 43, 44, and 45.

Parasites

In general, aspirates and scrapings (never swabs) from cutaneous ulcers are submitted to the laboratory for diagnosis of only one parasitic infection, leishmaniasis, but occasionally for diagnosis of cutaneous amebiasis produced by Entamoeba histolytica, and even less often for Acanthamoeba. Because the techniques used for diagnosis of cutaneous leishmaniasis should be followed strictly, these are discussed later, under skin biopsy.

ASPIRATES AND SWAB SPECIMENS FROM WOUND INFECTIONS AND ABSCESSES

Microbiologic studies of aspirates or swab specimens obtained from wound infections and abscesses are useful for identifying the organisms responsible for post-traumatic and postoperative wounds, burn wounds, and bite wounds (human and animal), and identifying the agents that cause cutaneous and subcutaneous abscesses (see Table 62–5). Specimen collection and transport are similar for all organisms listed in the table, but processing is different for bacteria and for fungi and algae and, therefore, is discussed separately for these groups of organisms.

Collection, Transport, and Processing

Ideally, purulent material is aspirated with a needle and syringe and transported as described earlier for ulcerative lesions. If an aspirate cannot be obtained swab specimens of exudate collected from the deep portion of the lesion are acceptable. For routine bacterial culture two swab specimens are optimal, one to prepare a smear for staining with the Gram stain and one for culture. To recover anaerobes an additional swab specimen must be collected and placed in an anaerobic transport system. Additional swab specimens also should be collected for recovery of mycobacteria and fungi. All specimens should be delivered promptly to the laboratory and processed as soon as possible. If a delay in processing is unavoidable, specimens may be stored in the refrigerator, except those for recovery of anaerobes, which should be maintained at room temperature.

Table 62–5. Pathogens Detected by Microbiologic Studies of Specimens from Wound Infections and Abscesses

Organism	Chapter
Bacteria	
Staphylococcus aureus	28
Group A Streptococcus	28
Viridans streptococci	28
Enterococcus spp	28
Nocardia spp	29
Clostridium spp	30
Actinomyces spp	30
Peptostreptococcus spp	30
Pseudomonas aeruginosa	32
Enterobacteriaceae	34
Vibrio vulnificus	35
Aeromonas species	35
Eikenella corrodens	36
Pasteurella multocida	36
Capnocytophaga canimorsus	36
Anaerobic gram-negative bacilli	38
Mycobacterium spp	40
Fungi	
Candida spp	43
Cryptococcus neoformans	43
Trichosporon beigelii	43
Aspergillus spp	44
Pseudallescheria boydii	44
Fusarium spp	44
Zygomycetes	44
Alga	
Prototheca	47
Parasites	
Entamoeba histolytica	49

Bacteria

Processing specimens collected from wounds and abscesses for detection of bacteria differs for different organisms or groups of organisms and is discussed separately for each.

Bacteria Detected by Routine Culture. Processing specimens from wounds and abscesses for bacteria recovered by routine culture involves preparing a smear of the aspirate or swab for staining with the Gram stain and inoculating appropriate media for culture. For swab specimens transported in an aerobic collection device, sheep blood and MacConkey agar and thioglycolate broth are inoculated and incubated in ambient air. Incubation temperatures and times are described in Chapter 54. If the specimen is from a dog bite wound, chocolate agar also should be inoculated, and all plates should be incubated up to 4 days in an atmosphere of 5 to 7% carbon dioxide to assure recovery of Capnocytophaga canimorsus (Chapter 36)(10). Aspirates of purulent material and specimens that include a swab transported in an anaerobic collection device are handled similarly, but an anaerobic blood agar plate, incubated anaerobically for 48 hours, is added. When granules are present and when culture for Actinomyces is requested specifically, the anaerobic blood agar plate and the broth should be held 14 days. If thin, branching, beaded gram-positive bacilli characteristic of Nocardia are seen in the smear stained with the Gram stain, additional steps should be taken to ensure recovery of this organism.

Nocardia species. When culture of Nocardia is requested specifically and when typical organisms are seen in smears of specimens submitted for routine culture stained with the Gram stain, special media and culture conditions (see Table 54–4) must be used. Moreover, when organisms suggestive of Nocardia are visualized in a smear stained with the Gram stain (Plate IIIE), an additional smear should be stained with the modified acid-fact stain (Appendix, Procedure 7). Organism identification is reviewed in Chapter 29.

Mycobacterium species. Processing of specimens from wounds and abscesses for detection of species of Mycobacterium is identical to that described earlier for specimens from ulcers.

Fungi and Algae

Purulent material aspirated with a needle and syringe is optimal for detection of fungi and algae in wounds and abscesses. To transport the aspirate, the needle is removed, and the syringe is tightly capped and promptly delivered to the laboratory. Exudate collected on a swab and transported in modified Stuart's medium is acceptable, but swab specimens for culture of fungi should be discouraged because the organisms become entrapped in the fibers of the swab and are difficult to dislodge. Specimens may be refrigerated for a short time until they are processed.

Processing specimens from wounds and abscesses for detection of fungi and algae involves preparation of a smear for direct microscopic examination (as described earlier for ulcerative lesions and vesicles or pustules) and inoculation of appropriate media for culture. To isolate fungi, a primary planting medium such as brain-heart infusion, inhibitory mold, or SABHI agar containing antibiotics with and without cycloheximide, which inhibits growth of some potential pathogens (Pseudallescheria boydii and species of Prototheca), is inoculated and incubated as described in Chapter 54.

SKIN SLITS

Leprosy is diagnosed in persons with clinical manifestations consistent with the disease (Chapter 40) when acid-fast bacilli are observed in smears made from nasal secretions (Chapter 57) or from skin slits. Skin slits of cutaneous lesions or ear lobes are made by holding a fold of skin between the thumb and forefinger, squeezing lightly to avoid blood in the smear, and making a short, shallow slit with a razor or scalpel blade. The edge of the lesion is scraped lightly, and the material collected is spread on a glass slide. Smears are air-dried, heat-fixed, and stained with the auramine rhodamine or an acid-fast stain (see Appendix, Procedures 4–6). For adequate classification and for diagnosis of early disease, full-thickness biopsy specimens of the skin (epidermis and dermis) should be taken from the active border of the lesion (see below).

SKIN BIOPSY SPECIMENS

Microbiologic studies of biopsy specimens of cutaneous and subcutaneous lesions are useful for diagnosing many infections (see Table 62–6); in addition, specimens of normal skin may confirm a diagnosis of rabies. Specimen collection is similar for all known pathogens. Specimen processing, however, is different for viruses, bacteria, fungi and algae, and parasites, and is discussed separately for each group of organisms.

Collection, Transport, and Processing

In general, specimen collection involves obtaining an ample biopsy specimen from an active area of the lesion. Special requirements are discussed below for the individual organisms. Specimens should be placed in a sterile container and transported immediately to the laboratory, where a pathologist should examine the fresh tissue and divide the specimen appropriately for histologic and microbiologic studies.

Viruses

Processing biopsy tissue from skin lesions for detection of viruses is different for each virus listed in Table 62–6.

Molluscum contagiosum. Lesions of molluscum contagiosum usually are diagnosed by clinical appearance alone, but the diagnosis may be confirmed by histologic examination of the lesion. The characteristic histologic findings are described in Chapter 4 (see Fig. 4–1).

Table 62–6. Pathogens Detected by Microbiologic Studies of Biopsy Specimens from Cutaneous and Subcutaneous Lesions

Organism	Chapter
Viruses	
Molluscum contagiosum virus	4
Human papillomavirus	7
Rabies virus	16
Bacteria	
Erysipelothrix rhusiopathiae	29
Nocardia spp	29
Actinomyces spp	30
Mycobacterium spp	40
Fungi	
Candida spp	43
Cryptococcus neoformans	43
Trichosporon beigelii	43
Dematiaceous fungi	44
Aspergillus spp	44
Pseudallescheria boydii	44
Fusarium spp	44
Zygomyctes	44
Blastomyces dermatitidis	45
Coccidioides immitis	45
Paracoccidioides brasiliensis	45
Sporothrix schenckii	45
Loboa loboi	46
Alga	
Prototheca spp	47
Parasites	
Entamoeba histolytica	49
Cutaneous leishmania	51

Human papillomavirus. Lesions of human papillomavirus (HPV) usually are diagnosed by their clinical appearance, a diagnosis confirmed by histological examination of sections stained with hematoxylin and eosin (the typical histologic appearance is described in Chapter 7). HPV DNA may be detected in tissue by nucleic acid hybridization using a commercially available kit. The DNA probes provided with the kit are specific for a limited number of HPV serotypes (principally those associated with genital lesions) and, so, are not very useful for cutaneous lesions.

Rabies virus. For optimal detection of rabies virus antigen by direct immunofluorescence, a 6- to 8-mm full-thickness wedge or punch biopsy of the skin of the posterior neck above the hairline is obtained from an area that contains as many hair follicles as possible. The specimen should be placed fresh in a small vial with a small piece of moist gauze, frozen at $-70°$ C, and shipped on dry ice to the reference laboratory that will performing the test.

Bacteria

Processing of biopsy specimens of cutaneous and subcutaneous lesions for detection of bacteria differs for different organisms and is discussed separately for each of the bacteria listed in Table 62–6.

Erysipelothrix rhusiopathiae. The optimal specimen for recovery of E. rhusiopathiae from a cutaneous lesion is an aseptically collected full-thickness biopsy sample (because the bacteria lie deep in the tissue) obtained from the edge of the lesion. The tissue is homogenized in a small amount of broth with a sterile tissue grinder or mortar and pestle to give a 10 to 20% (weight per volume) suspension, which is used to prepare a smear for staining with the Gram stain and inoculation of media for culture. Sheep blood and MacConkey agar and thioglycolate broth are inoculated and incubated in ambient air. Incubation temperatures and times are described in Chapter 54. Identification of E. rhusiopathiae is reviewed in Chapter 29.

Nocardia species. To detect species of Nocardia in biopsy specimens from cutaneous and subcutaneous lesions, the tissue is homogenized as described for Erysipelothrix rhusiopathiae. The homogenate is used to prepare smears for staining with the Gram stain and with the modified acid-fast stain (Appendix, Procedure 7) and to inoculate media for culture (see Table 54–4).

Actinomyces species. To detect species of Actinomyces the tissue should be processed as rapidly as possible; if a delay is unavoidable it should be placed in an anaerobic transport system. Processing involves preparing a homogenate as described earlier for Erysipelothrix rhusiopathiae, used for preparation of a smear for staining with the Gram stain, and for inoculation of media for culture, as described earlier for bacteria detected by routine culture of wounds and abscesses.

Mycobacterium species. Processing of biopsies of cutaneous and subcutaneous lesions to detect species of Mycobacterium differs for different species. Mycobacterium leprae cannot be recovered in the clinical laboratory, and the diagnosis of leprosy is based on clinical manifestations plus consistent histologic findings in skin and subcutaneous tissue taken from the active border of a well-defined lesion (Chapter 40). The remaining mycobacteria associated with cutaneous lesions (listed earlier for ulcerative lesions) are identified by culture.

To recover mycobacteria the tissue is homogenized in a biologic safety cabinet, as described for Erysipelothrix rhusiopathiae. For specimens collected aseptically and believed not to be contaminated, the homogenate is used directly to prepare smears for staining with auramine rhodamine or an acid-fast stain (Appendix, Procedures 4–6) and to inoculate media for culture (Table 54–4; see Chapter 40). For contaminated specimens the homogenate is poured through sterile gauze into a 50-ml centrifuge tube to which an equal volume of 2% NaOH-N-acetyl-L cysteine is added. The solution is mixed and allowed to stand 20 minutes, after which 25 ml of phosphate buffer is added and mixed. The suspension is centrifuged at 3000 to 3600 g for 20 minutes, the supernatant is discarded, and the sediment is suspended in 1 to 2 ml of buffer and used to prepare a smear for staining (as above) and to inoculate media for culture.

Fungi and Algae

Processing tissue from cutaneous and subcutaneous lesions for detection of fungi and algae is similar for all organisms listed in Table 62–6 except Loboa loboi, which has not been cultured and is detected only by histologic examination of involved skin. A homogenate of the biopsy is prepared in a biologic safety cabinet, as described for Erysipelothrix rhusiopathiae, and processed for detection of fungi and algae in specimens from wounds and abscesses.

Parasites

In this section the sampling, processing, and laboratory diagnosis of cutaneous leishmaniasis (Chapter 51) is discussed. The steps followed to procure the proper samples are very important if a correct diagnosis of leishmaniasis is to be made.

Cutaneous leishmaniasis (also referred to as mucocutaneous, because the process may involve the nasopharyngeal mucosae as well) usually manifests as one ulcer, sometimes two, least often more. Samples should be taken from the most recent or the most active lesion. If the ucler shows signs of secondary infection the ulcer should be débrided, and cleaned and antibiotics should be given for 1 week. Samples for examination should be taken after the treatment.

Lesions should be cleaned thoroughly with 70% alcohol before taking samples for parasitologic examination. All extraneous material should be removed, in some instances after injecting a small amount of 1% lidocaine with epinephrine for the patient's comfort. These samples are taken:

Scrapings. For clean ulcers, scrapings from the bottom, using a blade, a brush, or other instruments, are used to prepare smears on clean glass slides, which then are dried, fixed, and stained (11). This technique allows a diagnosis in about half the cases. If the scrapings from the

SKIN, ADNEXA, AND SUBCUTANEOUS TISSUES

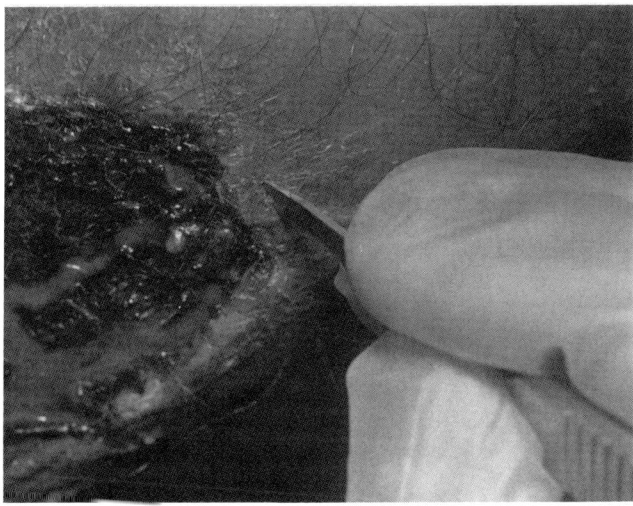

Fig. 62–1. Cutaneous leishmaniasis. Technique for obtaining scrapings from the skin slit at the border of the ulcer. Note where the cut is made and how deep the blade is inserted. (From Palma G and Gutierrez Y: Laboratory diagnosis of Leishmania. Clin Lab Med, *11*:909, 1991.)

bottom of the ulcer give negative results, scrapings from the border should be processed in a similar fashion.

Skin slit. The next sample, the skin slit, is made on the border of the ulcer, usually perpendicular to the center, with a scalpel blade. A cut about 5 mm long by 5 mm deep is made and blotted with sterile gauze until all bleeding stops (Fig. 62–1). With the blade or a spatula reintroduced into the slit, the walls of the slit are scraped (Fig. 62–2) and the tissue obtained is smeared on clean glass slides and processed as scrapings are (Fig. 62–3).

Biopsy and imprints. With local anesthesia a specimen is then taken, using a 4- or 5-mm disposable biopsy punch, of the border of the ulcer. The core is blotted on a clean paper towel and used to prepare imprint smears. Imprints are fixed and stained, as described for scrapings, and the tissue is sent to the surgical pathology laboratory for processing and examination (12).

Aspiration. Aspiration of the border of the ulcer is done with a syringe and needle (Fig. 62–4) to obtain material for preparation of smears to be stained with the Giemsa stain or any other hematologic stain. The smears are examined with a microscope, first under medium power to locate granulomas (seen as large masses of cells), high, dry to locate "suspicious" structures, and with oil immersion to confirm and diagnose leishmaniasis.

Study of samples in the manner described allows diagnosis of leishmaniasis, but the species of Leishmania cannot be identified because all are morphologically identical. If speciation is desired the samples must be cultured.

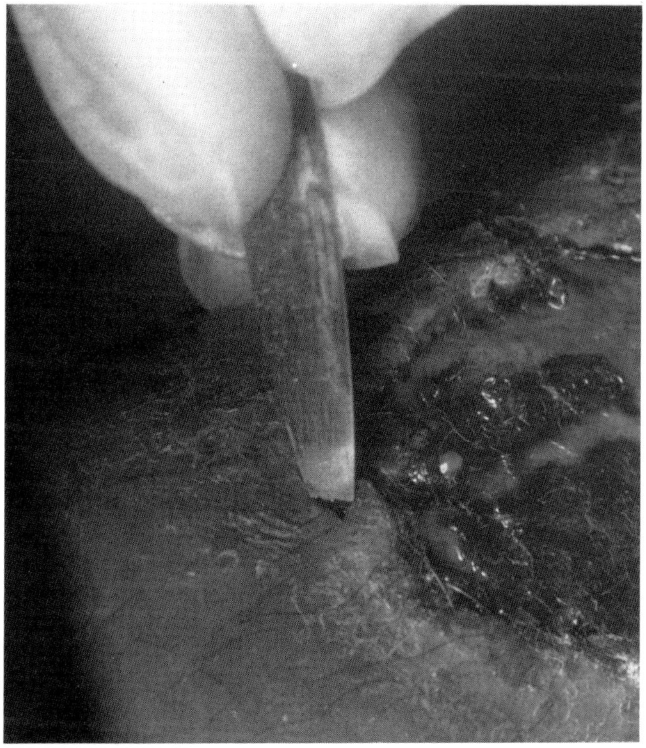

Fig. 62–2. Cutaneous leishmaniasis. Technique for obtaining scrapings from the skin slit at the border of the ulcer. After cutting, when bleeding has stopped, a stainless steel blade is inserted and the walls of the slit are scraped to obtain material. (From Palma G and Gutierrez Y: Laboratory diagnosis of Leishmania. Clin Lab Med, *11*:909, 1991.)

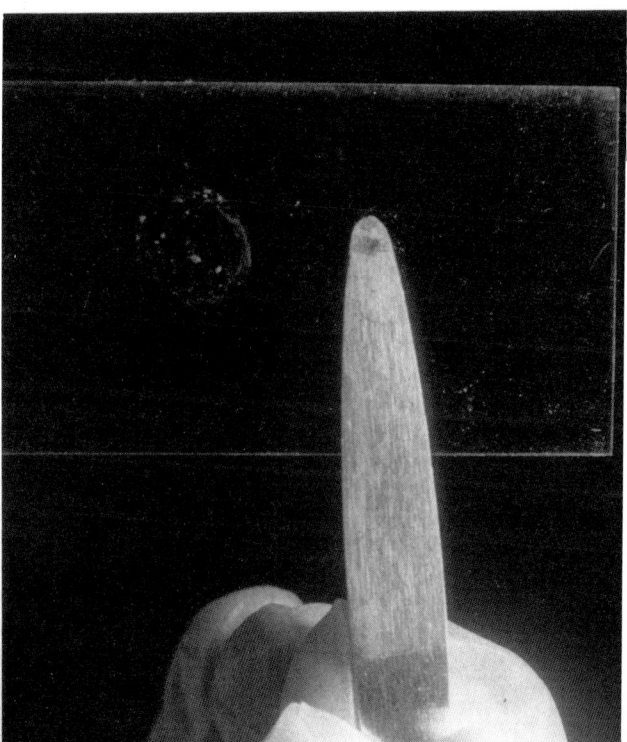

Fig. 62–3. Cutaneous leishmaniasis. The material obtained with the stainless steel blade is smeared on a glass slide. The smear is dried, fixed, and stained with Giemsa for examination. (From Palma G and Gutierrez Y: Laboratory diagnosis of Leishmania. Clin Lab Med, *11*:909, 1991.)

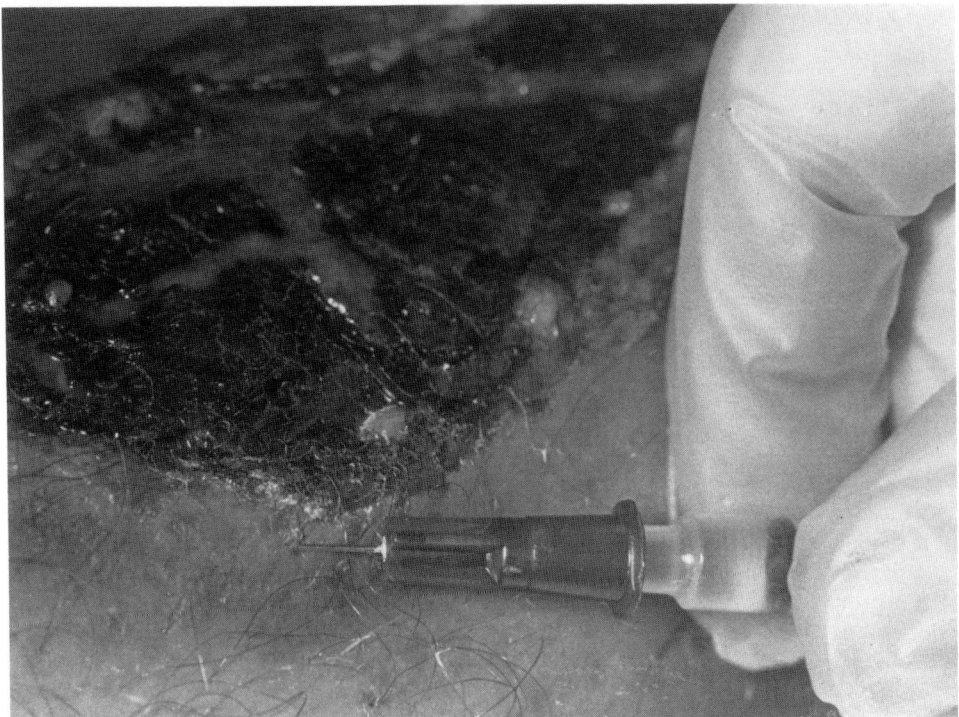

Fig. 62–4. Cutaneous leishmaniasis. Technique for obtaining material from the border of the ulcer for preparation of smears and culture. Note that the needle is inserted parallel to the border of the ulcer. (From Palma G and Gutierrez Y: Laboratory diagnosis of Leishmania. Clin Lab Med, *11*: 909, 1991.)

Cultures. Aspirates from the border of the ulcer and homogenized tissue fragments of biopsy samples are good for culture, but most clinical laboratories do not have the necessary media. Isolation of leishmaniae in culture is easy and allows the species to be identified by biochemical methods, a technique used for epidemiologic studies and for research purposes. Because culture is not required for good patient care, and because most clinical laboratory workers are not familiar with the technique, specimens received for isolation of Leishmania should be sent to a reference laboratory.

REFERENCES

1. Woods GL, and Mills RD: Effect of dexamethasone on detection of herpes simplex virus in clinical specimens by conventional cell culture and rapid 24-well plate centrifugation. J Clin Microbiol, *26*:1233, 1988.
2. Gleaves CA, Wilson DJ, Wold AD, and Smith TF: Detection and serotyping of herpes simplex virus in MRC-5 cells by use of centrifugation and monoclonal antibodies 16 h post-inoculation. J Clin Microbiol, *21*:29, 1985.
3. Woods GL, and Mills RD: Conventional tube cell culture compared with centrifugal inoculation of MRC-5 cells and staining with monoclonal antibodies for detection of herpes simplex virus in clinical specimens. J Clin Microbiol, *26*: 570, 1988.
4. Schmidt NJ, et al: Direct immunofluorescence staining for detection of herpes simplex and varicella zoster virus antigens in vesicular lesions and certain tissue specimens. J Clin Microbiol, *12*:651, 1980.
5. Zimmerman SJ, et al: Evaluation of a visual, rapid, membrane enzyme immunoassay for the detection of herpes simplex virus antigen. J Clin Microbiol, *29*:842, 1991.
6. Doyle RJ, Keller KF, and Ezzell JW: Bacillus. *In* Manual of Clinical Microbiology. 5th ed. Edited by A Balows, et al. Washington, DC, American Society for Microbiology, 1991.
7. Koneman EW, et al (eds): The aerobic gram-positive bacilli. *In* Color Atlas and Textbook of Diagnostic Microbiology. 3rd ed. Philadelphia, JB Lippincott, 1988.
8. Coyle MB, Hollis DG, and Groman NB: Corynebacterium spp. and other coryneform organisms. *In* Manual of Clinical Microbiology. 5th ed. Edited by A Balows, et al. Washington, DC, American Society for Microbiology, 1991.
9. Bodey GP, et al: Infections caused by Pseudomonas aeruginosa. Rev Infect Dis, *5*:279, 1983.
10. Brenner DJ, Hollis DG, Fanning GR, and Weaver RE: C. canimorsus sp. nov. (formerly CDC group DF-2), a cause of septicemia following dog bite, and C. cynodegmi sp. nov., a cause of localized wound infection following dog bite. J Clin Microbiol, *27*:231, 1989.
11. Palma G, and Gutierrez Y. Diagnosis of leishmania. Clin Lab Med, *11*:909, 1991.

Chapter 63

BODY CAVITIES

Specimens collected to identify organisms infecting the pericardial, pleural, or peritoneal cavity are handled similarly in the laboratory.

Microbiologic studies of pericardial fluid and tissue are useful for identifying organisms responsible for infectious pericarditis (Table 63–1). Viruses generally reach the pericardium via hematogenous spread from the myocardium and elicit a serous, serofibrinous, or serosanguineous effusion, which usually resolves without sequelae. Bacteria spread from a contiguous focus of infection in the chest or the heart or travel hematogenously from a distant focus of infection. Pyogenic bacteria elicit a purulent effusion, whereas the effusion of tuberculosis typically is serosanguineous. In both cases, the process heals with organization, and the resulting adhesions eventually may cause constrictive pericarditis. The clinical manifestations of acute infectious pericarditis vary with the infecting organism. In viral pericarditis the predominant symptom is retrosternal pain that radiates to the shoulder and neck and is aggravated by breathing and swallowing; fever is present in about 60% of cases. Persons with bacterial pericarditis have fever and dyspnea plus the manifestations of the underlying infection. Tuberculous pericarditis begins insidiously, with weight loss, night sweats, cough, dyspnea, and in as many as 80% of cases, chest pain.

Studies of pleural fluid and tissues are performed to identify the infectious causes of pleural effusions and empyema. Infectious agents reach the pleura by direct extension from an infection in the lung, mediastinum, pericardium, or cervical or subdiaphragmatic areas; via hematogenous or lymphatic spread from a distant focus of infection; or as a result of surgical or other trauma to the chest. Of the potential pathogens (see Table 63–1), Staphylococcus aureus, Streptococcus pneumoniae, and Streptococcus pyogenes are the most common causes of pleural empyema in otherwise healthy persons who have pneumonia (1). In patients with post-traumatic or nosocomial empyema, Staphylococcus aureus and gram-negative bacteria frequently are involved, and in immunocompromised hosts infection often is caused by fungi or gram-negative bacilli (1–3). The clinical manifestations of empyema typically reflect the underlying disease, but they may include chest pain, dyspnea, weight loss, chills, fever, or sweats.

Microbiologic studies of peritoneal fluid and tissue are useful for determining the organisms responsible for primary and secondary peritonitis and peritonitis associated with chronic ambulatory peritoneal dialysis. Primary peritonitis occurs spontaneously, with no evident intra-abdominal focus of infection. Bacteria are presumed to reach the peritoneal cavity via hematogenous or lymphatic spread, by transmural migration from the bowel lumen through an intact intestinal wall, or in women from the vagina through the fallopian tubes. In children, primary peritonitis is associated with postnecrotic cirrhosis, the nephrotic syndrome, or urinary tract infection, but it also occurs in the absence of predisposing disease (4–6). Primary peritonitis in adults most often is associated with alcoholic cirrhosis and ascites, but it may occur in association with other diseases that manifest with ascites, including postnecrotic cirrhosis, chronic active hepatitis, acute viral hepatitis, congestive heart failure, metastatic malignant disease, and systemic lupus erythematosus; rarely, there is no underlying disease (7–9). Of the organisms that may be involved (see Table 63–1), the most common are gram-negative bacilli, staphylococci, and Streptococcus pneumoniae in children and Escherichia coli, Klebsiella pneumoniae, Streptococcus pneumoniae, and enterococci in adults (4–6,9–11). Primary peritonitis in children is an acute illness characterized by fever, abdominal pain, nausea, vomiting, and diarrhea, whereas in adults with pre-existing ascites the process may be asymptomatic or begin insidiously, with fever that may or may not be accompanied by abdominal signs and symptoms.

Secondary peritonitis occurs as a complication of a disease or injury of the gastrointestinal tract: perforation of a peptic ulcer, appendicitis, diverticulitis, inflammatory bowel disease, suppurative cholecystitis, pancreatitis, intestinal neoplasms; traumatic perforation of the uterus, urinary bladder, stomach, small intestine, or colon; spontaneous perforation of an ulcer caused by Salmonella typhi, Mycobacterium tuberculosis, Entamoeba histolytica, or cytomegalovirus; gangrene of the bowel; septic abortion; or rupture of an intraperitoneal or visceral abscess. Infection often is polymicrobial and usually is caused by members of the normal bowel flora, particularly Escherichia coli, Bacteroides fragilis, enterococci, and other species of Bacteroides (9,12,13). Peritonitis associated with chronic peritoneal dialysis, in contrast, is caused by organisms of the normal skin flora, especially Staphylococcus epidermidis (14,15). Both types of peritonitis are manifested by abdominal pain, often accompanied by anorexia, nausea, and vomiting.

Collection, Transport, and Processing

Collection and transport of body fluids are similar for all potential pathogens. Specimen processing, however, is different for viruses, bacteria, fungi, and parasites and is discussed separately for each group of organisms.

Fluid is collected from the pericardial, thoracic, or peritoneal cavity by aspirating with a needle and syringe. A

Table 63–1. Pathogens Detected by Microbiologic Studies of Fluid and Tissue from Body Cavities

Organism	Pericardial	Pleural	Peritoneal	Chapter
Viruses				
Enteroviruses	X			13
Bacteria				
Chlamydia trachomatis		X	X	25
Mycoplasma pneumoniae	X			27
Staphylococcus aureus	X	X	X	28
Staphylococcus epidermidis			X	28
Group A Streptococcus		X	X	28
Streptococcus pneumoniae	X	X	X	28
Enterococcus spp			X	28
Corynebacterium spp			X	29
Nocardia spp		X		29
Clostridium spp			X	30
Actinomyces spp	X	X		30
Peptostreptococcus spp			X	30
Neisseria gonorrhoeae			X	31
Neisseria meningitidis	X			31
Pseudomonas spp		X	X	32
Legionella spp		X		33
Enterobacteriaceae	X	X	X	34
Haemophilus influenzae	X	X		36
Anaerobic gram-negative bacilli		X	X	38
Mycobacterium spp	X	X	X	40
Fungi				
Candida spp	X		X	43
Aspergillus spp	X	X		44
Histoplasma capsulatum	X	X		45
Coccidioides immitis	X	X		45
Parasites				
Entamoeba histolytica	X	X	X	49
Strongyloides stercoralis	X	X	X	50
Echinococcus granulosus	X	X	X	52
Microfilariae	X	X	X	52

volume of 1 to 5 ml is adequate for isolating most bacteria, but 10 to 15 ml is required for optimal recovery of mycobacteria and fungi, which generally are present in small numbers. Moreover, to diagnose peritonitis associated with chronic ambulatory peritoneal dialysis, collection of at least 50 ml of fluid is recommended (16). To transport the fluid, the air is expelled, the needle is removed, and the syringe is tightly capped with a sterile rubber stopper and delivered promptly to the laboratory. Alternatively, a portion of the fluid may be transferred to an anaerobic transport system. Biopsy specimens of pericardium, pleura, and peritoneum are obtained surgically and transported immediately to the laboratory in a sterile container. A pathologist should examine the fresh tissue and divide the specimen appropriately for histologic and microbiologic studies.

Viruses

Enteroviruses, primarily coxsackieviruses A and B, are among the most common causes of infectious pericarditis. These viruses may be detected in pericardial fluid, but because they are not recovered in all cases collection of throat washings and stool (which are more likely to yield the virus), in addition to pericardial fluid, for virus isolation from persons with pericarditis suspected to be enteroviral is strongly recommended. Other viruses (herpes, simplex virus, varicella-zoster virus, cytomegalovirus, Epstein-Barr virus, hepatitis B virus, mumps virus, and influenza virus) are infrequent agents of pericarditis and usually are not detected in pericardial fluid or tissue.

Pericardial fluid collected for detection of viruses should be delivered to the laboratory immediately or should be refrigerated for a short time and transported on wet ice. To ensure recovery of the enteroviruses, the specimen should be inoculated to MRC-5 and primary monkey kidney cells, as described in Chapter 54. Virus identification is discussed in Chapter 13.

Bacteria

Processing fluid and tissue from body cavities differs for detection of different bacteria or groups of bacteria and, therefore, is discussed separately for each.

Chlamydia trachomatis. C. trachomatis may cause peritoneal infection, primarily perihepatitis (called Fitz-Hugh-Curtis syndrome), in sexually active young women and pleural effusions in infants. To detect C. trachomatis in peritoneal or pleural fluid, cell culture must be performed. The fluid should be processed as soon as possible after it is collected, but if a delay is unavoidable it may be refrigerated up to 48 hours or stored at $-70°$ C for longer periods. Processing for cell culture is outlined in Procedure 8 of the Appendix.

Mycoplasma pneumoniae. M. pneumoniae is an uncommon cause of pericarditis and its detection in pericardial fluid occasionally may be requested. To isolate the organism the fluid is inoculated to a biphasic culture medium (several are available commercially) or to a vial of SP-4 broth, and the culture is incubated up to 3 weeks at $35°$ to $37°$ C. A nucleic acid probe for detection of M. pneumoniae is commercially available but currently is approved only for throat and sputum specimens. Given the prolonged culture time of M. pneumoniae, serologic studies for detection of specific immunoglobulin M (IgM) are recommended.

Bacteria Detected by Routine Culture. Processing fluid and tissue from body cavities involves preparing a smear for Gram staining and inoculating appropriate media for culture. Different methods may be used to detect bacteria in body fluids. One approach involves concentrating the specimen by centrifugation. The fluid is centrifuged at 1500 to 2500 g for at least 20 minutes, and the supernatant is removed, leaving about 0.5 ml, in which the sediment is mixed thoroughly and then used to prepare smears and inoculate media (described later). Alternatively, a small volume of fluid (about 0.5 ml) is removed before centrifugation and used to prepare a cytocentrifuged smear. Fluids also may be processed by directly inoculating a blood culture system (Chapter 58), saving 0.5 to 1.0 ml for preparation of a smear for staining with the Gram stain, an approach shown to be especially useful for detection of bacteria in peritoneal fluid (18,19).

Tissue is homogenized in broth with a sterile tissue grinder or a mortar and pestle, and the resulting suspension is used to prepare smears and inoculate media. Sheep blood, MacConkey, and chocolate agar (incubated in an atmosphere of 5 to 7% carbon dioxide), thioglycolate broth (incubated in ambient air), and anaerobic blood agar (incubated anaerobically) are the recommended primary planting media. Incubation temperature and times are discussed in Chapter 54. When culture for Actinomyces is requested, the anaerobic blood agar plate and the broth should be held 2 weeks. Moreover, if long, thin, beaded, branching, gram-positive bacilli characteristic of Nocardia (Plate IIIE) are seen in the smear stained with the Gram stain, steps should be taken to ensure recovery of Nocardia (see below).

Nocardia species. Processing fluid to detect species of Nocardia involves centrifugation (as previously described) and using the sediment to prepare smears for staining with the Gram and with the modified acid-fast stain (if organisms characteristic of Nocardia, described earlier, are seen in the smear stained with the Gram stain) and to inoculate media for culture. Tissue is homogenized (as previously discussed), and the suspension is used to prepare smears for staining and to inoculate media for culture. Appropriate media and culture conditions are outlined in Table 54–4.

Legionella species. Species of Legionella are rarely recovered from pleural fluid. When detection of Legionella is requested, the fluid sediment (prepared as described earlier for bacteria detected by routine culture) should be cultured as outlined in Table 54–4. Moreover, a smear of the sediment may be prepared for direct fluorescent antibody staining (as discussed for sputum specimens in Chapter 57).

Mycobacterium species. Fluid specimens submitted for detection of mycobacteria are concentrated by centrifuging at 3000 to 3600 g for 30 minutes. The supernatant is removed, and the sediment is resuspended in 1 to 2 ml of buffer and used to prepare a smear for staining with auramine rhodamine or an acid-fast stain (Appendix, Procedures 4–6) and to inoculate media for culture as outlined in Table 54–4 and described in more detail in Chapter 40. Tissue is homogenized in about 2 ml of buffer (as previously described), and the suspension is used to prepare smears for staining and to inoculate media for culture.

Fungi

Processing of fluids and tissues from body cavities for detection of fungi involves direct microscopic examination and inoculation of appropriate media for culture. Fluids should be concentrated by centrifugation at 1500 to 2500 g for 3 minutes. The supernatant is removed, leaving 1.5 to 2.0 ml, in which the sediment is thoroughly mixed. Tissues are homogenized in broth, as described earlier for bacteria detected by routine culture.

The fluid sediment and tissue homogenate may be examined directly by performing a potassium hydroxide preparation (Appendix, Procedure 19) or making a smear for staining with the Gram, calcofluor white, Congo red, or Gomori's methenamine silver stain. Ideally, 0.5 to 1.0 ml of sediment or homogenate is inoculated to primary fungal planting media such as inhibitory mold or SABHI agar (Chapter 54), but a smaller volume is acceptable. Culture conditions are described in Chapter 54.

Parasites

Body fluids rarely are collected for detection of parasites, because a clear suspicion of a parasitic infection involving serosal cavities is rare. Dissemination of Entamoeba histolytica into the pericardium, pleural cavity, or peritoneum occurs occasionally, owing to rupture of an abscess of the liver (into the peritoneal, pleural, or pericardial cavity) or the lungs (into the pleural or pericardial cavity) or of amoebic ulcers (into the peritoneal cavity). Rarely is the diagnosis made in the microbiology laboratory; sometimes in the surgical pathology laboratory; often at the autopsy table. Occasionally Toxoplasma gondii may be detected in smears of body cavity fluids.

The other parasitic infection diagnosed by examination of body cavity fluids is hydatid cyst, also due to rupture of a cyst into a viscus contiguous to the cavity in question. The fluid collected is usually as clear as distilled water and contains hydatid sand (see Chapter 52). Rarely, the fluid shows bacterial growth because of superimposed infection.

In persons with a filarial infection examination of wet preparations of body cavity fluid may demonstrate the microfilariae. By the same token, in patients with hyperinfection with Strongyloides larvae may be detected in body cavity fluids.

REFERENCES

1. Roberts WC, and Spray TL: Clinical and morphological spectrum of pericardial heart disease. Curr Probl Cardiol, *2*:1, 1977.
2. Vianna NJ: Nontuberculous bacterial empyema in patients with and without underlying disease. JAMA, *215*:69, 1971.
3. Caplan ES, et al: Empyema occurring in the multiply traumatized patient. J Trauma, *24*:785, 1984.
4. Lemmer JH, Botham MJ, and Orringer MD: Modern management of adult thoracic empyema. J Thorac Cardiovasc Surg, *90*:849, 1985.
5. Nohr CW, and Marshall DG: Primary peritonitis in children. Can J Surg, *27*:179, 1984.
6. McDougal WS, Izant RJ, and Zollinger RM, Jr: Primary peritonitis in infancy and childhood. Ann Surg, *181*:310, 1975.
7. Speck WT, Dresdale SS, and McMillan RW: Primary peritonitis and the nephrotic syndrome. Am J Surg, *127*:267, 1974.
8. Conn HO, and Fessel JM: Spontaneous bacterial peritonitis in cirrhosis: Variations on a theme. Medicine, *50*:161, 1971.
9. Conn HO: Spontaneous bacterial peritonitis, multiple revisitations. Gastroenterology, *70*:455, 1976.
10. Levison ME, and Bush LM: Peritonitis and other intra-abdominal infections. *In* Principles and Practice of Infectious Diseases. 3rd ed. Edited by GL Mandell, RG Douglas, Jr, and JE Bennett. New York, Churchill Livingstone, 1990.
11. Wilcox CM, and Dismukes WE: Spontaneous bacterial peritonitis: A review of pathogenesis, diagnosis and treatment. Medicine, *66*:447, 1987.
12. Hoefs JC, and Runyon BA: Spontaneous bacterial peritonitis. Dis a Month, *31*(9):1, 1985.
13. Lorber B, and Swenson RM: The bacteriology of intra-abdominal infections. Surg Clin North Am, *55*:1346, 1975.

14. Swenson RM, et al: The bacteriology of intra-abdominal infections. Arch Surg, *109*:398, 1974.
15. Vas S: Microbiological aspects of peritonitis. Peritoneal Dial Bull, *1*(Supp):S11, 1981.
16. Rubin SJ: Continuous ambulatory peritoneal dialysis: Dialysate fluid cultures. Clin Microbiol Newslett, *63*:3, 1984.
17. Dawson MS, et al: Total volume culture technique for the isolation of micro-organisms from continuous ambulatory peritoneal dialysis patients with peritonitis. J Clin Microbiol, *22*:391, 1985.
18. Savoia MC, and Oxman MN: Myocarditis, pericarditis, and mediastinitis. *In* Principles and Practice of Infectious Diseases. 3rd ed. Edited by GL Mandell, RG Douglas, Jr, and JE Bennett. New York, Churchill Livingstone, 1990.
19. Luce E, et al: Improvement in the bacteriologic diagnosis of peritonitis with the use of blood culture media. Trans Am Soc Artif Intern Organs, *28*:259, 1982.
20. Woods GL, and Washington JA II: Comparison of methods for processing dialysate in suspected continuous ambulatory peritoneal dialysis—associated peritonitis. Diagn Microbiol Infect Dis, *7*:155, 1987.

Chapter 64

MUSCULOSKELETAL SYSTEM

Specimens collected to identify organisms responsible for infections of the musculoskeletal system include samples from muscle (including tissue, aspirated purulent material, or a swab specimen from the involved site), joint fluid and synovial tissue, and biopsy specimens of bone.

MUSCLE, ASPIRATED PURULENT MATERIAL, AND SWAB SPECIMENS

Infections involving skeletal muscle are uncommon but may be caused by many organisms (Table 64–1). Bacterial infections of muscle usually are associated with a penetrating wound, vascular insufficiency in an extremity, or a contiguous focus of infection such as an abscess in the skin or the subcutaneous tissue, a decubitus ulcer, or osteomyelitis. Primary bacterial infections and those resulting from hematogenous spread from a distant focus of infection are rare. Four patterns of muscle infection are reviewed briefly: pyomyositis, clostridial myonecrosis, nonclostridial myositis, and psoas abscess.

Pyomyositis, a primary muscle abscess almost always caused by Staphyloccocus aureus, occurs at all ages, predominantly in the tropics (1). The infection, preceded by trauma in up to 50% of cases, usually has a subacute onset with pain in the involved muscle (most frequently a lower extremity or trunk muscle), followed by swelling, induration, and fever. Rarely, group A Streptococcus causes a fulminant form of pyomyositis accompanied by bacteremia and toxemia and associated with a high mortality rate (2).

Clostridial myonecrosis (gas gangrene) is a rapidly progressive, life-threatening infection of skeletal muscle that occurs in association with both muscle injury and contamination with soil or other foreign material that contains spores of Clostridium perfringens or other species of Clostridium (Chapter 30): traumatic injuries such as compound fractures, penetrating war wounds, and surgical wounds (especially following manipulation of the bowel or biliary tract); and with vascular insufficiency in an extremity (3–5). Occasionally, gas gangrene develops in the absence of an external wound, particularly infections caused by Clostridium septicum in persons with a hematologic malignancy or carcinoma of the colon (6). Symptoms (described in Chapter 30) typically begin 2 to 3 days after an injury, though they may become apparent within several hours. The infection progresses rapidly and is fatal if not appropriately treated.

Four entities are included in the pattern of infection termed nonclostridial myositis. (1) Anaerobic streptococcal myonecrosis, an interstitial myositis caused by anaerobic streptococci and group A Streptococcus or Staphyloccocus aureus, begins 3 to 4 days after an injury, with swelling, cutaneous erythema, and a seropurulent discharge, followed by pain. Gas is present in the tissue, and the involved muscles are discolored. Untreated, the infection progresses to frank gangrene with shock. (2) Synergistic nonclostridial anaerobic myonecrosis (also called synergistic necrotizing cellulitis) is a severe infection primarily involving the subcutaneous tissue and fascia that produces secondary changes in the adjacent skin and muscle. (3) Infected vascular gangrene is a mixed infection, typically in persons with diabetes mellitus, commonly produced by species of Proteus, Bacteroides, and anaerobic streptococci. The infection, which remains localized to an area of arterial insufficiency (and, subsequently, devitalization of tissue) is characterized by gas formation, unpleasant smell, and purulent drainage. (4) Myonecrosis produced by Aeromonas hydrophila is a rapidly progressive infection resembling gas gangrene that typically follows trauma in fresh water (7).

Psoas abscesses most frequently result from direct extension of an intra-abdominal infection; thus, members of the normal bowel flora (see Table 2–1) are the most common agents. Psoas abscess also may complicate tuberculous or pyogenic vertebral osteomyelitis, often caused by Staphylococcus aureus. The infection is manifested by fever, lower abdominal or back pain, and pain referred to the hip or knee.

Biopsy specimens of muscle for diagnosis of parasitic infections, especially trichinosis, are studied in the surgical pathology laboratory. Other parasitic infections diagnosed in such specimens are cysticercosis, sparganosis, some filarial worms, and hydatid cysts.

Optimally, to identify the agent of an infection of skeletal muscle, a tissue specimen should be obtained by biopsy. If muscle cannot be obtained, purulent material should be aspirated from the involved site. A swab specimen collected from the infected areas is the least desirable sample for microbiologic studies. Specimen collection and transport are similar for all potential pathogens, but processing differs and is discussed separately for bacteria, fungi, and parasites. Viruses, such as influenza A virus, may cause myositis, but generally they are not detected in muscle and are not discussed further here.

Collection, Transport, and Processing

A biopsy specimen of the affected muscle is obtained and immediately transported in a sterile container to the laboratory. If the muscle appears necrotic the surgeon who collects the specimen should place a separate fragment of muscle in an anaerobic transport device. Fresh tissue should be examined by a pathologist and divided appropriately for histologic (Fig. 64–1) and microbio-

Table 64–1. Pathogens Detected by Microbiologic Studies of Infected Muscle

Organism	Chapter
Bacteria	
Staphylococcus aureus	28
Group A Streptococcus	28
Microaerophilic streptococci	28
Bacillus spp	29
Clostridium spp	30
Actinomyces spp	30
Pseudomonas mallei	32
Pseudomonas pseudomallei	32
Enterobacteriaceae	34
Vibrio vulnificus	35
Aeromonas spp	35
Anaerobic gram-negative bacilli	38
Mycobacterium tuberculosis	40
Fungi	
Candida spp	43
Cryptococcus neoformans	43
Aspergillus spp	44

logic studies. A portion should be placed in an anaerobic transport device if a separate sample was not received for anaerobic culture.

Purulent material should be aspirated from the site of infection with a needle and syringe. To transport the aspirate the air is expelled, the needle is removed, and the syringe is tightly capped and promptly delivered to the laboratory. Swab specimens collected from the area of involvement must be placed in an anaerobic transport system.

Bacteria

Processing muscle specimens for detection of bacteria differs for different groups of organisms and is discussed separately for each.

Bacteria Detected by Routine Culture. Muscle biopsy specimens collected for bacterial culture are homogenized in a small amount of broth with a sterile tissue grinder or a mortar and pestle to make a 10 to 20% (weight per volume) suspension. Optimally, this is performed in an anaerobic glove box; but if this is not possible, the tissue should be processed rapidly in a biologic safety cabinet. Processing the muscle homogenate, aspirated purulent material, or a swab specimen involves preparing a smear for staining with Gram stain and inoculating appropriate media for culture. Sheep blood and MacConkey agar and thioglycolate broth are incubated in ambient air, and an anaerobic blood agar plate is incubated anaerobically. Incubation temperature and times discussed in Chapter 54 are appropriate; however, when granules are present and when culture for Actinomyces is requested, the anaerobic blood agar plate and broth should be incubated 2 weeks.

Mycobacterium species. To process muscle biopsy specimens for detection of mycobacteria a homogenate (prepared as described earlier) is poured through sterile gauze into a 50-ml centrifuge tube, to which an equal amount of 2% NaOH-N-acetyl-L cysteine is added. The suspension is mixed and allowed to stand 20 minutes. Phosphate buffer (25 ml) is added, and the suspension is mixed and centrifuged at 3000 to 3600 g for 20 minutes. The supernatant is decanted, and the sediment is suspended in 1 to 2 ml of buffer and is used to prepare smears for staining with auramine rhodamine or acid-fast stain (Appendix, Procedures 4–6) and for inoculation of appropriate media for culture (Table 54–4 and Chapter 40).

Aspirates and swabs are transferred to a sterile 50-ml centrifuge tube containing 10 ml of sterile, filtered distilled water. The specimen is mixed on a vortex mixer and allowed to stand 20 minutes. The swab is removed (if present) and the suspension is processed as described for sputum in Procedure 27 in the Appendix.

Fungi

A muscle biopsy specimen collected for detection of fungi is homogenized as described for bacteria. Processing tissue homogenates and aspirates (swab specimens should be discouraged for fungal culture) involves direct microscopic examination of a potassium hydroxide preparation (Appendix, Procedure 19) or a smear stained with the Gram, calcofluor white, Congo red, or Gomori's methenamine silver stain (Chapter 42) and inoculation of media such as inhibitory mold and SABHI agar containing antibiotics, with and without cycloheximide. Culture conditions are outlined in Chapter 54.

SYNOVIAL FLUID AND SYNOVIAL BIOPSIES

Microbiologic studies of joint fluid are useful in determining the organism responsible for infectious arthritis (Table 64–2) and in most cases identify the pathogen. Occasionally cultures of joint fluid are negative and studies of synovial tissue are necessary, a situation most likely to occur in cases of chronic granulomatous monarticular arthritis caused by species of Mycobacterium, fungi, or algae. Several viruses—parvovirus B19, hepatitis B virus, mumps virus, rubella virus, certain alphaviruses, and lymphocytic choriomeningitis virus—are associated with arthritis; but because infections with these organisms are

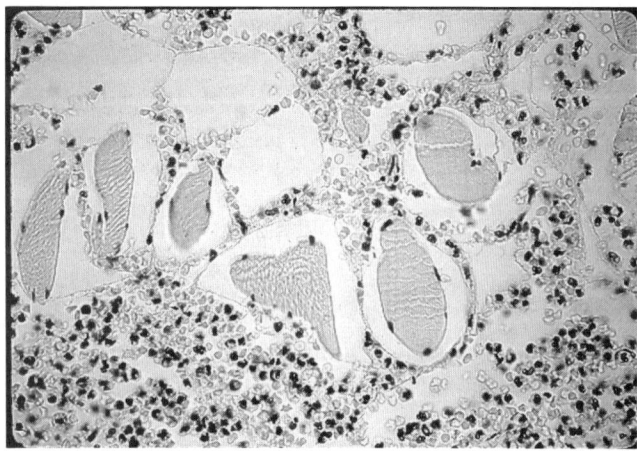

Fig. 64–1. Section of gangrenous muscle shows myonecrosis and acute inflammatory infiltrate (hematoxylin and eosin, × 100).

Table 64–2. Pathogens Detected by Microbiologic Studies of Synovial Fluid and Synovial Tissue

Organism	Chapter
Bacteria	
Staphylococcus aureus	28
Staphylococcus epidermidis*	28
β-Hemolytic streptococci	28
Streptococcus pneumoniae	28
Viridans streptococci*	28
Corynebacterium spp*	29
Clostridium spp	30
Actinomyces spp	30
Propionibacterium spp*	30
Peptostreptococcus spp	30
Neisseria gonorrhoeae	31
Branhamella catarrhalis	31
Pseudomonas spp	32
Moraxella osloensis	32
Kingella kingae	32
Brucella spp	33
Enterobacteriaceae	34
Haemophilus spp	36
Pasteurella multocida	36
Capnocytophaga spp	36
Eikenella corrodens	36
Anaerobic gram-negative bacilli	38
Borrelia burgdorferi	39
Mycobacterium spp	40
Fungi	
Candida spp	43
Cryptococcus neoformans	43
Pseudallescheria boydii	44
Blastomyces dermatitidis	45
Coccidioides immitis	45
Sporothrix schenckii	45
Algae	
Prototheca spp	47

* Usually associated with infections involving joints with prostheses.

not diagnosed by microbiologic studies of joint fluid or synovial tissue, viruses are not discussed further.

Infectious arthritis usually results from hematogenous spread from a distant focus of infection but may develop by direct extension of a contiguous infection, such as osteomyelitis, or may be associated with intra-articular injections. Bacterial (also called suppurative) arthritis is monarticular in about 90% of cases, and in both adults and children the knee is the joint most often affected, followed by the hip (8,9). Except in infections caused by Neisseria gonorrhoeae the wrist and the interphalangeal joints of the hand are involved infrequently. The bacteria usually responsible for infection vary with the age of the patient (9–12). Group B Streptococcus, Staphylococcus aureus, and gram-negative bacilli are most common in infants younger than 1 month, and Haemophilus influenzae type b is the predominant pathogen in children younger than 2 years. Staphylococcus aureus accounts for most cases of suppurative arthritis in children older than 2 years and in adults, although in adults under 30 years the primary pathogen is Neisseria gonorrhoeae. Typically, suppurative arthritis is manifested by fever and symptoms localized to the involved joint, such as pain on motion, limitation of motion, and swelling. The joint fluid appears turbid or, infrequently, serosanguineous and in up to 50% of cases has a leukocyte count over 100,000 cells per microliter, usually with over 90% neutrophils.

Chronic granulomatous monarticular arthritis may be caused by mycobacteria or fungi. Mycobacterial infections are chronic and may also involve tendon sheaths, producing the carpal tunnel syndrome, particularly Mycobacterium kansasii infection (13). Mycobacterium tuberculosis most commonly produces infections in the knee, followed by the hip, ankle, and wrist (14). Fungal arthritis is another chronic, indolent process, which most frequently involves the knee, progressing over months and occasionally years, often without fever (15–17).

Joints with prostheses become infected by spread of the organism from a contiguous wound, by introduction of the organism during placement of the prosthesis, or by hematogenous spread from a distant focus of infection. Staphylococcus epidermidis is the most common agent, followed by Staphylococcus aureus and facultative gram-negative bacilli (18). Joint pain is the most consistent manifestation of the infection; fever, swelling, and drainage from the wound or from a cutaneous sinus occur in fewer than 50% of cases. The clinical presentation, however, varies with the infecting pathogen. Infections produced by Staphylococcus epidermidis are indolent, whereas Staphylococcus aureus, facultative gram-negative bacilli, and β-hemolytic streptococci often produce fulminant infections, occasionally associated with septic shock.

Specimen collection, transport, and processing are similar for all potential pathogens. Borrelia burgdorferi is detected in synovial fluid or tissue in fewer than 25% of cases of Lyme arthritis by using culture techniques not available routinely in the clinical laboratory. Because most clinical laboratories do not have the capability to detect B. burgdorferi, and because Lyme disease usually is diagnosed serologically, the organism is not discussed further here.

Collection, Transport, and Processing

Synovial fluid is collected aseptically by aspirating with a needle and syringe. To transport the aspirate the air is expelled, the needle is removed, and the syringe is tightly capped and delivered promptly to the laboratory, where it is maintained at room temperature until processed. Synovial tissue is obtained surgically and transported immediately to the laboratory in a sterile container. A pathologist should examine the fresh tissue and divide it appropriately for histologic and microbiologic studies.

Processing synovial fluid for detection of bacteria involves preparing a smear for staining with the Gram stain and inoculating appropriate media for culture. Purulent specimens are processed directly, whereas fluid that does not appear grossly purulent should be concentrated by centrifugation at 1500 to 2500 g for 15 to 20 minutes. The supernatant is decanted and the sediment is used to prepare smears and to inoculate media. Synovial tissue is homogenized, as described earlier for muscle, and the homogenate is used to prepare smears and to inoculate media.

Chocolate and sheep blood agar (incubated in an atmosphere of 5 to 7% carbon dioxide) and thioglycolate broth (incubated in ambient air) are inoculated routinely. An anaerobic blood agar plate should be added if anaerobes are suspected. When isolation of Brucella is specifically requested, media and culture conditions outlined in Table 54–4 should be followed.

When cultures for mycobacteria are requested, smears for staining with auramine rhodamine or an acid-fast stain (Appendix, Procedures 4–6) are prepared directly from a purulent sample, from the sediment of a centrifuged fluid, or from a tissue homogenate, and appropriate media are inoculated (Table 54–4, and Chapter 40). Specimens submitted for detection of fungi or algae are processed as described earlier for muscle specimens. A smear is prepared for direct microscopic examination, and appropriate media are inoculated (Chapters 42 and 54). If infection with Prototheca is suspected media without cycloheximide must be included, because cycloheximide inhibits growth of the organism.

BONE

Microbiologic studies of bone biopsy specimens are important for identifying the pathogens of osteomyelitis (Table 64–3). Specimen collection, transport, and processing are similar for all potential pathogens.

Osteomyelitis develops as a result of hematogenous spread from a distant focus of infection, direct extension of a contiguous infection, or vascular insufficiency. Hematogenous osteomyelitis typically affects children and persons aged 50 years and older (19). In children the long bones of the extremities and the humerus are involved most often, whereas vertebral osteomyelitis is the most frequent presentation in adults. Staphylococcus aureus is the most common pathogen, although the prevalence of infections caused by facultative gram-negative bacilli is increasing. In persons with sickle cell anemia species of Salmonella account for the majority of cases (20). In children acute osteomyelitis begins abruptly, with high fever—and pain and swelling at the site of involvement. The most consistent manifestation of acute hematogenous osteomyelitis in adults is pain, and about 50% of affected persons experience fever and chills.

Osteomyelitis secondary to direct extension from a contiguous infection most often is associated with a surgical procedure (such as open reduction of a fracture), but it may be associated with soft tissue infection or with organisms, particularly Pasteurella multocida, introduced via an animal bite. This form of osteomyelitis is most common in persons 50 years and older and usually involves the long bones of the lower extremity, although any bone may be affected. Infections often are mixed: Staphylococcus aureus, facultative gram-negative bacilli, anaerobes, and mycobacteria, especially Mycobacterium fortuitum-chelonae, have been isolated.

Osteomyelitis associated with vascular insufficiency affects persons older than 50 years who have diabetes mellitus or severe atherosclerosis, and typically it involves the small bones of the feet. Infections usually are mixed. Staphylococcus aureus and Staphylococcus epidermidis are the most common isolates, but facultative gram-negative bacilli and anaerobes are encountered frequently.

Collection, Transport, and Processing

Samples of bone obtained surgically are transported immediately to the laboratory in a sterile container. A pathologist should examine the fresh specimen and divide it appropriately for histologic and microbiologic studies. If culture for anaerobes is requested, a fragment should be placed in an anaerobic transport system.

Processing bone for detection of bacteria and fungi involves direct microscopic examination and culture. Although preparing a homogenate is difficult, grinding small pieces of bone in broth with a sterile tissue grinder or a mortar and pestle should be attempted. Ideally, when culture for anaerobes is requested specimens are handled in an anaerobic chamber; but if such a chamber is not available the sample should be processed rapidly in a biologic safety cabinet.

Routine processing to detect bacteria includes using the homogenate to prepare a smear for Gram staining and to inoculate sheep blood and MacConkey agar and thioglycolate broth (incubated in ambient air) and anaerobic blood agar (incubated anaerobically). Incubation temperatures and times are discussed in Chapter 54. When culture for Actinomyces is requested the anaerobic plate and the broth should be incubated 2 weeks. To isolate species of Brucella, which must be requested specifically, media and culture conditions outlined in Table 54–4 should be followed.

When culture for mycobacteria is requested, the homogenate is used to prepare a smear for staining with auramine rhodamine or an acid-fast stain and to inoculate media for culture (see Table 54–4 and Chapter 40). To detect fungi, smears are prepared and media are inoculated as described for muscle.

REFERENCES

1. Levin MJ, Gardner P, and Waldvogel FA: "Tropical" pyomyositis. An unusual infection due to Staphylococcus aureus. N Engl J Med, *284*:196, 1971.

Table 64–3. Pathogens That Produce Osteomyelitis Detected by Microbiologic Studies of Bone

Organism	Chapter
Bacteria	
Staphylococcus aureus	28
Group B Streptococcus	28
Actinomyces spp	30
Peptostreptococcus spp	30
Pseudomonas spp	32
Brucella spp	33
Enterobacteriaceae	34
Haemophilus spp	36
Pasteurella multocida	36
Eikenella corrodens	36
Anaerobic gram-negative bacilli	38
Mycobacterium spp	40
Fungi	
Candida spp	43
Blastomyces dermatitidis	45
Coccidioides immitis	45

2. Yoder EL, Mendez J, and Khatib R: Spontaneous gangrenous myositis induced by Streptococcus pyogenes: Case report and review of the literature. Rev Infect Dis, 9:382, 1987.
3. Altemeier WA, and Fullen WD: Prevention and treatment of gas gangrene. JAMA, 217:806, 1971.
4. Bornstein DL, et al: Anaerobic infections: Review of current experience. Medicine, 43:207, 1964.
5. Hatheway CL: Toxigenic clostridia. Clin Microbiol Rev, 3:66, 1990.
6. Kornbluth AA, Danzig JB, and Bernstein LH: Clostridium septicum infection and associated malignancy: Report of 2 cases and review of the literature. Medicine, 68:30, 1989.
7. Davis WA, Kane JG, and Garagusi VF: Human Aeromonas infections: A review of the literature and case report of endocarditis. Medicine, 57:267, 1978.
8. Jackson MA, and Nelson JD: Etiology and medical management of acute suppurative bone and joint infections in pediatric patients. J Pediatr Orthop, 2:313, 1982.
9. Cooper C, and Cawley MID: Bacterial arthritis in an English health district: A 10-year review. Ann Rheum Dis, 45:458, 1986.
10. Nelson JD, and Koontz WC: Septic arthritis in infants and children: A review of 117 cases. Pediatrics, 38:966, 1966.
11. Ward JR, and Atcheson SG: Infectious arthritis. Med Clin North Am, 61:313, 1977.
12. Sharp JT, et al: Infectious arthritis. Arch Intern Med, 139:1125, 1979.
13. Sutker WL, Lankford LL, and Tompsett R: Granulomatous synovitis: The role of atypical mycobacteria. Rev Infect Dis, 1:729, 1979.
14. Berney S, Goldstein M, and Bishko F: Clinical and diagnostic features of tuberculous arthritis. Am J Med, 53:36, 1972.
15. Bayer AS, and Guze LB: Fungal arthritis. I. Candida arthritis: Diagnostic and prognostic implications and therapeutic considerations. Semin Arthritis Rheum, 8:142, 1978.
16. Bayer AS, and Guze LB: Fungal arthritis. II. Coccidioidal synovitis: Clinical diagnostic, therapeutic, and prognostic considerations. Semin Arthritis Rheum, 8:200, 1979.
17. Bayer AS, Scott VJ, and Guze LB: Fungal arthritis. III. Sporotrichal arthritis. Semin Arthritis Rheum, 9:66, 1979.
18. Brause BD: Infections with prostheses in bones and joints. In Principles and Practice of Infectious Diseases. 3rd ed. Edited by GL Mandell, RG Douglas, Jr, and JE Bennett. New York, Churchill Livingstone, 1990.
19. Norden CW: Osteomyelitis. In Principles and Practice of Infectious Diseases. 3rd ed. Edited by GL Mandell, RG Douglas, Jr, and JE Bennett. New York, Churchill Livingstone, 1990.
20. Engh C, et al: Osteomyelitis in the patient with sickle cell disease. J Bone Joint Surg, 53A:1, 1971.

Appendix

APPENDIX

PROCEDURE 1. HEMADSORPTION PROCEDURE FOR DETECTION OF HEMADSORBING VIRUSES

1. Test cell cultures of primary monkey kidney cells inoculated with a respiratory tract specimen: nasopharyngeal wash, aspirate, or swab, throat wash or swab, sputum, bronchoalveolar lavage fluid, lung tissue.
2. After 3 to 5 days' incubation, aspirate the maintenance medium from the cell culture, and add 0.2 ml of a 0.4% suspension of fresh guinea pig red blood cells (prepared from a 10% suspension in Alsever solution).
3. Place the tube horizontally at 4° C for 30 minutes, then rotate vigorously to dislodge nonspecifically absorbed erythrocytes.
4. Observe monolayer for adsorption of red blood cells under low-power objective of a light microscope (inverted microscopes are not suitable).
5. Adsorption of erythrocytes (see Fig. 10–4) indicates that the monolayer is infected with a hemadsorbing virus (influenza A virus, influenza B virus, the parainfluenza viruses, mumps virus).

PROCEDURE 2. CENTRIFUGATION CULTURE FOR DETECTION OF CYTOMEGALOVIRUS (CMV) EARLY NUCLEAR ANTIGEN

1. Shell vials containing circular glass coverslips seeded with MRC-5 cells are purchased or prepared in the laboratory; 24-well plates are prepared in the laboratory by placing a sterile coverslip in each well and seeding each coverslip with MRC-5 cells.
2. Specimens to be evaluated for the presence of CMV include urine, throat swab or wash, buffy coat, bronchoalveolar lavage fluid, endocervical swab specimens, and various tissues (liver, lung, brain, biopsy specimens of gastrointestinal ulcers).
3. Remove maintenance medium from shell vial or 24-well plate. Inoculate 2 shell vials or individual wells with 0.2 ml of each sample (for buffy coats inoculate 3 vials or wells with 0.3 ml).
4. Centrifuge 45 minutes at 700 g and add 1 ml of maintenance medium.
5. Incubate 16 to 18 hours at 37° C in 5 to 7% carbon dioxide.
6. Remove medium and fix coverslips in acetone (shell vials) or methanol (24-well plates).
7. Remove fixative and wash coverslips with phosphate-buffered saline.
8. Stain coverslips with monoclonal antibodies to the immediate early nuclear antigen of CMV (commercially available).
9. Wash coverslips and stain with fluorescein-labeled conjugate (commercially available).
10. Wash coverslips, mount on microscope slides, and view with epifluorescent microscope.
11. Interpretation: A specimen is positive for CMV if one or more intranuclear inclusions are observed (Fig. 5–9).

PROCEDURE 3. GRAM STAIN

1. The Gram stain is used for direct examination of smears prepared from clinical material (sputum, cerebrospinal fluid, other body fluids, imprints or homogenates of tissues, and purulent material or drainage from abscesses or wounds) or from isolated bacterial colonies.
2. Drop (if liquid) or roll (if on a swab) the material to be examined onto the surface of a clean microscope slide. Allow it to dry or heat on a slide warmer at 60° C for 10 minutes to kill any organisms that may be present. Allow the slide to cool. (Alternatively the smear may be fixed in methanol or ethanol for a few minutes).
3. Flood the slide with crystal violet and let it stand without drying for 30 seconds.
4. Rinse with tap water.
5. Flood the slide with iodine and let it stand without drying for 60 seconds.
6. Rinse with tap water.
7. Decolorize with acetone-alcohol (95% ethanol) decolorizer until no violet color washes off (about 10 seconds), and rinse with tap water.
8. Flood the slide with safranin and let it stand without drying for 30 to 60 seconds. Rinse with tap water and allow the smear to air dry.
9. Examine under oil immersion. Gram-positive bacteria (and fungi) appear dark blue; gram-negative bacteria appear pink to red (see Plates IB and IC).

PROCEDURE 4. ZIEHL-NEELSEN ACID-FAST STAIN

1. Prepare a smear directly from clinical specimens submitted for recovery of mycobacteria or after concentration (see Chapter 57 and Procedure 27), from radiometric culture bottles that yield a positive reading, or from colonies growing on mycobacterial culture media. Positive (prepared from a suspension of acid-fast bacilli such as Mycobacterium tuberculosis H37Rv) and negative (prepared from a suspension of non–acid-fast organisms such as Staphylococcus aureus or Escherichia coli) control slides should be included each time clinical specimens are stained.

2. Heat-fix slides at 65° to 75° C (on a hotplate) until dry.
3. Place on the slide a piece of filter paper slightly larger than the smear.
4. Flood smear with carbolfuchsin stain reagent (commercially available) and steam-heat slides gently by flaming from below the rack with a gas burner (or staining the slides directly on a special hotplate); allow stain to remain on the slides 4 to 5 minutes without heat (or 15 minutes if an electric staining rack is used).
5. Remove filter paper; rinse slides with deionized water; tilt to drain.
6. Decolorize with acid alcohol (95% ethanol and 3.0% hydrochloric acid) for 2 to 3 minutes.
7. Rinse slides with deionized water; tilt to drain.
8. Flood slides with methylene blue reagent (commercially available) for 1 minute.
9. Rinse with deionized water; air-dry.
10. Examine under oil immersion for the presence of acid-fast bacilli—organisms that retain carbolfuchsin and stain red (Color Plate ID, IE).

PROCEDURE 5. KINYOUN STAIN

1. Prepare a smear directly from clinical specimens submitted for recovery of mycobacteria or after concentrating the specimen (see Chapter 57 and Procedure 27) from radiometric culture bottles that yield a positive reading, or from colonies growing on mycobacterial culture media. Positive (prepared from a suspension of acid-fast bacilli such as Mycobacterium tuberculosis H37Rv) and negative (prepared from a suspension of non–acid-fast bacilli such as Staphylococcus aureus or Escherichia coli) control slides should be included each time clinical specimens are stained.
2. Heat-fix slides at 65° to 75° C (on hotplate) until dry.
3. Flood slides with Kinyoun's carbolfuchsin reagent (commercially available) and allow to stand 3 to 5 minutes at room temperature.
4. Rinse slide with deionized water; tilt to drain.
5. Decolorize with acid-alcohol for 2 to 3 minutes or until no more color appears in the washing; rinse with deionized water.
6. Flood slide with methylene blue counterstain and allow to stand 4 minutes (or with malachite green and allow to stand 30 seconds).
7. Rinse with distilled water; tilt to drain; air-dry.
8. Examine under oil immersion for acid-fast bacilli—organisms that retain carbol fuchsin and stain red (Plate ID, IE).

PROCEDURE 6. AURAMINE RHODAMINE FLUOROCHROME STAIN

1. Prepare a smear directly from clinical specimens submitted for recovery of mycobacteria or after concentration (see Chapter 57 and Procedure 27). Positive (prepared from a suspension of acid-fast bacilli such as Mycobacterium tuberculosis H37Rv) and negative (prepared from a suspension of non-acid fast organisms such as Staphylococcus aureus or Escherichia coli) control slides should be included each time clinical specimens are stained.
2. Heat-fix slides at 65° to 75° C until dry.
3. Flood slide with auramine rhodamine reagent and allow to stand at room temperature 15 to 20 minutes.
4. Rinse with deionized water; tilt slide to drain.
5. Decolorize with acid alcohol (70% ethanol and 0.5% hydrochloric acid) for 2 to 3 minutes.
6. Rinse with deionized water; tilt slide to drain.
7. Flood slide with 0.5% potassium permanganate and allow to stand 2 to 4 minutes.
8. Rinse with deionized water; air dry.
9. Examine at 250× magnification for yellow or golden yellow fluorescence, indicating the presence of mycobacteria.

PROCEDURE 7. MODIFIED ACID-FAST STAIN*

1. Test colonies demonstrating morphology typical of Nocardia (see text) and specimens demonstrating thin, beaded, branching gram-positive bacilli in smears stained with the Gram stain. Include a positive (Nocardia asteroides) and negative (Actinomadura madurai) control with each specimen or groups of specimens stained.
2. Prepare a smear of the colony or specimen and the controls on a microscope slide; allow to air-dry; heat-fix on slide warmer at 65° to 75° C until dry.
3. Flood slide with Kinyoun's carbolfuchsin, staining for 3 minutes. Rinse with tap water.
4. Decolorize with 2% sulfuric acid for 1 minute.
5. Counterstain with methylene blue for 30 seconds.
6. Rinse with tap water; air-dry.
7. Examine for patially acid-fast organisms, appearing as reddish to purple filaments (Plate IF); non–acid-fast organisms are blue only.

PROCEDURE 8. CELL CULTURE FOR ISOLATION OF CHLAMYDIA TRACHOMATIS

1. Specimens appropriate for isolating Chlamydia trachomatis include endocervical, urethral, conjunctival, rectal, and nasopharyngeal swab specimens; tracheobronchial, endometrial, and lymph node aspirates; bronchoalveolar lavage fluid; and tissue (fallopian tube, lung). All specimens should be received in transport medium (such as 2-sucrose phosphate) and maintained at 4° C (or at −70° C if prolonged storage [> 72 hours] prior to processing is necessary).
   a. Remove the swab from the transport medium.
   b. Homogenize all specimens by mixing on a vortex mixer or sonicating for 3 minutes.
2. Shell vials containing circular glass coverslips seeded with McCoy cells (or BGM cells) may be purchased or prepared in house.
3. Remove medium from cell monolayers; inoculate two shell vials (or wells) with 1 ml of each specimen; centrifuge at 2500 to 3000 g at 30 to 35° C for 1

---
* The modified acid-fast stain also is called partial acid-fast stain.

hour; incubate at 37° C for 2 hours; aspirate specimen; add 1 ml growth medium (Earle's modified essential medium containing 5 to 10% fetal calf serum, additional glucose [0.056M], and L-glutamine [2 mM], and cycloheximide [0.5 to 1.5 μg/ml]).
4. Incubate at 37° C in 5% carbon dioxide for 48 hours.
5. Aspirate medium; fix coverslips in methanol; stain with fluorescein-conjugated monoclonal antibodies to Chlamydia trachomatis.
6. Mount coverslips on microscope slides; view with an epifluorescent microscope.
7. Specimens with one or more positively fluorescing intracytoplasmic inclusions are positive for Chlamydia trachomatis.

PROCEDURE 9. CATALASE TEST

1. Test isolated colonies of gram-positive cocci to differentiate staphylococci from streptococci.
2. Transfer a small amount of the colony (preferably grown on a medium that does not contain blood) with a loop or sterile wooden stick onto a clean, dry glass slide, and cover the growth with 1 drop of 3% hydrogen peroxide.
3. Observe for the evolution of gas bubbles, indicating a positive result (see Fig. 28–1).
4. Isolates of staphylococci are catalase positive and produce many bubbles. Isolate of streptococci are catalase negative and do not yield visible bubbles. Isolates of streptococci grown on a medium containing blood may yield a very weak positive reaction, owing to the presence of contaminating red blood cells, which contain catalase. These weak reactions should be compared to the reaction of a small amount of blood-containing agar and 3% hydrogen peroxide. If the results of the colony and the agar are similar, the catalase test is considered negative; but if the catalase reaction of the colony is stronger, the isolate is considered catalase positive.

PROCEDURE 10. SLIDE COAGULASE (CLUMPING FACTOR) TEST

1. Test isolates of catalase-positive, gram-positive cocci.
2. On a clean, dry glass microscope slide place 1 drop each of rabbit plasma (with EDTA or citrate) and sterile distilled water or sterile saline.
3. Using a loop, straight wire, or wooden stick, emulsify a portion of an isolated colony in the sterile water (or saline) and then in the rabbit plasma.
4. Observe for clumping. If clumping occurs in both drops, the organism autoagglutinates and the slide coagulase test cannot be used for identification. Isolates that cause clumping in the rabbit plasma and a smooth, homogeneous suspension in water or saline are Staphylococcus aureus. Isolates that produce a smooth, homogenous suspension in both drops are coagulase-negative staphylococci.

PROCEDURE 11. TUBE COAGULASE TEST

1. Test isolates of catalase-positive, gram-positive cocci.
2. Aliquot rabbit plasma with EDTA in 0.5 ml amounts in 13 mm by 100 mm glass or plastic tubes.
3. Emulsify growth from an isolated colony in the plasma and incubate 1 to 4 hours at 35° to 37° C.
4. Observe for the presence of a gel or clot that cannot be resuspended by gentle shaking. If no clot forms after 4 hours incubate the tube overnight at room temperature.
5. Organisms that clot are Staphylococcus aureus, whereas those that fail to clot the plasma within 24 hours are considered coagulase negative and must be identified by other methods (see text).

PROCEDURE 12. DISK-DIFFUSION TEST FOR NOVOBIOCIN RESISTANCE

1. Test colonies of coagulase-negative Staphylococcus isolated from urine.
2. Prepare an inoculum of the isolate by suspending colonies in 2 ml of sterile physiologic saline or broth to a density equal to a 0.5 McFarland turbidity standard.
3. Using a cotton swab spread the bacterial inoculum on the surface of a Mueller-Hinton agar plate.
4. Place a 5 μg novobiocin disk on the inoculated plate.
5. Incubate the plate overnight in ambient air at 35° C.
6. Measure the zone of inhibition of growth around the disk. A zone diameter of ≤16 mm indicates novobiocin resistance, and the isolate presumptively is named Staphylococcus saprophyticus. Isolates that yield diameters greater than 16 mm are susceptible to novobiocin and therefore not S. saprophyticus.

PROCEDURE 13. BACITRACIN SUSCEPTIBILITY TEST

1. Test colonies of Streptococcus (smaller than 0.5 mm diameter) surrounded by a wide zone of β hemolysis (2 to 4 times the diameter of the colony) isolated from the throat.
2. Inoculate one quadrant or half of a 5% sheep blood agar plate with a pure culture of the organism to be tested by heavily streaking the entire surface.
3. Place a 0.04-U bacitracin disk in the center of the inoculum and incubate overnight in air or 5 to 10% carbon dioxide at 35° C.
4. Examine for a zone of inhibition of growth around the bacitracin disk (Plate IID). The presence of any zone indicates bacitracin susceptibility, and the isolate presumptively is named group A Streptococcus.

PROCEDURE 14. RAPID HIPPURATE HYDROLYSIS TEST

1. Test colonies of Streptococcus (larger than 0.5 mm diameter) surrounded by a narrow zone of β hemolysis (less than twice the diameter of the colony).
2. Heavily inoculate a tube containing 0.4 ml of a 1% sodium hippurate solution with a pure culture of the organism to be tested, making a milky suspension. Inoculate a positive (group B Streptococcus) and a negative (group A Streptococcus) control at the same time.
3. Incubate the capped tubes 2 hours at 35° C.

4. Add 0.2 ml ninhydrin reagent and reincubate for an additional 15 minutes. A deep purple color change indicates hippurate hydrolysis, and the isolate presumptively is named group B Streptococcus.

PROCEDURE 15. CAMP TEST

1. Test colonies of Streptococcus (larger than 0.5 mm diameter) surrounded by a narrow zone of β hemolysis (less than twice the diameter of the colony).
2. Inoculate a streak of β toxin–producing Staphylococcus aureus down the center of a 5% sheep blood agar plate.
3. Inoculate straight lines of the isolates to be tested plus a group B Streptococcus (positive control) and a group A Streptococcus (negative control) in straight lines perpendicular to the staphylococcal streak, stopping just before the staphylococcal line.
4. Incubate plates at 35° to 37° C overnight in ambient air. Isolates that produce an arrowhead-shaped zone of enhanced hemolysis at the juncture between the Streptococcus and the Staphylococcus (Plate IIIA) are CAMP positive. Approximately 95% of isolates of group B Streptococcus, as well as rare strains of other groups, are CAMP positive.

PROCEDURE 16. OPTOCHIN SENSITIVITY

1. Test colonies of α-hemolytic streptococci that are mucoid or show a central depression.
2. Streak an isolated colony on a quandrant of a sheep blood agar plate.
3. Aseptically apply an optochin disk onto the center of the streaked area.
4. Invert the plate and incubate in ambient air for 18 hours at 35° C.
5. A zone of inhibition at least 14 mm surrounding a 6-mm diameter disk or a zone at least 16 mm surrounding a 10-mm disk is positive, and the isolate presumptively is called Streptococcus pneumoniae (Plate IIE).

PROCEDURE 17. SCREEN FOR PENICILLIN-RESISTANT STREPTOCOCCUS PNEUMONIAE

1. Test isolates of Streptococcus pneumoniae recovered from sterile body sites.
2. Emulsify colonies from overnight growth on a blood agar plate into Mueller-Hinton broth, and adjust the turbidity to equal that of a 0.5 McFarland standard.
3. Inoculate growth from the broth onto Mueller-Hinton agar supplemented with 5% sheep blood, and place a 1-μg oxacillin disk on the inoculated surface.
4. Incubate at 35° C in ambient air for 18 to 24 hours (incubation in 5 to 7% carbon dioxide is not necessary except for rare strains that grow poorly or not at all without carbon dioxide).
5. Measure zones of inhibition of growth. Penicillin-susceptible isolates of Streptococcus pneumoniae have a zone size of at least 20 mm; isolates that are resistant or relatively resistant to penicillin have a zone of 19 mm or less. (This test does not distinguish between resistant and relatively resistant isolates.)

PROCEDURE 18. POTASSIUM HYDROXIDE (KOH) SOLUBILITY TEST FOR DISTINGUISHING GRAM-POSITIVE AND GRAM-NEGATIVE BACTERIA

1. Test isolates of bacteria, especially anaerobes, that yield Gram stain results that are difficult to interpret.
2. Place 2 drops of a 3% KOH solution on a glass microscope slide.
3. Stir a loopful of bacterial growth in a circular motion in the KOH solution for 30 seconds and then raise the loop, observing for a string of the mixture to follow the loop.
4. Interpretation: The reaction is positive if stringing occurs, indicating that the organism is gram negative, and negative if stringing is not observed, indicating a gram-positive organism.

PROCEDURE 19. POTASSIUM HYDROXIDE (KOH) PREPARATION FOR IDENTIFICATION OF FUNGAL ELEMENTS

1. The technique is used to visualize fungal elements in skin, hair, nails, sputum, or vaginal secretions.
2. Place a fragment of the skin, hair, or nail or smear a small amount of sputum or vaginal secretions on a glass slide.
3. Add 1 drop of 10% KOH (commercially available), coverslip, and gently heat (do not boil) by passing two or three times through a flame.
4. Let the slide stand 10 to 20 minutes (until clearing is complete), and observe it under low and high power for hyphae, arthroconidia, and yeasts.

PROCEDURE 20. TEASE MOUNT PREPARATION

1. This technique is used to visualize the microscopic features of a mature fungal colony.
2. Place one drop of lactophenol cotton blue (commercially available) on a glass side.
3. With a flamed and cooled stiff wire inoculating needle bent at a 90-degree angle, cut out a small portion of an isolated colony (including a small amount of the supporting agar) from an area intermediate between the center and the periphery.
4. Place the portion of the colony in the lactophenol cotton blue; tease the hyphae apart with a second needle; coverslip, applying gentle pressure to disperse the growth and agar; and examine microscopically.

PROCEDURE 21. SCOTCH TAPE PREPARATION

1. This technique is used to visualize the microscopic features of a mature fungal colony.
2. Using unfrosted, clear cellophone tape, press the sticky side gently but firmly to the surface of the

colony at a point intermediate between the center and the periphery.
3. Place a drop of lactophenol cotton blue on a microscope slide.
4. Stick one end of the tape to the surface of the slide to one side of the stain; stretch the tape over the slide, lowering it so that the mycelium is permeated with the stain; stick the opposite end of the tape to the slide, avoiding formation of air bubbles, and examine microscopically.

PROCEDURE 22. GERM TUBE TEST

1. The germ tube test is used to differentiate isolates of Candida albicans from other yeasts.
2. Suspend a small portion of an isolated colony of the yeast to be tested in 0.5 ml of rabbit, sheep, calf, or normal human serum.
3. Incubate 2 hours at 35° C.
4. Place a drop of the yeast-serum suspension on a microscope slide, coverslip, and examine under low power for germ tubes—appendages half the width and three to four times the length of the cell from which they arise (see Fig. 43–7), indicating the isolate is Candida albicans. Isolates of yeasts that do not form germ tubes must be identified by other tests (see text).

PROCEDURE 23. INOCULATION OF CORNMEAL–TWEEN 80 AGAR FOR IDENTIFICATION OF YEASTS

1. Inoculation of cornmeal–Tween 80 agar is used to identify yeasts isolated from clinical specimens.
2. With an inoculating wire pick an isolated colony of the yeast to be tested and inoculate a plate of cornmeal agar containing 1% Tween 80 by making three parallel cuts about $\frac{1}{2}$ inch apart at a 45-degree angle to the medium.
3. Cover a portion of the streaks with a sterile coverslip, and incubate the plate at 30° C for 48 hours.
4. Examine the plate microscopically, preferably through the coverslip, for blastoconidia, arthroconidia, pseudohyphae, and hyphae.

PROCEDURE 24. CALCOFLUOR WHITE STAIN

A. Preparation of stain:
1. Stock cellufluor white (1%): 1 g in 100 ml of distilled water.
2. Stock Evans blue (0.5%): Add 0.05 g to 10 ml distilled water.
B. Procedure:
1. Prepare working solution of stain by adding 1 ml of stock cellufluor white, 1 ml of stock Evans blue, and 8 ml of distilled water.
2. Prepare smear of cornea or other tissue suspected of having Acanthamoeba cysts.
3. Place 1 drop of stain working solution and cover with a coverglass.
4. Examine using fluorescence microscope.

PROCEDURE 25. TRICHROME STAIN FOR FECAL SMEARS

A. Preparation of stain: The trichrome stain is made of 0.6 g of chromotrope 2R, 0.3 g of light-green SF, and 0.7 g of phosphotungstic acid. Mix the dry components with 0.1 ml of glacial acetic acid and allow to stand 30 minutes. Dilute with 100 ml of distilled water.
B. Procedure:
1. Make fecal smears from the PVA-fixed stool sample and allow to dry.
2. Wash in 70% alcohol with enough iodine to give a yellow color, 1 to 5 minutes.
3. Wash in two changes of 70% alcohol 2 to 5 minutes each.
4. Stain in trichrome stain 10 minutes.
5. Differentiate in acid alcohol (mix 99 parts 90% alcohol with 1 part glacial acetic acid) 2 to 3 seconds.
6. Rinse in absolute alcohol several times.
7. Dehydrate in absolute alcohol, two changes, 2 to 5 minutes each.
8. Clear and mount.

PROCEDURE 26. GIEMSA STAIN

A. Preparation of stain: The Giemsa stock stain solution (commercially available) is diluted 1:10 in phosphate buffer (pH 7.0 to 7.2) just before each batch of slides is stained.
B. Procedure for thin smears:
1. Fix slide 1 minute in methyl alcohol.
2. Allow slides to dry thoroughly.
3. Stain for 10 minutes.
4. Rinse in buffer solution a couple of times.
5. Allow to dry thoroughly in vertical position.
6. Examine under the microscope.
C. Procedure for thick smears:
1. Stain slide directly (do not fix in alcohol) in vertical position (use Coplin jar) for 10 minutes.
2. Rinse in buffer twice.
3. Allow to dry in vertical position.
4. Examine under the microscope.

PROCEDURE 27. N-ACETYL-L CYSTEINE (NALC)–SODIUM HYDROXIDE (NaOH) PROCEDURE TO LIQUEFY, DECONTAMINATE, AND CONCENTRATE SPECIMENS FOR DETECTION OF MYCOBACTERIA

1. This technique is used to decontaminate and concentrate sputum, urine, and gastric lavage specimens for detection of mycobacteria. All work should be performed in a biologic safety cabinet.
2. A maximum of 10 ml of specimen is placed in a 50-ml conical centrifuge tube. An equal volume of 2% NaOH-NALC is added and mixed thoroughly by tightening the cap and mixing on a vortex mixer for 15 to 30 seconds.
3. The mixture is allowed to stand at room temperature for 15 minutes (decontamination).

4. To the mixture 30 ml of phosphate buffer (pH 6.8) is added, and the tubes are capped and inverted to mix.
5. Tubes are centrifuged at 3000 to 3600 g for 15 minutes or at 2000 to 2500 g for 20 minutes.
6. The supernatant is decanted, and the sediment is resuspended in 1 to 2 ml of sterile water or buffer and used to inoculate appropriate media (see Chapter 40) and to prepare smears for staining (see Procedures 4–6).

PROCEDURE 28. ACID-WASH TREATMENT OF CONTAMINATED SPECIMENS TO ENHANCE RECOVERY OF LEGIONELLA SPECIES

1. This procedure is used to process sputum specimens, other potentially contaminated clinical specimens, and water samples for detection of Legionella.
2. Prepare stock solutions of 0.2 N hydrochloric acid (50 ml) and 0.2 N potassium chloride (50 ml).
3. To prepare the working solution add 5.3 ml of the HCl stock solution and 25 ml of the KCl stock solution to 100 ml of distilled water, adjust the pH to 2.2, and filter-sterilize.
4. Dispense 0.9 ml of working solution into small, sterile, screw-capped tubes containing sterile glass beads and store in the refrigerator (stable for 6 months).
5. To process a specimen add 0.1 ml of sample to the tube containing the acid wash (0.9 ml), mix on a vortex mixer, and allow to stand 4 minutes. Mix again and inoculate 3 drops each onto nonselective and selective buffered charcoal–yeast extract agar plates.

PROCEDURE 29. SCOTCH TAPE TECHNIQUE FOR ENTEROBIUS

1. A transparent, 1″ by 4″ piece of Scotch tape is used to cover a glass slide, wrapping the ends around the ends of the slide and making a small tab at one end by folding the tape on itself.
2. When ready to use pull the tab from the slide, leaving the opposite end attached to the slide to expose the sticky side of the tape.
3. Wrap the nonsticky side of the tape around the end of a wooden tongue blade leaving the sticky side out.
4. Holding the glass slide and the tongue blade together, gently apply the sticky side of the tape to the perianal area.
5. Retrieve and fold the tape back to the glass slide, pressing slightly to secure it.
6. Examine under the microscope for eggs and adults of Enterobius.

PROCEDURE 30. STOOL CONCENTRATION: FORMALIN–ETHYL ACETATE

1. Mix well 2 ml of fresh stool in saline solution to make about 10 ml.
2. Strain the mixed sample through two layers of gauze and collect in a 15-ml conical centrifuge tube.
3. Centrifuge at 650 g for 1 to 2 minutes.
4. Decant supernatant to leave 1.5 ml of sediment. If too little, add more feces. If too large resuspend in saline, mix, and discard a portion. Repeat centrifugation.
5. Add about 9 ml of formalin at 10% and allow to stand 5 minutes, longer if necessary to save until later. Note: Stool already fixed in formalin can be processed in formalin directly to save the saline step.
6. Add 3 ml of ethyl acetate and shake the tube well for about 30 seconds.
7. Centrifuge at 450 to 500 g for 1 minute.
8. Four layers are formed: (1) ethyl acetate, (2) plug of debris, (3) formalin, (4) sediment.
9. Free the plug with applicator stick and decant carefully leaving the sediment.
10. With a pipette mix the sediment and prepare unstained and iodine-stained slides for examination under the microscope.

PROCEDURE 31. MODIFIED ACID-FAST STAIN FOR CRYPTOSPORIDIUM

1. Prepare slides. If fresh stools are used fix with heat. If PVA-fixed specimens are used, make smear and let it dry.
2. Stain with carbolfuchsin, 1 minute.
3. Rinse with tap water.
4. Rinse with 95% ethanol.
5. Decolorize with 10% sulfuric acid until no color comes off.
6. Rinse with tap water.
7. Counterstain with brilliant green, 1 minute.
8. Rinse with tap water.
9. Air-dry, mount with permount, and examine under the microscope.

PROCEDURE 32. BAERMANN CONCENTRATION FOR STRONGYLOIDES LARVAE

1. A 6-inch diameter funnel with a round metal mesh placed halfway into the funnel and 6 to 8 inches of rubber tubing attached to the bottom, is used.
2. On the metal mesh, place two to three layers of gauze.
3. Put a clamp on the rubber tubing and fill the funnel with distilled water up to the gauze layer.
4. Place a generous amount of stool sample on the gauze.
5. Let stand about 2 hours.
6. Open the clamp and collect 10 to 12 ml of water in a centrifuge tube.
7. Centrifuge at 500 g for 2 minutes.
8. Decant, prepare slides with the sediment, and examine for Strongyloides larvae.

PROCEDURE 33. SEDIMENTATION FOR SCHISTOSOMA

1. Mix thoroughly 5 to 10 ml of stool in 10 to 20 ml of water.
2. Strain the suspension through four layers of gauze into a conical sedimentation flask.
3. Sediment 1 hour and decant supernatant.
4. Refill flask with water, allow to sediment 45 minutes, and decant supernatant.
5. Repeat step 4 until supernatant is clear.
6. After last sedimentation decant slowly to leave sediment undisturbed.
7. Remove 1 or 2 drops of sediment from the middle and bottom layers. Transfer to a glass slide, and examine under the microscope.

INDEX

Page numbers in *italics* indicate figures; numbers followed by "t" indicate tables.

Abscess
  abdominal, anaerobic gram-negative bacteria and, 357
  genitourinary, specimens from, 608
  ocular, specimens from, 555–556
  of brain. *See* Brain abscess
  of liver. *See* Liver abscess specimens
  pancreatic. *See* Pancreatic abscess specimens
  spinal, epidural, Staphylococcus aureus and, 220
  splenic, specimens from, 582
Abscess and empyema material, 547–548
Acanthamoeba, 502–503, *503*
N-Acetyl-L cysteine (NALC)-sodium hydroxide (NaOH) procedure, to liquefy, decontaminate, and concentrate specimens for identification of Mycobacteria, 635–636
Acid-fast stains, 175
  modified, for Cryptosporidium, 636
  partial, 632
Acid-wash treatment, to enhance recovery of contaminated specimens of Legionella, 636
Acinetobacter, 286–287
  clinical manifestations of, 287
  epidemiology of, 286
  laboratory diagnosis of, organism identification and, 289
  pathogenesis of, 287
  treatment of, 290
Acquired immunodeficiency syndrome (AIDS), Mycobacterium avium-intracellulare and, 383, 384
Acridine orange, 175
Actinobacillus, 343–344
  epidemiology and pathogenesis of, 343
  laboratory diagnosis of, 343–344
  treatment of, 344
Actinobacillus actinomycetemcomitans, 343–344
Actinobacillus israelii, 343
Actinomadura, 249
  laboratory diagnosis of, 249
Actinomyces, 262–263
  clinical manifestations of, 263
  epidemiology of, 262–263
  in gastrointestinal tissue specimens, 593
  in skin biopsy specimens, 616
  laboratory diagnosis of, 264, 264t
  pathogenesis and pathology of, 263, *263*

Actinomyces israelii, 262
  laboratory diagnosis of, 264
  treatment of, 265
Actinomyces meyeri, 262
Actinomyces naeslundii, 262
Actinomyces odontolyticus, 262
  laboratory diagnosis of, 264
Actinomyces viscosus, 262
Actinomycetoma, Nocardia brasiliensis and, 248
Actinomycosis, 262–263
  abdominal, 262, 263
  cervicofacial, 262, 263
  pelvic, 262–263
  thoracic, 262, 263
Acyclovir, in herpesvirus infections, 59
Adenitis
  cervical, tuberculous, 381–382
  mesenteric, Yersinia pseudotuberculosis and, 315
Adeno-associated viruses, 76
  diagnosis of, 76
Adenoviruses, 65–68
  classification of, 65, 65t
  clinical manifestations of, 67, 67t
  epidemiology of, 65
  laboratory diagnosis of, 67–68, *68*
  pathogenesis and pathologic changes and, 65, 67, *67*
  replication of, 65
  structure of, 65, *66*
  treatment and prevention of, 68
Adhesins, 21, 21t
Adsorption, viruses and, 36, 36t
Aedes, 535
Aerococcus, 231
  laboratory diagnosis of, 233–234
Aeromonas, 332–333
  clinical manifestations of, 332–333
  epidemiology and pathogenesis of, 332
  in stool and rectal swab specimens, 590
  laboratory diagnosis of, 333
    organism identification and, 333
  treatment of, 333
Aeromonas hydrophila, 332
Aeromonas veronii, 332
Aerotolerance test, 258–259
Afipia, 401–402
Afipia felis, 401–402
  clinical manifestations and pathology of, 402
  epidemiology of, 401–402
  in conjunctival specimens, 554

  in liver tissue specimens, 598
  in lymph node specimens, 581
  laboratory diagnosis of, 402
  treatment and prevention of, 402
African Burkitt's lymphoma, Epstein-Barr virus and, 53, 54
Agar dilution, anaerobe susceptibility testing and, 180
Agrobacterium tumefaciens, 287
AIDS dementia complex, 155
Alanine aminotransferase (ALT), hepatitis A virus and, 110
Alcaligenes, 287
  laboratory diagnosis of, organism identification and, 289
Alcaligenes faecalis, 287
  laboratory diagnosis of, organism identification and, 289
Alcaligenes xylosoxidans, 287
Algae, 407. *See also specific organisms*
  in aspirates from wound infections and abscesses, 614t, 615
  in skin biopsy specimens, 615t, 616
  specimen handling and, 542
Allergies, mites producing, 530
Alphaviruses, 129–130, 130t
  laboratory diagnosis of, 132
Amantadine, orthomyxoviruses and, 100
Amastigotes, 498–499, *499*
Amblyomma americanum, 532
Amblyomma maculatum, 532
Amebae, 470
  blood and tissue, 501–503
  intestinal, *474*, 474–477, *475*
Amebiasis
  extraintestinal, 477, *477*
  intestinal, *476*, 476–477
Amino acid decaboxylation and dihydrolation, Enterobacteriaceae and, 321–322, *322*
Amniotic fluid specimens, 608
Anaerobes. *See also specific anaerobes*
  gram-negative, 357–360, 358t
    clinical manifestations of, 357–358
    epidemiology of, 357
    laboratory diagnosis of, 358–359, 359t
    pathogenesis of, 357
    treatment of, 359–360
  gram-positive
    identification of, 258–262
    non-spore-forming, 262–265
    susceptibility testing of, 179–180
  gram-positive cocci, 265
    clinical manifestations of, 265
    epidemiology and pathogenesis of, 265

639

Anaerobes (Continued)
    laboratory diagnosis of, 265
    treatment of, 265
Anaerobiospirillum succiniciproducens, 374–375
Anal infection, herpes simplex virus and, 49
Anaplora, 533–534, *534*
Angiomatosis, bacillary, Rochalimaea henselae and, 208
Angiostronglyoidiasis, abdominal, *519*, 520
Angiostrongylus cantonensis, 518–520, *519*
Angiostrongylus costaricensis, *519*, 520
Anisakis, 489
Annelloconidia, 409, *410*
Anopheles, 535
Anterior chamber specimens, 555–556
Anthrax, 239
    cutaneous, 239
    pulmonary, 239
Antifungal agents, susceptibility testing and, 413t, 413–414
Antigen detection, bacteria and, 176–177
Antimicrobial agents
    resistance to, 22–23
    selection and reporting of, 180, 181t, 182, 182t
Antiviral agents, 41, 41t
    in herpesvirus infections, 59
    in human immunodeficiency virus types 1 and 2, 157–158
    susceptibility testing and, 41
Apicomplexa, 470
    blood and tissue, 503–509
    intestinal, 478–480
Aplastic crisis, parvovirus B19 and, 75
Arachnida, 530–533. *See also specific organisms*
Arcanobacterium haemolyticum, 247
    in throat specimens, 565
Arenaviruses, 141–143
    classification of, 141
    replication of, 141
    structure of, 141, *142*
Argasidae, 531–532, *533*
Arthralgia, rubella virus and, 132
Arthritis
    Borrelia burgdorferi and, 370
    Candida and, 417
    Erysipelothrix rhusiopathiae and, 243
    rubella virus and, 132
    Yersinia and, 315
Arthroconidia, 409, 411
Arthropods, 530–536. *See also specific organisms*
Ascaridia, 471
Ascaris lumbricoides, 485, *486*, 487
Ascocarp, 411
Ascospores, 411
Asian hemorrhagic fever, Hantaan virus and, 139
Aspartate aminotransferase (AST), hepatitis A virus and, 110
Aspergillosis
    cutaneous, 432
    disseminated, 433
    pulmonary, necrotizing, 432
Aspergillus, 430–434, *431*, 431t
    clinical manifestations of, *432*, 432–433, *433*
    epidemiology of, 431
    laboratory diagnosis of, 439–440, *440*, *441*, 441t
    pathogenesis and pathology of, 431, *431*, *432*
Aspergillus flavus, 432, 439–440

Aspergillus fumigatus, 432, 439–440
Aspergillus niger, 432–433
Astroviruses, 163
    clinical manifestations of, 163
    epidemiology of, 163
    structure of, 163, *164*
Atmosphere, for bacterial culture, 541–542
Atypical measles, 90
Auramine rhodamine stain, 175, 632
Automated blood culture systems, *576*, 576–577, *577*
Auxotypine, 276

B cells, activation of, 13–14
B virus. *See* Cercopithecine herpes virus 1 (B virus)
Babesia, 508–509, *509*
Bacillus, 239–240
    clinical manifestations of, 240, 241t
    epidemiology of, 239
    laboratory diagnosis of, 240–241
    pathogenesis of, 239–240
    treatment and prevention of, 241
Bacillus anthracis, 239
    clinical manifestations of, 239
    epidemiology of, 239
    in aspirates and swab specimens from cutaneous ulcers, 613
    laboratory diagnosis of, 240–241
    pathogenesis of, 239
Bacillus cereus, laboratory diagnosis of, 241
Bacillus mycoides, laboratory diagnosis of, 241
Bacitracin susceptibility test, 633
Bacteremia
    anaerobic gram-negative bacteria and, 358
    Anaerobiospirillum succiniciproducens and, 374
    Campylobacter fetus subspecies fetus and, 352
    Chromobacterium violaceum and, 345
    Clostridium tertium and, 258
    enterococcus and, 231
    Erysipelothrix rhusiopathiae and, 243
    Haemophilus influenzae and, 338
    Neisseria meningitidis and, 271
    Pseudomonas aeruginosa and, 284
    Salmonella and, 314
    Staphylococcus aureus and, 219, 223
    Streptococcus agalactiae and, 228
    Yersinia and, 315
Bacteria, 173–182, *174*. *See also specific organisms*
    classification of, 173
    gram-negative, potassium hydroxide test for distinguishing gram-positive bacteria from, 634
    gram-positive, potassium hydroxide test for distinguishing gram-negative bacteria from, 634
    in amniotic fluid specimens, 608
    in anterior chamber, vitreous cavity, and ocular abscess specimens, 555
    in aspirates and swab specimens from cutaneous ulcers, 613
    in aspirates from wound infections and abscesses, 614t, 614–615
    in blood specimens, 574–577, *576*, *577*
    in body cavity specimens, 620t, 620–621
    in bone marrow specimens, 580, 580t
    in brain abscess and empyema specimens, 548
    in brain tissue specimens, 549

    in bronchial washing, protected specimen brush, and bronchoalveolar lavage specimens, 569–570
    in cerebrospinal fluid, 545t, 545–546
    in corneal specimens, 554–555
    in endomyocardial biopsy specimens, 579
    in fluid and swab specimens from vesicles, bullae, and pustules, 612
    in gastric contents specimens, 585–586
    in gastrointestinal tissue specimens, 592–593
    in liver and pancreas abscess specimens, 595
    in liver tissue specimens, 598
    in lymph node specimens, 581
    in middle ear fluid, 557–558
    in muscle specimens, 624, 624t
    in nasopharyngeal and nasal specimens, 562–563
    in oropharyngeal ulcer specimens, 559
    in products of conception, 608
    in sinus aspirates, 556
    in skin biopsy specimens, 615t, 616
    in sputum and tracheal aspirates, 566–568, 567
    in stool and rectal swab specimens, 588–590, 589t, 590t
    in throat specimens, 564–565
    in transbronchial and open lung biopsy specimens, 571
    in urethral swab specimens, 605–606
    in urine specimens, 601t, 601–603, *602*
    in vaginal specimens, 604–605
    laboratory diagnosis of, 175–182
        antigen detection in, 176–177
        culture in, 175–176, 176t
        future technology in, 177
        microscopy in, 175
        nucleic acid probes in, 177
        serologic tests in, 177
    specimen handling and, 539–542, 541t, *542*
    structure of, 173–174
    susceptibility testing and, 177–182
        anaerobes and, 179–180
        bactericidal activity and, 182
        broth dilution and, *177*, 177–178
        disk diffusion and, 178–179, *179*
        β-lactamase detection in, 179, *180*
        selection and reporting of antimicrobial agents and, 180, 181t, 182, 182t
        therapeutic drug monitoring and, 182
    toxins produced by, 21–22, 22t
Bactericidal activity, tests of, 182
Bacteroides distasonis, treatment of, 359
Bacteroides fragilis
    clinical manifestations of, 357, 358
    laboratory diagnosis of, 359
    pathogenesis of, 357
    treatment of, 359
Bacteroides gracilis
    laboratory diagnosis of, 359
    treatment of, 359
Bacteroides thetaiotaomicron
    clinical manifestations of, 357
    treatment of, 359
Bacteroides ureolyticus
    laboratory diagnosis of, 359
    treatment of, 359
Baermann concentration, for Strongyloides larvae, 636
Bairnsdale ulcer, 386
Balantidium coli, 477–478, *478*
Bartonella bacilliformis, 210
    in blood specimens, 577

INDEX

Bartonellosis, 210
  clinical manifestations of, 210
  epidemiology of, 210
  laboratory diagnosis of, 210
  pathogenesis of, 210
  treatment of, 210
Basidiospores, 411
Basophils, 12
BCG vaccine, 394–395
Bejel, 364
Bifidobacterium, laboratory diagnosis of, 264
Bifidobacterium dentium, 263
Bile specimens, 596, 596t
Biliary tract, trematodes and, 520–522
Bilirubin, hepatitis A virus and, 111
Biologic false-positive nontreponemal reactions, 366
BK virus. See Polyomavirus
Black piedra, 429
Blastocystis hominis, 480, 481
Blastomyces dermatitidis
  laboratory diagnosis of, 453–455, 453–455
  treatment of, 458
Blastomyces dermatitidis, 447–448
  clinical manifestations of, 448
  epidemiology of, 447
  pathogenesis and pathology of, 447, 448
Blastomycosis, 447–448
  cutaneous, 448
  of bone, 448
  pulmonary, 448
    treatment of, 458
  South American, 451–452
Blastoschizomyces, treatment of, 423
Blastoschizomyces capitatus, 419
  laboratory diagnosis of, cellular structure and colony characteristics in, 421
Blepharoconjunctivitis, Pseudomonas aeruginosa and, 284
Blood specimens, 573–578, 574t
  bacteria and fungi in, 574–577
  collection, transport, and processing of, 573
  parasites in, 578
  viruses in, 573–574
Blood vessels, trematodes and, 523–525, 524–526
Body cavity specimens, 619–621, 620t
  bacteria in, 620t, 620–621
  collection, transport, and processing of, 619–620
  fungi in, 620t, 621
  parasites in, 620t, 621
  viruses in, 620, 620t
Bone
  Blastomyces dermatitidis and, 448
  Cryptococcus neoformans and, 418
  specimens of, 626, 626t
    collection, transport, and processing of, 626
Bone marrow specimens, 580, 580t
Bordatella bronchiseptica, 287
Bordatella parapertussis, laboratory diagnosis of, 299
Bordetella pertussis, 297, 297–299
  clinical manifestations of, 298
  epidemiology of, 297, 297
  in nasopharyngeal and nasal specimens, 563
  laboratory diagnosis of, 298–299
  pathogenesis of, 297–298
  treatment and prevention of, 299
Bornholm disease. See Pleurodynia
Borrelia, 367–373
  in blood specimens, 577
  laboratory diagnosis of, 371–372

Borrelia burgdorferi, 367–370
  clinical manifestations of, 369–370
  epidemiology of, 368–369, 369
  in cerebrospinal fluid, 546
  laboratory diagnosis of, 371–372
  pathogenesis and immunology and, 369
  treatment of, 372
Borrelia recurrentis, 370
Botulism, 253–254
  foodborne, 253, 254
  infant, 254, 258
  wound, 254
Bouba, 364
Boutonneuse fever, 200–201
Brain, herpes simplex virus and, 49
Brain abscess
  actinomycosis and, 263
  anaerobic gram-negative bacteria and, 357
  specimens from, 547–548
    bacteria in, 548
    fungi in, 548
    parasites in, 548
  Staphylococcus aureus and, 220
Brain tissue specimens, 548–549
  bacteria in, 549
  fungi in, 549
  parasites in, 549
  viruses in, 549
Branhamella catarrhalis, 272–277
  laboratory diagnosis of, 272–277, 273t
    chromogenic enzyme substrate tests and, 275–276
    commercial carbohydrate degradation kits and, 275
    conventional biochemical tests and, 274–275
    immunologic tests and, 276
    microscopic features and colony characteristics and, 272–273, 274t
    organism identification and, 274
    susceptibility testing and, 277
Bronchial washing specimens, 569–570
  bacteria in, 569–570
  fungi in, 570
  parasites in, 570
  viruses in, 569
Bronchitis, Chlamydia pneumoniae and, 188
Bronchoalveolar lavage specimens, 569–570
  bacteria in, 569–570
  fungi in, 570
  parasites in, 570
  viruses in, 569
Broth dilution
  anaerobe susceptibility testing and, 180
  bacterial susceptibility testing and, 177, 177–178
Broth disk elution, anaerobe susceptibility testing and, 180
Brucella
  in blood specimens, 577
  in cerebrospinal fluid, 546
  in endomyocardial biopsy specimens, 579
  in liver tissue specimens, 598
Brucella abortus, 295, 296
Brucella canis, 295
Brucella melitensis, 295, 296
Brucella neotomae, 295
Brucella ovis, 295
Brucella suis, 295, 296
Brucellosis, 295–297
  clinical manifestations of, 295, 296t
  epidemiology of, 295
  laboratory diagnosis of, 296, 296t
  pathogenesis of, 295
  treatment and prevention of, 296–297

Brugia, 514, 514, 535
Buba, 364
Bunyaviridae, 535
Bunyaviruses, 138–140
  classification of, 138
  clinical manifestations of, 138–139
  epidemiology of, 138
  replication of, 138
  structure of, 138
Bursitis, olecranon, Prototheca and, 463
Buruli ulcer, 386
N-Butyl deoxynojirimycin, in human immunodeficiency virus types 1 and 2, 158

Calciviruses, 122
  clinical manifestations of, 122
  epidemiology of, 122
  laboratory diagnosis of, 122
  structure of, 122, 122
  treatment of, 122
Calcofluor white stain, 635
California encephalitis virus, 138
Calymmatobacterium granulomatis, 400
  clinical manifestations and pathology of, 400
  epidemiology of, 400
  in genital ulcer specimens, 607
  laboratory diagnosis of, 400
  treatment of, 400
CAMP test, 634
Campylobacter
  in gastrointestinal tissue specimens, 593
  in stool and rectal swab specimens, 590
  treatment of, 353
Campylobacter fetus subspecies fetus, 351–352
  clinical manifestations of, 352
  epidemiology of, 352
  laboratory diagnosis of, 353
  pathogenesis of, 352
Campylobacter jejuni, 350–351
  clinical manifestations of, 351
  epidemiology of, 350
  incubation of, 541
  laboratory diagnosis of, 352–353
  pathogenesis and pathology of, 350–351
Candida, 415–417
  clinical manifestations of, 416, 416–417, 417
  epidemiology of, 415
  laboratory diagnosis of
    cellular structure and colony characteristics in, 419, 420
    serologic tests in, 423
  pathogenesis and pathology of, 415–416, 416
  treatment of, 423
Candida albicans, 415
  laboratory diagnosis of, 421, 421
Candida guilliermondii, 415
Candida kefyr, 415
Candida krusei, 415
Candida parapsilosis, 415
Candida tropicalis, 415
Candidiasis, mucocutaneous, 416
  treatment of, 423
Capillaria philippinensis, 488–489, 489
Capnocytophaga, 344–345
  epidemiology, pathogenesis, and clinical manifestations of, 344
  laboratory diagnosis of, 344
  treatment of, 345

Capnocytophaga canimorsus, 344, 345
Capnocytophaga gingivalis, 344, 345
Capnocytophaga ochracea, 344, 345
Capnocytophaga sputigena, 344, 345
Capsid, of viruses, 33
Carate, 364–365
Carbohydrate degradation tests, 274–275
Carbuncle, Staphylococcus aureus and, 219
Carcinoma, nasopharyngeal, Epstein-Barr virus and, 54
Cardiac murmurs, viridans streptococci and, 229
Cardiobacterium hominis, 345
    laboratory diagnosis of, 345
    treatment of, 345
Cardiovascular system, Pseudomonas aeruginosa and, 284
Carrier state, of human immunodeficiency virus types 1 and 2, 153–154
Carrión's disease, 535
Castanospermine, in human immunodeficiency virus types 1 and 2, 158
Cat-scratch disease, 401–402
    conjunctival specimens and, 554
Cat-scratch fever bacillus. See Afipia felis
Catalase test, 633
Cell lines, for viral culture, 39, 40t
Cell-mediated immunity, 15–19
    mononuclear phagocytes and, 16
    natural killer cells and, 18–19
    T-lymphocytes and, 16–18, 17
Cell wall, bacterial, 173–174
Cellulitis
    Aeromonas and, 332–333
    aspirates from, 612, 612t
    Pseudomonas aeruginosa and, 283
    Streptococcus pyogenes and, 226
Central nervous system. See also Brain abscess
    Acanthamoeba and, 502
    actinomycosis and, 263
    Aspergillus and, 433, 433
    Candida and, 416
    measles virus and, 90
    mumps virus and, 87, 88
    picornaviruses and, 107–108
    Pseudomonas aeruginosa and, 284
    Rocky Mountain spotted fever and, 199
    specimens from, 544–549
        abscess and empyema material, 547–548
        brain tissue, 548–549
        cerebrospinal fluid, 544–547, 545t
    Staphylococcus aureus and, 220
    Toxoplasma gondii and, 504
Centrifugation culture
    adenoviruses and, 68
    cytomegalovirus and, 57, 57
    for detection of cytomegalovirus early nuclear antigen, 631
    herpes simplex virus and, 56
    of orthomyxoviruses, 100
Cercopithecine herpes virus 1 (B virus), 55
    clinical manifestations of, 55
    structure, epidemiology, and pathogenesis of, 55
    treatment of, 59
Cerebrospinal fluid specimens, 544–547, 545t
    bacteria in, 545–546
    fungi in, 546
    parasites in, 546–547
    viruses in, 544–545
Cervical adenitis, tuberculous, 381–382
Cestodes. See also specific organisms
    blood and tissue, 525–529
    intestinal, 491–495, 492

Chagas' disease, 500–501, 501
Chancre, of syphilis, 362–364
Chancroid, 338–339
Chandipura virus, 123
Cheyletiella blakei, 530
Cheyletiella parasitovorax, 530
Cheyletiella yasguri, 530
Chickenpox. See Varicella-zoster virus
Children
    human immunodeficiency virus types 1 and 2 in, 154–155, 155t
    paracoccidioidomycosis in, 452
Chlamydia, 184–191
    classification of, 184
    replication of, 184–185, 185
    structure of, 184
    treatment of, 191
Chlamydia pneumoniae, 187–188
    clinical manifestations of, 188
    epidemiology of, 188
    laboratory diagnosis of, 188t, 190–191
    pathogenesis of, 188
Chlamydia psittaci, 187
    clinical manifestations of, 187
    epidemiology of, 187
    laboratory diagnosis of, 190
    pathogenesis and pathology of, 187
Chlamydia trachomatis, 185–187
    cell culture for isolation of, 632–633
    classification of, 185, 185t
    epidemiology and clinical manifestations of, 185–187
    in body cavity specimens, 620
    in conjunctival specimens, 553
    in genital ulcer specimens, 607
    in lymph node specimens, 581
    in middle ear fluid, 557
    in nasopharyngeal and nasal specimens, 563
    in stool and rectal swab specimens, 588
    in throat specimens, 564
    in urethral swab specimens, 605
    in urine specimens, 601
    in vaginal specimens, 604
    laboratory diagnosis of, 188t, 188–190, 189t
    pathology of, 185
Chlamydoconidia, 409, 410
Chloramphenicol
    in boutonneuse fever, 201
    in murine typhus, 202
    in Rocky Mountain spotted fever, 200
    in scrub typhus, 203
Cholera, 329–330
    treatment and prevention of, 332
Chromobacterium violaceum, 345–346
    clinical manifestations of, 345
    epidemiology and pathogenesis of, 345
    laboratory diagnosis of, 345–346
    treatment of, 346
Chromoblastomycosis, 428t, 428–429
    clinical manifestations of, 428–429
    epidemiology of, 428
    pathology of, 428, 429
    treatment of, 442–443
Chromogenic enzyme substrate tests, 275–276
Ciliates, 470, 477–478, 478
Ciprofloxacin, in boutonneuse fever, 201
Citrate utilization, Enterobacteriaceae and, 321
Citrobacter, 317–318
    features of, 324
    treatment and prevention of, 325
Citrobacter amalonaticus, 317
Citrobacter diversus, 317–318

Citrobacter freundii, 317
    features of, 324
Clinical pathologist, role of, 3
Clonorchis sinensis, 521–522, 522
Clostridium, 253–258
    laboratory diagnosis of, 258, 258t
    treatment and prevention of, 262
Clostridium baratii, 258
Clostridium bifermentans, 258
Clostridium botulinum, 253–254
    clinical manifestations of, 254
    epidemiology of, 253–254
    in stool and rectal swab specimens, 588
    laboratory diagnosis of, 260
    pathogenesis of, 254
    treatment and prevention of, 261
Clostridium butyricum, 258
Clostridium difficile, 257–258
    clinical manifestations of, 257–258
    epidemiology of, 257
    in gastrointestinal tissue specimens, 593
    in stool and rectal swab specimens, 588–589
    laboratory diagnosis of, 260–261
    pathogenesis of, 257
    treatment and prevention of, 262
Clostridium haemolyticum, 253
Clostridium histolyticum, 253, 258, 259
Clostridium novyi, 253, 258
Clostridium perfringens, 256–257, 259
    clinical manifestations of, 256–257
    epidemiology of, 256
    in stool and rectal swab specimens, 589
    laboratory diagnosis of, 260
    pathogenesis of, 256
    treatment and prevention of, 262
Clostridium ramosum, 258, 259
    treatment of, 262
Clostridium septicum, 258
Clostridium sordellii, 258
Clostridium sporogenes, 258
Clostridium tertium, 253, 258, 259
    treatment of, 262
Clostridium tetani, 254–256
    clinical manifestations of, 255–256
    epidemiology of, 254–255, 255
    laboratory diagnosis of, 260, 261t
    pathogenesis of, 255
    treatment and prevention of, 261–262
Clumping test, 633
Coagglutination, bacteria and, 176
Coccidioides immitis, 450–451
    clinical manifestations of, 451
    dimorphic, 458
    epidemiology of, 450–451
    laboratory diagnosis of, 456, 456–457
    pathogenesis and pathology of, 451, 451
Coccidioidomycosis, 450–451
    cutaneous, 451
    treatment of, 458
Coccobacilli, fastidious, 293–302
Colds, coronaviruses and, 102
Colitis
    pseudomembranous, Clostridium difficile and, 257–258
        treatment of, 262
    Shigella and, 311
Colorado tick fever virus, 116
    clinical manifestations of, 116
    epidemiology and pathogenesis of, 116
    laboratory diagnosis of, 118
    treatment and prevention of, 119
Complement, 7t, 7–9
    activation of, 7, 8, 9
    role in nonspecific defense, 7, 9, 9t, 10t

Complement fixation, orthomyxoviruses and, 100
Concentration, parasites in blood specimens and, 578
Condyloma acuminatum, human papillomavirus and, 71
Congenital rubella syndrome, 131–132, 132t
Congenital varicella, 50
Conidiobolus, 436
Conjunctival specimens, 551–554, 552t
  bacteria in, 552t, 553–554
    collection, transport, and processing of, 551
  fungi in, 552t, 554
  parasites in, 552t, 554
  viruses in, 551, 552t, 553
Conjunctivitis
  Haemophilus influenzae and, 338
  hemorrhagic, chronic, 109
  in neonate, Neisseria gonorrhoeae and, 270
  inclusion, Chlamydia trachomatis and, 186–187
Corneal specimens, 554–555
    collection, transport, and processing of, 554
Corneal ulcers, Pseudomonas aeruginosa and, 284
Cornmeal-tween 80 agar, inoculation of, for identification of yeasts, 635
Coronaviruses, 102–103
    classification of, 102
    clinical manifestations of, 102
    epidemiology of, 102
    laboratory diagnosis of, 102–103
    structure and replication of, 102, 103
    treatment of, 103
Corynebacterium, 244
    in aspirates and swab specimens from cutaneous ulcers, 613
    laboratory diagnosis of, 246t, 246–247
    treatment and prevention of, 247
Corynebacterium bovis, 246
Corynebacterium diphtheriae, 244–245
    clinical manifestations of, 245
    epidemiology of, 244
    in throat specimens, 565
    laboratory diagnosis of, 246–247, 247
    pathogenesis of, 244–245, 245
    treatment and prevention of, 247
Corynebacterium group D2, 245
    laboratory diagnosis of, 247
Corynebacterium jeikeium, 245
    laboratory diagnosis of, 247
Corynebacterium minutissimum, 246
Corynebacterium pseudodiphtheriticum, 246
Corynebacterium pseudotuberculosis, 246
Corynebacterium ulcerans, 245–246
Corynebacterium xerosis, 246
Coxiella burnetii. See Q fever
Coxsackieviruses, clinical manifestations of, 107, 108, 109
Creutzfeldt-Jakob disease, in brain tissue specimens, 549. See also Prions
Crimean-Congo hemorrhagic fever virus, 140
    clinical manifestations of, 140
    epidemiology of, 140
    laboratory diagnosis of, 140
    treatment and prevention of, 140
Cryptococcus neoformans, 417–418
    clinical manifestations of, 418
    epidemiology of, 417
    laboratory diagnosis of, 421–422
        cellular structure and colony characteristics in, 419–420, 421

pathogenesis and pathology of, 417–418
    treatment of, 423
Cryptosporidium
    in stool and rectal swab specimens, 592
    modified acid-fast stain for, 636
Cryptosporidium parvum, 478–479, 479
Cul de sac aspirate, 608
Culex, 535
Culicoides, 535
Culicoides austeni, 535
Culicoides furens, 535
Culicoides grahami, 535
Culicoides phlebotomus, 535
Culture. See also Media
    criteria for specimens unsuitable for, 540
    for isolation of Chlamydia tracnomatis, 632–633
    of bacteria, 175–176, 176t
    of fungi, 412–413
    viral, 39–41, 40t, 41t
        handling of, 539, 540t
Cutaneous infection, herpes simplex virus and, 49
Cyanobacterium-like organisms, 464, 464
Cyst
    hydatid, 526–529
        alveolar, 528–529
        unilocular, 527, 527–528, 528
    phaeomycotis, 429, 430
Cystic fibrosis, Pseudomonas aeruginosa and, 284
Cysticercosis, 526, 526
Cystitis, Candida and, 416
Cytokines, biologic properties of, 16, 17t
Cytomegalovirus (CMV), 51–53
    clinical manifestations of, 52, 52–53
    epidemiology of, 51
    laboratory diagnosis of, 57, 57–58, 58
    pathogenesis of, 51–52
    prevention of, 60
    structure of, 51
    treatment of, 59
Cytomegalovirus early nuclear antigen, centrifugation culture for detection of, 631
Cytopathic effect (CPE)
    of adenoviruses, 67–68, 68
    of cytomegalovirus, 57, 57
    of herpes simplex virus, 56, 56
    of varicella-zoster virus, 56, 57
    parainfluenza virus and, 91–92
Cytopathic effect (CPE) of rhinoviruses, 112, 113
Cytoplasmic structures, bacterial, 174
Cytospin preparations, cytomegalovirus and, 57, 58

Defense mechanisms. See Nonspecific defenses; Specific defenses
Demodex brevis, 530
Demodex folliculorum, 530
Dendritic cells, 16
Dengue virus, 134–135
    clinical manifestations of, 134–135
    epidemiology of, 134
    laboratory diagnosis of, 137
    pathogenesis of, 134
Dermacentor andersoni, 196, 532
Dermacentor variabilis, 196, 198, 532
Dermanyssus gallinae, 530
Dermatitis, mites producing, 530
Dermatomycosis, 429
Dermatophilus, 249

Dermatophilus congoliensis, laboratory diagnosis of, 249
Dermatophytes, 426–428
    clinical manifestations of, 426–428, 427t
    epidemiology of, 426, 427t
    laboratory diagnosis of, 436–437, 437, 437t, 438
    pathogenesis of, 426, 427t
    treatment of, 442
Dermatophytosis, 426–427
Devil's grippe. See Pleurodynia
Diarrhea
    Aeromonas and, 333
    Clostridium difficile and, 257–258
        treatment of, 262
    Clostridium perfringens and, 256, 257
    Giardia lamblia and, 472–473
    Pseudomonas aeruginosa and, 284
    Salmonella and, 313
    Shigella and, 311
    Vibrio parahaemolyticus and, 330
Dichuchwa, 364
Dideoxycytidine, in human immunodeficiency virus types 1 and 2, 157–158
Dideoxyinosine (ddI), in human immunodeficiency virus types 1 and 2, 157–158
Dientamoeba fragilis, 473, 474
Differential media, 175
Diphtheria. See Corynebacterium diphtheriae
Diphtheria-tetanus toxoid vaccine (DTP), 262, 299
Diphyllobothrium, 494–495, 495
Diptera, 534–536
Dipylidium canium, 494, 495
Direct detection methods, for viruses, 41
Direct mounts, parasites in blood specimens and, 578
Dirofilariae immitis, 516, 517
Disk-diffusion test
    bacterial susceptibility testing and, 178–179, 179
    for novobiocin resistance, 633
Disseminated intravascular coagulation, in Rocky Mountain spotted fever, 198
DNA probes, Chlamydia trachomatis and, 190
DNA synthesis, viruses and, 36, 38
Donovanosis, Calymmatobacterium granulomatis and, 400
Doxycycline
    in boutonneuse fever, 201
    in epidemic louse-borne typhus, 202
    in murine typhus, 202
    in Rocky Mountain spotted fever, 199
Duck embryo vaccine, 127
Duodenal aspirate specimens, 586
    collection, transport, and processing of, 586
Duvenhage virus, 126
Dye uptake assay, antiviral agent susceptibility testing and, 41
Dysentery, Shigella and, 311

Eastern encephalitis virus, 129–130
    clinical manifestations of, 130
    epidemiology of, 129
    pathogenesis of, 130, 130
Ebola virus. See Filoviruses
Echinococcus granulosus, 526, 527, 527–528, 528
Echinococcus multilocularis, 526
Echinococcus oligarthrus, 526
Echinococcus vogeli, 526

Echoviruses, clinical manifestations of, 107–109
Ecthyma gangrenosum, Pseudomonas aeruginosa and, 283–284
Edmonston B vaccine, 93
Egress, by viruses, 38
Ehrlichia canis, 203, 204
Ehrlichia chaffeensis, 203–205
Ehrlichia equi, 203
Ehrlichia ewingii, 203
Ehrlichia phagocytophilia, 203
Ehrlichia platys, 203
Ehrlichia risticii, 204
Ehrlichioses, 203–205
  human, 203–204
    clinical manifestations of, 204
    epidemiology of, 203–204
    laboratory diagnosis of, 204
    pathogenesis of, 204
    treatment of, 204
  sennetsu, 205
Eikenella corrodens, 346
  clinical manifestations of, 346
  epidemiology and pathogenesis of, 346
  laboratory diagnosis of, 346
  treatment of, 346
Electron microscopy
  direct detection of viruses and, 41
  rotavirus and, 118
Embolism, cerebral, viridans streptococci and, 229
Empyema, specimens from, 547–548
  bacteria in, 548
  fungi in, 548
  parasites in, 548
Encephalitis
  Acanthamoeba and, 502
  herpes simplex virus and, 49
  picornaviruses and, 107
  polioviruses and, 107
  rubella virus and, 132
  subacute, human immunodeficiency virus types 1 and 2 and, 155
Encephalomyocarditis, neonatal, picornaviruses and, 109
Encephalopathy
  lymphocytic choriomeningitis virus and, 141
  spongiform. See Prions
Endarteritis, obliterative, Treponema pallidum subspecies pallidum and, 362, *362*
Endocardial vegetations, 578–579
Endocarditis
  Aspergillus and, 433, *433*
  Candida and, 416
  enterococcus and, 230–231
  Erysipelothrix rhusiopathiae and, 243
  Haemophilus and, 339
  in Q fever, 206–207
  Staphylococcus aureus and, 219
  viridans streptococci and, 229
Endocervical swab specimens, 606, 606t
  collection, transport, and processing of, 606
Endometrial specimens, 607–608
Endomyocardial biopsies, 579t, 579–580
  bacteria in, 579
  fungi in, 579–580
  parasites in, 580
  viruses in, 579
Endophthalmitis
  Candida and, 417
  Staphylococcus epidermidis and, 222
Endospores, bacterial, 174
Endotoxin, 21, 174

Enrichment media, 175
Entamoeba histolytica, 475–477
Enteric fever, Salmonella and, 313, *313*, 314
Enteritis necroticans, Clostridium perfringens and, 256
Enterobacter, treatment and prevention of, 325
Enterobacter aerogenes, 317
  features of, 324
Enterobacter agglomerans, 317
  features of, 324
Enterobacter cloacae, 317
  features of, 324
Enterobacter sakazakii, features of, 324
Enterobacteriaceae, 307–325, 308t. *See also specific organisms*
  laboratory diagnosis of, 318t, 318–322
  tests for identification and, 318–322, 319t
Enterobius, Scotch tape procedure for, 636
Enterobius vermicularis, 482, *483*
Enterococci, 230–231
  clinical manifestations of, 230–231
  epidemiology and pathogenesis of, 230
  laboratory diagnosis of, 232–233, *233*
  susceptibility testing and, 234
  treatment of, 234
Enterococcus durans, 230
Enterococcus faecalis, 230
Enterococcus faecium, 230
Enterocolitis
  Salmonella and, 314
  Yersinia and, 315
Enterovirus 72. *See* Hepatitis A virus
Enteroviruses, 105–106. *See also specific viruses*
  clinical manifestations of, 107–108, 109
  epidemiology of, 105–106
  in cerebrospinal fluid, 544, 545t
  laboratory diagnosis of, 111–112, *112*, 112t
  pathogenesis of, 106
Entomophthorales, 434
Entomophthoramycosis conidiobolae, 435, 436
Envelope, of viruses, 33, 36
Enzyme-linked immunosorbent assays (ELISA), 276
  adenoviruses and, 68
  bacteria and, 177
  Chlamydia trachomatis and, 190
  direct detection of viruses and, 41
  fungi in cerebrospinal fluid and, 546
  respiratory syncytial virus and, 93
  rotavirus and, 118
  Treponema pallidum subspecies pallidum and, 367
Eosinophils, 11–12
  development and structure of, 11, 12t
  role in host defense, 11–12, *13*
Epidemics, of influenza, 99
Epidermodysplasia verruciformis, human papillomavirus and, 71
Epidermophyton floccosum, 436, 437
Epididymo-orchitis, mumps virus and, 88
Epiglottitis, Haemophilus influenzae and, 338
Epstein-Barr virus (EBV), 53–54
  clinical manifestations of, 54, 54t
  epidemiology of, 53
  laboratory diagnosis of, 58t, 58–59, 59t
  pathogenesis of, 53–54
  replication of, 53
  structure of, 53
  treatment of, 59
Erysipelas, Streptococcus pyogenes and, 226–227

Erysipelothrix rhusiopathiae, 243
  clinical manifestations of, 243
  epidemiology of, 243
  in skin biopsy specimens, 616
  laboratory diagnosis of, 243
  pathogenesis of, 243
Erythema chronicum migrans (ECM), Borrelia burgdorferi and, 369, 370
Erythema infectiosum, parvovirus B19 and, 75
Erythema nodosum, Yersinia and, 315
Eschar, of boutonneuse fever, 200
Escherichia coli, 307, 309t, 309–310
  enterohemmorhagic (EHEC), 307, 309, 323
  enteroinvasive (EIEC), 307–308, 323
  enteropathogenic (EPEC), 307, 309
  enterotoxigenic (ETEC), 307, 323
  features of, 322–323
  in stool and rectal swab specimens, 589
  treatment and prevention of, 324–325
  uropathogenic, 309–310
Escherichia fergusonii, 307
Escherichia hermannii, 307
Escherichia vulneris, 307
Esophageal brushing specimens, 585
  collection, transport, and processing of, 585
Esophagitis, herpes simplex virus and, 49, *49*
Ethanol spore test, anaerobes and, 259
Eubacterium, 263
  laboratory diagnosis of, 264
Eubacterium lentum, 263
Exanthema subitum, human herpesvirus 6 and, 54
Exanthems, picornaviruses and, 108
Exotoxins, 21–22, 22t
Eye
  Acanthamoeba and, 502–503
  Candida and, 417
  conjunctival specimens and, 551–554, 552t
  collection, transport, and processing of, 551
  corneal specimens and, 554–556
  herpes simplex virus and, 49
  nonspecific defense and, 5
  Rhinosporidium seeberi and, 461

Fasciola, 520–521, *521*
Fasciola gigantica, 520
Fasciola hepatica, 520, *521*
Fasciolopsis buski, 489–490, *490*
Fecal smears, trichrome stain for, 635
Fetus
  cytomegalovirus and, 52
  mumps virus and, 88
  parvovirus B19 and, 75–76
  rubella virus and, 131–132
  Streptococcus agalactiae and, 227
  syphilis and, 364, 367
  Toxoplasma gondii and, 504–505
Filariae, 512–516. *See also specific organisms*
  zoonotic, 516, *517*
Filariasis, lymphatic, 535
  Brugia and, 514, *514*
  Wuchereria bancrofti and, 512–514, *513*
Filoviruses, 144–145
  clinical manifestations of, 144–145
  epidemiology of, 144
  laboratory diagnosis of, 145
  pathogenesis and pathology of, 144
  replication of, 144
  structure of, 144
  treatment and prevention of, 145
Filth flies, 536
Fimbriae, bacterial, 174

INDEX

Fine-needle aspirates, from respiratory tract, 570
Flagella, bacterial, 174
Flagellates
    blood and tissue, 497
    intestinal, 470
    nonpathogenic, 474
Flaviviruses, 134–137, 135t
    classification of, 134
    structure and replication of, 134
Flavobacterium, 287
    clinical manifestations of, 287
    epidemiology and pathogenesis of, 287
    treatment of, 290
Flavobacterium glenum, 287
Flavobacterium meningosepticum, 287
    laboratory diagnosis of, organism identification and, 289
Fleas, 534, 534, 535
Flies, 535–536, 536
Flora, normal, as nonspecific defense, 5, 6t
Flow cytometry, bacteria and, 177
Fluorescent treponemal antibody-absorption (FTA-ABS) test, 365, 366
Folliculitis, Staphylococcus aureus and, 219
Food poisoning
    bacteria associated with, in stool and rectal swab specimens, 588
    bacteria in gastric contents specimens and, 585–586
    Clostridium botulinum and, 253–254
    Clostridium perfringens and, 256–257
        treatment of, 262
    Staphylococcus aureus and, 221
Formalin-ethyl acetate, stool concentration and, 636
Fort Bragg fever, 373
Foscarnet, in herpesvirus infections, 59
Frambesia, 364
Francisella tularensis, 293–295
    clinical manifestations of, 294
    epidemiology of, 293
    in aspirates and swab specimens from cutaneous ulcers, 613
    in conjunctival specimens, 553
    in liver tissue specimens, 598
    in lymph node specimens, 581
    in sputum and tracheal aspirates, 567
    laboratory diagnosis of, 294
    pathogenesis and pathology of, 293–294
    treatment and prevention of, 294–295
Fulminant hepatitis, 80, 81
Fungemia, Malassezia and, 418–419
Fungi, 407–414. *See also specific organisms*
    antifungal agents and susceptibility testing and, 413t, 413–414
    classification of, 407–408
    dematiaceous, 428–430
        laboratory diagnosis of, 438, 438t, 439, 440
        treatment of, 442–443
    dimorphic, 447–458. *See also specific organisms*
        laboratory diagnosis of, 453t, 453–458, 454t
        morphologic appearance of, 408
        treatment of, 458
    fine structure of, 409
    in anterior chamber, vitreous cavity, and ocular abscess specimens, 555
    in aspirates and swab specimens from cutaneous ulcers, 614
    in aspirates from wound infections and abscesses, 614t, 615
    in blood specimens, 574–575

in body cavity specimens, 620t, 621
in bone marrow specimens, 580, 580t
in brain abscess and empyema specimens, 548
in brain tissue specimens, 549
in bronchial washing, protected specimen brush, and bronchoalveolar lavage specimens, 570
in cerebrospinal fluid, 545t, 546
in corneal specimens, 554–555
in endomyocardial biopsy specimens, 579–580
in esophageal brushing specimens, 585
in fluid and swab specimens from vesicles, bullae, and pustules, 612
in gastrointestinal tissue specimens, 593
in liver and pancreas abscess specimens, 595–596
in liver tissue specimens, 598
in lymph node specimens, 581–582
in muscle specimens, 624, 624t
in nasopharyngeal and nasal specimens, 563
in oropharyngeal ulcer specimens, 559
in sinus aspirates, 556–557
in skin biopsy specimens, 615t, 616
in sputum and tracheal aspirates, 568
in transbronchial and open lung biopsy specimens, 571
in urine specimens, 603
laboratory diagnosis of, 411t, 411–413
    culture in, 412–413
    direct microscopic examination in, 411–412, 412
    serologic tests in, 413
morphologic appearance of, 408–409
reproduction of, 409–411
    asexual, 409, 410, 411
    sexual, 411
specimen handling and, 542
Fusarium, 433–434
    laboratory diagnosis of, 442, 442
Fusarium sporotrichoides, 433–434
Fusobacterium
    clinical manifestations of, 358
    laboratory diagnosis of, 359
    pathogenesis of, 357
Fusobacterium necrophorum
    in throat specimens, 565
    pathogenesis of, 357, 358
Fusobacterium nucleatum, laboratory diagnosis of, 359

Ganciclovir, in herpesvirus infections, 59
Gardnerella vaginalis, 399–400
    clinical manifestations of, 399
    epidemiology and pathogenesis of, 399
    laboratory diagnosis of, 399–400
    treatment of, 400
Gas gangrene
    Clostridium and, 258
    Clostridium perfringens and, treatment of, 262
Gas-liquid chromatography, anaerobes and, 259
Gastric contents specimens, 585–586
Gastritis, Helicobacter pylori and, 354
Gastroenteritis
    Anaerobiospirillum succiniciproducens and, 374
    Campylobacter jejuni and, 350, 351, 352
    Plesiomonas shigelloides and, 333
    Vibrio parahaemolyticus and, treatment and prevention of, 332

viruses associated with, in stool and rectal swab specimens, 587–588
Gastrointestinal tract. *See also specific disorders*
    Campylobacter jejuni and, 350
    Candida and, 416, *416*
    coronaviruses and, 102
    nonspecific defense and, 7
    Pseudomonas aeruginosa and, 284
    specimens from, 585–594
        duodenal aspirates, 586
        esophageal brushings, 585
        gastric contents, 585–586
        stool and rectal swabs, 586–592, 587t
        tissues, 592t, 592–594
Genital infection
    Chlamydia trachomatis and, 186
    herpes simplex virus and, 49
Genital mycoplasmas, 215–216
Genitourinary tract
    abscess material and, 608
    amniotic fluid specimens and, 608
    cul de sac aspirate and, 608
    endocervical swab specimens and, 606, 606t
    endometrial tissue or swab specimens and, 607–608
    needle aspirates of kidney and, 603
    nonspecific defense and, 7
    products of conception and, 608
    ulcer specimens and, 607
    urethral swab specimens and, 605–606
    urine specimens and, 600–603
    vaginal specimens and, 604–605
    vesicle fluid or swab specimens and, 606–607
Genome
    bacterial, 174
    viral, 33
Germ tube test, 635
Gerstmann-Straussler syndrome. *See* Prions
Giardia lamblia, 472–473, *473*
    in duodenal aspirate specimens, 586
Giemsa stain, 175, 635
Gingivitis
    ulcerative, acute necrotizing, 374–375
    Vincent's, 374–375
Gingivostomatitis, herpes simplex virus and, 48–49
Glanders, Pseudomonas mallei and, 285
Glomerulonephritis, Streptococcus pyogenes and, 225, 226, *226*, 227
Glossina, 536
Glucose fermentation, Enterobacteriaceae and, 318–319, *320*
Gnats, 535
Gohn lesion, in tuberculosis, 380, *380*
Gonorrhea, 268–270
    anorectal, 269–270
    disseminated, 270
    urogenital, 269
Gram-negative bacilli
    Centers for Disease Control group DF-3, 346–347
    Centers for Disease Control group EF-4, 346
    Centers for Disease Control group HB-5, 346–347
    facultative, 336–347
    fastidious, 293–302
    nonfastidious, glucose-nonfermenting, 281–290, 282t
        laboratory diagnosis of, 287–290, 288t
        prevention of, 290
        treatment of, 290

Gram-negative bacteria
 anaerobic. See Anaerobes, gram-negative; specific organisms
 potassium hydroxide test for distinguishing gram-positive bacteria from, 634
Gram-positive bacteria
 anaerobic. See Anaerobes, gram-positive
 potassium hydroxide test for distinguishing gram-negative bacteria from, 634
Gram-positive cocci, anaerobic. See Anaerobes, gram-positive cocci
Gram stain, 175, 631
 anaerobes and, 259
 bacteria in cerebrospinal fluid detected by, 545–546
Granulocytes. See specific granulocytes
Granuloma
 Blastomyces dermatitidis and, 447
 in Q fever, 206, 206
 Mycobacterium kansasii and, 384
Granuloma inguinale, Calymmatobacterium granulomatis and, 400
Green-nail syndrome, Pseudomonas aeruginosa and, 283
Ground itch, 484
Gummas, 364

Haemophilus, 336–342
 classification of, 336
 laboratory diagnosis of, 339t, 339–341
 susceptibility testing and, 341
Haemophilus aphrophilus, 339
 laboratory diagnosis of, organism identification and, 341
Haemophilus ducreyi, 338–339
 clinical manifestations of, 339
 epidemiology of, 338
 in genital ulcer specimens, 607
 in lymph node specimens, 581
 laboratory diagnosis of, organism identification and, 341
 pathogenesis and pathology of, 338–339
 treatment and prevention of, 342
Haemophilus haemolyticus, 339
Haemophilus influenzae, 336–338
 capsular serotypes, clinical manifestations of, 338
 epidemiology of, 336–337
 in throat specimens, 565
 laboratory diagnosis of, organism identification and, 340t, 340–341
 pathogenesis of, 337
 treatment and prevention of, 342, 342t
 type B, clinical manifestations of, 337–338
 unencapsulated, clinical manifestations of, 338
Haemophilus influenzae biotype aegyptius, clinical manifestations of, 338
Haemophilus parahemolyticus, 339
Haemophilus parainfluenzae, 339
 laboratory diagnosis of, organism identification and, 341
Haemophilus paraphrophilus, 339
 laboratory diagnosis of, organism identification and, 341
Hair specimens, 610–618
 collection, transport, and processing of, 610
Hand-foot-and-mouth disease, picornaviruses and, 108
Hansen's disease. See Leprosy
Hansenula, 419
 laboratory diagnosis of, cellular structure and colony characteristics in, 421
 treatment of, 423

Hansenula anomala, 419
Hansenula polymorpha, 419
Hantaan virus, 139
Hantavirus, 139
 clinical manifestations of, 139
 epidemiology of, 139
 pathogenesis of, 139
Haverill fever, 400–401
Head and neck infections, anaerobic gram-negative bacteria and, 357–358
Heart
 mumps virus and, 87
 Toxoplasma gondii and, 504
Helicobacter, 353–355
Helicobacter pylori, 353–355
 clinical manifestations of, 354
 epidemiology of, 353
 in gastrointestinal tissue specimens, 593
 laboratory diagnosis of, 354, 354–355
 pathogenesis of, 353
 treatment of, 355
Helminths, 470–471. See also specific organisms
 blood and tissue, 512–529
 intestinal, 482–495
Hemadsorption procedure, for detection of hemadsorbing viruses, 631
Hemagglutination treponemal tests for syphilis (HATTS), 365, 366
Hemorrhage-hepatitis syndrome, neonatal, picornaviruses and, 109
Hemorrhagic fever. See also Crimean-Congo hemorrhagic fever virus
 filoviruses and, 144–145
 Hantaan virus and, 139
Hemorrhagic necrosis, Aspergillus and, 433, 433
Hepatitis δ virus (HDV), 81
 laboratory diagnosis of, 81
Hepatitis δ virus antigen (HDAg), 81
Hepatitis A virus (enterovirus 72), 109–111
 clinical manifestations of, 110, 110–111
 epidemiology of, 109–111
 laboratory diagnosis of, 112
 pathogenesis of, 110
 prevention of, 113, 113t
 structure of, 109
Hepatitis B core antigen (HBcAg), 77, 80
Hepatitis B e antigen (HBeAg), 77, 80, 81
Hepatitis B immune globulin (HBIG), 82, 83
Hepatitis B surface antigen (HBsAg), 77, 80, 81
Hepatitis B virus, 81–82, 82t
 treatment and prevention of, 82–83, 83t
Hepatitis B virus (HBV), 77–81
 clinical manifestations of, 79–81, 80, 81
 epidemiology of, 77–79, 79, 79t
 fulminant hepatitis and, 80, 81
 pathogenesis of, 79
 persistent infection and, 80
 replication of, 77
 structure of, 77, 78
Hepatitis C virus (HCV), 163–165
 clinical manifestations of, 164–165
 epidemiology of, 164
 laboratory diagnosis of, 165
 pathogenesis of, 164
 structure and replication of, 164
 treatment and prevention of, 165
Hepatitis E virus (HEV), 165
 clinical manifestations of, 165
 epidemiology of, 165
 laboratory diagnosis of, 165
 structure of, 165
 treatment and prevention of, 165

Herpangina, picornaviruses and, 108
Herpes labialis, 49
Herpes simplex virus (HSV), 46, 48–49
 clinical manifestations of, 48–49, 49
 epidemiology of, 48
 in genital ulcer specimens, 607
 in urethral swab specimens, 605
 laboratory diagnosis of, 55–56, 56, 56t
 pathogenesis of, 48, 48
 prevention of, 60
 structure of, 48
 treatment of, 59
Herpes zoster, 50–51
Herpesviruses, 46–60. See also specific viruses
 classification of, 46
 laboratory diagnosis of, 55t, 55–59
 prevention of, 60
 replication of, 46
 structure of, 46, 47
 treatment of, 59
Heterophile antibodies, Epstein-Barr virus and, 58, 58t
Heterophyes heterophyes, 490–491, 491
Hippurate hydrolysis test, rapid, 633–634
Histiocytic necrotizing lymphadenitis, human herpesvirus 6 and, 54–55
Histoplasma capsulatum
 dimorphic, 458
 laboratory diagnosis of, 455, 455–456
Histoplasma capsulatum var capsulatum, 448–450
 clinical manifestations of, 449–450
 epidemiology of, 448–449
 pathogenesis and pathology of, 449
Histoplasma capsulatum var duboisii, 450
 clinical manifestations of, 450
 epidemiology of, 450
 pathology of, 450
Histoplasmosis, 448–450
 disseminated, 449, 450
 excessive fibrosis and, 449
 pulmonary
  acute, 449
  chronic, 449, 450
 treatment of, 458
Hookworms, 483–485, 484
Host defenses. See also Nonspecific defenses; Specific defenses
 disruption, evasion, and inactivation of, 22
Human diploid cell rabies virus, 127
Human herpesvirus 6 (HHV-6), 54–55
 clinical manifestations of, 54–55
 epidemiology of, 54
 structure of, 54
 treatment of, 59
Human immunodeficiency virus (HIV) types 1 and 2, 148–158
 clinical manifestations of, 153t, 153–156, 154, 155t
 epidemiology of, 149–152, 150, 150t, 151
 laboratory diagnosis of, 156, 156–157, 157t
 pathogenesis of, 152–153
 prevention of, 158
 replication of, 149, 149
 structure of, 148, 148–149
 treatment of, 157–158
Human papillomavirus (HPV), 70–72, 71t
 clinical manifestations of, 71–72
 epidemiology of, 70
 in conjunctival specimens, 553
 in gastrointestinal tissue specimens, 592
 in skin biopsy specimens, 616
 in urethral swab specimens, 605
 laboratory diagnosis of, 73, 73

pathogenesis of, 70–71, *71*
replication of, 70
structure of, 70
treatment of, 73
Human T-cell leukemia virus types I and II, 146–148
  clinical manifestations of, 147–148
  epidemiology of, 147
  laboratory diagnosis of, 156
  pathogenesis of, 147
  structure and replication of, 146–147
  treatment of, 157
Humoral immunity, 12–15
  B-cell activation and, 13–14
  immunoglobulin structure and, 13, 13t, *14*, 14t
  role in host defense, 14–15, 15t
Hyaline septate moulds, 430
  laboratory diagnosis of, 439–442
  treatment of, 443–444
Hydatid cyst, 526–529
  alveolar, 528–529
  unilocular, *527*, 527–528, *528*
Hydrogen sulfide production, Enterobacteriaceae and, 322
Hymenolepis diminuta, 494, *494*
Hymenolepis nana, *493*, 493–494

Id reactions, dermatophytes and, 428
Immune disorders
  antibody production and, 15, 15t
  cell-mediated, 20t
Immune globulin, hepatitis A virus and, 113, 113t
Immunity. *See* Cell-mediated immunity; Humoral immunity
Immunoglobulin(s), structure of, 13, 13t, *14*, 14t
Immunologic tests, 276
Immunosuppressed patients, cytomegalovirus in, 53
Impetigo
  Pseudomonas aeruginosa and, 283
  Staphylococcus aureus and, 219
  Streptococcus pyogenes and, 225, 227
India ink preparation, fungi in cerebrospinal fluid and, 546
Indole, Enterobacteriaceae and, 321
Infant
  botulism and, 254, 258
  Chlamydia trachomatis and, 186–187
  cytomegalovirus and, 52
  pertussis in, 298
Infectious diseases
  epidemiology of, 23
  pathogenesis of, 23
Infectious mononucleosis
  complications of, 54, 54t
  Epstein-Barr virus and, 53–54
  heterophile-negative, 52
  human herpesvirus 6 and, 54
Infective dose, 20
Inflammatory infiltrate, Treponema pallidum subspecies pallidum and, 362
Influenza, vesiculovirus and, 123
Influenza A virus. *See* Orthomyxoviruses
Influenza B virus. *See* Orthomyxoviruses
Insecta, 533–536. *See also specific organisms*
Interstitial pneumonitis, cytomegalovirus in, *52*, 53
Intertrigo, Candida and, 416
Intestine
  myiasis and, 536
  schistosomiasis and, 523, *524*

Intravascular catheter tips, 578
Isospora belli, 479–480, *480*
Israeli spotted fever, 200
Ixididae, 531–532, *533*

Jamestown Canyon virus, 138
Janeway lesions, viridans streptococci and, 229
Japanese encephalitis virus, 136–137
  clinical manifestations of, 137
  epidemiology of, 137
  laboratory diagnosis of, 137
  pathogenesis of, 137
JC virus. *See* Polyomavirus
Joint prostheses, infected
  Staphylococcus aureus and, 220
  Staphylococcus epidermidis and, 222
Junin virus, 142–143
  clinical manifestations of, 142–143
  epidemiology and epizootology of, 142
  laboratory diagnosis of, 143, 143t
  pathogenesis of, 142
  treatment and prevention of, 143

Kala-azar, 499, *500*
Kaposi's sarcoma, human immunodeficiency virus types 1 and 2 and, 155
Keratitis
  Acanthamoeba and, 502–503
  mycotic, 429
    Aspergillus and, 433
Kidney, needle aspirates of, 603
Kingella denitrificans, 287
  laboratory diagnosis of, organism identification and, 290
Kingella indologenes, 287
Kingella kingae, 287
  laboratory diagnosis of, organism identification and, 290
  treatment of, 290
Kinyoun stain, 175, 632
Klebsiella, features of, 324
Klebsiella oxytoca, 316, 317
  features of, 324
Klebsiella ozaenae, 316, 317
  in nasopharyngeal and nasal specimens, 563
Klebsiella pneumoniae, 316–317
  features of, 324
Klebsiella rhinoscleromatis, 316, 317
Kligler's iron agar (KIA), Enterobacteriaceae and, 318–319, 322
Knott's concentration, parasites in blood specimens and, 578
Kurthia bessonii, 244
Kuru. *See* Prions

LaCrosse virus, 138–139
β-Lactamase detection, 179, *180*
  anaerobe susceptibility testing and, 180
Lactobacillus, 243–244, 263
  laboratory diagnosis of, 264
Lactococcus garviae, 231
Langerhans cells, 16
Larva migrans, 536
Larval migrans, visceral, 517–518, *519*
Lassa virus, 141–142
  clinical manifestations of, 142
  epidemiology and epizootology of, 141–142
  pathogenesis of, 142
Latex agglutination
  bacteria and, 176

  in cerebrospinal fluid, 546
  fungi and, in cerebrospinal fluid, 546
Legionella, 299–302, 300t
  acid-wash treatment of contaminated specimens to enhance recovery of, 636
  clinical manifestations of, 301
  epidemiology of, 300
  in body cavity specimens, 621
  in sputum and tracheal aspirates, 567–568
  laboratory diagnosis of, 301–302, 302t
  pathogenesis and pathology of, 300–301
  treatment and prevention of, 302
Legionella birminghamensis, 300
Legionella bozemanii, 300
Legionella cincinnatiensis, 300
Legionella dumoffi, 300
Legionella feeleii, 300
Legionella hackeliae, 300
Legionella micdadei, 299, 300
Legionella pneumophila, 299, 300, 301
Legionella wadsworthii, 300
Legionnaires' disease, 300–302
Leishmania, 497–499
Leishmania aethiopica, 497–498
Leishmania chagasi, 499
Leishmania donovani, 499
Leishmania infantum, 499
Leishmania mexicana, 497–498
Leishmania venezuelensis, 497–498
Leishmaniasis, 497–499, 535
  cutaneous, 497–499, *498*, *499*
  visceral, 499, *500*
Lepromin test, 389–390
Leprosy, 387–390
  borderline, 388–389
  indeterminate, 388
  lepromatous, 388, *388*
  tuberculoid, 388, *388*
Leptomyxid amoeba, 502–503
Leptospira biflexa, 373
Leptospira interrogans, 373
  in blood specimens, 577
  in urine specimens, 603
Leptospirosis, 373–374
  anicteric, 373–374
  clinical manifestations of, 373–374
  epidemiology of, 373
  laboratory diagnosis of, 374
  pathogenesis and pathology of, 373
  treatment and prevention of, 374
Leuconostoc, 231
  laboratory diagnosis of, 233, 233t
Leukemia, human T-cell leukemia virus types I and II and, 147
Leukoencephalopathy, multifocal, progressive, polyomavirus and, 72–73
Lice, 533–534, *534*
  and typhus, epidemic, 202
Lipopolysaccharide (LPS), bacterial, 173
Listeria monocytogenes, 241–243
  clinical manifestations of, 242
  epidemiology of, 241–242
  in liver tissue specimens, 598
  in stool and rectal swab specimens, 588
  laboratory diagnosis of, 242t, 242–243, 243t
  pathogenesis of, 242
  treatment of, 243
Listeriosis. *See* Listeria monocytogenes
Liver
  herpes simplex virus and, 49, *49*
  schistosomiasis and, 523–524
Liver abscess specimens, 595–596, 596t
  bacteria in, 595
  collection, transport, and processing of, 595

Liver abscess specimens (*Continued*)
  fungi in, 595–596
  parasites in, 596
Liver tissue specimens, 597, 597–599
  bacteria in, 598
  collection, transport, and processing of, 597
  fungi in, 598
  parasites in, 598–599
  viruses in, 597–598
Loa loa, 514–515, *515*, 536
Loboa loboi, 460
  clinical manifestations of, 460
  epidemiology of, 460
  laboratory diagnosis of, 461
  pathology of, 460, *461*
  treatment of, 461–462
Lobomycosis, 460
Loeffler's syndrome, 484–485
  Ascaris lumbricoides and, 485
Louse-borne typhus, epidemic, 202
Lutzomia, 535
Lyme disease, 368–370
Lymph node specimens, 580–582, 581t
  bacteria in, 581
  collection, transport, and processing of, 581
  fungi in, 581–582
  parasites in, 582
Lymphadenitis
  cervical, Mycobacterium avium-intracellulare and, 384
  necrotizing, histiocytic, human herpesvirus 6 and, 54–55
Lymphadenopathy, human immunodeficiency virus types 1 and 2 and, 154
Lymphocytic choriomeningitis virus, 141
  clinical manifestations of, 141
  epidemiology and epizootology of, 141
  pathogenesis of, 141
Lymphogranuloma venereum, Chlamydia trachomatis and, 186
Lymphoma
  African Burkitt's, Epstein-Barr virus and, 53, 54
  human T-cell leukemia virus types I and II and, 147
  non-Hodgkin's, human immunodeficiency virus types 1 and 2 and, 155
Lysine iron agar (LIA), Enterobacteriaceae and, 321–322
Lysis-centrifugation blood culture system, 576
Lyssavirus, 123–127. *See also* Rabies virus

Machupo virus, 142–143
  clinical manifestations of, 142–143
  epidemiology and epizootology of, 142
  laboratory diagnosis of, 143, 143t
  pathogenesis of, 142
  treatment and prevention of, 143
Macroconidia, 409, *410*
Mailing, of infectious material, 543
Major histocompatibility complex, 16–17
Mal de pinto, 364–365
Malaria, *505*, 505–508, 535
Malassezia, 418–419
  clinical manifestations of, 418–419
  epidemiology of, 418
  pathogenesis of, 418
Malassezia furfur, 418–419
  laboratory diagnosis of, cellular structure and colony characteristics in, 420–421
  treatment of, 423
Malassezia pachydermatis, 418

Malta fever, 295
Mansonella, 515–516, *516*
Mansonella ozzardi, 515, 516, *516*
Mansonella perstans, 515, 516, *516*
Mansonella streptocerca, 515, 516
Mansonia, 535
Mantoux test, 389
Marburg virus. *See* Filoviruses
Mastitis, Staphylococcus aureus and, 219
Measles
  atypical, 90
  3-day. *See* Rubella virus
Measles virus, 88–90
  clinical manifestations of, 90
  epidemiology of, 88–89, *89*
  in brain tissue specimens, 549
  laboratory diagnosis of, 92
  pathogenesis of, 89–90, *90*
  prevention of, 93–94, 94t
  structure of, 88
Media
  for bacterial culture, 540–541, 541t
  for fungal culture, 542
  for viral culture, 39
Melioidosis, 285–286
Meningeal symptoms, mumps virus and, 88
Meningitis
  aseptic
    human immunodeficiency virus types 1 and 2 and, 155
    picornaviruses and, 107
  Aspergillus and, 433
  cerebrospinal fluid specimens and, 544
  Cryptococcus neoformans and, treatment of, 423
  epidemic, Neisseria meningitidis and, 270, *270*
  Escherichia coli and, 310
  Haemophilus influenzae and, 337
  lymphocytic choriomeningitis virus and, 141
  mumps virus and, 88
  Neisseria meningitidis and, 270–271
  neonatal, Pseudomonas aeruginosa and, 284
  Plesiomonas shigelloides and, 333
  Pseudomonas aeruginosa and, 284
  pyogenic
    Staphylococcus aureus and, 220
    Streptococcus pneumoniae and, 228–229
Meningococcemia, Neisseria meningitidis and, 271
Meningoencephalitis
  chronic, picornaviruses and, 109
  Cryptococcus neoformans and, 418
  eosinophilic, Angiostrongylus cantonensis and, 518–520, *519*
  Naegleria fowleri and, 501–502, *502*
  Neisseria meningitidis and, 271
Methyl red test, Enterobacteriaceae and, 320–321
Microbes
  disruption, evasion, and inactivation of host defenses by, 22
  elaboration of toxins and enzymes and, 21–22, 22t
  infective dose and, 20
  penetration of anatomic barriers by, 20–21
  resistance to antimicrobial agents, 22–23
  surface characteristics of, 21, 21t
    endotoxin and, 21
Microbial factors, 19–23
Micrococcaceae, 218–225, 219t
Microhemagglutination-Treponema pallidum (MHA-TP) test, 365–366

Microimmunofluorescence test, Chlamydia pneumoniae and, 190
Microscopy
  bacteria and, 175
  laboratory diagnosis of fungi and, 411–412, *412*
Microspora, 470, 480, 509
Microsporium canis, 426
Microsporum audouinii, 436
Middle ear drainage fluid, 557t, 557–558
  collection, transport, and processing of, 557
Minimum bactericidal concentration (MBC), 182
Mites, 530–531
MMU 18006 vaccine, 119
Mokola virus, 126
Molluscum contagiosum
  clinical manifestations of, 44
  epidemiology and pathogenesis of, 44
  in conjunctival specimens, 551
  in skin biopsy specimens, 615
Monoclonal antibodies
  bacteria and, 175
  direct detection of viruses and, 41
Monocyte/macrophage cell, 16
Mononuclear phagocytes, 16
  development, structure, and activation of, 16
  role in host defense, 16, 17t
Moraten vaccine, 93–94
Moraxella, 287
  laboratory diagnosis of, organism identification and, 289–290
  treatment of, 290
Mosquitoes, 534–535, *535*
Motility, Enterobacteriaceae and, 322
Moulds, 426–444. *See also specific organisms*
  hyaline septate, 430
    laboratory diagnosis of, 439–442
    treatment of, 443–444
  laboratory diagnosis of, 436t, 436–442
  morphologic appearance of, 408, *408*, *409*
  treatment of, 442–444
Mucorales, 434
Mucormycosis, 435–436
  central nervous system, 436
  cutaneous, 435
  gastrointestinal, 435–436
  pulmonary, 435
  rhinocerebral, 435
Mucous membranes, Rhinosporidium seeberi and, 461
Mumps virus, 87–88
  clinical manifestations of, 88, 88t
  epidemiology of, 87
  laboratory diagnosis of, 92
  pathogenesis of, 87–88
  prevention of, 93
  structure of, 87
  treatment of, 93
Murine typhus, 201–202
Musca domestica, 536
Muscidae, 536
Muscle(s)
  actinomycosis and, 263
  Pseudomonas mallei and, 285
Muscle specimens, 623–624, 624t
  bacteria in, 624, 624t
  collection, transport, and processing of, 623–624, *624*
  fungi in, 624, 624t
Myalgia, epidemic. *See* Pleurodynia

Mycetoma, 430
  clinical manifestations of, 430
  epidemiology of, 430
  pathology of, 430
Mycobacteria, 175, 378–395. *See also specific organisms*
  N-acetyl-L cysteine (NALC)-sodium hydroxide (NaOH) procedure to liquefy, decontaminate, and concentrate specimens for identification of, 635–636
  laboratory diagnosis of, 389–393
    culture and, 391t, 391–392, *392, 393*
    microbial stains and, 390, 390t
    organism identification in, 390t, 390–393
    skin testing in, 389–390
  nontuberculous, 382, 382t
  rarely pathogenic, 386–387
  susceptibility testing and, 392–393
  treatment of, 393, 394t
  tuberculous, 378–382
Mycobacterium
  in aspirates and swab specimens from cutaneous ulcers, 613
  in aspirates from wound infections and abscesses, 615
  in blood specimens, 577
  in body cavity specimens, 621
  in cerebrospinal fluid, 546
  in gastric contents specimens, 586
  in gastrointestinal tissue specimens, 593
  in liver and pancreas abscess specimens, 595
  in liver tissue specimens, 598
  in lymph node specimens, 581
  in muscle specimens, 624
  in skin biopsy specimens, 616
  in sputum and tracheal aspirates, 568
  in stool and rectal swab specimens, 590
  incubation of, 541
Mycobacterium africanum, 382
Mycobacterium asiaticum, 387
Mycobacterium avium-intracellulare (MAI), 382–384
  clinical manifestations of, 383–384
  epidemiology of, 382–383
  pathogenesis and pathology of, 383, *383*
Mycobacterium bovis, 381–382
Mycobacterium flavescens, 387
Mycobacterium fordonae, 386
Mycobacterium fortuitum-chelonae complex, 384–385
  clinical manifestations of, 385
  epidemiology of, 384
  pathology of, 385
Mycobacterium haemophilum, 386
Mycobacterium kansasii, 384
  clinical manifestations of, 384
  epidemiology of, 384
  pathology of, 384
Mycobacterium leprae, 387–390
  clinical manifestations of, *388*, 388–389
  epidemiology of, 387
  in nasopharyngeal and nasal specimens, 563
  pathogenesis of, 387–388
  prevention of, 395
Mycobacterium malmoense, 385
Mycobacterium marinum, 386
Mycobacterium neoaurum, 387
Mycobacterium nonchromogenicum, 387
Mycobacterium paratuberculosis, 387
Mycobacterium scrofulaceum, 384
Mycobacterium shimoidei, 387
Mycobacterium simiae, 385–386
Mycobacterium smegmatis, 387
Mycobacterium szulgai, 382, 385
Mycobacterium terrae-triviale complex, 387
Mycobacterium thermoresistible, 387
Mycobacterium tuberculosis, 378–381
  clinical manifestations of, 380–381, 381t
  epidemiology of, 378–379, *379*
  in brain abscess and empyema specimens, 548
  in conjunctival specimens, 554
  in oropharyngeal ulcer specimens, 559
  in urine specimens, 603
  pathogenesis of, 379–380
  pathology of, 380, *380*
  prevention of, 393–395
Mycobacterium ulcerans, 386
  clinical manifestations of, 386
  epidemiology of, 386
  pathology of, 386
Mycobacterium xenopi, 385
  clinical manifestations of, 385
  epidemiology of, 385
  pathology of, 385
Mycoplasma hominis, 215–216
  clinical manifestations of, 215
  epidemiology of, 215
  laboratory diagnosis of, 215–216
  treatment and prevention of, 216
Mycoplasma pneumoniae, 214–215
  clinical manifestations of, 215
  epidemiology of, 214
  in body cavity specimens, 620
  in endomyocardial biopsy specimens, 579
  in sputum and tracheal aspirates, 567
  in throat specimens, 564–565
  pathogenesis and pathology of, 214–215
Mycoses. *See* Fungi; *specific fungi*
Myelopathy
  human T-cell leukemia virus types I and II and, 147–148
  progressive, chronic, human T-cell leukemia virus types I and II and, 147–148
  vacuolar, human immunodeficiency virus types 1 and 2 and, 155
Myiasis, 536, *536*
  cutaneous, 536, *536*
  of eyes, intestine, and urogenital tract, 536
  of wounds, ulcers, and moribund flesh, 536
Myocarditis, Corynebacterium diphtheriae and, 245
Myonecrosis
  Clostridium perfringens and, 256
  Clostridium septicum and, 258
Myopericarditis, picornaviruses and, 109

Naegleria fowleri, 501–502, *502*
Nail specimens, 610
  collection, transport, and processing of, 610
Nairovirus, 140
Nanophyetus salmincola, 490, *490*
Nasal disease, Rhinosporidium seeberi and, 461
Nasal specimens, 561–563, 562t
  bacteria in, 562–563
  collection, transport, and processing of, 561–563
  fungi in, 563
  parasites in, 563
  viruses in, 561–562, 562t
Nasopharyngeal carcinoma, Epstein-Barr virus and, 54
Nasopharyngeal specimens, 561–563, 562t
  bacteria in, 562–563
  collection, transport, and processing of, 561–563
  fungi in, 563
  parasites in, 563
  viruses in, 561–562, 562t
Natural killer (NK) cells, 18–19
  role in host defense, 19, 19t
Necrotizing fasciitis, type II, Streptococcus pyogenes and, 227
Neisseria, 268–272
  laboratory diagnosis of, 272–277, 273t
    chromogenic enzyme substrate tests and, 275–276
    commercial carbohydrate degradation kits and, 275
    conventional biochemical tests and, 274–275
    direct detection tests and, 276
    immunologic tests and, 276
    microscopic features and colony characteristics and, 272–273, 274t
    organism identification and, 273–274
    typing of isolates and, 276
  susceptibility testing and, 276–277
Neisseria cinerea, 271–272
  laboratory diagnosis of, 275–276
Neisseria denitrificans, laboratory diagnosis of, 276
Neisseria elongata, 271–272
  laboratory diagnosis of, organism identification and, 273
Neisseria flavescens, 271–272
Neisseria gonorrhoeae, 268–270
  clinical manifestations of, 269–270
  epidemiology of, 268–269
  in stool and rectal swab specimens, 589
  in throat specimens, 565
  in urethral swab specimens, 605–606
  in urine specimens, 603
  in vaginal specimens, 604
  laboratory diagnosis of, 274, 275t, 275–276
    microscopic features and colony characteristics and, 272, 273t
    organism identification and, 273, 274
  pathogenesis of, 269
  penicillinase-producing strains of, 269
  prevention and control of, 277
  structure of, 268
  susceptibility testing and, 276–277
  tetracycline-resistant strains of, 269
  treatment of, 277
Neisseria lactamica, 271
  laboratory diagnosis of, 275
Neisseria meningitidis, 270–271
  clinical manifestations of, 271
  epidemiology of, *270*, 270–271
  laboratory diagnosis of, 275, 276
    microscopic features and colony characteristics and, 272
  pathogenesis of, 271
  prevention and control of, 277
  structure of, 270
  susceptibility testing and, 277
Neisseria mucosa, 271–272
Neisseria perflava, laboratory diagnosis of, 276
Neisseria polysaccharea, 271–272
  laboratory diagnosis of, 275
Neisseria sicca, 271–272
  laboratory diagnosis of, microscopic features and colony characteristics and, 272–273
Neisseria subflava, 271–272
Nematodes, 470–471. *See also specific organisms*

Nematodes (*Continued*)
  blood and tissue, 512–520
  in sputum and tracheal aspirates, 568–569
  intestinal, 482–489
Neonate
  bacteremia in, Escherichia coli and, 310
  herpes simplex virus infection in, 48
  listeriosis in, 242
  meningitis in
    Escherichia coli and, 310
    Pseudomonas aeruginosa and, 284
  picornaviruses and, 109
  Streptococcus agalactiae and, 228
  tetanus in, 256
    prevention of, 262
Neurosyphilis
  late, 362, 363
  meningovascular, 362, 363
  parenchymatous, 362, 363
Neutrophils, 9–11
  development, structure, and activation of, 9–10, 10t
  role in host defense, 10–11, *11*, 12t
Nitrate reduction, Enterobacteriaceae and, 319–320
o-Nitrophenyl-β-D-galactopyranoside (ONPG) test, 274
  Enterobacteriaceae and, 321
Nocardia, 248–250
  clinical manifestations of, 248–249
  in aspirates from wound infections and abscesses, 615
  in body cavity specimens, 621
  in brain abscess and empyema specimens, 548
  in liver tissue specimens, 598
  in skin biopsy specimens, 616
  laboratory diagnosis of, 249, 249t
  pathogenesis and pathology of, 248
  treatment of, 249–250
Nocardia asteroides, 248–249
  in sputum and tracheal aspirates, 567
Nocardia brasiliensis, 248
Nocardia cariae (Nocardia otitidiscavarium), 248
Nocardia transvalensis, 248
Nocardiopsis, 249
  laboratory diagnosis of, 249
Nocardiosis. *See* Nocardia
Non-A, non-B hepatitis virus, 163–165. *See also* Hepatitis C virus; Hepatitis E virus
Non-Hodgkin's lymphoma, human immunodeficiency virus types 1 and 2 and, 155
Nonselective media, 175–176, 176t
Nonspecific defenses, 5–12
  complement and, 7t, 7–9
    activation of, 7, *8*, *9*
    role in host defense, 7, 9, 9t, 10t
  granulocytes and, 9–12
    basophils and, 12
    eosinophils and, 11–12
    neutrophils and, 9–11
  physical barriers and secretions as, 5–9
    eyes and, 5
    gastrointestinal tract and, 7
    genitourinary tract and, 7
    normal flora and, 5, 6t
    respiratory tract and, 5–7
    skin and, 5
Nontreponemal tests, 365
North Asian tick typhus, 200
Norwalk-like viruses, 163

Norwalk virus, 163, *164*
  clinical manifestations of, 163
  laboratory diagnosis of, 163
  structure of, 163
  treatment of, 163
Novobiocin, disk-diffusion test for resistance to, 633
Nucleic acid hybridization, direct detection of viruses and, 41
Nucleic acid probes, 276
  bacteria and, 177

Ocular abscesses, specimens from, 555–556
  collection, transport, and processing of, 555
Oculomycosis
  endogenous, Aspergillus and, 433
  extension, Aspergillus and, 433
Oerskovia, laboratory diagnosis of, 249
Oerskovia turbata, 249
Oerskovia xanthineolytica, 249
Oligella, laboratory diagnosis of, organism identification and, 289–290
Oligella urethralis, 287
Onchocerca volvulus, 514, *515*, 536
Onychomycosis, 429
  Candida and, 416
Open lung biopsy specimens, 570–571
  bacteria in, 571
  fungi in, 571
  parasites in, 571
  viruses in, 570–571
Ophthalmia neonatorum, Neisseria gonorrhoeae and, 270
Opistorchis, 521–522
Optichin sensitivity, test for, 634
Orbivirus, 116, 117t
Orfloxacin, in boutonneuse fever, 201
Oriental spotted fever, 200
Ornithonyssus bacoti, 530
Orofacial infection specimens, 558, 558t
Orofacial lesions, herpes simplex virus and, 49
Oropharyngeal ulcer specimens, 558t, 558–559
Oroya fever, 210, 535
Orthomyxoviruses, 97–101
  classification of, 97
  clinical manifestations of, 99
  epidemiology of, 98–99
  laboratory diagnosis of, 99–100, *100*
  pathogenesis of, 99
  replication of, 97–98
  structure of, 97, *98*, 98t
  treatment and prevention of, 100–101
Orthoreoviruses, 116
Osler's nodes, viridans streptococci and, 229
Osteomyelitis
  Candida and, 416–417
  Mycobacterium fortuitum-chelonae and, 385
  Staphylococcus aureus and, 220
Otitis externa, Pseudomonas aeruginosa and, 284
Otitis media, Pseudomonas aeruginosa and, 284
Otomycosis, 432–433
Oxidase test, Enterobacteriaceae and, 318
Oxyurida, 471

Paecilomyces, 434, 442
Pancreatic abscess specimens, 595–596, 596t
  bacteria in, 595

  collection, transport, and processing of, 595
  fungi in, 595–596
  parasites in, 596
Pandemics, of influenza, 99
Panencephalitis, sclerosing, subacute
  cerebrospinal fluid and, 545
  measles virus and, 90
Papanicolaou stain, herpes simplex virus and, 55, 56t
Papillomatosis, respiratory, 71–72
Papovaviruses, 70–74. *See also specific viruses*
Pappataci fever, 535
Paracoccidioides brasiliensis, 451–452
  clinical manifestations of, 452
  epidemiology of, 451–452
  laboratory diagnosis of, 457
  pathogenesis and pathology of, 452, *452*
Paracoccidioidomycosis, 451–452
  juvenile, 452
Paragonimus, *522*, 522–523
Paragonimus westermani, 522
Parainfluenza viruses, 85–87
  clinical manifestations of, 87
  epidemiology of, 85–86
  laboratory diagnosis of, 91–92, *92*
  pathogenesis of, 86–87
  structure of, 85
  treatment of, 93
Paralysis
  picornaviruses and, 107–108
  polioviruses and, 107
  tick, 532–533
Paramyxoviruses, 85–94
  classification of, 85
  replication of, 85, *86*
  structure of, 85, *86*
Paraparesis, spastic, tropical, human T-cell leukemia virus types I and II and, 147–148
Parapsilosis, 416
Parasites, 469–471. *See also specific organisms*
  classification of, 470–471
  diagnosis of, 469–470
  in anterior chamber, vitreous cavity, and ocular abscess specimens, 555–556
  in aspirates and swab specimens from cutaneous ulcers, 614
  in blood specimens, 578
  in body cavity specimens, 620t, 621
  in bone marrow specimens, 580, 580t
  in brain abscess and empyema specimens, 548
  in brain tissue specimens, 549
  in bronchial washing, protected specimen brush, and bronchoalveolar lavage specimens, 570
  in cerebrospinal fluid, 545t, 546–547
  in corneal specimens, 555
  in endomyocardial biopsy specimens, 580
  in gastrointestinal tissue specimens, 594
  in liver and pancreas abscess specimens, 596
  in liver tissue specimens, 598–599
  in lymph node specimens, 582
  in middle ear fluid, 558
  in nasopharyngeal and nasal specimens, 563
  in orofacial infection specimens, 558
  in oropharyngeal ulcer specimens, 559
  in sinus aspirates, 557
  in skin biopsy specimens, 615t, 616–618, *617*, *618*
  in sputum and tracheal aspirates, 568–569

INDEX

in stool and rectal swab specimens, 590–591
in transbronchial and open lung biopsy specimens, 571
in urine specimens, 603
in vaginal specimens, 605
life cycles of, 469
specimen handling and, 542–543
Parateneses, 529
Paronychia, Candida and, 416
Partial acid-fast stain, 632
Particle agglutination tests, bacteria and, 176–177
Particle assembly, viruses and, 36, 38
Parvovirus B19, 75–76
clinical manifestations of, 75–76
diagnosis of, 76
epidemiology of, 75
pathogenesis of, 75
treatment and prevention of, 76
Parvoviruses, 75–76
classification of, 75
structure and replication of, 75
Pasteurella, 342–343
Pasteurella multicida
clinical manifestations of, 342–343
epidemiology and pathogenesis of, 342
laboratory diagnosis of, 343
treatment of, 343
Pediculus humanus capitis, 533, *534*
Pediculus humanus humanus, 533, *534*
Pediococcus, laboratory diagnosis of, 233t, 233–234
Pediococcus acidilactici, 231
Pelvic infections, anaerobic gram-negative bacteria and, 358
Pelvic inflammatory disease (PID), Neisseria gonorrhoeae and, 269
Penetration, by viruses, 36
Penicillium, 434, 442
Peptic ulcer disease, Helicobacter pylori and, 353
Peptostreptococcus anaerobius, 265
Peptostreptococcus magnus, 265
Peptostreptococcus micros, 265
Peptostreptococcus prevotii, 265
Perianal infection, herpes simplex virus and, 49
Periodontitis, juvenile, Actinobacillus and, 343
Peripheral neuropathy, human immunodeficiency virus types 1 and 2 and, 155
Peritonitis, Candida and, 417
Pertussis, 297–299
Petechiae
conjunctival, viridans streptococci and, 229
cutaneous, viridans streptococci and, 229
Neisseria meningitidis and, 271
Phaeophyphomycosis, 429–430
cutaneous, 429
subcutaneous, 429, *430*
superficial, 429
treatment of, 443
systemic, 430
Phagocytosis, by neutrophils, 10
Pharyngitis
Chlamydia pneumoniae and, 188
herpes simplex virus and, 48–49
lymphonodular, picornaviruses and, 108
Streptococcus pyogenes and, 225, 226
Phenylalanine deaminase production, Enterobacteriaceae and, 322
Phialoconidia, 409, *410*

Phlebitis, intracranial, suppurative, Staphylococcus aureus and, 220
Phlebotomus, 535
Phlebotomus fever, 535
Phlebovirus, 139
Phthirius pubis, 533, *534*
Pian, 364
Picornaviruses, 105–113
classification of, 105, 106t
clinical manifestations of, 107–109, 108t
replication of, 105
structure of, 105, *106*
Piedra, black, 429
Pili, bacterial, 174
Pinta, 364–365
treatment of, 367
Pinworn, 482, *483*
Piry virus, 123
Pityriasis versicolor, treatment of, 423
Plagellates, 472–474
Plague, 315–316
bubonic, 316
pneumonic, 316
sylvatic, 316
treatment and prevention of, 325
urban (domestic), 316
prevention of, 325
Plaque reduction assay, antiviral agent susceptibility testing and, 41
Plasmodium, *505*, 505–508
eighteen to thirty-six hours, 507–508
first six hours, *506*, 506–507
six to eighteen hours, 507, *507*
thirty-six to forty-eight hours, 508, *508*
three weeks or more, 508, *508*
Plasmodium falciparum, 505, 506, 507, 508
Plasmodium malariae, 505, 506, 507, 508
Plasmodium ovale, 505, 506, 507–508
Plasmodium vivax, 505, 506, 507, 508
Plesiomonas shigelloides, 333–334
clinical manifestations of, 333–334
epidemiology and pathogenesis of, 333
in stool and rectal swab specimens, 590
laboratory diagnosis of, 334
organism identification and, 334
treatment of, 334
Pleurodynia, picornaviruses and, 108
Pleuropulmonary infections, anaerobic gram-negative bacteria and, 358
Pneumocystis carinii, *509*, 509–511, *510*
in bronchial washing, protected specimen brush, and bronchoalveolar lavage specimens, 570
in sputum and tracheal aspirates, 568
Pneumonia
Aspergillus and, 432
Candida and, 416, *417*
Chlamydia pneumoniae and, 188
community-acquired
Klebsiella pneumoniae and, 316–317
Staphylococcus aureus and, 220
Streptococcus pneumoniae and, 228
coronaviruses and, 102
Francisella tularensis and, 294
in Q fever, 207
measles virus and, 90
Mycoplasma pneumoniae and, 215
nosocomial, Staphylococcus aureus and, 220
orthomyxoviruses and, 99
Pneumocystis carinii and, 509, 510–511
Pseudomonas aeruginosa and, 284
Streptococcus agalactiae and, 228
Pneumonitis
Ascaris lumbricoides and, 485

hookworms and, 484–485
interstitial
Chlamydia trachomatis and, 187
cytomegalovirus in, *52*, 53
Poliomyelitis, nonparalytic, 107
Polioviruses, 106–107
clinical manifestations of, 107
epidemiology of, 107
pathogenesis of, 107
prevention of, 112–113
Polyclonal antibodies, bacteria and, 175
Polymerase chain reaction, bacteria and, 177
Polymorphonuclear leukocytes, Blastomyces dermatitidis and, 447
Polymorphonuclear neutrophils (PMN). See Neutrophils
Polyomavirus, 72–73
clinical manifestations of, 72–73
epidemiology of, 72
in brain tissue specimens, 549
laboratory diagnosis of, 73
pathogenesis and histologic appearance of, *72*, *72*, *73*
structure and replication of, 72
treatment of, 74
Pontiac fever, 301
Porphyromonas, treatment of, 359–360
Postoperative infections, Mycobacterium fortuitum-chelonae and, 385
Potassium hydroxide (KOH) solubility test
anaerobes and, 259
for distinguishing gram-positive and gram-negative bacteria, 634
for identification of fungal elements, 634
Poxviruses, 43–45
classification of, 43, 43t
laboratory diagnosis of, *44*, 44–45
structure and replication of, 43
treatment and prevention of, 45
Pregnancy, listeriosis during, 242
Prevotella, treatment of, 359–360
Prevotella denticola, laboratory diagnosis of, 359
Prevotella intermedia
laboratory diagnosis of, 359
pathogenesis of, 357
Prevotella loescheii, laboratory diagnosis of, 359
Prevotella melaninogenica
laboratory diagnosis of, 359
pathogenesis of, 357
Prevotella oralis, pathogenesis of, 357
Prions, 165–168
clinical manifestations of, 167–168
epidemiology of, 167
laboratory diagnosis of, 168
pathogenesis and pathology of, 167
structure and replication of, 16–167, *166*
treatment and prevention of, 168
Products of conception, 608
Progressive multifocal leukoencephalopathy (PML), polyomavirus and, 72–73
Propionibacterium, 263
laboratory diagnosis of, 264–265
Propionibacterium acnes, 263–264
treatment of, 265
Propionibacterium avidium, 263
Propionibacterium granulosum, 263
Prospect Hill virus, 139
Protected specimen brush specimens, 569–570
bacteria in, 569–570
fungi in, 570
parasites in, 570
viruses in, 569

Proteus mirabilis, 317
  features of, 324
Proteus vulgaris, 317
  features of, 324
  treatment and prevention of, 325
Prototheca, 463–464
  clinical manifestations of, 463
  epidemiology of, 463
  laboratory diagnosis of, 463–464
  pathogenesis and pathology of, 463, 464
  treatment of, 464
Protozoa, 470. *See also specific organisms*
  blood and tissue, 497–511
  intestinal, 472–481
Providencia
  features of, 324
  treatment and prevention of, 325
Pseudallescheria boydii, 433
  laboratory diagnosis of, 440–441, *442*
Pseudoappendicular syndrome, Yersinia and, 315
Pseudomembranous colitis, Clostridium difficile and, 257–258
  treatment of, 262
Pseudomonas, 281, 283t, 283–286
Pseudomonas aeruginosa, 281, 283–284
  clinical manifestations of, 283–284
  epidemiology of, 281, 283, 283t
  in aspirates and swab specimens from cutaneous ulcers, 613
  in gastrointestinal tissue specimens, 593
  laboratory diagnosis of, organism identification and, 288–289
  pathogenesis of, 283, 283t
  treatment of, 290
Pseudomonas cepacia, 281, 285
  clinical manifestations of, 285
  epidemiology of, 285
  laboratory diagnosis of, organism identification and, 289
  pathogenesis of, 285
  treatment of, 290
Pseudomonas mallei, 285
  clinical manifestations of, 285
  epidemiology of, 285
  laboratory diagnosis of, organism identification and, 289
  prevention of, 290
  treatment of, 290
Pseudomonas pseudomallei, 285–286
  clinical manifestations of, 286
  epidemiology of, 285–286
  laboratory diagnosis of, organism identification and, 289
  prevention of, 290
Pseudoterranova, 489
Psittacosis, Chlamydia psittaci and, 187
Psychodopygus, 535
Pulex irritans, 534, *534*
Pulmonary complications, of orthomyxoviruses, 99
Pulmonary disease
  Aspergillus and, 432
  Blastomyces dermatitidis and, 448
  Chlamydia psittaci and, 187
  Cryptococcus neoformans and, 418
  Mycobacterium avium-intracellulare and, 383
  Mycobacterium fortuitum-chelonae and, 385
  Mycobacterium kansasii and, 384
  Mycobacterium xenopi and, 385
  Nocardia and, 248
  Pasteurella multicida and, 343

  picornaviruses and, 108
  Pseudomonas mallei and, 285
  Pseudomonas pseudomallei and, 286
  respiratory syncytial virus and, 91
  Rocky Mountain spotted fever and, 199
  Toxoplasma gondii and, 504
  trematodes and, *522*, 522–523
Purified protein derivative (PPD) test, 389
Puumala virus, 139
Pyelonephritis
  Candida and, 416
  Staphylococcus aureus and, 220
Pyoderma. *See* Impetigo

Q fever, *205*, 205–208
  clinical manifestations of, 207
  epidemiology of, 206
  laboratory diagnosis of, 207
  pathogenesis of, *206*, 206–207
  treatment of, 207–208
Queensland tick typhus, 200

Rabies-related viruses, 126
Rabies virus, 123–127
  clinical manifestations of, 125–126
  epidemiology of, 124–125, *125*, 125t
  in conjunctival specimens, 553
  in skin biopsy specimens, 616
  laboratory diagnosis of, 126
  pathogenesis and pathology of, 125, *126*
  prevention of, 127, 127t
  structure of, 124
  treatment of, 126
Rapid hippurate hydrolysis test, 633–634
Rash
  dermatophytes and, 428
  Francisella tularensis and, 294
  in Rocky Mountain spotted fever, 198–199
  Neisseria meningitidis and, 271
  rubella virus and, 132
Rat-bite fever
  Spirillum minus and, 375
  Streptobacillus moniliformis and, 401
Recombinant IFN-α, in human immunodeficiency virus types 1 and 2, 158
Recombinant soluble CD4 preparations, in human immunodeficiency virus types 1 and 2, 157, 158
Rectal swab specimens, 586–592, 587t
  bacteria in, 588–590, 589t, 590t
  collection, transport, and processing of, 591–592
  parasites in, 590–591
  viruses in, 587–588
Reiter's syndrome, Yersinia and, 315
Relapsing fever, 370t, 370–371
  clinical manifestations of, 371, 371t
  epidemiology of, 370–371
  laboratory diagnosis of Borrelia in, 372
  pathogenesis and pathology of, 371
  treatment of, 372–373
Reoviruses, 116–119
Respiratory papillomatosis, 71–72
Respiratory syncytial virus (RSV), 90–91
  clinical manifestations of, 91
  epidemiology of, 91
  laboratory diagnosis of, 92–93, *93*
  pathogenesis of, 91
  prevention of, 94
  structure of, 90
  treatment of, 93

Respiratory tract. *See also* Pulmonary disease
  bronchial washing, protected specimen brush, and bronchoalveolar lavage specimens and, 569–570
  fine-needle aspirates and, 570
  nasopharyngeal and nasal specimens and, 561–563, 562t
  nonspecific defense and, 5–7
  Pseudomonas aeruginosa and, 284
  sputum and tracheal aspirates and, 565–569, 566t
  throat specimens and, 563–565, 564t
  transbronchial and open lung biopsy specimens and, 570–571
  transtracheal aspirates and, 569
Retroviruses, 146–158. *See also* Human immunodeficiency virus; Human T-cell leukemia virus types I and II
  classification of, 146, 147t
  replication of, 146
  structure of, 146
Rhabditida, 470
Rhabdoviruses, 123–127
  classification of, 123, 124t
  structure and replication of, 123, *124*
Rheumatic fever, Streptococcus pyogenes and, 225, 226, 227, *227*, 227t
Rhinosporidiosis, 460–461
  mucocutaneous, 461
  nasal, 461
  ocular, 461
  treatment of, 462
Rhinosporidium seeberi, 460–461
  clinical manifestations of, 461
  epidemiology of, 460
  in conjunctival specimens, 554
  laboratory diagnosis of, 461
  pathology of, 460–461, *461*
Rhinoviruses, 111
  clinical manifestations of, 111
  epidemiology of, 111
  laboratory diagnosis of, 112, *113*
  pathogenesis of, 111
  structure of, 111
Rhipicephalus sanguineus, 196
Rhizomucor, 434
Rhizopus, 434
Rhodamine, 175
Rhodococcus equi, 249
  laboratory diagnosis of, 249
Rhodotorula, 419
  laboratory diagnosis of, cellular structure and colony characteristics in, 421
  treatment of, 423
Rickettsia akari, 530
Rickettsia conorii, 200–201
Rickettsia prowazekii, 201, 202
Rickettsia rickettsii, 196, 198, 199
Rickettsia tsutsugamushi, 202–203, 530
Rickettsia typhi, 201, 534
Rickettsiae, 194–210, 195t. *See also specific organisms*
  Bartonellosis and, 210
  classification of, 194, 195t
  ehrlichioses and, 203–205
  Q fever and, *205*, 205–208
  Rochalimaea infections and, 208–210
  spotted fevers and, 196–201
  structure and physiology of, 194–196, *196*, *197*
  typhus fever and, 201–202
Rickettsialpox, 200
Rift Valley fever virus, 139
  clinical manifestations of, 139
  epidemiology of, 139
  pathogenesis of, 139

Rimantidine, orthomyxoviruses and, 100
River blindness, 514, *515*
Rochalimaea henselae, 208–210
　laboratory diagnosis of, 209
　pathology of, *208*, 208–209, *209*
　treatment of, 210
Rochalimaea quintana, 208
Rocky Mountain spotted fever, 196–200
　clinical manifestations of, *198*, 198–199
　laboratory diagnosis of, 199, 199t
　pathogenesis of, 198
　treatment of, 199–200
Roseola infantum, human herpesvirus 6 and, 54
Rotavirus, 116–119, *117*
　clinical manifestations of, 118
　epidemiology of, 117
　laboratory diagnosis of, 118–119
　pathogenesis of, 117–118
　structure of, 116–117, 117t
　treatment and prevention of, 119
Rothia dentocariosa, 247–248
Rubella virus, 130–133
　clinical manifestations of, 132, 132t
　epidemiology of, 131, *131*
　laboratory diagnosis of, 132–133
　pathogenesis of, 131–132
　structure of, 130–131
Rubivirus. *See* Rubella virus

Saccharomyces, treatment of, 423
Saccharomyces cerevisiae, 419
　laboratory diagnosis of, cellular structure and colony characteristics in, 421
St. Louis encephalitis virus, 135–136
　clinical manifestations of, 136
　epidemiology of, 136
　laboratory diagnosis of, 137
　pathogenesis of, 136
Salivary glands, mumps virus and, 87, 88
Salmonella, 311–314
　clinical manifestations of, 314
　epidemiology of, 312–313
　features of, 323
　in gastrointestinal tissue specimens, 593
　in liver tissue specimens, 598
　pathogenesis of, *313*, 313–314
　treatment and prevention of, 325
Salmonella anatum, 313
Salmonella choleraesuis, 313
Salmonella hirschfeldii, 312, 314
Salmonella paratyphi A, 312, 314
Salmonella schottmuelleri, 312, 314
Salmonella sendai, 312
Salmonella typhi, 311, 312, 313, 314
　features of, 323
　treatment and prevention of, 325
Salmonella typhimurium, 314
Salmonellosis, 312–313
　nontyphoidal, 312
Sandflies, 535
Sarcocystis, 480
Sarcoma, Kaposi's, human immunodeficiency virus types 1 and 2 and, 155
Scabies, 530–531, *531*, *532*
Scalded skin syndrome, Staphylococcus aureus and, 220
Scaroptes scabei, 530–531, *532*
Schistosoma
　in stool and rectal swab specimens, 592
　sedimentation for, 637
Schistosoma haematobium, 314, 523, 524, 525, *525*
Schistosoma japonicum, 523, *524*, 525, *525*

Schistosoma mansoni, 523, *524*, 525
Schistosoma mekongi, 523
Schistosomiasis, 523–525, *524–526*
Schlichter test, 182
Scopulariopsis, 434, 442
Scotch tape preparation, 634–635
Scotch tape procedure, for Enterobius, 636
Scrapie. *See* Prions
Scrofula, 381–382
Scrub typhus, 202–203
Sedimentation, for Schistosoma, 637
Selective media, 175
Seoul virus, 139
Sepsis, Neisseria meningitidis and, 271
Septic shock syndrome, Staphylococcus aureus and, 219
Septicemia
　Aeromonas and, 333
　Pseudomonas mallei and, 285
　Vibrio vulnificus and, 330–331
Serologic tests
　bacteria and, 177
　fungi and, 413
　serum for, 582t, 582–583
Serotyping, 276
Serratia marcescens, 317
　features of, 324
Serum bactericidal test, 182
Serum specimens, 582t, 582–583
Shanghai fever, Pseudomonas aeruginosa and, 284
Shigella, 307, 310–311
　in gastrointestinal tissue specimens, 593
　treatment and prevention of, 325
Shigella dysenteriae, 310, 311
Shigella flexneri, 310, 311
　features of, 323
Shigella sonnei, 310
Shigellosis, 310–311
　clinical manifestations of, 311
　pathogenesis of, 311
Shingles, 50–51
Simian vacuolating agent-40 (SV40)-PML viruses. *See* Polyomavirus
Simuliidae, 535–536
Sinus aspirates, 556t, 556–557
　collection, transport, and processing of, 556–557
Sinusitis, Chlamydia pneumoniae and, 188
Siti, 364
Skin
　anaerobic gram-negative bacteria and, 358
　as nonspecific defense, 5
　aspirates and swab specimens from ulcers of, 612t, 612–614
　　bacteria in, 613
　　collection, transport, and processing of, 613
　　fungi in, 614
　　parasites in, 614
　aspirates and swab specimens from wound infections and abscesses and, 614t, 614–615
　　bacteria in, 614t, 614–615
　　collection, transport, and processing of, 614, 614t
　　fungae and algae in, 614t, 615
　biopsy specimens from, 615t, 615–618
　　bacteria in, 615t, 616
　　collection, transport, and processing of, 615
　　fungi and algae in, 615t, 616
　　parasites in, 615t, 616–618
　　viruses in, 615t, 615–616
　Blastomyces dermatitidis and, 448

　Borrelia burgdorferi and, 369
　Candida and, 416
　Coccidioides immitis and, 451
　Cryptococcus neoformans and, 418
　dermatophytes and, treatment of, 442
　Erysipelothrix rhusiopathiae and, 243
　fluid and swab specimens from vesicles, bullae, and pustules and, 611t, 611–612
　　bacteria in, 612
　　collection, transport, and processing of, 611
　　fungi in, 612
　　viruses in, 611–612
　Histoplasma capsulatum var duboisii and, 450
　in pinto, 365
　in yaws, 364
　mites and, 530–531, *531*, *532*
　Mycobacterium fortuitum-chelonae and, 385
　Mycobacterium haemophilum and, 386
　Mycobacterium marinum and, 386
　Mycobacterium ulcerans and, 386
　Mycoplasma pneumoniae and, 215
　myiasis and, 536, *536*
　Nocardia and, 248
　Prototheca and, 463
　Rhinosporidium seeberi and, 461
　schistosomiasis and, 523
　scrapings from, 610–611, 611t
　　collection, transport, and processing of, 610–611
　　parasites in, 616–617
　skin slit specimens and, 615
Slide coagulase test, 633
Slime layer, 174
Smallpox virus, 43–44
　epidemiology and pathogenesis of, 43–44
Soft tissue infections, anaerobic gram-negative bacteria and, 358
Sparganosis, *528*, 529
Specific defenses, 12–19
　cell-mediated immunity and, 15–19
　　mononuclear phagocytes and, 16
　　natural killer cells and, 18–19
　　role in host defense, 19, 19t
　　T lymphocytes and, 16–18, *17*
　humoral immunity and, 12–15
　　B-cell activation and, 13–14
　　immunoglobulin structure and, 13, 13t, *14*, 14t
　　role in host defense, 14–15, 15t
Specimen(s). *See also specific sources*
　viral, collection and transport of, 38–39, 39t, 40t
Specimen handling, 539–543
　bacterial specimens and, 539–542, 541t, *542*
　fungal and algal specimens and, 542
　mailing infectious material and, 543
　parasitic specimens and, 542–543
　viral specimens and, 539, 540t
Sphingobacterium multivorum, 287
Spinal abscess, epidural, Staphylococcus aureus and, 220
Spirillum minus, 375
Spirochetes, 361–375. *See also specific organisms*
　anaerobic, 374–375
Spirometra, 529
Spirurida, 471
Spleen
　abscess specimens from, 582
　infarcts of, viridans streptococci and, 229
　schistosomiasis and, 523–524

Sporothrix schenckii, 452–453
    clinical manifestations of, 452–453
    dimorphic, 458
    epidemiology of, 452
    laboratory diagnosis of, 457, 457–458
    pathology of, 452
Sporotrichosis, 452–453
    extracutaneous, 453
    lymphocutaneous, 453
    treatment of, 458
Sputum specimens, 565–569, 566t
    bacteria in, 566–568, 567
    collection, transport, and processing of, 566
    fungi in, 568
    parasites in, 568–569
    viruses in, 566
Staphylococci, 218–222
    epidemiologic typing and, 224
    laboratory diagnosis of, 222–223, 223t
        coagulase-negative species and, 223, 224
    susceptibility testing and, 223–224
    treatment of, 225
Staphylococcus aureus, 218–221
    clinical manifestations of, 219–221, 220t, 221
    epidemiologic typing and, 224
    epidemiology of, 218
    identification of, 222–223, 223t
    in nasopharyngeal and nasal specimens, 563
    pathogenesis of, 218–219
Staphylococcus epidermidis, 221–222
    clinical manifestations of, 222
    epidemiologic typing and, 224
    epidemiology of, 221
    pathogenesis of, 221–222
Staphylococcus intermedius, 222
Staphylococcus saprophyticus, 222
    clinical manifestations of, 222
    epidemiology and pathogenesis of, 222
Stomatococcus mucilaginosus, 222
    identification of, 223
    susceptibility testing and, 223–224
Stool concentration, formalin-ethyl acetate and, 636
Stool specimens, 586–592, 587t
    bacteria in, 588–590, 589t, 590t
    collection, transport, and processing of, 591–592
    parasites in, 590–591
    viruses in, 587–588
Streptobacillus moniliformis, 400–401
    clinical manifestations of, 401
    epidemiology and pathogenesis of, 400–401
    laboratory diagnosis of, 401
    treatment of, 401
Streptococci, 225–230. See also Enterococcus
    group A, 225–227
        in throat specimens, 565
        prevention of, 234–235
    group B, 227–228
        in vaginal specimens, 604–605
    group C, 230, 230t
    group G, 230, 230t
    laboratory diagnosis of, 231t, 231–234
        cellular structure and, 231
        colony characteristics and, 231
        β-hemolytic species and, 231–232, 232
        α- and Γ-hemolytic species and, 232–233, 233
    susceptibility testing and, 234
    treatment of, 234
    viridans, 229–230
        clinical manifestations of, 229–230

epidemiology and pathogenesis of, 229, 229t
Streptococcus adjacens, 230
Streptococcus agalactiae, 227–228
    clinical manifestations of, 228
    epidemiology of, 227–228
    pathogenesis of, 228
Streptococcus anginosus, 229, 230
Streptococcus defectivus, 230
Streptococcus faecalis, 230
Streptococcus faecium, 230
Streptococcus pneumoniae, 228–229
    clinical manifestations of, 228–229
    epidemiology of, 228
    pathogenesis of, 228
    penicillin-resistant, screen for, 634
    prevention of, 235
Streptococcus pyogenes, 219, 225–227
    clinical manifestations of, 226–227, 227, 227t
    epidemiology of, 225
    pathogenesis of, 225–226, 226
Streptomyces, 249
    laboratory diagnosis of, 249
Strongylidae, 470–471
Strongyloides, Baermann concentration for, 636
Strongyloides fuelleborni, 488, 488
Strongyloides stercoralis, 486, 487, 487–488
    in duodenal aspirate specimens, 586
    in stool and rectal swab specimens, 592
Subacute sclerosing panencephalitis (SSPE), measles virus and, 90
Subcutaneous disease
    Nocardia and, 248
    Pseudomonas mallei and, 285
Sudan virus. See Filoviruses
Susceptibility testing. See also specific organisms
    antiviral agents and, 41
    bacteria and. See Bacteria, susceptibility testing and
    fungi and, 413t, 413–414
SV40 (simian vacuolating agent-40)-PML viruses. See Polyomavirus
Synovial specimens, 624–626, 625t
    collection, transport, and processing of, 625–626
Syphilis, 361–364
    cardiovascular, 363–364
    congenital, 364, 367
    endemic, 364
        treatment of, 367
    late, 362, 363
    latent, 362, 363
    primary, 361, 362–363
    secondary, 361, 362, 363
    tertiary, late, 363
    treatment of, 367
Syphonaptera, 534, 534, 535

T lymphocytes, 16–18, 17
    development, structure, and activation of, 17–18, 18
    major histocompatibility complex and, 16–17
    role in host defense, 18
Tabanidae, 536
Tabes dorsalis, 363
Tache noire, 200
Taenia saginata, 491–492
Taenia solium, 492–493, 493, 525–526
Tease mount preparation, 634
Testes, mumps virus and, 88

Tetanus, 254–256
    cephalic, 255–256
    generalized, 256
    local, 255–256
    neonatal, 256
        prevention of, 262
    otogenous, 256
Tetanus immune globulin, 262
Tetracycline
    in boutonneuse fever, 201
    in murine typhus, 202
    in Rocky Mountain spotted fever, 199
Therapeutic drug monitoring, 182
Thick smears, parasites in blood specimens and, 578
Thin smears, parasites in blood specimens and, 578
Throat specimens, 563–565, 564t
    collection, transport, and processing of, 564
Thrombocytopenia, immune-mediated, rubella virus and, 132
Thrush, Candida and, 416
Tick(s), 531–533, 533
Tick paralysis, 532–533
Tinea capitis, 426, 427, 427t
Tinea corporis, 427t, 427–428
Tinea cruris, 427t, 428
Tinea nigra, 429
Tinea pedis, 426, 427, 427t
Tissue specimens, gastrointestinal, 592t, 592–594
    bacteria in, 592–593
    fungi in, 593
    parasites in, 594
    viruses in, 592
Togaviruses, 129–133
    classification of, 129
    group B. See Flaviviruses
    replication of, 129
    structure of, 129
Torulopsis glabrata, 415
Toxic shock-like syndrome, type II, 227
Toxic shock syndrome (TSS)
    diagnosis of, 223
    Staphylococcus aureus and, 219, 220t, 220–221, 221
Toxocara, 517–518, 519
Toxoplasma gondii, 503–505, 504
    in bronchial washing, protected specimen brush, and bronchoalveolar lavage specimens, 570
Tracheal aspirates, 565–569, 566t
    bacteria in, 566–568, 567
    collection, transport, and processing of, 566
    fungi in, 568
    parasites in, 568–569
    viruses in, 566
Tracheobronchitis, Mycoplasma pneumoniae and, 215
Trachoma, Chlamydia trachomatis and, 186
Transbronchial biopsy specimens, 570–571
    bacteria in, 571
    fungi in, 571
    parasites in, 571
    viruses in, 570–571
Transcription, viruses and, 36, 38
Transtracheal aspirates, 569
Trematodes. See also specific organisms
    blood and tissue, 520–525
        biliary, 520–522
        of blood vessels, 523–525, 524–526
        pulmonary, 522, 522–523
    intestinal, 489–491

INDEX

Trench fever, 208
Treponema
　anaerobic species of, 374
　　laboratory diagnosis of, 365–367
　　　direct microscopy in, 365
　　　serologic tests in, 365–367, 367t
　　treatment and prevention of, 367
Treponema carateum, 364–365
　clinical manifestations of, 365
　epidemiology and pathogenesis of, 365
Treponema pallidum, 361
　in cerebrospinal fluid, 546
　in conjunctival specimens, 554
　in genital ulcer specimens, 607
　in oropharyngeal ulcer specimens, 559
Treponema pallidum subspecies endemicum, 364
　clinical manifestations of, 364
　epidemiology of, 364
Treponema pallidum subspecies pallidum, 361–364
　clinical manifestations of, 362–364
　epidemiology of, 361, 362
　pathogenesis and pathology of, 361–362, 362
Treponema pallidum subspecies pertenue, 364
　clinical manifestations of, 364
　epidemiology of, 364
Treponemal tests, 365–366
Trichinella spiralis, 516–517, 518
Trichinellosis, 516–517, 518
Trichistrongylus, 488, 488
Trichomonas vaginalis, 473–474, 474
　in urethral swab specimens, 606
Trichophyton, 436, 437
Trichophyton mentagrophytes, 436
Trichophyton verrucosum, 426
Trichosporon, treatment of, 423
Trichosporon beigelii, 419
　laboratory diagnosis of, cellular structure and colony characteristics in, 421
Trichrome stain, for fecal smears, 635
Trichuris trichura, 482–483, 484
Trichuroidea, 471
Triple sugar iron agar (TSIA), Enterobacteriaceae and, 318–319
Trypanosoma brucei gambiense, 499–500
Trypanosoma brucei rhodesiense, 499–500
Trypanosoma cruzi, 500–501, 501
Trypanosoma rangeli, 501
Trypanosomiasis
　African, 499–500, 536
　American, 500–501, 501
Tryptophan deaminase production, Enterobacteriaceae and, 322
Tube coagulase test, 633
Tuberculin skin test, 389
Tuberculosis, 378–381
　extrapulmonary, 381, 381t
　pulmonary, 380–381
Tularemia, 293–295
　glandular, 294
　oculoglandular, 294
　oropharyngeal, 294
　ulceroglandular, 294
Tunga penetrans, 534, 535
Tympanocentesis fluid, 557t, 557–558
　collection, transport, and processing of, 557
Typhlitis, Pseudomonas aeruginosa and, 284
Typhoid fever, Salmonella and, 312
Typhoid vaccine, 325

Typhus, 201–202
　louse-borne, epidemic, 202
　murine, 201–202
　scrub, 202–203
　sylvatic, 202

Ulcer(s)
　corneal, Pseudomonas aeruginosa and, 284
　cutaneous. See Skin
　genital, specimens from, 607
　myiasis and, 536
　oropharyngeal, specimens from, 558–559
　peptic, Helicobacter pylori and, 353
Uncoating, in viruses, 36
Unconventional viruses. See Prions
Ureaplasma urealyticum, 215, 216
　clinical manifestations of, 215
　epidemiology of, 215
　in urethral swab specimens, 605
　laboratory diagnosis of, 216
　treatment and prevention of, 216
Urease production, Enterobacteriaceae and, 321
Urethral swab specimens, 605–606
Urinary tract infection
　Candida and, 416
　enterococcus and, 230
　Escherichia coli and, 309–310
　Gardnerella vaginalis and, 399
　Klebsiella and, 317
　Pseudomonas aeruginosa and, 284
　schistosomiasis and, 524, 525
　Staphylococcus aureus and, 220
　Staphylococcus epidermidis and, 222
Urine specimens, 600–602
　bacteria in, 601t, 601–603, 602
　collection, transport, and processing of, 600–601
　fungi in, 601t, 603
　parasites in, 601t, 603
　viruses in, 601, 601t
Urogenital tract. See also Urinary tract infection
　myiasis and, 536

Vaccines
　Bordetella pertussis and, 299
　brucellosis and, 296–297
　Haemophilus influenzae and, 342
　hepatitis B, 82
　human immunodeficiency virus types 1 and 2 and, 158
　measles virus and, 93–94, 94t
　mumps virus and, 93
　Mycobacterium tuberculosis and, 394–395
　orthomyxoviruses and, 100–101
　pneumococcal, 235
　poliovirus and, 112–113
　rabies virus and, 127
　rotavirus and, 119
　rubella virus and, 133
　Salmonella and, 325
　Yersinia and, 325
Vaccinia virus, epidemiology and pathogenesis of, 44
Vaginal specimens, 604–605
　bacteria in, 604–605
　parasites in, 605
Vaginitis, Candida and, 415
Vaginosis, Gardnerella vaginalis and, 399
Vancomycin disk susceptibility test, anaerobes and, 259

Varicella-zoster immune globulin (VZIG), 60, 60t
Varicella-zoster virus (VZV), 50–51
　clinical manifestations of, 50–51
　epidemiology of, 50
　laboratory diagnosis of, 56–57, 57
　pathogenesis of, 50
　prevention of, 60, 60t
　structure of, 50
　treatment of, 59
Variola, 43–44
　epidemiology and pathogenesis of, 43–44
VDRL test, 365, 366–367
Venezuelan encephalitis virus, 129–130
　clinical manifestations of, 130
　epidemiology of, 129–130
　pathogenesis of, 130
Verruca plana, human papillomavirus and, 71
Verruca plantaris, human papillomavirus and, 71
Verruca vulgaris, human papillomavirus and, 71
Verruga peruana, 210, 535
Vesicle fluid or swab specimens, urogenital, 606–607
Vesiculovirus, 123, 124t
　clinical manifestations of, 123
　epidemiology of, 123
　laboratory diagnosis of, 123
　treatment of, 123
Vibrio
　in stool and rectal swab specimens, 590
　laboratory diagnosis of, 331–332
　　organism identification and, 331–332
　treatment and prevention of, 332
Vibrio cholerae, 329–330, 330t
　clinical manifestations of, 330
　epidemiology of, 329
　laboratory diagnosis of, organism identification and, 331–332
　pathogenesis of, 329–330
　treatment and prevention of, 332
Vibrio furnisii, laboratory diagnosis of, organism identification and, 332
Vibrio metschnikovii, laboratory diagnosis of, organism identification and, 332
Vibrio mimicus, laboratory diagnosis of, organism identification and, 332
Vibrio parahaemolyticus, 330
　treatment and prevention of, 332
Vibrio vulnificus, 330–331
　laboratory diagnosis of, organism identification and, 332
　treatment and prevention of, 332
Vibrionaceae, 329–334, 330t. See also specific organisms
Viruses, 33–41, 34. See also specific viruses and viral groups
　antiviral agents and, 41
　classification of, 33, 34t
　DNA, 34t, 35
　　transcription, DNA synthesis, particle assembly, and egress of, 36, 38
　hemadsorbing, hemadsorption procedure for, 631
　in amniotic fluid specimens, 608
　in anterior chamber, vitreous cavity, and ocular abscess specimens, 555
　in blood specimens, 573–574
　in body cavity specimens, 620, 620t
　in bone marrow specimens, 580, 580t
　in brain tissue specimens, 549
　in bronchial washing, protected specimen brush, and bronchoalveolar lavage specimens, 569

Viruses (*Continued*)
  in cerebrospinal fluid, 544–545, 545t
  in corneal specimens, 554–555
  in endomyocardial biopsy specimens, 579
  in esophageal brushing specimens, 585
  in fluid and swab specimens from vesicles, bullae, and pustules, 611–612
  in gastrointestinal tissue specimens, 592
  in liver tissue specimens, 597–598
  in middle ear fluid, 557
  in nasopharyngeal and nasal specimens, 561–562, 562t
  in oropharyngeal ulcer specimens, 558–559
  in products of conception, 608
  in sinus aspirates, 556
  in skin biopsy specimens, 615t, 615–616
  in sputum and tracheal aspirates, 566
  in stool and rectal swab specimens, 587–588
  in throat specimens, 564
  in transbronchial and open lung biopsy specimens, 570–571
  in urethral swab specimens, 605
  in urine specimens, 601
  laboratory diagnosis of, 38–41. *See also specific viruses and viral groups*
    cell culture and, 39–41, 40t, 41t
    direct detection methods and, 41
    poxviruses and, 44, 44–45
    specimen collection and transport and, 38–39, 39t, 40t
  nonproductive infections and, 38
  poxviruses, 43–45
  productive infections and, 36, *37*, 38
    adsorption and, 36, 36t
    penetration and, 36
    transcription, synthesis, particle assembly, and egress and, 36, 38
    uncoating and, 36
  replication of, 36–38. *See also specific viruses and viral groups*
    nonproductive infections and, 38
    poxviruses and, 43
    productive infections and, 36, *37*, 38
    structure of, 46
  RNA, 34t, *35*
    transcription, RNA synthesis, particle assembly, and egress of, 38
  specimen handling and, 539, 540t
  structure of, 33, 36, *36. See also specific viruses and viral groups*
    capsid and, 33
    envelope and, 33, 36
    genome and, 33
    herpesviruses and, 46, *47*
    poxviruses and, 43
  Vitreous cavity specimens, 555–556
    specimens from, 555
  Voges-Proskauer test, Enterobacteriaceae and, 320–321

Wart(s)
  common, human papillomavirus and, 71
  flat, human papillomavirus and, 71
  genital, human papillomavirus and, 71
  plantar and palmar, human papillomavirus and, 71
Warthin-Starry silver stain, 175
Waterhouse-Friderichsen syndrome, 271
WC3 vaccine, 119
Weeksella zoohelcum, 287
Weil-Felix serologic test, Rocky Mountain spotted fever and, 199
Weil's disease, 373–374
Western blot, human immunodeficiency virus types 1 and 2 and, 156, 157t
Western encephalitis virus, 129–130
  clinical manifestations of, 130
  epidemiology of, 129
  pathogenesis of, 130
Wet mount preparations, 175
Whooping cough, 297–299
Wistar RA27/3 vaccine, 133
Wound(s), myiasis and, 536
Wound infection
  Aeromonas and, 332–333
  aspirates from, 614t, 614–615
    bacteria in, 614t, 614–615
    fungae and algae in, 614t, 615
  Pasteurella multicida and, 342–343
  Vibrio vulnificus and, 331
Wuchereria, 535
Wuchereria bancrofti, 512–514, *513*

Xanthomonas maltophilia, 281, 286
  clinical manifestations of, 286
  epidemiology of, 286
  laboratory diagnosis of, organism identification and, 289
  pathogenesis of, 286
  treatment of, 290
Xylohypha bantiana, 430

Yaws, 364
  treatment of, 367
Yeasts, 415–423. *See also specific organisms*
  inoculation of cornmeal-tween 80 agar for identification of, 635
  laboratory diagnosis of, 419–423, 420t
    cellular structure and colony characteristics and, 419–421
    identification and, 421–422
    serologic tests in, 422–423
  morphologic appearance of, 408
  treatment of, 423
Yellow fever virus, 135
  clinical manifestations of, 135
  epidemiology of, 135, *136*
  laboratory diagnosis of, 137
  pathogenesis of, 135
Yersinia
  features of, 323–324
  treatment and prevention of, 325
Yersinia enterocolitica, 314–315
  clinical manifestations of, 315
  epidemiology of, 314–315
  features of, 323
  in gastrointestinal tissue specimens, 593
  in stool and rectal swab specimens, 590
  incubation of, 541
  pathogenesis of, 315
  treatment and prevention of, 325
Yersinia pestis, 315–316, 534
  clinical manifestations of, 316
  epidemiology of, 316
  features of, 323–324
  pathogenesis of, 316
  prevention of, 325
Yersinia pseudotuberculosis, 314–315
  clinical manifestations of, 315
  epidemiology of, 314–315
  features of, 323–324
  pathogenesis of, 315
  treatment and prevention of, 325

Zaire virus. *See* Filoviruses
Zidovudine (AZT), in human immunodeficiency virus types 1 and 2, 157, 158
Ziehl-Neelsen stain, 175, 631–632
Zygomycetes, 434–436
  clinical manifestations of, 435–436
  epidemiology of, 434
  laboratory diagnosis of, 442, *443*
  pathogenesis and pathology of, 434–435, *435*
  treatment of, 444
Zygospores, 411